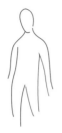

CECIL ESSENTIALS OF MEDICINE

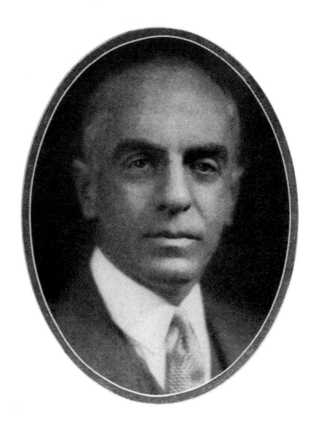

Russell L. Cecil, M.D.

The Editors thought it appropriate that readers of *Cecil Essentials of Medicine* understand why the book has commemorated the name of Dr. Cecil. These comments are particularly apt for today's readers, inasmuch as the first edition of *Cecil Essentials of Medicine* was published in 1986, 21 years after Dr. Cecil's death.

Dr. Cecil was born in 1882 and received his M.D. degree from the Medical College of Virginia in 1906. After training in Berlin and Vienna and at Johns Hopkins Hospital (Baltimore) and Presbyterian Hospital (New York), Dr. Cecil joined the faculty of Cornell University Medical College in 1915, where he spent the remainder of his career.

Dr. Cecil realized that the subject of internal medicine was too large in scope to be encompassed by a book written by a single individual and that advances in internal medicine were occurring at a rapidly accelerating pace. These tenets provided the basic motif for *The Cecil Textbook of Medicine,* first published in 1927: a comprehensive textbook written by distinguished experts and revised frequently in order to maintain currency.

Dr. Cecil's major clinical interests were in infectious diseases, particularly the pneumonias, and in rheumatologic diseases, particularly arthritis. He developed one of the first arthritis clinics in the United States, was a founding member of the American Rheumatism Association (ARA), and served as President of the ARA in 1937. His *Textbook of Medicine* rapidly became a standard throughout the world. He served as the sole Editor of *The Cecil Textbook of Medicine* for the first seven editions.

The Editors of *Essentials,* together with W.B. Saunders Company, have recognized the contributions of this exceptional clinician, scholar, and author by maintaining his name on the title of *Cecil Essentials of Medicine.*

T. E. Andreoli, Editor-in-Chief

C. C. J. Carpenter

R. C. Griggs

J. Loscalzo

EDITOR-IN-CHIEF

Thomas E. Andreoli, M.D., M.A.C.P.

Professor and *The Nolan Chair*
Department of Internal Medicine
University of Arkansas College of Medicine
Little Rock, Arkansas

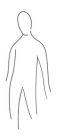

CECIL ESSENTIALS OF MEDICINE FIFTH EDITION

....

EDITORS

Charles C. J. Carpenter, M.D., M.A.C.P.

Professor of Medicine
Director, International Health Institute
Brown University School of Medicine
Providence, Rhode Island

Robert C. Griggs, M.D.

Edward A. and Alma Vollertsen Rykenboer Professor of Neurophysiology
Chair, Department of Neurology
University of Rochester School of Medicine and Dentistry
Rochester, New York

Joseph Loscalzo, M.D., Ph.D.

Wade Professor and Chair
Department of Medicine
Boston University School of Medicine
Physician-in-Chief
Boston Medical Center
Director, Whitaker Cardiovascular Institute
Boston, Massachusetts

W.B. Saunders Company

A Harcourt Health Sciences Company
PHILADELPHIA LONDON NEW YORK ST. LOUIS SYDNEY TORONTO

W.B. SAUNDERS COMPANY
A Harcourt Health Sciences Company

The Curtis Center
Independence Square West
Philadelphia, Pennsylvania 19106

Library of Congress Cataloging-in-Publication Data

Cecil essentials of medicine / [edited by] Thomas E. Andreoli, Charles C. J. Carpenter, Robert C. Griggs, Joseph Loscalzo.—5th ed.

p. cm.

Includes bibliographical references and index.

ISBN 0–7216–8179–4

1. Internal medicine.   I. Title: Essentials of medicine.   II. Andreoli, Thomas E.
   III. Cecil, Russell L. (Russell La Fayette).
   [DNLM: 1. Internal Medicine.   WB 115 C388 2001]

RC46.C42   2001   616—dc21   99-089413

Senior Developmental Editor: Lynne Gery
Senior Production Manager: Linda Garber
Manuscript Editor: Anne Ostroff
Illustration Specialist: Lisa Lambert

Cecil Essentials of Medicine   ISBN 0–7216–8179–4

Printed in the United States of America

Last digit is the print number: 9   8   7   6   5   4   3   2   1

This edition of *Cecil Essentials of Medicine* is dedicated to two former Editors:

Fred Plum, one of the founding Editors, who recognized the need for a compact textbook of Internal Medicine. Fred brought to *Cecil Essentials of Medicine* clarity in writing and a crisp logic in setting priorities for the content of the text.

J. Claude Bennett, an Editor for the third and fourth editions of this book. Claude brought to *Cecil Essentials of Medicine* his customary incisiveness and ecumenical knowledge of internal medicine.

We thank both of you.

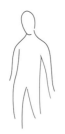

CONTRIBUTORS

Introduction to Molecular Medicine

Joseph Loscalzo, M.D., Ph.D.
Wade Professor and Chair, Department of Medicine, Boston University School of Medicine; Physician-in-Chief, Boston Medical Center; Director, Whitaker Cardiovascular Institute, Boston, Massachusetts

Decision-Making in Medical Practice

Susan S. Beland, M.D.
Associate Professor, Department of Internal Medicine, Division of General Internal Medicine, University of Arkansas College of Medicine, Little Rock, Arkansas

Awny S. Farajallah, M.D.
Assistant Professor, Department of Internal Medicine, Division of General Internal Medicine, University of Arkansas College of Medicine, Little Rock, Arkansas

Cardiovascular Disease

Eric H. Awtry, M.D.
Instructor in Medicine, Boston University School of Medicine; Director of Education, Section of Cardiology, Boston Medical Center, Boston, Massachusetts

Joseph Loscalzo, M.D., Ph.D.
Wade Professor and Chair, Department of Medicine, Boston University School of Medicine; Physician-in-Chief, Boston Medical Center; Director, Whitaker Cardiovascular Institute, Boston, Massachusetts

Lisa A. Mendes, M.D.
Assistant Professor of Medicine, Boston University School of Medicine; Staff Cardiologist, Boston Medical Center, Boston, Massachusetts

Pulmonary and Critical Care Medicine

Kenneth L. Brigham, M.D.
Ralph and Lulu Owen Professor of Pulmonary Medicine and Director, Center for Lung Research and Division of Allergy, Pulmonary and Critical Care Medicine, Vanderbilt University School of Medicine, Nashville, Tennessee

Bonnie S. Slovis, M.D.
Assistant Professor of Medicine and Director, Outpatient Medicine, Division of Allergy, Pulmonary and Critical Care Medicine, Vanderbilt University School of Medicine, Nashville, Tennessee

Renal Disease

Sameh R. Abul-Ezz, M.D.
Associate Professor of Internal Medicine, Division of Nephrology, University of Arkansas College of Medicine, Little Rock, Arkansas

Thomas E. Andreoli, M.D., M.A.C.P.
Professor and *The Nolan Chair*, Department of Internal Medicine, University of Arkansas College of Medicine, Little Rock, Arkansas

Yousri M. H. Barri, M.D.
Assistant Professor of Internal Medicine, Division of Nephrology, University of Arkansas College of Medicine, Little Rock, Arkansas

Dinesh K. Chatoth, M.D.
Assistant Professor of Internal Medicine, Division of Nephrology, University of Arkansas College of Medicine, Little Rock, Arkansas

Sudhir V. Shah, M.D.
Professor of Internal Medicine and Director, Division of Nephrology, University of Arkansas College of Medicine, Little Rock, Arkansas

Mary Jo Shaver, M.D.
Assistant Professor of Internal Medicine, Division of Nephrology, University of Arkansas College of Medicine, Little Rock, Arkansas

Gastrointestinal Disease

Edgar Achkar, M.D.
Vice Chairman, Department of Gastroenterology, Cleveland Clinic Foundation, Cleveland, Ohio

Aaron Brzezinski, M.D.
Staff Gastroenterologist, Center for Inflammatory Bowel Disease, Department of Gastroenterology, Cleveland Clinic, Cleveland, Ohio

Carol A. Burke, M.D.
Director, Center for Colon Cancer and Polyps, Department of Gastroenterology, Cleveland Clinic, Cleveland, Ohio

Darwin L. Conwell, M.D.
Director, Pancreas Clinic, Department of Gastroenterology, Cleveland Clinic Foundation, Cleveland, Ohio

Gary W. Falk, M.D.
Director, Center for Swallowing and Esophageal Disorders, Department of Gastroenterology, Cleveland Clinic Foundation, Cleveland, Ohio

Joel E. Richter, M.D.
Chairman, Department of Gastroenterology, Cleveland Clinic Foundation, Cleveland, Ohio

Edy E. Soffer, M.D.
Director, Center for Lower GI Motility Disorders, Department of Gastroenterology, Cleveland Clinic Foundation, Cleveland, Ohio

John J. Vargo II, M.D.
Department of Gastroenterology, Cleveland Clinic Foundation, Cleveland, Ohio

Gregory Zuccaro, Jr., M.D.
Head, Section of GI Endoscopy, Department of Gastroenterology, Cleveland Clinic Foundation, Cleveland, Ohio

Diseases of the Liver and Biliary System

Gary A. Abrams, M.D.
Assistant Professor of Medicine, Division of Gastroenterology and Hepatology, University of Alabama School of Medicine, Birmingham, Alabama

Miguel R. Arguedas
Senior Fellow, Gastroenterology and Hepatology, Department of Medicine, Division of Gastroenterology and Hepatology, University of Alabama School of Medicine, Birmingham, Alabama

Michael B. Fallon, M.D.
Assistant Professor of Medicine, Division of Gastroenterology and Hepatology, University of Alabama School of Medicine, Birmingham, Alabama

Brendan M. McGuire, M.D.
Assistant Professor of Medicine, Division of Gastroenterology and Hepatology, University of Alabama School of Medicine, Birmingham, Alabama

Hematologic Disease

Nancy Berliner, M.D.
Arthur and Isabel Bunker Associate Professor of Medicine and Genetics, Yale University School of Medicine, New Haven, Connecticut

Jill Lacy, M.D.
Associate Professor of Medicine, Section of Medical Oncology, Yale University School of Medicine, New Haven, Connecticut

Henry M. Rinder, M.D.
Assistant Professor, Department of Laboratory Medicine and Internal Medicine (Hematology), Yale University; Director, Coagulation Laboratory, and Associate Director, Hematology Laboratories, Yale–New Haven Hospital, New Haven, Connecticut

Eunice S. Wang, M.D.
Fellow, Department of Hematology-Oncology, Memorial Sloan Kettering Cancer Institute, New York, New York

Oncologic Disease

Christopher E. Desch, M.D.
Clinical Associate Professor of Medicine, Virginia Commonwealth University, Medical College of Virginia; Medical Director, Virginia Cancer Treatment Centers, Richmond, Virginia

Jennifer J. Griggs, M.D.
Senior Instructor of Medicine, Division of Hematology/Oncology, University of Rochester School of Medicine, Rochester, New York

Metabolic Disease

Peter N. Herbert, M.D.
Clinical Professor of Medicine, Yale University School of Medicine; Chief of Staff and Senior Vice President for Medical Affairs, Yale–New Haven Hospital, New Haven, Connecticut

Endocrine Disease

Philip Barnett, M.D., Ph.D.
Associate Professor of Medicine, University of California, Los Angeles, School of Medicine; Director, Diabetes Program, Cedars-Sinai Medical Center, Los Angeles, California

Glenn D. Braunstein, M.D.
Professor of Medicine, University of California, Los Angeles, School of Medicine; Chairman, Department of Medicine, Cedars-Sinai Medical Center, Los Angeles, California

Theodore C. Friedman, M.D., Ph.D.
Assistant Professor of Medicine, University of
California, Los Angeles, School of Medicine; Staff
Endocrinologist, Cedars-Sinai Medical Center, Los
Angeles, California

Vivien Herman-Bonert, M.D.
Associate Professor of Medicine, University of
California, Los Angeles, School of Medicine;
Clinical Coordinator, Pituitary Clinic, Cedars-Sinai
Medical Center, Los Angeles, California

Women's Health

Sally L. Hodder, M.D.
Associate Professor of Medicine, Case Western
Reserve University School of Medicine; Staff
Physician, University Hospitals of Cleveland,
Cleveland, Ohio

Ame L. Taylor, M.D.
Associate Professor of Medicine, Division of
Cardiology, and Vice Chair, Women's Health
Programs, Case Western Reserve University School
of Medicine; Attending Physician, University
Hospitals of Cleveland, Cleveland, Ohio

Diseases of Bone and Bone Mineral Metabolism

F. Richard Bringhurst, M.D.
Associate Professor of Medicine, Harvard Medical
School, Endocrine Unit; Chief of Staff,
Massachusetts General Hospital, Boston,
Massachusetts

Joel S. Finkelstein, M.D.
Associate Professor of Medicine, Harvard Medical
School, Endocrine Unit; Massachusetts General
Hospital, Boston, Massachusetts

Margaret P. Seton, M.D.
Instructor in Medicine, Harvard Medical School,
Arthritis Unit; Massachusetts General Hospital,
Boston, Massachusetts

Musculoskeletal and Connective Tissue Disease

Joseph Korn, M.D.
Professor of Medicine and Biochemistry, Arthritis
Center, Boston University School of Medicine,
Boston, Massachusetts

Peter A. Merkel, M.D., M.P.H.
Assistant Professor of Medicine, Boston University
School of Medicine, Boston, Massachusetts

Robert W. Simms, M.D.
Associate Professor of Medicine and Clinical
Director, Section of Rheumatology, Boston
University School of Medicine, Boston,
Massachusetts

Infectious Disease

Charles C. J. Carpenter, M.D., M.A.C.P.
Professor of Medicine and Director, International
Health Institute, Brown University School of
Medicine, Providence, Rhode Island

Michael M. Lederman, M.D.
Professor of Medicine, Case Western Reserve
University School of Medicine; Attending
Physician, University Hospitals of Cleveland,
Cleveland, Ohio

Robert A. Salata, M.D.
Professor of Medicine, Vice-Chairman, Department
of Medicine, and Chief, Division of Infectious
Diseases, Case Western Reserve University;
Attending Physician and Consultant and Medical
Director, Hospital Epidemiology and Infection
Control, University Hospitals of Cleveland,
Cleveland, Ohio

Neurologic Disease

Timothy J. Counihan, M.D., MRCPI
Assistant Professor of Neurology, University of
Rochester School of Medicine, Rochester, New
York

Jennifer J. Griggs, M.D.
Senior Instructor of Medicine, Division of
Hematology/Oncology, University of Rochester
School of Medicine, Rochester, New York

Robert C. Griggs, M.D.
Edward A. and Alma Vollertsen Rykenboer Professor
of Neurophysiology, and Chair, Department of
Neurology, University of Rochester School of
Medicine and Dentistry, Rochester, New York

Frederick J. Marshall, M.D.
Assistant Professor of Neurology and Chief, Geriatric
Neurology Unit, Department of Neurology,
University of Rochester School of Medicine and
Dentistry, Rochester, New York

Roger P. Simon, M.D.
Robert Stone Dow Chair in Neurology and Director,
Neurobiology Research, Legacy Health Systems,
Portland, Oregon

The Aging Patient

David A. Lipschitz, M.D., Ph.D.
Professor and Chairman, *Donald W. Reynolds*
Department of Geriatrics, University of Arkansas
College of Medicine, Little Rock, Arkansas

Robert J. Reis, M.D.
Professor of Geriatrics, University of Arkansas
College of Medicine, Little Rock, Arkansas

Dennis H. Sullivan, M.D.
Associate Professor of Geriatrics, University of
  Arkansas College of Medicine, Little Rock,
  Arkansas

Substance Abuse

Jeffrey L. Clothier, M.D.
Associate Professor of Psychiatry, University of
  Arkansas College of Medicine; Chief, Ambulatory
  Mental Health Service, John L. McClellan VA
  Hospital, Little Rock, Arkansas

Timothy E. Holcomb, M.D.
Associate Professor of Internal Medicine, University
  of Arkansas College of Medicine; Associate Chief
  of Staff for Primary Care, John L. McClellan VA
  Hospital, Little Rock, Arkansas

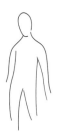

PREFACE

The fifth edition of *Cecil Essentials of Medicine,* like the preceding editions, is a succinct and yet comprehensive textbook of internal medicine that considers the biologic basis for understanding disease processes, the clinical characteristics of diseases, and the compassionate and rational approaches to the diagnosis and treatment of diseases commonly encountered by practitioners of internal medicine and the medical subspecialties. Thus, this book is intended primarily for medical students; house officers; practitioners of general medicine, internal medicine and other subspecialties, and other medical disciplines; and other persons involved either in preventive medicine or in caring for patients.

This fifth edition of *Essentials* has been revised extensively. Two new Editors, Robert C. Griggs and Joseph Loscalzo, have replaced J. Claude Bennett, an Editor for the third and fourth editions, and Fred Plum, one of the founding Editors of *Essentials.* Three new sections have been added: Molecular Medicine; Evidence-Based Medicine; and Women's Health. The Oncology section has been expanded. New authors have rewritten seven sections entirely, and the remaining sections have been revised exhaustively with regard to both content and timeliness. As with the fourth edition, this edition utilizes four-color illustrations extensively. Finally, expansion of tabular material and algorithms enabled us to make the fifth edition of *Essentials* more readable and yet approximately 10% smaller than the preceding edition.

We are deeply grateful to a number of individuals. The legacy of both Claude Bennett and Fred Plum, to whom this edition is dedicated, remains. Dr. Susan S. Beland, Associate Professor of Internal Medicine at the University of Arkansas, reviewed all the content for this edition.

We also thank Ms. Lynne Gery, Manager, Developmental Editors, and Ms. Lisette Bralow, Executive Publisher, Medical Books, both of the W.B. Saunders Company, who contributed their customary excellence in the design and preparation of the fifth edition of *Essentials.* Mr. Leslie E. Hoeltzel, Emeritus Manager, Developmental Editors, assisted with prior editions of *Essentials* and with the initial planning for this edition. Finally, we thank our very able secretarial staff, Ms. Clementine M. Whitman (Little Rock); Ms. Barbara S. Ryan (Providence); Ms. Katherine A. Seropian (Boston); and Ms. Shirley E. Thomas (Rochester).

THE EDITORS

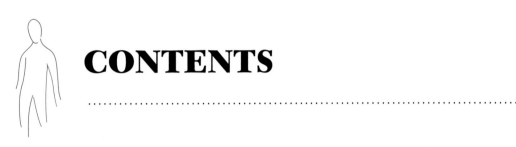

CONTENTS

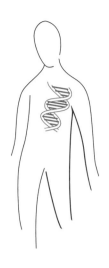

Introduction to Molecular Medicine

1 THE MOLECULAR BASIS OF HUMAN DISEASE

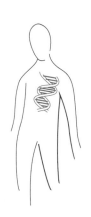

1

THE MOLECULAR BASIS OF HUMAN DISEASE

Joseph Loscalzo

Medicine has evolved dramatically over the past century from a healing art in which standards of practice were established on the basis of personal experience, passed on from one practitioner to the next, to a rigorous intellectual discipline steeped in the scientific method. The application of the scientific method has led to major advances in the fields of physiology, microbiology, biochemistry, and pharmacology; these advances served as the basis for the diagnostic and therapeutic approaches to illness in common use by physicians through most of the twentieth century. Since the 1980s, the understanding of the molecular basis of genetics has expanded dramatically, and advances in this field have identified new and exciting dimensions for defining the basis of "conventional" genetic diseases (e.g., sickle cell disease) as well as the basis of complex genetic traits (e.g., hypertension). The molecular basis for the interaction between genes and environment has also begun to be defined. Armed with a variety of sensitive and specific molecular techniques, the contemporary physician can now begin not only to understand the molecular underpinning of complex pathobiologic processes but also to identify individuals at risk for common diseases. Understanding modern medicine therefore requires an understanding of molecular genetics and the molecular basis of disease. This introductory chapter offers an overview of this complex and rapidly evolving topic and attempts to summarize principles of molecular medicine that will be highlighted in specific sections throughout the book.

Deoxyribonucleic Acid and the Genetic Code

All of the information needed to form an organism is contained within the nucleus of every cell within that organism. This information is encoded by a double-stranded, linear polymer of deoxyribonucleic acid (DNA) that constitutes the genome of the organism. DNA is made up of a linear backbone of deoxyribose sugars linked between the fifth carbon of one pentose ring and the third carbon of the next pentose ring through a (5'-3') phosphodiester bond (Fig. 1–1). Each deoxyribose phosphate monomer is covalently bound to one of four nucleic acid bases: the purines adenine (A) and guanine (G) and the pyrimidines cytosine (C) and thymine (T). The deoxyribose phosphate backbone forms the outer portion of a double-stranded helix of the polymer, in the center of which the bases pair through complementary hydrogen bonds. The thermodynamics of association dictate that only adenine can pair with thymidine and only cytosine can pair with guanine.

In the human genome, there are approximately 6×10^9 nucleotides, or 3×10^9 pairs of nucleotides, that associate in the double helix. All of the specificity of DNA is determined by the base sequence, and this sequence is stored in duplicated form in the double helical structure, which facilitates correction of sequence errors and provides a mechanistic basis for replication of the information during cell division. The base sequence of a single strand of DNA serves as a template for replication, which is accomplished by the action of DNA-dependent DNA polymerases that unwind the double helical DNA and copy each single strand with remarkable fidelity.

DNA is localized to the nucleus, where the polymers are tightly compressed in association with chromatin proteins into chromosomes. In human cells, there are 23 pairs of chromosomes, each of which contains a unique sequence and, therefore, unique genetic information. All cell types except for gametocytes contain this duplicate, diploid number of genetic units, half of which is referred to as a *haploid number*. The genetic information contained in chromosomes is separated into discrete functional elements, known as *genes*. A gene is defined as a unit of base sequence that encodes a specific polypeptide sequence. There are an estimated 50,000 to 100,000 genes in the human haploid genome, and these are interspersed among regions of sequence that do not code for protein and whose function is as

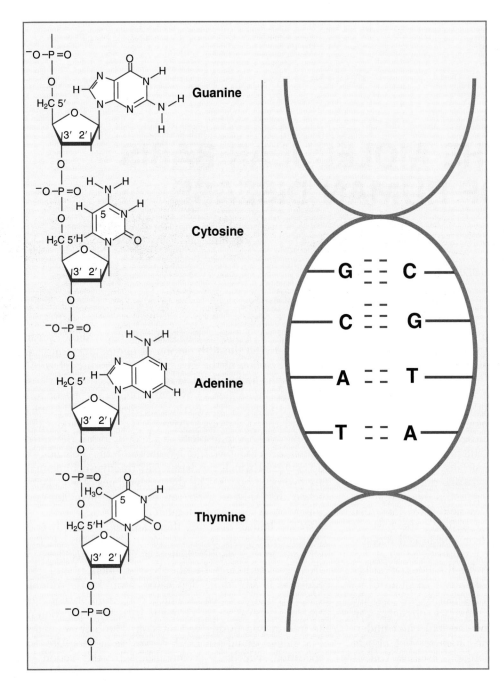

FIGURE 1–1 DNA structure. The structures of each nucleotide are given on the left side of the figure with the specific base denotation listed next to each nucleotide. The hydrogen-bonded bases are shown paired in a turn of the double helix on the right side of the figure, where three dashed lines connote three hydrogen bonds between guanine (G) and cytosine (C) bases and two dashed lines connote two hydrogen bonds between adenine (A) and thymine (T) bases.

yet unknown. The average chromosome contains 3000 to 5000 genes, and these range in size from approximately 1 kilobase (kb) to 2 megabases (Mb).

The precise location of genes on a chromosome is important for defining the likelihood that a portion of one chromosome will interchange, or cross over, with the corresponding portion of its complementary chromosome when genetic recombination occurs during meiosis (Fig. 1–2). During meiotic recombination, genetic loci or alleles that have been acquired from one parent interchange with those acquired from the other parent to produce new combinations of alleles, and the likelihood that alleles will recombine during meiosis varies as a function of their linear distance from one another in the chromosomal sequence. This recombination probability (or distance) is commonly quantitated in centimorgans: 1 centimorgan is defined as the chromosomal distance over which there is a 1% chance that two alleles will undergo a crossover event during meiosis. Crossover events serve as the basis for mixing parental base sequence during development and thereby promoting genetic diversity among offspring. Analysis of the tendency for specific alleles to be inherited together (linkage analysis) indicates that the recombination distance in the human genome is approximately 3000 centimorgans.

Protein synthesis occurs in the cytoplasm, and in order to transfer the information contained in nuclear DNA to the ribosomal site of protein synthesis, an intermediate molecular species, known as messenger ribonu-

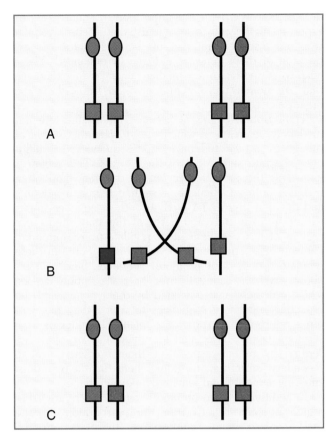

FIGURE 1–2 Crossing over and recombination. *A,* Two diploid chromosomes are shown, one pair from each parent (red and blue), with two genomic loci denoted by the circles and squares. *B,* Crossing over of one haploid chromosome from each parent. *C,* The resulting recombination of chromosomal segments now redistributes one haploid locus, denoted by squares, from one diploid pair to another.

cleic acid (mRNA), has evolved. There are two structural differences that distinguish RNA from DNA: the polymeric backbone is made up of ribose sugars linked by phosphodiester bonds, and the base composition is different in that uracil is substituted for thymine. Messenger RNA is produced in the nucleus by the action of DNA-dependent RNA polymerase, which copies the

"antisense" strand of the DNA double helix to synthesize a single strand of mRNA that is identical to the "sense" strand of the DNA double helix in a process called *transcription* (Fig. 1–3). Because a typical gene contains coding sequence (exons) that are linearly interrupted by stretches of noncoding sequences (introns), the resulting immature mRNA must next undergo splicing in order to link directly one exonic sequence to the next. The resulting mature mRNA then exits the nucleus and enters the cytoplasm to begin the process of translation, or conversion of the base code to polypeptide.

Protein synthesis or translation of the mRNA code occurs on ribosomes, which are macromolecular complexes of proteins and ribosomal RNA located in the cytoplasm. Translation involves the conversion of the linear code of a triplet of bases (the codon) into the corresponding amino acid. There are 64 possible triplet combinations that a 4-base code generates ($4 \times 4 \times 4$), and these correspond to 20 different amino acids, many of which are encoded by more than one base triplet (Table 1–1). To decode mRNA, an adapter molecule known as transfer RNA (tRNA) recognizes the codon in mRNA and associates with that codon through the 3-base anticodon that it bears; in addition, each tRNA is charged with a unique amino acid that corresponds to the anticodon. Enzymes on the ribosome then link amino acids through the synthesis of a peptide bond (Fig. 1–4), releasing the tRNA in the process. Consecutive linkage of amino acids in the growing polypeptide chain represents the terminal event in the conversion of information contained within the nuclear DNA sequence into mature protein (DNA → RNA → protein).

Regulation of Gene Expression

The information contained in the genome is, in essence, functionally meaningless without some mechanism for the regulation of its expression. The timing, duration, localization, and magnitude of gene expression are all important elements in the complex tapestry of cell form and function governed by the genome. The principal regulatory step in gene expression occurs at the level

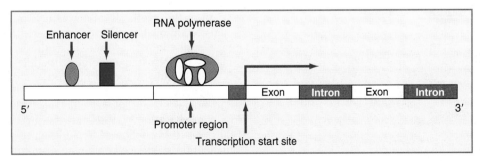

FIGURE 1–3 Transcription. Genomic DNA is shown with enhancer and silencer sites located 5′ upstream of the promoter region, to which RNA polymerase is bound. The transcription start site is shown downstream of the promoter region, and this site is followed by exonic sequences interrupted by intronic sequences; the former sequences are transcribed ad seriatim by the RNA polymerase.

TABLE 1–1   The Genetic Code

First	Second				Third
	U	**C**	**A**	**G**	
U	Phe	Ser	Tyr	Cys	U
	Phe	Ser	Tyr	Cys	C
	Leu	Ser	STOP	STOP	A
	Leu	Ser	STOP	Trp	G
C	Leu	Pro	His	Arg	U
	Leu	Pro	His	Arg	C
	Leu	Pro	Gln	Arg	A
	Leu	Pro	Gln	Arg	G
A	Ile	Thr	Asn	Ser	U
	Ile	Thr	Asn	Ser	C
	Ile	Thr	Lys	Arg	A
	Met	Thr	Lys	Arg	G
G	Val	Ala	Asp	Gly	U
	Val	Ala	Asp	Gly	C
	Val	Ala	Glu	Gly	A
	Val	Ala	Glu	Gly	G

A = adenine; Ala = alanine; Arg = arginine; Asn = asparagine; C = cytosine; Cys = cysteine; G = guanine; Gln = glutamine; Glu = glutamic acid; Gly = glycine; His = histidine; Ile = isoleucine; Leu = leucine; Lys = lysine; Met = methionine; Phe = phenylalanine; Pro = proline; Ser = serine; Thr = threonine; Trp = tryptophan; Tyr = ?

of gene transcription. The transcription of information contained in genomic DNA into mRNA (transcripts) is performed by a specific DNA-dependent RNA polymerase.

Regulation of transcription is a complex process that occurs at several levels (see Fig. 1–3). Of importance is that the expression of many genes is only marginally regulated, if at all, and these are known as "housekeeping," or constitutively expressed, genes. They typically yield protein products that are essential for normal cell function or survival and thus must be maintained at a specific steady-state concentration under all circumstances. Many other genes, in contrast, are not expressed or are only modestly expressed under basal con-

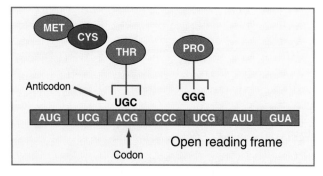

FIGURE 1–4 Translation. The open reading frame of a mature mRNA is shown with its series of codons. tRNA molecules are shown with their corresponding anticodons, charged with their specific amino acid. A short, growing polypeptide chain is depicted. A = adenine; C = cytosine; CYS = cysteine; G = guanine; MET = methionine; PRO = proline; THR = threonine; U = uracil.

ditions; however, with the imposition of some stress or exposure of the cell to an agonist that elicits a cellular response distinct from that of the basal state, the expression of these genes is induced or enhanced. These adaptive responses often mediate changes in phenotype that are homeostatically protective to the cell or the organism.

Transcription begins at a transcription start site immediately upstream of which (i.e., toward the 5′ end of the gene) are located nucleotide sequences that influence the rate and extent of the process. This region is known as the *promoter region* of the gene and often includes both an element of sequence rich in adenine and thymine (the TATA box) and other sequence motifs within approximately 100 bases of the start site. These regions of DNA sequence that regulate transcription are known as *cis*-acting regulatory sequences. Some of these regulatory regions of promoter sequence bind proteins known as *trans*-acting factors, or transcription factors, which are themselves encoded by other genes, and the *cis*-acting regulatory sequences to which they bind are often referred to as *response elements*. Families of transcription factors have been identified and are often described by unique aspects of their predicted protein secondary structure, including helix-turn-helix motifs, zinc-finger motifs, and leucine-zipper motifs.

In addition to gene promoter regions, there are other regions at some distance from the transcription start site that increase gene transcription; these regions are known as *enhancer sites*. Enhancer sites are distinct from promoter sites in that they can exist at distances quite remote from the start site, either upstream or downstream (i.e., beyond the 3′ end of the gene), and without clear orientation requirements. *Trans*-acting factors bind to these enhancer sites and are believed to alter the tertiary structure or conformation of the DNA in a manner that facilitates the binding and assembly of the transcription-initiation complex at the promoter region, perhaps in some cases by forming a broad loop of DNA in the process. Biochemical modification of selected promoter or enhancer sequences, such as methylation of CpG-rich sequences, can also modulate transcription; methylation typically serves to suppress transcription. The terms *silencer* and *suppressor* elements refer to *cis*-acting nucleotide sequences that reduce or shut off gene transcription and do so through association with *trans*-acting factors that recognize these specific sequences.

After the synthesis of immature mRNA in the nucleus, additional regulatory steps yield the mature message and, ultimately, protein synthesis. The initial, immature mRNA first undergoes modification at both the 5′ and 3′ ends. A special nucleotide structure called the *cap* is added to the 5′ end to increase ribosomal binding and enhance translational efficiency. The 3′ end undergoes modification by nuclease cleavage of approximately 20 nucleotides, followed by addition of a length of polynucleotide sequence containing a uniform stretch of adenine bases, the so-called polyA tail that stabilizes the mRNA.

In addition to these changes that occur uniformly in all mRNAs, other, more selective modifications can also occur. Because each gene contains both exonic and intronic sequences and the immature mRNA is transcribed without regard for exon-intron boundaries, this immature message must be edited in a way that splices all exons together in appropriate sequence. The process of splicing, or removal of intronic sequences to produce the mature mRNA, is an exquisitely choreographed event that involves the intermediate formation of a spliceosome, which contains a loop or lariat-like structure that includes the intron targeted for removal. Only after splicing has concluded is the mature mRNA able to exit the nucleus, enter the cytoplasm, and begin to be translated at the ribosome. Alternative splicing pathways (i.e., alternative exonic assembly pathways) for specific genes serve as yet another site for transcriptional regulation.

The precise sequence of a mature mRNA can be converted to a complementary DNA (cDNA) sequence through the use of reverse transcriptase, an enzyme that synthesizes DNA by using RNA as a template. The development of this approach has revolutionized molecular genetics in that cDNAs are chemically more stable than is mRNA, cDNAs can be cloned and their gene products expressed in cell culture systems, and the sequences of cDNAs can be modified or mutated to yield different gene products with different biochemical actions.

The mature mRNA contains elements of untranslated sequence at both the 5′ and 3′ ends that can regulate translation. Currently, less is known about the determinants of translational regulation than is known about transcriptional regulation. Because translation occurs at a fairly invariant rate among all mRNA species, the stability or half-life of a specific mRNA also serves as another point of regulation of gene expression. The 3′-untranslated region of mRNAs contains regions of sequence that dictate the susceptibility of the message to nuclease cleavage and degradation; stability appears to be sequence-specific and, in some cases, dependent on trans-acting factors that bind to the mRNA.

Genetic Variation, Population Diversity, and Genetic Polymorphisms

A stable, heritable change in DNA is defined as a mutation. This strict contemporary definition does not depend on the functional relevance of the sequence alteration and implicates a change in primary DNA sequence. Considered in historical context, mutations were first defined on the basis of identifiable changes in the heritable phenotype of an organism. As biochemical phenotyping became more precise in the mid-twentieth century, investigators demonstrated that many proteins exist in more than one form in a population, and these forms were viewed as a consequence of variations in the gene coding for that protein (allelic variation). With advances in DNA sequencing methods, the concept of mutation

evolved from one that could be appreciated only by identifying differences in phenotype to one that could be quite precisely defined at the level of changes in the structure of DNA. Although most mutations are stably transmitted from parents to offspring, some are genetically lethal and thus cannot be passed on. In addition, the discovery of regions of the genome that contain sequences that repeat in tandem a highly variable number of times (tandem repeats) suggests that some mutations are less stable than others. These tandem-repeats are described further later in this chapter.

The molecular nature of mutations is quite varied (Table 1–2). A mutation can involve the deletion, insertion, or substitution of a single base, all of which are referred to as *point mutations*. Substitutions can be further classified as "silent" when the amino acid encoded by the mutated triplet does not change, as "missense" when the amino acid encoded by the mutated triplet changes, and as "nonsense" when the mutation leads to premature termination of translation (stop codon). On occasion, point mutations can alter the processing of immature mRNA by producing alternate splice sites or eliminating a splice site. When a single- or double-base deletion or insertion occurs in an exon, a frameshift mutation results, leading to premature termination of translation. The other end of the spectrum of mutations includes large deletions of an entire gene or a set of contiguous genes; deletion, duplication, and translocation of a segment of one chromosome to another; or duplication or deletion of an entire chromosome.

Each individual possesses two alleles for any given gene locus, one from each parent. Identical alleles define homozygosity and nonidentical alleles define heterozygosity for any gene locus, and the heritability of these alleles follows typical mendelian rules. With a clearer

TABLE 1–2 The Molecular Basis of Mutations

Type	Example
Point Mutations	
Deletion	α-Thalassemia
Insertion	
Substitution	
Silent	Cystic fibrosis
Missense	Sickle cell anemia
Nonsense	Cystic fibrosis
Large Mutations (Gene or Gene Cluster)	
Deletion	Duchenne's muscular dystrophy
Insertion	Factor VIII deficiency (hemophilia A)
Duplication	Duchenne's muscular dystrophy
Inversion	Factor VIII deficiency
Expanding triplet	Huntington's disease
Very Large Mutations (Chromosomal Segment or Chromosome)	
Deletion	Turner's syndrome (45, XO)
Duplication	Trisomy 21
Translocation	XX male [46X,t(X;Y)]*

* Translocation onto an X chromosome of a segment of a Y chromosome that bears the locus for testicular differentiation.

understanding of the molecular basis of mutations and of allelic variation, their distribution in populations can now be analyzed quite precisely by following specific DNA sequences. Differences in DNA sequences studied within the context of a population are referred to as *genetic polymorphisms,* and these polymorphisms underlie the diversity observed within a given species and among species. Analyses of multiple genetic polymorphisms in the human genome reveal that there is a remarkable variation among individuals at the level of the sequence of genomic DNA. With each generation of a species, the frequency of polymorphic changes in a gene is 10^{-4} to 10^{-7}; thus, in view of the number of genes in the human genome, between 0.5% and 1.0% of the base sequence of the human genome is polymorphic. In this context, a mutation can now be defined as a specific type of allelic polymorphism that causes a functional defect in a cell or organism. Despite the high prevalence of benign polymorphisms in a population, the prevalence of harmful mutations is comparatively rare because of selective pressures that eliminate the most harmful mutations from the population (lethality) and the variability within genomic sequence of susceptibility to polymorphic change: Some portions of the genome are remarkably stable and free of polymorphic variation, whereas other portions are highly polymorphic, the persistence of variation within which is a consequence of the functional benignity of the sequence change. In other words, polymorphic differences in DNA sequence between individuals can be divided into those producing no effect on phenotype, those causing benign differences in phenotype (normal genetic variation), and those producing adverse consequences in phenotype (mutations); the last group can be further subdivided into the polymorphic mutations that alone are able to produce a functionally abnormal phenotype (monogenic disease; e.g., sickle cell anemia) and those that alone are unable to do so but in conjunction with other mutations can produce a functionally abnormal phenotype (complex disease traits; e.g., essential hypertension).

Polymorphisms are more common in noncoding regions of the genome than in coding regions, and one common type of these involves the tandem repetition of short DNA sequences a variable numbers of times. If these tandem repeats are long, they are termed *variable number tandem repeats;* if short, they are termed *short tandem repeats.* During mitosis, the number of tandem repeats can change, and the frequency of this kind of replication error is high enough to make alternative lengths of the tandem repeats common in a population; however, the rate of change in length of the tandem repeats is low enough to make the size polymorphism useful as a stable genotypic trait in families. In view of these features, polymorphic tandem repeats are quite useful in determining the familial heritability of specific genomic loci (vide infra). Polymorphic tandem repeats are sufficiently prevalent along the entire genomic sequence that they can serve as genetic markers for specific genes of interest through an analysis of their linkage to those genes during crossover and recombination events.

Genes and Human Disease

Human genetic diseases can be divided into three broad categories: those that are caused by a mutation in a single gene (monogenic disorders, or mendelian traits), those that are caused by mutations in more than one gene (polygenic disorders, or complex disease traits), and those that are chromosomal in nature. In all three groups of disorders, environmental factors can contribute to the phenotypic expression of the disease by modulating gene expression or unmasking a biochemical abnormality that has no functional consequences in the absence of a stimulus or stressor. Classical monogenic disorders include sickle cell anemia, familial hypercholesterolemia, and cystic fibrosis; of importance is that these genetic diseases can be produced exclusively by a single specific mutation (e.g., sickle cell anemia) or by any one of several mutations (e.g., familial hypercholesterolemia and cystic fibrosis) in a given family (genetic heterogeneity). Of interest is that some of these disorders evolved to protect the host: for example, sickle cell anemia as protection against falciparum malaria and cystic fibrosis as protection against cholera. Examples of polygenic disorders or complex disease traits include type I (insulin-dependent) diabetes mellitus, atherosclerotic cardiovascular disease, and essential hypertension. A common example of a chromosomal disorder is the presence of an extra chromosome 21 (trisomy 21). The overall frequency of monogenic disorders is approximately 1%; that of polygenic disorders, approximately 60% (including disorders with a genetic substrate that develops later in life); and that of chromosomal disorders, approximately 0.5%. Of importance is that chromosomal abnormalities are frequent causes of spontaneous abortion and malformations.

Contrary to the view held by early geneticists, few phenotypes are entirely defined by a single genetic locus. Thus, monogenic disorders are comparatively uncommon; however, they are still useful as a means to understanding some basic principles of heredity. Monogenic disorders are of three types: autosomal dominant, autosomal recessive, or X-linked. *Dominance* and *recessiveness* refer to the nature of the heritability of a genetic trait and correlate with the number of alleles affected at a given locus. If a mutation in a single allele determines the phenotype, the mutation is said to be dominant; that is, the heterozygous state conveys the clinical phenotype to the individual. In contrast, if a mutation is necessary at both alleles to determine the phenotype, the mutation is said to be recessive; that is, only the homozygous state conveys the clinical phenotype to the individual. Dominant or recessive mutations can lead to either a loss or a gain of function of the gene product. If the mutation is present on the X chromosome, it is defined as X-linked (which in females can, by definition, be viewed only as dominant or recessive; otherwise, it is autosomal. The importance of identifying a potential genetic disease as inherited by one of these three mechanisms is that if one of these patterns of inheritance is present, the disease must involve a single genomic abnormality that leads to an abnormality in a single protein. Classically identified genetic diseases are produced by mutations that affect coding (exonic) sequences. There are, however, mutations in intronic and other untranslated regions of the genome that may disturb the function or expression of specific genes; examples of diseases with these types of mutations include myotonic dystrophy and Friedreich's ataxia.

An individual with a dominant monogenic disorder typically has one affected parent and a 50% chance of transmitting the mutation to his or her offspring. In addition, men and women are equally likely to be affected and equally likely to transmit the trait to their offspring. The trait cannot be transmitted to offspring by two unaffected parents. In contrast, an individual with a recessive monogenic disorder typically has parents who are clinically normal; affected parents, each heterozygous for the mutation, have a 25% chance of transmitting the clinical phenotype to their offspring but a 50% chance of transmitting the mutation to their offspring (i.e., producing an unaffected carrier).

Notwithstanding the clear heritability of common monogenic disorders (e.g., sickle cell anemia), the clinical expression of the disease in an individual with a phenotype expected to produce the disease may vary. *Variability in clinical expression* is defined as the range of phenotypic effects observed in individuals carrying a given mutation; *penetrance* refers to a smaller subset of individuals with variable clinical expression of a mutation, being defined as the proportion of individuals with a given genotype who manifest any clinical phenotypic features of the disorder. There are three principal determinants of variability in clinical expression or incomplete penetrance of a given genetic disorder: environmental factors, offsetting effects of other genetic loci, and random chance.

Genetic disorders affecting a unique pool of DNA, mitochondrial DNA, have been identified. Mitochondrial DNA is unique in that it is inherited only from the mother. In addition, mutations in mitochondrial DNA can vary among mitochondria within a given cell and within a given individual (heteroplasmy). Examples of genetic disorders based in the mitochondrial genome are the Kearns-Sayre syndrome and Leber's hereditary optic neuropathy. The list of known mitochondrial genomic disorders is growing rapidly, and there may also be mitochondrial contributions to a large number of common polygenic disorders.

Gene Mapping

Identifying the gene or genes responsible for a specific disease phenotype requires an understanding of the topology of the human genome. Early attempts at mapping the genome involved visualization of chromosomal bands by standard cytogenetic analysis and correlating a specific gene locus to sites identified by banding patterns. More recent mapping strategies involve correlating a specific gene locus to chromosomal positions identified with molecular markers (unique sequences). The process of gene mapping involves identifying the relative order and distance of specific loci along the genome. Maps can be of two types: genetic and physical. Genetic maps identify the genomic location of specific genetic loci by a statistical analysis based on the frequency of recombination events of the locus of interest with other known loci. Physical maps identify the genomic location of specific genetic loci by a direct measurement of the distance along the genome at which the locus of interest is located in relation to one or more defined markers.

The process of gene mapping was greatly facilitated by the discovery and application of restriction endonucleases to the identification of unique sequences within the genome. Restriction endonucleases are enzymes, first identified in bacteria in the 1970s, that cleave nuclear DNA; they were termed *restriction enzymes* because they limited the entry of foreign DNA into bacteria by their nuclease-degrading activity. What makes restriction enzymes interesting is their specificity: They do not cleave DNA randomly but, rather, do so on the basis of their recognition of highly specific nucleotide sequences in the DNA polymer. More than 200 restriction endonucleases have been identified to date, and their specificity and cleavage mechanisms range widely. Some cleave double-stranded DNA at the same position in each complementary strand, creating "blunt" ends; others cleave at different positions in each complementary strand, creating free ends in each strand that are uncomplexed, so-called "sticky" ends. The frequency of cleavage depends on the frequency of the restriction sequence recognized by the specific restriction endonuclease, which decreases as a function of the length of the sequence.

Analysis of the products of restriction endonuclease digestion of DNA by gel electrophoresis yields so-called restriction maps, or patterns of DNA fragments. Because of the differences in genomic sequence that arise as a consequence of normal biologic variation or sequence polymorphisms, the resulting restriction fragment length polymorphisms (RFLPs) differ among individuals and are inherited according to mendelian principles. These polymorphisms can serve as genetic markers for specific loci in the genome. One of the most useful types of RFLPs for localization of genetic loci within the genome is that produced by tandem repeats of sequence. The repeating unit in a tandem repeat can be short (up to four nucleotides, so-called short tandem repeats [STRs]) or long (hundreds of bases in length). Tandem repeats arise through "slippage" or stuttering of the DNA polymerase during replication in the case of STRs; longer variations arise through unequal crossover events. STRs are distributed throughout the genome and are highly polymorphic. Of importance is that these markers have two different alleles at each locus that are derived from each parent; thus, the origins of the two chromosomes can be discerned through this analysis.

The use of highly polymorphic tandem repeats that occur throughout the genome as genomic markers has provided a basis for mapping specific gene loci through establishing the association or linkage with selected

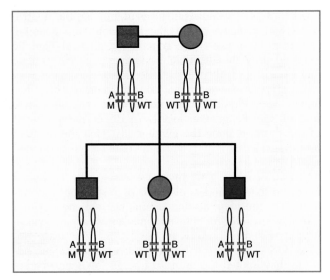

FIGURE 1–5   Linkage analysis. Analysis of the association (genomic contiguity) of a mutation (M) and a polymorphic allelic marker (A) shows close linkage in that the mutation segregates with the A allele, while the wild type gene locus (WT) associates with the B allele.

markers. Linkage analysis is predicated on a simple principle: the likelihood that a crossover event will occur during meiosis decreases the closer the locus of interest is to a given marker. The extent of genetic linkage can be ascertained for any group of loci, one of which may contain a disease-producing mutation (Fig. 1–5). Because recombination frequencies are not homogeneous throughout the entire genome, the genetic map does not precisely correlate with the physical map for a specific locus. Physical mapping requires the use of alternative molecular techniques, such as cutting the DNA into large fragments with restriction endonucleases that cleave the DNA at a paucity of sites, separating these large fragments by a special type of electrophoresis (pulse-field gel electrophoresis), and annealing the DNA fragments to complementary DNA probes that contain a sequence of interest for a given marker by hybridization on an agarose gel (Southern blot). The ongoing Human Genome Project, begun in the mid-1980s, represents an international effort to characterize the human genome completely, including the construction of its detailed genetic and physical maps with identification and characterization of all genes.

Identifying Mutant Genes

Once the physical localization of a gene of interest has been determined, the gene itself can be identified and sequenced. The size, complexity, and individual variability in DNA sequence have previously posed barriers to the precise molecular identification of specific genes. With the advent of recombinant DNA technology, wherein small DNA fragments are isolated, inserted into the nucleic acid from another biologic source, or vector,

and propagated in a prokaryotic or eukaryotic cell system (i.e., cloned), the identification of specific genetic sequences was greatly facilitated. In positional cloning approaches, this recombinant DNA technology is used to isolate and determine the precise sequence of a specific gene according to its location in the genome. Of importance is that this approach does not depend on knowing the function of the gene product.

Deducing the identity of a specific gene sequence believed to cause a specific human disease requires that mutations in the gene of interest be identified. If the gene believed to be responsible for the disease phenotype is known, its sequence can be determined by conventional cloning and sequencing strategies, and the mutation can be identified. A variety of techniques are currently available for detecting mutations. Mutations that involve insertion or deletion of large segments of DNA can be detected by Southern blot, in which the isolated DNA is annealed to a radioactively labeled fragment of complementary DNA sequence after incubation of the DNA with a specific restriction endonuclease that cleaves the DNA sequence of interest at specific sites to produce smaller fragments that can be monitored by agarose gel electrophoresis; shifts in mobility on the gel in comparison to wild-type sequence become apparent as a function of changes in the molecular size of the fragment. Alternatively, the polymerase chain reaction (PCR) can be used to identify mutations (Fig. 1–6). In this approach, small oligonucleotides (20 to 40 bases in length) complementary to regions of DNA that bracket the sequence of interest, one complementary to each strand of the double-stranded DNA, are synthesized and serve as primers for the amplification of the DNA sequence of interest. These primers are added to the DNA solution; the temperature of the solution is increased to dissociate the individual DNA strands and is then reduced to permit annealing of the primers to their template sites; and a thermolabile DNA polymerase is added to synthesize new DNA in the 5′-to-3′ direction from the primer annealing sites. The temperature is then increased to dissociate duplex structures, after which it is reduced so that another cycle of DNA synthesis can occur. Several temperature cycles (up to 40) are used to amplify progressively the concentration of the sequence of interest, which can be identified as a PCR product by agarose gel electrophoresis with a fluorescent dye. The product can be isolated and sequenced to identify the suspected mutation.

If the gene is large and the site of the mutation—especially if it is a point mutation—is unknown, other methods can be used to identify the likely mutated site in the exonic sequence. One approach that is commonly used involves scanning the gene sequence for mutations that alter the structural conformation of short complexes between parent DNA and PCR products, leading to a shift in mobility on a nondenaturing agarose gel (single-strand conformational polymorphism). A single base substitution or deletion can change the conformation of the complex in comparison with wild-type complexes, and yield a shift in mobility. Sequencing this comparatively small region of the gene then facilitates precise identification of the mutation.

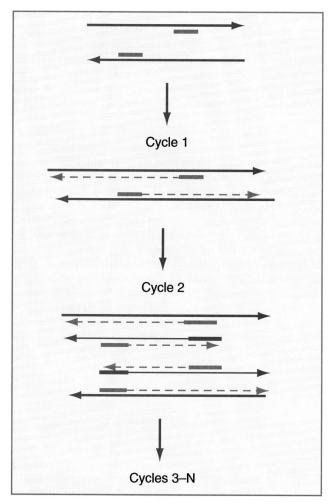

FIGURE 1-6 Polymerase chain reaction. Two cycles of a polymerase chain reaction are shown; the templates are denoted by the arrows and the primers by thick, short bars. Products of the reaction are depicted as dashed arrows.

Cycle 1

Cycle 2

Cycles 3–N

When the gene believed to cause the disease phenotype is unknown, its likely position on the genome has not been identified, or only limited mapping information is available, a candidate gene approach can be used to identify the mutated gene. In this strategy, potential candidate genes are identified on the basis of analogy to animal models or by analysis of known genes that map to the region of the genome for which limited information is available; the candidate gene is then analyzed for potential mutations. Of importance is that regardless of the approach used, mutations identified in candidate genes should always be correlated with functional changes in the gene product, because some mutations in exonic sequence could be functionally silent, representing a polymorphism without phenotypic consequences. Functional changes in the gene product can be evaluated through the use of cell culture systems to assess protein function by expressing the mutant protein through transiently transfecting the cells with a vector that carries the complementary DNA coding for the gene of interest and incorporating the mutation of interest. Alternatively, unique animal models can be developed in which the mutant gene is incorporated in the male pronucleus of oocytes taken from a superovulating impregnated female to produce an animal that overexpresses the mutant gene (a transgenic animal or an animal with more than the usual number of copies of a given gene) or in which the gene of interest is disrupted and the gene product is not synthesized (a gene "knockout" animal or an animal with half [heterozygote] or none [homozygote] of the usual number of a given gene).

Molecular Diagnostics

The application of molecular methods to human genetics has clearly revolutionized the field. Through the use of what have rapidly become straightforward, standardized techniques, the one or more mutations responsible for a particular disease phenotype can be readily identified, even when the specific disease gene or gene product may not be known. Through the use of approaches that incorporate linkage analysis and PCR, simple point mutations can be precisely localized and characterized. At the other end of the spectrum of genetic changes that underlie disease, chromosomal translocations, deletions, or duplications can be identified by conventional cytogenetic methods. Large deletions that can incorporate many kilobase pairs and many genes can now be visualized with fluorescence in situ hybridization, a technique in which a large segment of cloned DNA is labeled with a fluorescent tag and hybridized to chromosomal DNA; with deletion of the segment of interest from the genome, the chromosomal DNA fails to fluoresce in the corresponding chromosomal location.

The power of molecular techniques extends beyond their use in defining the precise molecular basis of an inherited disease. By exploiting the exquisite sensitivity of the polymerase chain reaction to amplify rare nucleic acid sequences, it is possible to diagnose rapidly a range of infectious diseases for which unique sequences are available. In particular, infections caused by fastidious or slow-growing organisms can now be rapidly diagnosed, as is the case for *Mycobacterium tuberculosis*. The presence of genes conferring resistance to specific antibiotics in microorganisms can also be verified by PCR techniques. The sequencing of the entire genome of organisms such as *Escherichia coli, M. tuberculosis,* and *Treponema pallidum* now offers unparalleled opportunities to monitor the epidemiology of infections, follow the course of acquired mutations, tailor antibiotic therapies, and develop unique gene-based therapies (vide infra) for infectious agents for which conventional antibiotic therapies are ineffective or marginally effective.

Advances in molecular medicine have also revolutionized the approach to the diagnosis and treatment of neoplastic diseases, as well as the understanding of the mechanisms of carcinogenesis. According to current views, a neoplasm arises from the clonal proliferation of a single cell that is transformed from a regulated, quiescent state into an unregulated growth phase. DNA damage accumulates in the parental tumor cell, as a result of either exogenous factors (e.g., radiation exposure) or heritable determinants. In early phases of carcinogenesis, certain of the genomic changes may impart intrinsic genetic instability that potentiates the likelihood of additional damage. One class of genes that become activated during carcinogenesis are oncogenes, which are primordial genes that normally exist in the mammalian genome in an inactive (proto-oncogene) state but, when activated, promote unregulated cell proliferation through activation of specific intracellular signaling pathways.

Molecular methods based on the acquisition of specific tumor markers, unique DNA sequences that result from oncogenetic markers of larger chromosomal abnormalities (translocations or deletions that promote oncogenesis) are now broadly applied to the diagnosis of malignancies. These methods can be used to establish the presence of specific tumor markers and oncogenes in biopsy specimens, to monitor the presence or persistence of circulating malignant cells after completion of a course of chemotherapy, and to identify the development of genetic resistance to specific chemotherapeutic agents. In addition, future studies will, through the use of conventional linkage analysis as well as candidate gene approaches, enable the identification of individuals with a heritable predisposition to malignant transformation. Many of these specific topics are discussed in later chapters.

There are, of course, many other applications of molecular medicine techniques in addition to these applications in infectious diseases and oncology. Molecular methods can be used to sort out genetic differences in metabolism that may modulate pharmacologic responses in a population of individuals (e.g., slow vs. rapid acetylators), address specific forensic issues such as paternity or criminal culpability, and approach epidemiologic analysis on a precise genetic basis.

Genetic Therapies

A principal goal of current molecular strategies is to restore normal gene function to individuals with genetic mutations. Methods to do so are currently primitive, and a number of obstacles must be surmounted for this approach to be successful.

The principal problems are that it is not easy to deliver a complete gene into a cell, and persistent expression of the new gene cannot be ensured because of variability in its incorporation in the genome and consequent variability in its regulated expression. Many approaches have been used to date, and none has been completely successful; they include packaging the complementary DNA in a viral vector, such as an attenuated adenovirus, and utilizing the cell's ability to take up the virus as a means for the complementary DNA to gain access to the cell; delivering the complementary DNA by means of a calcium phosphate–induced perturbation of the cell membrane; and encapsulating the complementary DNA in a liposome that can fuse with the cell membrane and thereby deliver the complementary DNA.

Once the complementary DNA has been successfully delivered to the cell of interest, the magnitude and durability of expression of the gene product are important variables. The magnitude of expression is determined by the number of copies of complementary DNA taken up by a cell and the extent of their incorporation in the genome of the cell; the durability of expression appears to be dependent partly on the antigenicity of the sequence and protein product.

Notwithstanding these technical limitations, gene therapy has been used to treat adenosine deaminase deficiency successfully, which suggests that the principle on which the treatment is based is reasonable. Clinical trials of gene therapy for cystic fibrosis and familial hypercholesterolemia are ongoing.

Promising Advances

The rapid and extraordinary evolution of molecular biology and genetics since 1980 has opened the way for the new era of molecular medicine. No longer will the physician be limited in the ability to define the fundamental basis of a clinical phenotype; nor will complex phenotypes elude appropriate diagnosis. Ultimately, patterns of gene expression, complex interactions between genes and between genes and environmental factors, and unique therapeutic approaches will be defined for a given individual. Individualized responses to specific therapies are also likely to be regulated by the genome (pharmacogenomics), which will lead to uniquely tailored pharmacologic and genetic therapies. This level of biomedical science is primitive; in view of what has been achieved thus far, the future holds great promise for more rapid and successful approaches to specific genetic disorders and the many other diseases that have a genetic basis for their expression.

REFERENCES

Housman D: Human DNA polymorphisms. N Engl J Med 1995; 332: 318–320.
Korf B: Molecular diagnosis. N Engl J Med 1995; 332:1218–1220, 1499–1502.
Ross DW: *Introduction to Molecular Medicine*, 2nd ed. New York: Springer, 1996.

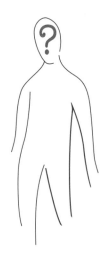

Decision-Making in Medical Practice

2 EVIDENCE-BASED MEDICINE

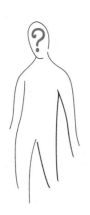

2

EVIDENCE-BASED MEDICINE

Awny S. Farajallah • Susan S. Beland

The diagnosis and treatment of individual patients involve clinical experience and skills on the part of the physician and knowledge of scientific information obtained through clinical trials. Since the 1960s, research has provided impressive new techniques for health care that can strain the ability of a society to fund and provide such services. Critical appraisal of both new and traditional diagnostic and treatment modalities is thus needed.

Traditionally, much of daily practice was based on informal learning and a tradition of knowledge transfer from experienced clinicians to trainees and colleagues. This approach, however, is increasingly being supplanted by rigorous analysis of the scientific underpinnings of clinical logic. Electronic databases and Internet technology enable collation and dissemination of information to help identify which techniques are supported by clinical trials. *Evidence-based medicine* (EBM) attempts to offer preferred strategies to clinicians based on published clinical science and to provide optimal clinical care to patients with the resources available to the health care system.

EBM is the practice of evaluating, critiquing, and applying recent research information to individual practice. It should complement the physician's clinical skills and experience. The practice of EBM requires the application of new skills, a process that includes identifying the problem and searching for the necessary information to solve that problem based on the best evidence available. EBM also involves informing the patient of the basis for care and then having him or her participate in the decision-making process. The requirements of EBM are outlined in Table 2–1.

Once a thorough history and physical examination have been completed, the first step in EBM is the formulation of the clinical question. This question can be about the origin of a particular disorder, the value of a diagnostic test, the optimal outcome, or the efficacy of a therapeutic modality. Clinical questions can also include the economic value of a certain therapy or the value of a specific clinical finding. A well-designed clinical question is formed with the following four elements:

1. The patient or problem: identifying and describing the medical problem in question and focusing on searchable terms.
2. Intervention (a diagnostic procedure or treatment): asking which particular intervention is indicated.
3. Comparison of interventions (if necessary): determining the alternatives.
4. Outcomes: predicting the prognosis or outcome from the intervention.

For example, a patient with hepatitis C and cirrhosis undergoes an esophagogastroduodenoscopy and is found to have grade III esophageal varices. He has never had hematemesis. As you inform the patient of the finding, he asks you whether any treatment is available to prevent him from bleeding. Applying the elements of the clinical question to the available information, the question would comprise the following:

The patient or problem: grade III esophageal varices.
Intervention: the value of oral propranolol.
Comparison of interventions: ligation or sclerotherapy of varices.
Outcome: prevention of gastrointestinal bleeding.

Narrowing the clinical problem to such simple terms makes it easier to conduct a literature search.

Searching for Relevant Information

Accessing the vast body of medical information presents two medical challenges: finding the relevant information and keeping up with the literature. The options for finding information include asking experts, searching in textbooks, and performing computer-assisted searches.

TABLE 2–1   Requirements of Evidence-Based Medicine

Understanding the pathophysiology of disease
Having competence in diagnostic clinical skills
Identifying the clinical problem
Searching for the relevant information
Determining the validity of the information
Applying the information to patients
Including the patient in the decision-making process

TABLE 2–2   Types of Research Studies

Primary Studies	Secondary Studies
Randomized control	Meta-analysis
Case-control	Clinical practice guidelines
Cohort studies	Decision analysis
Cross-sectional	Cost-effectiveness analysis
Case series	
Case report	

The last approach can be the most effective because it enables searches of large databases of published articles. MEDLINE, the Cochrane database of systematic reviews, and other Internet sites that teach EBM are available. Some of these sources compile the research results of several trials and present them in a concise format that summarizes the best evidence about the clinical question. After the applicable articles have been retrieved, the process of critically appraising the articles and assessing their validity and applicability for a particular patient starts.

Critical Appraisal of the Literature

Research studies are conducted in several different ways (Table 2–2). *Primary studies* can have several designs. In *randomized controlled studies*, participants in the trial are randomly assigned to one intervention or another. Both groups are monitored for a specified period, and the data are analyzed in terms of specific outcomes defined at the outset of the study. This type of study allows rigorous assessment of a single variable in a defined patient group, has a prospective design that potentially eradicates bias by comparing two otherwise similar groups, and allows for meta-analysis. However, these studies are expensive and time consuming. An example of such a randomized controlled study is one designed to assess the value of bupropion versus nicotine patches, or the combination of both, in smoking cessation. *Cohort studies* have two or more groups of people selected on the basis of differences in their exposure to a particular agent. These groups are monitored to see how many in each group develop a disease or other specific outcome. *Case-control studies* involve patients with a particular disease or condition who are identified and matched with control patients. The controls can be patients with another disease or persons from the general population. In *cross-sectional surveys*, a representative sample of subjects is interviewed, examined, or otherwise studied to gain answers to a specific clinical question. *Case reports* describe the medical history of a single patient. When medical histories of more than one patient with a particular condition are described together to illustrate one aspect of the disease process, the term *case series* is used.

Secondary (integrative) studies attempt to summarize and draw conclusions from primary studies. In EBM, *meta-analyses* are considered the best sources of information. Meta-analyses use statistical techniques to combine and summarize the results of primary studies. By combining the results from many trials, meta-analyses are able to estimate the magnitude of the effect of an intervention or risk factor, as well as to evaluate previously unanswered questions by performing subgroup analyses. The use of meta-analysis has provoked some controversy. Some investigators believe that these analyses may be as reliable as randomized controlled trials, whereas others believe that the technique should be used only to generate hypotheses, rather than to test them. However, in the absence of a large, randomized controlled study, a meta-analysis of multiple, smaller studies may be the best source of information with which to answer a specific question.

Clinical practice guidelines attempt to summarize diagnostic and treatment strategies for common clinical problems to assist the physician with specific circumstances. These guidelines are usually published by medical organizations, such as the American College of Physicians, and government agencies, such as the Agency for Health Care Policy and Research. To avoid misapplication of clinical recommendations, guidelines should clearly state to which specific patients and conditions they apply; this concept is termed *clinical applicability*. *Clinical flexibility* allows the clinician to interpret and apply the recommendations according to the patient's unique situation. Applying the techniques of EBM to clinical guidelines aids the physician in individualizing the guidelines on the basis of the patient's unique situation.

Decision analysis uses the results of primary studies to generate probability trees to aid both health professionals and patients in making choices about clinical management. *Cost-effectiveness analysis* evaluates whether a particular course of action is an effective use of resources. The process of determining the validity and applicability of the information begins after the literature search is complete.

Evaluating Evidence About Diagnostic Tests

Four types of diagnostic tests are used. *Screening tests* are performed on apparently healthy people to distinguish those who have a disease from those who do not.

Case-finding tests assess patients for disorders that are unrelated to the reasons they came to the physician. A *diagnostic test* is specifically ordered to determine the cause of a patient's illness. An *achievement of treatment goal test* is done to assess the efficacy of a specific therapeutic modality. A critical feature of all these tests is that the investigator who interprets the results should be blinded as to whether the patients have the disease.

When the efficacy of a new diagnostic test is assessed, the critical issues are as follows: (1) Does it have something to offer that the currently accepted test does not, and (2) does the test provide additional information that alters the *posttest probability*, which is the ability of the test to distinguish patients with and without the target diagnosis? The investigator should also compare the posttest probability with the *pretest probability*, which is the clinical assessment of diagnostic possibilities before the test is ordered. If a new test is to be useful, it will offer information that improves the posttest probability and also will add data that alter the pretest probability. This information then aids the physician in evaluating subsequent patients with the target diagnosis.

Published values exist for some pretest probabilities, but more often these values are derived from the physician's clinical experience and are influenced by the practice setting. For instance, an obese African-American woman from the rural south presents with fatigue, blurry vision, frequent vaginal yeast infections, and a strong family history of diabetes. On the basis of these features, she would have a high pretest probability of having type 2 diabetes. If a new diagnostic test is available for the diagnosis of diabetes, a comparison can be done on the posttest probabilities expected from the standard test (fasting blood glucose) and the new test. Ideally, the new test will offer greater diagnostic accuracy.

Sensitivity and specificity are important parameters to consider in evaluating a diagnostic test. *Sensitivity* is an index of the diagnostic test's ability to detect the disease when it is present. *Specificity* is the ability of the diagnostic test to identify correctly the absence of the disease. These parameters are calculated by the use of a 2 × 2 table (Table 2–3). An additional parameter, the *likelihood ratio*, which uses both sensitivity and specificity, gives even a better indication of the test's performance.

$$\text{Likelihood ratio} = \frac{\text{Sensitivity}}{1 - \text{Specificity}}$$

After determining the validity of the diagnostic test, the investigator should determine whether the test is applicable to the patient in question and whether it is affordable and accurate in a particular setting. If the diagnostic test requires special devices or skills that are not available in the practice facility, then the results provided can be inaccurate. Most important, an assessment should be made about whether the test will change the management offered or decrease the need for the use of other tests.

TABLE 2–3 Schematic Outcomes of a Diagnostic Test (2 × 2 Table)

Test Result	Disease Present	Disease Absent
Positive	True positive a	False positive b
Negative	False negative c	True negative d

Positive predictive value (true-positive rate) = a/(a + b)
Negative predictive value (false-positive rate) = d/(c + d)
Sensitivity = a/(a + c); those patients with the disease who have a positive test
Specificity = d/(b + d); those patients without the disease who have a negative test

Evaluation of Evidence About Outcome

Outcome can be described *qualitatively* (what is likely to happen) or *temporally* (over what period a particular event would happen) (Table 2–4). To evaluate evidence about prognosis, patients should be enrolled at an early and uniform point (*inception cohort*). The pathways by which patients are enrolled in the study sample should be analyzed to see whether the results are applicable to patients in a particular practice.

All study subjects enrolled should be accounted for at the end of the follow-up period, and their clinical status should be known. The loss to follow-up of 10% or more of the original inception cohort raises questions about the validity of the trial.

Once the validity of the information is ascertained, the investigator should assess the likelihood of this particular outcome over time, because every disease process has separate outcomes at certain stages of the disease. The last step is to apply the valid information to the particular patient or problem in question.

Evaluating Evidence About Treatment

This evaluation is one of the most common problems facing physicians. The validity of new treatments being developed, as well as that of traditional treatments used

TABLE 2–4 Evaluation of Evidence About Outcome

Are patients enrolled at an early point in the disease?
How are the patients enrolled?
Are all patients accounted for at the end of the study time?
Are researchers blinded to other features of the patients?
Does this outcome occur at all stages of the disease process?
Is the information applicable to my patient?

for years, needs to be assessed. For example, how long should antimicrobial agents be administered to patients for pneumonia after these patients have been discharged from the hospital? What is the value of plasmapheresis in the management of thrombotic thrombocytopenic purpura? The first step in evaluating prospective treatments is to assess whether the information is derived from a properly conducted randomized controlled study. Every patient who entered the trial must be accounted for at the end of the study. Patients who are lost to follow-up often have different outcomes. If the conclusion of the trial does not change after the lost patients are accounted for, the study is considered more valid. Another point is whether patients were analyzed in their original randomized groups even if they did not undergo the intervention in question. This concept is termed an *intention-to-treat* analysis. A description of whether both groups were treated differently with regard to other interventions (cointerventions) should be included.

The next step is to assess the importance of the data provided. This step includes certain simple statistical calculations applied to the available results. The first is relative risk reduction (RRR):

$$RRR = \frac{\text{Incidence of outcome in control group} - \text{Incidence of outcome in study group}}{\text{Incidence of outcome in control group}}$$

For example, the Diabetes Control and Complication Trial investigated the effect of tight control of blood glucose in patients with type 1 diabetes on the development and progression of long-term complications. The study involved more than 1400 patients, with half randomly assigned to intensive treatment and half to conventional therapy. In this study, 3.4% of the patients in the conventional treatment group and 2.2% in the intensive treatment group developed microalbuminuria, a 35% decrease in the occurrence of microalbuminuria in the primary prevention group:

$$RRR = \frac{0.034 - 0.022}{0.034} \times 100 = 35\%$$

The greater the RRR, the more effective is the therapy. However, RRR does not take into account the baseline risk of the patients entering the trial and thus does not differentiate between large and small effects.

Another way of assessing the outcome is by calculating the *absolute risk reduction* (ARR), which gives the absolute difference in rates between the two groups. The ARR is defined as the number (X) that had the ill effect in the control group minus the number (Y) in the treatment group (i.e., ARR = X − Y). According to the foregoing example, the ARR for the development of microalbuminuria is 0.034 − 0.022 = 0.012, or 1.2%. Another valuable calculation is the *number needed to treat*, which represents the number of patients who need to be treated to prevent a single outcome event. This is the inverse of the ARR [i.e., 1/(X − Y)]. The lower the number needed to treat, the more clinically relevant is the treatment. Again, according to the example, to prevent 1 patient from developing microalbuminuria, 83 patients with diabetes would have to be treated with intensive therapy (1/[X − Y] = 1/0.012 = 83).

As before, assessment of the applicability of this information to a particular patient should be done by taking into account whether the patient in question has the same characteristics as the patients included in the study. Similarly, evidence about the side effects, the cause, or the value of a particular clinical sign in diagnosis can be assessed.

Including the Patient in the Decision Process

Searching for the best evidence and applying it has the ultimate goal of providing better care to a particular patient or a group of patients. The process of EBM should also involve informing the patient of the available options and offering options based on strong evidence. Using a certain therapy or implementing a diagnostic test may be inconvenient, or the patient may develop a certain side effect that he or she is not willing to accept. Involvement of patients in the decision-making process requires good communication and adequate resources for patient education.

REFERENCES

Center for Evidence Based Medicine: http://cebm.jr2.ox.ac.uk
Cochrane Collaboration: http://hiru.mcmaster.ca/cochrane/default.html
Diabetes Control and Complications Trial Research Group: The effect of intensive treatment of diabetes on the development and progression of long-term complications in insulin-dependent diabetes mellitus. N Engl J Med 1993; 329:977–986.
Douglas JE, Leischow SJ, Nides MA, et al: A controlled trial of sustained-release bupropion, a nicotine patch, or both for smoking cessation. N Engl J Med 1999; 340:685–691.
Evidence-Based Medicine Working Group. Users' guide to the medical literature series. JAMA 1992–1999; vols 268, 270–275, 277, 279, 281, 282.
Sackett DL, Richardson WS, Rosenberg W, et al: Evidence-Based Medicine: How to Practice and Teach EBM. Edinburgh: Churchill Livingstone, 1998.
Sarin SK, Gurwant LS, Kumar M, et al: Comparison of endoscopic ligation and propranolol for the primary prevention of variceal bleeding. N Engl J Med 1999; 340:988–993.

SECTION III

Cardiovascular Disease

3

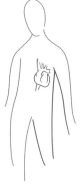

STRUCTURE AND FUNCTION OF THE NORMAL HEART AND BLOOD VESSELS

Eric H. Awtry • Joseph Loscalzo

Microscopic Anatomy

Cardiac tissue (myocardium) is composed of several cell types that together produce the organized contraction of the heart. Specialized myocardial cells comprise the cardiac electrical system (conduction system) and are responsible for the generation of an electrical impulse and organized propagation of that impulse to cardiac muscle fibers (myocytes), which, in turn, respond by mechanical contraction. Atrial and ventricular myocytes are specialized, branching muscle cells connected end-to-end by intercalated discs. These thickened regions of the cell membrane (sarcolemma) aid in the transmission of mechanical tension between cells. The sarcolemma has functions similar to other cell membranes, including maintenance of ionic gradients, propagation of electrical impulses, and provision of receptors for neural and hormonal inputs. In addition, the sarcolemma is intimately involved with the coupling of myocardial excitation and contraction through small transverse tubules (T-tubules) that extend from the sarcolemma into the intracellular space. The myocytes contain several other organelles, including the nucleus; the multiple mitochondria responsible for generating the energy required for contraction; an extensive network of intracellular tubules called the sarcoplasmic reticulum, which functions as the major intracellular storage site for calcium; and myofibrils, the contractile elements of the cell. Each myofibril is made up of repeating units called sarcomeres, which are in turn composed of overlapping thin actin filaments and thick myosin filaments and their regulatory proteins troponin and tropomyosin (Fig. 3–1).

Gross Anatomy

The heart is composed of four chambers, two atria and two ventricles, which form two separate pumps arranged side by side and in series (Fig. 3–2). The atria are low-pressure capacitance chambers that function mainly to store blood during ventricular contraction (systole) and then fill the ventricles with blood during ventricular relaxation (diastole). The two atria are separated by a thin interatrial septum. The ventricles are higher-pressure chambers responsible for pumping blood through the lungs and to the peripheral tissues. Because the pressure generated by the left ventricle is higher than that generated by the right, the left ventricular myocardium is thicker than the right. The two ventricles are separated by the interventricular septum, which is a membranous structure at its superior aspect and a thick, muscular structure at its mid- and distal portions.

The atria and ventricles are separated by the atrioventricular (AV) valves. The mitral valve is a bileaflet valve that separates the left atrium and ventricle. The tricuspid valve is trileaflet and separates the right atrium and ventricle. The ventricular aspects of these valves are attached by strong chords (chordae tendineae) to the papillary muscles of their respective ventricle. These papillary muscles are extensions of normal myocardium that project into the ventricular cavities and are important for optimal valve closure. The semilunar valves separate the ventricles from the arterial chambers: the aortic valve separates the left ventricle from the aorta, and the pulmonic valve separates the right ventricle from the pulmonary artery. These valves do not have chordae.

21

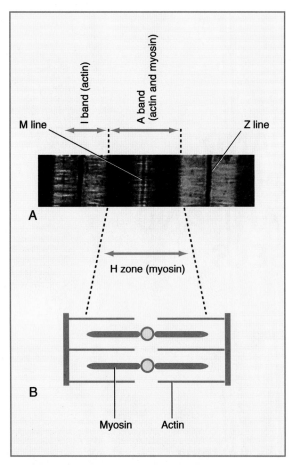

FIGURE 3–1 *A,* A sarcomere as it appears under the electron microscope. *B,* Schematic of the location and interaction of actin and myosin (see text).

Rather, they are fibrous valves whose edges coapt closely, thus allowing for adequate valve closure. Each of the four valves is surrounded by a fibrous ring, or annulus, that forms part of the structural support of the heart. When open, the valves allow free flow of blood across them and into the adjacent chamber or vessel. When closed, the valves effectively prevent the backflow of blood into the preceding chamber.

The heart is surrounded by the thin, double-layered pericardium. The visceral pericardium is adherent to the heart and constitutes its outer surface, or *epicardium.* This is separated from the parietal pericardium by the pericardial space, which normally contains less than 50 mL of fluid. The parietal pericardium has attachments to the sternum, vertebral column, and diaphragm, which serve to stabilize the heart in the chest. Normal pericardial fluid lubricates contact surfaces and limits direct tissue surface contact during myocardial contraction. In addition, the normal pericardium modulates interventricular interactions during the cardiac cycle.

The Circulatory Pathway

Deoxygenated blood drains from peripheral tissues and enters the right atrium through the superior and inferior

venae cavae (see Fig. 3–2). Blood draining from the heart itself enters the right atrium through the coronary sinus. This blood mixes in the right atrium during ventricular systole and then flows across the tricuspid valve and into the right ventricle during ventricular diastole. When the right ventricle contracts, blood is ejected across the pulmonic valve and into the main pulmonary artery, which then bifurcates into the left and right pulmonary arteries as these branches enter their respective lungs. After multiple bifurcations, blood flows into the pulmonary capillaries where carbon dioxide is exchanged for oxygen across the alveolar-capillary membrane. Oxygenated blood then drains from the lungs into the four pulmonary veins, which empty into the left atrium. During ventricular diastole, this blood flows across the open mitral valve and into the left ventricle. With ventricular contraction, the blood is ejected across the aortic valve and into the aorta and is subsequently delivered to the various organs, where oxygen and nutrients are exchanged for carbon dioxide and metabolic wastes.

The heart itself receives blood through the left and right coronary arteries (Fig. 3–3). These are the first arterial branches of the aorta and originate in outpouchings of the aortic root called the sinuses of Valsalva. The left main coronary artery originates in the left sinus of Valsalva and is a short vessel that bifurcates into the left

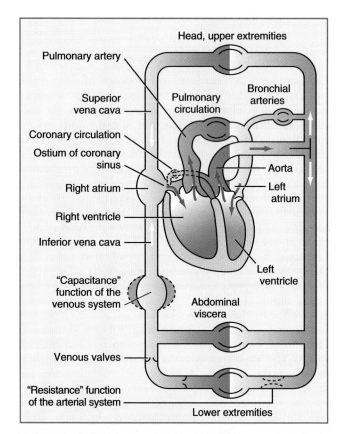

FIGURE 3–2 Schematic representation of the systemic and pulmonary circulatory systems. The venous system contains the greatest amount of blood at any one time and is highly distensible, accommodating a wide range of blood volumes (high capacitance). The arterial system comprises the aorta, arteries, and arterioles. Arterioles are small muscular arteries that regulate blood pressure by changing tone (resistance).

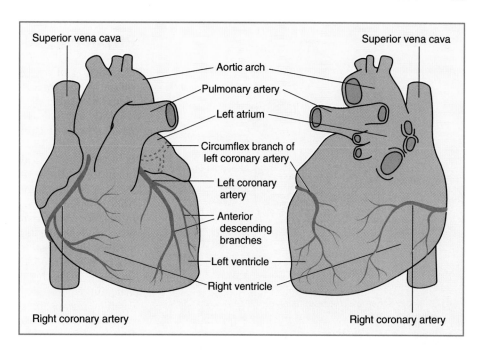

FIGURE 3–3 Major coronary arteries and their branches.

anterior descending (LAD) and the left circumflex (LCx) coronary arteries. The LAD travels across the surface of the heart in the anterior interventricular groove toward the cardiac apex. It supplies blood to the anterior and anterolateral left ventricle through its diagonal branches and to the anterior two thirds of the interventricular septum through its septal branches. The LCx passes posteriorly in the left AV groove (between the left atrium and left ventricle) and supplies blood to the lateral aspect of the left ventricle through obtuse marginal branches, as well as gives off branches to the left atrium. The right coronary artery (RCA) originates in the right sinus of Valsalva and courses down the right AV groove to a point where the left and right AV grooves and the inferior interventricular groove meet, the "crux" of the heart. The RCA gives off atrial branches to the right atrium and acute marginal branches to the right ventricle. The blood supply to the diaphragmatic and posterior aspects of the left ventricle varies. In 85% of individuals, the RCA bifurcates at the crux into the posterior descending coronary artery (PDA), which travels in the inferior interventricular groove to supply blood to the inferior left ventricular wall and the inferior third of the interventricular septum, and the posterior left ventricular (PLV) branches, which supply the posterior left ventricle. This is termed a *right dominant circulation*. In 10% of individuals, the RCA terminates before reaching the crux and the LCx supplies the PLV and PDA. This is termed a *left dominant circulation*. In the remaining individuals, the RCA gives rise to the PDA and the LCx gives rise to the PLV in a so-called *codominant circulation*. The blood supply to the sinoatrial node may originate from the RCA (60%) or the LCx (40%), while the dominant artery supplies the AV node.

Small vascular channels, called collaterals, interconnect the normal coronary arteries. These vessels are nonfunctional in the normal myocardium because there is no pressure gradient across them. However, in the setting of severe stenosis or complete occlusion of a coronary artery, the pressure in the vessel distal to the stenosis decreases and a gradient develops across the collateral vasculature, resulting in flow through the collateral vessel. The development of collaterals is directly related to the severity of the coronary stenosis and may be stimulated by ischemia, hypoxia, and a variety of growth factors. Over time, these vessels may reach up to 1 mm in luminal diameter and are almost indistinguishable from similarly sized, normal coronary arteries.

The majority of the venous drainage from the heart occurs through the coronary sinus, which runs in the AV groove and empties into the right atrium. A small amount of blood from the right side of the heart drains directly into the right atrium through the thebesian veins and small anterior myocardial veins.

The Conduction System

The electrical impulse that initiates cardiac contraction originates in the sinoatrial (SA) node, a collection of specialized pacemaker cells measuring 1 to 2 cm in length located high in the right atrium between the superior vena cava and the right atrial appendage (Fig. 3–4). The impulse then spreads through the atrial tissue through preferential internodal tracts reaching the AV node. This structure consists of a meshwork of cells located at the inferior aspect of the right atrium between the coronary sinus and the septal leaflet of the tricuspid valve. Both the SA node and the AV node are richly innervated by sympathetic and parasympathetic neurons, allowing for neural regulation of the heart rate.

The AV node provides the only normal electrical connection between the atria and ventricles. After an electrical impulse enters the AV node, conduction tran-

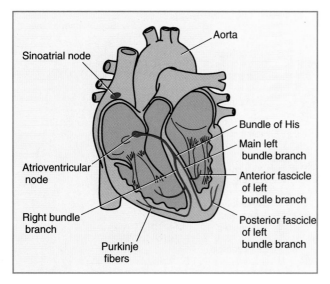

FIGURE 3–4   Schematic representation of the cardiac conduction system.

siently slows and then proceeds to the ventricles by means of the His-Purkinje system. The His bundle extends from the AV node down the membranous interventricular septum to the muscular septum, where it divides into the left and right bundle branches. The right bundle branch is a discrete structure that extends along the interventricular septum and enters the moderator band on its way toward the anterolateral papillary muscle of the right ventricle. The left bundle branch is less distinct, consisting of an array of fibers organized into an anterior fascicle, which proceeds toward the anterolateral papillary muscle of the left ventricle, and a posterior fascicle, which proceeds posteriorly in the septum toward the posteromedial papillary muscle. Both the right and left bundle branches terminate in Purkinje cells, which are large cells with well-developed intercellular connections allowing for the rapid propagation of electrical impulses. These cells then directly stimulate myocytes.

Neural Innervation

The normal myocardium is richly innervated by the autonomic nervous system. Sympathetic nerve terminals are located throughout the atria and ventricles, where an increase in sympathetic activity results in increased force of myocardial contraction. The parasympathetic system innervates the atria by means of the vagus nerve but has few projections to the ventricles. The SA and AV nodes are densely innervated by both sympathetic and parasympathetic neurons, allowing for neural regulation of the heart rate. Increases in sympathetic tone lead to an increase in the heart rate and shortened conduction time through the AV node. Increases in parasympathetic tone lead to decreases in the heart rate and slower conduction through the AV node.

Physiology of Contraction

Contraction of myocytes begins with electrical depolarization of the sarcolemma, resulting in an influx of calcium into the cell through channels in the T tubules (Fig. 3–5). This initial calcium entry stimulates the rapid release of large amounts of calcium from the sarcoplasmic reticulum into the cell cytosol. The calcium then binds to the calcium-binding troponin subunit (troponin C) on the actin filaments of the sarcomere, resulting in a conformational change in the troponin-tropomyosin complex. This change facilitates the actin-myosin interaction, which results in cellular contraction. As the wave of depolarization passes, the calcium is rapidly and actively resequestered in the sarcoplasmic reticulum, where it is stored by various proteins, including calsequestrin, until the next wave of depolarization occurs. Calcium is also extruded from the cytosol by various calcium pumps in the sarcolemma. The force of myocyte contraction can be regulated by the amount of free calcium released into the cell by the sarcoplasmic reticulum: more calcium allows for greater actin-myosin interaction, producing a stronger contraction.

The energy for myocyte contraction is derived from adenosine triphosphate (ATP), which is generated by oxidative phosphorylation of adenosine diphosphate (ADP) in the abundant mitochondria of the cell. ATP is required both for calcium influx and for force generation by actin-myosin interaction. During contraction, ATP promotes dissociation of myosin from actin, thereby permitting the sliding of thick filaments past thin filaments as the sarcomere shortens. Under normal circumstances, fatty acids are the preferred energy source, although glucose can also be used as a substrate. These substrates must be constantly delivered to the heart through the blood stream because there are minimal energy stores in the heart itself. Myocardial metabolism is aerobic and, thus, requires a constant supply of oxygen. Under anaerobic conditions, glycolysis and lactate may serve as a source of ATP, although in insufficient quantities to sustain the working heart.

Circulatory Physiology and the Cardiac Cycle

The cardiac cycle is a repeating series of contractile and valvular events during which the valves open and close in response to pressure gradients between different cardiac chambers (Fig. 3–6). This cycle can be divided into systole, the period of ventricular contraction, and diastole, the period of ventricular relaxation. With the onset of ventricular contraction, the pressure in the ventricles increases and exceeds that in the atria, at which time the AV valves close. Intraventricular pressure continues to rise, initially without a change in ventricular volume (isovolumic contraction), until the intraventricular pressures exceed the pressures in the aorta and pulmonary artery, at which time the semilunar valves open and

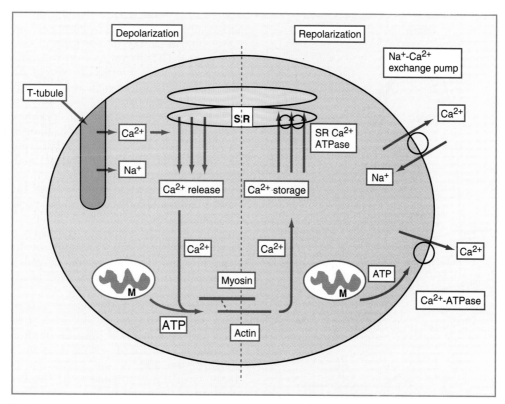

FIGURE 3–5 Calcium dependence of myocardial contraction. Electrical depolarization of the myocyte results in an influx of Ca²⁺ into the cell through channels in the T tubules. This initial phase of calcium entry stimulates the release of large amounts of Ca²⁺ from the sarcoplasmic reticulum (SR). The Ca²⁺ then binds to the troponin-tropomyosin complex on the actin filaments, resulting in a conformational change that facilitates the binding interaction between actin and myosin. In the presence of adenosine triphosphate (ATP), the actin-myosin association is cyclically dissociated as the thick and thin filaments slide past each other, resulting in contraction. During repolarization, the Ca²⁺ is actively pumped out of the cytosol and sequestered in the SR. M = mitochondrion.

ventricular ejection of blood occurs. With the onset of ventricular relaxation, the pressure in the ventricles falls until the pressure in the arterial chambers exceeds that in the ventricles, and the semilunar valves close. Ventricular relaxation continues, initially without a change in ventricular volume (isovolumic relaxation). When the pressure in the ventricles falls below the pressure in the atria, the AV valves open and a rapid phase of ventricular filling occurs as blood in the atria empties into the ventricles. At the end of diastole, active atrial contraction augments ventricular filling. This augmentation is particularly important in patients with poor ventricular function and is lost in patients with atrial fibrillation.

In the absence of valvular disease, there is no impediment to flow from the ventricles to the arterial beds and the systolic arterial pressure rises sharply to a peak. During diastole, the arterial pressure gradually falls as blood flows distally and elastic recoil of the arteries occurs. This response contrasts to the pressure response in the ventricles during diastole, which gradually increases as blood enters the ventricles from the atria. Atrial pressure can be directly measured in the right atrium, whereas left atrial pressure is often obtained indirectly by occluding a small pulmonary artery branch and measuring the pressure distally (the pulmonary cap-

illary "wedge" pressure). An atrial tracing is shown in Figure 3–6 and is composed of several pressure waves. The *a wave* represents atrial contraction. As the atria subsequently relax, the atrial pressure falls and the *x descent* is noted on the pressure tracing. The x descent is interrupted by a small *c wave*, which is generated as the AV valve bulges toward the atrium during ventricular systole. As the atria fill from venous return the *v wave* is seen, after which the *y descent* appears as the AV valves open and blood from the atria empties into the ventricles. The normal ranges of pressures in the various cardiac chambers are shown in Table 3–1.

Cardiac Performance

The amount of blood ejected by the heart each minute is referred to as the cardiac output (CO) and is the product of the stroke volume (SV = the amount of blood ejected with each ventricular contraction) and the heart rate (HR):

$$CO = SV \times HR.$$

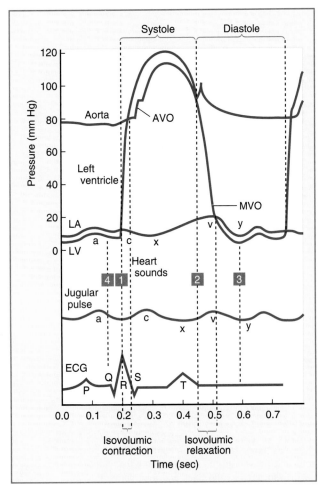

The cardiac index (CI) is the CO divided by the body surface area, is measured in liters per minute per square meter, and is a way of normalizing CO to body size. The normal CO at rest is 5 to 6 L/min, although this value can increase fourfold to sixfold during strenuous exercise as a result of increases in heart rate (chronotropy) and SV (inotropy).

The SV is a measure of the mechanical function of the heart and is affected by preload, afterload, and contractility (Table 3–2). *Preload* is the volume of blood in the ventricle at the end of diastole and is primarily a reflection of venous return. Within limits, as the preload increases, the ventricle stretches and the ensuing ventricular contraction becomes more rapid and forceful. This phenomenon is known as the Frank-Starling relationship. Because ventricular volume is not easily measured, ventricular filling pressure (ventricular end-diastolic pressure, atrial pressure, or pulmonary capillary wedge pressure) is frequently used as a surrogate measure of preload.

Afterload is the force against which the ventricles must contract to eject blood. The arterial pressure is often used as a practical measure of afterload, although, in truth, afterload is determined by the intraventricular pressure, the size of the ventricular cavity, and the thickness of the ventricular walls (Laplace's law). Thus, afterload is increased in the setting of systemic hypertension or stenosis of the aortic valve but may be equally increased in the setting of ventricular dilation or ventricular hypertrophy.

Contractility, or inotropy, although difficult to define, represents the force of ventricular contraction indepen-

FIGURE 3–6 Simultaneous electrocardiogram (ECG) and pressure tracings obtained from the left atrium (LA), left ventricle (LV), and aorta, and the jugular venous pressure during the cardiac cycle. For simplification, right-sided pressures have been omitted. Normal right atrial pressure closely parallels that of the left atrium, and right ventricular and pulmonary artery pressures are timed closely with their corresponding left-sided heart counterparts, being reduced only in magnitude. The normal mitral and aortic valve closure precedes tricuspid and pulmonic valve closure, respectively, whereas valve opening reverses this order. The jugular venous pulse lags behind the right atrial pulse.

During the course of one cardiac cycle, note that the electrical events (ECG) initiate and therefore precede the mechanical (pressure) events and that the latter precede the auscultatory events (heart sounds) they themselves produce. Shortly after the P wave, the atria contract to produce the a wave; a fourth sound may succeed the latter. The QRS complex initiates ventricular systole, followed shortly by LV contraction and the rapid build-up of LV pressure. Almost immediately, LV pressure exceeds LA pressure, closing the mitral valve and producing the first heart sound. After a brief period of isovolumic contraction, LV pressure exceeds aortic pressure and the aortic valve opens (AVO). When the ventricular pressure once again falls below the aortic pressure, the aortic valve closes to produce the second heart sound and terminate ventricular ejection. The LV pressure decreases during the period of isovolumic relaxation until it drops below LA pressure and the mitral valve opens (MVO). A period of rapid ventricular filling commences, during which a third heart sound may be heard. See text for a discussion of the jugular venous pulse.

TABLE 3–1   Normal Values for Common Hemodynamic Parameters

Heart rate	60–100 beats per minute
Pressures	
Central venous	≤9 mm Hg
Right atrial	≤9 mm Hg
Right ventricular	
Systolic	15–30 mm Hg
End diastolic	≤9 mm Hg
Pulmonary artery	
Systolic	15–30 mm Hg
Diastolic	3–12 mm Hg
Pulmonary capillary	
wedge	≤12 mm Hg
Left atrial	≤12 mm Hg
Left ventricular	
Systolic	100–140 mm Hg
End diastolic	3–12 mm Hg
Aorta	
Systolic	100–140 mm Hg
Diastolic	60–90 mm Hg
Resistance	
Systemic vascular (SVR)	800–1500 dynes-sec/cm^{-5}
Pulmonary vascular (PVR)	30–120 dynes-sec/cm^{-5}
Cardiac output	4–6 L/min
Cardiac index	2.5–4 L/min

TABLE 3-2   **Factors Affecting Cardiac Performance**

Preload (left ventricular diastolic volume)	Total blood volume Venous tone (sympathetic tone) Body position Intrathoracic and intrapericardial pressure Atrial contraction Pumping action of skeletal muscle
Afterload (impedance against which the left ventricle must eject blood)	Peripheral vascular resistance Left ventricular volume (preload, wall tension) Physical characteristics of the arterial tree (e.g., elasticity of vessels or presence of outflow obstruction)
Contractility (cardiac performance independent of preload or afterload)	Sympathetic nerve impulses ⎫ Circulating catecholamines ⎬ Increased contractility Digitalis, calcium, other inotropic agents ⎪ Increased heart rate or postextrasystolic augmentation ⎭ Anoxia, acidosis ⎫ Pharmacologic depression ⎬ Decreased contractility Loss of myocardium ⎪ Intrinsic depression ⎭
Heart Rate	Autonomic nervous system Temperature, metabolic rate

dent of loading conditions. For example, an increase in contractility results in a stronger ventricular contraction even when the preload and afterload are kept constant. Contractility can be altered under normal conditions by direct stimulation from adrenergic nerves in the myocardium and by circulating catecholamines released from the adrenal glands. Several medications have important positive inotropic effects that can be exploited clinically, including digoxin and sympathomimetic amines (epinephrine, norepinephrine, dopamine). Other medications (e.g., β blockers, calcium channel antagonists) have negative inotropic effects and can decrease the strength of ventricular contraction.

Overall, ventricular systolic function is frequently quantified by the ejection fraction, which is the ratio of the SV to the end-diastolic volume, that is, the fraction of blood in the ventricle ejected with each ventricular contraction. The normal ejection fraction is approximately 60% and can be measured by invasive (contrast ventriculography) or noninvasive (echocardiography, radionuclide ventriculography) methods.

Clearly, systolic contraction is an important component of ventricular function; however, ventricular diastolic relaxation (lusitropy) also plays an important role in overall cardiac performance. Impaired relaxation (diastolic dysfunction), as occurs with ventricular hypertrophy or ischemia, results in a stiff, noncompliant ventricle, leading to impaired ventricular filling and an increased ventricular pressure for any given diastolic volume.

Physiology of the Coronary Circulation

The heart is an aerobic organ requiring a constant supply of oxygen to maintain normal function. Under normal conditions, the supply of oxygen delivered to the heart is closely matched to the amount of oxygen required by the heart (the myocardial oxygen consumption [MvO_2]). The main determinants of MvO_2 are heart rate, contractility, and wall stress. The wall stress, as determined by the law of Laplace, is directly related to the systolic pressure and the heart size:

Wall stress = (pressure × radius)/(2 × wall thickness).

Thus, the MvO_2 parallels changes in heart rate, blood pressure, contractility, and heart size. In general, oxygen delivery to an organ can be augmented by either increasing blood flow or by increasing oxygen extraction from the blood. For all practical purposes, the oxygen extraction by the heart is maximal at rest, and, thus, increases in MvO_2 must be met by increases in coronary blood flow.

Because of the compression of intramyocardial blood vessels during systole, the majority of coronary flow occurs during diastole. Therefore, diastolic pressure is the major pressure driving the coronary circulation. An important implication of this fact is that tachycardia, which primarily shortens the duration of diastole, results in reduced time for coronary flow, which occurs despite the increase in MvO_2 associated with increased heart rate. The systolic pressure has little impact on coronary blood flow except insofar as changes in blood pressure lead to changes in MvO_2.

Regulation of coronary blood flow occurs primarily through changes in coronary vascular resistance. In response to a change in MvO_2, the coronary arteries can dilate or constrict to allow for appropriate changes in coronary flow. Additionally, in the range of coronary perfusion pressures of 60 to 130 mm Hg, coronary blood flow is held constant by the process of autoregulation of the coronary arteries. This regulation of arterial resistance occurs at the level of the arterioles and is mediated by several factors. As adenosine triphosphate is metabolized during increased myocardial activity, adenosine is released and acts as a potent vasodilator. Decreased oxygen tension and increased carbon dioxide, as well as acidosis and hyperkalemia, all develop during increased myocardial metabolism and may also mediate coronary vasodilation.

The coronary arteries are innervated by the autonomic nervous system, and activation of sympathetic or parasympathetic neurons alters coronary blood flow by affecting changes in vascular tone. Parasympathetic innervation occurs through the vagus nerve and, through the neurotransmitter acetylcholine, results in vasodilation. Sympathetic neurons use norepinephrine as a neurotransmitter and may have opposing effects on the coronary vasculature. Stimulation of α receptors results in vasoconstriction, whereas stimulation of β receptors leads to vasodilation.

The ability of the coronary vasculature to mediate changes in blood flow through changes in vascular tone depends in large part on an intact, normally functioning endothelium. The endothelium produces several potent vasodilators, including endothelium-derived relaxing factor (EDRF) and prostacyclin. EDRF is likely to be nitric oxide or a compound containing nitric oxide and is released by the endothelium in response to acetylcholine, thrombin, ADP, serotonin, bradykinin, platelet aggregation, and an increase in shear stress. This latter stimulus accounts for the dilation of the coronary arteries in response to increases in blood flow in the setting of increases in MvO_2 (the so-called flow-dependent vasodilation).

Vasoconstricting factors, most notably endothelin, are also produced by the endothelium and also likely play a role in regulating vascular tone. The balance of these vasodilator and vasoconstriction factors may be important in conditions such as coronary vasospasm. Aside from influencing vascular tone, the endothelium has several other functions that have important implications for blood flow and tissue perfusion. These include maintenance of a nonthrombotic surface through inhibition of platelet activity, control of thrombosis and fibrinolysis, and modulation of the inflammatory response of the vasculature. It is likely that disturbances in these normal properties of the endothelium (*endothelial dysfunction*) play an important role in the pathophysiology of coronary atherosclerosis and thrombosis.

Physiology of the Systemic Circulation

The walls of the aorta and large arteries are rich in elastic fibers. With the ejection of blood during ventricular systole, these fibers allow the arteries to stretch and subsequently recoil, resulting in the gradual delivery of blood to the periphery. The large arteries branch to become progressively smaller arteries, then arterioles, the terminal regulatory branches of the arterial tree. The arterioles function as "resistance vessels," owing to the presence of muscular sphincters, and control the flow of blood to the capillary systems. The arterioles themselves are under dual regulatory control: centrally through the nervous system and locally by means of conditions in the immediate vicinity of the blood vessels. Both sympathetic and parasympathetic fibers innervate the vascular system. Stimulation of the α-adrenergic system results in vasoconstriction, whereas β-adrenergic or vagal stimulation results in vasodilation. Locally, low PO_2, high PCO_2, and acidosis result in vasodilation by directly causing relaxation of arteriolar sphincters. The systemic vascular resistance (SVR) is a measure of total vascular tone and is defined as the pressure drop across the peripheral capillary beds divided by the blood flow across the beds. In practice, this is calculated as the mean arterial pressure minus the right atrial pressure divided by the cardiac output and is normally in the range of 800 to 1500 dynes-sec/cm^{-5}.

Blood leaves the arterioles and flows into capillary systems, where oxygen and nutrients are delivered to cells and carbon dioxide and metabolic wastes are removed. The deoxygenated blood then drains into peripheral veins, which contain valves to prevent backflow. These veins have thinner walls than arteries and function as "capacitance vessels," able to accommodate a significantly larger volume of blood than the arterial system. With the aid of the pumping action of skeletal muscles and the respiratory motion of the chest wall, blood returns to the right atrium. This venous return can be altered by constriction or dilation of the peripheral veins. In addition to the venous drainage, a rich system of lymphatics helps to drain excess interstitial fluid from the periphery. The various lymphatic vessels drain into the thoracic duct and subsequently into the left brachiocephalic vein.

Physiology of the Pulmonary Circulation

Similar to the systemic circulation, the pulmonary circulation consists of a branching network of progressively smaller arteries, arterioles, capillaries, and veins. The pulmonary capillaries are separated from the alveoli by a thin alveolar-capillary membrane through which gas exchange occurs. Carbon dioxide thus diffuses from the capillary blood into the alveoli, and oxygen diffuses from the alveoli into the blood. The flow of blood to various lung segments is regulated by several factors, the most important being the partial pressure of oxygen in the alveoli. In this manner, blood is shunted toward well-ventilated lung segments and away from poorly ventilated segments. As a result of the extensive nature of the pulmonary capillary system and the distensibility of the pulmonary vasculature, the resistance across the pulmonary system (the pulmonary vascular resistance [PVR]) is approximately one-tenth that of the systemic circulation. Owing to these features, the pulmonary system is able to tolerate significant increases in blood flow with little or no rise in pulmonary pressure. Thus, intracardiac shunts (such as atrial septal defects) may be associated with normal pulmonary pressure.

The lung receives a dual blood supply. The pulmonary artery accounts for the vast majority of pulmonary blood flow; however, the lungs also receive oxygenated blood through the bronchial arteries. These vessels supply oxygen to the lung itself and drain into the bronchial veins. The bronchial veins drain partly into the pulmonary veins; thus, a small amount of deoxygenated blood normally enters the systemic circulation and accounts for a physiologic right-to-left shunt. In the normal setting, this shunt is insignificant, accounting for only 1% of total systemic blood flow.

Cardiovascular Response to Exercise

The response of the heart to exercise is multifaceted and involves many of the previously discussed mechanisms of circulatory control (Table 3–3). In anticipation of exercise, neural centers in the brain stimulate vagal withdrawal and increased sympathetic tone, resulting in an increase in the heart rate and contractility (thus, an increase in CO) before exercise ever starts. With exercise, sympathetic venoconstriction, augmented pumping action of skeletal muscles, and increased respiratory movements of the chest wall all result in an increase in venous return to the heart. Through the Frank-Starling mechanism, this results in an increase in contractility, thus augmenting CO. Sympathetic activation may also increase contractility; however, the majority of the increase in CO during exercise (up to four to six times normal) is a consequence of an increase in the heart rate. The peak heart rate that can be achieved is dependent on age and can be estimated by the following formula: maximal HR = $(220 - \text{age}) \pm (10-12)$ beats/min.

Local factors in exercising muscle cause arteriolar dilation, resulting in increased flow to capillary beds. This vasodilation results in decreased resistance to flow and, therefore, the SVR decreases with exercise. Despite this change in resistance, the systolic blood pressure rises, owing to the augmented CO as well as to sympathetic vasoconstriction, leading to the preferential shunting of

TABLE 3–3 Physiologic Responses to Exercise

Response	Mechanism
↑ Heart rate	↑ Sympathetic stimulation ↓ Parasympathetic stimulation
↑ Stroke volume	
↑ Contractility	↑ Sympathetic stimulation
↑ Venous return	Sympathetic-mediated venoconstriction
	Pumping action of skeletal muscles
	↓ Intrathoracic pressure with deep inspirations
	Arteriolar vasodilation in exercising muscle
↓ Afterload	Arteriolar vasodilation in exercising muscle (mediated chiefly by local metabolites)
↑ Blood pressure	↑ Cardiac output
	Vasoconstriction (sympathetic stimulation) of nonexercising vascular beds
↑ O_2 extraction	Shift in oxyhemoglobin dissociation curve due to local acidosis

blood away from nonexercising vascular beds. The diastolic blood pressure, by contrast, generally remains constant during exercise. The pulmonary system is able to tolerate the increased flow with only small increases in pulmonary pressure. The increase in heart rate and contractility result in a marked increase in MvO_2 (up to 300%), and coronary blood flow subsequently increases.

Various types of exercises have different effects on the circulatory system. The response described here occurs with isotonic exercises, such as running or biking. With isometric exercises, such as weight lifting, the predominant response is an increase in blood pressure, owing to an increase in peripheral vasoconstriction.

REFERENCES

Brown H, Kozlowski R: Physiology and Pharmacology of the Heart. Cambridge, UK: University Press, 1997.

Hurst JW, Anderson RH, Becker AE, et al: Atlas of the Heart. New York: McGraw-Hill, 1988.

Loscalzo J, Creager MA, Dzau VJ: Vascular Medicine: A Textbook of Vascular Biology and Diseases, 2nd ed. Boston: Little, Brown, 1996.

Opie LH: The Heart: Physiology from Cell to Circulation, 3rd ed. Philadelphia: Lippincott-Raven, 1998.

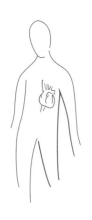

4

EVALUATION OF THE PATIENT WITH CARDIOVASCULAR DISEASE

Eric H. Awtry • Joseph Loscalzo

History

As with diseases of most organ systems, the ability of the physician to diagnose diseases of the cardiovascular system is in large part dependent on eliciting and interpreting the patient's clinical history. A thorough history may enable the physician to identify a patient's symptoms as characteristic of a specific cardiovascular disorder or exclude the presence of cardiovascular disease altogether. In addition, a complete history will reveal the presence of other systemic diseases that may have cardiovascular manifestations, identify existing risk factors that may be modified to prevent the future development of cardiovascular disease (see Chapter 9), enable the selection of appropriate further diagnostic testing (see Chapter 5), and allow the assessment of functional capacity and extent of cardiovascular disability. The patient should be asked about prior medical conditions, including childhood illnesses (e.g., rheumatic fever), as well as intravenous drug use, which may predispose to the development of valvular heart disease. Several cardiovascular disorders are inherited (e.g., hypertrophic cardiomyopathy, Marfan's syndrome, long Q-T syndrome), and a thorough family history may bring this potential to the examiner's attention.

The classic symptoms of cardiac disease include chest pain or discomfort, dyspnea, palpitations, syncope or presyncope, and edema. Although characteristic of heart disease, these symptoms are nonspecific and may also occur as a result of diseases of other organ systems (e.g., musculoskeletal, pulmonary, renal, or gastrointestinal). Furthermore, some patients with established cardiovascular disease may be asymptomatic or have atypical symptoms.

Chest pain is a frequent symptom and may be a manifestation of cardiovascular or noncardiovascular disease (Tables 4–1 and 4–2). Full characterization of the pain with regard to quality, quantity, frequency, location, duration, radiation, aggravating or alleviating factors, and associated symptoms may help to distinguish among various causes. Reversible myocardial ischemia due to obstructive coronary artery disease commonly results in episodic chest pain or discomfort (angina pectoris). Patients frequently deny having pain and, instead, describe a discomfort in their chest, referring to it as a "squeezing," "tightening," "pressing," or "burning" sensation, or as a "heavy weight" on their chest, and will commonly clench their fist over their chest while describing the discomfort (Levine's sign). Anginal discomfort is classically located substernally or over the left chest. It frequently radiates to the epigastrium, neck, jaw, or back and down the ulnar aspect of the left arm. Radiation to the right chest or arm is less common, whereas radiation above the jaw or below the epigastrium is not typical of cardiac disease. Angina is usually brought on by either physical or emotional stress, is mild to moderate in intensity, lasts 2 to 10 minutes, and resolves with rest or sublingual administration of nitroglycerin. It may occur more frequently in the morning, in cold weather, after a large meal, or after exposure to environmental factors, including cigarette smoke, and is frequently accompanied by other symptoms, such as dyspnea, diaphoresis, nausea, palpitations, or lightheadedness. Patients frequently report a stable pattern of angina that is predictably reproducible with a given amount of exertion. Unstable angina occurs when a patient reports a significant increase in the frequency or severity of angina or when angina occurs with progressively decreasing exertion or at rest. When anginal-type

TABLE 4–1   Cardiovascular Causes of Chest Pain

Condition	Location	Quality	Duration	Aggravating or Alleviating Factors	Associated Symptoms or Signs
Angina	Retrosternal region: radiates to or occasionally isolated to neck, jaw, shoulder, arms (usually left), or epigastrium	Pressure, squeezing, tightness, heaviness, burning, indigestion	<2–10 minutes	Precipitated by exertion, cold weather, or emotional stress; relieved by rest or nitroglycerin; variant (Prinzmetal's) angina may be unrelated to exertion, often early morning	Dyspnea S_3, S_4, or murmur of papillary dysfunction during pain
Myocardial infarction	Same as angina	Same as angina, although more severe	Variable; usually longer than 30 minutes	Unrelieved by rest or nitroglycerin	Dyspnea, nausea, vomiting, weakness, diaphoresis
Pericarditis	Left of the sternum; may radiate to neck or left shoulder, often more localized than pain of myocardial ischemia	Sharp, stabbing, knifelike	Lasts many hours to days; may wax and wane	Aggravated by deep breathing, rotating chest, or supine position; relieved by sitting up and leaning forward	Pericardial friction rub
Aortic dissection	Anterior chest; may radiate to back, interscapular region	Excruciating, tearing, knifelike	Sudden onset, unrelenting	Usually occurs in setting of hypertension or predisposition such as Marfan's syndrome	Murmur of aortic insufficiency; pulse or blood pressure asymmetry; neurologic deficit

pain occurs mainly at rest, it may be of a noncardiac origin or it may reflect true cardiac ischemia resulting from coronary spasm (Prinzmetal's or variant angina). The pain of an acute myocardial infarction may be similar to angina, although it is usually more severe and prolonged (>30 minutes).

The pain of acute pericarditis is usually sharper than anginal pain, is located to the left of the sternum, and may radiate to the neck or left shoulder. In contrast to angina, it may last hours, typically worsens with inspiration, and improves when the patient sits up and leans forward; it may be associated with a pericardial friction rub. Acute aortic dissection presents as severe, sharp, "tearing" pain that radiates to the back and may be associated with asymmetric pulses and a murmur of aortic insufficiency. Pulmonary emboli may present as the sudden onset of sharp chest pain that is worse on inspiration, is associated with shortness of breath, and may have an associated pleural friction rub, especially if a pulmonary infarction is present. A multitude of noncardiac conditions may also present as chest pain (see Table 4–2). In general, the clinical history and physical examination findings will help distinguish these causes from true cardiac chest pain.

Dyspnea, an uncomfortable, heightened awareness of breathing, is commonly a symptom of cardiac disease. In patients with decreased left ventricular function, signifi-

cant abnormalities of the aortic or mitral valves, or decreased myocardial compliance (i.e., left ventricular hypertrophy, acute ischemia), left-sided heart pressure increases and is transmitted through the pulmonary veins to the pulmonary capillary system, producing vascular congestion. This results in exudation of fluid into the alveolar space and impairs gas exchange across the alveolar-capillary membrane, producing the subjective sensation of dyspnea. Dyspnea frequently occurs on exertion; however, in patients with severe cardiac disease, it may be present at rest. Patients with heart failure commonly sleep on two or more pillows because the augmented venous return that occurs on assuming the recumbent position produces an increase in dyspnea (orthopnea). In addition, these patients report awakening 2 to 4 hours after the onset of sleep with dyspnea (paroxysmal nocturnal dyspnea), which is likely due to the central redistribution of peripheral edema in the supine position.

Dyspnea may be associated with diseases of the lungs or chest wall and is also seen in anemia, obesity, deconditioning, and anxiety disorders. In addition, the sudden onset of dyspnea, with or without chest pain, may be present with pulmonary emboli. It is sometimes difficult to distinguish cardiac from pulmonary causes of dyspnea, because both may produce resting or exertional dyspnea, orthopnea, or cough. Wheezing and hemopty-

TABLE 4-2   Noncardiac Causes of Chest Pain

Condition	Location	Quality	Duration	Aggravating or Alleviating Factors	Associated Symptoms or Signs
Pulmonary embolism (chest pain often not present)	Substernal or over region of pulmonary infarction	Pleuritic (with pulmonary infarction) or angina-like	Sudden onset; minutes to hours	Aggravated by deep breathing	Dyspnea, tachypnea, tachycardia; hypotension, signs of acute right-sided heart failure, and pulmonary hypertension with large emboli; pleural rub; hemoptysis with pulmonary infarction
Pulmonary hypertension	Substernal	Pressure; oppressive		Aggravated by effort	Pain usually associated with dyspnea, signs of pulmonary hypertension
Pneumonia with pleurisy	Located over involved area	Pleuritic		Aggravated by breathing	Dyspnea, cough, fever, bronchial breath sounds, rhonchi, egophony, dullness to percussion, occasional pleural rub
Spontaneous pneumothorax	Unilateral	Sharp, well-localized	Sudden onset, lasts many hours	Aggravated by breathing	Dyspnea; hyperresonance and decreased breath and voice sounds over involved lung
Musculoskeletal disorders	Variable	Aching, well localized	Variable	Aggravated by movement; history of exertion or injury	Tender to palpation or with light pressure
Herpes zoster	Dermatomal distribution	Sharp, burning	Prolonged	None	Vesicular rash appears in area of discomfort
Esophageal reflux	Substernal or epigastric; may radiate to neck	Burning, visceral discomfort	10–60 minutes	Aggravated by large meal, postprandial recumbency; relief with antacid	Water brash
Peptic ulcer	Epigastric, substernal	Visceral burning, aching	Prolonged	Relief with food, antacid	
Gallbladder disease	Right upper quadrant, epigastric	Visceral	Prolonged	Spontaneous or following meals	Right upper quadrant tenderness may be present
Anxiety states	Often localized over precordium	Variable; often location moves from place to place	Varies; often fleeting	Situational	Sighing respirations; often chest wall tenderness

sis are classically a result of pulmonary disease, although they are frequently present in the patient with pulmonary edema resulting from left ventricular dysfunction or mitral stenosis. True paroxysmal nocturnal dyspnea is, however, more specific for cardiac disease. In patients with coronary artery disease, dyspnea may be an "anginal equivalent," that is, the dyspnea occurs in a pattern consistent with angina but in the absence of chest discomfort.

Palpitation refers to the subjective sensation of the heart beating. Patients may describe a "fluttering or pounding" in the chest or a feeling that their heart "races" or "skips a beat." Common arrhythmic causes of palpitations include premature atrial or ventricular contractions, supraventricular tachycardia, ventricular tachycardia, and sinus tachycardia. Occasionally, patients report palpitations even when no rhythm disturbance is noted during monitoring, as occurs commonly in patients with anxiety disorders. The pattern of palpitations, especially when correlated to the pulse, may help narrow the differential diagnosis: rapid, regular palpitations are noted with supraventricular tachycardia or ventricular tachycardia; rapid, irregular palpitations are noted with atrial fibrillation; and "skipped beats" are noted with premature atrial or ventricular contractions.

Syncope is the transient loss of consciousness resulting from inadequate cerebral blood flow and may be the result of a variety of cardiovascular diseases (see Chapter 10). True syncope must be distinguished from primary neurologic causes of loss of consciousness (i.e., seizures) and metabolic causes of loss of consciousness (e.g., hypoglycemia, hyperventilation). Cardiac syncope occurs after an abrupt decrease in cardiac output, as may occur with acute myocardial ischemia, valvular heart disease (aortic or mitral stenosis), hypertrophic obstructive cardiomyopathy, left atrial tumors, tachyarrhythmias (ventricular, or less commonly supraventricular, tachycardias), or bradyarrhythmias (e.g., sinus arrest, atrioventricular block, Stokes-Adams attacks). Reflex vasodilation or bradycardia may also result in syncope (vasovagal syncope, carotid sinus syncope, micturition syncope, cough syncope, neurocardiogenic syncope), as may acute pulmonary embolism and hypovolemia. Because global, or at the very least bilateral, cortical ischemia is required to produce syncope, it rarely occurs as a result of unilateral carotid artery disease. However, syncope is occasionally the result of bilateral carotid artery disease and can also occur when disease of the vertebrobasilar system results in brain stem ischemia. Frequently, the cause of a syncopal episode cannot be determined; however, in those cases in which a cause is determined, the most important factor in establishing the diagnosis is obtaining an accurate history of the event.

Edema is a nonspecific symptom that commonly accompanies cardiac disease, as well as renal disease (e.g., nephrotic syndrome), hepatic disease (e.g., cirrhosis), and local venous abnormalities (e.g., thrombophlebitis, chronic venous stasis). When edema occurs as a result of cardiac disease, it reflects an increase in venous pressure. This alters the balance between the venous hydrostatic and oncotic forces, resulting in extravasation of fluid into the extravascular space. When this process

occurs due to elevated left-sided heart pressure, pulmonary edema results, whereas elevated right-sided heart pressure results in peripheral edema. Characteristically, the peripheral edema of heart failure is "pitting," that is, an indentation is left in the skin after pressure is applied to the edematous region. The edema is exacerbated by long periods of standing, is worse in the evening, improves after lying down, and may first be noted when a patient has difficulty in fitting into his or her shoes. The edema may shift to the sacral region after a patient lies down for several hours. When visible edema is noted, it is usually preceded by a moderate weight gain (i.e., 5 to 10 pounds), indicative of volume retention. As heart failure progresses, the edema may extend to the thighs and involve the genitalia and abdominal wall, and fluid may collect in the abdominal (ascites) or thoracic (pleural effusion) cavities.

Cyanosis is an abnormal bluish discoloration of the skin resulting from an increase in the level of reduced hemoglobin in the blood, and, in general, reflects an arterial oxygen saturation of 85% or less (normal arterial oxygen saturation: ≥95%). Central cyanosis presents as cyanosis of the lips or trunk and reflects right-to-left shunting of blood owing to structural cardiac abnormalities (e.g., atrial or ventricular septal defects) or pulmonary parenchymal or vascular disease (e.g., chronic obstructive pulmonary disease, pulmonary embolism, pulmonary arteriovenous fistula). Peripheral cyanosis may occur because of systemic vasoconstriction in the setting of poor cardiac output or may be a localized phenomenon resulting from venous or arterial occlusive or vasospastic disease (e.g., venous or arterial thrombosis, arterial embolic disease, Raynaud's disease). When cyanosis presents in childhood, it usually reflects congenital heart disease with right-to-left shunting of blood.

A myriad of other symptoms, many of them nonspecific, may occur with cardiac disease. Fatigue frequently occurs in the setting of poor cardiac output or may occur secondary to the medical therapy of cardiac disease from overdiuresis, aggressive blood pressure lowering, or use of β-blocking agents. Nausea and vomiting frequently occur during an acute myocardial infarction and may also reflect intestinal edema in the setting of right-sided heart failure. Anorexia and cachexia may occur in severe heart failure. The positional fluid shifts may result in polyuria and nocturia in patients with edema. In addition, epistaxis, hoarseness, hiccups, fever, and chills may reflect underlying cardiovascular disease.

ASSESSMENT OF FUNCTIONAL CAPACITY

In patients with cardiac disorders, their ability or inability to perform various activities (functional status) plays an important role in determining their extent of disability, deciding when to institute various therapies or interventions, assessing their response to therapy, as well as determining their overall prognosis. The New York Heart Association Functional Classification is a standardized method for the assessment of functional status (Table 4–3) and relates functional capacity to the presence or absence of cardiac symptoms during the performance of "usual activities." The Canadian Cardiovascular Soci-

TABLE 4–3   **Classification of Functional Status**

Class I	Uncompromised	Ordinary activity does not cause symptoms.* Symptoms only occur with strenuous or prolonged activity.
Class II	Slightly compromised	Ordinary physical activity results in symptoms; no symptoms at rest.
Class III	Moderately compromised	Less than ordinary activity results in symptoms; no symptoms at rest.
Class IV	Severely compromised	Any activity results in symptoms; symptoms may be present at rest.

*Symptoms refer to undue fatigue, dyspnea, palpitation, or angina in the New York Heart Association classification and refer specifically to angina in the Canadian Cardiovascular Society classification.

ety has provided a similar classification of functional status specifically in patients with angina pectoris. These are useful tools in that they allow a patient's symptoms to be classified and then compared with their symptoms at a different point in time.

Physical Examination

EXAMINATION OF THE JUGULAR VENOUS PULSATIONS

The examination of the neck veins allows for estimation of the right atrial pressure and also for identification of the venous waveforms. The right internal jugular vein is used for this examination because it more accurately reflects right atrial pressure than the external jugular or left jugular veins. With the patient lying at a 45-degree angle (higher in patients with elevated venous pressure, lower in patients with low venous pressure) with his or her head turned to the left, the vertical distance from the sternal angle (angle of Louis) to the top of the venous pulsation can be determined. Because the right atrium lies approximately 5 cm vertically below the sternal angle, distention of the internal jugular vein 4 cm above the sternal angle reflects a right atrial pressure of 9 cm H_2O. The normal right atrial pressure is 5 to 9 cm H_2O and is increased with congestive heart failure, tricuspid insufficiency or stenosis, and restrictive or constrictive heart disease. With inspiration, negative intrathoracic pressure develops, venous blood drains into the thorax, and the normal venous pressure falls; the opposite is true with expiration. This pattern is reversed (Kussmaul's sign) in the setting of right-sided heart failure, constrictive pericarditis, or restrictive myocardial disease. With right-sided heart failure, the elevated venous pressure results in passive congestion of the liver. Pressure applied over the liver for 1 to 3 minutes in this setting results in an increase in the jugular venous pressure (hepatojugular reflux).

The normal waveforms of the venous pulsation consist of the a, c, and v waves and the x and y descents; these are shown in Figure 4–1A and reflect events in the right side of the heart. The a wave results from atrial contraction. Subsequent atrial relaxation results in a decrease in the right atrial pressure, which is seen as the x descent. This descent is interrupted by the c wave,

generated by the bulging of the tricuspid valve cusps into the right atrium during ventricular systole. As the atrial pressure increases owing to venous return, the v wave is generated. This is normally smaller than the a wave and is followed by the y descent as the tricuspid valve opens and blood flows from the right atrium to the right ventricle during diastole.

Abnormalities of the venous waveforms reflect underlying structural, functional, or electrical abnormalities of the heart (see Fig. 4–1B–G). The a wave increases in any condition in which there is greater resistance to right atrial emptying (e.g., tricuspid stenosis, right ventricular hypertrophy, pulmonary hypertension). "Cannon a waves" are seen when the atrium contracts against a closed tricuspid valve, as occurs with complete heart block, junctional or ventricular rhythms, and occasionally with ventricular pacemakers. The a wave is absent in atrial fibrillation. In tricuspid regurgitation, the v wave is prominent and may merge with the c wave (cv wave), thus diminishing or eliminating the x descent altogether. The y descent is attenuated in tricuspid stenosis, owing to the impaired atrial emptying. In pericardial constriction and restrictive cardiomyopathy, as well as in right ventricular infarction, the y descent becomes rapid and deep and the x descent may also become prominent ("W" waveform). In pericardial tamponade, the x descent is prominent but the y descent is diminished or absent.

EXAMINATION OF THE ARTERIAL PULSE

The arterial blood pressure can be measured with the use of a sphygmomanometer. The cuff is applied to the upper arm, rapidly inflated to 30 mm Hg above the anticipated systolic pressure, and then slowly deflated (≤3 mm Hg/sec) while listening for the sounds produced by blood entering the previously occluded brachial artery (Korotkoff sounds). The pressure at which the first sound is heard (usually a clear, tapping sound) represents the systolic pressure. Diastolic pressure occurs at the point at which the Korotkoff sounds disappear. Normally, the pressure in both arms is the same (approximately 120/70 mm Hg), and the systolic pressure in the legs is 10 to 20 mm Hg higher. Asymmetric arm pressures can result from atherosclerotic disease of the aorta, aortic dissection, and stenosis of the innominate or subclavian arteries. Coarctation of the aorta and severe atherosclerotic disease of the aorta, femoral, or

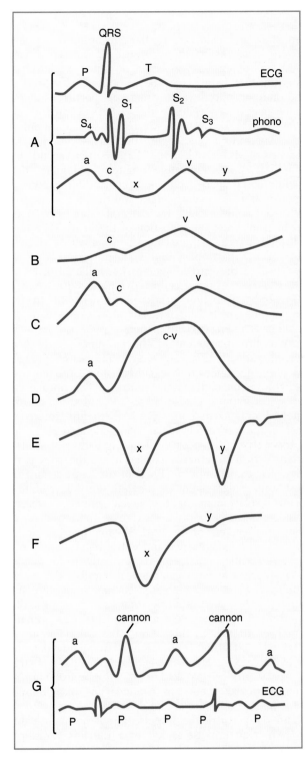

iliac arteries can result in a lower blood pressure in the legs than in the arms. Aortic insufficiency is frequently associated with a leg pressure greater than 20 mm Hg higher than the arm pressure (Hill's sign). Use of a cuff that is too large for a patient's arm will result in erroneously high pressure measurements. Likewise, a cuff that is too small results in erroneously low measurements.

The arterial examination should include an assessment of the carotid, radial, brachial, femoral, popliteal, posterior tibial, and dorsalis pedis pulses, although the carotid artery pulse most accurately reflects the central aortic pulse. The rhythm, strength, contour, and symmetry of the pulses should be noted. The normal arterial pulse (Fig. 4–2A) rises rapidly to a peak in early systole,

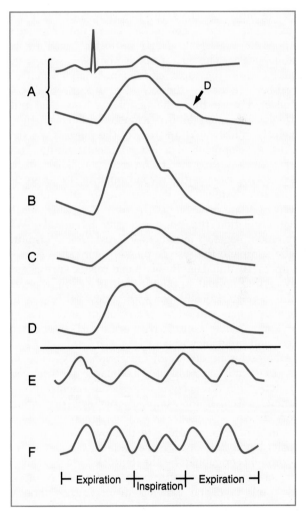

FIGURE 4–1 Normal and abnormal jugular venous pulse tracings. *A,* Normal jugular pulse tracing with simultaneous electrocardiogram (ECG) and phonocardiogram. *B,* Loss of the a wave in atrial fibrillation. *C,* Large a wave in tricuspid stenosis. *D,* Large c-v wave in tricuspid regurgitation. *E,* Prominent x and y descents in constrictive pericarditis. *F,* Prominent x descent and diminutive y descent in pericardial tamponade. *G,* Jugular venous pulse tracing and simultaneous ECG during complete heart block demonstrating "cannon waves" occurring when the atrium contracts against a closed tricuspid valve during ventricular systole.

FIGURE 4–2 Normal and abnormal carotid arterial pulse contours. *A,* Normal arterial pulse with simultaneous ECG. The dicrotic wave (D) occurs just after aortic valve closure. *B,* Wide pulse pressure in aortic insufficiency. *C,* Pulsus parvus et tardus (small amplitude with a slow upstroke) associated with aortic stenosis. *D,* Bisferious pulse with two systolic peaks, typical of hypertrophic obstructive cardiomyopathy or aortic insufficiency, especially if concomitant aortic stenosis is present. *E,* Pulsus alternans characteristic of severe left ventricular failure. *F,* Paradoxical pulse (systolic pressure decrease of greater than 10 mm Hg with inspiration), most characteristic of cardiac tamponade.

plateaus, and then falls. The descending pressure wave is interrupted by the dicrotic notch, related to aortic valve closure. This normal pattern is altered in a variety of cardiovascular disease states (see Fig. $4-2B-F$). The amplitude of the pulse increases in aortic insufficiency, anemia, pregnancy, and thyrotoxicosis and decreases in conditions such as hypovolemia, tachycardia, left ventricular failure, and severe mitral stenosis. Aortic insufficiency results in a "bounding" pulse (Corrigan's pulse or water-hammer pulse), owing to an increased pulse pressure (the difference between systolic and diastolic pressure), and is accompanied by a multitude of abnormalities in the peripheral pulses that reflect this increased pulse pressure. Aortic stenosis characteristically results in an attenuated carotid pulse with a delayed upstroke (pulsus parvus et tardus) and may be associated with a palpable thrill over the aortic area (the carotid shudder). A bisferious pulse is commonly felt in the presence of pure aortic regurgitation and is characterized by two systolic peaks. The first peak is the percussion wave, resulting from the rapid ejection of a large volume of blood early in systole; the second peak is the tidal wave, a reflected wave from the periphery. This bifid pulse may also be noted in hypertrophic cardiomyopathy in which the initial rapid upstroke of the pulse is cut short by the development of a left ventricular outflow tract obstruction resulting in a fall in the pulse. The reflected wave again produces the second impulse. In severe left ventricular dysfunction, the intensity of the pulse may alternate from beat to beat (pulsus alternans), and in atrial fibrillation the pulse intensity is variable. With inspiration, negative intrathoracic pressure is transmitted to the aorta and the systolic pressure normally decreases by up to 10 mm Hg. Pulsus paradoxus is an exaggeration of this normal inspiratory fall in systolic pressure and is characteristically seen with pericardial tamponade, although it may also occur as a result of severe obstructive lung disease, constrictive pericarditis, hypovolemic shock, and pregnancy.

Atherosclerotic disease of the peripheral vascular system frequently accompanies coronary atherosclerosis; therefore, the presence of peripheral vascular disease warrants a search for symptoms or signs of coronary artery disease and vice versa. When atherosclerosis occurs in a peripheral artery to the lower extremity and impairs blood flow distally, the patient may complain of intermittent cramping in the buttocks, thigh, calf, or foot (claudication). Severe peripheral vascular disease may result in digital ischemia or necrosis, without or with associated erectile dysfunction (Leriche's syndrome). The peripheral pulses should be palpated and the abdominal aorta assessed for enlargement in all cardiac patients; a pulsatile, expansile, periumbilical mass suggests the presence of an abdominal aortic aneurysm. With significant stenosis of the peripheral vasculature, the distal pulses may be diminished or absent and the blood flow through the stenotic artery may be audible (a *bruit*). With normal aging, the elastic arteries lose their compliance, and this change in physical property may obscure abnormal findings.

EXAMINATION OF THE PRECORDIUM

Inspection and palpation of the precordium may yield valuable clues as to the existence of cardiac disease. Chest wall abnormalities should be noted, such as pectus excavatum (which may be associated with Marfan's syndrome or mitral valve prolapse), pectus carinatum (which may be associated with Marfan's syndrome), and kyphoscoliosis (occasionally a cause of secondary pulmonary hypertension and right-sided heart failure). The presence of visible pulsations in the aortic (second right intercostal space, suprasternal notch), pulmonic (third left intercostal space), right ventricular (left parasternal region), and left ventricular (fourth–fifth intercostal space, left midclavicular line) regions should be noted and help to direct the palpation of the heart. Retraction of the left parasternal area may be seen with severe left ventricular hypertrophy, and systolic retraction of the chest wall at the cardiac apex or left axilla (Broadbent's sign) is characteristic of constrictive pericarditis.

Precordial palpation is best performed with the patient supine or in the left lateral position, with the examiner standing to the patient's right side. In this position, firm placement of the examiner's right hand over the patient's lower left chest wall places the fingertips over the region of the cardiac apex and the palm over the region of the right ventricle. The normal cardiac apical impulse is a brief, discrete impulse (approximately 1 cm) located in the fourth to fifth intercostal space in the left midclavicular line, generated as the left ventricle strikes the chest wall during early systole. In a patient with a structurally normal heart, the apex is the point of maximal impulse (PMI) of the heart against the chest wall. Enlargement of the left ventricle results in lateral displacement of the apical impulse, whereas chronic obstructive pulmonary disease may result in inferior displacement of the PMI. Volume overload states, such as aortic insufficiency and mitral regurgitation, produce ventricular enlargement primarily from dilation and result in a hyperdynamic apical impulse; that is, the impulse is brisk and increased in amplitude. Pressure overload states, such as aortic stenosis and long-standing hypertension, produce ventricular enlargement primarily from hypertrophy. In this setting, the apical impulse is sustained, and atrial contraction is frequently detected ("a palpable S_4"). Hypertrophic cardiomyopathy characteristically produces a double or triple apical impulse. Left ventricular aneurysms produce an apical impulse that is larger than normal and dyskinetic.

The right ventricular impulse is not normally palpable. When an impulse is felt over the left parasternal region, it usually reflects right ventricular hypertrophy or dilation. Aortic aneurysms may be palpable (or visible) in the suprasternal notch or the second right intercostal space. Pulmonary hypertension may produce a palpable systolic impulse in the left third intercostal space and may also be associated with a palpable pulmonic component of the second heart sound (P_2). Harsh murmurs originating from valvular or congenital heart disease may be associated with palpable vibratory sensations (thrills), as can occur with aortic stenosis, hypertrophic cardiomyopathy, and ventricular septal defects.

Auscultation

TECHNIQUE

Auscultation of the heart should ideally be performed in a quiet room with the patient in a comfortable position and the chest fully exposed. Certain heart sounds are better heard with either the bell or diaphragm of the stethoscope. Low-frequency sounds are best heard with the bell applied to the chest wall with just enough pressure to form a seal. As more pressure is applied to the bell, low-frequency sounds are filtered out. High-frequency sounds are best appreciated with the diaphragm firmly applied to the chest wall. In a patient with a normally situated heart, there are four major zones of cardiac auscultation. Aortic valvular events are best heard in the second right intercostal space. Pulmonary valvular events are best heard in the second left interspace. The fourth left interspace is ideal for auscultating tricuspid valvular events, and mitral valvular events are best heard at the cardiac apex or PMI. Because anatomic abnormalities, both congenital and acquired, can alter the location of the heart in the chest, the auscultatory areas may vary among patients. For instance, in patients with emphysema, the heart is shifted downward and heart sounds may be best heard in the epigastrium. In dextrocardia, the heart lies in the right hemithorax and the auscultatory regions are reversed. Additionally, auscultation in the axilla, supraclavicular areas, or over the thoracic spine may be helpful in some settings, and having the patient lean forward, exhale, or perform various maneuvers may help to accentuate particular heart sounds (see Table 4–6).

NORMAL HEART SOUNDS

The two major heart sounds heard during auscultation are termed S_1 and S_2. These are high-pitched sounds originating from valve closure. S_1 occurs at the onset of ventricular systole and corresponds to closure of the atrioventricular valves. It is usually perceived as a single sound, although occasionally its two components, M_1 and T_1, corresponding to closure of the mitral and tricuspid valves, respectively, can be appreciated. M_1 occurs earlier, is the louder of the two components, and is best heard at the cardiac apex. T_1 is somewhat softer and heard at the left lower sternal border. The second heart sound results from closure of the semilunar valves. The two components, A_2 and P_2, originating from aortic and pulmonic valve closure, respectively, can be easily distinguished. A_2 is usually louder than P_2 and is best heard at the right upper sternal border. P_2 is loudest over the second left intercostal space. During expiration, the normal S_2 is perceived as single. However, during inspiration, the augmented venous return to the right side of the heart and the increased capacitance of the pulmonary vascular bed result in a delay in pulmonic valve closure. In addition, the slightly decreased venous return to the left ventricle results in slightly earlier aortic valve closure. Thus, "physiologic splitting" of the second heart sound, with A_2 preceding P_2 during inspiration, is a normal respiratory event.

Occasionally, additional heart sounds may be heard in normal individuals. A third heart sound (see discussion later) can be heard in normal children and young adults, where it is referred to as a "physiologic S_3"; it is rarely heard after the age of 40. A fourth heart sound (S_4) is generated by forceful atrial contraction and is rarely audible in normal individuals.

A murmur is an auditory vibration usually generated either by abnormally increased flow across a normal valve or normal flow across an abnormal valve or structure. "Innocent" murmurs are always systolic murmurs, are usually soft and brief, and are by definition not associated with abnormalities of the cardiovascular system. They arise from flow across the normal aortic or pulmonic outflow tracts and are present in a large proportion of children and young adults. Murmurs associated with high-flow states (e.g., pregnancy, anemia, fever, thyrotoxicosis, exercise) are not considered innocent. These are termed *physiologic murmurs,* owing to their association with altered physiologic states. Diastolic murmurs are never "innocent" or "physiologic."

ABNORMAL HEART SOUNDS (Figures 4–3 and 4–4)

Abnormalities of S_1 and S_2 relate to abnormalities in their intensity (Table 4–4) or abnormalities in their respiratory splitting (Table 4–5). As noted, splitting of the S_1 is normal but not frequently noted. This splitting becomes more apparent with right bundle branch block or with Ebstein's anomaly of the tricuspid valve, owing to delay in closure of the tricuspid valve in these conditions. The intensity of S_1 is determined in part by the opening state of the atrioventricular valves at the onset of ventricular systole. If the valves are still widely open, as may occur with tachycardia or a short PR interval, S_1 will be accentuated. Conversely, in the presence of a long PR interval, the mitral valve drifts toward a closed position before the onset of ventricular systole and the subsequent S_1 is soft. The intensity of S_1 may vary in the presence of Mobitz I heart block, atrioventricular dissociation, and atrial fibrillation when the relationship between atrial and ventricular systole varies. In mitral stenosis with a pliable valve, the persistent pressure gradient at the end of diastole keeps the mitral valve leaflets relatively open and results in a loud S_1 at the onset of systole. In severe mitral stenosis when the mitral valve is heavily calcified and has decreased leaflet excursion, S_1 becomes faint or absent.

S_2 may be loud in systemic hypertension, owing to accentuated aortic valve closure (loud A_2), or in pulmonary hypertension, owing to accentuated pulmonic valve closure (loud P_2). When the aortic or pulmonary valves are stenotic, the force of valve closure is decreased and, thus, A_2 and P_2 become soft or inaudible. In this setting, S_2 may appear to be single; in the setting of aortic stenosis, prolonged left ventricular ejection narrows the normal splitting of S_2, and with severe aortic stenosis S_2 may become absent altogether as prolonged ejection

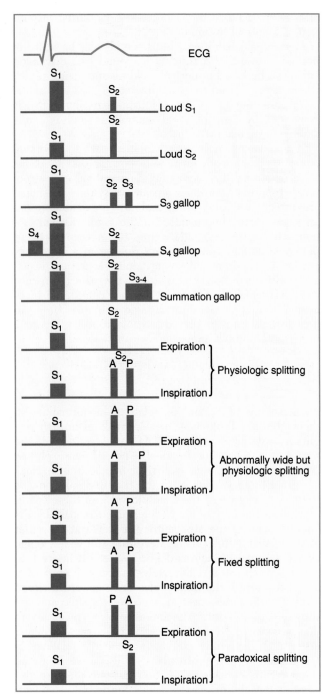

FIGURE 4-3 Abnormal heart sounds can be related to abnormal intensity, abnormal presence of a gallop rhythm, or abnormal splitting of S_2 with respiration.

splitting of S_2 is a reversal of the usual closure sequence of the aortic and pulmonic valves (i.e., P_2 precedes A_2). In this setting, there is a single S_2 with inspiration and splitting of S_2 with expiration. This occurs most commonly when there is delay in closure of the aortic valve either due to delay in electrical conduction to the left ventricle (e.g., left bundle branch block) or prolonged mechanical contraction of the left ventricle (e.g., aortic stenosis, hypertrophic cardiomyopathy).

The third heart sound, S_3 (also called the *ventricular diastolic gallop*), is a low-pitched sound occurring shortly after A_2 in mid-diastole and heard best at the cardiac apex with the patient in the left lateral position. A pathologic S_3 is distinguished from a physiologic S_3 only by the presence of underlying cardiac disease. It is frequently heard with ventricular systolic dysfunction from any cause and likely results either from blood entering the ventricle during the rapid filling phase of diastole or from the impact of the ventricle against the chest wall. Maneuvers that increase venous return accentuate S_3, and maneuvers that decrease venous return make the S_3 softer. An S_3 can also be heard in hyperdynamic states, where it likely results from excessive early diastolic filling. The left ventricular S_3 is best appreciated at the cardiac apex, whereas the right ventricular S_3 is heard best at the left lower sternal border and increases in intensity with inspiration. The timing of the S_3 is similar to the sound generated by atrial tumors ("tumor plop") and constrictive pericarditis ("pericardial knock") and can also be confused with the "opening snap" of a stenotic mitral valve.

The fourth heart sound, S_4 (also called the *atrial diastolic gallop*), is best heard at the cardiac apex with

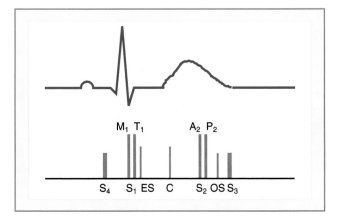

FIGURE 4-4 The relationship of extra heart sounds to the normal first (S_1) and second (S_2) heart sounds. S_1 is composed of the mitral (M_1) and tricuspid (T_1) closing sounds, although it is frequently perceived as a single sound. S_2 is composed of the aortic (A_2) and pulmonic (P_2) closing sounds, which are usually easily distinguished. A fourth heart sound (S_4) is soft and low pitched and precedes S_1. A pulmonic or aortic ejection sound (ES) occurs shortly after S_1. The systolic click (C) of mitral valve prolapse may be heard in midsystole or late systole. The opening snap (OS) of mitral stenosis is high pitched and occurs shortly after S_2. A tumor plop or pericardial knock occurs at the same time and can be confused with an OS or an S_3, which is lower in pitched and occurs slightly later.

and its accompanying murmur obscure P_2. Wide splitting of the S_2 with normal respiratory variation occurs when either pulmonic valve closure is delayed (e.g., right bundle branch block, pulmonic stenosis) or aortic valve closure occurs earlier owing to more rapid ejection of left ventricular volume (e.g., mitral regurgitation, ventricular septal defect). Fixed splitting of S_2 without respiratory variation is characteristic of atrial septal defects and also occurs with right ventricular failure. Paradoxical

TABLE 4–4   **Abnormal Intensity of Heart Sounds**

	S₁	A₂	P₂
Loud	Short PR Interval Mitral stenosis with pliable valve	Systemic hypertension Aortic dilation Coarctation of the aorta	Pulmonary hypertension Thin chest wall
Soft	Long PR interval Mitral regurgitation Poor left ventricular function Mitral stenosis with rigid valve Thick chest wall	Calcific aortic stenosis Aortic regurgitation	Valvular or subvalvular pulmonic stenosis
Varying	Atrial fibrillation Heart block		

the bell of the stethoscope. It is a low-pitched sound originating from the active ejection of blood from the atrium into a noncompliant ventricle, and is, therefore, not present in the setting of atrial fibrillation. It is commonly heard in patients with left ventricular hypertrophy from any cause (e.g., hypertension, aortic stenosis, hypertrophic cardiomyopathy) or acute myocardial ischemia and in hyperkinetic states. Frequently, the S₄ is also palpable at the cardiac apex. S₃ and S₄ are occasionally present in the same patient. In the presence of tachycardia or a prolonged PR interval, the S₃ and S₄ may merge to produce a summation gallop.

The opening of normal cardiac valves is not audible. However, abnormal valves may produce opening sounds. In the presence of a bicuspid aortic valve or in aortic stenosis with pliable valve leaflets, an "ejection sound" is audible as the leaflets open to their maximal extent. A similar ejection sound may originate from a stenotic pulmonic valve, and in this case, the ejection sound decreases in intensity with inspiration. These ejection sounds are high pitched, occur early in systole, and are frequently followed by the typical ejection murmur of aortic or pulmonic stenosis. Ejection sounds are also heard with systemic or pulmonary hypertension, the exact mechanism of which is not clear.

Ejection sounds heard in midsystole to late systole are referred to as systolic "clicks" and are most commonly associated with mitral valve prolapse. As the redundant mitral valve prolapses and reaches its maximal superior displacement, it produces a high-pitched click. Several clicks may be heard as various parts of the redundant valve prolapse. Frequently, the click is followed by a mitral regurgitant murmur. Maneuvers that decrease venous return cause the clicks to occur earlier in systole and the murmur to become longer (Table 4–6).

The opening of abnormal mitral or tricuspid valves can also be heard in the presence of rheumatic valvular stenosis when the sound is referred to as an *opening snap*. The "snap" is heard only if the valve leaflets are pliable and is generated as the leaflets abruptly dome during early diastole. The interval between S₂ and the opening snap is of diagnostic importance: as the stenosis worsens and the atrial pressure increases, the mitral valve opens earlier in diastole, and the interval between the S₂ and the opening snap shortens.

MURMURS

As stated previously, murmurs are a series of auditory vibrations generated when either abnormal blood flow across a normal cardiac structure or normal flow across an abnormal cardiac structure results in turbulent flow. These sounds are longer than the individual heart

TABLE 4–5   **Abnormal Splitting of S₂**

Single S₂	Widely Split S₂ with Normal Respiratory Variation	Fixed Split S₂	Paradoxically Split S₂
Aortic stenosis Pulmonic stenosis Systemic hypertension Coronary artery disease Any condition that can lead to paradoxical splitting of S₂	Right bundle branch block Left ventricular pacing Pulmonic stenosis Pulmonary embolism Idiopathic dilation of the pulmonary artery Mitral regurgitation Ventricular septal defect	Atrial septal defect Severe right ventricular dysfunction	Left bundle branch block Right ventricular pacing Angina, myocardial infarction Aortic stenosis Hypertrophic cardiomyopathy Aortic regurgitation

TABLE 4-6   **Effects of Physiologic Maneuvers on Auscultatory Events**

Maneuver	Major Physiologic Effects	Useful Auscultatory Changes
Respiration	↑ Venous return with inspiration	↑ Right heart murmurs and gallops with inspiration; splitting of S_2 (see Fig. 4–3)
Valsalva (initial ↑ BP, phase I; followed by ↓ BP, phase II)	↓ BP, ↓ venous return, ↓ LV size (phase II)	↑ HCM ↓ AS, MR MVP click earlier in systole, murmur prolongs
Standing	↓ Venous return ↓ LV size	↑ HCM ↓ AS, MR MVP click earlier in systole, murmur prolongs
Squatting	↑ Venous return ↑ Systemic vascular resistance ↑ LV size	↑ AS, MR, AI ↓ HCM MVP click delayed, murmur shortens
Isometric exercise (e.g., handgrip)	↑ Arterial pressure ↑ Cardiac output	↑ Gallops ↑ MR, AI, MS ↓ AS, HCM
Post PVC or prolonged RR interval	↑ Ventricular filling ↑ Contractility	↑ AS Little change in MR
Amyl nitrate	↓ Arterial pressure ↑ Cardiac output ↓ LV size	↑ HCM, AS, MS ↓ AI, MR, Austin Flint murmur MVP click earlier in systole, murmur prolongs
Phenylephrine	↑ Arterial pressure ↓ Cardiac output ↑ LV size	↑ MR, AI ↓ AS, HCM MVP click delayed, murmur shortens

↑ = increased intensity; ↓ = decreased intensity; AI = aortic insufficiency; AS = aortic stenosis; BP = blood pressure; HCM = hypertrophic cardiomyopathy; LV = left ventricle; MR = mitral regurgitation; MS = mitral stenosis; MVP = mitral valve prolapse; PVC = premature ventricular contraction.

sounds and can be described by their intensity, frequency (pitch), quality, duration, and timing in relation to systole or diastole. The intensity of a murmur is graded on a scale of 1 to 6 (Table 4–7). In general, murmurs of grade 4 or greater are associated with a palpable thrill. The loudness of a murmur does not necessarily correlate with the severity of the underlying abnormality. For instance, flow across a large atrial septal defect is essentially silent, whereas flow across a small ventricular septal defect is frequently associated with a loud murmur. Higher-frequency murmurs correlate with a higher velocity of flow at the site of turbulence. It is important to note the pattern or configuration of the murmur (e.g., crescendo, crescendo-decrescendo, decrescendo, plateau) (Fig. 4–5), the quality of the murmur (e.g., harsh, blowing, rumbling), as well as the location of maximal intensity and the pattern of radiation of the murmur. Various physical maneuvers may help to clarify the nature of a particular murmur (see Table 4–6).

Murmurs can be divided into three categories—sys-

tolic, diastolic, and continuous (Table 4–8)—and can result from abnormalities on the right or left side of the heart. Right-sided murmurs may become significantly louder after inspiration, owing to the resulting augmentation of venous return, whereas left-sided murmurs are relatively unaffected by respiration. Systolic murmurs can be further divided into ejection type murmurs and regurgitant murmurs. Ejection murmurs reflect turbulent flow across the aortic or pulmonic valve. They begin shortly after S_1, increase in intensity as the velocity of flow increases, and subsequently decrease in intensity as the velocity falls (crescendo-decrescendo). Examples of ejection-type murmurs include innocent murmurs, aortic sclerosis, aortic stenosis, pulmonic stenosis, and the murmur of hypertrophic cardiomyopathy. Innocent murmurs and aortic sclerotic murmurs are short in duration and do not radiate. The duration of aortic or pulmonic stenotic murmurs varies depending on the severity of the stenosis. With more severe stenosis, the murmur becomes longer and the time to peak intensity of the murmur lengthens (i.e., early-, mid-, and late-peaking murmur). The murmur of aortic stenosis is usually harsh, radiates to the carotid arteries, and at times may radiate to the cardiac apex (Gallavardin phenomenon). The murmur of hypertrophic cardiomyopathy may be confused with aortic stenosis, but it does not radiate to the carotids, and it is the only murmur that becomes louder with decreased venous return.

The classic regurgitant systolic murmurs of mitral (MR) and tricuspid regurgitation (TR) last throughout all of systole (holosystolic), are plateau in pattern, and terminate at S_2. With acute MR, the murmur may be limited to early systole and may be somewhat decre-

TABLE 4-7   **Grading System for Intensity of Murmurs**

Grade 1	Barely audible murmur
Grade 2	Murmur of medium intensity
Grade 3	Loud murmur, no thrill
Grade 4	Loud murmur with thrill
Grade 5	Very loud murmur; stethoscope must be on the chest to hear it; may be heard posteriorly
Grade 6	Murmur audible with stethoscope off the chest

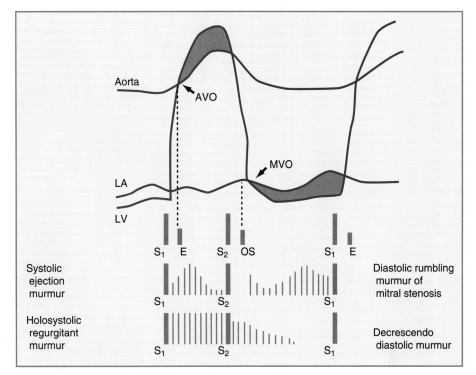

FIGURE 4–5 Abnormal sounds and murmurs associated with valvular dysfunction displayed simultaneously with left atrial (LA), left ventricular (LV), and aortic pressure tracings. AVO = Aortic valve opening; E = ejection click of the aortic valve; MVO = mitral valve opening; OS = opening snap of the mitral valve. The shaded areas represent pressure gradients across the aortic valve during systole or mitral valve during diastole, characteristic of aortic stenosis and mitral stenosis, respectively.

TABLE 4–8 Classification of Heart Murmurs

Timing	Class	Description	Characteristic Lesions
Systolic	Ejection	Begins in early systole; may extend to mid- or late systole Crescendo-decrescendo pattern Often harsh in quality	Valvular, supravalvular, and subvalvular aortic stenosis Hypertrophic cardiomyopathy Pulmonic stenosis Aortic or pulmonary artery dilation Malformed but nonobstructive aortic valve ↑ Transvalvular flow (e.g., aortic regurgitation, hyperkinetic states, atrial septal defect, physiologic flow murmur)
	Holosystolic	Extends throughout systole Relatively uniform in intensity	Mitral regurgitation Tricuspid regurgitation Ventricular septal defect
	Late	Variable onset and duration, often preceded by a nonejection click	Mitral valve prolapse
Diastolic	Early	Begins with A_2 or P_2 Decrescendo pattern with variable duration Often high-pitched, blowing	Aortic regurgitation Pulmonic regurgitation
	Mid	Begins after S_2, often after an opening snap Low-pitched "rumble" heard best with bell of stethoscope Louder with exercise and left lateral position Loudest in early diastole	Mitral stenosis Tricuspid stenosis ↑ Flow across atrioventricular valves (e.g., mitral regurgitation, tricuspid regurgitation, atrial septal defect)
	Late	Presystolic accentuation of mid-diastolic murmur	Mitral stenosis Tricuspid stenosis
Continuous		Systolic and diastolic components "Machinery murmurs"	Patent ductus arteriosus Coronary atrioventricular fistula Ruptured sinus of Valsalva aneurysm into right atrium or ventricle Mammary souffle Venous hum

scendo in pattern. When MR is secondary to mitral valve prolapse, it starts in midsystole to late systole and is preceded by a mitral valve click. Ventricular septal defects may also result in holosystolic murmurs, although a small muscular ventricular septal defect may have a murmur limited to early systole.

Early diastolic murmurs result from aortic or pulmonic insufficiency and are decrescendo in pattern. The duration of the murmur reflects chronicity: a short murmur is heard in acute aortic insufficiency, whereas chronic aortic insufficiency may produce a murmur throughout diastole. A Graham Steell murmur denotes a pulmonic insufficiency murmur in the setting of pulmonary hypertension. Mid-diastolic murmurs classically result from mitral or tricuspid stenosis, are low pitched, and are referred to as diastolic rumbles. Similar murmurs may be heard with obstructing atrial myxomas or in the presence of augmented diastolic flow across an unobstructed mitral or tricuspid valve, as occurs with an atrial or ventricular septal defect or with significant MR or TR. Severe, chronic aortic insufficiency may also produce a diastolic rumble, owing to premature closure of the mitral valve (Austin Flint murmur). Late diastolic murmurs reflect presystolic accentuation of the mid-diastolic murmurs, owing to augmented mitral or tricuspid flow after atrial contraction.

Continuous murmurs are murmurs that last throughout all of systole and continue into at least early diastole. These are referred to as "machinery murmurs" and are generated by continuous flow from a vessel or chamber with high pressure into a vessel or chamber with low pressure. A patent ductus arteriosus produces the classic continuous murmur.

OTHER CARDIAC SOUNDS

Pericardial rubs occur in the setting of pericarditis. They are coarse, scratching sounds heard best at the left sternal border with the patient leaning forward and holding his or her breath at end expiration. The classic rub has three components corresponding to atrial systole, ventricular systole, and ventricular diastole, although frequently only one or two of the components are audible. Localized irritation of the surrounding pleura may result in an associated pleural friction rub (pleuropericardial rub), which varies with respiration.

Continuous venous murmurs, or venous "hums," are almost universally present in children. They are also frequent in adults, especially during pregnancy, or in the setting of thyrotoxicosis or anemia. They are best heard at the base of the neck with the patient's head turned to the opposite direction and can be eliminated by gentle pressure over the vein.

PROSTHETIC HEART SOUNDS

Prosthetic valves produce characteristic auscultatory findings. Porcine or bovine bioprosthetic valves produce heart sounds that are similar to native valve sounds; however, because these valves are smaller than the native valves which they replace, they almost always have an associated murmur (systolic ejection murmur when placed in the aortic position, diastolic rumble when placed in the mitral position). Mechanical valves result in crisp, high-pitched sounds related to valvular opening and closure. With ball-in-cage valves (e.g., Starr-Edwards) the opening sound is louder than the closure sound. With all other mechanical valves (e.g., Bjork-Shiley, St. Jude), the closure sound is louder. These valves also produce an ejection-type murmur. It is important to listen for all of the expected prosthetic sounds in patients with prosthetic valves because dysfunction of these valves may first be suggested by a change in the intensity or quality of the heart sounds or the development of a new or changing murmur.

REFERENCES

Braunwald E: The history. *In* Braunwald E (ed): Heart Disease: A Textbook of Cardiovascular Medicine, 5th ed. Philadelphia: WB Saunders, 1997, pp 1–14.
Lembo N, Dell'Italia LJ, Crawford MH, et al: Bedside diagnosis of systolic murmurs. N Engl J Med 1988; 318:1572.
Perloff JK: Physical Examination of the Heart and Circulation, 2nd ed. Philadelphia: WB Saunders, 1990.

5

DIAGNOSTIC TESTS AND PROCEDURES IN THE PATIENT WITH CARDIOVASCULAR DISEASE

Lisa A. Mendes • Joseph Loscalzo

Chest Radiography

The chest x-ray film is an integral part of the cardiac evaluation and gives valuable information regarding structure and function of the heart, lungs, and great vessels. A routine examination includes posteroanterior and lateral projections (Fig. 5–1).

In the posteroanterior view, cardiac enlargement may be present when the transverse diameter of the cardiac silhouette is greater than half of the transverse diameter of the thorax. The heart may appear falsely enlarged when the heart is displaced horizontally, such as with poor inflation of the lungs, and if the film is an anteroposterior projection, which magnifies the heart shadow. Left atrial enlargement is suggested when the left-sided heart border is straightened or bulges toward the left. In addition, the main bronchi may be widely splayed and a circular opacity or "double density" within the cardiac silhouette may be seen. Right atrial enlargement may be present when the right-sided heart border bulges toward the right. Left ventricular enlargement results in downward and lateral displacement of the apex. A rounding of the displaced apex suggests ventricular hypertrophy. Right ventricular enlargement is best assessed in the lateral view and may be present when the right ventricular border occupies more than one third of the retrosternal space between the diaphragm and thoracic apex.

The aortic arch and thoracic aorta may become dilated and tortuous in patients with severe atherosclerosis, long-standing hypertension, and aortic dissection.

Dilation of the proximal pulmonary arteries may occur when pulmonary pressures are elevated and pulmonary vascular resistance is increased. Disease states associated with increased pulmonary artery flow and normal vascular resistance, such as atrial or ventricular septal defects, may result in dilation of the proximal and distal pulmonary arteries.

Pulmonary venous congestion secondary to elevated left-sided heart pressures results in redistribution of blood flow in the lungs and prominence of the apical vessels. Transudation of fluid into the interstitial space may result in fluid in the fissures and along the horizontal periphery of the lower lung fields (Kerley B lines). As venous pressures further increase, fluid collects within the alveolar space, which early on collects preferentially in the inner two thirds of the lung fields, resulting in a characteristic "butterfly" appearance.

Fluoroscopy or plain films may identify abnormal calcification involving the pericardium, coronary arteries, aorta, and valves. In addition, fluoroscopy can be instrumental in evaluating the function of mechanical prosthetic valves.

Specific radiographic signs of congenital and valvular disease are discussed in their respective sections.

Electrocardiography

The electrocardiogram (ECG) represents the electrical activity of the heart recorded by skin electrodes. This wave of electrical activity is represented as a sequence

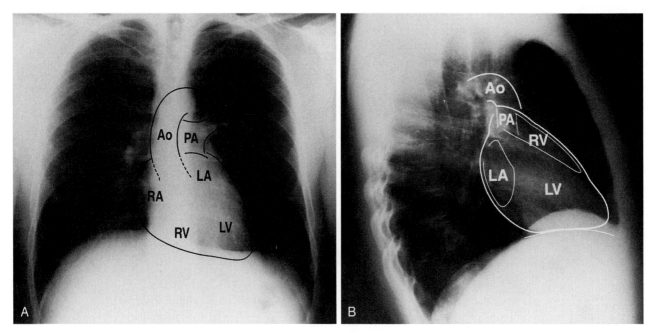

FIGURE 5–1   Schematic illustration of the parts of the heart, whose outlines can be identified on a routine chest radiograph. *A,* Posteroanterior chest radiograph. *B,* Lateral chest radiograph. Ao = aorta; PA = pulmonary artery; LA = left atrium; RA = right atrium; RV = right ventricle; LV = left ventricle.

of deflections on the ECG (Fig. 5–2). The horizontal scale represents time, such that at a standard paper speed of 25 mm/sec each small box (1 mm) represents 0.04 second and each large box (5 mm) represents 0.20 second. The vertical scale represents amplitude (10 mm = 1 mV). The heart rate can be estimated by dividing the number of large boxes between complexes (RR interval) into 300.

In the normal heart, the electrical impulse originates in the sinoatrial (SA) node and is conducted through the atria. Given that depolarization of the SA node is too weak to be detected on the surface ECG, the first, low-amplitude deflection on the surface ECG reflects atrial

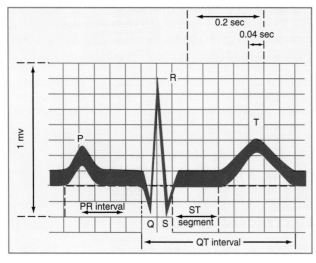

FIGURE 5–2   Normal electrocardiographic (ECG) complex with labeling of waves and intervals.

activation and is termed the *P wave.* The interval between the onset of the P wave and the next rapid deflection (QRS complex) is known as the PR interval and primarily represents the time it takes for the impulse to travel through the atrioventricular (AV) node. The normal PR segment ranges from 0.12 to 0.20 second. A PR interval greater than 0.20 second defines AV nodal block.

Once the wave of depolarization has moved through the AV node, the ventricular myocardium is depolarized in a sequence of four phases. First, the interventricular septum depolarizes from left to right. This is followed by depolarization of the right ventricle and inferior wall of the left ventricle, then the apex and central portions of the left ventricle, and finally, the base and the posterior wall of the left ventricle. Ventricular depolarization results in a high-amplitude complex on the surface ECG known as the QRS complex. The first downward deflection of this complex is the Q wave; the first upward deflection, the R wave; and the subsequent downward deflection, the S wave. In some individuals, a second upward deflection may be present after the S wave and is termed R *prime* (R′). Normal duration of the QRS complex is less than 0.10 second. Complexes greater than 0.12 second are usually secondary to some form of interventricular conduction delay.

The isoelectric segment after the QRS complex is the ST segment and represents a brief period during which there is little electrical activity in the heart. The junction between the end of the QRS complex and the beginning of the ST segment is the J point. The upward deflection after the ST segment is the T wave and represents ventricular repolarization. The QT interval, which reflects the duration of ventricular depolarization and repolarization, is measured from the onset of the

QRS complex to the end of the T wave. The QT interval varies with heart rate, but for rates between 60 and 100 beats/min, the normal QT interval ranges from 0.35 to 0.44 second. For heart rates outside this range, the QT interval can be corrected by the formula $QT_c = QT$ (sec)/RR interval$^{1/2}$ (sec). In some individuals, a low-amplitude U wave may be noted after the T wave, the etiology of which is unknown.

The standard electrocardiogram consists of 12 leads: six limb leads (I, II, III, aVR, aVL, aVF) and six chest or precordial leads (V_1 to V_6). The electrical activity recorded in each lead represents the direction and magnitude of the electrical force as seen from that particular lead position. Electrical activity directed toward a particular lead is represented as an upward deflection, and an electrical impulse directed away from a particular lead is represented as a downward deflection. Although the overall direction of electrical activity can be determined for any of the waveforms previously described, the mean QRS axis is the most clinically useful and is determined by examining the six limb leads. Figure 5–3 illustrates Einthoven's triangle and the polarity of each of the six limb leads of the standard ECG. Skin electrodes are attached to both arms and legs, with the right leg serving as the ground. Leads I, II, and III are bipolar leads and represent electrical activity between two leads: lead I represents electrical activity between the right and left arms (left arm positive), lead II between the right arm and left leg (left leg positive), and lead III between the left arm and left leg (left leg positive). Leads aVR, aVL, and aVF are designated the augmented leads. With these leads, the QRS will be positive or have a predominant upward deflection when the electrical forces are directed toward the right arm

for aVR, left arm for aVL, and left leg for aVF. These six leads form a hexaxial frontal plane of 30-degree arc intervals. The normal QRS axis ranges from − 30 to + 90 degrees. An axis more negative than − 30 defines left-axis deviation and an axis greater than + 90 defines right-axis deviation. In general, a positive QRS complex in leads I and aVF suggests a normal QRS axis between 0 and 90 degrees.

The six precordial leads (V_1 to V_6) are attached to the anterior chest wall. Electrical activity directed toward these leads results in a positive deflection on the ECG tracing. Leads V_1 and V_2 are closest to the right ventricle and interventricular septum, and leads V_5 and V_6 are closest to the anterior and anterolateral walls of the left ventricle. Normally, there is a small R wave in lead V_1 reflecting septal depolarization and a deep S wave reflecting predominantly left ventricular activation. From V_1 to V_6, the R wave becomes larger (and the S wave smaller) because the predominant forces directed at these leads originate from the left ventricle.

Abnormal ECG Patterns

CHAMBER ABNORMALITIES AND VENTRICULAR HYPERTROPHY

The P wave is normally upright in leads I, II, and F; inverted in aVR; and biphasic in V_1. Left atrial abnormality (defined as enlargement, hypertrophy, or increased wall stress) is characterized by a wide P wave in II (≥0.12 second) and a deeply inverted terminal component in V_1. Right atrial abnormality is present when the P waves in the limb leads are peaked and 2.5 mm or more in height.

Left ventricular hypertrophy may result in increased QRS voltage, slight widening of the QRS complex, late intrinsicoid deflection, left-axis deviation, and abnormalities of the ST-T segments. Multiple criteria with variable sensitivity and specificity for detecting left ventricular hypertrophy are available. The most frequently used criteria are given in Table 5–1.

Right ventricular hypertrophy is characterized by tall R waves in V_1 through V_3; deep S waves in leads I, L, V_5, and V_6; and right-axis deviation. In patients with chronically elevated pulmonary pressures, such as with chronic lung disease, a combination of ECG abnormalities reflecting right-sided pathology may be present and include right atrial abnormality, right ventricular hypertrophy, and right-axis deviation. In patients with acute pulmonary embolus, ECG changes may suggest right ventricular strain and include right-axis deviation; incomplete or complete right bundle branch block; S waves in I, II, and III; and T wave inversions in V_1 through V_3.

INTERVENTRICULAR CONDUCTION DELAYS

The ventricular conduction system consists of two main branches, the right and left bundles. The left bundle further divides into the anterior and posterior fascicles.

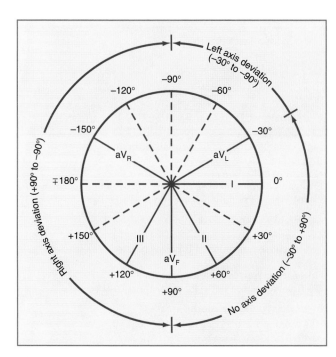

FIGURE 5–3 Hexaxial reference figure for frontal plane axis determination, indicating values for abnormal left and right QRS axis deviation.

TABLE 5–1   ECG Manifestations of Atrial Abnormalities and Ventricular Hypertrophy

Left Atrial Abnormality

P wave duration $\geq$ 0.12 sec
Notched, slurred P wave in leads I and II
Biphasic P wave in V_1 with a wide, deep, negative terminal component

Right Atrial Abnormality

P wave duration $\leq$ 0.11 sec
Tall, peaked P waves of $\geq$ 2.5 mm in leads II, III, and aV_F

Left Ventricular Hypertrophy

Voltage criteria
    R wave in $AV_L \geq$ 12 mm
    R wave in I $\geq$ 15 mm
    S wave in V_1 or V_2 + R wave in V_5 or $V_6 \geq$ 35 mm
Depressed ST segments with inverted T waves in the lateral leads
Left-axis deviation
QRS duration $\geq$ 0.09 sec
Left atrial enlargement

Right Ventricular Hypertrophy

Tall R waves over right precordium (R:S ratio in lead V_1, > 1.0)
Right-axis deviation
Depressed ST segments with inverted T waves in V_1–V_3
Normal QRS duration (if no right bundle branch block)

Conduction block can occur in either of the major branches or in the fascicles (Table 5–2).

Fascicular block results in a change in the sequence of ventricular activation but does not prolong overall conduction time (QRS duration remains < 0.10 second). Left anterior fascicular block is a relatively common ECG abnormality and is often associated with right bundle branch block. This conduction abnormality is present when there is extreme left axis deviation (< −45 degrees); the R wave is greater than the Q wave in leads I and aVL; and the S wave is greater than the R wave in leads II, III, and aVF. Left posterior fascicular block is uncommon but is associated with right-axis deviation (>90 degrees); small Q waves in leads II, III, and aVF; and small R waves in leads I and aVL.

In left bundle branch block, depolarization proceeds down the right bundle, across the interventricular septum from right to left, and then to the left ventricle. Characteristic ECG findings include a wide QRS complex ($\geq$0.12 second); a broad R wave in leads I, aVL, V_5, and V_6; a deep QS wave in leads V_1 and V_2; and ST depression and T wave inversion opposite the QRS deflection (Fig. 5–4). Given the abnormal sequence of ventricular activation with left bundle branch block, many ECG abnormalities, such as Q wave myocardial infarction and left ventricular hypertrophy, cannot be interpreted. However, left bundle branch block almost always indicates the presence of underlying myocardial disease. With right bundle branch block, the interventricular septum depolarizes normally from left to right,

and, therefore, the initial QRS deflection remains unchanged. As a result, ECG abnormalities such as Q wave myocardial infarction can still be interpreted. After septal activation, the left ventricle depolarizes, followed by the right ventricle. The ECG is characterized by a wide QRS complex; a large R′ wave in lead V_1 (rsR′); and deep S waves in leads I, L, and V_6 representing delayed right ventricular activation (see Fig. 5–4). Although right bundle branch block may be associated with underlying cardiac disease, it may also appear as a normal variant.

MYOCARDIAL ISCHEMIA AND INFARCTION

Myocardial ischemia and infarction may be associated with abnormalities of the ST segment, T wave, and QRS complex. Myocardial ischemia primarily affects repolarization of the myocardium and is often associated with horizontal or downsloping ST segment depression and T wave inversion. These changes may be transient, such as during an anginal episode or an exercise stress test, or may be long lasting in the setting of unstable angina or myocardial infarction. T wave inversion without ST segment depression is a nonspecific finding and must be correlated with the clinical setting. Localized ST segment elevation suggests more extensive myocardial injury and is often associated with acute myocardial infarction (Fig. 5–5). Vasospastic or Prinzmetal's angina may be associated with reversible ST segment elevation without myocardial infarction. ST elevation may occur in other settings not related to acute ischemia or infarction. Persistent, localized ST segment elevation in the

TABLE 5–2   ECG Manifestations of Fascicular and Bundle Branch Blocks

Left Anterior Fascicular Block

QRS duration $\leq$ 0.1 sec
Left-axis deviation (more negative than −45 degrees)
rS pattern in II, III, and aV_F
qR pattern in leads I and aV_L

Right Posterior Fascicular Block

QRS duration $\leq$ 0.1 sec
Right-axis deviation (+90 degrees or greater)
qR pattern in II, III, and aV_F
rS pattern in I and aV_L
Exclusion of other causes of right-axis deviation (chronic obstructive pulmonary disease, right ventricular hypertrophy)

Left Bundle Branch Block

QRS duration $\geq$ 0.12 sec
Broad, slurred or notched R waves in lateral leads (I, aV_L, V_5–V_6)
QS or rS pattern in anterior precordium
ST-T wave vectors opposite to terminal QRS vectors

Right Bundle Branch Block

QRS duration $\geq$ 0.12 sec
Large R′ wave in lead V_1 (rsR′)
Deep terminal S wave in V_6
Normal septal Q waves
Inverted T waves in V_1–V_2

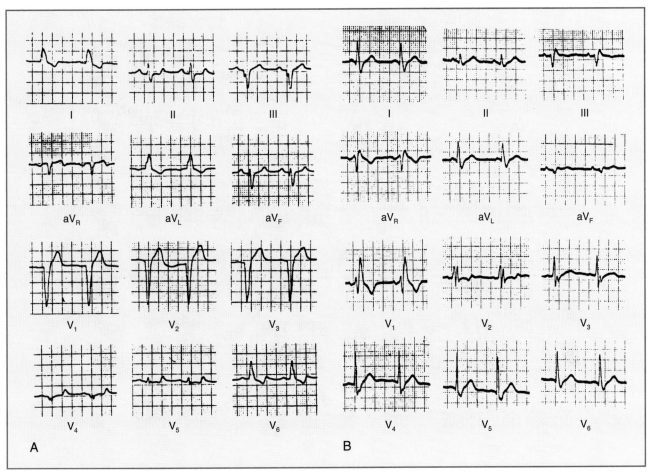

FIGURE 5-4 *A,* Left bundle branch block. *B,* Right bundle branch block. Criteria for bundle branch block are summarized in Table 5-2.

same leads as pathologic Q waves is consistent with a ventricular aneurysm. Acute pericarditis is associated with diffuse ST segment elevation and PR depression. Diffuse J point elevation in association with upward coving ST segments is a normal variant common among young men.

The presence of a Q wave is one of the diagnostic criteria used to verify a myocardial infarction. Infarcted myocardium is unable to conduct electrical activity, and, therefore, electrical forces will be directed away from the surface electrode overlying the infarcted region, resulting in a Q wave on the surface ECG. The area of infarction can, therefore, be localized by knowing which region of the myocardium each lead represents (Table 5–3). A pathologic Q wave has a duration of ≥0.04 second and/or a depth one-fourth or more the height of the corresponding R wave.

Not all myocardial infarctions will result in the formation of Q waves. In addition, small R waves can return many weeks to months after a myocardial infarction.

Abnormal Q waves, or "pseudoinfarction," may also be associated with nonischemic cardiac disease, such as cardiac amyloidosis, sarcoidosis, idiopathic or hypertrophic cardiomyopathy, myocarditis, and chronic lung disease.

ABNORMALITIES OF THE ST SEGMENT AND T WAVE

A number of drugs and metabolic abnormalities may affect the ST segment and T wave (Fig. 5–6). Hypokalemia may result in prominent U waves in the precordial leads and prolongation of the QT interval. Hyperkalemia may result in tall, peaked T waves. Hypocalcemia typically lengthens the QT interval, whereas hypercalcemia shortens it. A commonly used cardiac medication, digoxin, often results in diffuse, scooped ST segment depression. Minor or "nonspecific" ST segment and T wave abnormalities may be present and have no definable cause. In these instances, the physician must determine the significance of the abnormalities based on the clinical setting.

Long-Term Ambulatory ECG Recording

Ambulatory electrocardiography (Holter monitoring) is a widely used, noninvasive method to evaluate cardiac arrhythmias and conduction disturbances over an extended period of time and to detect electrical abnormalities that

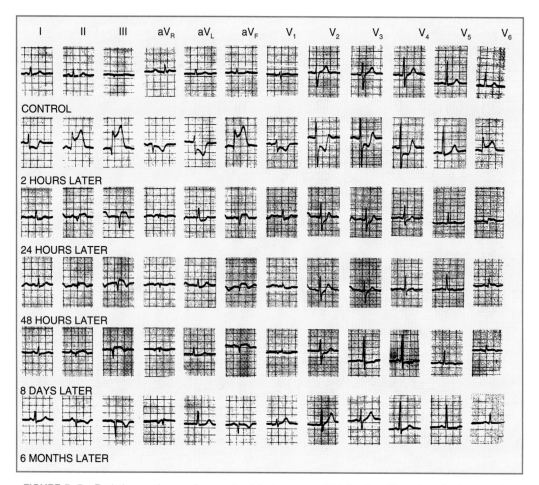

| I | II | III | aV_R | aV_L | aV_F | V₁ | V₂ | V₃ | V₄ | V₅ | V₆ |

CONTROL

2 HOURS LATER

24 HOURS LATER

48 HOURS LATER

8 DAYS LATER

6 MONTHS LATER

FIGURE 5–5 Evolutionary changes in a posteroinferior myocardial infarction. Control tracing is normal. The tracing recorded 2 hours after onset of chest pain demonstrated development of early Q waves, marked ST segment elevation, and hyperacute T waves in leads II, III, and aV_F. In addition, a larger R wave, ST segment depression, and negative T waves have developed in leads V₁ and V₂. These are early changes indicating acute posteroinferior myocardial infarction. The 24-hour tracing demonstrates evolutionary changes. In leads II, III, and aV_F, the Q wave is larger, the ST segments have almost returned to baseline, and the T wave has begun to invert. In leads V₁ to V₂ the duration of the R wave now exceeds 0.04 second, the ST segment is depressed, and the T wave is upright. (In this example, electrocardiographic [ECG] changes of true posterior involvement extend past V₂; ordinarily only V₁ and V₂ may be involved.) Only minor further changes occur through the 8-day tracing. Finally, 6 months later the ECG illustrates large Q waves, isoelectric ST segments, and inverted T waves in leads II, III, and aV_F and large R waves, isoelectric ST segment, and upright T waves in V₁ and V₂, indicative of an "old" posteroinferior myocardial infarction.

may be brief or transient. With this approach, ECG data from two to three surface leads are stored on a tape recorder worn by the patient for a minimum of 24 to 48 hours. The recorders have both patient-activated event markers and time markers so that any abnormalities can be correlated with the patient's symptoms or time of day. These data can then be printed in a standard, real-time ECG format for review.

For patients with intermittent or rare symptoms, an event recorder, which can be worn for several weeks, may be helpful in identifying the arrhythmia. The simplest device is a small, hand-held monitor that is applied to the chest wall when symptoms occur. The ECG is recorded and can later be transmitted by telephone to a monitoring center for analysis. A more sophisticated system uses a wrist recorder that allows continuous loop

storage of 4 to 5 minutes of ECG data from one lead. When the system is activated by the patient, ECG data preceding the event and for 1 to 2 minutes after the event are recorded and stored for further analysis. With both these devices, the patient must be physically able to activate the recorder during the episode to store the ECG data.

Stress Testing

Stress testing is an important noninvasive tool for evaluating patients with known or suspected coronary artery disease (CAD). The theoretical basis for this form of testing is that during exercise there is an increased de-

TABLE 5-3   ECG Localization of Myocardial Infarction

Infarct Location	Leads Depicting Primary ECG Changes	Likely Vessel* Involved
Inferior	II, III, AVF	RCA
Septal	V_1–V_2	LAD
Anterior	V_3–V_4	LAD
Anteroseptal	V_1–V_4	LAD
Extensive anterior	I, AVL, V_1–V_6	LAD
Lateral	I, AVL, V_5–V_6	CIRC
High lateral	I, AVL	CIRC
Posterior†	Prominent R in V_1	RCA or CIRC
Right ventricular‡	ST elevation, V_1 and, more specifically, V_4R in setting of inferior infarction	RCA

*This is a generalization; variations occur.
†Usually in association with inferior or lateral infarction.
‡Usually in association with inferior infarction.
CIRC = circumflex artery; LAD = left anterior descending coronary artery; RCA = right coronary artery.

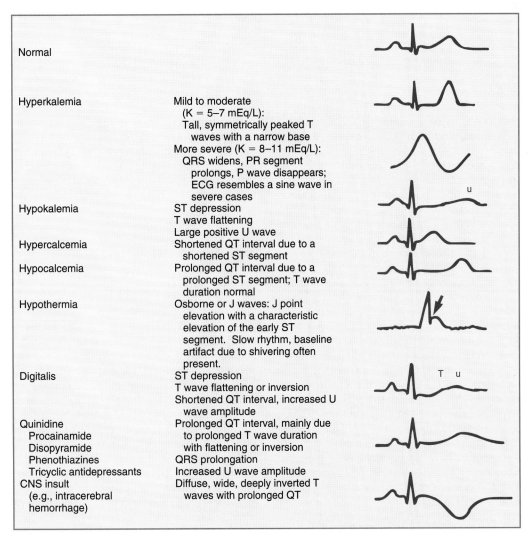

Normal	
Hyperkalemia	Mild to moderate (K = 5–7 mEq/L): Tall, symmetrically peaked T waves with a narrow base More severe (K = 8–11 mEq/L): QRS widens, PR segment prolongs, P wave disappears; ECG resembles a sine wave in severe cases
Hypokalemia	ST depression T wave flattening Large positive U wave
Hypercalcemia	Shortened QT interval due to a shortened ST segment
Hypocalcemia	Prolonged QT interval due to a prolonged ST segment; T wave duration normal
Hypothermia	Osborne or J waves: J point elevation with a characteristic elevation of the early ST segment. Slow rhythm, baseline artifact due to shivering often present.
Digitalis	ST depression T wave flattening or inversion Shortened QT interval, increased U wave amplitude

Quinidine
  Procainamide
  Disopyramide
  Phenothiazines
  Tricyclic antidepressants
	Prolonged QT interval, mainly due to prolonged T wave duration with flattening or inversion
	QRS prolongation
	Increased U wave amplitude

CNS insult (e.g., intracerebral hemorrhage)	Diffuse, wide, deeply inverted T waves with prolonged QT

FIGURE 5–6   Metabolic and drug influences on the electrocardiogram.

mand for oxygen by the working skeletal muscles that is met by an increase in heart rate and cardiac output. In patients with significant CAD, the increase in myocardial oxygen demand cannot be met by an increase in coronary blood flow. As a result, myocardial ischemia may occur, resulting in chest pain and characteristic ECG abnormalities. These changes combined with the hemodynamic response to exercise can give useful diagnostic and prognostic information in the cardiac patient.

The most frequent indications for stress testing include establishing a diagnosis of CAD in patients with chest pain, assessing prognosis and functional capacity in patients with chronic stable angina or after a myocardial infarction, evaluating exercise-induced arrhythmias, and assessing for ischemia after a revascularization procedure.

The most common form of stress testing uses continuous ECG monitoring while the patient walks on a treadmill. With each advancing stage, the speed and incline of the belt increases, thus increasing the amount of work the patient performs. Exercise testing may also be performed using a bicycle or arm ergometer. The stress test is deemed adequate if the patient achieves 85% of his or her maximal heart rate, which is equal to 220 minus the patient's age. Indications for stopping the test include achieving an adequate heart rate; developing worsening angina during exercise; or developing marked or widespread ischemic ECG changes, significant arrhythmias, or hypotension. The diagnostic accuracy of stress testing may be improved with adjunctive echocardiography or radionuclide imaging. Contraindications to stress testing include unstable angina, acute myocardial infarction, poorly controlled hypertension, severe aortic stenosis, and significant congestive heart failure.

The diagnostic accuracy of the exercise test is dependent on the pretest likelihood of CAD in a given patient and on the sensitivity and specificity of the test results in that patient population. Clinical features that are most useful at predicting important angiographic coronary disease before exercise testing include advanced age, male sex, and the presence of typical (vs. atypical) anginal chest pain. The accuracy of the exercise test is determined by the sensitivity, specificity, and predictive value, which are dependent on the population being studied and the ECG criteria used to define a positive test. The diagnostic accuracy of exercise testing is best in patients with an intermediate risk for CAD (30% to 70%) and when ischemic ECG changes are accompanied by chest pain during exercise. Exercise testing is least useful in diagnosing CAD in a patient with classic symptoms of angina because a positive test will not significantly increase the post-test probability of CAD, and a negative test would likely represent a false-negative result. Likewise, exercise testing in young patients with atypical chest pain may not be diagnostically useful given that an abnormal test result will likely represent a false-positive test and will not significantly increase the post-test probability of CAD.

The normal physiologic response to exercise is an increase in heart rate and systolic and diastolic blood pressures. The ECG will maintain normal T wave polarity, and the ST segment will remain unchanged or, if depressed, will have a rapid upstroke back to baseline. An ischemic ECG response to exercise is defined as (1) 1.5 mm of upsloping ST depression measured 0.08 second past the J point, (2) at least 1 mm of horizontal ST depression, or (3) 1.5 mm of downsloping ST segment depression measured at the J point. Given the large amount of artifact on the ECG that may occur with exercise, these changes must be present in at least three consecutive depolarizations. Other findings suggestive of more extensive CAD include early onset of ST depression (≤ 6 minutes); marked, downsloping ST depression (≥ 2 mm), especially if present in more than five leads; ST changes persisting into recovery for more than 5 minutes; and failure to increase systolic blood pressure to 120 mm Hg or more or a sustained decrease of 10 mm Hg or more below baseline.

The ECG is not diagnostically useful in the presence of left ventricular hypertrophy, left bundle branch block, Wolff-Parkinson-White syndrome, or chronic digoxin therapy. In these instances, nuclear or echocardiographic imaging may be helpful in demonstrating signs of ischemia. In patients unable to exercise, pharmacologic stress testing with myocardial imaging has been shown to have equal sensitivity and specificity for detecting CAD as exercise stress imaging. Intravenous dipyridamole is a coronary vasodilator that results in increased blood flow in normal arteries without significantly changing flow in diseased vessels. The resulting heterogeneity in blood flow can be detected by nuclear imaging techniques and the regions of myocardium supplied by diseased vessels identified. Another commonly used technique is dobutamine-stress echocardiography. Dobutamine is an inotropic agent that increases myocardial oxygen demand by increasing heart rate and contractility. The echocardiogram is used to monitor for ischemia, which is defined as new or worsening wall motion abnormalities during the infusion.

Echocardiography

Echocardiography is a widely used noninvasive technique in which sound waves are used to image cardiac structures and evaluate blood flow. Ultrasound waves are produced by a piezoelectric crystal housed in a transducer placed on the patient's chest wall. As the sound waves encounter structures with different acoustic properties, some of the ultrasound waves are reflected back to the transducer and recorded. Ultrasound waves emitted from a single, stationary crystal image a thin slice of the heart (M-mode), which can then be followed through time (Fig. 5–7). Two-dimensional imaging is created by steering the ultrasound beam across a 90-degree arc multiple times per second. This form of echocardiography is most commonly used to assess cardiac size, structure, and function.

Doppler echocardiography allows assessment of both direction and velocity of blood flow within the heart and great vessels. When ultrasound waves encounter moving red blood cells, the energy reflected back to the trans-

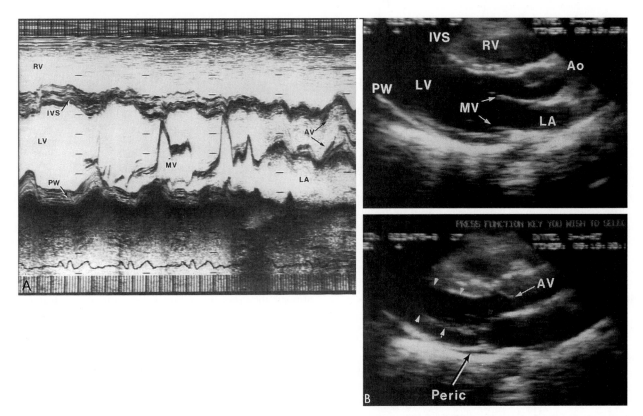

FIGURE 5-7 Portions of normal M-mode (*A*) and two-dimensional (*B*) echocardiograms. Ao = aorta; AV = aortic valve; IVS = interventricular septum; LA = left atrium; LV = left ventricle; MV = mitral valve; Peric = pericardium; PW = posterior LV wall; RV = right ventricle. The four white arrowheads in *B* indicate the left ventricular endocardium. (Courtesy of William F. Armstrong.)

ducer is altered. The magnitude of this change (Doppler shift) is represented as velocity on the echocardiographic display and can be used to determine if the blood flow is normal or abnormal (Fig. 5–8). In addition, the velocity of a particular jet of blood can be converted to pressure using the modified Bernoulli equation ($\Delta P \cong 4v^2$). This allows for the assessment of pressure gradients across valves or between chambers. Color Doppler imaging allows visualization of blood flow through the heart by assigning a color to the red blood cells based

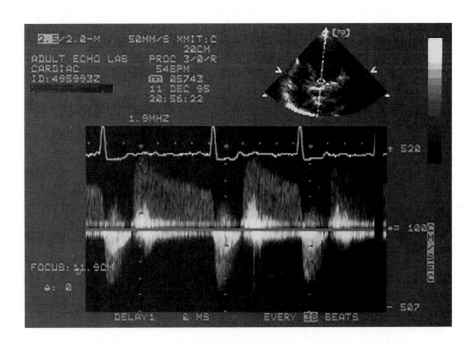

FIGURE 5-8 Doppler tracing in a patient with aortic stenosis and regurgitation. The velocity of systolic flow is related to the severity of obstruction.

on their velocity and direction. By convention, blood moving away from the transducer is represented in shades of blue and blood moving toward the transducer is represented in red. Color Doppler imaging is particularly useful in identifying valvular insufficiency and abnormal shunt flow between chambers.

Transesophageal echocardiography (TEE) allows two-dimensional and Doppler imaging of the heart through the esophagus by having the patient swallow a gastroscope with an ultrasound crystal at its tip. Given the close proximity of the esophagus to the heart, high-resolution images can be obtained, especially of the left atrium, mitral valve apparatus, and aorta. Transesophageal echocardiography is particularly useful in diagnosing aortic dissection, endocarditis, prosthetic valve dysfunction, and left atrial masses.

Nuclear Cardiology

Radionuclide imaging of the heart allows quantification of left ventricular size and systolic function, as well as myocardial perfusion. With radionuclide ventriculography, the patient's red blood cells are labeled with a small amount of a radioactive tracer (usually technetium 99m). Left ventricular function can then be assessed by one of two methods. With the first-pass technique, radiation emitted by the tagged red blood cells as they initially flow though the heart is detected by a gamma camera positioned over the patient's chest. With the gated equilibrium method, the tracer is allowed to achieve an equilibrium distribution throughout the blood pool before count acquisition begins. This second method improves the resolution of the ventriculogram. For both techniques, the gamma camera can be gated to the ECG, allowing for determination of the total emitted counts at end diastole (EDC) and end systole (ESC). Left ventricular ejection fraction (LVEF) can then be calculated as

$$LVEF = (EDC - ESC)/EDC.$$

If scintigraphic information is collected throughout the cardiac cycle, a computer-generated image of the heart can be displayed in a cinematic fashion, allowing for the assessment of wall motion.

Myocardial perfusion imaging is usually performed in conjunction with exercise or pharmacologic stress testing. Thallium 201 and technetium 99m sestamibi are the most frequently used radionuclides and are usually injected just before completion of the stress test. Planar or tomographic (single-photon emission computed tomography) images of the heart are obtained for visual qualitative analysis after stress and approximately 4 hours later (delayed images). In the normal heart, radioisotope is equally distributed throughout the myocardium. In patients with ischemia, a localized area of decreased uptake will occur after exercise but partially or completely fill in at rest (redistribution). A persistent defect at peak exercise and rest (fixed defect) is consist-

ent with myocardial infarction or scar. However, in some patients with fixed defects at 4 hours, repeat rest imaging at 24 hours or after reinjection of a smaller quantity of isotope will demonstrate improved uptake, indicating the presence of viable, but severely ischemic, myocardium.

Cardiac Catheterization

Cardiac catheterization is an invasive technique in which fluid-filled catheters are introduced percutaneously into the arterial and venous circulation. This allows for the direct measurement of intracardiac pressures and oxygen saturation and, with the injection of a contrast agent, visualization of the coronary arteries, cardiac chambers, and great vessels. Cardiac catheterization is generally indicated when a clinically suspected cardiac abnormality requires confirmation and its anatomic and physiologic importance needs to be quantified. Most often, catheterization will precede some type of beneficial intervention, such as coronary artery angioplasty, coronary bypass surgery, or valvular surgery. Although cardiac catheterization is generally safe (0.1% to 0.2% overall mortality rate), procedure-related complications such as vascular injury, renal failure, stroke, and myocardial infarction can occur.

An important objective during the cardiac catheterization is to document the filling pressures within the heart and great vessels. This is accomplished through use of fluid-filled catheters that transmit intracardiac pressures to a transducer that displays the pressure waveform on an oscilloscope. During a right-sided heart catheterization, pressures within the right atrium, right ventricle, and pulmonary artery are routinely measured in this manner. The catheter can then be advanced farther until it "wedges" in the distal pulmonary artery. The transmitted pressure measured in this location originates from the pulmonary venous system and is known as the pulmonary capillary wedge pressure. In the absence of pulmonary venous disease, the pulmonary capillary wedge pressure reflects left atrial pressure, and, similarly, if there is no significant mitral valve pathology, reflects left ventricular diastolic pressure. A more direct method of obtaining left ventricular filling pressures is to advance an arterial catheter into the left ventricular cavity. With these two methods of obtaining intracardiac pressures, each chamber of the heart can be assessed and the gradients across any of the valves determined (Fig. 5–9).

Cardiac output can be determined by one of two widely accepted methods: the Fick oxygen method and the indicator dilution technique. The basis of the Fick method is that total uptake or release of a substance by an organ is equal to the product of blood flow to that organ and the concentration difference of that substance between the arterial and venous circulation of that organ. If this method is applied to the lungs, the substance released into the blood is oxygen; and if no intrapulmonary shunts exist, pulmonary blood flow is equal

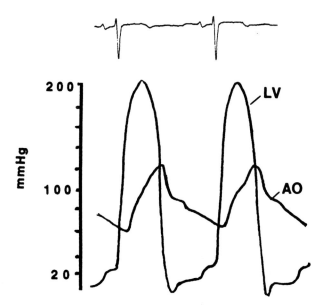

FIGURE 5-9   Electrocardiogram and left ventricular (LV) and aortic (AO) pressure curves in a patient with aortic stenosis. There is a pressure gradient across the aortic valve during systole.

to systemic blood flow or cardiac output. Thus, the cardiac output can be determined by the following equation:

$$\text{Cardiac output} = \text{O}_2\ \text{consumption}/(\text{arterial O}_2\ \text{content} - \text{venous O}_2\ \text{content}).$$

Oxygen consumption is measured in milliliters per minute by collecting the patient's expired air over a known period of time while simultaneously measuring oxygen saturation in a sample of arterial and mixed venous blood (arterial and venous O_2 content, respectively, measured in milliliters per liter). The cardiac output is expressed in liters per minute and then corrected for body surface area (cardiac index). The normal range of cardiac index is 2.6 to 4.2 L/min/m². Cardiac output can also be determined by the indicator dilution technique, which most commonly uses cold saline as the indicator. With this method, cold saline is injected into the blood and the resulting temperature change "downstream" is monitored. This generates a curve in which temperature change is plotted over time and the area under the curve represents cardiac output.

Detection and localization of intracardiac shunts can be performed by sequential measurement of oxygen saturation in the venous system, right side of the heart, and two main pulmonary arteries. In patients with left-to-right shunt flow, an increase in the oxygen saturation, or "step up," will occur as one samples from the chamber where arterial blood is mixing with venous blood. By using the Fick method for calculating blood flow in the pulmonary and systemic system, the shunt ratio can be calculated.

Left ventricular size, wall motion, and ejection fraction can be accurately assessed by injecting contrast into the left ventricle (left ventriculography). Aortic and mitral valve insufficiency can be qualitatively assessed during angiography by observing the reflux of contrast medium into the left ventricle and left atrium, respectively. The degree of valvular stenosis can be determined by measurement of pressure gradients across the valve and determination of cardiac output (Gorlin formula).

The coronary anatomy can be defined by injecting contrast medium into the coronary tree. Atherosclerotic lesions appear as narrowings of the internal diameter (lumen) of the vessel. A hemodynamically important stenosis is defined as 70% or more narrowing of the luminal diameter. However, the hemodynamic significance of a lesion can be underestimated by coronary angiography, particularly in settings where the atherosclerotic plaque is eccentric or elongated.

Biopsy of the ventricular endomyocardium can be performed during cardiac catheterization. With this technique, a bioptome is introduced into the venous system through the right internal jugular vein and guided into the right ventricle by fluoroscopy. Small samples of the endocardium are then sampled for histologic evaluation. The primary indication for endomyocardial biopsy is the diagnosis of rejection after cardiac transplantation.

Right-Sided Heart Catheterization

A right-sided heart catheterization can be performed at the bedside with a balloon-tipped, pulmonary artery (Swan-Ganz) catheter. This technique allows for serial measurements of right atrial, pulmonary artery, and pulmonary capillary wedge pressures, as well as cardiac output by thermodilution (Fig. 5–10). It is particularly useful in the critically ill patient for assessing volume status and differentiating cardiogenic from noncardiogenic pulmonary edema. In addition, the pulmonary artery catheter may be helpful in diagnosing certain cardiac conditions, such as pericardial tamponade, constrictive pericarditis, right ventricular infarction, and ventricular septal defect, and in monitoring the response to various treatments, such as diuretic therapy, inotropic agents, and vasopressors (Table 5–4).

Other Procedures

Computed tomography (CT) and magnetic resonance imaging (MRI) are new techniques that have greatly advanced our ability to diagnose cardiovascular disease noninvasively. Great vessel morphology and chamber size can be accurately assessed with both of these methods and, in contrast to echocardiography, are not limited by the presence of lung disease or chest wall deformity. These tests are most frequently used to diagnose aortic aneurysm and acute aortic dissection but are also sensitive methods for defining congenital abnormalities and detecting pericardial thickening associated with constric-

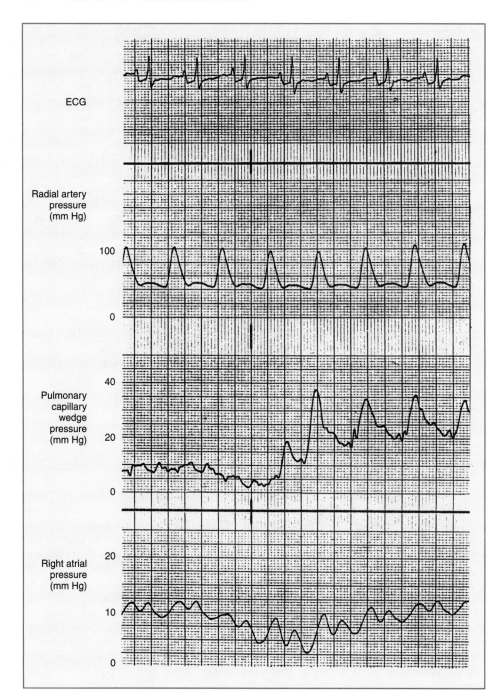

ECG

Radial artery pressure (mm Hg)

Pulmonary capillary wedge pressure (mm Hg)

Right atrial pressure (mm Hg)

FIGURE 5–10   Electrocardiogram (ECG) and Swan-Ganz flotation catheter recordings. The left portion of tracing three was obtained with the balloon inflated, yielding the pulmonary arterial wedge pressure. The left portion of tracing three was recorded with balloon deflated, depicting the pulmonary arterial pressure. In this patient, the pulmonary arterial wedge pressure (left ventricular filling pressure) is normal and the pulmonary artery pressure is elevated because of lung disease.

tive pericarditis. Ultrafast CT (contrast medium–enhanced electron beam CT) provides complete cardiac imaging in real time and is the most accurate noninvasive method for quantifying left ventricular volume and ejection fraction. However, given the radiation exposure, lack of machine portability, and expense, it is not routinely used in clinical practice for this purpose. Both ultrafast CT and MRI are able to visualize and quantitate the extent of coronary artery calcification, which has been shown to be a sensitive method for detecting the presence of significant CAD. Very recently, ultrafast CT has also been shown to be a useful method of assessing the extent of CAD. However, at the current time, coro-

nary angiography remains the gold standard for localizing and quantifying the severity of CAD.

Magnetic resonance angiography (MRA) is a noninvasive method of studying the vasculature, especially in patients who have contraindications to standard contrast angiography. This technique has become particularly popular in the evaluation of renovascular and lower extremity disease.

Positron emission tomography (PET) is a noninvasive method of detecting myocardial viability. In patients with left ventricular dysfunction, the presence of metabolic activity in a region of myocardium supplied by a severely stenotic coronary artery suggests viable tissue,

TABLE 5-4　Differential Diagnosis Using a Bedside Balloon Flow-Directed (Swan-Ganz) Catheter

Disease State	Thermodilution Cardiac Output	PCW Pressure	RA Pressure	Comments
Cardiogenic shock	↓	↑	nl or ↓	↑ Systemic vascular resistance
Septic shock (early)	↑	↓	↓	↑ Systemic vascular resistance; myocardial dysfunction can occur late
Volume overload	nl or ↑	↑	↑	
Volume depletion	↓	↓	↓	
Noncardiac pulmonary edema	nl	nl	nl	
Pulmonary heart disease	nl or ↓	nl	↑	↑ PA pressure
RV infarction	↓	↓ or nl	↑	
Pericardial tamponade	↓	nl or ↑	↑	Equalization of diastolic RA, RV, PA, and PCW pressure
Papillary muscle rupture	↓	↑	nl or ↑	Large v waves in PCW tracing
Ventricular septal rupture	↑	↑	nl or ↑	Artifact due to RA → PA sampling of thermodilution technique; O$_2$ saturation higher in PA than RA; may have large v waves in PCW tracing

nl = Normal; PA = pulmonary artery; PCW = pulmonary capillary wedge; RA = right atrium; RV = right ventricle; ↑ = increased; ↓ = decreased.

which may regain more normal function after revascularization.

Noninvasive Vascular Testing

Assessment for the presence and severity of peripheral vascular disease is an important component of the cardiovascular evaluation. One of the simplest tests to detect the presence of hemodynamically important arterial disease is measurement and comparison of the systolic blood pressure in the upper and lower extremities. Normally, the systolic pressure in the thigh is similar to that in the brachial artery. An ankle-to-brachial pressure ratio (ankle-brachial index) of less than or equal to 0.9 is abnormal. Patients with claudication usually have an index ranging from 0.5 to 0.8, and patients with rest pain have an index less than 0.5. In some patients, measurement of the ankle-brachial index after treadmill exercise may be helpful in identifying the importance of borderline lesions. Normally, exercise results in increased blood flow to the upper and lower extremities, owing to a decrease in peripheral vascular resistance, and the ankle-brachial index remains unchanged. If a hemodynamically important lesion is present, the increase in systolic blood pressure in the arm is not matched by an increase in blood pressure in the leg. As a result, the ankle-brachial index will decrease, the magnitude of which is proportional to the severity of the stenosis.

Once significant vascular disease in the extremities has been identified, plethysmography can be used to determine the location and severity of the disease. With this method a pneumatic cuff is positioned on the leg or thigh and, when inflated, temporarily obstucts venous return. Volume changes in the limb segment below the cuff are converted to a pressure waveform, which can then be analyzed. The degree of amplitude reduction in the pressure waveform corresponds to the severity of arterial disease at that level.

Doppler ultrasound uses reflected sound waves to identify and localize stenotic lesions in the peripheral arteries. This test is particularly useful in patients with severely calcified arteries where pneumatic compression is not possible and ankle-brachial indices are inaccurate. In combination with real-time imaging (duplex imaging), this technique is very useful in interrogating specific arterial segments and bypass grafts for stenotic or occlusive lesions.

REFERENCES

ACC/AHA Guidelines for Cardiac Catheterization and Cardiac Catheterization Laboratories. J Am Coll Cardiol 1991; 18:1149–1182.

Chou T: Electrocardiography in Clinical Practice, 2nd ed. Philadelphia: WB Saunders, 1986.

Ellestad M: Stress Testing—Principles and Practice, 3rd ed. Philadelphia: FA Davis, 1986.

Weyman A: Principles and Practice of Echocardiography, 2nd ed. Philadelphia: Lea & Febiger, 1994.

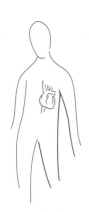

6

HEART FAILURE AND CARDIOMYOPATHY

Lisa A. Mendes • Joseph Loscalzo

Heart failure occurs when an abnormality of cardiac function fails to provide adequate blood flow to meet the metabolic needs of the body's tissues and organs. Heart failure can result from a large number of heterogeneous disorders (Table 6–1). One of the most common causes is idiopathic cardiomyopathy, which, strictly defined, is a primary myocardial disease of unknown etiology. However, in the clinical setting, the term *cardiomyopathy* may be used to refer to myocardial dysfunction that is the result of a known cardiac or systemic disease. These "secondary" cardiomyopathies may be related to a number of disorders, but in the United States they are most often the result of ischemic heart disease. Ventricular dysfunction can also result from excessive pressure overload, such as with long-standing hypertension or aortic stenosis, or volume overload, such as aortic insufficiency or mitral regurgitation. Diseases that result in infiltration and replacement of normal myocardial tissue, such as amyloidosis and hemochromatosis, can result in both abnormal ventricular filling as well as emptying. Diseases of the pericardium, such as chronic pericarditis or pericardial tamponade, can impair cardiac function without directly affecting the myocardial tissue. Long-standing tachyarrhythmias have been associated with myocardial dysfunction, especially in children. In addition, an individual with underlying myocardial or valvular disease will often develop heart failure with the acute onset of an arrhythmia. Finally, there are multiple metabolic abnormalities (thiamine deficiency, thyrotoxicosis), drugs (alcohol, doxorubicin), and toxic chemicals (lead, cobalt) that can impair cardiac performance.

Forms of Heart Failure

Heart failure can be classified as systolic or diastolic, high output or low output, left- or right-sided, and acute or chronic. Systolic heart failure refers to the inability of the heart to contract strongly enough to provide adequate blood flow to the periphery. This is the primary abnormality in idiopathic cardiomyopathy. Diastolic dysfunction occurs when there is abnormal relaxation of the myocardium, resulting in reduced filling of the ventricle, and is associated with such diseases as hypertrophic cardiomyopathy, cardiac amyloidosis, and sarcoidosis. High-output failure, which can occur with severe anemia or thyrotoxicosis, results when the heart is unable to meet the abnormally elevated metabolic demands of the peripheral tissues. Low-output failure is characterized by insufficient forward output both at rest and during times of increased metabolic demand. Cardiac dysfunction may predominantly affect the left ventricle, as with a large anterior myocardial infarction, or the right ventricle, as with an acute pulmonary embolus; however, in many disease states, both ventricles will be impaired (biventricular heart failure). Acute heart failure usually refers to the situation in which an individual who is completely asymptomatic before the onset of heart failure symptoms decompensates when there is an acute injury to the heart, such as myocardial infarction or rupture of a heart valve. Chronic heart failure refers to an individual whose symptoms have developed over a long period of time, often when there is preexisting cardiac disease. However, a patient with myocardial dysfunction from any cause may be well compensated for long periods of time and develop heart failure symptoms only after an acute insult, such as an arrhythmia or infection.

Adaptive Mechanisms in Heart Failure

A number of compensatory changes occur in the cardiovascular system to maintain adequate blood flow to the vital organs of the body. These include changes in left ventricular volume and pressure through the Frank-Star-

TABLE 6–1   Causes of Congestive Heart Failure and Cardiomyopathy

Idiopathic
Idiopathic dilated cardiomyopathy
Idiopathic restrictive cardiomyopathy
Idiopathic hypertrophic cardiomyopathy

Coronary Artery Disease
Acute ischemia
Left ventricular aneurysm
Ischemic cardiomyopathy

Pressure Overload
Hypertension
Aortic stenosis

Volume Overload
Mitral regurgitation
Aortic insufficiency

Toxins
Ethanol
Cocaine
Doxorubicin (Adriamycin)

Metabolic-Endocrine
Thiamine deficiency
Diabetes
Thyrotoxicosis

Infiltrative
Amyloidosis
Hemochromatosis

Inflammatory
Viral myocarditis

ling mechanism, ventricular remodeling, and neurohormonal activation.

In the normal heart, cardiac output can be augmented by increasing the stroke volume or heart rate. Stroke volume is dependent on the contractile state of the myocardium, left ventricular filling (preload), and resistance to left ventricular emptying (afterload). According to the Frank-Starling Law (Fig. 6–1), stroke volume can be increased with minimal elevation in left ventricular pressure as long as contractility is normal and there is no impedance to outflow. In the failing heart with depressed intrinsic contractility (see Fig. 6–1, curve A), small increases in stroke volume result in significantly higher left ventricular filling pressures. When left ventricular pressure approaches 20 mm Hg, pulmonary edema may occur. A similar relationship is seen with diastolic function. In this case, myocardial contractility may be normal but the "stiff" noncompliant ventricle impairs diastolic filling. As a result, small increases in left ventricular volume result in a marked increase in left ventricular filling pressure, which can lead to pulmonary congestion.

The failing heart may also undergo changes in left ventricular size, shape, and mass to maintain adequate forward flow. This process is known as remodeling and occurs in response to myocyte loss, such as after a myocardial infarction, or to hemodynamic overload, such as aortic or mitral valve insufficiency. The initial response is usually hypertrophy of the viable myocytes, primarily through an increase in cell length, and ventricular dilatation, which helps to maintain cardiac output and minimize wall stress. However, if the hypertrophy is inadequate to normalize wall stress, a vicious cycle is established. Overstretching of the myocytes can lead to an increase in myocyte death, ventricular dilatation, development of a spherical left ventricular cavity, and further elevation in wall stress.

The mechanical changes are triggered, in part, by activation of several neurohormonal systems. The renin-angiotensin-aldosterone system helps maintain cardiac output and tissue perfusion by stimulating arterial vasoconstriction through production of angiotensin II and expansion of intravascular volume by retaining sodium and water. In addition, release of vasopressin will also promote free water absorption by the kidney. The sympathetic nervous system helps maintain tissue perfusion by increasing arterial tone, as well as increasing heart rate and ventricular contractility.

However, activation of these systems is associated with several deleterious effects, including elevation in ventricular filling pressures, which may result in pulmonary and/or systemic edema, depression of cardiac function secondary to an increase in peripheral vascular resistance, and stimulation of myocardial hypertrophy and left ventricular remodeling. It is these maladaptive changes that are responsible for many of the signs and symptoms associated with congestive heart failure and that provide the rationale for treatment.

Evaluation and Treatment of Patients with Heart Failure

The history and physical examination are an integral part of the diagnosis of heart failure and in the determination of its underlying or precipitating cause. One of the cardinal manifestations of left ventricular heart failure is dyspnea, which is related to elevation in pulmonary venous pressure. In patients with chronic heart failure, shortness of breath initially occurs with exertion but may progress to occur at rest. Cardiac dyspnea is often worsened by the recumbent position (orthopnea) when increased venous return further elevates pulmonary venous pressure. Paroxysmal nocturnal dyspnea occurs after several hours of sleep and is probably due to central redistribution of edema. If heart failure is predominantly systolic with low cardiac output, the patient may complain primarily of fatigue due to diminished blood flow to the exercising muscles. In some instances, heart failure is slow to progress and the patient may unknowingly restrict his or her activities. Thus, the history should not only include an assessment of the patient's symptoms but also his or her level of activity (functional capacity). Many patients will complain of peripheral edema, usually involving the lower extremities, which commonly worsens during the day and decreases overnight with elevation of the legs. In patients with

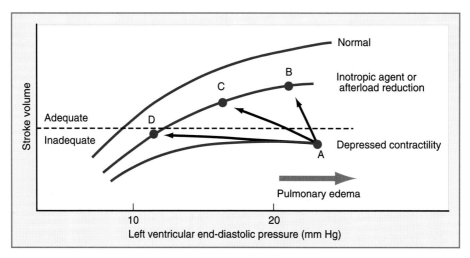

FIGURE 6–1 Normal and abnormal ventricular function curves. When the left ventricular end-diastolic pressure is greater than 20 mm Hg (A), pulmonary edema often occurs. The effect of diuresis or venodilatation is to move leftward along the same curve, with a resultant improvement in pulmonary congestion with minimal decrease in cardiac output. The stroke volume is poor at any point along this depressed contractility curve; thus, therapeutic maneuvers that would raise it more toward the normal curve would be necessary to improve cardiac output significantly. Unlike the effect of diuretics, that of digitalis or arterial vasodilator therapy in a patient with heart failure is to move the patient into another ventricular function curve intermediate between the normal and depressed curves. When the patient's ventricular function moves from A to B by the administration of one of these agents, the left ventricular end-diastolic pressure may also decrease because of improved cardiac function; further administration of diuretics or venodilators may shift the patient farther to the left along the same curve from B to C and eliminate the risk of pulmonary edema. A vasodilating agent that has both arteriolar and venous dilating properties (e.g., nitroprusside) would shift this patient directly from A to C. If this agent shifts the patient from A to D because of excessive venodilatation or administration of diuretics, the cardiac output may fall too low, even though the left ventricular end-diastolic pressure would be normal (10 mm Hg) for a normal heart. Thus, left ventricular end-diastolic pressures between 15 and 18 mm Hg are usually optimal in the failing heart, to maximize cardiac output but avoid pulmonary edema.

severe, long-standing heart failure, the edema can involve the thighs and abdomen and ascites may develop.

Many of the physical findings of heart failure are related to the neurohormonal changes that help compensate for the reduced cardiac output. An increased heart rate may be present as a result of increased sympathetic tone. The pulse pressure may be narrowed secondary to peripheral vasoconstriction. If left ventricular filling pressures are elevated, crackles may be heard on auscultation of the lung fields. Elevation in right-sided filling pressures will result in distended neck veins. If the liver is also congested, firm pressure applied to the right upper quadrant will cause the jugular veins to become further engorged (hepatojugular reflux). Palpation of the precordium may reveal left ventricular enlargement. A third heart sound or gallop is consistent with systolic dysfunction and can be generated from the left or right ventricle. A fourth heart sound suggests a noncompliant ventricle but is not specific for heart failure. The murmurs of both mitral and tricuspid regurgitation are common in patients with congestive heart failure and may become accentuated during an acute decompensation. As stated earlier, peripheral edema is a common finding on physical examination and may be related to elevation in venous pressure and/or increased sodium and water retention. In bedridden patients, the edema may predominantly be in the presacral region.

The electrocardiogram in patients with congestive

heart failure is not specific, but it may provide insight into the etiology of the cardiac dysfunction, such as prior myocardial infarction, left ventricular hypertrophy, or significant arrhythmias. The chest radiograph may show chamber enlargement and signs of pulmonary congestion (Fig. 6–2). Treatment of heart failure will result in improvement of the vascular congestion on the chest radiograph, but these changes may lag 24 to 48 hours behind clinical improvement. Certain blood chemistries may be altered in the patient with heart failure. The serum sodium concentration may be low, owing to increased water retention with activation of the renin-angiotensin system. Renal function may be impaired secondary to intrinsic kidney disease and/or reduced perfusion secondary to renal artery vasoconstriction and low cardiac output. Hepatic congestion is common with right-sided heart failure and may result in elevated liver enzyme levels.

Because many of the signs and symptoms of heart failure may also occur with pulmonary disease, differentiating between these two disease processes may be difficult. Initial therapy will often be directed at both potential pulmonary and cardiac causes until further testing can be performed. In addition, pulmonary edema may be secondary to noncardiac causes, such as severe infection, drug toxicity, or neurologic injury. This syndrome, termed *adult respiratory distress syndrome* (ARDS), can be differentiated from cardiogenic pulmo-

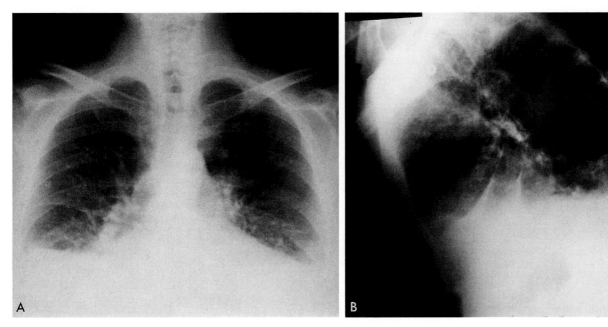

FIGURE 6–2 Posteroanterior chest radiographs showing cardiomegaly (*A*) and pulmonary vascular congestion typical of pulmonary edema (*B*).

nary edema by the presence of a low or normal pulmonary capillary wedge pressure.

Peripheral edema may also occur in disease states other than congestive heart failure. Renal disease, especially nephrotic syndrome, cirrhosis, and severe venous stasis disease, may be associated with peripheral edema.

Treatment

Treatment of congestive heart failure should be directed not only at relieving the patient's symptoms but also at treating the underlying or precipitating causes (Table 6–2). Patients should be educated about the importance of compliance with medical therapy, as well as dietary salt and fluid restriction. Rhythm disturbances, such as atrial fibrillation, may precipitate congestive heart failure and may require specific therapy. Treatment of active coronary artery disease or valvular disease may improve heart failure symptoms. In addition, correction of concomitant medical problems may help to stabilize heart function.

TABLE 6–2 Precipitants of Heart Failure

Dietary (sodium and fluid) indiscretion
Noncompliance with medications
Development of cardiac arrhythmia
Uncontrolled hypertension
Superimposed medical illness (pneumonia, renal dysfunction)
New cardiac abnormality (acute ischemia, acute valvular insufficiency)

NONPHARMACOLOGIC TREATMENT

All patients with heart failure should be instructed to restrict sodium intake to approximately 2 g/day. Fluid intake should also be limited to avoid hyponatremia. Weight reduction in the obese patient helps to reduce the workload of the failing heart. In addition, a supervised exercise cardiac rehabilitation program can help reduce heart failure symptoms and improve functional capacity in select patients.

PHARMACOLOGIC TREATMENT
Diuretics

Salt and water retention is common in congestive heart failure secondary to activation of the renin-angiotensin-aldosterone system. Diuretics help promote renal excretion of sodium and water and provide rapid relief of pulmonary congestion and peripheral edema. Loop diuretics, such as furosemide, are the preferred agents in the treatment of symptomatic heart failure. In patients refractory to high doses of these agents, diuretics that block sodium absorption at different sites within the nephron may be beneficial. Spironolactone may also provide unique benefit to some patients with heart failure.

It is important to note that diuretic therapy will lower intracardiac filling pressures and, thus, cardiac output through the Frank-Starling mechanism. In most patients, this change is well tolerated. However, in some patients, the reduced cardiac output will result in decreased renal perfusion and a rise in the blood urea nitrogen and creatinine level.

Vasodilators

A number of vasodilators have been shown to reverse the peripheral vasoconstriction that occurs in congestive heart failure. The most important group of vasodilator agents is the angiotensin-converting enzyme (ACE) inhibitors. These agents help improve heart failure symptoms, in part, by blocking production of angiotensin II and reducing afterload. In addition, ACE inhibitors have been shown to reduce mortality in patients with both symptomatic and asymptomatic left ventricular dysfunction. The major side effects of ACE inhibitors include hypotension, hyperkalemia, and azotemia. Cough may occur in approximately 10% of patients and is related to increased bradykinin levels associated with ACE inhibitor use.

Hydralazine in combination with oral nitrates has also been shown to reduce mortality in patients with symptomatic congestive heart failure, although not to the degree of ACE inhibitors. This combination provides an alternative to the patient who is ACE-inhibitor intolerant or may require additional therapy for blood pressure control.

A new class of agents, the angiotensin II receptor antagonists, prevent the binding of angiotensin II to its receptor. This has the theoretic advantage of blocking the effects of angiotensin II produced in the bloodstream, as well as at the tissue level. In addition, the angiotensin II receptor blockers do not interfere with bradykinin metabolism and, therefore, are not associated with cough. Several small studies comparing ACE inhibitors to angiotensin II blockers suggest that these two classes of agents may be equally effective in reducing morbidity and mortality in heart failure patients. However, until long-term studies are completed, angiotensin II receptor blockers should be reserved for those patients intolerant of ACE inhibitors or hydralazine and nitrates.

The negative inotropic effects of the calcium channel blockers and their activation of the sympathetic nervous system make these agents less attractive in the treatment of patients with congestive heart failure. In particular, several studies have shown worsening of heart failure symptoms in patients treated with nifedipine. Other calcium channel blockers, such as diltiazem, have been shown to improve symptoms and functional capacity without a deleterious effect on survival in patients with idiopathic dilated cardiomyopathy. Amlodipine has been studied in patients with both ischemic and nonischemic cardiomyopathy and also has not been associated with an increased cardiac morbidity and mortality. In addition, patients with nonischemic cardiomyopathy treated with amlodipine may have a modest survival benefit. Further studies with these agents are necessary before general recommendations regarding their use in heart failure patients can be made.

Inotropic Agents

This class of agents helps relieve heart failure symptoms by increasing ventricular contractility. The oldest and most commonly used agent in this class is digoxin, which has been associated with symptomatic improvement in heart failure in patients with systolic dysfunction. However, a recent trial found no significant improvement in survival among patients randomized to digoxin compared with patients treated with placebo.

There was a small reduction in death secondary to heart failure, but this was counterbalanced by a slight increase in death secondary to arrhythmias. In general, digoxin therapy should be considered in the patient with left ventricular systolic dysfunction who remains symptomatic after treatment with an ACE inhibitor and diuretic. There is no evidence that digoxin should be administered to the patient with asymptomatic left ventricular dysfunction. In addition, digoxin may be harmful in patients with infiltrative cardiomyopathies, such as amyloidosis.

Several other classes of oral inotropic agents have recently been evaluated for treatment of congestive heart failure, such as milrinone, vesnarinone, and xamoterol. All these agents have been associated with increased mortality with long-term use.

β Blockers

As previously discussed, many of the symptoms associated with heart failure are related to activation of several neurohormonal systems, including the sympathetic nervous system. Release of catecholamines may initially help to maintain blood pressure and cardiac output but, in the long term, increase cardiac work and may induce further myocardial injury. β-Blocker therapy may, therefore, be beneficial in patients with congestive heart failure by counteracting the chronic effects of sympathetic stimulation. In one study, the use of metoprolol in patients with dilated cardiomyopathy was associated with an improvement in heart failure symptoms and functional capacity. A new β blocker, carvedilol, has been shown to improve symptoms and reduce mortality in patients with reduced left ventricular function, especially those with mild-to-moderate functional impairment. This agent differs from other currently available β blockers in that it is also an antioxidant and α blocker, additional properties that may be beneficial in heart failure patients. Therapy with carvedilol should be considered in a patient who has been stabilized on ACE inhibitor, diuretic, and digoxin but who remains mildly to moderately impaired (New York Heart Association classes II to III).

Anticoagulation

Thrombosis and thromboemboli occur in patients with congestive heart failure secondary to stasis of blood, intracardiac thrombi, and atrial arrhythmias. Although long-term warfarin therapy remains controversial, certain patients may benefit from its use, including patients with chronic atrial fibrillation or flutter, patients with definite mural thrombi noted by echocardiography or ventriculography, and patients in sinus rhythm with left ventricular ejection fractions less than 20%.

Refractory Heart Failure

Despite adequate medical therapy, many patients with congestive heart failure will fail to have significant improvement in their symptoms. In these instances, therapy with intravenous inotropic agents for 24 to 96 hours, often with hemodynamic monitoring (Swan-Ganz catheter), may be necessary to stabilize the patient. One commonly used agent is dobutamine, which enhances contractility of the heart and reduces peripheral vasoconstriction through stimulation of β_2 receptors. Amrinone is an intravenous phosphodiesterase inhibitor that has similar effects on contractility and afterload. Administration of these agents will often promote diuresis, especially when given concomitantly with intravenous loop diuretics. If these agents do not produce a satisfactory response, dopamine given in doses ranging from 2 to 5 μg/kg/min may facilitate diuresis by stimulating renal dopaminergic receptors.

If heart failure is accompanied by hypotension, higher doses of dopamine may be necessary. With doses of more than 5 μg/kg/min, dopamine can increase heart rate and peripheral vascular resistance through stimulation of β_1 and α receptors. Although this dose range of dopamine may help to stabilize blood pressure, the increase in afterload may have further deleterious effects on the failing heart. In addition, dopamine may provoke arrhythmias that may lead to further hemodynamic instability. If hypotension persists despite dopamine doses greater than 15 μg/kg/min, mechanical assist devices, such as the intra-aortic balloon pump, should be considered as a means to stabilize the patient.

In patients who cannot be weaned from pharmacologic or mechanical support, or in ambulatory patients with severe functional impairment refractory to medical therapy, cardiac transplantation should be considered as a means to improve symptoms and prolong survival (see Chapter 12).

Cardiovascular Assist Devices

The most commonly used mechanical support device is the intra-aortic balloon pump. This device can be inserted percutaneously through the femoral artery and advanced into the descending thoracic aorta. Inflation of the balloon occurs during diastole such that perfusion pressure in the proximal aorta and coronary arteries is enhanced. Deflation, which occurs just before the onset of systole, greatly reduces aortic impedance and thus significantly reduces afterload. This device is particularly useful in stabilizing patients with severe coronary disease before percutaneous or surgical revascularization. In addition, this device may provide hemodynamic support in patients with severe mitral regurgitation or acquired ventricular septal defect before surgical repair. In patients with refractory congestive heart failure, the intra-aortic balloon pump may serve as a temporizing measure until cardiac transplantation can be performed.

In addition to the intra-aortic balloon pump, there are several short-term ventricular assist devices that provide hemodynamic support after coronary revascularization or in patients awaiting cardiac transplantation. These devices are placed percutaneously or through a sternotomy incision and can be used to support either ventricle. Blood is collected from the right or left atrium into an extracorporeal reservoir and then actively pumped back into the pulmonary or systemic circulation by the assist device. These units have been used to provide hemodynamic support for several days to weeks. A similar device, which is implantable, may be used for a longer period of time and allows the patient to ambulate.

Acute Pulmonary Edema

In patients with the acute onset of pulmonary edema, initial management should be directed at improving oxygenation and providing hemodynamic stability. Standard therapy includes supplemental oxygen and an intravenous loop diuretic. Sublingual or intravenous nitroglycerin helps reduce preload through venodilatation and may provide symptomatic relief in patients with ischemic as well as nonischemic ventricular dysfunction. Intravenous morphine acts in a similar manner but must be used with caution given its depressive effects on respiratory drive. In patients with severe hypertension or congestive heart failure related to aortic or mitral regurgitation, an arterial vasodilator, such as nitroprusside, may be helpful in reducing afterload.

Evaluation of the patient's response to treatment requires frequent assessment of blood pressure, heart rate, end-organ perfusion, and oxygen saturation. In patients with persistent hypoxia or respiratory acidosis, mechanical ventilation may be necessary for support. Pulmonary artery catheterization may be helpful in documenting filling pressures, cardiac output, and peripheral vascular resistance and in monitoring the response to therapy. In patients with refractory pulmonary edema, an inotropic agent or an intra-aortic balloon pump may be necessary.

Diastolic Dysfunction

Diastolic dysfunction occurs when there is abnormal relaxation of the left ventricle, which impairs filling and results in elevated left ventricular, left atrial, and pulmonary venous pressures. Diastolic filling abnormalities may contribute to heart failure symptoms in patients with reduced left ventricular function. However, up to one third of all cases of congestive heart failure are directly related to diastolic dysfunction with minimal impairment of left ventricular systolic function.

The causes of diastolic dysfunction include acute ischemia associated with coronary artery disease, chronic hypertension, and aortic stenosis, especially in the presence of left ventricular hypertrophy, and hypertrophic and infiltrative cardiomyopathies (Table 6–3). In addition, diastolic dysfunction may occur in the elderly and in diabetics, even in the absence of significant coronary artery disease or left ventricular hypertrophy.

The most common symptom associated with diastolic dysfunction is dyspnea on exertion. However, in some patients, symptoms may be abrupt in onset and are associated with acute pulmonary edema. The diagnosis of diastolic dysfunction can be made by echocardiography or radionuclide ventriculography by demonstrating

TABLE 6-3 Causes of Diastolic Dysfunction

Acute ischemia
Chronic hypertension
Severe aortic stenosis
Infiltrative cardiomyopathy (e.g., amyloid)
Hypertrophic cardiomyopathy

normal left ventricular systolic function in a patient with classic signs and symptoms of congestive heart failure. Echocardiography may also help identify possible causes, such as left ventricular hypertrophy, regional wall motion abnormalities suggestive of coronary disease, valve abnormalities, and infiltrative myocardial diseases.

Treatment of diastolic dysfunction should focus on identifying and correcting the underlying cause, such as ischemia or hypertension. Pharmacologic therapy with β blockers and calcium channel blockers may be helpful in this setting by slowing heart rate, thus increasing the time for ventricular filling, decreasing myocardial oxygen demand in patients with coronary artery disease, and lowering blood pressure. Patients with diastolic dysfunction are sensitive to changes in left ventricular filling

pressures. Therefore, diuretics and nitrates should be used with caution because the decrease in preload may result in reduced left ventricular filling, a decrease in cardiac output, and hypotension. New data suggest that ACE inhibitors may also be helpful by lowering systemic blood pressure and by improving myocardial relaxation. Inotropic agents, such as digoxin, are generally not helpful in the management of isolated diastolic dysfunction and, in some instances, such as cardiac amyloidosis, may be harmful.

REFERENCES

ACC/AHA Task Force: Guidelines for the evaluation and management of heart failure. Circulation 1995; 92:2764.

Bonow RO, Udelson JC: Left ventricular diastolic dysfunction as a cause of congestive heart failure: Mechanisms and management. Ann Intern Med 1992; 117:502.

Cohn JN, Johnson G, Ziesche S, et al: A comparison of enalapril with hydralazine-isosorbide dinitrate in the treatment of chronic congestive heart failure. N Engl J Med 1991; 325:303.

Digitalis Investigation Group: The effect of digoxin on mortality and morbidity in patients with heart failure. N Engl J Med 1997; 336:525.

Packer M, Bristow MR, Cohn JN, et al, for the US Carvedilol Heart Failure Study Group: The effect of carvedilol on morbidity and mortality in patients with chronic heart failure. N Engl J Med 1996; 334:1349.

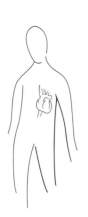

7

CONGENITAL HEART DISEASE

Lisa A. Mendes • Joseph Loscalzo

General Considerations

Congenital heart disease is defined as an abnormality of cardiac structure or function that is present at birth. Approximately 0.8% of all live births are complicated by congenital cardiac abnormalities not including bicuspid aortic valve and mitral valve prolapse (see Chapter 8), which are more prevalent, 2% and 5%, respectively. Congenital cardiac defects may result from genetic abnormalities, environmental factors, or a combination of both. The impact of the defect on cardiac function depends on the circulatory changes that result. Many abnormalities may be detected at birth as a result of the hemodynamic changes that occur during the transition from the fetal to neonatal circulation (patent ductus arteriosus [PDA], transposition of the great arteries). Other defects may not be apparent clinically until childhood or young adulthood, when the hemodynamic consequences of the lesion may become manifest (bicuspid aortic valve). Finally, some abnormalities may go undetected throughout life (small atrial septal defect [ASD]) or may resolve spontaneously (small muscular ventricular septal defect [VSD]). This chapter focuses on the most common congenital abnormalities detected in adults and includes lesions whose natural history permits long-term survival and on abnormalities in which surgical correction during infancy and childhood permits survival into adulthood.

Fetal and Transitional Circulations

Understanding the potential hemodynamic consequences of congenital heart disease requires a knowledge of the fetal circulation and the changes that occur after birth. During *fetal life,* gas exchange occurs across the placenta while the lungs receive minimal blood flow secondary to the high pulmonary vascular resistance. Oxygenated blood returning from the placenta bypasses the liver through the ductus venosus and enters the inferior vena cava. Blood in the inferior vena cava mixes with blood returning from the lower extremities and liver and then enters the right atrium, where it is shunted across the foramen ovale to the left atrium and left ventricle. Blood returning through the superior vena cava is directed into the right ventricle. Given the high pulmonary vascular resistance in utero, blood ejected from the right ventricle is shunted into the descending thoracic aorta through the ductus arteriosus. Blood ejected from the left ventricle supplies the head and upper extremities. Any remaining blood flows into the thoracic aorta, where it joins the large stream of blood from the ductus arteriosus and flows to the lower extremities and the placenta.

At *birth,* inflation of the lungs results in a dramatic fall in pulmonary vascular resistance. As a result, blood returning from the inferior and superior vena cava now flows into the right ventricle and is ejected into the pulmonary circulation. The increased volume of blood returning to the left atrium results in a rise in left atrial pressure and closure of the foramen ovale. The combination of increased arterial oxygenation and changes in local production of prostaglandins results in constriction of the ductus arteriosus. The ductus becomes functionally closed approximately 72 hours after birth and anatomically closed in 4 to 8 weeks.

Congenital Aortic Stenosis

Congenital left ventricular outflow obstruction may occur at the valvular, subvalvular, or supravalvular level. *Valvular stenosis* is most often secondary to a *bicuspid aortic valve,* which is present in approximately 2% of the population and occurs more frequently in males than in females. Associated cardiovascular abnormalities can occur in $\leq 20\%$ of affected persons and include coarctation of the aorta and PDA. Bicuspid aortic valves rarely cause significant obstruction during infancy and early childhood. However, their abnormal structure results in turbulent flow that leads to leaflet injury, thickening, calcification, and ultimately, narrowing of the orifice.

Although a few patients with bicuspid aortic stenosis remain asymptomatic throughout life, most affected persons develop symptoms during the fifth and sixth decades of life. As with acquired aortic stenosis, chest pain, syncope, and congestive heart failure are the most frequent presenting symptoms. Complications of bicuspid aortic valves include sudden death, which may occur during periods of rest or exertion, and infective endocarditis, which often leads to significant aortic regurgitation. In rare cases, aortic regurgitation is the predominant abnormality associated with a bicuspid aortic valve.

The physical examination of a patient with a stenotic bicuspid aortic valve is similar to that of patients with acquired aortic stenosis and is usually characterized by an ejection-quality murmur at the left sternal border (Table 7–1). If the leaflets are still pliable, an early systolic ejection click may be appreciated as the leaflets open. The murmur of aortic insufficiency may be present, especially if the patient has a history of endocarditis.

The diagnosis of bicuspid aortic valve and the degree of stenosis and/or regurgitation are usually made by two-dimensional and Doppler echocardiography. Treatment of patients with significant obstruction or insufficiency is outlined in Chapter 8. Children and young adults with significant stenosis may have improvement with percutaneous valvuloplasty, especially when calcification of the valve cusps is minimal. In older patients, or those patients with significant leaflet calcification, aortic valve replacement remains the treatment of choice.

Other causes of congenital left ventricular outflow tract obstruction are much less common. *Subaortic stenosis* is often first diagnosed in adulthood and is characterized by the presence of a discrete, fibrous diaphragm that encircles the left ventricular outflow tract between the mitral annulus and the basal interventricular septum. Patients with this defect have a characteristic outflow murmur but not the systolic ejection click appreciated in patients with bicuspid aortic valves. *Supravalvular stenosis* is a rare form of outflow obstruction and is characterized by variable degrees of ascending aortic root stricture. This abnormality is usually diagnosed in childhood and is associated with hypercalcemia and multiple skeletal, vascular, and developmental abnormalities.

Coarctation of the Aorta

Coarctation of the aorta is a fibrotic narrowing of the aortic lumen usually located distal to the left subclavian artery in the region of the ligamentum (ductus) arteriosus. The defect is more common in men than in women (2:1), and approximately 25% of patients have

TABLE 7–1 **Findings in Selected Uncomplicated Cardiac Defects**

Type	Physical Findings	Electrocardiogram	Chest Radiogram
Congenital aortic stenosis	Decreased carotid upstroke Sustained apical impulse Single S_2, S_4 Systolic ejection murmur	LV hypertrophy	Poststenotic aortic dilatation Prominent LV
Coarctation of aorta	Delayed femoral pulses Reduced blood pressure in the lower extremities Findings associated with bicuspid aortic valve	LV hypertrophy	Poststenotic aortic dilatation Prominent ascending aorta LV enlargement
Pulmonic valve stenosis	RV lift Pulmonic ejection sound Systolic ejection murmur at left sternal border RV S_4, widely split S_2, soft P_2	RV hypertrophy RA abnormality	Poststenotic dilatation of the main or left pulmonary artery RA and RV enlargement
Tetralogy of Fallot	Usually cyanotic Possible clubbing Prominent ejection murmur at left sternal border Soft or absent P_2	RV hypertrophy RA abnormality	Boot-shaped heart Small pulmonary artery Normal pulmonary vasculature
Ebstein's anomaly	Acyanotic or cyanotic Increased jugular venous pressure Prominent v wave Systolic murmur at sternal border, increases with inspiration	RA abnormality Right bundle branch block PR prolongation Ventricular preexcitation	Enlarged RA Normal pulmonary vasculature

LA = left atrium; LV = left ventricle; RA = right atrium; RV = right ventricle.

an associated bicuspid aortic valve. The most common extracardiac abnormality is an aneurysm of the circle of Willis.

Coarctation produces obstruction to left ventricular outflow and results in a rise in blood pressure in the proximal aorta and great vessels relative to the distal aorta and lower extremities. The development of left ventricular hypertrophy helps to maintain normal stroke volume in the presence of increased afterload. Most cases of coarctation remain undiagnosed until adulthood, when a work-up for secondary causes of hypertension may reveal the abnormality. If the condition is left untreated, more than two thirds of patients will develop left ventricular dysfunction and congestive heart failure by the fourth decade of life. Other complications include aortic dissection or rupture, stroke secondary to chronic hypertension or spontaneous rupture of cerebral aneurysms, and endocarditis that may involve the coarctation or an associated bicuspid aortic valve.

Clinically, most patients with coarctation have upper extremity hypertension with forceful carotid and upper extremity pulses (see Table 7–1). The pulses in the lower extremities are typically weak and delayed relative to the carotid upstroke. An ejection-quality murmur may be heard if a bicuspid aortic valve is present. A systolic murmur originating from the coarctation is typically heard over the left upper back. Older adults may have findings of heart failure.

In infants and children, the diagnosis of coarctation may be made by two-dimensional and Doppler echocardiography. However, in adults, magnetic resonance imaging and cardiac catheterization are the preferred methods for defining the location of the coarctation and the anatomy of the arch vessels. Surgical repair in adults is recommended at the time of diagnosis, although only approximately 50% of patients become normotensive after the procedure. Restenosis of the aorta may occur postoperatively, although in many instances this recurrent stenosis may be dilated with percutaneous techniques. Endocarditis prophylaxis is recommended for the rest of the patient's life regardless of prior repair.

Pulmonic Valve Stenosis

Pulmonic valve stenosis is the most common cause of obstruction to right ventricular outflow and usually occurs as an isolated congenital lesion. The pressure-overloaded state created by fusion of the pulmonary leaflets results in right ventricular hypertrophy. Some patients develop discrete hypertrophy of the infundibulum beneath the pulmonic valve, further contributing to outflow obstruction.

Unless the valve is severely stenotic at birth, most affected persons live a normal life until adolescence or young adulthood. The development of symptoms depends on the severity of the stenosis and right ventricular function. Patients with mild to moderate stenosis are usually asymptomatic and rarely have complications associated with the defect. Patients with moderate to severe obstruction often present with progressive fatigue

and dyspnea. If right ventricular dysfunction occurs, symptoms and signs of right-sided heart failure may be present.

On physical examination, the patient with severe stenosis has a right ventricular lift on palpation of the precordium (see Table 7–1). The S_1 sound is usually normal and is followed by an opening click that becomes louder with expiration. The P_2 sound becomes softer and delayed as the severity of the stenosis increases. The characteristic murmur of pulmonic stenosis is a systolic ejection murmur heard best at the left upper sternal border and increased with inspiration. As with aortic stenosis, a late peaking murmur indicates more severe stenosis. A prominent jugular venous *a* wave and right-sided S_4 sound may also be present in patients with severe obstruction to right ventricular outflow.

For patients with mild to moderate pulmonic stenosis, therapy is limited to endocarditis prophylaxis. Symptomatic patients with severe obstruction (peak gradient >50 mm Hg) require surgical repair of the valve that includes separation of the fused commissures and resection of the infundibulum if significant hypertrophy is present. Valve replacement is rarely necessary. In children and adults with isolated pulmonic stenosis, percutaneous balloon valvuloplasty is a suitable therapeutic option that offers results comparable to those achieved with surgery.

Tetralogy of Fallot

Tetralogy of Fallot is the most common cyanotic congenital heart lesion in adults and may present to the physician before or, more commonly, after corrective or palliative surgery (see Table 7–1). The tetralogy has four components, which include right ventricular outflow obstruction secondary to pulmonic valve or infundibular stenosis, membranous VSD, overriding aorta across the VSD, and right ventricular hypertrophy secondary to right ventricular outflow obstruction. The VSD is usually large and allows blood flow to be shunted from the right ventricle to the systemic circulation. The degree of right-to-left shunt flow depends on the degree of right ventricular outflow obstruction. If pulmonic stenosis is mild, right-to-left shunt flow is minimal, and the patient remains acyanotic (*pink tetralogy*). More commonly, the pulmonic stenosis is severe, and a large volume of poorly oxygenated blood is shunted into the systemic circulation, with resulting *cyanosis*. The degree of cyanosis is worsened with exercise, when the fall in systemic vascular resistance increases the degree of right-to-left shunt flow.

Complications of tetralogy include severe erythrocytosis, paradoxical emboli, bacterial endocarditis, and ventricular arrhythmias. Surgical correction of tetralogy is usually performed during infancy or childhood and involves relief of right ventricular obstruction and patch closure of the VSD. In patients surviving to adulthood, corrective surgery should still be undertaken, but the operative risk is higher secondary to the presence of right ventricular dysfunction. Palliative surgery involves the creation of a shunt between the systemic and pulmonary circulation (i.e., descending aorta to left pulmonary artery window). This procedure results in increased pulmonary blood flow and improved oxygenation of the systemic blood. Although such procedures often result in long-term palliation of hypoxia, several complications can occur. Patients may outgrow their shunts, or the shunts may spontaneously close and may lead to progressive cyanosis. If the shunt is too large, then the increased volume of blood into the pulmonary circulation and left heart may result in pulmonary congestion. If the condition is left uncorrected, irreversible pulmonary vascular obstruction may develop. Patients presenting with progressive cyanosis after palliative surgery must undergo cardiac catheterization before surgical repair to assess for irreversible pulmonary vascular obstruction. All patients with tetralogy, even if the condition has been surgically corrected, should receive endocarditis prophylaxis.

Atrial Septal Defect

ASD is one of the most common congenital defects in adults and occurs more frequently in women than men by a ratio of 3:1. Defects are classified according to their location within the interatrial septum. The most common ASD is the *ostium secundum defect* that involves the fossa ovalis and may be associated with mitral valve prolapse. *Ostium primum defects* involve the atrioventricular junction and are associated with mitral and tricuspid leaflet abnormalities and high VSDs. *Sinus venosus defects* are located in the superior septum and may be associated with partially anomalous pulmonary venous drainage into the superior vena cava or right atrium.

In patients with uncomplicated ASD (i.e., normal pulmonary vascular resistance), blood is shunted from the left to the right atrium, the magnitude of which depends on both the size of the defect and the compliance of the left and right ventricles. If the defect is small, increased blood flow to the right atrium is minimal, and no significant hemodynamic compromise of the right heart occurs. If the defect is large, the right atrium and right ventricle dilate to accommodate the increased volume of shunted blood (Fig. 7–1). Pressure in the pulmonary artery increases secondary to the increased volume of blood, but with the exception of extremely large, long-standing defects, pulmonary vascular resistance usually remains normal.

Most patients with ASD are asymptomatic until adulthood. When symptoms do develop, they are usually secondary to right ventricular dysfunction and include fatigue, dyspnea, and poor exercise tolerance. Older patients may decompensate when left ventricular filling pressures increase (which can occur with active ischemia or poorly controlled hypertension) and more blood is shunted from the left atrium to the already volume-overloaded right heart. *Atrial fibrillation* is a common rhythm disturbance in patients with ASD, especially pa-

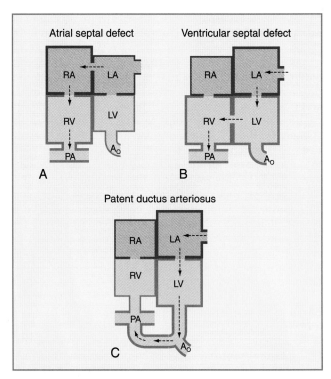

FIGURE 7–1 Diagram illustrating the three types of shunt lesions that commonly survive until adulthood and their effects on chamber size. *A*, Uncomplicated atrial septal defect (ASD) demonstrating left-to-right shunt flow across the interatrial septum and resulting in dilatation of the right atrium (RA), right ventricle (RV), and pulmonary artery (PA). *B*, Uncomplicated ventricular septal defect resulting in dilatation of the RV, left atrium (LA), and left ventricle (LV). *C*, Uncomplicated patent ductus arteriosus resulting in dilatation of the LA, LV, and PA. (Reprinted with permission from Liberthson RR, Waldman H: Congenital heart disease in the adult. *In* Kloner RA [ed]: The Guide to Cardiology, 3rd ed. Greenwich, CT: Le Jacq Communications, 1991, pp 24–47. Copyright 1991 by Le Jacq Communications, Inc.)

tients over 50 years of age. Irreversible pulmonary vascular obstruction with resultant right-to-left shunting and cyanosis (*Eisenmenger's complex*) is uncommon and occurs in fewer than 5% of patients with ASD.

On physical examination, a prominent right ventricular pulsation may be heard along the left sternal border secondary to a dilated, hyperdynamic right ventricle (Table 7–2). The S_2 sound is widely split and fixed because right ventricular volume overload results in a prolonged ejection period and delayed closure of the pulmonic valve. An ejection-quality murmur that increases with inspiration is commonly heard at the left sternal border and is secondary to increased blood flow across the pulmonic valve. If severe pulmonary vascular obstruction develops, the P_2 sound becomes loud, the splitting of S_2 narrows, and a right ventricular gallop may be heard.

The diagnosis of ASD is usually made with two-dimensional and color Doppler echocardiography. In particular, transesophageal imaging allows for excellent visualization of the interatrial septum, as well as associated congenital defects such as anomalous pulmonary veins, VSDs, and mitral leaflet abnormalities. Additional

TABLE 7–2 Findings in Uncomplicated Shunt Lesions

Type	Physical Findings	Electrocardiogram	Chest Radiograph
Atrial septal defect	Parasternal RV impulse Widely and fixed split S_2 Ejection murmur across pulmonic valve	Right bundle branch block Left axis deviation with ostium primum defect	Large pulmonary artery Increased pulmonary markings
Ventricular septal defect	Hyperdynamic precordium Holosystolic left parasternal murmur, ±thrill	LV and RV hypertrophy	Cardiomegaly Prominent pulmonary vasculature
Patent ductus arteriosus	Hyperdynamic apical impulse Continuous "machinery" murmur	LV hypertrophy	Prominent pulmonary artery Enlarged LA and LV

LA = left atrium; LV = left ventricle; RV = right ventricle.

information pertaining to right ventricular size and function and the degree of shunt flow can also be assessed with this technique. Cardiac catheterization is useful in older patients to confirm the severity of the defect, to assess pulmonary artery pressure and pulmonary vascular resistance, and to evaluate for concomitant coronary artery disease before surgical repair. Patients with pulmonary-to-systemic shunt ratios greater than 1.5 to 2 should undergo closure of the defect.

Surgical closure of the ASD remains the treatment of choice for patients with large defects. Ideally, the defect should be closed during childhood; however, repair of the defect in early adulthood usually leads to complete recovery of right ventricular size and function. After the fourth decade, symptoms are usually significantly improved after surgical repair. However, some degree of right ventricular dysfunction may persist. Percutaneous closure of secundum ASDs is under investigation. Complications, which have limited approval of this procedure, include embolization of the closure device to the venous or arterial system, thromboemboli, and atrial perforation.

Ventricular Septal Defect

VSD is a common congenital abnormality in newborns and is present in approximately 1 in 500 normal births. However, this defect is rarely encountered in adults because nearly 50% of VSDs close spontaneously during childhood, and most large defects are surgically corrected at an early age.

VSDs are classified according to their location within the interventricular septum. Most VSDs involve the membranous or muscular portion of the interventricular septum, and, if small, they often close spontaneously during childhood. In these patients, associated cardiac abnormalities are unusual. A less common type of VSD involves the atrioventricular canal and is often associated with ostium primum ASDs, as well as with mitral and tricuspid leaflet abnormalities. This type of VSD is common in patients with Down's syndrome. High (supracristal) membranous VSDs are located beneath the aortic annulus and often lead to aortic valve incompetence.

In patients with uncomplicated VSDs, oxygenated blood from the left ventricle is shunted across the defect into the right ventricle. If the defect is small, right ventricular size and function are normal, and pulmonary vascular resistance does not increase. If the defect is large, the right ventricle dilates to accommodate the increased volume, and pulmonary blood flow increases (see Fig. 7–1). If the condition is uncorrected, pulmonary vascular obstruction may develop and may lead to pulmonary artery hypertension, reversal of the interventricular shunt, and systemic desaturation and cyanosis (*Eisenmenger's syndrome*).

The clinical course of a patient with VSD depends on the size of the defect. Most small defects spontaneously close, or, if they are still present in adulthood, they are usually not associated with any significant hemodynamic complications. Large defects are usually detected and repaired during infancy. Affected individuals with uncorrected defects who survive to adulthood may present with signs and symptoms of right-sided heart failure. If pulmonary vascular obstruction with Eisenmenger's physiology develops, cyanosis and clubbing of the fingers may be present. All patients with VSD (or repaired VSD with residual shunt flow) are at risk of bacterial endocarditis that usually involves the right ventricular outflow tract.

On physical examination, the patient with an uncomplicated VSD has a hyperdynamic precordium and a palpable thrill along the left sternal border (see Table 7–2). The murmur is usually holosystolic and is best heard at the left sternal border. In general, small defects are associated with loud murmurs because of the significant pressure gradient between the left and the right ventricle. As pulmonary hypertension develops and left-to-right shunt flow decreases, the murmur may soften, and a loud P_2 sound may be present.

Two-dimensional and Doppler echocardiography are useful in diagnosing VSDs, as well as in assessing right ventricular size and function and associated cardiac abnormalities. Cardiac catheterization is often necessary before surgical repair to document the severity of shunt flow and to determine pulmonary artery pressure and pulmonary vascular resistance. Patients with Eisenmenger's physiology and net right-to-left shunt flow are not surgical candidates. Surgical closure of the VSD with sutures or a prosthetic patch is recommended for patients with left-to-right shunt flow greater than 2 to 1 without evidence of irreversible pulmonary hypertension.

Patent Ductus Arteriosus

The ductus arteriosus functionally closes several hours after birth and anatomically closes within 4 to 8 weeks thereafter. PDA is more common in infants who are premature or are born at high altitude. PDA is more common in women than in men, and it may be associated with other cardiac abnormalities such as coarctation and VSD.

Failure of the ductus arteriosus to close results in a persistent communication between the aorta and pulmonary artery. The hemodynamic consequences of this communication depend on the size of the ductus. If the defect is small, pulmonary artery resistance remains normal, and blood flows from the aorta to the pulmonary circulation. When the ductus is large, blood flow through the pulmonary circulation and returning to the left side of the heart is significantly increased, resulting in left ventricular volume overload and pulmonary congestion (see Fig. 7–1). Persistence of a large PDA may result in pulmonary vascular obstruction with Eisenmenger's physiology. When pulmonary vascular resistance exceeds systemic vascular resistance, shunt flow reverses from the pulmonary artery to the thoracic aorta. Such patients often have cyanosis of the lower extremities with clubbing of the toes, whereas the upper extremities are usually normal in color without evidence of clubbing of the fingers. This *differential cyanosis* is secondary to shunting of poorly oxygenated blood from the pulmonary artery to the aorta distal to the left subclavian artery, whereas well-oxygenated blood from the left ventricle is supplied to the head and upper limbs.

Most patients with small PDAs are asymptomatic and survive into adulthood without developing significant hemodynamic complications. If PDA is not corrected during childhood, many adults with a large ductus develop symptoms of left-sided heart failure. If pulmonary vascular obstruction should develop, Eisenmenger's physiology with right-sided heart failure may occur.

The characteristic physical examination finding of uncomplicated PDA is a loud, continuous, machinery-like murmur best heard in the left infraclavicular region (see Table 7–2). If the PDA is large, the left ventricle may be enlarged, and signs of pulmonary congestion may be present. If Eisenmenger's physiology complicates the course, signs of pulmonary hypertension may be present, and the ductus murmur may diminish in intensity.

The diagnosis of PDA is usually confirmed with two-dimensional and Doppler echocardiography. Cardiac catheterization is often performed before surgical closure to confirm the presence of the PDA and to exclude irreversible pulmonary vascular obstruction. Surgical closure of a PDA is indicated in most patients unless serious comorbid illness or irreversible pulmonary hypertension is present. All patients with known PDA should receive endocarditis prophylaxis.

Other Congenital Abnormalities

Several uncommon congenital abnormalities are compatible with survival into adulthood. *Ebstein's anomaly* is characterized by apical displacement of the tricuspid valve into the right ventricle. As a result, the basal portion of the right ventricle forms part of the right atrium and leaves a small functional right ventricle. The tricuspid leaflets are often dysplastic, and the leaflets may partially adhere to the interventricular septum or right ventricular free wall, often with significant tricuspid regurgitation. The degree of right ventricular dysfunction depends on the size of the "functioning" right ventricle and the severity of the tricuspid regurgitation. A patent foramen ovale or ostium secundum ASD is present in >50% of patients and may result in right-to-left shunt flow as right atrial pressure increases. Supraventricular arrhythmias are common in Ebstein's anomaly, as is ventricular preexcitation associated with Wolff-Parkinson-White syndrome.

Inversion of the ventricles and abnormal positioning of the great arteries characterize congenitally corrected *transposition of the great arteries (L-transposition)*. In this anomaly, the anatomic right ventricle lies on the left and receives oxygenated blood from the left atrium. Blood is ejected into an anteriorly displaced aorta. The anatomic left ventricle lies on the right and receives venous blood from the right atrium and ejects it into the posteriorly displaced pulmonary artery. The clinical course of patients with corrected transposition depends on the severity of other intracardiac anomalies. When the abnormality is an isolated lesion, many persons survive into adulthood without symptoms. In some persons, the systemic ventricle (anatomic right ventricle) may fail, and pulmonary congestion may result. Associated anomalies include atrioventricular nodal block, VSD, and Ebstein's anomaly.

Congenital anomalies of the coronary arteries are not uncommon and may be asymptomatic or associated with myocardial ischemia. The left circumflex or left anterior descending artery may arise from the right sinus of Valsalva and is usually not associated with abnormalities of myocardial perfusion. Either coronary artery may arise from the right sinus and may pass between the pulmonary trunk and the aorta. This abnormality may result in myocardial ischemia, infarction, or sudden death in young adults, especially during exertion. *Coronary artery fistulas* with drainage into the right ventricle, vena cava, or pulmonary vein may be associated with myocardial ischemia if a significant amount of coronary blood flow is shunted into the venous system. Diagnosis of these abnormalities is made by coronary angiography.

REFERENCES

Liberthson RR: Congenital Heart Disease Diagnosis and Management in Children and Adults. Boston: Little, Brown, 1989.
Perloff JK, Child JS: Congenital Heart Disease in Adults. Philadelphia: WB Saunders, 1991.

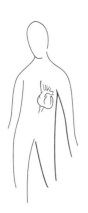

8

ACQUIRED VALVULAR HEART DISEASE

Lisa A. Mendes • Joseph Loscalzo

Aortic Stenosis

Aortic stenosis can be congenital or acquired in origin (Table 8–1). The most common congenital abnormality is the bicuspid aortic valve. Significant narrowing of the orifice usually occurs during middle age after years of turbulent flow through the valve results in leaflet injury, thickening, and calcification. Rheumatic aortic stenosis results from fusion of the leaflet commissures and is usually associated with mitral valve disease. The most common cause of aortic stenosis in adults is degenerative or senile aortic stenosis, which usually occurs in patients older than the age of 65. Aortic stenosis is more common in men than women.

In patients with aortic stenosis, the outflow obstruction gradually increases over many years, resulting in left ventricular hypertrophy. This response allows the left ventricle to generate and maintain a large pressure gradient across the valve without a reduction in stroke volume. However, left ventricular hypertrophy results in increased diastolic wall stiffness such that greater intracavitary pressure is required to maintain left ventricular filling.

Patients with severe aortic stenosis may be asymptomatic for many years despite the presence of severe obstruction. The cardinal symptoms associated with aortic stenosis are angina, syncope, and congestive heart failure. Angina can occur in the absence of epicardial coronary artery disease because of the increased oxygen demand of the hypertrophied ventricle and decreased coronary blood flow secondary to elevated left ventricular diastolic pressure. Syncope may result from transient arrhythmias but more commonly occurs with exertion when the cardiac output is insufficient to maintain arterial pressure in the presence of exercise-induced peripheral vasodilation. Dyspnea may result from diastolic dysfunction associated with the noncompliant, hypertrophied left ventricle or may signal the onset of systolic dysfunction that may develop late in the course of this disease. Once patients with severe aortic stenosis develop symptoms, the prognosis is poor unless surgical correction is undertaken. Previous studies have shown that the mean survival after the onset of symptoms is approximately 2 years in patients with heart failure, 3 years in patients with syncope, and 5 years in patients with angina (Fig. 8–1).

On physical examination, the patient with aortic stenosis may have a laterally displaced, sustained apical impulse secondary to left ventricular hypertrophy (Table 8–2). A palpable S_4 may also be present if the patient is in sinus rhythm. The A_2 component of S_2 may be soft or absent owing to decreased mobility of the aortic cusps. The presence of an S_4 is indicative of a noncompliant left ventricle. The murmur of aortic stenosis is a harsh, crescendo-decrescendo murmur that is best heard over the right sternal border and often radiates to the neck. As the obstruction increases, the "peak" of the murmur occurs later in systole. If left ventricular dysfunction develops, the murmur may decrease in intensity secondary to a reduction in stroke volume. The carotid impulse is often diminished in intensity and delayed (pulsus parvus et tardus) (Fig. 8–2), although in the elderly these changes may be present secondary to intrinsic vascular disease in the absence of significant aortic stenosis.

The principal electrocardiographic finding in aortic stenosis is left ventricular hypertrophy. Echocardiography is useful both to determine the etiology of the aortic stenosis and to quantitate the degree of obstruction. By using Doppler techniques, the mean gradient and valve area can be estimated. Patients with severe stenosis will usually undergo cardiac catheterization both to confirm the presence of severe aortic stenosis and to determine if concomitant coronary artery disease is present. A valve area less than or equal to 0.7 cm² defines critical aortic stenosis (normal valve area 3 cm²) and is usually associated with a mean transvalvular gradient of more than 50 mm Hg when normal left ventricular function is present. One should note that in patients with reduced systolic function, the mean gradi-

TABLE 8-1 Major Causes of Valvular Heart Disease in Adults

Aortic Stenosis
Bicuspid aortic valve
Rheumatic
Degenerative

Aortic Regurgitation
Bicuspid aortic valve
Endocarditis
Rheumatic
Aortic root dilatation

Mitral Stenosis
Rheumatic

Mitral Regurgitation
Chronic
Mitral valve prolapse
Left ventricular dilatation
Rheumatic
Endocarditis

Acute
Papillary muscle dysfunction (ischemia)
Papillary muscle or chordal rupture
Endocarditis
Prosthetic valve dysfunction

Tricuspid Regurgitation
Functional (annular dilatation)
Tricuspid valve prolapse
Endocarditis

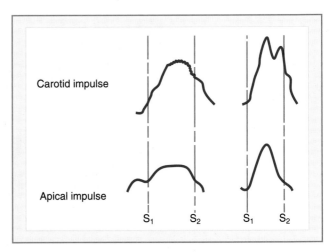

FIGURE 8-2 Diagrammatic depiction of carotid and apical impulses with aortic stenosis *(left panel)* and aortic regurgitation *(right panel)*. (See text for more information.)

can result in significant clinical and hemodynamic improvement. Balloon aortic valvuloplasty is a percutaneous technique in which a balloon catheter is positioned across the aortic valve. Inflation results in fracture and/or separation of the fused and calcified cusps. This procedure is most effective in young patients with noncalcified congenital aortic stenosis and is rarely used in adult patients with calcific aortic stenosis, owing to the high restenosis rate (~30% at 6 months).

ent may be low despite the presence of severe aortic stenosis.

Treatment in most adults with symptomatic aortic stenosis is surgical replacement of the valve. The operative risk and prognosis are best in patients with preserved left ventricular systolic function. However, surgery should still be considered in patients with left ventricular dysfunction because relief of the obstruction

Aortic Regurgitation

Aortic regurgitation (AR) may be secondary to primary disease of the aortic leaflets, the aortic root, or both (see Table 8–1). Abnormalities of the aortic leaflets may be secondary to rheumatic disease, congenital abnormalities, or prior endocarditis. In addition, AR is commonly a consequence of degenerative and bicuspid aortic stenosis. Aortic root pathology associated with annular and root dilatation may result in separation and/or prolapse of the leaflets.

With chronic AR, the left ventricle must accommodate the normal inflow from the left atrium in addition to the aortic regurgitant volume. As a result, the left ventricle dilates and hypertrophies to maintain normal effective forward flow and minimize wall stress. As the AR progresses, these changes in left ventricular size and wall thickness may be insufficient to maintain normal left ventricular filling pressures, and irreversible myocyte damage may occur. As a result, the left ventricle will dilate further and systolic function and effective stroke volume will decrease.

Clinically, patients with chronic, severe AR may be asymptomatic for long periods of time secondary to the compensatory changes in the left ventricle. When symptoms do develop, they are primarily related to an elevation in left ventricular filling pressures and include dyspnea on exertion, orthopnea, and paroxysmal nocturnal

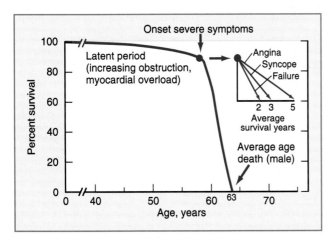

FIGURE 8-1 Natural history of aortic stenosis without surgical therapy. (Reproduced with permission from Ross J Jr, Braunwald E: Aortic stenosis. Circulation 1968; 38[Suppl V]:61. Copyright 1968, American Heart Association.)

TABLE 8-2 **Characteristic Physical, ECG, and Chest Radiographic Findings in Chronic Acquired Valvular Heart Disease**

	Physical Findings*	ECG	Radiograph
Aortic stenosis	Pulsus parvus et tardus (may be absent in older patients or with associated aortic regurgitation); carotid "shudder" (coarse thrill) Ejection murmur radiates to base of neck; peak late in systole if stenosis severe Sustained but not markedly displaced LV impulse A_2 decreased, S_2 single or paradoxically split S_4 gallop, often palpable	LV hypertrophy; left bundle branch block also common Rare heart block from calcific involvement of conduction system	LV prominence without dilation Poststenotic aortic root dilation Aortic valve calcification
Aortic regurgitation	Increased pulse pressure Bifid carotid pulses Rapid pulse upstroke and collapse LV impulse hyperdynamic and displaced laterally Diastolic decrescendo murmur; duration related to severity Systolic flow murmur S_3G common	LV hypertrophy, often with narrow deep Q waves	LV and aortic dilation
Mitral stenosis	Loud S_1 Opening snap (OS) (S_2-OS interval inversely related to stenosis severity) S_1 not loud, and OS absent if valve heavily calcified Signs of pulmonary arterial hypertension	Left atrial abnormality Atrial fibrillation common RV hypertrophy pattern may develop if associated pulmonary arterial hypertension	Large LA: double-density, posterior displacement of esophagus, elevation of left mainstem bronchus Straightening of left heart border due to enlarged left appendage Small or normal size LV Large pulmonary artery Pulmonary venous congestion
Mitral regurgitation	Hyperdynamic LV impulse S_3 Widely split S_2 may occur Holosystolic apical murmur radiating to axilla (murmur may be atypical with acute mitral regurgitation, papillary muscle dysfunction, or mitral valve prolapse—see text)	Left atrial abnormality LV hypertrophy Atrial fibrillation	Enlarged LA and LV Pulmonary venous congestion
Mitral valve prolapse	One or more systolic clicks—often midsystolic—followed by late systolic murmur Auscultatory findings dynamic—see text Patients may exhibit tall thin habitus, pectus excavatum, straight back syndrome	Often normal Occasionally ST segment depression and/or T wave changes in inferior leads	Depends on degree of valve regurgitation and presence or absence of those abnormalities
Tricuspid stenosis	Jugular venous distention with prominent a wave if sinus rhythm Tricuspid OS and diastolic rumble at left sternal border—may be overshadowed by concomitant mitral stenosis Tricuspid OS and rumble increased during inspiration	Right atrial abnormality Atrial fibrillation common	Large RA
Tricuspid regurgitation	Jugular venous distention with large regurgitant (systolic) wave Systolic murmur at left sternal border, increased with inspiration Diastolic flow rumble RV S_3 increased with inspiration Hepatomegaly with systolic pulsation	RA abnormality Findings often related to cause of the tricuspid regurgitation	RA and RV enlarged Findings often related to cause of the tricuspid regurgitation

* Findings are influenced by the severity and chronicity of the valve disorder.
ECG = electrocardiogram; LA = left atrium; LV = left ventricle; RA = right atrium; RV = right ventricle.

dyspnea. Many patients will describe chest or head pounding secondary to the hyperdynamic circulation. If effective cardiac output is reduced, the patient may complain primarily of fatigue and weakness. As with aortic stenosis, angina may occur in patients with AR even in the absence of epicardial coronary artery disease secondary to elevated left ventricular filling pressures and reduced coronary perfusion pressure.

On physical examination, patients with severe AR have a widened pulse pressure (difference between the systolic and diastolic pressures), owing to runoff of blood back into the left ventricle (see Table 8–2). The pulse is usually bounding with a rapid upstroke and quick collapse (Corrigan's or water-hammer pulse) (see Fig. 8–2). The cardiac impulse is hyperdynamic and displaced laterally and inferiorly. The murmur of AR is a high-pitched, decrescendo diastolic murmur best heard at the left sternal border with the patient sitting up and leaning forward. Asking the patient to hold his or her breath at end-expiration while the hands are held behind the head may also improve the ability to auscultate the murmur of AR. A systolic ejection murmur is often heard secondary to increased forward flow across the aortic valve. An S_3 gallop may be present, especially if the patient has developed heart failure symptoms. A low-pitched, diastolic murmur (Austin Flint murmur) may be heard at the apex and confused with the murmur of mitral stenosis. This sound is thought to be secondary to the incomplete opening of the mitral leaflets (functional mitral stenosis) secondary to elevated left ventricular filling pressures.

The natural history of chronic AR is variable. Many patients with moderate to severe AR will remain asymptomatic for many years and generally have a favorable prognosis. Other patients may have progression of AR severity and develop left ventricular dysfunction and congestive heart failure symptoms. Echocardiography is a useful tool to follow the progression of disease and optimize the timing of surgery. Prior studies have shown that patients at high risk are those with left ventricular end-systolic diameters greater than 50 mm or an ejection fraction less than 50%. Therefore, patient with known moderate to severe AR should be monitored regularly with noninvasive testing to detect early signs of cardiac (i.e., left ventricular) decompensation.

Treatment of patients with moderate to severe AR should include vasodilator therapy, such as nifedipine or angiotensin-converting enzyme (ACE) inhibitors, because these agents unload the left ventricle and may slow the progression of myocardial dysfunction. Prior studies suggest that the greatest benefit with these agents is noted in symptomatic patients with significant left ventricular enlargement (left ventricular end-diastolic diameter >65 mm). However, vasodilator therapy in asymptomatic patients with moderate to severe AR may prolong the asymptomatic period.

Valve replacement surgery should be considered in symptomatic patients or those with evidence of left ventricular dysfunction. In patients with reduced left ventricular ejection fraction of short duration (<14 months), valve replacement usually results in significant improvement in ventricular function. If left ventricular dysfunction has been present for a prolonged period of time, permanent myocardial damage may occur. Although such patients should not be excluded from surgery, their long-term prognosis remains poor.

As compared with chronic AR, acute AR is a medical emergency that often requires immediate surgical intervention. The causes of acute AR include infective endocarditis, traumatic rupture of the aortic leaflets, aortic root dissection, and acute dysfunction of a prosthetic valve. Acute AR results in hemodynamic instability because the left ventricle is unable to dilate to accommodate the increased diastolic volume, resulting in decreased effective forward flow. Left ventricular and left atrial pressures rise quickly, leading to pulmonary congestion.

Patients with acute AR often present with symptoms and signs of cardiogenic shock. The patient is usually pale with cool extremities, owing to peripheral vasoconstriction. The pulse is weak and rapid, and the pulse pressure is normal or decreased. The murmur of acute AR is low pitched and short, owing to rapid equilibration of aortic and left ventricular pressures during diastole. An S_3 gallop is often present. Echocardiography is useful to assess AR severity and determine its etiology and can be performed at the bedside quickly in an acutely ill patient.

The medical treatment of acute AR includes vasodilator therapy and diuretics if the blood pressure is stable. In hemodynamically compromised patients, inotropic support and vasopressors may be necessary. For most patients with acute AR, urgent valve replacement remains the treatment of choice.

Mitral Stenosis

Mitral stenosis (MS) occurs when thickening and immobility of the mitral leaflets impede flow from the left atrium to the left ventricle. The most common cause of MS is rheumatic fever, although rarely, congenital abnormalities, carcinoid disease, and connective tissue disorders may lead to obstruction of the mitral valve. Two thirds of patients with MS are women. The pathologic changes that occur with rheumatic MS include fusion of the leaflet commissures, and thickening, fibrosis, and calcification of the mitral leaflets and chordae. These changes occur over many years before dysfunction becomes hemodynamically important.

The initial hemodynamic change that occurs with MS is elevation in left atrial pressure created by obstruction to left ventricular inflow (Fig. 8–3). This pressure change is transmitted back to the pulmonary venous system and may result in pulmonary congestion. Initially, this change may only occur at more rapid heart rates, such as with exercise or atrial arrhythmias, when higher left atrial pressures develop during the shortened diastolic period. As the MS becomes more severe, left atrial pressure remains elevated even at normal heart rates, and symptoms related to elevated pulmonary venous pressures may be present at rest. Chronic elevations in pulmonary venous pressures may lead to an

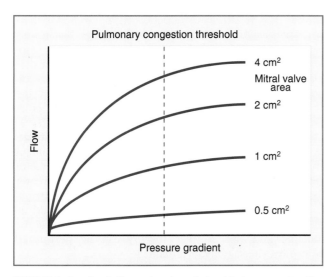

FIGURE 8–3 Graph illustrating the relationship between the diastolic gradient across the mitral valve and flow through the mitral valve. As the mitral valve becomes more stenotic, the pressure gradient across the mitral valve must increase to maintain flow into the left ventricle. When the mitral valve area is 1.0 cm² or less, the flow rate into the left ventricle cannot be significantly increased despite a markedly elevated pressure gradient across the mitral valve. (Adapted from Wallace AG: Pathophysiology of cardiovascular disease. *In* Smith LH Jr, Thier SO [eds]: Pathophysiology: The Biological Principles of Disease. The International Textbook of Medicine, vol 1. Philadelphia, WB Saunders, 1981, p 1192.)

Labels on figure: Pulmonary congestion threshold; Flow; Pressure gradient; Mitral valve area; 4 cm²; 2 cm²; 1 cm²; 0.5 cm²

increase in pulmonary vascular resistance and pulmonary arterial pressures. If the MS is not corrected, irreversible changes in the pulmonary vasculature may occur, and signs and symptoms of right-sided heart failure may develop. In contrast, left ventricular filling pressures are usually normal or low with mild to moderate MS. As the stenosis becomes severe, filling of the left ventricle is impaired and stroke volume and cardiac output are reduced.

Patients with MS of rheumatic etiology usually become symptomatic during the third or fourth decades of life. Dyspnea and orthopnea are the most common presenting symptoms, although some patients may have sudden hemoptysis secondary to rupture of the dilated bronchial veins (pulmonary apoplexy) or blood-tinged sputum associated with pulmonary edema. Peripheral embolism from left atrial thrombus may also occur even in the absence of atrial fibrillation. In long-standing, severe MS, patients may develop peripheral edema secondary to elevated right-sided pressures and right ventricular dysfunction. Compression of the left recurrent laryngeal nerve by a severely dilated left atrium may result in hoarseness (Ortner's syndrome).

On physical examination, S_1 is loud early in the course of mitral stenosis because leaflets remain fully open throughout diastole and then quickly close (see Table 8–2). As the leaflets become more calcified and immobile, S_1 will become softer or completely absent. The opening snap is a high-pitched sound following the S_2 and reflects the abrupt mitral valve opening. As the MS becomes more severe, the interval between the S_2

and opening snap becomes shorter because left atrial pressure exceeds left ventricular pressure earlier in diastole. The characteristic low-pitched rumbling murmur of mitral stenosis is best heard at the left ventricular apex with the patient in the left lateral decubitus position. The murmur is loudest in early diastole when rapid ventricular filling occurs. If sinus rhythm is present, the murmur may increase in intensity after atrial contraction (presystolic accentuation). In some patients, the murmur may only be heard at times of increased blood flow through the mitral valve, such as after exercise. If pulmonary artery pressures are elevated, a palpable P_2 may be detected at the upper left sternal border. On auscultation, the pulmonic component of S_2 is prominent and a right-sided gallop may be present.

Echocardiography is a useful tool to assess the pathology of the mitral apparatus as well as the severity of the stenosis. The characteristic rheumatic deformity observed with two-dimensional imaging is doming of the anterior mitral valve leaflet, which is secondary to fusion of the commissures. In addition, the mobility of the leaflets and the extent of valvular calcification can be assessed and used to determine treatment options. Doppler techniques allow calculation of the mitral valve area and the transvalvular gradient. More recently, transesophageal echocardiography has become a useful tool for studying the mitral apparatus and examining the left atrium for thrombus before percutaneous valvuloplasty.

The severity of mitral stenosis and associated hemodynamic changes can also be evaluated with cardiac catheterization. Measurement of the cardiac output and transvalvular gradient can be used to calculate the valve area by means of the Gorlin formula. A normal mitral valve area is 4 to 6 cm², and critical mitral stenosis is defined as a valve area less than 1 cm².

Patients with mild to moderate mitral stenosis can usually be managed medically. Heart rate control is imperative in these patients because more rapid rates reduce the length of the diastolic filling period. This is especially true in patients with atrial fibrillation, in whom loss of atrial contraction may further reduce left ventricular filling. Anticoagulant therapy is indicated for patients with atrial fibrillation and those patients with sinus rhythm who have had prior embolic events or who have moderate to severe mitral stenosis. Diuretics are useful in relieving pulmonary congestion and signs of right-sided heart failure. All patients should be instructed on the importance of endocarditis prophylaxis.

Patients with severe symptoms (classes III to IV) and moderate to severe MS should be considered for a percutaneous or surgical intervention. Percutaneous balloon valvuloplasty is a new technique in which a balloon catheter positioned across the mitral valve is inflated, resulting in separation of the fused cusps. Optimal short- and long-term results are obtained in patients with pliable, noncalcified leaflets and chords, minimal mitral regurgitation, and no evidence of left atrial thrombus. A surgical option in this same group of patients is open mitral valve commissurotomy. With direct visualization of the mitral valve, the surgeon is able to debride the valve, separate the fused cusps, and remove left atrial thrombi. Although the valve remains abnormal, this procedure is associated with a low operative mortality and a good hemodynamic result and may spare the patient from a valve replacement for many years. If mitral commissurotomy is not an option, then valve replacement with a bioprosthetic or mechanical prosthesis can be performed.

Mitral Regurgitation

Mitral regurgitation (MR) can result from abnormalities of the mitral leaflets, annulus, chordae, or papillary muscles (see Table 8–1). The most common leaflet abnormality resulting in chronic MR is myxomatous degeneration of the mitral valves, such as mitral valve prolapse and rheumatic heart disease.

With chronic MR, the left ventricle dilates to compensate for the increased regurgitant volume. However, in contrast to aortic insufficiency, the increased volume is ejected into the low-pressure left atrium. Thus, left ventricular wall stress and pressure remain normal. If the left atrium dilates sufficiently to accommodate the increased volume, left atrial and pulmonary venous pressures will remain normal. As the MR progresses, myocyte damage may occur, resulting in further left ventricular dilatation, elevation in diastolic filling pressures, and a reduction in left ventricular systolic function. As left atrial and pulmonary venous pressures increase, pulmonary congestion may occur.

Patients with chronic compensated MR are usually asymptomatic and have normal functional capacity. When symptoms do occur, left ventricular systolic function is usually depressed. Patients may initially complain of fatigue and dyspnea with exertion secondary to reduced cardiac output and elevation in pulmonary venous pressures. If the MR remains untreated, pulmonary hypertension and right-sided heart failure may occur.

MR characteristically produces a holosystolic murmur best heard at the apex and radiating to the axilla and back (see Table 8–2). If an eccentric, anteriorly directed jet of MR is present, an ejection quality murmur may be present and confused with an aortic outflow murmur. If the MR is secondary to mitral valve prolapse, a midsystolic click may be present, followed by a late systolic murmur. MR associated with rheumatic mitral disease may be accompanied by heart sounds typical of MS.

Echocardiography is a useful noninvasive method for defining mitral valve pathology and assessing left ventricular size and function. Doppler techniques are useful in grading the severity of MR, although eccentric jets may underestimate the degree of regurgitation. MR can also be assessed during cardiac catheterization by estimating the amount of contrast medium that is ejected into the left atrium during left ventriculography. In addition, left ventricular size and systolic function can be quantitated, filling pressures can be measured, and the coronary anatomy defined.

The medical treatment of patients with compensated chronic MR is afterload reduction with vasodilator therapy, such as ACE inhibitors or hydralazine. The timing of surgery is difficult because the development of symptoms often indicates the presence of left ventricular dysfunction and irreversible myocardial damage. In addition, mitral valve replacement with disruption of the chordal apparatus often results in further left ventricular dilatation and decline in systolic function.

Echocardiographic parameters that identify patients at risk for a poor response to mitral valve replacement are those with a left ventricular end-diastolic diameter greater than 70 mm, an end-systolic diameter greater than 45 mm, and a low-normal or reduced left ventricular ejection fraction. Patients with known MR should be followed with yearly studies to monitor left ventricular function and size so that surgery can be performed before irreversible myocyte damage.

In many patients, the mitral valve may be repaired, thus avoiding many of the potential complications associated with valve replacement. With this surgery, sections of redundant leaflet can be excised, leaflets debrided, and chordae shortened. If MR is secondary to annular dilatation, a prosthetic ring (annuloplasty) can be sewn into the annulus to reduce the size of the orifice and increase the degree of leaflet coaptation. The advantage of this procedure is that preservation of the mitral apparatus helps maintain normal left ventricular geometry and function. In addition, long-term anticoagulation is not necessary in most patients in sinus rhythm. Valve repair is generally not indicated if the mitral valve is heavily calcified or disrupted secondary to papillary muscle disease or endocarditis. In these instances, valve replacement is the procedure of choice.

Acute MR is usually a life-threatening condition that can result from a variety of papillary muscle, chordal, and leaflet abnormalities (see Table 8–1). Patients with acute MR usually become acutely ill because the left atrium does not dilate to accommodate the regurgitant volume. As a result, left atrial and pulmonary venous pressures abruptly increase, resulting in pulmonary congestion. In addition, the decrease in stroke volume and cardiac output results in an increase in systemic vascular resistance, and, as a consequence, an increase in the severity of the MR. Patients usually present with the acute onset of pulmonary edema and signs of cardiogenic shock. On auscultation, the MR murmur is often a soft, low-pitched sound in early systole resulting from rapid equilibration of left ventricular and left atrial pressures. Afterload reduction with either an intravenous vasodilator, such as nitroprusside, or an intra-aortic balloon pump may help stabilize the patient before urgent valve replacement surgery.

Mitral Valve Prolapse

Mitral valve prolapse (MVP) is the most common congenital valvular abnormality, affecting 4% to 5% of the population. Although MVP can be seen in all ages and in both sexes, epidemiologic studies suggest that the prevalence is greater in women than men. MVP is inherited as a autosomal dominant trait with variable penetrance. Thirty percent to 50% of first-degree relatives will be affected.

MVP is present when there is superior displacement in ventricular systole of one or both mitral valve leaflets across the plane of the mitral annulus toward the left atrium. Primary or classic MVP occurs when there is myxomatous degeneration of the mitral valve without evidence of systemic disease. Secondary MVP is also characterized by myxomatous degeneration of the mitral apparatus, but in the presence of a recognizable systemic or connective tissue disease, such as Marfan's syndrome or systemic lupus erythematosus. Functional MVP results from structural abnormalities of the mitral annulus or papillary muscles, but the mitral leaflets are anatomically normal.

Most patients with MVP are asymptomatic. However, a variety of nonspecific symptoms have been associated with MVP, such as chest pain, palpitations, dizziness, and anxiety (MVP syndrome). These symptoms are not related to the mitral leaflet abnormalities but are thought to be secondary to neuroendocrine or autonomic dysfunction. MVP may be associated with variable degrees of mitral regurgitation. If severe mitral regurgitation is present, cardiac symptoms as previously described may be present.

The characteristic physical examination finding in MVP is the midsystolic click followed by a late systolic murmur (see Table 8–2). The auscultatory findings of MVP can be subtle and are greatly affected by changes in left ventricular volume. Maneuvers that reduce left ventricular volume will result in prolapse of the redundant leaflets earlier in systole; as a result, the click will occur earlier in systole and the MR murmur will sound more holosystolic. If left ventricular volume is increased, the click will be heard late in systole, followed by a short systolic murmur. The diagnosis of MVP is usually confirmed by echocardiography, which allows examination of the mitral apparatus and the MR severity.

Most patients with mild prolapse and insignificant MR are asymptomatic and require no specific intervention other than endocarditis prophylaxis. However, in some individuals the MR may progress such that serial examinations and echocardiograms are necessary to monitor MR severity and left ventricular function. Middle-aged and older men and patients with asymmetric prolapse are at highest risk for developing complications from MVP, such as severe MR and endocarditis. MR that acutely worsens may be related to rupture of the chordae tendineae. Cardiac arrhythmias, especially supraventricular tachycardia, are associated with MVP. Sudden death in the absence of hemodynamically significant MR is rare.

All patients with MVP and evidence of structural leaflet abnormalities and/or MR should receive endocarditis prophylaxis. Symptomatic arrhythmias should be treated as discussed in Chapter 10. For patients with severe MR, mitral valve repair or replacement may be indicated as discussed earlier.

Tricuspid Stenosis

Tricuspid stenosis is most often rheumatic in origin and is usually associated with mitral and/or aortic disease. Other rare causes include carcinoid syndrome, congenital valve abnormalities, and leaflet tumors or vegetations.

Similar to mitral stenosis, tricuspid stenosis is more common in women than men and tends to be a slowly progressive disease. Patients generally present with symptoms and signs of right-sided heart failure, such as fatigue, abdominal bloating, and peripheral edema. On physical examination, a prominent jugular venous a wave may be present if the patient is in sinus rhythm and may be confused with an arterial pulsation. In addition, a palpable presystolic pulsation coinciding with atrial contraction may be felt on palpation of the liver. On auscultation, the findings of tricuspid stenosis may not be detected secondary to the presence of mitral and aortic valve disease. However, an opening snap may be audible at the left sternal border followed by a soft, high-pitched diastolic murmur. In contrast to MS, the murmur of tricuspid stenosis is shorter in duration and accentuated with inspiration.

The diagnosis of tricuspid stenosis can be diagnosed by echocardiography or right-sided heart catheterization. Because the right heart is a low-pressure system, the mean gradient across the tricuspid valve may be quite small (5 mm Hg), yet still clinically important.

Tricuspid Regurgitation

Tricuspid regurgitation (TR) is most often secondary to dilatation of the right ventricle and tricuspid annulus that may occur with right-sided heart failure of any etiology. Other causes include endocarditis, carcinoid syndrome, congenital abnormalities, and chest wall trauma.

In the absence of pulmonary hypertension, TR is usually well tolerated. However, if right ventricular dysfunction is present, patients will usually have symptoms of right-sided heart failure. On physical examination, the jugular veins are distended and a prominent v wave is usually present. Hepatic congestion is common and is often associated with a palpable systolic pulsation. The murmur of TR is high-pitched and pansystolic and is best heard along the sternal border. Maneuvers that increase venous return, such as inspiration or leg raising, accentuate the murmur and are helpful in differentiating TR from MR or aortic outflow tract murmurs. If the TR is acute, the murmur is usually soft and present only during early systole.

TR related to pulmonary hypertension and right ventricular dysfunction will usually significantly improve with treatment of the underlying cause. In patients with persistent symptoms despite treatment, repair of the tricuspid annulus (annuloplasty) may restore tricuspid valve competence. In individuals with primary leaflet pathology, tricuspid valve replacement may be necessary.

Pulmonic Stenosis and Regurgitation

Pulmonic stenosis is most often congenital in origin and is discussed further in Chapter 7. Rheumatic deformity of the pulmonic valve is rare and is usually not associated with hemodynamically important obstruction.

Pulmonic regurgitation is most often the result of dilatation of the annulus secondary to pulmonary hypertension of any cause. Symptoms are usually related to the primary disease and in most cases are secondary to right ventricular heart failure. In this setting, the murmur of pulmonic regurgitation is a high-pitched, blowing murmur best heard at the second left intercostal space (Graham Steell murmur). In the absence of pulmonary hypertension, the murmur is usually low pitched and occurs late in diastole. Treatment is usually directed at the underlying cause of the pulmonary hypertension. Rarely, and usually in the setting of congenital pulmonic regurgitation, the valve will need to be replaced, owing to intractable right-sided heart failure.

Multivalvular Disease

Multivalvular disease is common, especially in patients with rheumatic heart disease. Often, regurgitant lesions, such as tricuspid and pulmonic regurgitation, are the result of another valve lesion, such as MS in association with pulmonary hypertension. In general, symptoms are most often related to the most proximal valve lesion. However, the severity of each individual lesion may be difficult to assess clinically, and, therefore, careful evaluation with right- and left-sided heart catheterization is necessary to assess valve function before any planned surgery. Failure to correct all significant valvular lesions may result in a poor clinical result. Double valve replacement is associated with a higher operative and long-term mortality than single valve replacement.

Rheumatic Heart Disease

Acute rheumatic fever (ARF) is the sequela of group A hemolytic streptococcal infection. The etiology of the disease is thought to be secondary to an abnormal immunologic response to the streptococcal infection. ARF usually occurs in children 4 to 9 years of age, with boys and girls being equally affected. Although the prevalence of this disease has significantly decreased in the United States over the past several decades, it still poses a major health care problem in many developing

nations, and endemic outbreaks have been identified even in the United States.

ARF is characterized by a diffuse inflammation of the heart (pancarditis). An exudative pericarditis is common and often results in fibrosis and obliteration of the pericardial sac. Constrictive pericarditis is rare. The myocardium is often infiltrated with lymphocytes and areas of necrosis may occur. The characteristic histologic finding in the myocardium is the Aschoff body, which is a confluence of monocytes and macrophages surrounded by fibrous tissue. Valvulitis is characterized by verrucous lesions on the leaflet edge, which are composed of cellular infiltrates and fibrin. The mitral valve is most frequently involved, followed by the aortic valve. Involvement of the tricuspid or pulmonic valve is rare. Valvulitis can be recognized by the presence of a new insufficiency murmur. Aortic and mitral stenosis do not occur for many years, when progression of the fibrosis results in restricted leaflet mobility.

ARF usually presents as an acute, febrile illness 2 to 4 weeks after a streptococcal pharyngitis. Because the diagnosis of ARF cannot be made by laboratory tests, guidelines based on symptoms and the physical examination have been established (modified Jones criteria) (Table 8–3). A diagnosis of ARF can be made if two major, or one major and two minor, criteria are present after a recent, documented streptococcal pharyngitis. Major criteria include evidence of carditis (pleuritic chest pain, friction rub, heart failure, MR), polyarthritis, chorea, erythema marginatum, and subcutaneous nodules. Minor criteria include fever, arthralgia, and a previous history of rheumatic fever or known rheumatic heart disease.

Once the diagnosis is established, a course of therapy with penicillin is indicated to eradicate the streptococcal infection. Salicylates are effective for the treatment of fever and arthritis. Corticosteroids and immunosuppressive therapy have not been proved beneficial in the management of the carditis. Heart failure should be treated with standard therapy.

Recurrent attacks of rheumatic fever are common, especially during the first 5 to 10 years after the primary illness. Rheumatic fever prophylaxis should be continued during this period, and for 10 years in patients with a high exposure rate to streptococcal infection (health care professionals, child-care workers, military recruits). Patients with significant rheumatic heart disease should

TABLE 8–3   Revised Jones Criteria

Major Criteria
Carditis (pleuritic chest pain, friction rub, heart failure)
Polyarthritis
Chorea
Erythema marginatum
Subcutaneous nodules
Minor Criteria
Fever
Arthralgia
Previous rheumatic fever or known rheumatic heart disease

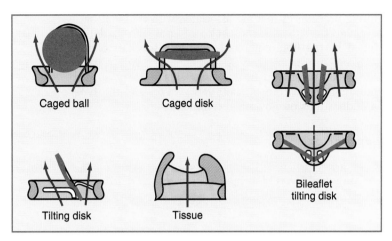

FIGURE 8-4   Designs and flow patterns of major categories of prosthetic heart valves: caged ball, caged disk, tilting disk, bi-leaflet tilting disk, and bioprosthetic (tissue) valves. Whereas flow in mechanical valves must course along both sides of the occluder, bioprostheses have a central flow pattern. (Reprinted with permission from Schoen FJ, et al: Bioengineering aspects of heart valve replacement. Ann Biomed Eng 10:97–128, 1982, Pergamon Press, Ltd.; and Schoen FJ: Pathology of cardiac valve replacement. *In* Morse D, Steiner RM, Fernandez J [eds]: Guide to Prosthetic Cardiac Valves. New York, Springer-Verlag, 1985, p 208. Copyright Springer-Verlag, Inc., 1985.)

receive prophylaxis indefinitely given the high rate of recurrence in these individuals. The recommended therapy for prophylaxis is an intramuscular injection of 1.2 million U of benzathine penicillin monthly. Alternatively, oral penicillin or erythromycin may be used. Noncompliance with these agents reduces the effectiveness of this mode of therapy.

Prosthetic Heart Valves

Two types of artificial heart valves are available for use in the atrioventricular and aortic positions: mechanical valves (tilting disc and bileaflet) and tissue valves (bioprostheses) (Fig. 8–4). The mechanical valves have a favorable hemodynamic profile and are extremely durable. However, mechanical valves carry a high thromboembolic risk, and require long-term anticoagulation. Bioprosthesis use is less likely to be complicated by thromboembolic disease, but the durability of the valve is less than with mechanical valves, especially in young patients. The type of prosthesis used in a particular patient is dependent on multiple factors, including the patient's age, suitability for long-term anticoagulation, and valve position.

Replacement of a diseased valve with an artificial valve results in a new set of potential risks and complications with the prosthesis. All valve prostheses result in some degree of stenosis because the effective valve orifice is smaller than that of the native valve. Thrombosis or calcification of the prosthetic valve can result in pros-

thetic dysfunction and hemodynamically important stenosis. Prosthetic valve insufficiency can result from perivalvular leaks in the area of the sewing ring. With bioprosthetic valves, deterioration of the prosthetic valve leaflets can lead to valve insufficiency as well as stenosis. Hemolysis is a frequent complication of the older mechanical valves (ball-cage, disk-cage) and can occur with present-day prostheses if there is turbulent flow associated with prosthetic valve dysfunction, especially regurgitation. Endocarditis remains a potential complication in all patients with prosthetic valves. The guidelines for endocarditis prophylaxis are given later.

Evaluation of prosthetic valve function is best performed with two-dimensional and Doppler echocardiographic techniques. Transesophageal echocardiography is particularly useful in studying prosthetic valves when thrombosis or endocarditis is suspected. Mechanical valves can be assessed with fluoroscopy to determine if leaflet excursion is normal.

Endocarditis Prophylaxis

Patients with valvular heart disease and prosthetic heart valves are at increased risk for developing endocarditis (Table 8–4) (see Chapter 100). The role of antibiotic prophylaxis is to prevent infection of the abnormal valve

TABLE 8-4   Cardiac Conditions in Which Antibiotic Prophylaxis Is Recommended

Prosthetic heart valves
Previous bacterial endocarditis
Rheumatic and other acquired valvular dysfunction
Most congenital cardiac malformations
Hypertrophic cardiomyopathy
Mitral valve prolapse with thickened leaflets or mitral regurgitation

TABLE 8-5   Dental and Surgical Procedures in Which Endocarditis Prophylaxis Is Recommended

Dental procedures known to induce gingival bleeding, including professional cleaning
Tonsillectomy and/or adenoidectomy
Surgery involving intestinal or respiratory mucosa
Sclerotherapy for esophageal varices
Cystoscopy
Gallbladder surgery
Urinary tract surgery if urinary tract infection is present
Incision and drainage of infected tissue
Vaginal hysterectomy

during procedures that are associated with transient bacteremia (Table 8–5). The choice of antibiotics is determined by the flora commonly found in the part of the body being instrumented. All patients with known valve disease or prosthetic heart valves should carry a card indicating the nature of their valve lesion and the type of endocarditis prophylaxis recommended.

REFERENCES

Bonow RO, Lakatos E, Maron BJ, et al: Serial long-term assessment of the natural history of asymptomatic patients with chronic aortic regurgitation and normal left ventricular ventricular systolic function. Circulation 1991; 84:1625–1635.

Cohen DJ, Kuntz RE, Gordon SPF, et al: Predictors of long term outcome after percutaneous balloon valvotomy. N Engl J Med 1992; 327:1329–1335.

Enriquez-Sarano M, Schaff HV, Orszulak TA, et al: Valve repair improves the outcome of surgery for mitral regurgitation. Circulation 1995; 91:1022–1028.

Gaasch WH, John RM, Aurigemma GP: Managing asymptomatic patients with chronic mitral regurgitation. Chest 1995; 108:842–847.

Prevention of Bacterial Endocarditis: Recommendations by the American Heart Association by the Committee on Rheumatic Fever, Endocarditis, and Kawasaki Disease. JAMA 1997; 277:1794–1801.

Vongpatanasin W, Hillis LD, Lange RA: Prosthetic heart valves. N Engl J Med 1996; 335:407–416.

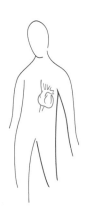

9

CORONARY HEART DISEASE

Eric H. Awtry • *Joseph Loscalzo*

Epidemiology

Coronary heart disease is the leading cause of death in most industrialized nations, including the United States. In addition, this disease results in significant morbidity, disability, and loss of productivity and is the leading cause of health care expenditure. The clinical spectrum of coronary heart disease ranges from silent (asymptomatic) ischemia to chronic stable angina, unstable angina, acute myocardial infarction, ischemic cardiomyopathy, and sudden cardiac death. With the advent of newer medical therapies, as well as interventional and surgical techniques, the mortality rate from coronary heart disease has gradually decreased over the past several decades. Nonetheless, almost 900,000 people have a myocardial infarction each year in the United States alone. Of these, approximately 225,000 die, mostly of arrhythmias or heart failure. Many risk factors for the development of coronary heart disease have been identified. Current recommendations for the early detection of these risk factors and aggressive therapies aimed toward risk factor modification may further decrease the burden of this disease.

Pathophysiology of Atherosclerosis

The clinical syndromes of coronary heart disease are overwhelmingly the result of underlying atherosclerosis of the epicardial coronary arteries. This process is present to some degree at almost all ages and in both men and women; however, its extent in any given individual varies depending in part on genetic background, risk factors, and local hemodynamic conditions. Injury to the vascular endothelium is the initiating event. The normal endothelium is an important modulator of vascular tone, producing vasoactive substances, such as pros-

tacyclin and endothelium-derived relaxing factor, and is also intricately involved in the local control of intravascular thrombosis. Hypertension, hypercholesterolemia, cigarette smoking, and local hemodynamic abnormalities produce endothelial injury leading to impaired endothelium-dependent vasodilation and a local prothrombotic state (endothelial dysfunction). Endothelial dysfunction is the earliest measurable abnormality in atherosclerotic vessels. This injury results in the accumulation of macrophages (derived from circulating monocytes) and lipids (predominantly low-density lipoproteins) at the site of vascular injury. The low-density lipoproteins are oxidized and are ingested by the macrophages, producing foam cells. Aggregates of these foam cells compose the earliest visible lesion of atherosclerosis, the fatty streak.

The release of enzymes and toxic substances by macrophages produces endothelial denudation, resulting in the adhesion of platelets to the injury site. As the plaque matures, growth factors derived from platelets and macrophages stimulate the migration and proliferation of smooth muscle cells and fibroblasts, resulting in formation of either a fibrotic lesion of the intima or a fibrous cap over a lipid-rich core. With further growth of the plaque, the vessel lumen is compromised and blood flow through the vessel is impaired (Fig. 9–1). The hemodynamic significance of a plaque varies depending on length and morphology of the lesion; however, a 70% decrease in the luminal diameter of a coronary artery is generally adequate to limit blood flow in the presence of increased demand (e.g., exercise) and a 90% stenosis may limit flow in the resting state. The inability of the affected coronary artery to augment blood flow in this setting results in the clinical pattern of stable angina.

As lipid accumulates in the macrophages, cell necrosis occurs, leaving a free lipid pool in the core of the plaque. Activated macrophages and mast cells release metalloproteinase enzymes (e.g., collagenase, gelatinase) that break down interstitial matrix proteins, and T lymphocytes in the plaque elaborate cytokines (e.g., inter-

79

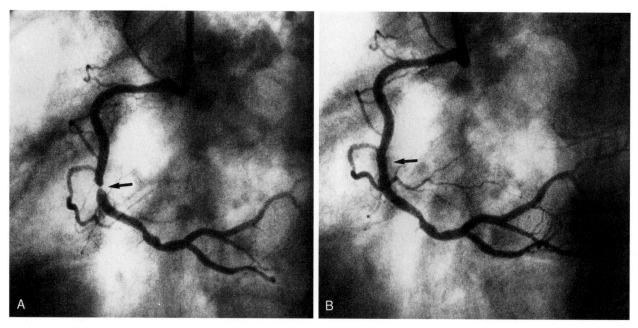

FIGURE 9–1   Angiograms of the right coronary artery. *A,* There is a discrete stenosis of the middle segment of the artery *(arrow). B,* The same artery is shown after successful balloon angioplasty of the stenosis and placement of an intracoronary stent.

feron-γ) that inhibit the formation of interstitial collagen by vascular smooth muscle cells. Thus, a vulnerable plaque is formed with a lipid-laden core and a weakened fibrous cap. Such plaques are prone to fissure or rupture, especially in the presence of increased shear force (increased intraluminal pressure). Disruption of the *vasa vasorum,* the nutrient vessels of the vascular wall, also increases the likelihood of plaque rupture.

Plaque rupture frequently occurs at the margin, or shoulder region, of the plaque. Fissuring in this region results in the exposure of highly thrombogenic collagen and lipid to the circulation, with the resultant formation of intraluminal thrombus. Activated platelets mediate vasoconstriction and further thrombus propagation, abruptly compromising coronary blood flow. The severity of plaque rupture and extent of thrombosis are reflected clinically in the spectrum of acute coronary syndromes, including unstable angina, non–Q wave myocardial infarction, and Q wave myocardial infarction.

Risk Factors

Epidemiologic studies have identified multiple factors that increase the probability of the development of atherosclerosis in a given individual (Table 9–1). Advanced age, male sex, and a family history of premature atherosclerosis are considered nonmodifiable risk factors. The prevalence of coronary artery disease (CAD) increases with advancing age. At any given age, the prevalence of CAD in men is higher than that in women, and, on average, it tends to become manifest about 10 years later in women than in men. This is at least in part due

to the protective effects of estrogen, as evidenced by the marked increase in CAD in postmenopausal women, and the blunting of this effect by the administration of exogenous estrogens during the postmenopausal period. A family history of premature atherosclerosis (occurring in men before age 55 and women before age 65) increases the risk of atherosclerosis in an individual, likely as a result of both environmental factors (i.e., dietary habits, smoking habits) and a heritable predisposition to the disease.

Other risk factors are largely modifiable, and treat-

TABLE 9–1   Risk Factors for Coronary Artery Disease

Nonmodifiable Risk Factors
Age
Male sex
Family history of premature coronary artery disease
Modifiable, Independent Risk Factors
Hyperlipidemia
Hypertension
Diabetes mellitus/glucose intolerance
Smoking
Other Risk Factors
Obesity
Physical inactivity
Hyperhomocysteinemia
Elevated lipoprotein a
Elevated fibrinogen levels
Decreased fibrinolytic activity (elevated plasminogen activator inhibitor)

ment of these factors may decrease the risk of developing atherosclerosis. Lipids play a central role in the atherosclerotic process, and elevated levels of cholesterol (primarily low-density lipoprotein cholesterol) are associated with accelerated disease. Elevated triglycerides may also be an independent risk factor for CAD, especially in women. High-density lipoproteins, on the other hand, appear to serve a protective function and are inversely related to the risk of CAD. Large-scale trials of lipid-lowering therapy have clearly demonstrated the effectiveness of cholesterol reduction in both primary and secondary prevention of CAD. Guidelines have thus been developed that provide defined lipid level goals in patients with established CAD and in those with risk factors for the disease.

Hypertension, defined as a systolic blood pressure greater than 140 mm Hg or a diastolic blood pressure greater than 90 mm Hg, significantly increases the risk of atherosclerotic heart disease. This risk increases proportionally with the extent of blood pressure elevation, and aggressive treatment of hypertension effectively reduces the risk. Diabetes mellitus clearly increases both the risk of developing CAD and the mortality associated with CAD. In the absence of overt diabetes, insulin resistance and hyperinsulinemia are associated with an increased incidence of CAD, possibly through alterations in lipid metabolism and increased platelet aggregation. In addition, diabetes frequently coexists with other risk factors, including dyslipidemia and hypertension. Cigarette smoke has adverse effects on the lipid profile, clotting factors, and platelet function and is associated with a twofold-to-threefold increase in the risk of CAD. A measurable reduction in the incidence of myocardial infarction occurs as early as 12 months after cessation of smoking.

Several other factors have been recognized as contributing to atherosclerotic risk. Lipoprotein(a) is identical to low-density lipoprotein with the addition of an apo(a) molecule. It has structural homology with plasminogen and appears to interfere with the generation of plasmin, thus predisposing to thrombotic complications of atherosclerosis. Elevated levels of homocysteine are clearly associated with an increased risk of coronary, cerebral, and peripheral vascular disease. The mechanism likely involves both endothelial injury and an increased propensity for thrombosis. Elevated homocysteine levels can be effectively treated in many individuals with dietary folate supplementation; however, the effect of treating elevated lipoprotein(a) or homocysteine levels on the incidence of cardiovascular events remains to be determined.

Nonatherosclerotic Causes of Cardiac Ischemia

Although atherosclerosis is by far the most common disease affecting the coronary arteries, it is by no means the only one. Several nonatherosclerotic processes may affect the coronary arteries and produce acute coronary insufficiency. Acute embolization down a coronary artery may occlude blood flow and produce myocardial ischemia and infarction. The most common sources of such emboli include infectious endocarditis, mural thrombi in the left atrium or ventricle, thrombi from prosthetic valves, intracardiac tumors, and paradoxical emboli from the venous system across an atrial or ventricular septal defect. Chest wall trauma may result in coronary injury and in situ thrombosis. Mediastinal radiation may result in fibrosis of the coronary arteries and produce myocardial infarction. Aortic dissection may propagate to the aortic root and occlude a coronary artery at its origin. Coronary artery dissection may occur during cardiac catheterization and rarely may be a spontaneous event.

Several forms of arteritis may involve the coronary arteries, including syphilis, Takayasu's arteritis, polyarteritis nodosa, systemic lupus erythematosus, and giant cell arteritis. These syndromes may result in obstruction, occlusion, or thrombosis of the coronary arteries. Kawasaki's disease (mucocutaneous lymph node syndrome) is a systemic disease, and its most prominent manifestation is coronary vasculitis with resultant coronary aneurysms. Spontaneous in situ coronary thrombosis may occur in the setting of hematologic disorders (e.g., polycythemia vera, disseminated intravascular coagulation, sickle cell anemia), and several congenital coronary anomalies may predispose to coronary insufficiency. Spontaneous coronary spasm, with or without underlying coronary artery disease, may induce myocardial ischemia. Cocaine use may result in myocardial ischemia and infarction through several mechanisms, including coronary spasm and thrombosis, and may accelerate atherosclerosis.

In 10% to 20% of patients with suspected angina and 3% of patients with myocardial infarction, normal epicardial coronary arteries are documented at arteriography (syndrome X). These patients tend to be young, are more commonly women, have minimal cardiac risk factors, and have a relatively good prognosis. The anginal pain tends to be atypical. Coronary spasm, thrombosis, or embolism has been suggested as the cause in many of these patients. More recently, microvascular or small-vessel disease has been implicated. The small resistance vessels in these patients, which are not visualizable by coronary arteriography, appear to have reduced vasodilatory capability. This dysfunction may lead to true ischemia; exercise-related abnormalities on echocardiography and nuclear scintigraphy have been noted in some patients. Some patients respond to treatment with usual antianginal medications, although in general, these drugs are much less effective than in patients with atherosclerotic CAD.

Furthermore, myocardial ischemia may result from a mismatch of the myocardial oxygen supply and demand. The increased myocardial oxygen demand associated with increases in heart rate, left ventricular wall stress, or left ventricular mass may outstrip the maximal possible oxygen supply in such settings as thyrotoxicosis, aortic stenosis, aortic insufficiency, tachyarrhythmias, and sepsis. Decreased oxygen delivery can occur as a result of acute blood loss, hypotension, anemia, or carbon monoxide poisoning.

Pathophysiology and Consequences of Myocardial Ischemia

Myocardial ischemia is a state of decreased perfusion during which the oxygen supply to the myocardium is insufficient to meet its metabolic demands. This imbalance results in the manifestations of CAD. In the normal state, oxygen in the blood is maximally extracted by the heart and an increase in myocardial oxygen demand (secondary to increased heart rate, wall stress, or contractility) must therefore be met by a proportional increase in myocardial blood flow. This autoregulatory function occurs at the level of the arterioles, is dependent on autonomic tone and an intact, functioning endothelium, and results in coronary vasodilation in response to increased demands. Atherosclerosis alters endothelial function and may impair the ability of the vessel to dilate. In the presence of a fixed stenosis in a coronary artery, the distal vessel may be maximally or near-maximally dilated in the resting state. During periods of increased demand, the stenosed artery will have limited ability to dilate further (decreased coronary vasodilator reserve), resulting in supply-demand mismatch and subsequent ischemia. Acute coronary thrombosis secondary to a ruptured atherosclerotic plaque, acute coronary spasm, or coronary emboli may limit coronary flow to such an extent that ischemia occurs in the resting state. Furthermore, normal augmentation of coronary blood flow in normal coronary arteries may still be insufficient in the face of marked increases in myocardial oxygen demand.

During ischemia, the first demonstrable abnormality of cardiac function is impaired myocardial relaxation (diastolic dysfunction), which is followed by impairment of contraction (systolic dysfunction). Chest pain and ischemic electrocardiographic (ECG) changes occur relatively late in the ischemic response. If the ischemia is transient, the dysfunction may be short lived. More prolonged ischemia may produce myocardial stunning, hibernation, or infarction. Myocardial stunning refers to a prolonged period (hours to days) of reversible myocardial dysfunction after an ischemic event. Hibernation occurs in the setting of chronic ischemia, presumably when oxygen delivery is adequate to maintain myocardial viability but inadequate to maintain normal function. The clinical importance of this concept is that restoration of blood flow to the involved myocardium may result in improved ventricular function.

The extent of myocardial injury after occlusion of blood flow to a given myocardial territory depends largely on the duration of the occlusion and the presence or absence of collateral vessels. After as little as 15 to 20 minutes of coronary occlusion, infarction occurs, as evidenced by irreversible cellular injury and necrosis. The longer the period of ischemia, the larger the area of necrosis. Blood flow increases in pre-existing collateral vessels within seconds of coronary occlusion and helps to limit infarct extent. In arteries with gradually developing stenoses, sufficient collaterals may develop to prevent irreversible myocardial injury even with the development of a complete occlusion. In contrast, after acute plaque rupture with thrombotic occlusion at the site of a previously insignificant stenosis, collateral circulation does not have sufficient time to develop and extensive infarction ensues. If a large area of ischemia develops, sufficient enough contractile dysfunction may occur to result in decreased stroke volume, decreased cardiac output, and increased intraventricular pressure, resulting in heart failure. When 20% to 25% of the myocardium is involved, heart failure is usually present. With loss of 40% or more of the myocardium, cardiogenic shock develops.

Owing to limited energy expenditure, conduction tissue is more resistant to ischemia than is contractile tissue. Nonetheless, the conduction system of the heart is susceptible to ischemic injury. Ischemia results in altered ionic transport, altered autonomic tone, and structural injury to the conduction system, resulting in a variety of ischemia-induced arrhythmias and conduction abnormalities.

Angina Pectoris

Angina pectoris (Table 9–2) is classically described as a visceral discomfort in the chest that is a result of transient myocardial ischemia. Importantly, many patients deny actual pain but instead describe substernal chest discomfort that may radiate to their back, neck, jaw, arms, or epigastrium. Discomfort above the jaw or below the epigastrium is usually not angina pectoris. Angina occurs in the setting of a flow-limiting coronary stenosis and in response to an increase in myocardial oxygen demand due to physical or emotional stress. Some patients also note angina on exposure to cold air or after a large meal. The discomfort may be associated with dyspnea, diaphoresis, nausea, or palpitations. Most patients can identify a level of exertion that will reproduce the discomfort, such as climbing a flight of stairs or walking up an incline. Such effort-related angina usually comes on gradually, lasts less than 15 minutes, and resolves rapidly with rest or with the sublingual administration of nitroglycerin.

The physical examination of a patient with angina may be entirely normal both between and during ischemic episodes. Nonetheless, signs of cardiovascular disease are frequently present. These include abnormal pulses, arterial bruits, cutaneous signs of peripheral vascular disease, and evidence of increased venous pressure (crackles, elevated jugular venous pressure, edema). During an anginal episode, patients are often hypertensive and tachycardic. A transient S_4 may be heard as a result of an ischemia-induced decrease in ventricular compliance. Transient signs of left ventricular systolic dysfunction (S_3, pulmonary congestion) may be present if a large territory of myocardium is involved in the

TABLE 9-2 **Angina Pectoris**

Type	Pattern	ECG	Usual Coronary Abnormality	Medical Therapy
Stable	Chronic unchanged pattern of precipitation and relief Induced by physical activity or emotional stress; lasts 5–10 min, relieved by rest or sublingual nitroglycerin	Baseline often normal or nonspecific ST-T changes, or signs of prior myocardial infarction ST segment depression or T wave inversion during angina	≥70% stenosis due to atherosclerotic plaque in one or more coronary arteries	Aspirin Sublingual nitroglycerin Anti-ischemic medications*
Unstable	Recent increase in angina frequency or severity, especially with rest pain; new-onset angina if at low activity level; angina after a myocardial infarction May last longer and be less responsive to sublingual nitroglycerin	As with stable angina, although changes during discomfort may be more pronounced Occasionally, ST segment elevation during discomfort	Fissured plaque with platelet and fibrin-thrombus contribute to stenosis	Aspirin, heparin (e.g., aPTT 1.5–2 × normal) Anti-ischemic medications
Prinzmetal's or variant angina	Typically unpredictable rest pain, often in early morning hours	Transient ST segment elevation during pain (ST segment depression and/or T wave inversion can also occur)	Coronary artery spasm at a region of fixed but often nonstenotic lesion; can also occur in angiographically normal vessel	Calcium channel blockers Nitrates Aspirin

* Long-acting nitrates, β-adrenergic blocking drugs, calcium channel–blocking drugs—see text.
aPTT = activated partial thromboplastin time.

ischemic process. Apical murmurs are occasionally heard during an anginal episode and presumably result from ischemic papillary muscle dysfunction causing mitral regurgitation.

The ECG in patients with angina may be normal between episodes or may reveal either nonspecific ST-T wave changes or evidence of underlying cardiac disease (e.g., left ventricular hypertrophy, prior infarction). During an anginal episode, the ECG classically demonstrates ST segment depression (Fig. 9–2). T wave inversion may also develop during angina; in patients with inverted T waves on their resting ECG, normalization of the T waves may occur during angina (pseudonormalized T waves). Rarely, transient ST segment elevation may be seen; this characteristically occurs in vasospastic angina (see later). The ST segment and T waves changes usually rapidly return to normal after resolution of the ischemia. The persistence of ECG changes predicts a poorer prognosis.

Angina is considered stable when it exists as a chronic pattern of predictable exertional discomfort. It is considered "unstable" when there is a significant change in the frequency, severity, or duration of the episodes, or when it occurs with decreasing levels of exertion. Unstable angina can be further classified on the basis of its severity and the clinical circumstances under which it occurs. Class I refers to new-onset, severe, or accelerated angina without episodes of rest angina. Class II and class III refer to rest angina occurring within the preceding month or the preceding 48 hours, respectively. Further subclassification divides unstable angina into that which is the result of a secondary cause such as anemia or hypotension (subclass A), that which occurs in the absence of secondary causes (subclass B), and that which occurs within 2 weeks of a documented myocardial infarction (subclass C). Patients with unstable angina have an increased risk of myocardial infarction and death and frequently warrant hospital admission, intensive medical therapy, and consideration for revascularization procedures.

EVALUATION OF THE PATIENT WITH ANGINA

When patients present with the classic symptoms described earlier, the diagnosis is straightforward. Unfortunately, not all patients have classic symptoms and instead may present with isolated dyspnea on exertion or atypical chest pain as their anginal equivalent or may have no symptoms at all during an ischemic episode (silent ischemia). Pain that is sharp, stabbing, fleeting, or exacerbated by breathing or movement of the upper extremities is usually not angina. The differential diagnosis of chest pain is reviewed in Chapter 4. The presence or absence of cardiac risk factors is important to

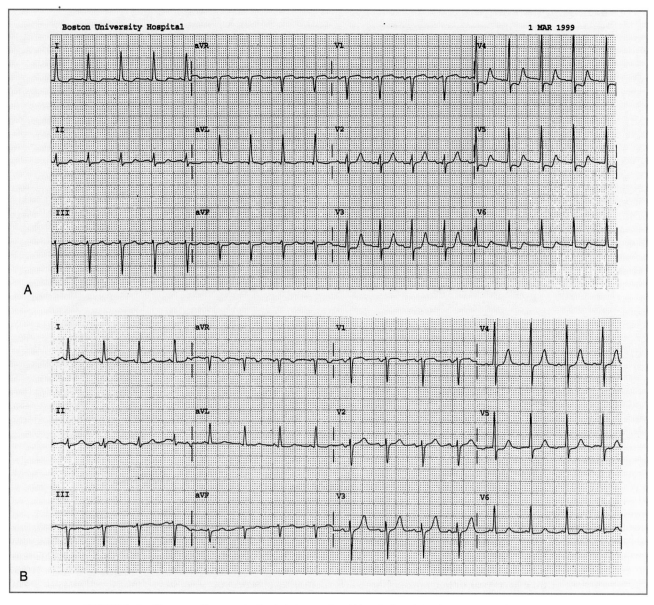

FIGURE 9–2   Electrocardiogram obtained during angina *(A)* and after the administration of sublingual nitroglycerin and subsequent resolution of angina *(B)*. During angina in this patient, there is transient ST segment depression and T wave abnormalities.

note but does not define or exclude the diagnosis of angina.

For patients in whom the diagnosis is not clear, exercise or pharmacologic stress testing may clarify the diagnosis by reproducing the patient's symptoms and demonstrating objective evidence of ischemia. Stress testing may also be useful in patients with chronic stable angina for determination of exercise capacity, documentation of the effectiveness of medication, and for risk stratification (i.e., identifying patients at high risk in whom more aggressive therapy is warranted) (Fig. 9–3). Patients with unstable angina are not appropriate candidates for stress testing until their symptoms have been stabilized. For patients who are able to ambulate, routine exercise treadmill testing is appropriate and gives much more physiologic information than pharmacologic stress test-

ing does (see Chapter 5). In nonambulatory patients or patients with very limited exercise capacity, pharmacologic stress testing with dobutamine, dipyridamole, or adenosine may give similar diagnostic information but cannot yield information regarding exercise capacity or hemodynamic response to exercise.

In a patient with a normal resting ECG, routine stress testing with ECG monitoring is usually sufficient. However, in patients with baseline abnormalities on their ECG (e.g., nonspecific ST abnormalities, left ventricular hypertrophy, left bundle branch block) and in patients taking digoxin, the specificity of exercise-induced ST-T wave changes is diminished. In these patients, imaging with echocardiography or nuclear scintigraphy improves both the sensitivity and specificity of stress testing, however, at significantly increased cost.

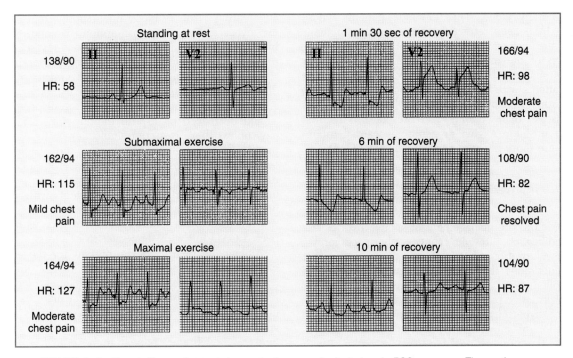

FIGURE 9–3 Treadmill exercise test demonstrating a markedly ischemic ECG response. The resting ECG was normal. The test was stopped on reproduction of angina at a relatively low work load, accompanied by ST segment depression in lead II and ST segment elevation in lead V_2. These changes worsened early in recovery and resolved after administration of sublingual nitroglycerin. Only leads II and V_2 are shown; however, ischemic changes were seen in 10 of 12 recorded leads. Severe atherosclerotic disease of all three coronary arteries was documented at subsequent cardiac catheterization.

Exercise-induced ECG changes in women are less specific than in men; for this reason many physicians perform exercise testing with imaging in all women.

Electron-beam or ultrafast computed tomography (CT) has also been used for the detection of CAD. The absence of calcification on CT strongly correlates with the absence of significant coronary atherosclerosis, and the presence of coronary calcification is diagnostic of coronary atherosclerosis, although the extent of disease cannot be predicted by this test. In addition, the prognostic importance of coronary calcification on CT is yet to be determined.

The two most important predictors of survival in patients with chronic CAD are left ventricular function and the extent of myocardium at risk. A poor prognosis is predicted by left ventricular dysfunction, as evidenced by either the presence of congestive heart failure on examination or a depressed ejection fraction on echocardiography or ventriculography. In addition, the greater the degree of dysfunction, the worse the prognosis. The presence of a large area of jeopardized myocardium can be demonstrated by identifying large or multiple stress-induced abnormalities on echocardiogram or nuclear scanning. Exercise-induced ECG changes are relatively specific for identifying the presence of ischemic myocardium but are not very accurate in determining its location or extent. Nonetheless, poor prognostic markers have been identified with stress testing and include ischemic ECG changes (ST depression) occurring early in exercise, occurring in multiple leads, and persisting several minutes after the completion of exercise, as well as an associated drop in blood pressure.

Cardiac catheterization with coronary angiography allows visual assessment of the extent and severity of coronary disease, factors that also relate directly to prognosis. The anatomic information thus obtained must be interpreted in light of functional information (e.g., stress testing) because the anatomic severity of a given coronary stenosis does not necessarily correlate with the physiologic significance of the lesion. Coronary angiography carries with it a small, albeit not insignificant, risk, and is expensive. Nonetheless, the risk-benefit analysis of catheterization favors the procedure in many patients with angina (Table 9–3), either as a diagnostic test when the diagnosis cannot be made by noninvasive testing or to define the coronary anatomy in patients for whom revascularization will improve prognosis over

TABLE 9–3 Indications for Coronary Angiography in Patients with Stable Angina Pectoris

Unacceptable angina despite medical therapy (for consideration of revascularization)
High-risk results of noninvasive testing
Angina in the setting of depressed left ventricular function
As a diagnostic test in patients for whom noninvasive testing is either not possible or nondiagnostic

medical therapy alone. These include patients whose symptoms have been refractory to medications, patients in whom medical management is limited by intolerable side effects of the medications, and patients with poor prognostic markers by clinical features or noninvasive testing. Patients with chronic stable angina who undergo cardiac catheterization are more likely to have more diffuse disease than patients who present for the first time with unstable angina or acute myocardial infarction, who are more likely to have single-vessel CAD.

MEDICAL MANAGEMENT OF STABLE ANGINA

The approach to the management of angina involves risk factor modification, lifestyle changes, pharmacotherapy, and revascularization. In addition, other concurrent medical conditions that may precipitate angina should be controlled (e.g., anemia, congestive heart failure, chronic obstructive pulmonary disease, hyperthyroidism). Control of hypertension, diabetes, and hyperlipidemia and cessation of smoking are of utmost importance in controlling the progression of disease in patients with coronary atherosclerosis, and guidelines for aggressive risk factor reduction have been established (Table 9–4). In obese patients, attainment of ideal body weight may help control hypertension, diabetes, and hyperlipidemia and may raise the threshold for the onset on angina. Patients should be instructed on dietary changes, and evaluation by a nutritionist may be helpful. Exercise is frequently limited by angina; however, regular activity at a level that is tolerated should be encouraged and helps to maintain physical conditioning. Isometric exercises such as weight lifting and high-intensity activities (especially in the cold, such as skiing, shoveling snow) are not advisable, but many patients with stable angina may perform vigorous activities, including moderate physical exertion at work.

As previously noted, the pathophysiology of angina is one of supply-demand mismatch. Therapy for angina is, therefore, aimed at diminishing this mismatch by either augmenting coronary blood flow (supply) or by decreasing myocardial oxygen consumption (demand). Coronary blood flow can be improved by various revascularization procedures (see later). Pharmacologic therapy is directed at controlling the major determinants of myocardial oxygen consumption (i.e., heart rate and wall stress). All patients with known or suspected CAD should be placed on aspirin therapy (75–325 mg each day) unless there is a contraindication to its use. Owing principally to its ability to suppress the platelet-dependent thrombotic response to atherosclerotic plaque rupture, aspirin has been shown to decrease myocardial infarction and mortality rates in patients with angina or prior myocardial infarction and may also decrease the risk of myocardial infarction in patients without suspected CAD but with significant risk factors.

Among the pharmacologic options for the control of symptoms in patients with chronic stable angina, nitrates, β blockers, and calcium channel blockers are most commonly used (Table 9–5). Unlike aspirin and lipid-lowering therapy, none of these agents has convincingly been shown to decrease mortality in these patients, although they appear to be equally effective in controlling symptoms. The choice of a particular agent must be individualized, and factors such as left ventricular function, hypertension, and concomitant lung disease must be taken into consideration. When a single agent fails to control angina, combination therapy is usually effective. If combinations are used, careful monitoring for signs of orthostatic hypotension or progressive heart block is mandatory, especially with the combination of β blockers and calcium channel blockers. In patient with refractory symptoms despite aggressive medical therapy, cardiac catheterization is indicated.

The effectiveness of organic nitrates for controlling angina has been recognized for over a century, and these medications remain the most prescribed antianginal therapy in patients with chronic angina. The effect of nitrates is mediated through relaxation of vascular smooth muscle. Dilation of arterioles results in a drop in systemic vascular resistance and, therefore, decreased

TABLE 9–4   Goals of Risk Factor Modification

Risk Factor	Goal
Dyslipidemia	
Increased LDL	
In patients with CAD	LDL < 100 mg/dL
Without CAD, with ≥2 CRF	LDL < 130 mg/dL
Without CAD, with <2 CRF	LDL < 160 mg/dL
Increased triglycerides	TG < 200 mg/dL
Decreased HDL	HDL > 35 mg/dL
Hypertension	Systolic blood pressure < 140 mm Hg
	Diastolic blood pressure < 90 mm Hg
Smoking	Complete cessation
Obesity	<120% of ideal body weight for height
Sedentary lifestyle	30–60 minutes of moderate-intensity activity (e.g., walking, jogging, cycling) three to four times per week

CAD = coronary artery disease; CRF = cardiac risk factors; HDL = high-density lipoprotein; LDL = low-density lipoprotein; TG = triglycerides.

TABLE 9–5 Medications for Angina Pectoris

Drug Class	Examples	Physiologic Antianginal Effect	Side Effects	Comments
Organic nitrates	Available in sublingual, topical, intravenous, and oral preparations	↓ Preload > afterload Coronary vasodilation	Headache, flushing, orthostasis	Tolerance develops with continuous use
β-Adrenergic blocking agents	Metoprolol, atenolol, propranolol, nadolol	↓ Heart rate ↓ Blood pressure ↓ Contractility	Bradycardia, hypotension, bronchospasm, depression	May worsen heart failure and AV conduction Avoid in vasospastic angina
Calcium channel–blocking agents				
Phenylalkylamines Benzothiazepines	Verapamil Diltiazem	Both classes produce: ↓ Heart rate ↓ Blood pressure ↓ Contractility Coronary vasodilation	Bradycardia, hypotension; Constipation with verapamil	May worsen heart failure and AV conduction
Dihydropyridines	Nifedipine, amlodipine	↓ Blood pressure Coronary vasodilation	Hypotension, reflex tachycardia	Short-acting formulations may aggravate angina

AV = atrioventricular.

afterload. There is a more profound effect on the venous system, where venodilation results in venous pooling, decreased venous return, and, therefore, decreased preload. These effects significantly reduce myocardial oxygen consumption and, thereby, decrease angina. Nitrates also have a dilatory effect on epicardial coronary arteries, with resultant augmentation of coronary blood flow. This effect is minimal, however, in extensively diseased coronary arteries. In addition, nitrates increase blood flow through collateral vessels. The most common side effects of nitrates are a result of vascular relaxation and include headaches and orthostasis. Several formulations are available and useful in particular situations. Sublingual nitroglycerin tablets are effective for the acute treatment of anginal episodes and as prophylactic therapy before an activity that is likely to provoke angina. Topical and oral formulations are effective for the chronic management of stable angina, whereas intravenous nitroglycerin is appropriate therapy for unstable angina. The chronic use of nitrates results in tolerance, an effect that can be minimized by allowing for a daily nitrate-free period (removing topical nitrate preparations during sleeping hours or prescribing oral nitrates such that they are not dosed around the clock). Sublingual nitroglycerin for acute anginal episodes is usually taken every 5 minutes until relief of symptoms or until a third tablet must be taken. Anginal episodes that persist after treatment with three sublingual nitroglycerin tablets usually require medical evaluation. Intravenous nitroglycerin is frequently used to treat unstable angina and myocardial infarction.

β-Adrenergic blocking drugs are competitive inhibitors of catecholamine β receptors and act to reduce myocardial oxygen demand by reducing heart rate, blood pressure, and contractility. These agents are effective in controlling anginal symptoms (especially exercise-induced symptoms) and decrease mortality and reinfarction after myocardial infarction. Four β blockers have been approved for the treatment of angina (atenolol, metoprolol, nadolol, and propranolol) and differ in their lipid solubility, duration of action, and β-receptor selectivity. β₁ receptors predominate in the heart where they mediate increases in heart rate, contractility, and atrioventricular conduction. β₂ receptors mediate bronchodilation and vasodilation. Blockade of β₁ receptors produces several beneficial cardiac effects, whereas β₂-receptor blockade may produce bronchospasm and increase peripheral vasoconstriction. Atenolol and metoprolol are β₁ selective at low doses; however, at the moderate-to-high doses frequently used in clinical practice, all β blockers lose their selectivity. The most common side effects include bradycardia, hypotension, bronchospasm, fatigue, and sexual dysfunction. Lipophilic agents (propranolol, metoprolol) cross the blood-brain barrier and may produce central nervous system effects (e.g., lethargy, depression, nightmares). β blockers may exacerbate congestive heart failure in patients with systolic dysfunction and may worsen underlying conduction system abnormalities; therefore, they should be used with caution in this patient population. In addition, these agents may result in a mild increase in triglycerides and a mild decrease in HDL cholesterol.

Calcium ions play a critical role in myocardial and vascular smooth muscle contraction, as well as in the genesis of the cardiac action potential (see Chapter 10). Blockade of these effects with calcium antagonists results in a blunting of the heart rate, decreased contractility, and peripheral vasodilation, all of which decrease myocardial oxygen demand. In addition, coronary vasodilation occurs, resulting in augmented coronary blood flow, especially if coronary spasm is present. There are three major classes of calcium antagonists. The dihydropyridines (e.g., nifedipine) have predominantly vasodilatory properties with little or no depressant effect on heart rate, contractility, or atrioventricular conduction. In fact, the marked vasodilation may lead to a reflex tachycardia, an effect that limits the use of short-acting nifedipine preparations for the treatment of CAD. Long-acting nifedipine and newer (second generation) dihydropyridines, such as amlodipine, may be less problematic in this regard. The phenylalkylamines (e.g., verapamil) reduce the heart rate, slow atrioventricular conduction, depress contractility, and have less of an effect on peripheral vascular tone than the dihydropyridines. They may be problematic in patients with depressed systolic function or underlying conduction system disease. The benzothiazepines (e.g., diltiazem) have less vasodilatory action than the dihydropyridines and less myocardial suppressant action than the phenylalkylamines. The particular agent used must, therefore, be individualized for a particular patient.

MEDICAL MANAGEMENT OF UNSTABLE ANGINA

Patients who present with unstable angina represent a particularly high-risk group with progression to myocardial infarction in up to 15% of cases and 1-year mortality rates as high as 10%. For this reason, these patients warrant hospital admission and aggressive antianginal therapy. The pathophysiology of unstable angina appears to relate to acute activation or rupture of an unstable atherosclerotic plaque, platelet activation and aggregation with resultant vasospasm and nonocclusive thrombus formation, and a resultant reduction in oxygen supply. This is in contrast to chronic stable angina, which tends to occur during periods of increased myocardial oxygen demand superimposed on a stable atherosclerotic coronary plaque.

Similar pharmacologic therapies are used for unstable angina as for chronic stable angina, although intravenous nitroglycerin is frequently employed in the place of oral preparations. Rest (for 24 to 48 hours), analgesics, and supplemental oxygen therapy are frequently prescribed. β blockers and calcium channel blockers are similarly effective, and the choice depends on patient characteristics. Aspirin has been shown to decrease mortality and myocardial infarction rates in patients with unstable angina, and the addition of intravenous heparin to aspirin reduces recurrent ischemic events (death, recurrent angina, or infarction) more than does treatment with aspirin alone. Many physicians choose to treat unstable angina patients with 2 to 3 days of intravenous heparin therapy to allow for plaque stabilization. With aggressive medical therapy, 80% of patients will have their conditions stabilize by 48 hours. Continuing aspirin therapy after stopping heparin is mandatory because recurrent ischemic events increase if aspirin is withheld. In patients with aspirin allergies, other platelet-inhibiting drugs, such as ticlopidine or clopidogrel, appear to be effective.

Because of the central role of thrombus in unstable angina, studies of other antithrombotic agents have been undertaken in these patients. Surprisingly, thrombolytic therapy has not been shown to be beneficial for the treatment of unstable angina and may, in fact, be detrimental. Low-molecular-weight heparins (e.g., enoxaparin) have similar antithrombotic effects as unfractionated heparin but have several potential advantages. They have greater bioavailability than standard heparin, achieve a reliable anticoagulant effect for a given dose, have a lower incidence of thrombocytopenia, and do not require monitoring of the activated partial thromboplastin time. Several studies suggest that these agents may be more effective than unfractionated heparin in the treatment of unstable angina, resulting in lower rates of recurrent ischemic events and lesser need for revascularization procedures. The final common pathway of platelet aggregation involves the cross-linking of platelets by fibrinogen, an action mediated by the glycoprotein IIb/IIIa receptor. Blockade of this receptor by monoclonal antibodies (abciximab) or by receptor antagonists (e.g., tirofiban, lamifiban, sibrafiban) results in more complete platelet inhibition than with aspirin and may decrease the rate of recurrent ischemic events when added to aspirin and heparin for the treatment of unstable angina. In addition, these agents significantly decrease the rate of ischemic complications in patients with unstable angina who undergo percutaneous revascularization procedures. It is likely that these newer agents will play a significant role in the medical management of unstable angina in the future.

Because of the high-risk nature of these patients, many physicians opt for early cardiac catheterization and coronary revascularization if possible (see later discussion). Others reserve this procedure for patients who fail to stabilize with medical management or have high-risk markers on noninvasive testing. For patients with severe, refractory angina, intra-aortic balloon pump counterpulsation can be used as a bridge to revascularization. By reducing left ventricular afterload and augmenting diastolic coronary perfusion pressure, the intra-aortic balloon pump counterpulsation decreases myocardial oxygen demand while increasing oxygen delivery and thus is an effective treatment for angina.

REVASCULARIZATION IN PATIENTS WITH ANGINA

In patients for whom medical therapy does not effectively control anginal symptoms and in patients with high-risk markers clinically (unstable angina, angina associated with heart failure, or poor exercise capacity) or by noninvasive testing (depressed left ventricular function, high-risk stress test results), revascularization plays an important therapeutic role. Several modalities for revascularization of diseased coronary arteries now exist, including surgical revascularization (coronary artery bypass graft surgery [CABG]) and catheter-based percutaneous techniques (percutaneous transluminal coronary angioplasty [PTCA] and related interventional techniques). Careful selection of patients for a given procedure is critical.

With advances in technology and increasing operator

experience, percutaneous revascularization can now be achieved with high success rates and at relatively low risk. More than 400,000 percutaneous revascularization procedures are performed each year in the United States alone. PTCA involves passing a deflated balloon retrograde through the femoral artery, up the aorta, and into the diseased coronary artery. The balloon is then positioned across the stenotic area and inflated under pressure. This results in fracture of the atherosclerotic plaque and disruption of the vessel intima. The vessel lumen can be successfully dilated in greater than 90% of cases. Because of the local vessel trauma, coronary artery dissection may result from angioplasty, and acute thrombosis complicates this procedure in 2% to 8% of cases. This complication can be a catastrophic event, resulting in acute myocardial infarction and the need for emergent CABG in approximately 4% and 3% of patients, respectively. In addition, repeat angiography demonstrates restenosis of the lesion in up to 40% to 50% of patients by 6 months after the procedure; however, clinical complications resulting from this process (i.e., recurrent ischemia) occur in less than one third of these patients. Restenosis is a complex process but involves elastic recoil of the artery, vascular remodeling, and hyperplasia of the vascular intima.

Developments with coronary stents have revolutionized interventional cardiology. A stent is a metallic mesh mounted on an angioplasty balloon and deployed at the lesion site by balloon inflation. The stent remains embedded in the arterial wall and results in a much larger vessel lumen than that attainable by balloon angioplasty (see Fig. 9–1). Stents can be used to treat procedure-related dissections, resulting in a decreased need for emergent CABG (<1%). Stents significantly decrease the rate of restenosis (20%) and can be used to treat atherosclerotic disease of bypass grafts. Other interventional techniques include rotational and directional atherectomy and coronary laser therapy. These techniques have a role in specific patients with long, calcified, or eccentric atherosclerotic plaques, although in most patients, balloon angioplasty with or without stenting results in satisfactory results.

Large studies performed in the 1970s established the effectiveness of CABG surgery both for control of anginal symptoms and, in some patients, for mortality benefit. The surgery involves the anastomosis of a segment of saphenous vein or radial artery to the ascending aorta with subsequent anastomosis of the distal aspect of the vascular graft to the diseased coronary artery distal to the stenosed segment. Anastomosis of the distal aspect of the internal mammary arteries to the affected coronary artery is also frequently employed. These procedures effectively bypass the occlusive atherosclerotic lesions, allowing blood to flow freely to the distal coronary arteries. Patients with greater degrees of symptoms, greater ischemic burden, and more severe angiographic coronary disease demonstrate the greatest benefit. Compared with medical therapy, surgery decreases mortality in patients with left main CAD and in patients with depressed left ventricular systolic function and either three-vessel CAD or two-vessel CAD with one of the stenoses being in the proximal left anterior descending

coronary artery. Most centers can perform CABG with a perioperative mortality of 1% to 2% and a perioperative myocardial infarction rate of less than 3%.

Both percutaneous and surgical revascularization techniques are superior to medical therapy for the treatment of anginal symptoms. As noted, CABG may also decrease mortality in a subset of these patients; this effect has not been convincingly shown with percutaneous procedures. The effectiveness of either modality is similar when employed in the setting of chronic stable angina or unstable angina; however, the risks and complications of both modalities are somewhat greater in patients with unstable angina. Surgery is more invasive and has a slightly higher periprocedural mortality rate, but it is also more effective for symptom control and requires fewer repeated procedures than does PTCA. There is no significant difference in cost between the two approaches when repeat procedures are taken into account.

In patients with a significant stenosis of the left main coronary artery (>50% luminal narrowing), percutaneous revascularization is currently not an option and surgery is warranted. This is also true for most patients with severe multivessel CAD and depressed left ventricular systolic function. In most patients with single-vessel disease, percutaneous revascularization is the modality of choice. Studies comparing the two approaches to revascularization in patients with multivessel disease and preserved ventricular function (ejection fraction, >50%) demonstrate no difference in mortality after 1 to 5 years of follow-up, except in diabetic patients who fare better with CABG. Thus, the approach to revascularization must be tailored to the individual patient.

Unfortunately, neither percutaneous nor surgical revascularization techniques halt the underlying atherosclerotic process, and progressive atherosclerosis occurs with new stenoses developing at previously uninvolved sites in both native coronary arteries and in bypass grafts. As many as 50% of saphenous vein grafts are occluded by 10 years after grafting. The rate is significantly lower with arterial conduits (left or right internal mammary artery or radial artery grafts). Aspirin used in the postoperative period and continued for at least 1 year may increase the rate of graft patency. If stenosis does develop in a bypass graft, PTCA or stenting is frequently effective, although restenosis rates are higher than for native vessels. Repeat bypass surgery is also possible, although the surgical risks are somewhat higher than with a first operation.

VARIANT ANGINA

In addition to fixed coronary stenoses, angina may also be precipitated by dynamic coronary obstruction. This is the result of coronary artery spasm, which may occur either at the site of an atherosclerotic plaque (Prinzmetal's angina) or in the setting of angiographically normal coronary arteries (pure vasospastic angina). The spasm tends to involve a proximal coronary artery but may be more diffuse. The clinical syndrome is similar to usual angina; however, patients describe the discomfort as a pain, and episodes tend to occur at rest, frequently in the morning hours, and are associated with profound, transient ST elevation on the ECG (Fig. 9–4). Marked ischemia may develop and may precipitate ventricular tachyarrhythmias and sudden cardiac death; however, progression to myocardial infarction is relatively uncommon. Patients may not have the usual cardiac risk factors, although smoking is frequent and cocaine use may precipitate an attack. During cardiac catheterization, coronary vasospasm may be provoked after intracoronary infusion of ergot alkaloids (ergonovine) or acetylcholine. Hyperventilation may also be used as a provocative test for coronary vasospasm with a sensitivity of more than 90%. Variant angina can be treated with vasodilators, specifically nitrates and vasodilating calcium channel blockers. Nonselective β blockers are contraindicated in true vasospastic angina because blockade of the vasodilatory effects of β_2-receptor stimulation may result in unopposed α-adrenergic vasoconstriction. Similarly, aspirin may exacerbate vasospastic angina by inhibiting the production of naturally occurring vasodilatory prostaglandins.

Pure vasospastic angina is unusual; most coronary vasospasm occurs at the site of a nonocclusive atherosclerotic plaque. Similarly, angina occurring as a result of pure, fixed, obstructive, atherosclerotic coronary artery disease is uncommon, because most stenotic atheromatous vessel segments manifest some degree of vasospastic response.

Acute Myocardial Infarction

Acute myocardial infarction (AMI) may initially be indistinguishable from angina. However, the chest discomfort is usually more severe; more prolonged (>30 minutes); frequently associated with dyspnea, nausea, and diaphoresis; and not relieved with rest or sublingual nitroglyc-

erin. The intensity of these symptoms varies greatly, and approximately 20% of AMIs may go undetected because the symptoms are mild, atypical, or absent altogether. These so-called silent infarctions may occur more commonly in patients with diabetes. Elderly patients frequently present with atypical symptoms and may not seek medical care until many hours after the onset of an AMI when they present with symptoms of heart failure. In patients with a history of angina, AMI is frequently preceded by accelerating or rest angina. Unusually heavy physical or emotional stress, as well as the physiologic stress of surgery, may precipitate AMI. A circadian pattern of AMIs has been noted, with the majority of infarctions occurring between the hours of 6 a.m. and noon. This pattern may relate to the normal morning increases in circulating catecholamines or increased platelet aggregability.

Unstable angina and AMI are two points in the spectrum of acute coronary syndromes. These syndromes reflect underlying atherosclerotic coronary disease complicated by acute plaque rupture and superimposed coronary thrombosis. If the thrombus significantly limits or completely occludes blood flow in the affected vessel, ischemia develops. If the blood flow is rapidly restored (<20 minutes) due to spontaneous clot lysis or resolution of associated vasospasm, then myocardial necrosis usually does not occur; this is the syndrome of unstable angina. If blood flow is not restored and ischemia persists for greater than approximately 20 minutes, necrosis of the myocardium supplied by the occluded artery begins and may progress to full-thickness (transmural) infarction within several hours unless reperfusion occurs; this is the syndrome of acute myocardial infarction.

The patient presenting with an AMI generally appears uncomfortable and distressed. The heart rate is frequently increased, owing to increased catecholamines or heart failure, although bradycardia may occur secondary to an increase in vagal tone or the development of

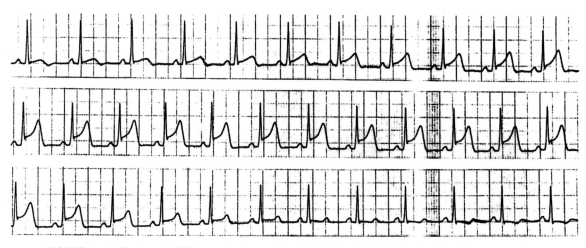

FIGURE 9–4 Continuous ECG recording in a patient with Prinzmetal's (variant) angina. Spontaneous onset of chest discomfort began during the *top strip* accompanied by transient ST segment elevation. By the *bottom strip* (several minutes later), both discomfort and ST elevation have resolved.

heart block (common with infarctions of the inferior ventricular wall). Blood pressure may also be mildly elevated. The cardiac examination may be normal, although an S_4 is frequently heard and reflects an ischemia-induced increase in myocardial stiffness. An apical murmur of mitral regurgitation may occur as a result of ischemia of the posterolateral papillary muscle. Evidence of pulmonary congestion is frequently present and may reflect elevated left ventricular filling pressure secondary to decreased myocardial compliance or may derive from acute or pre-existing systolic dysfunction. If a large area of myocardium is involved and significant systolic dysfunction is present, frank pulmonary edema may occur and a prominent S_3 may be heard. As with anginal syndromes, evidence of coexisting valvular and vascular disease is frequently present.

In patients presenting with chest pain, an ECG should be immediately obtained because it is frequently diagnostic in the setting of AMI, aids in determining appropriate treatment plans, and allows identification of associated rhythm or conduction abnormalities. AMIs can be divided into two groups on the basis of their associated ECG findings, a distinction that has both pathophysiologic and prognostic implications. Q wave myocardial infarction (previously referred to by the pathologically inaccurate term *transmural infarction*) refers to an AMI in which pathologic Q waves (>0.04 msec in duration and more than one-third the height of the associated R wave) develop on the surface ECG. These infarctions result from complete thrombotic occlusion of the coronary artery and may first be manifest on the ECG by symmetrically peaked (hyperacute) T waves. These peaked T waves resolve after several minutes as the characteristic ST segment elevation develops (Fig. 9–5; also see Fig. 5–5 and Table 5–3). Non–Q

wave myocardial infarctions (previously termed *subendocardial infarctions*) occur as a result of high-grade, but nonocclusive, thrombi and are an intermediate syndrome between unstable angina and Q wave myocardial infarctions. These infarctions are associated with ST segment depression and/or T wave inversions on the ECG and do not evolve pathologic Q waves (Fig. 9–6). Patients with Q wave myocardial infarctions in general have a larger area of myocardium at risk and have a higher in-hospital mortality rate than patients with non–Q wave infarctions; however, over the course of the year after an infarction, the mortality of non–Q wave infarctions increases, approaching that of Q wave infarctions. Despite the importance of ECG findings, the first ECG is nondiagnostic in about 50% of patients with AMI. The diagnostic yield increases significantly with serial ECGs. The echocardiogram may be helpful in such cases by demonstrating either normal or abnormal ventricular wall motion.

Myocardial necrosis results in myocyte disruption and the subsequent release of specific myocardial enzymes into the bloodstream. These can be measured by serial phlebotomy. The World Health Organization criteria for the diagnosis of an AMI mandate that at least two of the following three findings be present: ischemic-type chest discomfort, evolution of ECG changes, and a rise and fall in serum markers of myocyte necrosis. Because 20% of AMIs are clinically unapparent (silent) and initial ECGs are nondiagnostic in approximately 50% of cases of infarction, serologic identification of myocyte necrosis has become an important diagnostic tool. Several serum markers have been identified, each with a different pattern of rise after an AMI (Fig. 9–7). The MB isoenzyme of creatine kinase (CK-MB) begins to enter the blood stream within 4 to 8 hours after the

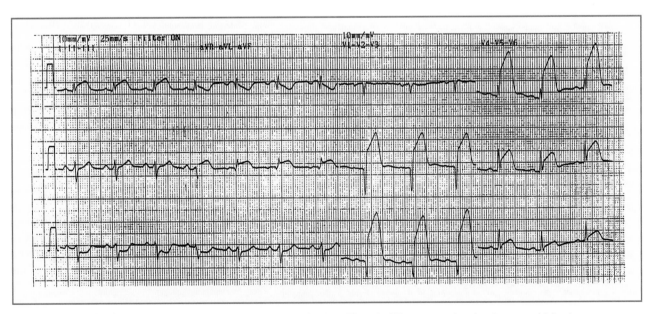

FIGURE 9–5 Acute anterolateral myocardial infarction. There is ST segment elevation (current of injury) across the precordial leads (V_2–V_6) and in leads I and aVL. Reciprocal ST segment depression is seen in the inferior leads (leads II, III, and aVF). Deep Q waves have developed in leads V_2 and V_3.

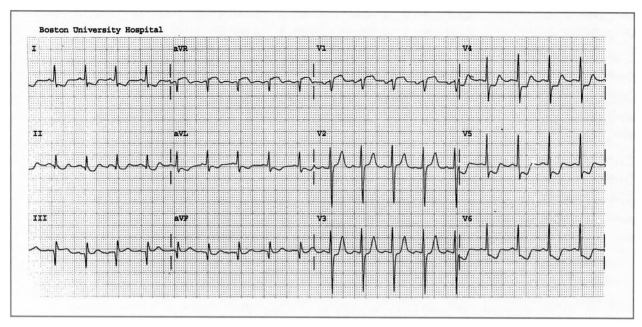

Boston University Hospital

FIGURE 9–6 Marked ST segment depression in a patient with prolonged chest pain due to an acute non–Q wave myocardial infarction. One to 3 mm of ST segment depression is seen in leads V_4 to V_6 and in leads I and aVL. The patient was known to have had a prior Q wave inferior myocardial infarction.

onset of an AMI. The level usually peaks at about 24 hours and returns to normal within several days. The CK-MB is relatively specific for cardiac injury; however, it may also be elevated in other settings, including after

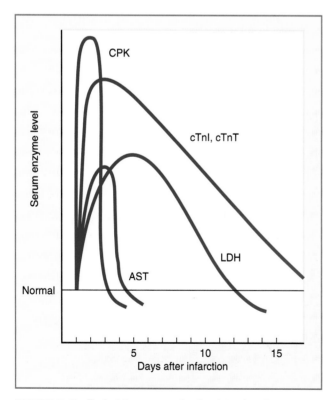

FIGURE 9–7 Typical time course for the detection of enzymes released after myocardial infarction. AST = serum aspartate aminotransferase; CPK = creatine kinase; cTnI = cardiac troponin I; cTnT = cardiac troponin T; LDH = lactate dehydrogenase.

significant skeletal muscle injury, following vigorous exercise, and with pulmonary embolism. Cardiac isoforms of serum lactate dehydrogenase and aspartate aminotransferase have also been used to diagnose AMI; however, these enzyme measurements have been supplanted by the development of tests for cardiac troponins.

Troponins are a complex of proteins that regulate the calcium-mediated actin-myosin interaction in muscle. Troponin C binds calcium, troponin T binds to tropomyosin, and troponin I binds to the actin filament and inhibits its interaction with myosin. These proteins are found in both cardiac and skeletal muscle, and exist in several isoforms depending on their tissue of origin. These different forms can be detected by specific antibody-based assays. Because these proteins are not detected in blood under usual circumstances, even small amounts of myocardial necrosis will produce a positive test. Assays measuring cardiac troponin T or I (cTnT or cTnI) have been developed. These isoforms begin to rise in peripheral blood within 3 to 4 hours after the onset of an AMI, and reach 95% to 99% sensitivity and specificity by 10 hours. Furthermore, they remain detectable for 10 to 14 days after the acute event, allowing for the diagnosis of AMI even more than a week after its onset. Through use of this assay, many patients who previously would have been diagnosed with unstable angina are now identified as having had a small myocardial infarction. These patients appear to have a worse prognosis than similar patients with unstable angina but without an increase in serum troponin.

TREATMENT OF ACUTE MYOCARDIAL INFARCTION

The importance of time in the treatment of AMI cannot be overemphasized because the extent of the infarcted myocardium increases with increased duration of coronary artery occlusion. The highest rate of mortality occurs in the first hours after onset of an infarction, and most deaths are arrhythmic in origin. The most important delay in treatment results from patient denial of the symptoms or failure to recognize the symptoms, leading to significant delays in seeking medical care. Over 50% of all deaths from AMI occur before hospital presentation. Educating the general population in this regard has the potential to modify the mortality of this disease. The institution of medical therapy in the field by trained emergency medical personnel capable of identifying and treating life-threatening arrhythmias improves the survival of patients with AMI.

Initial hospital care involves establishing the diagnosis of AMI (usually by identifying the presence of characteristic changes on a 12-lead ECG) and instituting therapy aimed at decreasing ischemia, controlling hemodynamic instability, and relieving symptoms. All patients should be placed on continuous ECG monitoring to allow identification and early treatment of malignant arrhythmias. Those patients who are not already on aspirin therapy should be given soluble aspirin to chew (160 to 325 mg), an intervention that significantly reduces mortality. Supplemental oxygen should be administered, as should sublingual nitroglycerin, provided hypotension is not present. Physical activity should be limited during the first 12 to 24 hours, and stool softeners should be instituted to prevent constipation and excessive straining. Liberal use of intravenous morphine (2 to 4 mg as needed) is appropriate for the adequate control of pain and anxiety. Intravenous infusion of nitroglycerin is frequently required to treat persistent ischemia and also may be effective in treating acute hypertension and ischemic pulmonary edema.

Patients who present with an AMI are frequently tachycardic and hypertensive as a response to increased sympathetic tone, which further increases the myocardial oxygen demand and exacerbates the ischemic process. This situation is frequently improved by adequate analgesia alone; however, persistent elevation of the heart rate should be treated with intravenous β blockers unless hypotension, significant pulmonary congestion, or

significant conduction disease is present. Bradycardia is occasionally present (most commonly with inferior myocardial infarctions) and results from enhanced vagal tone and/or sinus node ischemia. If the bradycardia is symptomatic, atropine (0.5 mg IV) should be administered. Patients who present with mild pulmonary congestion are frequently not volume overloaded; in fact, owing to their tachypnea and diaphoresis, they may be somewhat volume depleted. Care must be taken in the management of such patents because aggressive treatment with diuretics may precipitate hypotension. Frequently, simply treating the ischemia will resolve the pulmonary congestion. Although prophylactic treatment with antiarrhythmic agents is not indicated, they should be rapidly available if significant arrhythmias develop.

Reperfusion Therapy

The management of the patient with an ST elevation type of acute myocardial infarction has been revolutionized by the development of modalities to reestablish blood flow in the occluded culprit coronary artery, specifically thrombolytic therapy and percutaneous revascularization. Perhaps the most important component of the initial evaluation of these patients is identifying those who are candidates for these reperfusion therapies. Timely restoration of blood flow has been definitively proven to decrease the mortality associated with an AMI.

The goal of thrombolytic therapy is to lyse occlusive coronary thrombi and, thus, reinstate adequate coronary blood flow (Fig. 9–8). Eligibility for thrombolytic therapy requires that the patient have ischemic-type chest pain, show ECG evidence of an acute infarction (ST elevation), and have no contraindication to thrombolysis (Tables 9–6 and 9–7). Randomized trials have also shown benefit in patients presenting with ischemic chest pain and a left bundle branch block pattern on the ECG. Patients with non–ST segment elevation AMIs or with unstable angina do not appear to benefit from thrombolytic therapy and, in fact, may have a higher mortality with thrombolysis. Time is a primary consideration in determining the appropriateness of thrombolytic

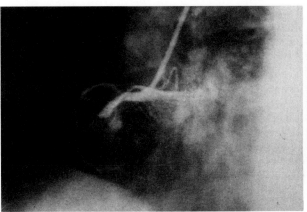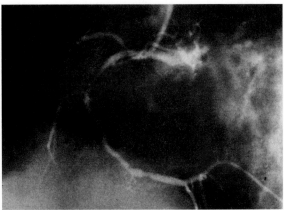

FIGURE 9–8   Right coronary artery angiogram in a patient with acute inferior myocardial infarction. The *left panel* demonstrates total obstruction of the right coronary artery. The *right panel* depicts restoration of flow 90 minutes after the intravenous administration of tissue-type plasminogen activator.

TABLE 9-6 Selection Criteria for Thrombolytic Therapy in Acute Myocardial Infarction

1. Chest pain consistent with acute myocardial infarction
2. ECG changes:
   ST segment elevation $\geq$1 mm in two or more contiguous limb leads or $\geq$2 mm in two or more contiguous precordial leads
   New or presumed new left bundle branch block
   ST segment depression with prominent R wave in leads V_2–V_3 *if* believed to represent posterior infarction
3. Time from onset of symptoms:
   <6 hours: most beneficial
   6–12 hours: less benefit but worthwhile if continued ischemic pain
   >12 hours: little apparent benefit unless "stuttering" course with ongoing chest pain
4. Age—"physiologic" age more important than chronologic age:
   <75 years: definite benefit
   >75 years: benefit less clear cut

TABLE 9-7 Contraindications for Thrombolytic Therapy in Acute Myocardial Infarction

Absolute

Aortic dissection
Acute pericarditis
Any active bleeding*
Previous cerebral hemorrhage
Intracranial neoplasm
Cerebral aneurysm or arteriovenous malformation

Relative

Bleeding diathesis/coagulopathy
Major surgery, puncture of a noncompressible vessel, head or major body trauma within 2–4 weeks
Nonhemorrhagic stroke or gastrointestinal hemorrhage within 6 months
Proliferative retinopathy
Severe uncontrolled hypertension (SBP > 180 mm Hg, DBP > 95 mm Hg)
Prolonged cardiopulmonary resuscitation
Pregnancy

* Does not include menstrual bleeding.

therapy. Patients presenting within 6 hours of symptom onset have a clear benefit with treatment, and the benefit is greater the earlier they are treated. Patients presenting 6 to 12 hours after symptom onset may benefit, especially if a stuttering pattern of chest pain has been present and ongoing ischemia is suspected. After 12 hours, there is no clear benefit of thrombolytic therapy.

Contraindications to thrombolytic therapy are listed in Table 9–7 and identify patients who have an unacceptably high risk of bleeding complications. The most important potential complication of thrombolysis is intracranial hemorrhage. This risk is significantly increased in patients with a prior history of hemorrhagic stroke, uncontrolled hypertension, body weight less than 70 kg, and advanced age (>65 years). The risk varies among different thrombolytic agents, being somewhat higher with tissue-type plasminogen activator than with streptokinase, and may increase slightly with the concomitant use of anticoagulants. The overall incidence of intracranial hemorrhage after thrombolysis is 0.5%. Age is not a contraindication to thrombolytic therapy; although very elderly patients (age, >75 years) have a higher risk of intracranial hemorrhage with thrombolytic therapy, they also have a very high mortality risk from an AMI.

Several thrombolytic agents have been approved for use in AMI, including streptokinase (SK) and tissue-type plasminogen activator (tPA) (Table 9–8). Anisoylated plasminogen-streptokinase activator complex (APSAC) is also available, as are several newer tPA-like agents, although these are less frequently used. Although slight differences in their effectiveness and bleeding complications have been reported, the particular choice of agent is much less important than the timely decision to administer a thrombolytic. Streptokinase can result in acute allergic reactions and is frequently associated with mild hypotension, although rarely significant enough to warrant interruption of the infusion. Antibodies to SK

develop within days of administration; therefore, SK should not be given to patients who have previously received it. Tissue-type plasminogen activator is significantly more expensive than SK and is associated with a higher rate of intracranial hemorrhage (0.7% vs 0.5%); however, it is also more clot specific and is not associated with a generalized lytic state.

Overall, thrombolytic therapy decreases the rate of mortality from AMI by about 22%. Angiographic studies comparing thrombolytic regimens have demonstrated that restoration of blood flow in the culprit artery is faster and more complete with tPA than with SK, and this appears to translate into a decreased mortality rate with tPA, especially when it is given as a "front-loaded"

TABLE 9-8 Accelerated (Front-Loaded) Tissue-Type Plasminogen Activator and Streptokinase Regimens Utilizing Intravenous Heparin as Tested in the GUSTO Trial

Streptokinase (SK)	Tissue-Type Plasminogen Activator (tPA)
Aspirin $\geq$160 mg	Aspirin $\geq$160 mg
SK: 1.5 million units IV over 60 min	tPA: 15-mg bolus IV, followed by 0.75 mg/kg body weight (not to exceed 50 mg) over 30 min, followed by 0.5 mg/kg (not to exceed 35 mg) over 60 min
Heparin 5000-unit bolus IV, then 1000 units/hr*	Heparin 5000-unit bolus IV, then 1000 units/hr*

* Adjusted by PTT determinations.
IV = intravenous.

regimen consisting of an initial bolus followed by infusion therapy. In the landmark GUSTO trial, tPA produced a significant 1% absolute mortality reduction when compared with SK. The majority of this benefit occurred in younger patients (<70 years of age) presenting within 4 hours of the onset of an anterior infarction. In older patients, patients presenting more than 4 hours after symptom onset, and with infarctions in territories other than the anterior wall, the difference between thrombolytic agents is minimal.

Aspirin therapy is an obligatory adjuvant to thrombolysis irrespective of the thrombolytic agent used and demonstrates an additive benefit on mortality as well as a decrease in recurrent ischemic events. Intravenous heparin therapy (administered for 48 hours) has been demonstrated to maintain patency of the effected coronary artery after thrombolysis with tPA, but similar benefits of heparin have not been demonstrated with other agents. Heparin may also increase the risk of bleeding complications.

The use of percutaneous revascularization techniques as the primary modality for establishing coronary reperfusion in patients with AMI (primary angioplasty) has gained increased acceptance. This approach has the highest probability of establishing normal coronary blood flow, and has been shown in several studies to decrease recurrent ischemic events and possibly decrease mortality in comparison with thrombolytic therapy for AMI. However, these results are likely reproducible only in centers where the procedure can be performed promptly and with highly experienced staff. In hospitals without on-site angioplasty facilities, the time inherent in transferring a patient to another institution for primary PTCA results in unacceptable delays in attaining coronary reperfusion; thus, in this setting, thrombolytic therapy should be used. Primary PTCA plays an important role in patients with contraindications to thrombolysis and appears particularly beneficial in patients with cardiogenic shock. Patients who fail to show improvement after thrombolytic therapy or who have recurrent ischemia after initial successful thrombolysis are also candidates for percutaneous revascularization. The use of glycoprotein IIb/IIIa inhibitors (i.e., abciximab) to block platelet aggregation may decrease the rate of ischemic complications after primary percutaneous revascularization procedures for AMI.

Additional Therapies

The patient with an ST elevation AMI should receive early treatment with intravenous β blockers (metoprolol, 5 mg every 5 minutes for a total dose of 15 mg, as tolerated), followed by oral therapy, provided that no contraindication exists. Such treatment decreases mortality in this population. Calcium channel blockers do not have a clear role in the management of patients with ST elevation AMIs and should be used with extreme care in patients with depressed ventricular function. Short-acting nifedipine preparations are contraindicated, owing to reflex tachycardia and increased mortality associated with their use in this setting. Angiotensin-converting enzyme inhibitors substantially decrease the mortality of

AMI and should be instituted early in the postinfarction period unless contraindications exist. Nitrates do not clearly alter mortality in patients with AMI; nonetheless, intravenous nitroglycerin is a reasonable therapy for patients with ongoing ischemia and/or pulmonary congestion.

Treatment of Non–ST Segment Elevation Myocardial Infarction

Patients with a non–Q wave myocardial infarction in general do not have total occlusion of the infarct-related coronary artery. Thrombolytic therapy has not been shown to be of benefit in these patients and in several studies has been associated with a higher mortality. Medical management is otherwise similar to that with Q wave infarctions and involves aspirin, β blockers, nitrates, oxygen, and analgesia. Oral diltiazem may decrease the risk of reinfarction in patients with preserved ventricular function, but as with AMIs with ST segment elevation, the routine use of calcium channel blocking agents in patients with depressed ventricular function is not recommended. Angiotensin-converting enzyme inhibitors are indicated in patients with depressed ventricular function. Intravenous heparin had been shown in the prethrombolytic era to decrease the mortality of AMI and should be administered to patients who are not candidates for reperfusion therapy, as well as to patients who are at a high risk of thromboembolic complications (e.g., patients with atrial fibrillation, intraventricular thrombus, or large anterior infarctions).

Patients with non–Q wave myocardial infarction have smaller infarctions and lower in-hospital mortality rates than do patients with Q wave myocardial infarction. Despite this, the mortality at 1 year after infarction is no different and relates to a higher rate of recurrent infarction in the non–Q wave group. Non–Q wave events may thus be viewed as an incomplete infarction. Because of the increased risk of recurrent infarction in these patients, aggressive approaches to treatment have frequently been applied with early catheterization and consideration of percutaneous or surgical revascularization. Data from studies in the 1990s, however, suggest that a more conservative approach with aggressive medical therapy and risk stratification with noninvasive modalities may be an equally effective, and perhaps safer, approach to these patients.

COMPLICATIONS

Arrhythmias and Conduction Abnormalities

Most complications of AMI can be divided into structural, mechanical, or electrical problems (Table 9–9). Cardiac arrhythmias are frequent occurrences in AMI and may be asymptomatic or result in profound hemodynamic compromise. Symptomatic arrhythmias always warrant treatment, whereas asymptomatic arrhythmias can frequently be managed conservatively. Most of these arrhythmias are a direct result of the ischemic process; however, other reversible aggravating factors such as

TABLE 9-9   Complications of Acute Myocardial Infarction

Mechanical
Left ventricular failure
Right ventricular failure
Cardiogenic shock

Structural
Free wall rupture
Ventricular septal defect
Papillary muscle rupture with acute mitral regurgitation

Electrical
Arrhythmias
  Bradyarrhythmias
  Ventricular ectopy
  Tachyarrhythmias (ventricular, supraventricular)
  Sudden cardiac death
Conduction abnormalities
  First-, second-, and third-degree heart block
  Bundle branch and fascicular blocks

Other
Pericarditis, Dressler's syndrome

electrolyte disturbances, hypoxemia, and medication toxicity must be excluded.

Premature ventricular complexes, ventricular couplets, and short runs of nonsustained ventricular tachycardia (NSVT) have an increased incidence in the peri-infarction period. Such ectopy can effectively be suppressed with antiarrhythmic agents; however, in the absence of symptoms, treatment does not appear to be justified. The presence of frequent ventricular ectopy does not predict the development of more malignant arrhythmias, and empirical antiarrhythmic therapy is associated with a higher mortality rate. Accelerated idioventricular rhythms ("slow VT") frequently occur after successful coronary reperfusion and also do not require specific treatment.

Most deaths from AMI are arrhythmic and result from sustained ventricular tachycardia (VT) or ventricular fibrillation. A significant proportion of the decreased mortality from AMI seen in the past two decades has resulted from the development of continuous cardiac monitoring and effective therapies for ventricular tachyarrhythmias. Ventricular fibrillation and hemodynamically unstable VT should be treated with immediate electrical defibrillation (200 to 360 joules), after which it is reasonable to administer intravenous antiarrhythmic medications (e.g., lidocaine, procainamide) for 6 to 24 hours. Sustained, hemodynamically stable VT can be treated first with antiarrhythmic agents, with electrical cardioversion reserved for persistent arrhythmias. Recurrent VT refractory to usual antiarrhythmics and cardioversion may respond to intravenous amiodarone. Polymorphic VT is usually a marker of recurrent or persistent ischemia, and aggressive anti-ischemic treatment is warranted. When sustained VT or ventricular fibrillation occurs in the first 48 hours after an AMI, it does not portend the same poor prognosis as it does

when it occurs later in the post-AMI period. Transient supraventricular tachyarrhythmias occur in approximately one third of patients with an AMI; atrial fibrillation accounts for almost one half of these common arrhythmias. The rapid heart rate may exacerbate ischemia and precipitate hemodynamic compromise. Prompt electrical cardioversion is indicated in such cases. β blockers are usually effective for controlling the rate of atrial fibrillation, provided there is no contraindication to their use. Calcium channel–blocking agents are also effective but should be avoided in patients with heart failure. These arrhythmias are discussed at length in Chapter 10.

Bradyarrhythmias also frequently complicate AMI. Sinus bradycardia occurring in the first 4 to 6 hours after AMI usually results from the stimulation of cardiac vagal efferent receptors or is a result of medications. Sinus bradycardia occurring more than 6 hours after the onset of an AMI is usually a manifestation of sinus node dysfunction or atrial ischemia and is frequently transient. Unless accompanied by hemodynamic instability or malignant ventricular escape rhythms, sinus bradycardia should simply be observed. If treatment is necessary, intravenous atropine should be administered, aiming for a heart rate of about 60 beats/min and resolution of symptoms. Temporary pacing is rarely required.

Ischemia and infarction can result in injury to the conduction system, thus producing various degrees of heart block. Ischemia of the AV node can result in first-degree heart block and Mobitz I second-degree heart block (Wenckebach). These rhythms are most commonly associated with inferior myocardial infarction and do not appear to affect survival. Mobitz II second-degree heart block is a rare complication of AMI (<1% of cases of AMI) and usually results from injury to the His-Purkinje system in the setting of extensive anterior myocardial infarction. It has a significant rate of progression to complete (third degree) heart block and is an indication for temporary transvenous or transcutaneous pacing. Complete heart block occurs in 5% to 15% of AMI, and, owing to the dual blood supply to the conduction system (from left anterior descending and right coronary artery septal branches), may occur with either inferior or anterior infarction. When it occurs in the setting of an inferior MI, the block is usually at the level of the AV node, is associated with stable escape rhythms, and tends to be transient (several days). When associated with an anterior infarction, the His-Purkinje system is usually involved, there are frequently unstable ventricular escape rhythms, and the mortality is high. Block in one or more branches of the conduction system (e.g., left anterior or posterior fascicular block, right or left bundle branch block) occurs in 5% to 10% of AMI and is more common with anterior than with inferior infarction. First-degree heart block and Wenckebach block rarely require therapy; however, when they are associated with symptomatic bradycardia, administration of intravenous atropine is warranted. Pacing is almost never required. Similarly, patients with isolated left anterior or posterior fascicular block (LAFB, LPFB) or right bundle branch block (RBBB) do not require specific therapy. Temporary pacing is suggested in patients with new bifascicular blocks (e.g., LBBB, or RBBB with either

LAFB or LPFB), Mobitz II second-degree heart block, and complete heart block.

Pump Failure

Patients with anterior AMI are frequently hemodynamically unstable with systemic hypotension, pulmonary congestion, or both. In patients with isolated hypotension in the absence of pulmonary congestion, hypovolemia and medication effects must be excluded. Careful fluid administration may lead to substantial improvement. The development of pulmonary congestion indicates a poorer prognosis. Isolated congestion in the absence of hypotension may relate to decreased ventricular compliance or systolic ventricular dysfunction and responds to treatment with vasodilators (nitroglycerin) and diuretics. Patients with both hypotension and pulmonary congestion frequently require treatment with inotropic agents (dopamine, dobutamine) and vasodilators in an attempt to augment cardiac output and unload the heart. Cardiogenic shock is defined by the presence of increased ventricular filling pressures, decreased cardiac output, systemic hypotension, and vital organ hypoperfusion (e.g., confusion, oliguria, cool extremities). These patients usually have large infarcts involving greater than 40% of the left ventricle and have a mortality rate in excess of 70%. Inotropic agents and vasodilators may be effective; however, these patients frequently require placement of an intra-aortic balloon pump for stabilization, although this therapy has not yet been shown to improve survival. Studies suggest that patients with cardiogenic shock may benefit from acute PTCA, possibly reducing mortality by 20% to 50%. Thrombolysis may be relatively ineffective in these patients because the decreased coronary perfusion pressure results in inadequate delivery of the thrombolytic agent to the site of coronary occlusion.

Because of the difficulties in managing patients with severe heart failure, hemodynamic monitoring with a right-sided balloon-tipped catheter (Swan-Ganz catheter) is frequently employed. The left-sided heart filling pressure (pulmonary capillary wedge pressure), central venous pressure, cardiac output, and systemic vascular resistance can be determined and used to guide therapy (normal pressures are shown in Table 3–1). Owing to the increased stiffness of ischemic myocardium, the ideal pulmonary capillary wedge pressure in patients with an AMI is higher than normal, usually in the range of 16 to 20 mm Hg. Pressures higher than this are associated with pulmonary edema. The Swan-Ganz catheter may also be useful in identifying mechanical complications of AMI (see later).

Right Ventricular Infarction

Inferior myocardial infarctions are frequently associated with right ventricular infarctions because the blood supply to both these territories is derived from the right coronary artery. Isolated right ventricular infarctions are rare. Right ventricular infarctions result in the clinical picture of hypotension, clear lungs (normal pulmonary capillary wedge pressure), and elevated jugular venous

pressure (high right-sided heart pressure). In the absence of hemodynamic measurements, right ventricular infarction may be confused with hypovolemia or acute pulmonary edema. Acute right ventricular failure may be associated with a prominent y descent in the atrial pressure tracing (Fig. 9–9), a positive Kussmaul's sign, and an increased paradoxical pulse, all mimicking pericardial disease. The presence of a right ventricular infarction complicating an inferior myocardial infarction places the patient in a much higher mortality group. The diagnosis of right ventricular infarction can be made by demonstrating ST segment elevation in the right precordial leads (greater than 0.1 mm of elevation in V_4R). For this reason, right-sided ECG leads should be obtained in all patients with inferior infarctions. The treatment of hypotension in patients with right ventricular infarction often requires excessive volume repletion as well as inotropic agents (dobutamine). Diuretic and vasodilator therapy may provoke hypotension. Over time, right ventricular function often improves, possibly related to the protective effects of the thebesian circulation.

Mechanical Complications

Mechanical complications of an AMI include papillary muscle rupture, ventricular septal defect (VSD), and

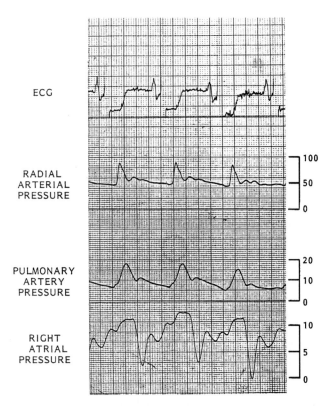

FIGURE 9–9 Electrocardiogram (ECG), arterial, and Swan-Ganz bedside catheter recordings in a patient with right ventricular infarction. Hypotension is present, and cardiac output estimated by thermodilution (not shown) is reduced. The pulmonary artery pressures are normal. There is elevation of the right atrial pressure with a prominent y descent.

ventricular free wall rupture. Patients with these complications frequently present with hemodynamic collapse. Papillary muscle rupture results in acute mitral regurgitation. The sudden increase in volume in the left atrium results in a marked increased in left atrial pressure, resulting in acute pulmonary edema. Because of its single blood supply from the RCA, the posteromedial papillary muscle is more commonly involved than the anterolateral papillary muscle, and this event usually occurs in the setting of an inferior myocardial infarction. A loud, apical holosystolic murmur may be heard but becomes faint as hypotension ensues. The diagnosis may be suggested by the presence of large v waves in the pulmonary capillary wedge tracing. Echocardiography is diagnostic of this complication. Development of an acute VSD may complicate both anterior and inferior infarctions. It is usually heralded by the appearance of a new, harsh systolic murmur at the left lower sternal border and may be difficult to differentiate from acute mitral regurgitation. The diagnosis can be confirmed by detecting an increase ("step-up") in oxygen saturation of the blood from the right atrium to the right ventricle, reflecting shunting of oxygenated blood from the left to the right ventricle. Doppler echocardiography allows visualization of the abnormal flow. Both an acute VSD and papillary muscle rupture can result in cardiogenic shock. Treatment includes inotropic agents, vasodilators, and intra-aortic balloon pump counterpulsation. These in general are temporizing measures while preparing the patient for emergency cardiac surgery to repair the VSD or ruptured papillary muscle. Free wall rupture of the left ventricle results in hemopericardium, cardiac tamponade, and electromechanical dissociation. Survival is uncommon and depends on prompt recognition and surgical repair. These mechanical complications of AMI most commonly occur between 3 and 5 days after the acute event, are associated with very high mortality rates, and, as a group, account for approximately 15% of mortality from AMI. Thrombolytic therapy appears to hasten the appearance of these complications but does not clearly increase their incidence.

A pseudoaneurysm (or false aneurysm) develops when a free wall rupture occurs but is sealed over by the pericardium and the development of organized thrombus and hematoma. Over time, this area bulges outward, maintaining continuity with the left ventricular cavity through a narrow neck. The wall of the pseudoaneurysm contains no myocardium, only pericardium, and can potentially rupture. In contrast, a true aneurysm represents an area of infarcted myocardium that has become thinned and dilated through a process of ventricular remodeling. Angiotensin-converting enzyme inhibitors and early reperfusion limit this remodeling process and, thus, may limit aneurysm formation. True aneurysms have a wide base, their walls always contain some myocardial elements, and they rarely rupture. Both true and false aneurysms frequently contain thrombus and are a potential source of systemic emboli. Mural thrombi develop in almost half of patients with anterior apical Q wave AMI, even in the absence of aneurysm formation. Anticoagulation of these patients with intravenous heparin followed by oral warfarin for 3 to 6 months reduces the risk of embolic events.

Transmural myocardial infarction causes localized pericardial irritation, and the resultant pericardial friction rub is a common occurrence in the peri-infarction period. Similarly, echocardiography detects pericardial effusions in nearly 25% of post-MI patients. The majority of these patients do not develop symptoms of pericarditis, and tamponade is distinctly rare. Occasionally, pericardial pain does occur and can be confused with recurrent ischemic chest pain. Dressler's syndrome comprises an inflammatory, probably immunologic, pericarditis associated with systemic symptoms such as fevers and malaise, and with leukocytosis and elevated erythrocyte sedimentation rate on laboratory examination. It is relatively uncommon and develops 1 to 2 months after an AMI. High-dose aspirin is the optimal therapy. Corticosteroids and nonsteroidal anti-inflammatory agents are relatively contraindicated in the first month after an AMI, owing to their interference with myocardial healing.

POSTINFARCTION MANAGEMENT

In patients who survive an AMI, prolonged bed rest may be detrimental and early ambulation is encouraged. Activity is progressively increased after the first 24 to 36 hours, usually under the guidance of a structured, stepwise cardiac rehabilitation program. After an uncomplicated AMI, patients may be ready to be discharged home after 4 to 7 days. Before discharge, a submaximal exercise test should be performed to identify patients at high risk of recurrent ischemic events. These patients should be considered for cardiac catheterization and revascularization. Aggressive risk factor modification should be pursued, with lipid-lowering therapy instituted when appropriate and counseling of patients with regard to dietary changes, smoking cessation, and medication compliance. After discharge, patients may gradually increase their activity levels over the course of several weeks. A standard, symptom-limited exercise test is generally obtained at 4 to 6 weeks after an AMI to evaluate exercise capacity, effectiveness of medications, and ischemic threshold. Enrollment in a formal cardiac rehabilitation program may be beneficial for many patients, not only by incorporating exercise into their daily activities but also by monitoring patients for early signs of recurrent ischemia, by providing information regarding risk factor modification, and by providing emotional support for patients during the recovery phase of their illness.

REFERENCES

ACC/AHA guidelines for the management of patients with acute myocardial infarction. J Am Coll Cardiol 1996; 28:1328–1428.

ACC/AHA guidelines for coronary angiography. J Am Coll Cardiol 1987; 10:935–950.

ACC/AHA guidelines for percutaneous transluminal coronary angioplasty. Circulation 1993; 88:2988–3007.

ACC/AHA guidelines and indications for coronary bypass surgery. J Am Coll Cardiol 1991; 17:543–589.

AHCPR Clinical Practice Guidelines: Unstable angina: Diagnosis and treatment. Bethesda, MD: U.S. Public Health Service, 1994.

Fibrinolytic Therapy Trialists Collaborative Group: Indications for fibrinolytic therapy in suspected acute myocardial infarction. Lancet 1994; 343:311–321.

Fuster V, Badiman L, Badiman JJ, Chesebro JH: The pathogenesis of coronary artery disease and the acute coronary syndromes: I and II. N Engl J Med 1992; 326:242–250, 310–318.

GUSTO Investigators: An international randomized trial comparing four thrombolytic strategies for acute myocardial infarction. N Engl J Med 1993; 329:673–682.

10

CARDIAC ARRHYTHMIAS

Eric H. Awtry • Joseph Loscalzo

The myocyte cellular membrane (sarcolemma) is a phospholipid bilayer that contains multiple channels allowing for the selective movement of charged particles (ions) into or out of the cell. The electrical gradients and ionic currents thus produced result in the maintenance of a resting electrical potential across the cellular membrane and the production of an action potential in response to the electrical depolarization of the cell. Within cardiac tissue, the depolarization is rapidly propagated from cell to cell with the aid of specialized intercellular connections (intercalated discs). Specialized cells in the heart promote the generation and regulation of electrical impulses and the rapid conduction of these impulses to the myocardium, thus allowing the millions of cardiac cells to function as a single, organized, synchronous unit. Abnormalities anywhere within this system may result in the abnormal generation or propagation of electrical impulses, resulting in abnormal cardiac rhythms (arrhythmias) or abnormal electrical conduction (heart block). Advances in the understanding of the genesis of these disorders have spurred the development of more effective pharmacologic and nonpharmacologic therapies.

Mechanisms of Arrhythmogenesis

THE CARDIAC ACTION POTENTIAL AND NORMAL CARDIAC CONDUCTION

The electrical activity of a single cardiac cell can be recorded with the aid of a microelectrode and demonstrates that the resting potential of a myocyte is -80 to -90 mV. This resting potential is maintained by the accumulation of potassium inside the cell and the removal of sodium from the cell by the energy-requiring Na^+,K^+-ATPase. When a myocyte is depolarized to a certain threshold level (threshold potential), an action potential is produced as a result of a complex series of ionic shifts (Fig. 10–1A). The action potential can be divided into five phases. Phase 0 is the rapid initial depolarization and is mediated by an increased permeability of the sarcolemma to sodium ions. This is followed by phase 1, an early, rapid, repolarization resulting from the movement of potassium out of the cell. The plateau phase (phase 2) of the action potential is mainly determined by the inward movement of calcium ions, but also by the movement of sodium, chloride, and potassium ions. Phase 3 constitutes the repolarization phase of the action potential and is the result of the movement of potassium ions out of the cell. Phase 4 of the action potential represents the outward flow of potassium and the inward flow of sodium and results in the gradual depolarization of the cell from resting to threshold potential (see Fig. 10–1B). During the action potential and shortly thereafter there is a period of time during which an adequate depolarizing stimulus fails to elicit an action potential. This is termed the *absolute refractory period* and is most closely related to the duration of phase 3 of the action potential.

The appearance of the action potential of sinus and atrioventricular (AV) nodal cells is different from that of the typical myocyte. The normal resting potential of these cells is higher (-60 mV), the initial upstroke of depolarization is slower and calcium dependent, and the phase 4 depolarization is much more pronounced. The slope of the phase 4 depolarization determines the rate at which a cell will spontaneously depolarize (automaticity) until it reaches threshold potential, thus generating an action potential that is then propagated to surrounding cells. The sinus node usually has the fastest phase 4 depolarization and thus functions as the normal pacemaker of the heart, producing a rate of contraction (heart rate) of 60 to 100 beats/min. If the sinus node fails, the AV node has the next fastest pacemaker rate (approximately 50 beats/min). The ventricular myocytes have slow phase 4 depolarization and produce a heart rate of 30 to 40 beats/min if higher pacemakers fail. When a lower pacemaker focus appropriately fires in the setting of slowing of the higher focus, the firing is termed an *escape beat* (if single) or an *escape rhythm* (if sustained).

The autonomic nervous system has important effects on the generation and propagation of cardiac impulses.

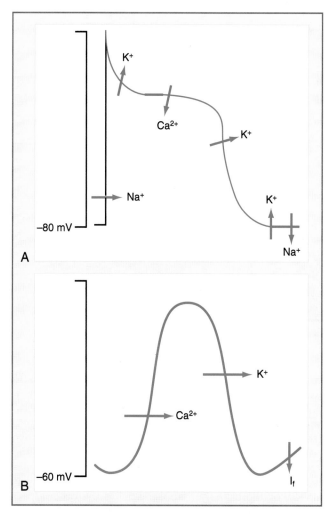

FIGURE 10-1 Genesis of the cardiac action potential. *A*, Ventricular action potential with predominant ionic currents. *B*, Sinus node action potential with predominant ionic currents. See text for details. Ca^{2+} = calcium; K^+ = potassium; Na^+ = sodium; I_f = hyperpolarization-activated current; mV = millivolt.

The sinus and AV nodes are the most richly innervated regions of the heart and are most affected by changes in autonomic tone. Sympathetic stimulation, either directly from sympathetic nerve endings in the heart or indirectly by means of circulating catecholamines, increases the heart rate by increasing the rate of phase 4 depolarization and also increases intercellular conduction velocity. Parasympathetic stimulation has the opposite effects. Vagal tone is, in part, controlled by the baroreceptors of the carotid sinus, which are located at the bifurcation of the internal and external carotid arteries and respond to increases in blood pressure by increasing vagal output, with a resulting decrease in heart rate and AV nodal conduction velocity.

The normal cardiac impulse starts at the sinoatrial node, passes through the atria to the AV node where it slows, and then continues down the His-Purkinje system to the ventricular myocardium, where the wave of depolarization terminates because there is no further tissue to depolarize. Further conduction occurs only after a new impulse is formed in the sinoatrial node.

GENERATION OF ABNORMAL RHYTHMS

Although the exact mechanism of a given arrhythmia may not be known, most arrhythmias can be described as either abnormalities of impulse formation or abnormalities of impulse conduction (Table 10–1). Abnormalities of impulse formation result in an inappropriately fast firing rate of either the normal sinus pacemaker cells or an ectopic pacemaker focus. This may occur in the absence of a specific stimulus, but more frequently it occurs in the setting of ischemic or otherwise diseased myocardium and is likely the result of increased phase 4 depolarization (increased automaticity). Singular premature atrial or ventricular depolarizations may arise by this mechanism. Some sustained rhythms, including ectopic atrial tachycardia, accelerated junctional or idioventricular rhythms, and some forms of ventricular tachycardia (VT), may also result from increased automaticity.

A second form of abnormal impulse formation is triggered automaticity, which occurs in the setting of abnormal afterdepolarizations. These afterdepolarizations are oscillations of the membrane potential that may reach threshold level, thus generating a subsequent action potential. They do not occur spontaneously but, rather, are triggered by prior activation of the heart. Afterdepolarizations that occur during the action potential are termed *early afterdepolarizations*. Early afterdepolarizations occur during slow heart rates or after a brief pause, are exacerbated by hypokalemia or potassium channel blockade, are associated with QT prolongation on the surface electrocardiogram (ECG), and likely account for the mechanism of drug-induced torsades de pointes, a form of polymorphic VT. *Delayed afterdepolarizations* occur after the membrane has completely repolarized, are more pronounced at fast heart rates, are facilitated by intracellular calcium overload, and account for the mechanism underlying most digoxin-toxic rhythms.

Abnormalities of impulse conduction may result in delayed or accelerated conduction and form the substrate for *reentry*, the most common mechanism of clinically important arrhythmias. Delayed conduction through the AV node or His-Purkinje system may result in transient or persistent heart block and may be associated with symptomatic bradycardia. Occasionally, conduction from the atria to the ventricles does not follow the usual route through the AV node but occurs by means of an abnormal bridge of myocardial tissue, a so-called accessory pathway or bypass tract. These bypass tracts are able to conduct impulses faster than the AV node and result in premature depolarization (preexcitation) of the ventricles that manifest as characteristic ECG abnormalities and reentrant tachyarrhythmias (see later).

Reentry provides a mechanism whereby the initial wave of depolarization can be propagated continuously in a reciprocating fashion. For reentry to occur, several conditions must be met. First, there must be two distinct conducting pathways. Second, there must be unidirectional block in one pathway. Third, there must be slower conduction down the other pathway. These conditions can be met when either an anatomic obstruction

TABLE 10-1 Genesis of Arrhythmias

Mechanism of Arrhythmia	Examples
Disorders of Impulse Formation	
Increased automaticity	Premature atrial, junctional, and ventricular complexes
	Ectopic atrial tachycardia
	Accelerated junctional rhythm
	Accelerated idioventricular rhythm
	Parasystole
	Some forms of ventricular tachycardia (RVOT)
Triggered automaticity	Early afterdepolarizations (torsades de pointes)
	Delayed afterdepolarizations (digoxin-toxic rhythms)
Disorders of Impulse Conduction	
Heart block	Sinus node exit block
	First-, second-, and third-degree AV block
Reentry	AV nodal reentrant tachycardia
	AV reentrant tachycardia using an accessory pathway (WPW)
	Atrial fibrillation
	Atrial flutter
	Most forms of ventricular tachycardia
	Ventricular flutter and fibrillation

AV = atrioventricular; RVOT = right ventricular outflow tract; WPW = Wolff-Parkinson-White.

to conduction occurs in one pathway or a functional block occurs because of differences in the properties of conduction and refractoriness of the pathways. For example, in Figure 10–2 two distinct pathways are present. Pathway A conducts rapidly but has a relatively long refractory period. Pathway B conducts slowly but has a shorter refractory period. In the usual state (see Fig. 10–2A), an impulse enters the two pathways by means of a proximal common pathway. Conduction occurs rapidly down pathway A and, once reaching the distal common pathway, continues distally as well as proceeding retrograde up pathway B until it intercepts the slow antegrade impulse traveling down this pathway and is extinguished. The surface ECG may appear normal without evidence of the dual pathways. If a premature depolarization occurs, it also enters the two pathways through the proximal common pathway. If it occurs early enough, it is unable to conduct down pathway A, because of the long refractory period of this path (see Fig. 10–2B). The impulse therefore travels down pathway B (which has the short refractory period) and reaches the distal common pathway, where it continues distally. However, because pathway B conducts relatively slowly, by the time the impulse reaches the distal aspect of pathway A, this path is no longer refractory and the impulse rapidly conducts in a retrograde direction up pathway A, reenters the loop by means of pathway B, and conducts retrograde up the proximal common pathway. If the reentrant circuit is in the AV node, the resulting surface ECG demonstrates a premature com-

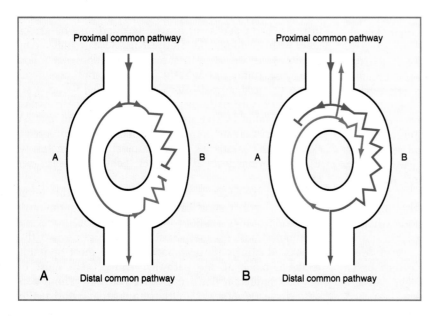

FIGURE 10–2 Mechanism of reentry. Reentry requires two distinct pathways with disparate conductive and repolarizing properties. In A an impulse enters the two pathways and conducts rapidly down pathway A and slowly down pathway B. When it reaches the distal common pathway, it proceeds distally as well as traveling retrograde up pathway B where it is extinguished, owing to collision with the antegrade depolarization in this pathway. In B a premature depolarization enters the pathways but is blocked in pathway A, owing to the slow repolarization of this pathway. The impulse travels down pathway B (slow conducting, rapidly repolarizing) to the distal common pathway, where it proceeds distally as well as traveling up pathway A, which by then is fully repolarized and able to conduct in a retrograde fashion, allowing the impulse to re-enter the loop and produce the reciprocating rhythm.

In figure: Proximal common pathway ... A ... B ... Distal common pathway (A). Proximal common pathway ... A ... B ... Distal common pathway (B).

plex initiating a tachycardia, and retrograde P waves may be seen.

Reentry can occur at any point along the normal conduction system, including the sinoatrial node, the AV node, and atrial or ventricular myocardium. It may occur in a small focus of cardiac tissue such as the AV node (a microreentrant circuit) or involve anatomically distinct pathways such as bypass tracts (a macroreentrant circuit).

Approach to the Patient with Suspected Arrhythmias

Many, if not most, arrhythmias occur intermittently, and patients present to their physician having had an "episode" but without an arrhythmia occurring at the time of evaluation. Therefore, the suspicion that an arrhythmic problem exists, as well as the necessity and urgency of further evaluation, must frequently be determined by the history alone. Palpitations, syncope, presyncope, dizziness, chest pain, and symptoms of heart failure are the most common complaints of patients with arrhythmic disorders. Palpitations are an awareness of a rapid or irregular heart beat. Characterizing the pattern (regular or irregular, intermittent or continuous) and rate of palpitations by having patients tap their fingers on a table to the rhythm of the palpitations may help to determine their etiology. For instance, occasional "skipped beats" are likely the result of premature atrial or ventricular beats, whereas periods of rapid, irregular heart beats may be reflective of paroxysmal atrial fibrillation. The perception of palpitations does not invariably correlate with arrhythmias: some patients have tachyarrhythmias without palpitations whereas other patients have palpitations without tachyarrhythmias. Correlation between the symptoms and an arrhythmia can only be confirmed by simultaneously recording the ECG and documenting the symptoms (see later). Syncope is the sudden, transient loss of consciousness. Obtaining a complete history of the events immediately preceding and after a syncopal episode will suggest the diagnosis in the majority of patients for whom a diagnosis is eventually determined (see later). Chest pain may be a manifestation of palpitations or may represent arrhythmia-induced cardiac ischemia. Dizziness and presyncope are often noncardiac in origin, although they may be a result of either bradyarrhythmias or tachyarrhythmias. These rhythms may also precipitate or exacerbate congestive heart failure. A prior history of cardiac disease is important to elicit. Patients with palpitations or syncope and a history of cardiomyopathy or prior myocardial infarction frequently have ventricular tachyarrhythmias, whereas patients with valvular heart disease or hypertension frequently develop atrial fibrillation. A family history of cardiac disease (e.g., dilated or hypertrophic cardiomyopathy, bypass tracts, sudden cardiac death, long QT syndrome) is important to note.

In addition to noting the pulse rate and rhythm, a thorough examination is useful for identifying evidence of underlying cardiac disease. When patients are examined during an arrhythmic episode, several clues to the nature of the arrhythmia may be present. Evidence of AV dissociation suggests a ventricular arrhythmia and includes variable intensity of S_1 (because of variations in the PR interval), intermittent cannon a waves in the jugular venous pulsation (because of contraction of the right atrium against a closed tricuspid valve), and a cacophony of sounds (as a result of atrial systole occurring during various parts of the cardiac cycle generating intermittent S_3 and S_4). The S_2 may become widely or paradoxically split if a bundle branch block develops during an arrhythmia. Nonetheless, these findings are not diagnostic of a ventricular source of the arrhythmia as bundle branch blocks and, rarely, AV dissociation may occur during supraventricular tachyarrhythmias as well.

The ECG taken during the arrhythmia is usually diagnostic. If P waves are not well seen, moving the arm leads to a parasternal position (Lewis leads) or using an esophageal electrode (placed 40 cm into the esophagus by means of a nasogastric tube) may help to discern atrial activity. In patients who present with a hemodynamically stable tachyarrhythmia, carotid sinus massage or pharmacologic therapy with adenosine or verapamil may slow or block conduction in the AV node and allow the underlying rhythm to be identified. Carotid sinus massage is performed with the patient in the supine position by applying light pressure for 5 to 10 seconds over the carotid impulse at the angle of the jaw. A successful test should result in slowing of the ventricular rate (Fig. 10–3). If no effect is noted, massage can be performed over the contralateral carotid impulse. This test should not be performed if carotid bruits are present. Unfortunately, many patients present after the arrhythmia has resolved. Nonetheless, clues may be present on the resting ECG. A delta wave is diagnostic of Wolff-Parkinson-White (WPW) syndrome, which is associated with AV reentrant arrhythmias and atrial fibrillation. Evidence of prior myocardial infarction raises the suspicion of ventricular tachyarrhythmias.

Because of the intermittent nature of arrhythmias, prolonged recording devices are more effective than a single ECG in electrocardiographically capturing an arrhythmia. Ambulatory ECG (Holter) monitors continuously record the rhythm and are useful in patients who have frequent episodes of presumed arrhythmic symptoms. Patient-activated event monitors, or loop recorders, can be worn for weeks at a time and continuously monitor the patient's heart rhythm. If symptoms occur, the patient activates the device, which then permanently records the rhythm for several minutes before and after the event. This type of monitor is useful if the patient has infrequent symptoms. Both of these devices are useful in diagnosing arrhythmias, determining the relationship (if any) of the patient's symptoms to an arrhythmia, monitoring the efficacy of antiarrhythmic therapy, and evaluating artificial pacemaker function. If a patient's symptoms are exertionally related, formal exercise testing may be useful.

Head-up tilt table testing is performed by strapping a patient to the tilt table, then tilting the table 60 to 80

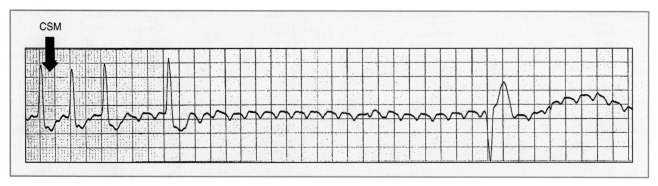

FIGURE 10-3 Carotid sinus massage (CSM) during atrial flutter with resultant unmasking of the underlying flutter waves.

degrees vertically for 15 to 60 minutes. In patients with suspected *neurocardiogenic syncope,* this procedure may reproduce their symptoms. The presumed mechanism involves a postural decrease in ventricular filling, resulting in increased sympathetic activity with a consequent increase in the force of ventricular contraction. This increased contraction is sensed by mechanoreceptors in the heart that reflexly increase vagal tone and withdraw sympathetic tone, which results in hypotension and bradycardia. The sensitivity of the test is approximately 85% with a relatively low false-positive rate (<15%). The diagnostic yield of this test may be increased by the administration of intravenous isoproterenol.

Invasive electrophysiologic (EP) studies are performed by recording the electrical activity of the heart through electrodes strategically positioned in the right atrial and ventricular chambers. This test may be useful in a group of patients in whom conduction disorders of the sinus or AV node are suspected. The results may help determine the mechanism of heart block and the need for permanent pacemaker implantation. More commonly, EP studies are used to evaluate patients with documented tachyarrhythmias or with syncope for which a tachyarrhythmia is suspected as the cause. Both supraventricular and ventricular tachyarrhythmias may be reproduced by programmed electrical stimulation. Repeated testing can be used to assess the effectiveness of pharmacologic therapy for suppressing tachyarrhythmias. EP studies may also be therapeutic. If the source of the arrhythmia is identified, an electrical current can be used to ablate the abnormal focus or pathway and prevent recurrences of the arrhythmia.

Management of Cardiac Arrhythmias

When initiating treatment of an arrhythmia, several clinical factors should be considered, including the nature of the specific arrhythmia, the setting in which the arrhythmia occurred, the consequences of the arrhythmia, and the potential risks of therapy. Certain arrhythmias (e.g., VT) can cause hemodynamic instability or sudden cardiac death and warrant aggressive treatment to pre-

vent recurrences. Other arrhythmias are hemodynamically stable but produce intolerable symptoms (e.g., palpitations, dizziness) and likewise should be suppressed. Certain arrhythmias may not be a problem acutely but warrant treatment to prevent long-term complications (e.g., stroke prevention in atrial fibrillation). The situation in which an arrhythmia occurs may dictate the need for therapy. For example, ventricular fibrillation (VF) occurring in the setting of an acute myocardial infarction is unlikely to recur if the underlying ischemic process is treated and warrants no specific therapy for the arrhythmia itself. Conversely, VF occurring in the absence of acute ischemia is likely to recur and requires aggressive therapy. Arrhythmias that are tolerated well and require no therapy in patients with structurally normal hearts may not be tolerated at all in patients with depressed left ventricular systolic function or valvular heart disease and may require aggressive therapy in these settings. Some arrhythmias are secondary to an underlying disease process. Metabolic abnormalities (hypokalemia, hypomagnesemia, hypoxia, hyperthyroidism) and acute illness (congestive heart failure, sepsis, anemia) may precipitate arrhythmias, as may emotional upset, certain foods or beverages (caffeine-containing products, alcohol), and both prescription (digoxin, theophylline, antiarrhythmic agents) and nonprescription (decongestants, certain antibiotics, cocaine) drugs. Although treatment of arrhythmias associated with these conditions may be warranted acutely, long-term therapy is not required, provided that the inciting factor is removed or controlled.

Asymptomatic arrhythmias are difficult clinical problems. Some, such as ventricular premature contractions (VPCs) and nonsustained ventricular tachycardia (NSVT), may be markers of underlying heart disease and, although benign themselves, may progress to more malignant arrhythmias. Treatment with antiarrhythmic medications in this case has not been shown to decrease mortality, and, in fact, some agents are associated with increased mortality because of their proarrhythmic side effects. The presence of symptoms is clearly important in deciding whether to treat an arrhythmia. In asymptomatic cases, the risks of the arrhythmia must be compared with the risks of therapy before institution of an antiarrhythmic agent.

PHARMACOLOGIC THERAPY

Antiarrhythmic medications work by interfering with various aspects of myocardial depolarization or repolarization and can be classified based on their particular mechanism of action. The most frequently used classification system is the Vaughn Williams classification, which categorizes these drugs on the basis of their in vitro EP effects on normal Purkinje fibers (Table 10–2). This classification is a helpful construct; however, several limitations to its interpretation and use exist. First, it is not clear that the in vivo effects of a drug in a specific class are the same as those seen in vitro. Second, a given drug may have properties of more than one class. Third, drugs in the same class may differ somewhat in their modes of action, side effect profile, and clinical effectiveness for treating a given arrhythmia. Nonetheless, the classification remains a useful communication tool.

Several general points are worth noting in regard to antiarrhythmic agents. Many drugs are given as a standard dose, whereas others are titrated depending on clinical effect. Therapeutic blood levels of many drugs have been established; however, the absolute concentration of the agent in the patient's blood is a much less useful guide to therapy than is the clinical effectiveness of the drug and the presence or absence of side effects. The therapeutic-to-toxic ratio of most antiarrhythmic agents is small so that at therapeutically effective doses, toxic side effects are common. Knowledge of the metabolism of these agents is important. Most are metabolized by either the kidney or the liver (Table 10–3), and dosages must be decreased in patients with renal or hepatic dysfunction to avoid toxicity. Many of these agents have negative inotropic effects and, even at nontoxic levels, noncardiac side effects are common. These drugs frequently interact with other medications and may interfere with nonpharmacologic modes of therapy. For example, quinidine and amiodarone increase the serum digoxin level and augment the anticoagulant effect of warfarin. In addition, quinidine increases the amount of energy required for an artificial pacemaker to pace the heart effectively (pacing threshold), whereas amiodarone increases the amount of energy required to defibrillate the heart effectively (defibrillation threshold). For this reason, artificial pacemakers and implantable cardioverter-defibrillators (ICDs) need to be checked after the institution of antiarrhythmic agents.

Table 10–3 and Table 10–4 summarize the important characteristics of the most commonly used antiarrhythmic agents. An in-depth discussion of each agent is beyond the scope of the chapter; however, several points warrant specific mention.

Class IA antiarrhythmic agents block sodium channels to a moderate degree and are useful for the long-term oral treatment of both supraventricular and ventricular arrhythmias. Procainamide is also available in an intravenous preparation and is useful for the acute management of these arrhythmias. These agents prolong the conduction time and the effective refractory period of most cardiac tissues, including accessory pathways, and may be effective therapy for patients with AV nodal or atrioventricular reentrant tachycardias. Because these agents slow the spontaneous sinoatrial rate and can enhance conduction through the AV node through vagolytic effects, they can induce more rapid ventricular rates in patients with atrial flutter. Therefore, when they are used to treat atrial flutter, care must be taken to ensure that the ventricular rate is controlled with a β blocker, calcium channel blocker, or digoxin before instituting a type IA agent. Sixty percent to 70% of patients who receive procainamide develop antinuclear antibodies (specifically, antihistone antibodies), whereas a clinical lupus-like syndrome occurs in only 20% to 30%; this is reversible on stopping the drug. Disopyramide has significant negative inotropic effects and should be used with extreme caution (if at all) in patients with left ventricular dysfunction. As a result of its α-adrenergic blocking effects, quinidine may cause significant hypotension and may also produce syncope in 0.5% to 2% of patients as a result of QT prolongation and subsequent polymorphic VT. This proarrhythmic effect may also be seen with the other agents in this class.

TABLE 10–2   The Vaughn Williams Classification of Antiarrhythmic Drugs

Class	Physiologic Effect*	Examples
Class I	Block sodium channels; predominantly reduce the maximum velocity of the upstroke of the action potential (phase 0)	
IA	Intermediate potency blockade	Quinidine, procainamide, disopyramide
IB	Least potent blockade	Lidocaine, tocainide, mexiletine, phenytoin
IC	Most potent blockade	Flecainide, propafenone, moricizine
Class II	β-Adrenergic receptor blockade	Propranolol, metoprolol, atenolol
Class III	Potassium channel blockade (except ibutilide); predominantly prolong action potential duration	Amiodarone, sotalol, bretylium, ibutilide
Class IV	Calcium channel blockade	Verapamil, diltiazem

*Several agents have physiologic effects characteristic of more than one class.

TABLE 10-3   **Selected Characteristics of Antiarrhythmic Drugs**

Drug	Effect on Surface ECG	Effect on LV Function	Important Drug Interactions	Effect on Pacing and Defibrillation Thresholds	Major Route of Elimination
Quinidine	Prolongs QRS and QT	None	Increases digoxin level and warfarin effect. Heparin, verapamil, cimetidine increase quinidine level. Phenobarbital, phenytoin, rifampin decrease quinidine level	Increases PT and DT at high doses	Liver
Procainamide	Prolongs PR, QRS, and ST	Negative inotrope	Cimetidine, alcohol, amiodarone increase procainamide level	Increases PT at high doses	Liver and kidney
Disopyramide	Prolongs QRS and QT	Negative inotrope	Phenobarbital, phenytoin, rifampin all increase disopyramide level	Increases PT at high doses	Liver and kidney
Lidocaine	Shortens QT	None	Propranolol, metoprolol, cimetidine all increase lidocaine level	Increases DT	Liver
Tocainide	Shortens QT	None	Cimetidine decreases bioavailability of tocainide	?	Liver and kidney
Mexiletine	Shortens QT	None	Increases theophylline level. Phenobarbital, phenytoin, rifampin all decrease mexiletine level	Variable effects	Liver
Flecainide	Prolongs PR and QRS	Negative inotrope	Increases digoxin level	Increases PT; variable effect on DT	Liver and kidney
Propafenone	Prolongs PR and QRS	Negative inotrope	Increases digoxin, theophylline, cyclosporine levels; increases warfarin effect. Phenobarbital, phenytoin, rifampin decrease propafenone level. Cimetidine increases propafenone level	Increases PT; variable effect on DT	Liver
Moricizine	Prolongs PR and QRS	Negative inotrope	Decreases theophylline level. Cimetidine increases moricizine level	?	Liver
Amiodarone	Prolongs PR and QT; slows sinus rate	None	Increases digoxin and cyclosporine levels; increases warfarin effect	Increases DT	Liver
Sotalol	Prolongs PR and QT; slows sinus rate	Negative inotrope	Additive effects with other β-blockers	Decreases DT	Kidney
Bretylium	Prolongs PR and QR	None		?	Kidney
Ibutilide	Prolongs PR and QT	None	?	?	Kidney

ECG = electrocardiogram; LV = left ventricle; PT = pacing threshold; DT = defibrillation threshold; PR, QRS, and QT refer to their respective intervals on the surface electrocardiogram.

Class IB agents are weak sodium channel blockers. They are useful for treating ventricular tachyarrhythmias, but because they have minimal effects on the sinus or AV nodes they are not effective for supraventricular arrhythmias. Lidocaine is the most clinically useful drug in this class and is the initial intravenous drug of choice in patients with ventricular tachyarrhythmias. It appears particularly effective in ischemia-related arrhythmias; however, its prophylactic use during an acute infarction is not indicated and may increase mortality. Tocainide is an analogue of lidocaine that can be given orally. Its use is limited by the occasional development of agranulocytosis. Phenytoin is a potent antiepileptic that also has class IB antiarrhythmic properties. It is particularly effective in treating atrial and ventricular arrhythmias caused by digoxin toxicity. These agents have relatively little effect on hemodynamics, and clinically important proarrhythmia is rare.

TABLE 10-4 Common Side Effects of Selected Antiarrhythmic Drugs

Drug	Major Side Effects
Quinidine	Nausea, diarrhea, abdominal cramping
	Cinchonism: decreased hearing, tinnitus, blurred vision, delirium
	Rash, thrombocytopenia, hemolytic anemia
	Hypotension, "quinidine syncope"
Procainamide	Drug-induced lupus syndrome
	Nausea, vomiting
	Rash, fevers, hypotension, psychosis
Disopyramide	Anticholinergic: dry mouth, blurred vision, constipation, urinary retention, closed-angle glaucoma
	Hypotension
Lidocaine	CNS: dizziness, perioral numbness, paresthesias, altered consciousness, coma, seizures
Tocainide	Nausea, vomiting, granulocytosis
	CNS: dizziness, tremor, paresthesias, ataxia, confusion
Mexiletine	Nausea, vomiting
	CNS: dizziness, tremor, paresthesias, ataxia, confusion
Flecainide	Congestive heart failure
	CNS: blurred vision, headache, ataxia
Propafenone	Nausea, vomiting, metallic taste to food
Moricizine	Nausea, dizziness, headache
β-Blockers	Bronchospasm, bradycardia, fatigue, depression, impotence
	Congestive heart failure
Calcium channel blockers	Congestive heart failure, bradycardia, heart block, constipation
Amiodarone	Agranulocytosis, pulmonary fibrosis, hepatopathy, hyper- or hypothyroidism, corneal microdeposits, bluish discoloration of the skin, nausea, constipation, bradycardia
	Hypotension with intravenous administration
Sotalol	Same as β blockers
Bretylium	Orthostatic hypotension
	Transient hypertension, tachycardia, and worsening of arrhythmia (initial catecholamine release)
Ibutilide	Heart block, hypotension, nausea

CNS = central nervous system.

Class IC agents are potent blockers of sodium channels. They are effective therapy for both ventricular and supraventricular arrhythmias; however, the use of flecainide and moricizine to treat asymptomatic ventricular arrhythmias after myocardial infarction has proved to increase mortality, especially in patients with left ventricular dysfunction. Flecainide remains an effective and relatively safe therapy for supraventricular arrhythmias (especially paroxysmal atrial fibrillation) in patients with structurally normal hearts. Propafenone is similar to flecainide but with β-blocking effects and, therefore, may exacerbate bradycardia, heart block, heart failure, and bronchospasm.

The β blockers and nondihydropyridine calcium channel blockers constitute class II and class IV antiarrhythmic agents, respectively. These agents have been discussed at length in Chapter 9. The antiarrhythmic effectiveness of these drugs relates mainly to their ability to slow the rate of the sinus node and decrease conduction through the AV node. They are effective for controlling the rate of supraventricular tachycardias (SVTs), such as atrial fibrillation or atrial flutter, although they are not effective for converting these arrhythmias to normal sinus rhythm. Intravenous adminis-

tration of these agents may acutely terminate some supraventricular tachyarrhythmias, especially reentrant rhythms that use the AV node as one limb of the reentrant circuit (i.e., AV nodal and atrioventricular reentrant tachycardias). By virtue of their ability to selectively slow conduction in the AV node, these agents may increase conduction down a bypass tract and are contraindicated in patients with WPW syndrome and atrial tachyarrhythmias (atrial flutter or fibrillation or ectopic atrial tachycardia). These agents also are negatively inotropic and must be used with caution in patients with left ventricular dysfunction or overt heart failure.

Class III antiarrhythmic drugs prolong the action potential duration. Amiodarone is mainly a class III agent but has physiologic effects of all four classes. It is an effective therapy for a wide range of both supraventricular and ventricular arrhythmias and is safe to use in patients with left ventricular dysfunction. It is the drug of choice for the treatment of atrial fibrillation in patients with heart failure and is likely more effective than other antiarrhythmics in preventing recurrences of VT or VF. In addition, it may decrease arrhythmic death after myocardial infarction and in patients with nonischemic heart failure. Amiodarone may be administered intravenously for the acute treatment of refractory ventricular tachyarrhythmias. Its use has been somewhat limited by the fear of significant side effects, specifically pulmonary fibrosis; however, this appears to be a relatively rare complication when standard dosages are used. Sotalol has both class III and β-blocking effects. It is particularly effective for the treatment of ventricular tachyarrhythmias, but it is also effective for a number of supraventricular arrhythmias, including atrial fibrillation. Ibutilide is a new parenteral class III agent that is effective for the acute termination of atrial fibrillation of recent onset (<90 days), and it enhances the success of electrical cardioversion of this arrhythmia. All of these agents routinely prolong the QT interval and are potentially associated with an increased risk of torsades de pointes, although the incidence of this arrhythmia is quite low in patients given amiodarone. Bretylium causes an initial release of norepinephrine from nerve terminals and may result in transient hypertension and aggravation of arrhythmias. It subsequently prevents norepinephrine release and, thus, prevents arrhythmia recurrence. Bretylium is administered intravenously and is indicated for the treatment of life-threatening ventricular tachyarrhythmias when other agents have failed.

Several other antiarrhythmic agents that do not fit into the Vaughn Williams classification are worthy of mention. Adenosine is an endogenous nucleoside that, when given intravenously in pharmacologic dosages, results in profound, albeit transient, slowing of AV conduction and sinus discharge rate. Flushing, chest pain, and dyspnea commonly occur after adenosine injection but are short-lived because of the short half-life of this agent (approximately 6 seconds). Its main use is in the treatment of SVT: adenosine terminates more than 95% of AV nodal or AV reentrant tachycardias. During rapid atrial tachyarrhythmias, transient adenosine-induced heart block may help to unmask the underlying rhythm. Theophylline blocks the effects of adenosine, and dipyridamole potentiates its effects. Atropine blocks the effects of the vagus nerve on the heart and results in an increased sinus rate and faster conduction through the AV node. It is indicated for the treatment of symptomatic bradycardia. Digoxin enhances vagal tone and results in a slowing of the sinus rate and slowed conduction through the AV node. It is useful for controlling the ventricular response to an SVT and may also be effective in treating AV nodal and AV reentrant tachyarrhythmias.

NONPHARMACOLOGIC THERAPY OF BRADYARRHYTHMIAS: CARDIAC PACEMAKERS

Artificial cardiac pacemakers are devices that deliver a small electrical impulse to a localized region of the heart, causing the affected myocytes to depolarize to the threshold potential, thus initiating an action potential that then spreads to the remainder of the heart. These devices can be used temporarily to treat a transient bradyarrhythmia resulting from a reversible cause or can be implanted permanently to treat irreversible disorders of impulse formation or conduction that result in recur-

rent or persistent bradyarrhythmias. Temporary pacemakers can deliver the electrical impulse indirectly through the chest wall (transcutaneous pacing) or can be placed intravenously into the right side of the heart to deliver the impulse locally (transvenous pacing). Transcutaneous pacing requires higher energy to electrically "capture" the heart and, therefore, can be somewhat uncomfortable. In addition, some patients, especially obese individuals, cannot be effectively paced transcutaneously. Nonetheless, this can be an effective mode of pacing in most patients, may help to stabilize a patient who has an unstable bradyarrhythmia until a transvenous or permanent pacemaker can be inserted, and is useful to have as prophylaxis for acutely ill patients who are at high risk of developing significant bradyarrhythmias. Permanent pacemakers are usually inserted intravenously. The pulse generator is buried in a "pocket" created in the pectoral region of the chest wall, and the electrodes pass from the generator, through the cephalic or subclavian vein, and into the right atrium and/or ventricle, where they are anchored into place. Indications for temporary and permanent pacemaker insertion are listed in Table 10–5.

Current pacemakers allow for the tailoring of the pacemaker function to the specific needs of the patient. A code has been developed that describes these various functions. The first letter reflects the cardiac chamber being paced (V, ventricle; A, atrium; D, dual chamber/atrium and ventricle). The second letter reflects the chamber in which electrical activity is being sensed (V, ventricle; A, atrium; D, dual chamber/atrium and ventricle; O, none). The third letter reflects the response mode of the pacemaker. If the pacemaker senses the patient's own native beat it may respond by being inhibited (I), being triggered to fire at the same time as the native beat (T), or being triggered to fire after a sensed atrial event but inhibited by a sensed ventricular event (D). Newer pacemakers are also capable of sensing a patient's activity level (through temperature, vibration, or respiratory sensors) and changing their paced rate in response to a sensed increase in metabolic need. This is termed a *rate-responsive* mode and is indicated by an "R" after the first three letters. Examples of common pacing modes are listed in Table 10–6.

The choice of pacing mode depends on individual patient needs. Dual-chamber pacing maintains AV synchrony, which is an advantage because the timing of atrial contraction is important for the maximization of cardiac output. Therefore, AV synchronous pacing is very useful in patients with left ventricular dysfunction in whom loss of AV synchrony may result in the precipitation of heart failure. For patients who have structurally normal hearts or who have a pacemaker implanted for only occasional symptomatic bradyarrhythmias, the maintenance of AV synchrony is not as important and a single ventricular pacing electrode is sufficient.

Safeguards have been programmed into the pacemakers that limit the upper pacing rate, thus preventing rapid ventricular pacing in response to a supraventricular tachyarrhythmia. Newer pacemakers can detect the onset of an atrial tachyarrhythmia and switch to an appropriate pacing mode (mode switching). Pacemaker

TABLE 10-5 Indications for Pacemaker Insertion

Pacing is definitely indicated.	Acquired CHB with or without symptoms*
	Congenital CHB with symptoms
	Mobitz I (Wenckebach) second-degree heart block with symptomatic bradycardia
	Mobitz II second-degree heart block with symptomatic bradycardia
	Symptomatic sinus bradycardia (heart rate < 40)
	Symptomatic sinus bradycardia secondary to drug therapy for which there is no acceptable alternative
	Sinus node dysfunction with symptomatic bradycardia or life-threatening bradycardia-dependent arrhythmias
	Symptomatic carotid sinus sensitivity with >3-second pause after CSM
Pacing is probably indicated.	Congenital CHB with moderate bradycardia
	Asymptomatic Mobitz II second-degree heart block
	Bi- or trifascicular block with syncope that is attributed to transient CHB
	Transient CHB or Mobitz II second-degree heart block after an AMI
	Neurocardiogenic syncope with a positive tilt-table test
Pacing is not indicated.	Asymptomatic sinus bradycardia
	Asymptomatic sinus node dysfunction
	Bradycardia during sleep
	First-degree AV block
	Asymptomatic Mobitz I (Wenckebach) second-degree heart block
	Transient asymptomatic pause during atrial fibrillation
	RBBB with syncope or presyncope
	Asymptomatic > 3-second pause with CSM
	Recurrent syncope with negative tilt test or of undetermined cause

*Symptoms include syncope, dizziness, confusion, congestive heart failure, and decreased exercise tolerance. CSM = carotid sinus massage; CHB = complete heart block; AMI = acute myocardial infarction; RBBB = right bundle branch block.

TABLE 10-6 Common Pacemaker Modes

Pacemaker Type	Code	Chamber Paced	Chamber Sensed	Mode
Ventricular asynchronous	VOO	V	None	Continuous pacing
Ventricular demand	VVI	V	V	Ventricular pacing inhibited by spontaneous QRS
Atrial demand	AAI	A	A	Atrial pacing inhibited by spontaneous P wave
Atrial synchronous, ventricular inhibited	VDD	V	A, V	Ventricular pacing follows a sensed P wave after a preset AV delay; ventricular pacing inhibited by spontaneous QRS; no atrial pacing
AV sequential	DVI	A, V	V	Ventricular pacing follows atrial pacing after a preset AV delay; ventricular and atrial pacing inhibited by spontaneous QRS; no P wave sensing
Optimal sequential	DDD	A, V	A, V	Ventricular pacing follows sensed P waves or atrial pacing after a preset AV delay; ventricular pacing inhibited by spontaneous QRS; atrial pacing inhibited by spontaneous P wave
Rate responsive	VVIR	V	V	Same as VVI or DDD, but pacing rate increases with physiologic demand
	DDDR	A, V	A, V	

A = atrial; AV = atrioventricular; V = ventricular.

malfunction may be manifested as failure of a pacemaker impulse to depolarize the heart (failure to capture), abnormalities of sensing (oversensing or undersensing), or pacing at an abnormal rate. Many pacemakers decrease their pacing rate or change their pacing mode as the battery life is depleted.

NONPHARMACOLOGIC THERAPY OF TACHYARRHYTHMIAS

Direct Current Cardioversion and Defibrillation

Direct current cardioversion and electrical defibrillation are effective methods for treating atrial or ventricular tachyarrhythmias and are the methods of choice for terminating hemodynamically unstable tachyarrhythmias as well as stable tachyarrhythmias that are refractory to pharmacologic therapy. Cardioversion refers to the synchronized application of an electrical shock to the heart in an attempt to terminate a tachyarrhythmia. Synchronization of the shock to the QRS complex is a critical feature because the inadvertent administration of an electrical shock during ventricular repolarization (i.e., during the T wave) may precipitate ventricular fibrillation. Defibrillation refers to the asynchronous delivery of an electrical shock to terminate VF. Synchronization in this setting is not possible, because there is no organized ventricular activity (QRS) during VF.

There are small, although real, risks of electrical cardioversion. For this reason, several factors need to be addressed before elective procedures. Hyperkalemia should be excluded, as should a supratherapeutic digoxin level; cardioversion in the setting of digoxin toxicity may precipitate refractory ventricular arrhythmias. Adequate sedation is important and can usually be accomplished by the intravenous administration of benzodiazepines (e.g., midazolam) or short-acting anesthetic agents (e.g., propofol). Aspiration of gastric contents can occur because patients are unable to protect their airways during this type of sedation; therefore, patients should have fasted for at least 6 hours before the procedure. Minor cutaneous burns at the site of application of the electrical current are common, especially if multiple shocks are delivered. Even with appropriate synchronization, electrical cardioversion may precipitate VF, in which case immediate defibrillation is required. In patients with atrial fibrillation, systemic embolization of atrial thrombus may occur after conversion to normal sinus rhythm. Therefore, it is imperative that patients undergoing elective cardioversion of atrial fibrillation be adequately anticoagulated with warfarin for at least 3 weeks before and 3 weeks after electrical cardioversion.

The electrical shock is delivered through paddles applied to the patient's chest. These can be arranged either with both paddles placed on the anterior chest (one paddle at the upper sternal border and the other at the cardiac apex) or with one paddle anteriorly located over the right upper sternal border and the other posteriorly over the left interscapular region. Lubrication with electrolyte gel or the use of electrolyte pads improves contact and decreases burns. Atrial flutter can frequently be

converted to normal sinus rhythm with low-energy shocks (<50 joules), whereas atrial fibrillation frequently requires higher energy (100 to 360 joules). VT can be cardioverted with low-energy shocks (10 to 50 joules), but ventricular fibrillation should always be defibrillated with high-energy shocks ($\geq$200 joules). If the initial shock is not successful, the energy should be titrated up and several paddle positions tried before accepting failure. Many tachyarrhythmias recur after initially successful cardioversion. The administration of an antiarrhythmic agent may help to maintain sinus rhythm in these patients.

Radiofrequency Catheter Ablation and Automatic Implantable Cardioverter-Defibrillators

Because of the frequent recurrence of tachyarrhythmias despite pharmacologic therapy and the risk of proarrhythmia with most antiarrhythmic agents, several nonpharmacologic approaches to the chronic management of tachyarrhythmias have been developed. Radiofrequency catheter ablation involves the application of alternating current (AC) electrical energy in the radiofrequency range to a strategically chosen area of the endocardium. An arrhythmogenic focus or the pathway by which the arrhythmia is perpetuated can be identified (mapped), and a radiofrequency-induced lesion can be created at that site, thereby eliminating (i.e., ablating) the arrhythmia. Ablation is effective in eliminating supraventricular tachyarrhythmias caused by accessory pathways (e.g., WPW syndrome) or dual pathways in the AV node (see later discussion). The success rate of this procedure in curing these arrhythmias is greater than 95%. The success rate of ablation for atrial flutter is somewhat less (~90%). Ablation is associated with a relatively low risk of complications; inadvertent complete AV block occurs in less than 1% of cases. In patients with atrial fibrillation or atrial flutter that is refractory to attempts at cardioversion or pharmacologic rate control, production of iatrogenic complete heart block by ablation of the AV node and subsequent placement of a permanent ventricular pacemaker offers a definitive method of controlling the ventricular rate. Catheter ablation of VT is more difficult than for SVT but can be effective in selected patients. Patients with monomorphic VT in the absence of structural heart disease (e.g., right ventricular outflow tract VT, bundle branch reentry VT) are good candidates, and success can be expected in approximately 90% of these cases. Patients with VT related to prior myocardial infarction are difficult to treat with ablation, and such therapy should be attempted only if these patients have incessant VT despite antiarrhythmic therapy.

The automatic implantable cardioverter-defibrillator (AICD) is the antitachycardic equivalent of a pacemaker and is used for the treatment of ventricular tachyarrhythmias. Like the pacemaker, the AICD has a generator that is buried in the pectoral region and is connected to an electrode that is placed transvenously and anchored to the endocardium. The device monitors heart rate, not QRS morphology, and identifies a tachyarrhythmia as any rhythm that is faster than the rate programmed into the device. Thus, the current devices cannot distinguish an SVT with rapid ventricular response (including sinus tachycardia) from VT. Most AICDs have several possible therapeutic responses to a sensed tachyarrhythmic event. Relatively slow VT may be successfully terminated by pacing the ventricle at a faster rate (antitachycardia pacing). If this is not successful, the device may then deliver a 20- to 40-joule electrical discharge, which may be repeated several times at escalating energy levels in an attempt to terminate the tachyarrhythmia. Most of the current devices also have pacemaker capabilities in the event of a bradyarrhythmia.

The indications for the implantation of an AICD are continuously changing as trials demonstrate their effectiveness (or lack of effectiveness) in specific situations. They have been shown to decrease mortality compared with antiarrhythmic therapy in survivors of ventricular fibrillation or hemodynamically unstable VT. They also offer a mortality benefit in a subset of patients at high risk for arrhythmic events after a myocardial infarction. Antiarrhythmic therapy is often necessary after AICD implantation to decrease the frequency of ventricular tachyarrhythmic events or to control the rate of SVTs so that the number of shocks a patient receives from the device is limited. Given the effectiveness of radiofrequency ablation and AICDs, surgical therapy of tachyarrhythmias is rarely necessary. It is occasionally used after failed ablation in patients with accessory bypass tracts. In addition, in patients with refractory VT in the setting of a ventricular aneurysm, surgical aneurysmectomy may eliminate the arrhythmia, with a success rate of approximately 70%, and improve pharmacologic control of the arrhythmia in an additional 20%.

Specific Arrhythmias

SINUS NODAL RHYTHM DISTURBANCES

The sinus node is located high in the right atrium and depolarizes the atria in a superior-to-inferior direction, resulting in a P wave on the surface ECG that is positive in the inferior leads (II, III, aVF) and negative in aVR. *Normal sinus rhythm* denotes a rhythm that originates from the sinus node and has a rate between 60 and 100 beats/min in the awake, adult population. Normal sinus rates are faster in infants and children and decrease during sleep, at times dropping below 40 beats/min. The sinus node is heavily innervated by the autonomic nervous system; its rate increases in response to sympathetic stimulation and decreases in response to parasympathetic stimulation. These autonomic influences can result in cyclic variations in the heart rate (>10% variation) referred to as *sinus arrhythmia* (Fig. 10–4C). This variability is synchronized with the respiratory cycle and reflects an inspiratory reflex inhibition of vagal tone, resulting in a faster heart rate. Sinus arrhythmia is less common in older patients as a result of the normal age-related decrease in parasympathetic tone. In rare cases, a long cycle length (the interval between two P waves)

is sensed by the patient as a pause or palpitation. This rhythm is benign and requires no specific therapy.

Wandering atrial pacemaker is a variant of sinus arrhythmia in which the dominant pacemaker shifts from the sinoatrial node to other atrial or junctional sites. The surface ECG demonstrates variable P wave morphology and cyclical slowing of the heart rate as lower pacemakers take over. This rhythm is a normal variant in younger individuals, especially in athletes. Therapy is usually not necessary.

A sinus rhythm with a rate greater than 100 beats/min is referred to as *sinus tachycardia* (see Fig. 10–4A). This is usually either catecholamine-mediated in response to a physiologic state (e.g., exercise, anemia, hypotension, pain, fever, thyrotoxicosis) or pharmacologically induced by administration of exogenous stimulants or inhibitors of vagal tone (e.g., β agonists, catecholamines, theophylline, cocaine, caffeine, atropine). During exercise, the heart rate increases progressively to an age-predicted maximum that is roughly approximated by the formula 220 beats/min minus the patient's age. Therapy for sinus tachycardia involves treatment of the underlying cause. If a patient is symptomatic as a result of the tachycardia, treatment with β blockers is usually effective. A sinus rate less than 60 beats/min in an awake adult is considered *sinus bradycardia* (see Fig. 10–4B). It is common in young adults, especially well-trained athletes, and frequently occurs during sleep. It usually results from either increased parasympathetic tone (which may be triggered by gastrointestinal or genitourinary disorders, increased intracranial pressure, acute inferior myocardial infarction, or heightened sensitivity of the carotid baroreceptors) or decreased sympathetic tone (e.g., administration of β-blocking agents, hypothyroidism). If sinus bradycardia results in symptoms as a result of hypotension or results in bradycardia-mediated tachyarrhythmias, treatment is indicated. Vagally mediated bradycardia may respond to atropine. The β agonist isoproterenol is also effective. A temporary artificial pacemaker is rarely required. No drugs are effective and safe for the long-term treatment of this disorder; therefore, permanent pacemaker implantation is the treatment of choice in patients with chronic, symptomatic, sinus bradycardia.

A *sinus pause* may result from either failure of the sinus node to discharge (*sinus arrest*) or failure of the impulse generated by the sinus node to propagate beyond the perinodal tissue and depolarize the atria (*sinoatrial exit block*). These abnormalities are recognized on the surface ECG by the sudden absence of an expected P wave. In the case of sinoatrial exit block (a disorder of conduction), the pause related to the absent P wave is a multiple of the usual PP interval, whereas with sinus arrest (a disorder of impulse formation), the duration of the pause is unrelated to the usual cycle length. Excessive vagal tone, ischemia, infarction, or fibrosis of the sinoatrial node, and drugs, such as digoxin or antiarrhythmic agents, may all contribute to sinus pauses. Treatment is usually not necessary aside from identification and reversal of the inciting agent. Symptomatic pauses are treated the same as is symptomatic sinus bradycardia.

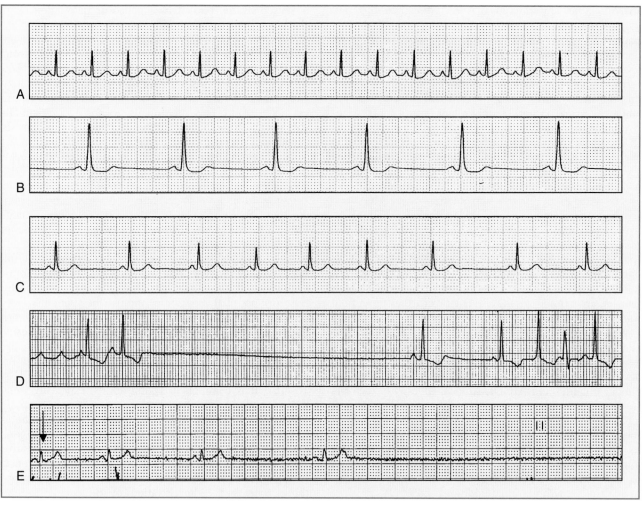

FIGURE 10–4 Sinus node disturbances. *A,* Sinus tachycardia at a rate of 123 beats/min. The subtle ST segment depression is a normal rate-related phenomenon. *B,* Sinus bradycardia at a rate of 49 beats/min in a patient receiving metroprolol. *C,* Sinus arrhythmia. The heart rate varies as a result of respiration-induced changes in vagal tone. *D,* Sick sinus syndrome. Coarse atrial fibrillation was followed by a prolonged spontaneous period of asystole before restoration of sinus rhythm (tachy-brady syndrome). *E,* Hypersensitivity carotid sinus syndrome. Gentle left carotid sinus massage *(arrow)* resulted in slowing of the sinus rate and, subsequently, a prolonged period of asystole. Normal sinus rhythm returned after a 6-second pause (not shown).

Differential conduction properties of cells in the sinus node and perinodal tissue supply the substrate for *sinus node reentrant tachycardia* to occur. This rhythm accounts for approximately 10% of supraventricular tachyarrhythmias and may be indistinguishable from sinus tachycardia except that it usually starts suddenly and after a premature atrial depolarization: it generally occurs at a rate of 110 to 140 beats/min. Maneuvers that increase vagal tone (Valsalva maneuver, carotid sinus massage) may terminate the tachycardia. Chronic treatment with digoxin, β blockers, or calcium channel blockers is usually effective. Radiofrequency ablation or modification of part of the sinus node is necessary in refractory cases.

Sinus node dysfunction and *sick sinus syndrome* are terms applied to a variety of conditions characterized by one or more of the following manifestations: (1) sinus pauses; (2) persistent sinus bradycardia, either relative or absolute; (3) intra-atrial and/or AV nodal conduction abnormalities; (4) SVTs (usually atrial flutter or fibrillation) either precipitating, or precipitated by, periods of bradycardia ("tachy-brady" or "brady-tachy" syndromes); and (5) failure of extranodal pacemakers to respond to bradycardia. Sick sinus syndrome (see Fig 10–4D) is often the result of degenerative changes in the sinus node and is aggravated by the use of cardioactive drugs such as β blockers, calcium channel blockers, and class III antiarrhythmic drugs. Symptoms are frequent and may reflect either tachycardia or bradycardia. Permanent pacemaker placement is warranted for symptomatic bradycardia and may be necessary to allow adequate therapy of tachyarrhythmias because agents aimed at controlling the tachycardia frequently precipitate bradycardiac episodes.

ATRIAL RHYTHM DISTURBANCES

Atrial premature complexes (APCs) result from the premature discharge of nonsinus atrial pacemakers and generate P waves on the surface ECG that are distinct from those generated by the sinus node (Fig. 10–5*B*). Depending on the site of origin of the APC and its timing with regard to the refractory period of the AV node, it may be associated with a normal, shortened, or prolonged PR interval or may fail to conduct to the ventricles altogether (a blocked APC), the most common cause of a pause on the surface ECG. APCs that do conduct to the ventricles may generate normal-appearing QRS complexes or complexes that are aberrantly conducted, as a result of impingement on the refractory period of the His-Purkinje system. These aberrant complexes are usually of a right bundle branch block pattern because of the longer refractory period of this bundle. If an APC occurs early enough, the wave of depolarization will "reset" the sinoatrial node and will result in a noncompensatory pause; that is, the RR interval surrounding the APC will be less than twice the normal RR interval. Late APCs do not reach the sinoatrial node before it spontaneously discharges and are therefore followed by a compensatory pause (the RR interval surrounding the APC equals twice the normal RR interval).

APCs occur in patients of all ages, with or without

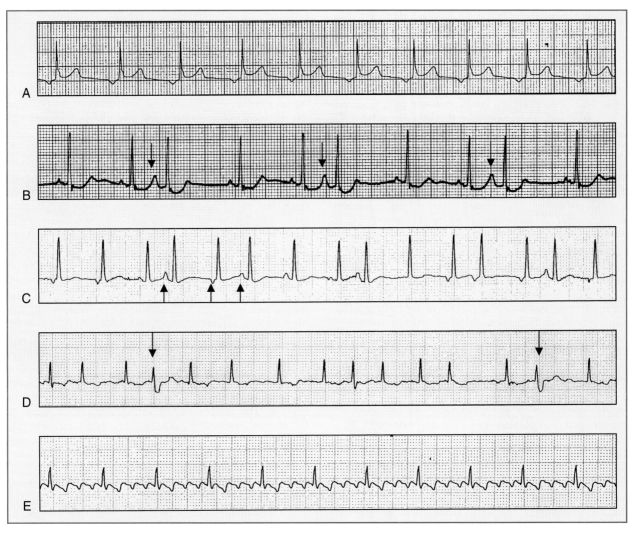

FIGURE 10–5 Atrial rhythm disturbances. *A,* Ectopic atrial rhythm. The P waves are inverted in this lead II rhythm strip, suggesting a low atrial focus of the arrhythmia. *B,* Atrial premature systoles. The premature P waves *(arrows)* conduct with a slightly longer PR interval. The premature complexes are followed by noncompensatory pauses (see text). *C,* Multifocal atrial tachycardia demonstrating an irregularly irregular rhythm at a rate of approximately 110 beats/min, with at least three different P wave morphologies *(arrows)* and without a dominant underlying rhythm. *D,* Atrial fibrillation. The rhythm is irregularly irregular without evidence of organized atrial electrical activity. The occasional wide complex beats *(arrows)* may represent premature ventricular complexes or aberrantly conducted supraventricular complexes. *E,* Atrial flutter. Flutter waves are seen as the discrete undulations of the baseline ("sawtooth pattern"). The conduction rate is 4 : 1, that is, four flutter waves for each QRS complex.

underlying cardiac disease, although their incidence is increased in certain cardiac (e.g., mitral valve disease, myocardial infarction, cardiomyopathy) and noncardiac (e.g., thyrotoxicosis, pulmonary disease) conditions. Smoking, alcohol, and caffeine may precipitate APCs. They are frequently asymptomatic and require no specific therapy other than treatment of the underlying disease or avoidance of precipitants. Symptomatic APCs usually produce palpitations or the sensation of skipped beats and can usually be controlled with β blockers. These APCs may also be the initiating factor for sustained tachyarrhythmias.

In *ectopic atrial tachycardias*, the wave of depolarization originates in a nonsinus atrial site, occurs at rates between 120 and 240 beats/min, and may be paroxysmal or sustained. The most common ectopic site is low in the right atrium, resulting in a negative P wave in the inferior leads on the surface ECG (II, III, aVF) (Fig. 10–5A). Most commonly, AV conduction is 1:1; however, when atrial tachycardia occurs with AV block, digoxin toxicity should be suspected. Atrial tachycardias are more likely to occur in patients with concomitant heart disease, including coronary artery disease, valvular disease, cardiomyopathies, cor pulmonale, and congenital heart disease. This type of arrhythmia may be difficult to treat. If it is a result of digoxin toxicity, withholding the agent or treating with digoxin-specific antibodies will lead to resolution of the arrhythmia. If it is not a result of digoxin toxicity, β blockers and calcium channel blockers are the mainstays of therapy with class I or class III antiarrhythmic agents reserved for refractory cases. Catheter ablation can eliminate this arrhythmia in 75% to 90% of cases.

Multifocal atrial tachycardia is an irregular rhythm defined by the presence of three or more P wave morphologies and a rate greater than 100 beats/min (see Fig. 10–5C). It occurs most commonly in patients with underlying lung disease; is also seen in the setting of an acute myocardial infarction, hypokalemia, or hypomagnesemia; and may be a precursor of atrial fibrillation. Aminophylline use may also be a contributing factor. Treatment is directed at the underlying disease. Rate control of this arrhythmia may be difficult, although verapamil is frequently effective.

Atrial fibrillation is the most common sustained supraventricular tachyarrhythmia (see Fig. 10–5D). It is the result of multiple reentrant loops continuously circulating in both atria, generating chaotic atrial depolarization with resultant ineffective atrial contraction, and bombarding the AV node at rates greater than 400 beats/min. Because of the conductive properties of the AV node, many of the impulses are blocked at this level. The resultant ventricular rhythm is irregularly irregular at rates between 120 and 170 beats/min. At rapid ventricular rates, the rhythm may appear to be regular, although careful measurements will disclose the irregularity. A truly regular ventricular rate in the setting of atrial fibrillation suggests the development of a junctional or ventricular rhythm, both of which may be a reflection of digoxin toxicity. Atrial fibrillation may be paroxysmal or chronic and may be the only arrhythmia present or be part of a more generalized rhythm distur-

bance (sick sinus syndrome). The surface ECG demonstrates an irregular ventricular pattern and the absence of organized atrial activity (i.e., no P waves present). Physical examination of a patient in atrial fibrillation reveals variation in the intensity of S_1, an irregular cardiac rhythm, and absence of a waves in the jugular venous pulsations. At the very short RR intervals, which occur intermittently during rapid heart rates, the minimal diastolic filling time and subsequent low stroke volume fail to produce a palpable pulse. A discrepancy may, therefore, exist between the auscultated heart rate and the palpable pulse rate, with the auscultated rate being a more accurate reflection of the true ventricular rate.

There is a clear association of atrial fibrillation with age, and a sharp increase in incidence is noted after the seventh decade of life. Atrial fibrillation may occur without any identifiable cardiac abnormality but is much more common in the setting of underlying cardiac disease, including valvular heart disease (especially rheumatic), heart failure, and ischemic cardiac disease. The most frequent predisposing cardiovascular condition for the development of atrial fibrillation is hypertension. Atrial fibrillation may also be precipitated by pericarditis, thyrotoxicosis, pulmonary emboli, pneumonia, and acute alcohol ingestion and occurs postoperatively in approximately one third of patients who undergo cardiac surgery. Atrial fibrillation is frequently asymptomatic or associated with only minor symptoms, such as palpitations. In patients with obstructive coronary artery disease, the rapid heart rate associated with the onset of atrial fibrillation may precipitate ischemia. In patients with aortic or mitral stenosis and in other patients who are dependent on the atrial contribution to cardiac output (e.g., patients with left ventricular hypertrophy, or with a dilated or hypertrophic cardiomyopathy), the loss of effective atrial contraction with the onset of atrial fibrillation may result in significant hemodynamic compromise. In addition, in patients with bypass tracts (see later), atrial fibrillation may result in extremely rapid ventricular rates with subsequent hemodynamic collapse.

The treatment of atrial fibrillation is threefold: (1) rate control, (2) prevention of thromboembolic complications, and (3) restoration and maintenance of sinus rhythm. The control of the ventricular rate is important for several reasons. Symptoms and hemodynamic compromise are more common at faster ventricular rates, and, as noted, the tachycardic response may induce ischemia in patients with coronary artery disease. In addition, the poorly controlled heart rate may result in the development of progressive ventricular dysfunction. The heart rate can usually be controlled with digoxin, β blockers, or calcium channel blockers. Occasionally, patients present with atrial fibrillation and a relatively slow ventricular rate in the absence of rate-lowering medications. This usually reflects significant underlying conduction system disease.

Because of the ineffective mechanical function of the atria during fibrillation, stasis of blood may occur, especially in the atrial appendages, and result in thrombus formation and subsequent thromboembolic events. In the absence of anticoagulation therapy, atrial fibrillation is associated with a 5% to 6% per year risk of embolic stroke. This risk is much higher in the setting of rheumatic valvular disease (>10%). Other clinical factors that increase the risk of stroke in patients with atrial fibrillation include prior stroke, diabetes, hypertension, heart failure, and increasing age. There is no difference in stroke rate between paroxysmal and chronic atrial fibrillation. Given this fact, any patient with persistent or intermittent atrial fibrillation despite therapy who does not have a contraindication to anticoagulation should be treated with warfarin therapy to maintain the international normalized ratio between 2.0 and 3.0.

Restoration of normal sinus rhythm is the best method of controlling the heart rate, limiting thromboembolic risk, and maximizing hemodynamic status. When atrial fibrillation is associated with hemodynamic compromise, electrical cardioversion (with 100 to 360 joules) is the treatment of choice. In hemodynamically stable patients with less than 48 to 72 hours of atrial fibrillation, the risk of thromboembolism is low and chemical or electrical cardioversion can be attempted without anticoagulation. The class Ia (quinidine, procainamide, disopyramide), class Ic (propafenone, flecainide), or class III (sotalol, amiodarone) agents may be effective in restoring sinus rhythm and for long-term maintenance therapy. However, the benefits of such therapy must be weighed against the risks of toxicity with these agents, and the probability of maintaining sinus rhythm must be taken into account. Patients with long-standing (>12 months) atrial fibrillation or with large atria are less likely to remain in sinus rhythm irrespective of antiarrhythmic therapy. Patients with more than 72 hours of atrial fibrillation, or in whom the duration of the arrhythmia is unknown, are at increased risk of having atrial thrombi and should be treated with rate control and anticoagulation for at least 3 weeks before an attempt at cardioversion. An alternative approach is to perform a transesophageal echocardiogram; if atrial thrombi are not present, cardioversion can be safely performed. Anticoagulation should be continued for at least 3 weeks after successful cardioversion because effective atrial contraction may be slow to return.

In rare cases, the ventricular rate cannot be controlled by pharmacologic means and catheter ablation of the AV node and permanent pacemaker implantation are necessary for adequate heart rate control. In refractory cases, surgery may be curative. The maze procedure involves making surgical lesions in the atria that interrupt reentrant circuits and may restore sinus rhythm in more than 90% of patients. This procedure may also be performed by radiofrequency ablation in the EP laboratory.

Atrial flutter is the result of a macroreentrant circuit producing atrial depolarization at a rate of 250 to 350 beats/min (see Fig. 10–5E). The most common ventricular rate is approximately 150 beats/min, as a result of 2:1 block at the AV node. Variable AV block or a Wenckebach pattern of AV block may result in an irregular pattern of ventricular depolarization. Higher degrees of block with resultant slow ventricular heart rates can occur when underlying conduction system disease is present or AV nodal blocking agents are used. As with

atrial fibrillation, this rhythm may be asymptomatic, although palpitations are frequent. At rapid ventricular rates, ischemia or hemodynamic compromise may occur. The ECG classically demonstrates an undulating baseline with a sawtooth pattern in the inferior leads (II, III, aVF) and without an isoelectric segment between the flutter waves. Vagal maneuvers may transiently worsen the AV block and make the flutter waves more obvious.

Atrial flutter may occur in patients with or without structural heart disease and may be precipitated by thyrotoxicosis, pericarditis, and alcohol ingestion. The same considerations noted earlier for the treatment of atrial fibrillation apply to the management of atrial flutter, although rate control is more difficult with atrial flutter and the thromboembolic risk is somewhat lower. When electrical cardioversion is used, relatively low-energy shocks are frequently effective (25 to 50 joules). When class Ia antiarrhythmic agents are used to convert atrial flutter to sinus rhythm, it is imperative that the ventricular rate is first controlled with either digoxin, β blockers, or calcium channel blockers. Class Ia agents may slow the flutter rate and augment AV nodal conduction, resulting in 1:1 conduction of flutter with very rapid ventricular rates. Radiofrequency catheter ablation of the reentrant flutter circuit is quite effective, resulting in the restoration of sinus rhythm in 90% to 95% of patients.

ATRIOVENTRICULAR NODAL (JUNCTIONAL) RHYTHM DISTURBANCES

If the atrial heart rate falls sufficiently, the AV node will emerge as the dominant pacemaker at a rate of 40 to 60 beats/min. This is termed a *junctional escape rhythm* (Fig. 10–6A, B). Occasionally, the junctional pacemaker may inappropriately overtake the atrial pacemaker for a single beat (premature junctional complex), for sustained periods of time at rates of 60 to 100 beats/min (accelerated junctional rhythm), or at rates greater than 100 beats/min (junctional tachycardia). These may accelerate gradually (nonparoxysmal rhythms) or occur suddenly (paroxysmal rhythms). The ECG with these junctional rhythms demonstrates a narrow-complex QRS identical to the normal sinus QRS. Evidence of retrograde atrial depolarization is frequently seen with an inverted P wave occurring either with a very short PR interval or immediately after the QRS complex. These rhythms are common in patients with inferior myocardial infarction or after cardiac surgery. Digoxin toxicity must also be excluded as a cause. Specific therapy of these rhythms is usually not necessary.

AV nodal reentrant tachycardia (AVNRT) is the most common paroxysmal SVT and is characterized by the sudden onset and termination of a narrow QRS complex, regular tachyarrhythmia at rates of 150 to 250 beats/min (see Fig. 10–6C). A wide QRS complex may occur if there is aberrant conduction in the His-Purkinje system. These rhythms may occur at any age; are somewhat more common in women; may occur in the absence of organic heart disease; may be short-lived or sustained; and may produce palpitations, chest pain, dyspnea, and presyncope. AVNRT is the result of a

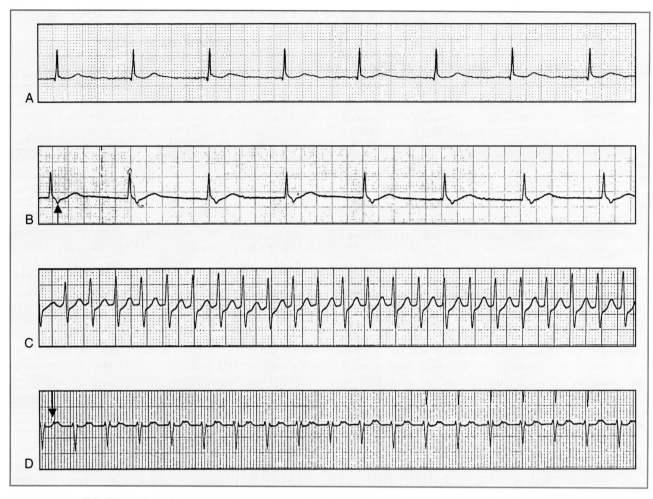

FIGURE 10-6   AV nodal rhythm disturbances. *A,* Junctional escape rhythm at a rate of 58 beats/min in a patient treated with digoxin and metoprolol for control of his underlying atrial fibrillation ("regularized atrial fibrillation"). *B,* Junctional escape rhythm at a rate of 50 beats/min demonstrating retrograde P waves after each QRS complex *(arrow). C,* AV nodal reentrant tachycardia at a rate of 185 beats/min. The retrograde P waves are hidden in the QRS complexes. *D,* Orthodromic atrioventricular reentrant tachycardia at a rate of 146 beats/min in a patient with Wolff-Parkinson-White syndrome. The retrograde P waves are clearly seen altering the normal T wave contour *(arrow).*

microreentrant circuit that utilizes two distinct pathways in the AV node. It is usually initiated by an APC that enters the reentrant circuit and uses the slow pathway as the antegrade limb and the fast pathway as the retrograde limb. The atria and ventricles depolarize almost simultaneously, with the retrograde P wave occurring in the terminal portion of the QRS or in the ST segment (short RP tachycardia). In rare cases (10%), the reentrant circuit travels in the opposite direction and the ventricles depolarize before the atria, resulting in a retrograde P wave that occurs after the T wave (long RP tachycardia). Vagal maneuvers (carotid sinus massage, Valsalva maneuver, coughing) may terminate an episode by causing a transient increase in AV nodal blockade. Adenosine (6 to 12 mg intravenously) terminates episodes in more than 95% of cases and is the treatment of choice if vagal maneuvers fail. In rare cases, direct current cardioversion is necessary. Intravenous β blockers, digoxin, or calcium channel blockers are also extremely effective acute therapy, and their oral formulations are

effective chronically. Class Ia, Ic, and III antiarrhythmic agents are useful in resistant cases. Radiofrequency catheter ablation of one limb of the reentrant circuit can cure AVNRT in more than 90% of cases, with a low risk of inducing complete heart block (<2%) and requiring the placement of a permanent pacemaker.

ATRIOVENTRICULAR RECIPROCATING ARRHYTHMIAS

Normally, the AV node is the only pathway that allows the wave of depolarization to conduct from the atria to the ventricles. However, anomalous bands of tissue (accessory pathways or bypass tracts) may exist and form an additional conduction pathway. The conductive properties of these bypass tracts differ from those of the AV node in that they can conduct at extremely rapid rates without developing conduction block (i.e., they do not manifest the decremental conduction property of normal conduction tissue). The bypass tracts may conduct in one direction only or may be bidirectional. These properties provide the substrate for macroreentrant arrhythmias using the bypass tract as one limb of the reentrant circuit and the AV node as the other. The WPW syndrome represents the most common accessory pathway and forms a direct connection from the atrial tissue to the ventricular myocardium (Fig. 10–7). Other pathways are less frequent and may connect the atrial tissue directly to the His-Purkinje system (Lown-Ganong-Levine or atrionodal pathway). The majority of patients with bypass tracts have otherwise anatomically normal hearts, although there is an increased incidence of accessory pathways in patients with Ebstein's anomaly of the right side of the heart.

When the bypass tract in WPW syndrome conducts in an antegrade fashion, preexcitation of the ventricles may occur; that is, an atrial depolarization will conduct to the ventricle more rapidly down the bypass tract than down the AV node and results in a short PR interval (<0.12 msec). The area of the ventricle at the site of the bypass tract is depolarized early, before the remainder of the ventricle is depolarized by means of the usual conduction pathways. The resultant QRS is a fusion complex created by ventricular activation through the two separate pathways. The extent of preexcitation is determined by the conductive properties of the pathways—as AV nodal conduction slows, a larger portion of the ventricle is preexcited through conduction down the bypass tract. With a "manifest" accessory pathway, the preexcitation can be identified on the surface ECG as a slurring of the initial portion of the QRS complex (the delta wave) and is diagnostic of WPW syndrome. The bypass tract may be located at various sites on the

left or right side of the heart, resulting in a variety of ECG manifestations. Occasionally, the accessory pathway cannot conduct antegrade so that ventricular preexcitation does not occur and there is no evidence of the bypass tract on the surface ECG (a concealed accessory pathway).

The most common arrhythmia in WPW syndrome is an *orthodromic* AV reentrant tachycardia (AVRT) in which the AV node is used as the antegrade limb of the circuit and the bypass tract as the retrograde limb. This results in a narrow-complex QRS on the surface ECG, unless aberrant conduction is present. A retrograde P wave may be noted, usually with a short RP interval. Less commonly, an *antidromic* AVRT may occur that uses the accessory pathway as the antegrade limb and the AV node as the retrograde limb. This results in complete preexcitation of the ventricles with a wide, bizarre QRS complex on the ECG. Because the AV node is an intrinsic component of both forms of AVRT, transient blockade of the AV node by vagal maneuvers or medications will interrupt the circuit and terminate the tachyarrhythmia. The incidence of atrial tachyarrhythmias, such as atrial fibrillation or flutter, is increased in patients with bypass tracts. When these arrhythmias occur, AV nodal–blocking drugs are contraindicated: in this setting, digoxin, β blockers, or calcium-channel blockers may result in slowing of conduction through the AV node with resultant preferential excitation of the ventricles through the accessory AV connection. Extremely rapid ventricular rates are possible and may precipitate hemodynamic collapse and sudden death.

In a patient with a delta wave noted on ECG but

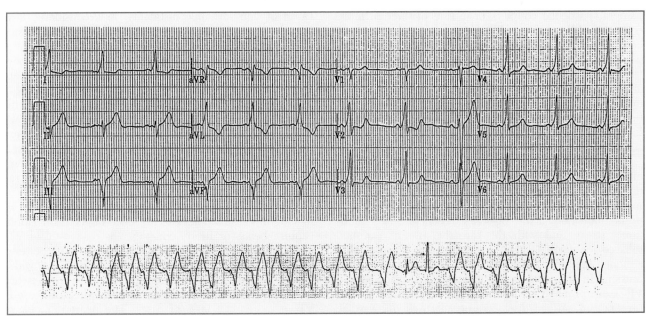

FIGURE 10–7   Wolff-Parkinson-White (WPW) syndrome. The upper tracing is a 12-lead electrocardiogram in a patient with WPW and reveals a short PR interval and slurring of the upstroke of the QRS complex in multiple leads (delta waves). The lower tracing demonstrates rapid atrial fibrillation in a patient with WPW. The irregular cycle lengths, wide QRS complexes with occasional normal QRS complexes, and very rapid rate should suggest the diagnosis of atrial fibrillation in the presence of an atrioventricular bypass tract.

without any symptoms, no specific therapy is required. In patients with frequent episodes of AVRT, chronic pharmacologic therapy with drugs that either slow conduction in the AV node (digoxin, β blockers, calcium channel blockers) or prolong the refractory period of the accessory pathway (class Ia, Ic, or III antiarrhythmic agents) is effective. Intravenous procainamide is the drug of choice for controlling the rate of atrial fibrillation or atrial flutter in patients with bypass tracts. Electrical cardioversion should be considered early in these patients. Radiofrequency catheter ablation of the accessory pathway has become the therapy of choice for symptomatic patients and has a success rate in excess of 95%.

VENTRICULAR RHYTHM DISTURBANCES

Ventricular premature complexes (VPCs) result from the spontaneous depolarization of the ventricular myocardium. The result is a QRS complex that is wide (>120 msec), has a bizarre morphology, and occurs earlier than expected. The repolarization phase is also abnormal and results in ST segment and T wave changes directed opposite the major deflection of the QRS complex. The wave of depolarization may conduct retrograde through the AV node, depolarize the atria, and result in a retrograde P wave on the surface ECG. Usually, this wave of depolarization does not reach the sinoatrial node before its spontaneous discharge and, thus, the sinus rate is unaffected. Most VPCs are, therefore, followed by a fully compensatory pause; that is, the RR interval surrounding the VPC is twice the normal RR interval (Fig. 10–8*B*). Occasionally, a VPC may occur without affecting the underlying sinus or ventricular rate (an interpolated VPC). VPCs may occur as single contractions, in pairs (a ventricular couplet), or in runs of three or more consecutive beats (i.e., VT). They may occur as every other complex (ventricular bigeminy), every third complex (ventricular trigeminy), and so on. They may be of uniform morphology (monomorphic) or vary in appearance (polymorphic). VPCs commonly have a fixed relationship to the preceding QRS complex. When this relationship varies, it suggests that there is a ventricular focus that is depolarizing at a rate independent of the sinus node, a so-called parasystolic focus.

VPCs occur with increased frequency in the presence of underlying heart disease (coronary artery disease, cardiomyopathy, mitral valve prolapse), advancing age, metabolic abnormalities (hypokalemia, hyperkalemia, hypoxia), infection, acute myocardial ischemia, and emotional stress, and with the excessive use of caffeine, tobacco, or alcohol. They are frequently asymptomatic, although they may produce palpitations and rarely hypotension. In the absence of underlying cardiac disease, VPCs are probably of no prognostic importance. In the presence of cardiac disease, especially ischemic cardiac disease, VPCs predict an increased risk of cardiac death. However, suppression of VPCs with antiarrhythmic agents has not been shown to improve mortality and, in fact, has been associated with an increase in cardiac death. Thus, VPCs should only be treated to control symptoms. β-Blocking agents may be effective in this regard, although class Ia or class III antiarrhythmic agents are occasionally necessary.

When the primary pacemakers fail or conduction of the atrial impulse to the ventricles is blocked (see later), the ventricular myocardium assumes the pacemaker role. The resultant ventricular escape rhythm is usually at a rate of 30 to 40 beats/min, but it may be faster at 60 to 100 beats/min (accelerated idioventricular rhythm [AIVR]) (see Fig. 10–8*A*). These escape rhythms should not be suppressed, because they may be the only remaining pacemaker activity available to the patient. AIVR may also occur if the automaticity of the ventricles is abnormally increased and overtakes the normal pacemaker rate despite normal impulse generation and conduction. This is frequently noted after successful reperfusion therapy for an acute myocardial infarction and does not necessitate treatment unless symptoms are present.

Ventricular tachycardia is defined as three or more consecutive ventricular depolarizations occurring at a rate of greater than 100 beats/min. The resulting QRS complexes on the surface ECG are aberrant, as described earlier for VPCs, and may be monomorphic or polymorphic (see Fig. 10–8*C, D*). Evidence of independent atrial activity may be present (AV dissociation); however, when retrograde conduction to the atria is present, AV dissociation is not seen. Occasionally, a normal sinus depolarization may be conducted to the ventricles before the pathologic ventricular depolarization occurs and results in a normal-appearing QRS complex (capture beat). If the atrial depolarization reaches the ventricles simultaneously with the spontaneous ventricular depolarization, a fusion complex will result. These abnormalities are pathognomonic for VT. When VT lasts for more than 30 seconds or requires termination because of hemodynamic instability, it is considered sustained; when it lasts less than 30 seconds, it is considered nonsustained.

When a wide-complex tachycardia occurs, it is important to determine whether it is VT or SVT with aberrancy because the therapeutic and prognostic implications differ significantly. When an SVT is associated with a narrow-complex QRS, the diagnosis is straightforward. However, when an SVT occurs in the setting of a preexisting bundle branch block, conducts aberrantly as a result of rate-related block in the His-Purkinje system, or conducts by means of an accessory pathway, the resulting QRS complex is wide and may be difficult to distinguish from VT. Several features may be helpful in making this distinction. The presence of AV dissociation, capture beats, or fusion complexes is diagnostic of VT. The absence of these findings is not helpful because they are present in less than 50% of cases. A wide-complex tachycardia occurring in the presence of ischemia or in a patient with known ischemic heart disease is VT in more than 90% of cases. The heart rate, blood pressure, and presence or absence of syncope do not differentiate these arrhythmias, whereas intermittent cannon a waves in the jugular venous pulsations suggest VT. If an abnormal QRS complex is present when the patient is in normal sinus rhythm and the QRS complex during the tachycardia is identical to this, the rhythm is

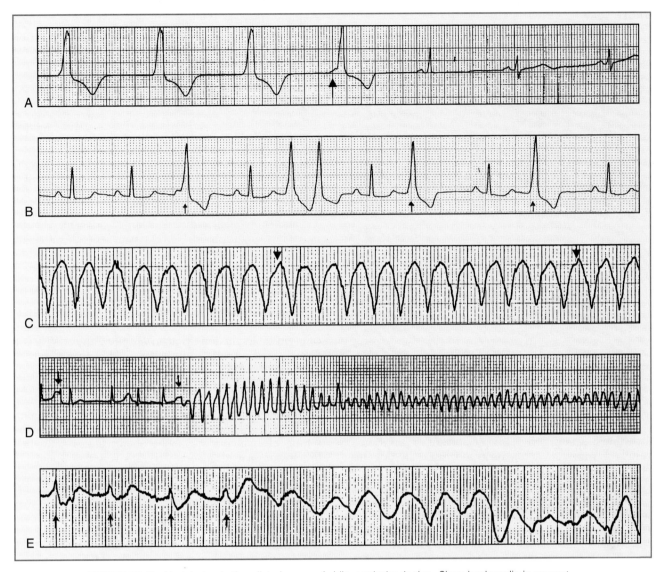

FIGURE 10–8   Ventricular rhythm disturbances. *A,* Idioventricular rhythm. Sinus bradycardia is present and allowed for the escape of an idioventricular rhythm at a rate similar to that of the sinus node. The fourth complex is preceded by a P wave, and the subsequent QRS is slightly narrower than those preceding it as a result of partial fusion of the ventricular and supraventricular impulses. The following QRS is also a fusion complex, after which sinus bradycardia with normal atrioventricular (AV) conduction returns. *B,* Multiple ventricular premature complexes *(arrows).* The wide complex beats are followed by fully compensatory pauses (see text). The fourth and fifth QRS complexes represent a ventricular couplet. *C,* Monomorphic ventricular tachycardia at a rate of 200 beats/min. The QRS complex is wide and p waves are seen to occasionally alter the QRS morphology *(arrows),* reflecting AV dissociation. *D,* Polymorphic ventricular tachycardia (torsades de pointes). (*Note:* the rhythm strip is at half the usual speed.) There is QT prolongation and several QRS complexes occur at the peak of the preceding T waves *(arrows)* with resultant induction of a wide-complex tachycardia that appears to rotate around the baseline. *E,* Ventricular fibrillation. An "agonal" rhythm is initially present *(arrows)* but deteriorates into ventricular fibrillation. The baseline is irregular without evidence of organized ventricular electrical activity.

likely SVT. Adenosine may be useful in determining the etiology: with SVT, adenosine-induced blockade of the AV node will reveal the atrial activity and may terminate the arrhythmia, whereas there is rarely any effect of adenosine on VT. Verapamil should never be used as a diagnostic test because it may precipitate ventricular fibrillation if the initial rhythm is VT. Table 10–7 lists the features that may help differentiate these arrhythmias from one another.

VT occurs most frequently in patients with underlying heart disease, including acute ischemia, prior infarction with scar formation, congestive cardiomyopathy, right ventricular dysplasia, and hypertrophic heart disease. The mechanism is usually reentry in the ventricular myocardium, although it may also arise in a diseased portion of the conduction system (e.g., bundle branch reentry). Metabolic abnormalities, such as hyperkalemia and hypoxia, and medications, such as digoxin and anti-

TABLE 10-7 **Features that May Differentiate VT from SVT with Aberrancy**

Features	Implications
Helpful Features	
Cannon a waves in jugular venous pulsations	Suggests VT
History of CAD	Suggests VT
First arrhythmia after AMI	Suggests VT
QRS duration > 0.16 sec	Suggests VT
Shift of axis from baseline	Suggests VT
QRS during tachycardia identical to QRS during sinus rhythm	Suggests SVT
Positive QRS concordance	Suggests VT
Presence of AV dissociation, capture beats, or fusion beats	Diagnostic of VT
Termination of arrhythmia with adenosine	Suggests SVT
Unhelpful Features	
Presenting symptom	
Blood pressure	
Heart rate	
Absence of AV dissociation	

AMI = acute myocardial infarction; AV = atrioventricular; CAD = coronary artery disease; SVT = supraventricular tachycardia; VT = ventricular tachycardia.

arrhythmic agents, may also precipitate VT, likely as a result of triggered automaticity. Occasionally, VT may occur spontaneously in the absence of an identifiable cause or underlying cardiac disease.

The acute treatment of hemodynamically stable VT involves the use of intravenous lidocaine. If this is not effective, procainamide or bretylium should be tried. Intravenous amiodarone has been shown to be extremely effective in the acute management of ventricular tachyarrhythmias. In patients with hemodynamic instability (hypotension, active ischemia, overt congestive heart failure), immediate synchronized electrical cardioversion should be performed. Relatively low energy shocks may be effective (10 to 50 joules), although as much as 360 joules is sometimes required. Digoxin-induced VT may be refractory to cardioversion or may degenerate to ventricular fibrillation. Phenytoin may be effective for this specific type of VT. Ventricular tachyarrhythmias that occur in the setting of acute ischemia or infarction respond to treatment of the ischemia and do not necessarily require prolonged antiarrhythmic therapy.

The appropriate chronic treatment of intermittent ventricular tachyarrhythmias is not as clear. Nonsustained VT is usually asymptomatic but is clearly a marker for increased cardiac mortality in certain populations with structural or ischemic heart disease. However, treatment of this arrhythmia has not been demonstrated to decrease mortality in most settings. Patients presenting with hemodynamically unstable VT or with recurrent sustained VT despite aggressive treatment of possible reversible precipitants (ischemia, metabolic abnormalities, drug toxicity, heart failure) require chronic antiar-

rhythmic therapy. Multiple pharmacologic agents have been used for this purpose, including quinidine, procainamide, disopyramide, propafenone, mexiletine, amiodarone, and sotalol. The risk of proarrhythmia must be taken into account in each patient. For patients with normal LV function, sotalol and amiodarone are the most effective agents. Amiodarone is the agent of choice for a patient with depressed ventricular function. Right ventricular outflow tract VT is a specific type of VT that occurs in young, otherwise healthy individuals, is frequently exercise induced, is associated with a left bundle branch block morphology on ECG, and is suppressible with verapamil. With improvements in interventional techniques, localization of the abnormal ventricular focus and subsequent radiofrequency ablation may be curative in many forms of VT. For patients with refractory arrhythmias, or arrhythmias associated with hemodynamic instability, placement of an AICD is indicated. Continued antiarrhythmic therapy may still be necessary to limit the frequency of delivered shocks.

Ventricular flutter is a form of monomorphic VT occurring at a rate of 300 beats/min and is a hemodynamically unstable rhythm. *Ventricular fibrillation* (VF) is a disorganized, chaotic, ventricular rhythm that results in ineffective ventricular contraction, rapid hemodynamic collapse, and death if not immediately terminated (see Fig. 10–8E). It is recognized on ECG by coarse undulations of the baseline without identifiable QRS complexes, ST segments, or T waves. It may occur in the setting of ischemia, metabolic abnormalities, and drug toxicity or may degenerate from VT, either spontaneously or after attempted cardioversion. Treatment with immediate nonsynchronized direct current shock at 200 to 360 joules is required in all cases. Several shocks may be required for termination of this arrhythmia, and concurrent treatment of precipitating causes is essential. Once the rhythm has been successfully terminated, an intravenous antiarrhythmic agent should be started to prevent recurrences. If VF is the result of an acute reversible cause, no chronic therapy is required. However, if VF occurs as a result of fixed underlying cardiac disease, implantation of an AICD is indicated.

Heart Block

Heart block refers to an impairment in impulse conduction (Fig. 10–9). The block may occur at any point in the conduction system, although it is most commonly recognized at the level of the AV node or His-Purkinje system. The incidence of heart block increases with age and may result from idiopathic fibrosis of the AV node, infarction of the AV node or His-Purkinje system, and calcification of the valvular annulus with impingement on the conduction system. Medications, either at therapeutic or toxic levels, may also result in various degrees of heart block.

Heart block at the level of the AV node is divided into several types. *First-degree AV block* refers to a prolongation of AV conduction time (PR interval >200 msec) but with eventual conduction of the atrial impulse

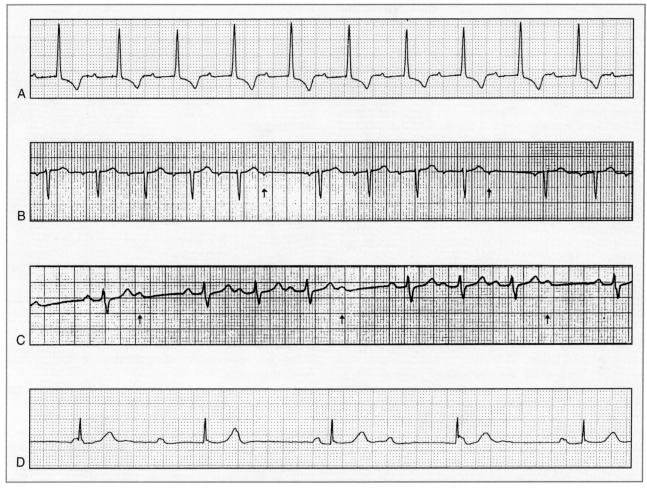

FIGURE 10–9 Heart block. *A,* First-degree atrioventricular (AV) block; the PR interval is prolonged. *B,* Second-degree AV block, type I (Wenckebach). There is progressive PR prolongation preceding a nonconducted P wave *(arrows).* *C,* Second-degree AV block, type II. Nonconducted P waves are seen *(arrows)* in the absence of progressive PR prolongation. *D,* Third-degree (complete) AV block with AV dissociation and a narrow-complex (AV nodal) escape rhythm.

to the ventricles (see Fig. 10–9A). *Second-degree AV block* refers to intermittent failure of the impulse to conduct from the atrium to the ventricles. This can be further divided into *Mobitz I second-degree heart block* (Wenckebach) (see Fig. 10–9B) in which there is a gradual prolongation of the PR interval until a nonconducted P wave occurs, and *Mobitz II second-degree heart block,* in which there is a sudden nonconducted P wave, or series of non-conducted P waves, without prior PR interval prolongation (see Fig. 10–9C). Mobitz I heart block usually reflects the effects of increased vagal tone on the AV node in the absence of structural disease of the node and is a benign rhythm that rarely causes symptoms. It commonly occurs at night, even in young patients with normal hearts. It may also occur in the setting of an acute inferior myocardial infarction, at which time it is usually transient, does not tend to progress to higher degrees of heart block, and rarely requires therapy. Mobitz II heart block usually reflects structural disease of the AV node or His-Purkinje system, may be associated with presyncope or syncope, and

may progress to higher degrees of heart block. It may also occur in the setting of an acute myocardial infarction (usually anterior), at which time it reflects ischemia or infarction of the conduction system, is associated with a high mortality rate, and requires at least temporary pacing. First- or second-degree AV block may also be the result of medications that affect the AV node (digoxin, β blockers, calcium channel blockers). When every other P wave is blocked (2:1 AV block), it cannot be determined whether the rhythm is Mobitz I or Mobitz II heart block because at least two consecutive conducted P waves are necessary to determine if progressive PR prolongation is present.

Complete or *third-degree heart block* is present when no atrial impulses conduct to the ventricles (see Fig. 10–9D). This may occur as a result of the processes noted earlier, may result from infiltrative (amyloid, sarcoid) or infectious diseases (endocarditis, Chagas' disease), may occur after cardiac surgery, and may also be a congenital condition. The clinical result of complete heart block depends on the response of the remainder of the conduction system to the disturbance. If the block occurs at the level of the AV node, the node will usually assume the pacemaker function and fire at a rate of 40 to 60 beats/min (junctional escape rhythm). If the block occurs in the His-Purkinje system, the ventricles will usually assume the pacemaker role and fire at a rate of 30 to 40 beats/min (ventricular escape rhythm). If no lower pacemaker fires, asystole will obviously result. Heart block may also occur at the level of the sinoatrial node but is difficult or impossible to diagnose on the surface ECG.

The treatment of heart block depends on the degree of block and the setting in which it occurs. First-degree AV block rarely, if ever, requires therapy. Mobitz I AV block requires treatment only if symptomatic and will usually respond to the administration of atropine. Mobitz II heart block usually requires at least temporary pacemaker placement. Acquired complete heart block warrants implantation of a permanent pacemaker. Congenital complete heart block has a good prognosis and does not generally require pacemaker implantation unless symptoms develop.

The term *AV dissociation* refers to the condition in which the atria and ventricles are depolarizing independently of each other. This occurs when the sinus rate falls below that of the lower subsidiary pacemaker (e.g., sinus bradycardia with a junctional escape rhythm), when a lower pacemaker focus accelerates pathologically to a rate faster than that of the sinus node (e.g., junctional tachycardia or VT), or when complete heart block is present. In the first two cases, the sinus rate is slower than the subsidiary pacemaker rate, whereas in complete heart block the sinus rate is faster than the escape rhythm. It is important to remember that AV dissociation is not synonymous with complete heart block; rather, complete heart block is a subset of AV dissociation.

Clinical Syndromes

LONG QT SYNDROME

The *long QT syndrome* refers to specific congenital and acquired abnormalities of repolarization that result in prolongation of the QT interval on the surface ECG (Table 10–8). Acquired forms are the result of various drugs or metabolic abnormalities. At least four separate genetic mutations account for the congenital forms of this disorder and do so by alterations in potassium or sodium channels. Congenital forms may be associated with deafness (Jervell and Lange-Nielsen syndrome) or occur in isolation (Romano-Ward syndrome). The significance of the long QT syndrome is its association with the development of a specific type of VT called *torsades de pointes*. This arrhythmia occurs in the setting of a prolonged QT interval, is usually initiated when a VPC occurs during the susceptible period of repolarization (i.e., at the peak of the T wave), and is characterized by a wide-complex tachyarrhythmia with QRS complexes of varying axis and morphology that appear to rotate

TABLE 10–8 Conditions Associated with Prolongation of the QT Interval

Condition	Examples
Congenital	Romano-Ward syndrome (without deafness)
	Jervell and Lange-Nielsen syndrome (with deafness)
Acquired	
Drugs	Class Ia and class III antiarrhythmic agents
	Tricyclic antidepressants
	Phenothiazines
	Antibiotics (macrolides, pentamidine, trimethoprim-sulfamethoxazole)
	Terfenadine (especially when combined with macrolides or antifungal agents)
Metabolic	Hypokalemia
	Hypocalcemia
	Hypomagnesemia
Other	Liquid protein diets

around the isoelectric baseline. Frequently these episodes are self-limited, although syncope and sudden death may occur.

The treatment of torsades de pointes differs from that of other forms of VT. Many antiarrhythmic agents will prolong the QT interval and exacerbate the arrhythmia. Intravenous magnesium (2 to 3 g) is effective in terminating this arrhythmia even in the presence of normal serum magnesium levels. Treatment with isoproterenol or temporary transvenous pacing at rates of 100 to 120 beats/min can effectively terminate the arrhythmia, presumably through tachycardia-induced shortening of the QT interval. Removal of the inciting agent is of paramount importance in acquired cases. Chronic treatment in patients with the congenital syndromes is with β-blocker therapy at the highest doses tolerated. Chronic pacemaker and/or AICD implantation is indicated in patients with recurrent arrhythmia despite β-blocker therapy. It is also important to screen family members of these patients to identify those at risk for this arrhythmia.

SYNCOPE

Syncope is defined as the sudden, transient loss of consciousness and may be the result of a variety of cardiac and noncardiac conditions (Table 10–9). Presyncope is a feeling of impending syncope without true loss of consciousness. Cardiovascular causes are responsible for the vast majority of cases and produce loss of consciousness by means of a drop in blood pressure with resultant bilateral cortical or brain stem hypoperfusion. Cerebrovascular disease is an uncommon cause of syncope unless bilateral carotid artery disease or vertebrobasilar disease is present.

The most important aspect of the approach to the patient with syncope is in obtaining a thorough history, both from the patient as well as from any witnesses to the episode. The conditions during which a syncopal

TABLE 10–9   Causes of Syncope

Cause	Features
Peripheral Vascular or Circulatory	
Vasovagal syncope (neurally mediated)	Prodrome of pallor, yawning, nausea, diaphoresis; precipitated by stress or pain; occurs when patient is upright, aborted by recumbency; fall in blood pressure without appropriate rise in heart rate
Micturition syncope	Syncope with urination (probably vagal)
Post-tussive syncope	Syncope after paroxysm of coughing
Hypersensitive carotid sinus syndrome	Vasodepressor and/or cardioinhibitory responses with light carotid sinus massage (see text)
Drugs	Orthostasis
	Occurs with antihypertensive drugs, tricyclic antidepressants, phenothiazines
Volume depletion	Orthostasis
	Occurs with hemorrhage, excessive vomiting or diarrhea, Addison's disease
Autonomic dysfunction	Orthostasis
	Occurs in diabetes, alcoholism, Parkinson's disease, deconditioning after a prolonged illness
Central Nervous System	
Cerebrovascular	Transient ischemic attacks and strokes are unusual causes of syncope; associated neurologic abnormalities are usually present
Seizures	Warning aura sometimes present, jerking of extremities, tongue biting, urinary incontinence, postictal confusion
Metabolic	
Hypoglycemia	Confusion, tachycardia, jitteriness before syncope; patient may be taking insulin
Cardiac	
Obstructive	Syncope is often exertional; physical findings consistent with aortic stenosis, hypertrophic obstructive cardiomyopathy, cardiac tamponade, atrial myxoma, prosthetic valve malfunction, Eisenmenger's syndrome, tetralogy of Fallot, primary pulmonary hypertension, pulmonic stenosis, massive pulmonary embolism
Arrhythmias	Syncope may be sudden and occurs in any position; episodes of dizziness or palpitations; may be a history of heart disease; brady- or tachyarrhythmias may be responsible—check for hypersensitive carotid sinus

episode occurs may suggest the etiology. For instance, syncope that occurs on arising from a lying or sitting position suggests orthostasis. Exercise-induced syncope suggests obstructive cardiac disease, such as aortic or mitral valve stenosis, or hypertrophic cardiomyopathy. Syncope during straining, coughing, or micturition is the result of Valsalva-induced decrease in venous return. A history of palpitations preceding the event suggests an arrhythmic cause. Syncope that occurs during emotional stress suggests a vasovagal episode. Certain features may suggest a noncardiac cause, including incontinence or tonic-clonic movements, which suggest seizure. Patients who suffer a cardiac syncopal episode usually regain consciousness rapidly (<5 minutes). Longer episodes of unresponsiveness suggest a noncardiac cause. Review of the patient's medications is important and may suggest drug-induced hypotension or arrhythmias as the cause of a syncopal episode.

The physical examination of a patient with syncope should include evaluation of orthostatic changes in the heart rate and blood pressure, a thorough cardiac examination to exclude significant murmurs, a neurologic examination, and carotid sinus massage when the history suggests carotid sinus sensitivity as the diagnosis. A 12-lead ECG should be obtained and may be diagnostic of the etiology of syncope (e.g., complete heart block) or reveal abnormalities that warrant further evaluation (e.g., prior myocardial infarction, conduction system disease, nonsustained VT, or a delta wave of WPW syndrome).

Further cardiac testing is useful in selected patients. An echocardiogram is not routinely indicated but is helpful in patients for whom a structural cardiac cause is suspected. A 24-hour Holter monitor or an event monitor may be helpful in evaluating for possible arrhythmias. In patients in whom ventricular tachyarrhythmias are suspected as the cause of syncope, a signal-averaged ECG (SAECG) may predict the ability to induce the arrhythmia during EP testing. The SAECG is a computerized technique that averages and filters multiple QRS complexes and is, thus, able to identify oscillations (*late potentials*) in the terminal portion of the QRS complex. These late potentials reflect regions of the myocardium with altered repolarization properties that provide the substrate for sustained ventricular arrhythmias. In patients with recurrent syncope without evidence of a structural or arrhythmic etiology and in patients in whom the history suggests vasovagal or neurocardiogenic syncope, tilt-table testing may be useful (see earlier). In patients in whom the history, ECG, SAECG, or Holter monitoring suggests a tachyarrhythmia or heart block as the cause of syncope, EP testing is indicated and may reproduce the arrhythmia or identify the level of heart block present. However, in patients with a normal resting ECG and no structural heart disease, the diagnostic yield of EP testing is so low that it is rarely useful. Fig. 10–10 offers a diagnostic approach to the patient with syncope. Despite all of these diagnostic modalities, in more than 30% of all cases of syncope, the cause remains unknown.

SUDDEN CARDIAC DEATH

Sudden death is commonly defined as a natural, unexpected death occurring within 1 hour of the onset of symptoms. Sudden death may be the result of a variety of cardiac and noncardiac diseases (Table 10–10), although cardiac causes are by far the most common. Sudden cardiac death (SCD) accounts for an estimated 300,000 deaths per year—over 50% of all deaths from cardiac causes—and is the leading cause of death among men aged 20 to 60. Ventricular tachyarrhythmias (VT and VF) occurring in the setting of ischemic heart disease account for the mechanism of death in the vast majority of these cases. Polymorphic VT occurring in the setting of the long QT syndrome, idiopathic causes

of VT in the absence of underlying heart disease, and rapid conduction of an SVT over an accessory bypass tract precipitating VT/VF account for other tachyarrhythmic causes of SCD. Bradyarrhythmias and pulseless electrical activity, a condition during which the electrical activity of the heart continues in the absence of mechanical contraction, account for only a small proportion of SCD.

Ischemic heart disease is present in at least 80% of patients who die suddenly of a cardiac cause, and as many as 75% of these patients have a prior history of a myocardial infarction. In the remainder, SCD is their first manifestation of ischemic heart disease. Nonetheless, only 20% of patients resuscitated from an episode of SCD have evidence of having had an acute transmural myocardial infarction at the time of the event. This is of prognostic importance—survivors of SCD that occurred in the setting of an acute myocardial infarction have a recurrence rate of less than 5% in the following year compared with a 30% recurrence rate in survivors in whom SCD occurred in the absence of an acute infarction.

The only effective treatment of an acute episode of SCD is immediate circulatory support with cardiopulmo-

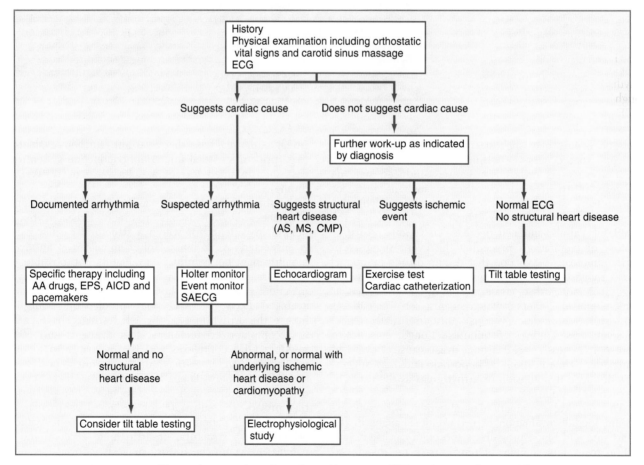

FIGURE 10–10 Diagnostic approach to the patient with syncope. ECG = electrocardiogram; AS = aortic stenosis; MS = mitral stenosis; CMP = cardiomyopathy; AA = antiarrhythmic; EPS = electrophysiologic study; AICD = automatic implantable cardioverter-defibrillator; SAECG = signal-averaged electrocardiogram.

TABLE 10–10   Causes of Sudden Cardiac Death

Noncardiac
  Central nervous system hemorrhage
  Massive pulmonary embolus
  Drug overdose
  Hypoxia secondary to lung disease
  Aortic dissection or rupture

Cardiac
  Ventricular tachycardia
  Bradyarrhythmias, sick sinus syndrome
  Aortic stenosis
  Tetralogy of Fallot
  Pericardial tamponade
  Cardiac tumors
  Complications of infective endocarditis
  Hypertrophic cardiomyopathy (arrhythmia or obstruction)
  Myocardial ischemia
    Atherosclerosis
    Prinzmetal's angina
    Kawasaki's arteritis

TABLE 10–11   Predictors of Sudden Cardiac Death After Myocardial Infarction

Decreased left ventricular ejection fraction
Residual ischemia
Complex ventricular ectopy (nonsustained ventricular tachycardia) on ambulatory ECG monitoring
Late potentials on signal averaged ECG
Absence of heart rate variability
Decreased carotid baroreceptor sensitivity
Prolonged QT on ECG
Induction of sustained monomorphic ventricular tachycardia with programmed electrical stimulation

nary resuscitation (see later) and establishment of an effective cardiac rhythm with electrical defibrillation. Once a stable rhythm has been restored, intravenous antiarrhythmic therapy (usually with lidocaine) should be instituted for the first 24 hours while determination of the precipitating cause is made. It cannot be assumed that VT/VF was the mechanism of SCD unless these rhythms were documented at the time of arrest; a thorough search for other possible causes is mandatory. In SCD survivors, a full cardiac evaluation should be performed to define cardiac function, identify the presence of reversible heart disease, and assess the risk of recurrent arrhythmias. Echocardiography can identify possible structural cardiac causes of SCD (aortic stenosis, hypertrophic cardiomyopathy) and allows assessment of left ventricular function. This is important prognostically—patients with depressed ventricular function have a higher likelihood of recurrent SCD, a poorer response to antiarrhythmic drug therapy, and a higher mortality rate than do those with normal ventricular function. Ambulatory ECG monitoring and stress testing are useful in documenting the frequency and severity of recurrent ventricular arrhythmias and in assessing residual ischemia. Patients in whom SCD was precipitated by an acute ischemic event do not necessarily require antiarrhythmic therapy; the main goal should be the control of ischemia. Cardiac catheterization and revascularization should be performed if possible.

In SCD survivors in whom the event occurred in the absence of an acute myocardial infarction, and in patients with recurrent ventricular tachyarrhythmias, antiarrhythmic therapy has been the mainstay of treatment. Various antiarrhythmic agents have been used, although trials during the 1990s suggest that sotalol and amiodarone are the most effective. The effectiveness of these agents in suppressing tachyarrhythmias can be assessed equally well with serial ambulatory ECG monitoring or serial EP studies. The AVID trial (Antiarrhythmics versus Implantable Defibrillators) has significantly changed the therapeutic approach to SCD survivors. This study was a randomized trial of antiarrhythmic therapy (primarily amiodarone) versus AICD implantation in patients with depressed ventricular function who had survived an episode of life-threatening ventricular tachyarrhythmia, and it demonstrated a mortality benefit with AICD therapy.

Perhaps the most effective method of treating SCD is by identifying those patients at highest risk and instituting therapy aimed at preventing its occurrence. In the post–myocardial infarction patient, several factors have been shown to be associated with an increased risk of SCD (Table 10–11). The occurrence of frequent complex ventricular ectopy in patients after an acute myocardial infarction is associated with a near tripling of the risk of subsequent SCD; however, attempts at suppression of these arrhythmias with antiarrhythmic agents have resulted in an increased mortality. Several studies have, however, demonstrated a decrease in overall mortality, as well as in SCD, in patients treated with β-blocking agents after a myocardial infarction. Therefore, these agents should be instituted in these patients unless there is a contraindication to their use. Post–myocardial infarction patients with left ventricular dysfunction, nonsustained VT on ambulatory ECG monitoring, and inducible monomorphic VT during EP testing have been demonstrated to have an improved survival with AICD implantation. Whether prophylactic AICDs will benefit other high-risk group remains to be seen.

Principles of Cardiopulmonary Resuscitation

Most cases of sudden cardiac death do not occur in the hospital and, thus, immediate medical therapy may not be available. Over two thirds of patients who suffer an out-of-hospital cardiac arrest die before ever reaching a hospital. Less than half of the remainder survive to hospital discharge. Basic cardiac life support (BCLS) performed by civilian bystanders may allow for circulatory and ventilatory support until trained medical personnel arrive and can institute advanced cardiac life support (ACLS) techniques. These interventions have significantly improved the probability of survival in SCD patients. The time interval between the onset of SCD and the institution of these lifesaving measures is critical. Ideally, BCLS should be instituted within 2 minutes of SCD and ACLS by 8 minutes. A delay of 5 minutes before cardiopulmonary resuscitation (CPR) is performed is associated with a very low survival rate.

On identifying a patient with presumed cardiac arrest, the rescuer should first establish that the patient is truly unresponsive. If so, help should immediately be summoned, including leaving the patient for 1 or 2 minutes to telephone for emergency medical care. Once help has been called for, or if no mechanism of obtaining help is available, the rescuer should check to see whether the patient is breathing and has a pulse. If the arrest is witnessed and the patient is pulseless, a precordial thump to the midsternum may be tried and occasionally will terminate a ventricular tachyarrhythmia. Subsequently, the "ABCDs" of resuscitation should be employed: airway, breathing, circulation, and defibrillation. The airway should be cleared of any obstruction and the tongue moved from the posterior pharynx by tilting the head back and lifting the chin. This maneuver occasionally results in the resumption of spontaneous breathing. If no breathing occurs, mouth-to-mouth breathing should be instituted, ideally with a barrier ventilation device. Two breaths are given while the chest is observed for evidence of adequate ventilation. If the patient remains pulseless after the initial ventilations, external cardiac compressions should be started. In the adult victim, compression of the lower half of the sternum by 3 to 5 cm (not over the xiphoid process) should be performed at a rate of 80 to 100 times per minute. If two rescuers are present, five compressions should be given, followed by one ventilation. If only one rescuer is present, the ratio of chest compressions to ventilations is 15:2. As soon as a defibrillator is available, it should be applied to the chest to determine if a ventricular tachyarrhythmia is present, and, if so, defibrillation should ensue, repetitively if necessary. This is the single most important treatment for patients with SCD. Time is of utmost importance; the probability of successful defibrillation decreases by about 10% per minute after the onset of cardiac arrest.

While these resuscitative efforts are underway, oxygen should be applied, tracheal intubation performed if necessary, and intravenous access established. Once the rhythm is identified, appropriate pharmacologic therapy should be instituted. Asystole should be treated with epinephrine (1 mg IV bolus every 3 to 5 minutes); transcutaneous pacing may be effective if instituted very early in the resuscitation. Bradycardia may respond to atropine (boluses of 0.5 mg IV every 5 minutes up to a maximal dose of 3 mg). If this is ineffective, the early use of transcutaneous pacing or intravenous catechol-amine infusion with dopamine (5 to 20 μg/min) or epinephrine (2 to 10 μg/min) should be considered. Isoproterenol is no longer suggested for the treatment of bradycardia because it markedly increases myocardial oxygen demands and may exacerbate ischemia. Ventricular tachyarrhythmias should be aggressively treated with a multimodal approach. Electrical defibrillation should be attempted early and repeated as often as necessary. Epinephrine boluses may increase the success rate of defibrillation. Intravenous lidocaine, bretylium, procainamide, and amiodarone may be given to help terminate ventricular tachyarrhythmias and prevent their recurrence.

Certain drugs may be useful for specific types of cardiac arrest. Ventricular tachyarrhythmias occurring in the setting of digoxin toxicity may be refractory to electrical cardioversion. Intravenous phenytoin may be effective in this setting. Intravenous sodium bicarbonate (1 mEq/kg) is indicated in cardiac arrest resulting from hyperkalemia or tricyclic antidepressant overdose, may be helpful after prolonged resuscitative efforts, but is not routinely indicated in all arrest situations.

Pulseless electrical activity (previously termed *electromechanical dissociation*) refers to the persistence of cardiac electrical activity in the absence of mechanical contraction. Causes include hypovolemia, cardiac tamponade, tension pneumothorax, hypothermia, massive pulmonary embolism, metabolic disturbances (hypoxia, hyperkalemia, acidosis), mechanical complications of an acute myocardial infarction, and drug overdoses (tricyclic antidepressants, digoxin, β blockers, calcium channel blockers). Empirical treatment is with epinephrine and atropine. Definitive therapy requires the identification and reversal of the precipitating cause. Emergency pericardiocentesis should be performed if cardiac tamponade is suspected.

REFERENCES

Antiarrhythmic versus Implantable Defibrillators (AVID) Investigators: A comparison of antiarrhythmic drug therapy with implantable defibrillators in patients resuscitated from near-fatal ventricular tachyarrhythmias. N Engl J Med 1997; 337:1576.

Dreifus LS (chairman): ACC/AHA Task Force. Guidelines for implantation of cardiac pacemakers and antiarrhythmic devices. J Am Coll Cardiol 1991; 18:1.

Falk RH, Podrid PJ: Atrial Fibrillation, Mechanisms and Management, 2nd ed. Philadelphia: Lippincott-Raven, 1997.

Ganz LI, Friedman PL: Supraventricular tachycardia. N Engl J Med 1995; 332:162.

Laupacis A, Albers G, Dalen JE, et al: Antithrombotic therapy in atrial fibrillation. Chest 1995; 108(Suppl):352S.

Morandy F: Radiofrequency catheter ablation as treatment for cardiac arrhythmias. N Engl J Med 1998; 340:534.

Podrid PJ, Kowey PR: Cardiac Arrhythmia. Mechanisms, Diagnosis, and Management. Baltimore: Williams & Wilkins, 1995.

Roden DM: Risks and benefits of antiarrhythmic therapy. N Engl J Med 1994; 331:785.

Zipes DP (chairman): ACC/AHA Task Force: Guidelines for intracardiac electrophysiological and catheter ablation procedures. J Am Coll Cardiol 1995; 26:555.

11

MYOCARDIAL AND PERICARDIAL DISEASE

Lisa A. Mendes • Joseph Loscalzo

Myocarditis

Myocarditis is an inflammatory disease of the myocardium. Although associated with a number of infectious and systemic diseases, myocarditis is most frequently the result of a viral infection, with coxsackievirus B and echovirus being the most frequently implicated infectious agents. However, any virus may replicate in the heart and induce myocardial inflammation. The true incidence of this disease is unknown because most cases resolve spontaneously and never reach medical attention. However, myocardial involvement has been reported to occur in 1% to 5% of patients with acute viral infections.

Myocardial damage is believed to be secondary to direct viral invasion of the myocytes, as well as to the immunologic response to the infection. Initially, replication of the virus in the myocytes leads to cell damage and death. At this early phase, the virus is eliminated primarily by humoral and cell-mediated immune processes, and, in most cases, myocardial inflammation promptly resolves. If this initial immune response fails to clear the viral agent, it has been hypothesized that an autoimmune response directed against the myocardium may be triggered, leading to further myocardial inflammation and injury.

The clinical presentation of myocarditis is quite variable. Many patients are asymptomatic and will have complete resolution of the myocarditis without complications. Others may present with nonspecific complaints typical of a viral syndrome, such as fever, malaise, and myalgias. Pleuritic chest pain secondary to pericardial inflammation is common, although some patients may have pain more typical of myocardial ischemia. If cardiac dysfunction is present, patients may present with symptoms of congestive heart failure and, in rare instances, cardiogenic shock. Life-threatening arrhythmias can occur in patients with myocarditis even in the presence of preserved left ventricular systolic function.

On physical examination, patients are often tachycardic. A pericardial friction rub may be heard if myopericarditis is present. If left ventricular dysfunction has resulted, patients may have signs of volume overload, including crackles on lung examination, distended neck veins, and peripheral edema. On auscultation, an S_3 gallop may be present, as well as murmurs of tricuspid and mitral regurgitation. The most common changes on the electrocardiogram are ST segment and T wave abnormalities, especially if pericardial involvement is present. Elevated levels of myocardial creatine kinase and troponin I, which signify myocardial necrosis, may be detected in the blood during the acute phase of the illness. Transthoracic echocardiography is useful to assess biventricular size and function. Endomyocardial biopsy of the right ventricle remains the gold standard for diagnosing myocarditis and is most useful when a treatable cause is found. Histologic evidence of myocardial inflammation and cellular necrosis are required to make a definitive diagnosis of myocarditis (Dallas criteria). Because of the patchy nature of the disease process and sampling errors with this procedure, a negative biopsy does not exclude the diagnosis of myocarditis.

The natural history of myocarditis is quite variable. Most patients with subclinical disease have complete resolution of myocardial inflammation without long-term sequelae. In some patients, depressed ventricular function may develop in the absence of symptoms and become manifested months to years later as a dilated cardiomyopathy. Of patients with myocarditis presenting with heart failure symptoms or serious arrhythmias, the 5-year survival is approximately 55%. Therapy is usually supportive and includes avoidance of exercise, electrocardiographic monitoring for arrhythmias, and treatment of heart failure (see Chapter 6). At present, there is no role for immunosuppressive therapy in the treatment of viral myocarditis. However, specific subgroups of patients, such as those with giant cell myocarditis, may benefit from this treatment. Finally, patients with myocarditis associated with a specific systemic illness may

127

TABLE 11-1   Classification of Cardiomyopathy

	Dilated (Congestive)	Hypertrophic	Restrictive
Symptoms	Dyspnea, orthopnea fatigue, leg edema	Dyspnea, angina, syncope after exertion, palpitations	Dyspnea, fatigue, leg edema
Characteristic cardiac physical findings	Cardiomegaly; S_3 and S_4 common; murmur of mitral and tricuspid regurgitation	Bifid apical impulse with palpable S_4; ejection murmur at LSB (increased with Valsalva); often associated mitral regurgitation murmur	Normal size or slightly enlarged heart; S_3 common; S_4; murmur of tricuspid or mitral regurgitation; elevated jugular venous pressure, inspiratory increase in venous pressure
Electrocardiogram	Sinus tachycardia; left bundle branch block common	Left ventricular hypertrophy; abnormal Q waves	Low voltage; abnormal Q waves; conduction abnormalities
Echocardiogram	Dilated cardiac chambers; generalized reduced ventricular wall motion and systolic function	Normal or small left ventricular cavity; left ventricular hypertrophy; asymmetric septal thickening; systolic anterior motion of anterior mitral valve leaflet	Thick walls, reduced systolic function; glistening appearance of left ventricle in amyloid
Treatment	Diuretics; unloading agents; digoxin	β-Adrenergic–blocking drugs or selected calcium channel–blocking drugs; sequential atrioventricular (DDD) pacing for selected patients with refractory symptoms; surgical septal myectomy for refractory obstructive symptoms	Treatment of underlying cause; diuretics

DDD = atrial synchronous ventricular pacemaker; LSB = left sternal border.

have improvement in the myocarditic process with treatment of the underlying disease.

Cardiomyopathy

Cardiomyopathy refers to a group of primary myocardial diseases of unknown etiology and can be divided into three broad categories: dilated, hypertrophic, and restrictive (Table 11–1).

DILATED CARDIOMYOPATHY

Dilated cardiomyopathy (DCM) is a cardiac condition characterized by chamber enlargement and impaired systolic function of one or both ventricles. By definition, the etiology of DCM is unknown. However, there are many diseases, toxins, and metabolic disorders that may produce myocardial damage similar to that of DCM (Table 11–2). In addition, familial transmission of DCM as an autosomal dominant trait with variable penetrance has been reported and is thought to affect 10% to 20% of a patient's first- and second-degree relatives.

Patients with DCM may be asymptomatic for many years despite severely impaired left ventricular function. However, most affected individuals will develop symptoms of congestive heart failure, which may be gradual

or abrupt in onset. In addition, patients may present with symptomatic atrial or ventricular arrhythmias as well as sudden cardiac death. The physical examination is typical of patients with heart failure and may reveal evidence of left and right ventricular dysfunction. The electrocardiogram may be completely normal but more

TABLE 11-2   Causes of Dilated Cardiomyopathy

Idiopathic
Toxin-induced
  Alcohol
  Anthracycline
  Cobalt
  Catecholamine
Radiation
Infectious
  Viral
  Parasitic (e.g., Chagas' disease)
Metabolic
  Starvation
  Thiamine deficiency (beriberi)
  Thyrotoxicosis
Sarcoidosis
Hemochromatosis
Peripartum or postpartum cardiomyopathy
Genetic

often demonstrates poor R wave progression and an intraventricular conduction delay, especially left bundle branch block. Two-dimensional and Doppler echocardiography is useful in assessing ventricular size and systolic function, as well as valve competency. Cardiac catheterization is performed primarily to exclude the presence of significant epicardial coronary artery disease, although, in selected patients, measurement of filling pressures may help guide pharmacologic therapy. Endomyocardial biopsy is usually reserved for those patients who are suspected of having a treatable cause of DCM.

Management of patients with DCM is similar to that for patients with congestive heart failure (see Chapter 6). The clinical outcome of patients with DCM has significantly improved with the use of angiotensin-converting enzyme inhibitors, and, more recently, β-blocker therapy. However, the prognosis in patients with advanced heart failure is poor, with 5-year mortality in excess of 50%.

HYPERTROPHIC CARDIOMYOPATHY

Hypertrophic cardiomyopathy (HCM) is a heterogeneous disorder characterized by variable degrees of left ventricular hypertrophy, normal or small left ventricular cavity size, and hyperdynamic systolic function. A subset of these patients has predominantly interventricular septal hypertrophy in association with anterior motion of the mitral leaflets and subvalvular left ventricular outflow tract obstruction, a condition denoted as hypertrophic obstructive cardiomyopathy. Reports suggest that HCM is quite common, affecting 1 in 500 individuals in the general population. Both familial (autosomal dominant) and sporadic forms of this disease can occur. In addition, there is a variant of HCM that is found in elderly, often female patients with hypertension. Prior molecular studies have determined that mutations in the genes coding for cardiomyocyte contractile proteins may be responsible for HCM. More than 50 different mutations affecting myosin heavy chains, myosin light chains, tropomyosin, and troponins have been described thus far. Notwithstanding the wide variety of genetic abnormalities, all are associated with a common phenotype that includes cardiomyocyte dysfunction, myofibril disarray, cardiomyocyte hypertrophy, and interstitial fibrosis.

HCM is characterized by the presence of a dynamic left ventricular outflow tract obstruction and diastolic dysfunction. The degree of outflow obstruction is quite variable and may develop within the mid cavity of the left ventricle or, more commonly, below the aortic valve. In the later presenting form, the left ventricular outflow tract is narrowed by the septal hypertrophy and, in some patients, is associated with anterior displacement of the mitral leaflets toward the interventricular septum. The resulting pressure gradient across the left ventricular outflow tract is highly dependent on physiologic and pharmacologic maneuvers that affect left ventricular volume (dynamic gradient). Maneuvers that reduce left ventricular volume, such as standing, the Valsalva maneuver, or sublingual nitroglycerin, further narrow the left ventricular outflow tract and increase the degree of obstruction. An increase in left ventricular volume that occurs with squatting or administration of intravenous fluids will expand the outflow tract and reduce the pressure gradient. Diastolic dysfunction is frequently present in patients with HCM, even in the absence of a significant outflow tract gradient, and is independent of the degree of left ventricular hypertrophy. Reduced compliance of the left ventricle results in elevated left ventricular end-diastolic and pulmonary venous pressures, leading to pulmonary congestion.

The clinical manifestations of HCM are also variable. Some patients with HCM are asymptomatic for many years, even if severe left ventricular outflow obstruction is present. Others may present with life-threatening arrhythmias or sudden cardiac death. However, the most frequent symptom in patients with HCM is dyspnea on exertion, which is secondary to diastolic dysfunction and elevation in left ventricular filling pressures. As the myocardial disease progresses, the left ventricle may begin to dilate, thus alleviating outflow obstruction. Dyspnea under these conditions may be secondary to both systolic and diastolic dysfunction. Ischemic chest pain can occur in the absence of epicardial coronary artery disease and is caused by increased oxygen demand by the hypertrophied ventricle and elevated wall tension reducing blood flow to the subendocardium. Syncope can result from severe obstruction to left ventricular outflow and concomitant reduced cardiac output, as well as arrhythmias. Syncope associated with vigorous exertion is not uncommon because the increase in left ventricular inotropy increases the degree of outflow tract obstruction. If the right ventricle is involved in the myopathic process, symptoms of right-sided heart failure may also be present.

The characteristic findings on cardiac examination are summarized in Tables 11-1 and 11-3. Patients with significant outflow tract obstruction typically have a harsh, crescendo-decrescendo systolic murmur heard best at the left sternal border that is intensified by maneuvers that decrease left ventricular volume. An S_4 secondary to increased ventricular stiffness is frequently heard and may be palpable at the apex. If left ventricular dysfunction has developed, an S_3 may be audible. The initial carotid upstroke is brisk but is followed by a midsystolic dip secondary to the development of left ventricular tract outflow obstruction. Late in systole, the carotid impulse rises again as the remaining blood in the left ventricle is ejected (bisferiens pulse). A prominent a wave signifying forceful atrial contraction may be seen on inspection of the neck veins.

The electrocardiogram in HCM typically demonstrates increased QRS voltage secondary to left ventricular hypertrophy. Prominent, abnormal Q waves are frequently present in the inferior and lateral leads and reflect depolarization of the hypertrophied septum. Two-dimensional echocardiography allows assessment of left ventricular function, the degree and location of the hypertrophy, and the severity of the systolic anterior motion of the mitral leaflets. Doppler techniques can be used to estimate the severity and location of left ventric-

TABLE 11–3　Effect of Selected Maneuvers on Dynamic Outflow Gradient and Murmur in Hypertrophic Cardiomyopathy

Maneuver	Mechanism	Effect on Gradient and Murmur
Valsalva (during strain)	↓ LV cavity size (↓ preload and ↓ afterload)	↑
Standing	↓ LV cavity size (↓ preload)	↑
Postextrasystolic beat	↑ Contractility, (also ↑ preload)	↑
Squatting	↑ LV cavity size (↑ preload and ↑ afterload)	↓
Isometric handgrip exercise	↑ afterload	↓

LV = left ventricle.

ular outflow tract obstruction and to monitor changes in the gradient during provocative maneuvers or after specific treatment. Echocardiography is also useful for screening family members of patients with HCM. On occasion, cardiac catheterization may be necessary to assess patients with HCM if the echocardiogram is inadequate to define the severity of obstruction or if evaluation for coronary artery disease is indicated.

Treatment of HCM is aimed at improving diastolic dysfunction and minimizing left ventricular outflow obstruction. Both β blockers and calcium channel blockers have been used extensively in this disease and have been shown to improve symptoms, especially dyspnea and chest pain. The beneficial effects of these medications are primarily related to heart rate slowing, which prolongs diastole and allows for increased passive ventricular filling. In addition, these drugs have a negative inotropic effect on myocardial function and help decrease the severity of left ventricular outflow tract obstruction. In patients with refractory symptoms from left ventricular outflow obstruction, insertion of a dual-chamber pacemaker may help relieve the obstruction and relieve symptoms. The mechanism of benefit with this therapy appears, in part, related to diminished inward systolic motion of the interventricular septum from asynchronous contraction of the right and left ventricles. This results in an increase in left ventricular outflow dimensions and a reduction in outflow obstruction. In selected patients with severely symptomatic obstructive HCM, left ventricular myomectomy to thin the proximal interventricular septum relieves left ventricular outflow tract obstruction and improves symptoms and long-term survival. For patients with atrial fibrillation, maintenance of sinus rhythm is best achieved with amiodarone, as outlined in Chapter 10. Patients presenting with life-threatening ventricular arrhythmias should undergo electrophysiologic evaluation. In selected patients, treatment with amiodarone or an automatic implantable defibrillator may be indicated. Endocarditis prophylaxis is indicated in all patients with HCM.

The clinical course of patients with HCM is unpredictable and independent of the presence or severity of left ventricular outflow tract obstruction. In general, clinical deterioration occurs slowly with the incidence of symptomatic cases, increasing with advancing age. Sudden death can occur at any time, even in an asymptomatic individual, and is the leading cause of death in this population. Treatment may improve symptoms and relieve the outflow tract obstruction but has not been shown to prolong survival.

RESTRICTIVE CARDIOMYOPATHY

Restrictive cardiomyopathy is a rare heart muscle disease that may affect both ventricles and is characterized by small ventricular cavity size, diastolic dysfunction, and elevated ventricular filling pressures. Systolic function is usually normal, especially early in the coarse of the disease. Restrictive cardiomyopathy may result from various systemic disorders, as well as exposure to several toxins and chest radiation (Table 11–4). Within the United States and Western Europe, this disease is most often secondary to amyloidosis (see later discussion).

Patients with restrictive cardiomyopathy usually present with symptoms and signs of congestive heart failure, which on presentation make this disease process indistinguishable from more common forms of cardiomyopathy. Signs of right-sided heart failure are usually prominent. The neck veins are distended and fail to collapse with inspiration or paradoxically rise (Kussmaul's sign) secondary to impaired emptying of blood from the right atrium into the right ventricle. Peripheral edema, an enlarged liver, and ascites are also frequently present. On cardiac examination, the apical impulse is

TABLE 11–4　Causes of Restrictive Cardiomyopathy

Myocardial

Noninfiltrative
　Idiopathic
　Scleroderma
Infiltrative
　Amyloid
　Sarcoid
　Gaucher's disease
Storage diseases
　Hemochromatosis

Endomyocardial

Endomyocardial fibrosis
Hypereosinophilic syndrome
Radiation

usually normal in location and intensity. An S_3 originating from the right or left ventricle is frequently present. In advanced cases, the carotid impulse may be diminished in amplitude secondary to reduced stroke volume.

The electrocardiogram may be normal in restrictive cardiomyopathy or only demonstrate nonspecific ST segment or T wave abnormalities. If the cardiomyopathy is secondary to an infiltrative process, such as amyloidosis, the QRS complexes may be diminished in amplitude (low voltage) and atrioventricular and interventricular conduction abnormalities may be present. Echocardiography is helpful in excluding more common causes of congestive heart failure, and the Doppler examination may demonstrate abnormalities in diastole that are typical of a restrictive process. However, right-sided heart catheterization is often necessary to confirm the diagnosis and differentiate this disease process from constrictive pericarditis (see later), which may present with similar clinical signs and symptoms. With both restrictive cardiomyopathy and constrictive pericarditis, early diastolic filling is unimpaired and is characterized by a rapid decline in ventricular pressure at the onset of diastole. This is followed by a rapid rise and leveling off of ventricular pressure through the remainder of diastole. This dip and plateau waveform is reflected in the atrial tracing as a rapid y descent followed by a rapid rise and plateau in atrial pressure. If sinus rhythm is present, a prominent a wave may be noted. Both left and right ventricular filling pressures are elevated, although with restrictive cardiomyopathy, left ventricular end-diastolic pressure usually exceeds right ventricular end-diastolic pressure by more than 5 mm Hg. This difference is accentuated with exercise and volume loading and may be the only finding that differentiates restrictive cardiomyopathy from constrictive pericarditis. In some cases, endomyocardial biopsy may reveal a specific cause of the restrictive cardiomyopathy when other tests are not diagnostic.

Treatment of restrictive cardiomyopathy in most cases is directed at relief of heart failure symptoms. Diuretics are useful for the management of systemic and venous congestion. However, an excessive reduction in ventricular filling pressures will reduce stroke volume and may result in symptomatic hypotension. Atrial fibrillation with loss of the atrial contribution to ventricular filling is often poorly tolerated in patients with restrictive cardiomyopathy. Sinus rhythm should be maintained whenever possible, although digoxin and many of the antiarrhythmic agents are potentially arrhythmogenic and should be used with caution, especially in patients with amyloidosis. Patients with life-threatening ventricular arrhythmias should undergo electrophysiologic evaluation and may require treatment with an automatic defibrillator.

Amyloidosis

Amyloidosis is a group of diseases characterized by the deposition of abnormal fibrillar proteins (amyloid) in tissues and organs throughout the body. Amyloidosis can be classified as primary, secondary, or familial depending on the type of precursor protein that forms the amyloid fibril.

Primary amyloidosis is a rare systemic disease caused by the abnormal production of immunoglobulin light chains by a plasma cell dyscrasia. Cardiac involvement is common in this disease and results in a restrictive cardiomyopathy because of the deposition of amyloid fibrils within the myocardium. Although diastolic dysfunction is common with cardiac amyloid, systolic dysfunction may also occur, especially late in the course of the disease. The electrocardiogram typically reveals low voltage of the QRS complexes. Abnormal Q waves, especially in the anterior leads, may simulate myocardial infarction. The echocardiogram often reveals increased wall thickness, small ventricular cavity size, enlarged atria, and thickened valve leaflets. The myocardium often has a sparkling, granular appearance that is thought to be secondary to myocardial infiltration with the abnormal protein. A diagnosis of cardiac amyloid in a patient with clinical and echocardiographic findings typical of this disease can often be established by detecting amyloid deposits in tissue obtained from a fat pad or rectal tissue biopsy. If such methods are inconclusive, myocardial biopsy may be required.

The prognosis of patients with primary cardiac amyloid is extremely poor, with a median survival of less than 6 months if symptoms of congestive heart failure are present. Chemotherapy with high-dose intravenous melphalan followed by autologous stem cell rescue has been shown to improve the manifestations of amyloid disease in patients without significant cardiac involvement. Current studies are now under way to determine if this therapy may be beneficial in selected patients with cardiac involvement.

Familial amyloid is a group of autosomal dominant diseases characterized by deposition of mutant proteins within the extracellular space. The most common form of this disease is caused by the production of an abnormal transthyretin, a protein predominantly synthesized in the liver. More than 50 different mutations in the transthyretin protein are associated with amyloid deposition, resulting primarily in peripheral and autonomic neuropathy and cardiomyopathy. A unique form of amyloid cardiomyopathy has been observed in the African-American population and is associated with a mutation in the transthyretin gene at position 122 (isoleucine substitutes for valine).

Senile amyloid is the most common cause of amyloid cardiomyopathy in the elderly and is highly prevalent in autopsy specimens from individuals in the eighth and ninth decades. The pathogenesis of this disease is poorly understood, but it appears to be caused by the deposition of amyloid fibrils composed of normal transthyretin. This disease does not carry the same grave prognosis as primary amyloid; however, the development of conduction disturbances, atrial arrhythmias, and congestive heart failure is not uncommon.

Secondary amyloid is caused by the deposition of serum amyloid protein (SAA) that is produced in response to chronic inflammation. Although rarely seen in developed nations secondary to the successful treatment of many chronic infectious diseases, secondary amyloid can still complicate other inflammatory illnesses, such as rheumatoid arthritis and inflammatory bowel disease. Patients with secondary amyloidosis usually present with signs of renal and hepatic involvement. Cardiac involvement is rare and, if present, rarely causes symptoms.

Pericardial Disease

ACUTE PERICARDITIS

Acute pericarditis results from inflammation of the visceral and parietal pericardium and is characterized by chest pain, a pericardial friction rub, and serial electrocardiographic changes. The cause of pericarditis in most cases is unknown but in many cases is presumed to be secondary to a viral infection. However, a variety of infectious agents, medications, and systemic diseases may result in pericarditis (Table 11–5).

The classic manifestation of pericarditis is pleuritic retrosternal chest pain, which is usually abrupt in onset, often sharp, and relieved with sitting up and leaning forward. On physical examination a pericardial friction rub may be heard during auscultation of the heart. The rub is a scratchy, superficial sound that typically has three components that correspond to movement of the heart during the cardiac cycle (ventricular systole, early ventricular diastole, and atrial contraction). The rub may be intermittent and variable in intensity with only one or two components audible. Because of the variable nature of the friction rub, its absence does not exclude the diagnosis of pericarditis.

The electrocardiographic changes that occur with acute pericarditis are secondary to inflammation of the underlying myocardium. The earliest changes in the electrocardiogram are sinus tachycardia and diffuse ST segment elevation with upward concavity that is not associated with reciprocal ST segment depression or the development of pathologic Q waves (Fig. 11–1). Associ-

TABLE 11–5 Causes of Pericarditis

Idiopathic
Viral (e.g., coxsackievirus B, echovirus, adenovirus, infectious mononucleosis, hepatitis B, acquired immunodeficiency syndrome)
Fungal (e.g., histoplasmosis)
Tuberculosis
Acute bacterial (purulent)
Acute myocardial infarction
Postpericardiotomy syndrome
Radiation
Neoplasm (e.g., metastatic lung or breast carcinoma; leukemia, lymphoma, melanoma)
Uremia
Autoimmune disorders (e.g., systemic lupus erythematosus, rheumatoid arthritis, scleroderma)
Drug reaction/hypersensitivity syndromes (e.g., procainamide, hydralazine)
Myxedema

ated inflammation of the atrial myocardium can result in PR segment depression. The ST segments return to baseline during the first few hours to days and are followed by diffuse T wave inversion. The electrocardiogram gradually normalizes over many days to weeks. In some patients, the T wave abnormalities may persist if chronic pericarditis develops. Sustained atrial and ventricular arrhythmias are uncommon in acute pericarditis.

Laboratory tests are directed at excluding specific causes of pericarditis and may include tuberculin skin testing, thyroid and renal function tests, antinuclear antibody, complement levels, rheumatoid factor, and human immunodeficiency virus serology, if appropriate. An elevated erythrocyte sedimentation rate or white blood cell count suggests active inflammation but is not helpful in identifying the causal agent. Viral serologic studies are usually low yield and do not alter therapy. If pericarditis is complicated by a pericardial effusion, an echocardiogram may detect the fluid and determine its hemodynamic significance (see discussion of pericardial effusion later). However, the absence of pericardial fluid does not exclude the diagnosis of pericardial inflammation.

The treatment of acute pericarditis is directed at management of the underlying cause and pain relief. For most patients with idiopathic or viral pericarditis, treatment with salicylates or nonsteroidal anti-inflammatory agents relieves the chest discomfort and helps resolve the pericardial inflammation. In rare instances, a short course of corticosteroids may be necessary to provide relief, but treatable causes of pericarditis should first be excluded. Anticoagulants should be avoided in patients with acute pericarditis because of the risk of development of a hemopericardium.

Most cases of pericarditis are self-limited and resolve within days to several weeks. Some individuals may develop a chronic, relapsing course that may require intermittent corticosteroid therapy or, in rare cases, pericardiectomy. Complications, such as pericardial tamponade or constrictive pericarditis, are rare (see later).

PERICARDIAL EFFUSION

Abnormal accumulation of fluid within the pericardial space can result from any cause of pericarditis (see Table 11–5). A pericardial effusion may be clinically silent or, if associated with increased intrapericardial pressure, may result in symptoms of pericardial tamponade. In the normal state, the pericardial sac contains less than 50 mL of fluid. If fluid accumulates slowly and the pericardium is allowed to stretch, this space can accommodate up to 2 L of fluid without a significant increase in pericardial pressure.

Patients with hemodynamically insignificant pericardial effusions are usually asymptomatic. Some patients may have a constant pressure in the chest or develop symptoms related to compression of adjacent structures, such as the esophagus or trachea. The physical examination in a patient with a small pericardial effusion is often normal. If the effusion is large, the heart sounds may be muffled. Compression of a segment of the left lung may result in decreased breath sounds and egophony beneath the angle of the scapula on auscultation

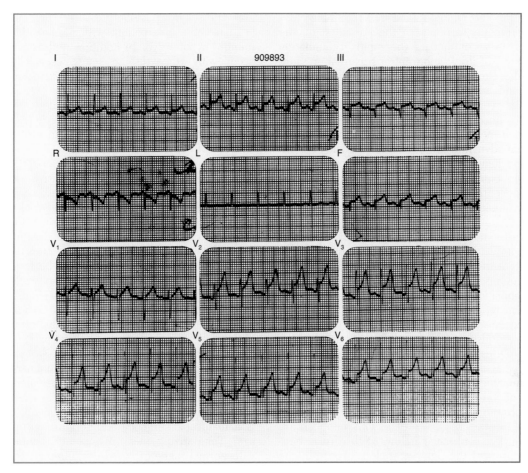

FIGURE 11–1 Typical electrocardiogram in pericarditis, showing diffuse ST segment elevation.

(Ewart's sign). On chest radiogram the cardiac silhouette may be enlarged and have a flask-shaped contour if at least 250 mL of fluid has accumulated within the pericardial sac (Fig. 11–2). When a large volume of pericardial fluid is present, the voltage of the QRS complexes may be diminished. In addition, the amplitude of the QRS complexes may vary from beat to beat (QRS alternans), an abnormality thought secondary to the heart's changing its electrical axis by "swinging" within the pericardial sac.

Echocardiography is the most useful test to diagnose the presence of a pericardial effusion. With this technique the size of the effusion can be estimated, the location of the fluid (i.e., loculated or circumferential) can be determined, and the hemodynamic significance of the effusion can be assessed. The work-up to determine the etiology of the pericardial effusion is similar to that for acute pericarditis. In general, drainage of the pericardial fluid for diagnostic purposes is usually of low yield and should be reserved for patients with symptomatic, persistent (>2 weeks) pericardial effusions, pericardial tamponade, or suspected purulent pericarditis.

CARDIAC TAMPONADE

The hemodynamic consequences of a pericardial effusion are dependent on the size of the effusion, the rate

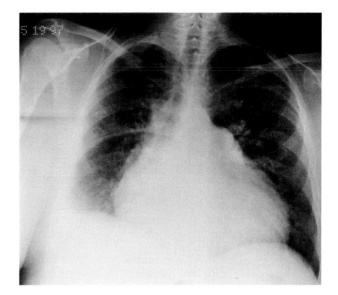

FIGURE 11–2 Posteroanterior chest radiograph from a patient with a large circumferential pericardial effusion. Note the flask-shaped contour of the cardiac silhouette.

at which the fluid accumulates, and the restraining characteristics of the pericardium. In the normal state, the pericardium can accommodate the rapid accumulation of 80 to 100 mL of fluid before intrapericardial pressure rises. If fluid accumulation is slow, the pericardium has time to expand and the intrapericardial pressure may remain normal even if a large volume of fluid is present. In both cases, once the intrapericardial pressure begins to rise, a small increase in pericardial volume can have significant hemodynamic consequences. Cardiac tamponade develops when further increases in pericardial pressure result in compression of the heart and reduced filling of the ventricles. As a result, venous pressures rise, stroke volume is reduced, and hypotension develops.

When cardiac tamponade develops slowly, the main presenting complaints are dyspnea and fatigue. In contrast, patients with acute tamponade are usually acutely ill with symptoms and signs of cardiogenic shock. On physical examination, tachycardia is usually present in attempts to maintain cardiac output. The jugular veins are distended because of elevated right ventricular diastolic pressure. Pulsus paradoxus, defined as a fall in the systolic blood pressure of more than 10 mm Hg with inspiration, is a characteristic finding in patients with cardiac tamponade (Fig. 11–3). Under normal conditions, filling of the right ventricle increases with inspiration when intrathoracic pressure is lowered. This results in distention of the right ventricle with minimal impingement on left ventricular inflow. With cardiac tamponade, expansion of the right ventricle is limited by the compressive effects of the pericardial fluid. As a result, the interventricular septum bulges into the left ventricular cavity to accommodate the increased volume of blood in the right ventricle. This further impedes left ventricular filling, leading to a reduction in stroke volume and a fall in systolic pressure. This finding may not be detectable in a patient with tamponade who is profoundly hypotensive. In addition, pulsus paradoxus may occur with other disease states, especially respiratory distress secondary to chronic obstructive lung disease or asthma.

The diagnosis of cardiac tamponade is based on clinical findings. However, echocardiography is a useful tool to verify the hemodynamic significance of a pericardial effusion. Because the right atrium and right ventricle are thin-walled low-pressure chambers, they are most susceptible to the effects of increased intrapericardial pressures. As a result, collapse of these chambers occurs when intrapericardial pressure exceeds right-sided filling pressures. Inversion of the right atrium for more than one third of the cardiac cycle and/or diastolic collapse of the right ventricle are findings consistent with tamponade physiology. Similar changes may be apparent for the left atrium if the effusion is located posteriorly. Despite the usefulness of echocardiography, right-sided heart catheterization may be necessary to document the hemodynamic importance of a pericardial effusion. Typical findings of tamponade include elevation and equalization of atrial and ventricular diastolic pressures. If the intrapericardial pressure is measured simultaneously, it is elevated and equal to atrial and ventricular filling pressures.

Cardiac tamponade with hemodynamic compromise is a medical emergency and requires immediate drainage. Temporizing measures include volume expansion with normal saline or blood. Vasopressors may be necessary to stabilize the patient while preparation for drainage is under way. If the effusion is large and circumferential, removal of the fluid percutaneously by the subxiphoid approach (pericardiocentesis) is often successful and quickly restores hemodynamic stability. If

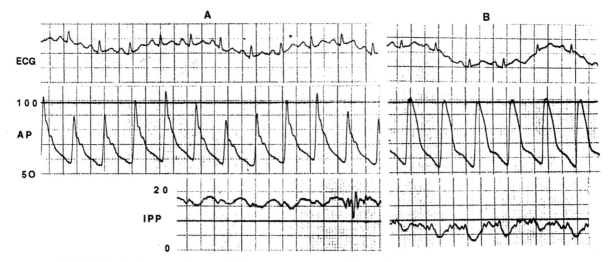

FIGURE 11–3 Electrocardiogram (ECG), systemic arterial and intrapericardial pressures (recorded in the catheterization laboratory) in a patient with cardiac tamponade. The left tracings (A) demonstrate sinus tachycardia and pulsus paradoxus. The intrapericardial pressure is elevated at about 15 mm Hg. After pericardiocentesis (B), the heart rate has slowed, the pulsus paradoxus is no longer present, and the elevated intrapericardial pressure has resolved.

the effusion is loculated or recurrent, surgical drainage with the formation of a pericardial "window" (pericardiotomy) may be necessary. Fluid and pericardial tissue should be examined for evidence of infection and malignancy.

PERICARDIAL CONSTRICTION

Constrictive pericarditis is a rare disorder that results from progressive scarring of the pericardium in response to prior injury. The most common causes include idiopathic pericarditis, chest radiation, cardiac surgery, and tuberculosis.

With classic constrictive pericarditis the scarring process is circumferential, leading to restricted diastolic filling of all four cardiac chambers. As with cardiac tamponade, atrial and ventricular diastolic pressures are elevated and equalized. However, in contrast to tamponade physiology in which ventricular filling is impaired throughout diastole, early diastolic filling in constrictive pericarditis is not impaired. This leads to rapid early filling of the ventricle secondary to elevated atrial pressure, followed by an abrupt rise and plateau in ventricular pressure during mid and late diastole as the ventricular volume reaches the limit set by the nondistensible pericardium.

Patients with mild to moderate constrictive pericarditis (elevation in venous pressures of 10 to 15 mm Hg) usually present with symptoms of right-sided heart failure, such as leg edema, abdominal fullness, and pain secondary to hepatic congestion. As the process becomes more severe and venous pressures exceed 20 mm Hg, symptoms of pulmonary congestion, such as exertional dyspnea, cough, and orthopnea, develop. If cardiac output is reduced, fatigue and muscle weakness may be the primary complaint.

On physical examination the jugular veins are distended and paradoxically rise with inspiration (Kussmaul's sign); this occurs because negative intrathoracic pressure is not transmitted to the pericardium in constrictive physiology. As a result, increased venous return cannot be accommodated by the right atrium and right ventricle, and the jugular veins become more distended. This sign is unusual in cardiac tamponade or restrictive cardiomyopathy, in which the jugular venous pressure may also be elevated. In these instances, negative intrathoracic pressure is transmitted to the pericardium, allowing increased, albeit limited, filling of the right ventricle during inspiration. For similar reasons, pulsus paradoxus is usually absent in constrictive pericarditis because inspiration does not result in an increase in right ventricular filling. Other findings include signs of right-sided heart failure, such as hepatomegaly, ascites, and peripheral edema. On cardiac examination, an early diastolic sound (pericardial knock) may be heard at the left sternal border and corresponds to cessation of early, rapid diastolic filling.

If constrictive pericarditis is of long standing or secondary to tuberculosis, a ring of pericardial calcification may be seen on chest radiography. Computed tomography and magnetic resonance imaging are useful techniques to measure pericardial thickness and detect other findings associated with constriction, such as dilation of the vena cavae and small right ventricular cavity size. More recently, measurement of pericardial thickening during transesophageal echocardiography was shown to correlate well with that obtained by computed tomography.

In most cases of constrictive pericarditis, right-sided heart catheterization is necessary to establish a diagnosis. Typical findings include elevation and equalization of atrial and ventricular diastolic pressures. A prominent y descent is commonly seen in the atrial pressure tracings and corresponds to rapid emptying of the atria early in diastole. Both the right and left ventricular diastolic pressures show an early diastolic fall in pressure, followed by a rapid rise and plateau during mid and late diastole ("square root sign") as additional filling is impaired by the noncompliant pericardium. As compared with restrictive cardiomyopathy, the left and right ventricular diastolic pressure tracings are nearly superimposable and do not separate with volume loading or exercise. In cases in which differentiation from restrictive cardiomyopathy is difficult, a pericardial or myocardial biopsy may be helpful.

Mild cases of constrictive pericarditis may be successfully treated with salt restriction and diuretics. However, in most symptomatic patients, surgical removal of the pericardium (pericardiectomy) is the treatment of choice. Operative mortality is high, ranging from 5% to 12% in series during the 1980s and 1990s. Among those patients who survive surgery, approximately 90% have symptomatic improvement. Those patients with severe functional impairment preoperatively (functional class III or IV), or who have incomplete removal of the pericardium, are at highest risk for a poor outcome after surgery.

EFFUSIVE-CONSTRICTIVE PERICARDITIS

Effusive-constrictive pericarditis is a variant of constrictive pericarditis and is characterized by myocardial constraint secondary to scarring of the visceral pericardium in association with a tense pericardial effusion. Patients usually present with symptoms and signs consistent with cardiac tamponade. However, after pericardiocentesis and restoration of the pericardial pressure to zero, the atrial and ventricular diastolic pressures remain high and equalized. In addition, the pressure waveforms become more typical of constrictive pericarditis, with the development of a prominent y descent in the atrial tracing and a "dip and plateau" pattern during ventricular diastole. Recognition of this process is important because pericardiocentesis may not significantly improve symptoms. In this setting, surgical removal of the parietal and visceral pericardium is the treatment of choice.

REFERENCES

Dec GW, Fuster V: Idiopathic dilated cardiomyopathy. N Engl J Med 1994; 331:1564–1575.

Falk RH, Comenzo RL, Skinner M: The systemic amyloidoses. N Engl J Med 1997; 337:898–909.

Fowler NO: Cardiac tamponade: A clinical or echocardiographic diagnosis? Circulation 1993; 87:1738–1741.

Kushwaha SS, Fallon JT, Fuster V: Restrictive cardiomyopathy. N Engl J Med 1997; 336:267–276.

Spirito P, Seidman CE, McKenna WJ, Maron BJ: The management of hypertrophic cardiomyopathy. N Engl J Med 1997; 336:775–785.

Vaitkus PT, Kussmaul WG: Constrictive pericarditis versus restrictive cardiomyopathy: A reappraisal and update of diagnostic criteria. Am Heart J 1991; 122:1431–1441.

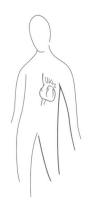

12

OTHER CARDIAC TOPICS

Lisa A. Mendes • Joseph Loscalzo

Cardiac Tumors

Primary cardiac tumors are extremely rare, with a prevalence of less than 0.3% in most pathologic series (Table 12–1). Myxoma is the most common primary tumor of the heart and is usually benign. These tumors are frequently isolated lesions, arising most often in the left atrium in the region of the fossa ovalis. Less commonly, myxomas may be detected in the right atrium, in the right or left ventricle, or in multiple sites within the heart. A familial pattern of myxomas can occur and is transmitted in an autosomal dominant manner. In these patients, multiple cardiac myxomas may be present in association with a constellation of extracardiac abnormalities, including pigmented nevi, cutaneous myxomas, breast fibroadenomas, and pituitary and adrenal gland disease. In addition, patients with familial myxoma may have recurrence of the tumor or tumors after surgical excision. Whether sporadic or familial, less than 10% of myxomas are malignant.

Symptoms associated with myxoma are usually related to embolization of tumor fragments and obstruction of the mitral valve. In addition, patients may present with a constellation of nonspecific symptoms and laboratory abnormalities, including fever, malaise, weight loss, anemia, and elevated erythrocyte sedimentation rate. The diagnosis is usually made by echocardiography, with the transesophageal approach being the most sensitive method for detecting small left atrial tumors. Given the propensity for embolization, most myxomas are surgically removed when diagnosed. Because tumors may recur, follow-up echocardiograms should be performed.

Other less common benign tumors include papillary fibroelastomas, fibromas, and rhabdomyomas. Fibroelastomas are pedunculated tumors with frondlike attachments that usually arise from the surface of the mitral and aortic valve leaflets. These tumors do not result in valve dysfunction but may be a source of systemic embolization. Fibromas most often arise within the interventricular septum and may be associated with arrhythmias or conduction disturbances. Rhabdomyomas are the most common cardiac tumors found in children and are often associated with tuberous sclerosis.

Cardiac lipomas may occur throughout the heart and pericardium. Whereas pericardial lipomas can be quite large, intramyocardial lipomas are small and often encapsulated. Surgical excision is the treatment of choice. Lipomatous hypertrophy of the interatrial septum should be considered in the differential of atrial masses. This lesion is a consequence of nonencapsulated adipose tissue hyperplasia and, while on occasion is found incidentally at autopsy, may be associated with supraventricular arrhythmias, conduction disturbances, and, in rare cases, sudden cardiac death.

Approximately one fourth of primary cardiac tumors are malignant, and most are often sarcomas. These tumors grow rapidly and often result in chamber obliteration and obstruction of blood flow. If there is involvement of the pericardium, a hemorrhagic effusion with pericardial tamponade may develop. The prognosis in affected individuals is poor; surgical excision is possible in rare cases. Irradiation and chemotherapy may provide palliative relief.

In contrast to primary cardiac tumors, metastatic disease involving the heart is common, occurring in up to one in five patients dying with malignancy. The most common tumors to metastasize to the heart are carcinomas of the lung, breast, and kidney; melanoma and lymphoma may also have cardiac involvement. Metastasis to the pericardium is common and often complicated by a hemorrhagic effusion and pericardial tamponade. Infiltration of the myocardium may result in conduction disturbances and arrhythmias. Intracavitary masses are unusual but may result from local tumor invasion or direct extension of the malignancy through the venous system (i.e., renal cell carcinoma may metastasize to the heart through the inferior vena cava). Treatment is directed at the underlying malignancy. If pericardial tamponade is present, immediate drainage will help stabilize the patient. Often, a pericardotomy is necessary to prevent reaccumulation of fluid within the pericardial sac. Surgical excision of an obstructing tumor mass is usually palliative.

TABLE 12-1 Examples of Tumors of the Heart and Pericardium

Primary	Metastatic
Benign	
Myxoma	Melanoma
Lipoma	Lung
Papillary fibroelastoma	Breast
Rhabdomyoma	Lymphoma
Fibroma	Renal cell
Malignant	
Angiosarcoma	
Rhabdomyosarcoma	
Mesothelioma	
Fibrosarcoma	

Traumatic Heart Disease

NONPENETRATING CARDIAC INJURIES

Blunt cardiac trauma accounts for approximately 10% of all traumatic heart disease (Table 12–2). Motion-related injuries secondary to abrupt body deceleration (motor vehicle accidents) and chest wall compression (steering wheel impact, athletic blow, cardiac resuscitative maneuvers) are the most common causes of blunt injury to the heart. Changes in the myocardium range from small ecchymotic areas in the subepicardium to transmural injury with myocardial hemorrhage and necrosis. Pericarditis is present in most patients and may be complicated by a tear or rupture of the pericardium or cardiac

TABLE 12-2 Cardiac Lesions From Nonpenetrating Trauma

Pericardium
Hematoma
Hemopericardium
Rupture
Pericarditis
Constriction (late complication)
Myocardium
Contusion
Intracavitary thrombus
Aneurysm/pseudoaneurysm
Rupture (free wall, septum)
Acute rupture (atrium, ventricle, septa)
Valves
Rupture (leaflets, chordae, papillary muscle)
Coronary Arteries
Laceration
Great Vessels
Aortic rupture

Adapted from Schick EC: Nonpenetrating cardiac trauma. Cardiol Clin 1995; 13:241–247.

tamponade. Less common complications include rupture of a papillary muscle or chordae tendineae and coronary artery laceration.

Patients most often present with precordial pain that is similar to that associated with myocardial infarction. However, musculoskeletal pain secondary to chest wall injury may confuse the clinical presentation. Congestive heart failure is unusual unless myocardial injury has been extensive or valve dysfunction has occurred. Life-threatening ventricular arrhythmias may occur with severe trauma and are a frequent cause of death in such patients. The electrocardiogram most often demonstrates nonspecific repolarization abnormalities or ST segment and T wave changes consistent with acute pericarditis. If myocardial injury is extensive, localized ST segment elevation and pathologic Q waves may be present. Elevation of the myocardial component of creatine kinase (CK-MB) is supportive of a diagnosis of cardiac contusion but is of limited diagnostic utility in patients with massive chest wall trauma because the CK-MB fraction may be elevated as a result of severe skeletal muscle injury. Newer markers of myocardial injury, such as troponin T and I, may be more specific for establishing a diagnosis of myocardial contusion. Echocardiography is a useful, noninvasive tool to assess for wall motion abnormalities, valve dysfunction, and the presence of hemodynamically significant pericardial effusion.

Treatment of patients with cardiac contusion is similar to that for myocardial infarction with initial observation and monitoring, followed by a gradual increase in physical activity. Anticoagulants and thrombolytic agents are contraindicated given the risk of hemorrhage into the myocardium and pericardial sac. Most patients who survive the initial injury will have partial or complete recovery of myocardial function. However, patients should be monitored for late complications that include aneurysm formation, free wall or papillary muscle rupture, and significant arrhythmias.

GREAT VESSEL INJURY

Rupture of the aorta is one of the most common cardiovascular injuries resulting from blunt chest wall trauma. In over 90% of the cases, rupture occurs in the descending thoracic aorta just distal to the origin of the subclavian artery. Most individuals die immediately of exsanguination. However, up to 20% of patients may survive the initial injury if the blood is confined within the aortic adventitia and surrounding mediastinal tissues (pseudoaneurysm). Characteristic symptoms and findings on presentation include chest and interscapular back pain, increased arterial pressure and pulse amplitude in the upper extremities, decreased pressure and pulse amplitude in the lower extremities, and mediastinal widening on the chest radiograph. Aortography is the test of choice to confirm the diagnosis, localize the site or sites of injury, and assess for subclavian and carotid artery involvement. More recently, transesophageal echocardiography has been used to screen patients with suspected rupture, although aortography is often still necessary to exclude the presence of great vessel involvement. Once the diagnosis is confirmed, urgent surgical correction is the only treatment option.

PENETRATING CARDIAC INJURIES

Penetrating cardiac injuries are frequently the result of physical violence secondary to bullet and knife wounds. Similar wounds may result from the inward displacement of bone fragments or fractured ribs secondary to blunt chest wall injury. Iatrogenic injuries may occur during placement of central venous catheters and wires.

With traumatic perforations, the right ventricle is the most frequently involved chamber, given its anterior location in the chest, and is often associated with pericardial laceration. Symptoms are related to the size of the wound and the nature of the concomitant pericardial injury. If the pericardium remains open, extravasated blood drains freely into the mediastinum and pleural cavity and symptoms are related to the resulting hemothorax. If blood loss is limited by the pericardial sac, pericardial tamponade results. In this situation, treatment includes emergent pericardiocentesis followed by surgical closure of the wound. Small penetrating wounds to the ventricles that are not associated with extensive cardiac damage are associated with the highest survival. Late complications include chronic pericarditis, arrhythmias, aneurysm formation, and ventricular septal defects.

Cardiac Surgery

CORONARY ARTERY BYPASS

Despite the effectiveness of current medical therapy for the treatment of coronary artery disease, many patients may require revascularization. Coronary artery bypass grafting (CABG) is an effective means of reducing or eliminating symptoms of angina pectoris. In addition, previous studies have shown that CABG may improve survival in certain subgroups of patients, including patients with angina refractory to medical therapy, patients with greater than 50% stenosis of the left main coronary artery, and patients with severe three-vessel coronary artery disease associated with left ventricular dysfunction. In addition, patients with two-vessel coronary artery disease in which a severe stenosis (>75%) is present in the proximal left anterior descending artery appear to benefit from CABG even if left ventricular function is normal.

Standard coronary artery bypass surgery is performed through a median sternotomy incision with cardiopulmonary bypass and cardioplegic arrest. Operative mortality is 1% or less in stable patients with normal left ventricular function, with the incidence of perioperative myocardial infarction and stroke ranging from 1% to 4%. An increase in adverse events is associated with advancing age, short stature, diabetes, unstable angina or recent myocardial infarction, and severely reduced left ventricular function. Overall survival at 10 years is approxi-

mately 80%, with recurrent or progressive angina occurring in approximately 50% of patients.

Long-term success of surgery is dependent on the type of conduit used during surgery (saphenous vein grafts versus internal mammary artery) and the progression of atherosclerotic disease in the native and graft vessels. The internal mammary artery is particularly resistant to atherosclerotic disease and has a patency rate of approximately 90% at 10 years. In comparison, venous grafts are subject to closure both during the immediate postoperative period (usually secondary to technical factors) and months to years after surgery secondary to intimal hyperplasia and progression of atherosclerosis. As a result, only 50% of venous grafts are patent 7 to 10 years after CABG. Aggressive lowering of LDL levels after CABG, as well as the administration of a daily aspirin, has been shown to reduce the incidence of venous graft occlusion. Most cases of recurrent angina can be managed successfully with medication, as outlined in Chapter 9. In some cases, percutaneous revascularization of a native vessel or graft will provide symptomatic relief. In patients with refractory symptoms not amenable to percutaneous revascularization, repeat CABG is an option; however, in this setting, it is associated with increased perioperative mortality and less satisfactory long-term control of angina.

VALVULAR SURGERY

Surgical repair or replacement of a diseased valve is dependent on multiple factors, including the type and severity of the valve lesion, the presence of symptoms, and the functional status of the left, and in some cases right, ventricle (see Chapter 8). In most adults, the diseased valve is usually replaced with a prosthesis, although some forms of valve disease, such as mitral valve prolapse or mitral stenosis without significant valvular or chordal calcification, may be amenable to repair. Because prosthetic heart valves are associated with a number of complications, including thrombosis, endocarditis, and hemolysis, the decision to proceed with valve surgery should be made only after the risks of valve replacement are weighed against the potential benefits of symptom relief and/or improved survival.

Valve surgery is performed in a similar manner to coronary artery bypass surgery, with most cases requiring a median sternotomy, cardiopulmonary bypass, and cardioplegic arrest. Operative mortality ranges from 1% to 8% for most patients with preserved left ventricular function and good exercise capacity. The risk of surgery increases with advancing age, depressed left ventricular ejection fraction, the presence of severe coronary artery disease, and replacement of multiple valves. Symptomatic patients usually have significant clinical improvement after valve surgery; however, long-term survival is strongly dependent on the patient's preoperative functional status.

CARDIAC TRANSPLANTATION

Over the last two decades, cardiac transplantation has become a life-saving treatment choice in patients with end-stage congestive heart failure. With advances in surgical techniques and immunosuppressive therapy, 1- and 5-year survival rates are approximately 85% and 75%, respectively. This is far superior to the 1-year survival in patients with advanced heart failure, which can be as high as 50%. Unfortunately, many patients suitable for cardiac transplantation die before surgery, as a result of the limited number of donor hearts available each year.

The major indications for cardiac transplantation are to prolong survival and improve the quality of life. Determining which patients are suitable for cardiac transplantation can be difficult because many patients may have clinical and hemodynamic improvement with intensification of medical therapy. In general, functional capacity as assessed by exercise stress testing with measurement of maximal oxygen consumption at peak exercise is the best predictor of which patients should be selected for cardiac transplantation. Those individuals with severely impaired exercise capacity (peak oxygen consumption less than 10 to 12 mL/min/kg, lower limit of normal 20 mL/min/kg) are most likely to experience a survival benefit from transplantation. Exclusion criteria include irreversible pulmonary vascular hypertension, malignancy, active infection, diabetes mellitus with end-organ damage, and advanced liver or kidney disease. Although advanced age is associated with a higher surgical and 1-year mortality, an age limit for cardiac transplantation is no longer enforced at most centers.

The procedure is performed through a median sternotomy incision. The posterior walls of the left and right atria with their venous connections are left in place and used to suture to the donor heart. The aorta and pulmonary artery are directly anastomosed to the recipient's great vessels. Immunosuppressive therapy is begun immediately after surgery and continued throughout the patient's life. Although new immunosuppressive agents are available, most regimens still include combinations of cyclosporine, azathioprine, and prednisone. Frequent complications during the first year include infection and rejection of the donor heart. In addition, hyperlipidemia and hypertension are common medical problems that may require treatment.

The major long-term complication is the development of coronary vasculopathy in the transplanted heart. In contrast to coronary artery atherosclerosis, which tends to be a focal process affecting primarily the proximal vessels, this disease is characterized by diffuse myointimal proliferation involving primarily the mid and distal segments of the coronary arteries. Although the etiology of this disease is not entirely known, it is thought to be secondary to an immune-mediated response directed against the donor vessels. Monitoring for this complication can be difficult because angina is not provoked in the denervated heart and standard exercise stress testing has a low sensitivity for detecting this disease. Coronary angiography is performed after transplantation and yearly thereafter to monitor for significant coronary artery narrowing. Unfortunately, the diffuse nature of the vasculopathy makes coronary angiography less accurate for the detection of this disease. Intracoronary ultrasound with measurement of the intimal layer and coronary artery lumen size is a new technique that appears to be more sensitive than coronary angiography for detection of this complication. Treatment options are limited, but aggressive management of hypercholesterolemia and the use of calcium channel blockers, specifically diltiazem, have been associated with a slowing of disease progression and a higher survival rate. Retransplantation is reserved for patients with severe, three-vessel coronary artery disease with reduced left ventricular function and congestive heart failure symptoms.

Noncardiac Surgery in the Cardiac Patient

Noncardiac surgery in patients with known cardiovascular disease may be associated with an increased risk of death or cardiac complications, such as myocardial infarction, congestive heart failure, and arrhythmias. To determine an individual patient's risk for a procedure, the consulting physician must have knowledge of the type and severity of the patient's cardiac disease, his or her co-morbid risk factors, and the type and urgency of surgery. In general, the preoperative evaluation and management of cardiac patients is similar to that in the nonoperative setting, with additional noninvasive and invasive testing targeted toward those high-risk patients in whom the results would affect treatment or outcome.

Estimation of a patient's perioperative risk can usually be determined by a careful clinical evaluation including a history, physical examination, and review of the electrocardiogram. Patients at highest risk for a perioperative cardiac event are those with a recent myocardial infarction (defined as greater than 7 days but less than or equal to 1 month), unstable or severe angina, decompensated congestive heart failure, significant arrhythmias, or severe valvular disease (Table 12–3). Predictors of moderate or intermediate cardiac risk include a history of stable angina, compensated heart failure, prior myocardial infarction, or diabetes mellitus. Advanced age, an abnormal electrocardiogram, low functional capacity, and poorly controlled hypertension are associated with cardiovascular disease but are not independent predictors of a perioperative cardiac event.

Risk associated with the type of surgery is highest in patients undergoing major emergency procedures, especially when performed in the elderly (Table 12–4). Cardiac complications are also common after vascular surgery, given that the prevalence of underlying coronary artery disease is high in this population of patients. In addition, any surgery associated with large volume shifts or blood loss may place increased demands on an already diseased heart. Procedures associated with the lowest risk in the cardiac patient are cataract extraction and endoscopy.

Once the clinical evaluation is complete and the type of surgery is known, the need for additional testing and treatment can be determined. If emergency surgery is contemplated, little in the way of cardiac assessment can be performed and recommendations may be directed at

TABLE 12-3 **Clinical Predictors of Increased Perioperative Cardiovascular Risk (Myocardial Infarction, Congestive Heart Failure, Death)**

Major

Unstable coronary syndromes
  Recent myocardial infarction (>1 week and ≤ 1 month)
  Unstable or severe angina (Canadian class III or IV)
Decompensated heart failure
Significant arrhythmias
  High-grade atrioventricular block
  Symptomatic ventricular arrhythmias
  Supraventricular arrhythmias with uncontrolled ventricular
    response
Severe valvular disease

Intermediate

Mild angina (Canadian class I or II)
Prior myocardial infarction
Compensated or prior congestive heart failure
Diabetes mellitus

Minor

Advanced age
Abnormal ECG (left ventricular hypertrophy, left bundle
  branch block)
Rhythm other than sinus
Low functional capacity (unable to climb one flight of stairs
  with a bag of groceries)
History of a stroke
Uncontrolled systemic hypertension

Adapted from ACC/AHA Task Force Report: Guidelines for perioperative cardiovascular evaluation for noncardiac surgery. J Am Coll Cardiol 1996; 27:910–948.

perioperative medical management and surveillance. If surgery is not urgent, then additional evaluation is based on the clinical assessment of risk and the type of surgery. Patients with major risk factors for cardiac complications should have surgery delayed until the cardiac condition can be treated and stabilized. Patients with intermediate predictors of cardiac risk scheduled for high-risk surgery should undergo noninvasive testing, such as exercise or pharmacologic stress testing, or echocardiography. The results of these tests will help determine future management, such as cardiac catheterization or intensification of medical therapy. Those patients scheduled for low or intermediate risk surgery, especially if the patient has good exercise capacity, should proceed with surgery with appropriate medical management and postoperative surveillance. Noncardiac surgery is generally safe for patients with minor or no clinical risk factors for cardiac complications, although some patients with poor functional capacity scheduled for high-risk operations may benefit from additional cardiac evaluation.

DISEASE-SPECIFIC APPROACHES

Coronary Artery Disease and Myocardial Infarction

Approximately 70% of postoperative myocardial infarctions occur within the first 6 days, with the peak inci-

dence between 24 and 72 hours. Mortality associated with noncardiac surgery has been reported as high as 30% to 40%, especially if associated with congestive heart failure or significant arrhythmias. Multiple stresses associated with surgery can provoke ischemia. Physiologic tachycardia and hypertension secondary to volume shifts, anemia, infection, and the stress of wound healing increase myocardial oxygen demand and may provoke ischemia. In addition, increased platelet reactivity during the postoperative period may increase the risk of coronary thrombosis and subsequent infarction.

Despite the high mortality associated with this perioperative myocardial infarction, few studies have examined the effects of anti-ischemic therapy on the prevention of this complication. Several small, uncontrolled trials have suggested that β blockers may reduce intraoperative ischemia. More recently, the use of atenolol before and after surgery was associated with a reduction in myocardial infarction and cardiac death, especially during the first 6 to 12 months after surgery. Although the data are limited, the use of a perioperative β blocker should be considered in all patients with suspected or known coronary artery disease unless there is a specific contraindication to its use. The data available on the usefulness of calcium channel blockers and nitrates are even more limited, but this approach may be appropriate for the treatment of symptomatic coronary disease in individuals who are not candidates for revascularization. Coronary angiography and revascularization should be reserved for individuals in whom this treatment would otherwise result in significant improvement in symptoms or long-term survival. In rare cases, revascularization may be indicated in high-risk patients undergoing major noncardiac surgery.

All patients with suspected or known cardiac disease should have routine electrocardiograms the first 3 days after surgery to monitor for ischemia. When the electro-

TABLE 12-4 **Cardiac Risk Stratification for Noncardiac Surgical Procedures**

High (reported cardiac risk >5%)

Emergent major operations, particularly in the elderly
Major vascular surgery, aortic aneurysm repair
Peripheral vascular surgery
Prolonged procedures associated with large fluid shifts and/
  or blood loss

Intermediate (reported cardiac risk <5%)

Carotid endarterectomy
Head and neck
Intraperitoneal and intrathoracic
Orthopedic
Prostate

Low (reported cardiac risk <1%)

Endoscopic procedures
Cataract extraction
Breast biopsy

Adapted from ACC/AHA Task Force Report: Guidelines for perioperative cardiovascular evaluation for noncardiac surgery. J Am Coll Cardiol 1996; 27:910–948.

cardiogram is inconclusive, measurement of troponin levels may be helpful to document an ischemic event. Treatment of a myocardial infarction in this setting is similar to that for the nonsurgical patient (see Chapter 9), although the use of anticoagulants and thrombolytic agents may be contraindicated in the immediate postoperative period. Special attention should be paid to correcting abnormalities that may provoke additional ischemia (i.e., hypoxia, anemia).

Congestive Heart Failure

Several studies have shown that decompensated heart failure is associated with increased perioperative cardiac complications. In these patients, surgery should be postponed until appropriate treatment is instituted and symptoms have been stabilized. If planned surgery is associated with large blood loss or fluid shifts, a pulmonary artery catheter may be helpful in managing the patient.

During the postoperative period, congestive heart failure most commonly occurs during the first 24 to 48 hours when fluid administered during surgery is mobilized from the extravascular space. However, heart failure may also result from myocardial ischemia and new arrhythmias. Initial management includes identification and treatment of the underlying cause. In addition, intravenous diuretics usually provide rapid relief of pulmonary congestion. If heart failure is complicated by hypotension or poor urine output, insertion of a pulmonary artery catheter may be helpful to guide additional therapy (see Chapter 6).

Valvular Heart Disease

Aortic and mitral stenosis are associated with the greatest risk for complications after noncardiac surgery. Patients with symptomatic, severe aortic stenosis should have valve replacement before noncardiac surgery. In patients with mild to moderate mitral stenosis, careful attention to volume status and heart rate control are necessary to optimize left ventricular filling and avoid pulmonary congestion. Patients with severe mitral stenosis should be considered for percutaneous valvuloplasty or mitral valve replacement before high-risk surgery. In patients with valve disease or prosthetic heart valves, prophylactic antibiotics should be recommended when appropriate.

Arrhythmias and Conduction Defects

Patients with symptomatic, high-grade conduction disturbances, such as third-degree atrioventricular (AV) block, have an increased risk of cardiac complications perioperatively and should have a temporary pacemaker inserted before surgery. Patients with first-degree AV block, Mobitz type I AV block, or bifascicular block (right bundle branch block and left anterior fascicular block) do not require prophylactic pacemaker insertion.

Atrial arrhythmias, such as atrial fibrillation, are common after surgery and usually are not associated with significant complications if the ventricular rate is well controlled. Ventricular premature beats and nonsustained ventricular tachycardia are also common after noncardiac surgery and do not require specific therapy unless associated with myocardial ischemia or heart failure. In most instances, treatment of the underlying cause (hypoxia, metabolic abnormalities, ischemia, volume overload) will result in significant improvement or resolution of the rhythm disturbance without specific antiarrhythmic therapy.

Cardiac Disease in Pregnancy

Pregnancy is associated with dramatic changes in the cardiovascular system that may result in significant hemodynamic stress to the patient with underlying heart disease. During a normal pregnancy, plasma volume increases an average of 50%, beginning in the first trimester and peaking between the 20th and 24th weeks of pregnancy. This change is accompanied by an increase in stroke volume, heart rate, and, accordingly, cardiac output. In addition, there is a concomitant fall in systemic vascular resistance and mean arterial pressure because of the effects of gestational hormones on the vasculature and the creation of a low-resistance circulation in the pregnant uterus and placenta. During labor, uterine contractions result in a transient increase of up to 500 mL of blood into the central circulation, resulting in a further increase in stroke volume and cardiac output. After delivery, intravascular volume and cardiac output increase further as compression of the inferior vena cava by the gravid uterus is relieved and extravascular fluid is mobilized. Symptoms and signs that may mimic cardiac disease often accompany these hemodynamic changes and include fatigue, reduced exercise tolerance, lower extremity edema, distention of the neck veins, an S_3 gallop, and new systolic murmurs. Differentiating symptoms from cardiac disease versus those attributable to a normal pregnancy can be difficult. Under such circumstances, echocardiography can be a safe and helpful noninvasive test to assess cardiac structure and function in the pregnant patient.

Many pregnant patients with known cardiac disease can complete a normal pregnancy and delivery without significant harm to the mother or fetus. However, certain cardiac conditions, including irreversible pulmonary hypertension, cardiomyopathy associated with severe heart failure, and Marfan's syndrome with a dilated aortic root, are associated with a high risk for cardiovascular complications and death. Under these circumstances, patients should be advised against having children. If pregnancy should occur, a first-trimester therapeutic abortion should be strongly recommended.

Specific Cardiac Conditions

MITRAL STENOSIS

Mitral stenosis secondary to rheumatic heart disease frequently occurs in young women of child-bearing age.

The physiologic increase in heart rate and cardiac output during pregnancy results in a significant increase in the gradient across the mitral valve and a rise in left atrial and pulmonary venous pressures. Congestive heart failure may develop as the pregnancy progresses through the second and third trimester or may occur more acutely with the onset of atrial fibrillation. The management of the patient with mitral stenosis depends on her prepregnant functional capacity and the severity of the valve obstruction. In general, patients with severely symptomatic mitral valve stenosis should have percutaneous or surgical correction of the valve before conception. Women with minimal symptoms (New York Heart Association class I to II) usually tolerate pregnancy and vaginal delivery well even if moderate to severe stenosis is present. Treatment includes salt restriction, diuretic therapy, and aggressive treatment of pulmonary infections. Patients who develop atrial fibrillation with a rapid ventricular response should be treated with AV nodal blocking agents and cardioversion if possible. Patients who develop refractory heart failure during pregnancy should be considered for mitral balloon valvuloplasty, because surgical commissurotomy or valve replacement may be associated with fetal demise.

AORTIC STENOSIS

Aortic stenosis in a pregnant woman is usually congenital in origin. Patients with significant outflow obstruction may develop angina or heart failure during the later portion of the pregnancy as cardiac output increases. Supportive therapy includes bed rest and prevention of hypovolemia. If these measures fail to control symptoms and the fetus is not near term, balloon valvuloplasty or aortic valve surgery should be considered to reduce the risk of maternal death.

MARFAN'S SYNDROME

Pregnant women with Marfan's syndrome are at increased risk of aortic dissection and rupture, especially during the third trimester and first postpartum month. Patients with an aortic root diameter greater than 40 mm are at greatest risk for this complication and should strongly consider therapeutic abortion during the first trimester. Women with an aortic root diameter less than 40 mm should have serial echocardiograms to monitor the size of the aortic root during pregnancy. In addition, restriction in physical activity and treatment with a β blocker may help prevent further dilatation of the aorta.

CONGENITAL HEART DISEASE

Survival to reproductive age is common in patients with corrected congenital defects. The risk of pregnancy in these patients is related to the completeness of the repair and the mother's functional capacity. Uncomplicated atrial or ventricular septal defects not associated with symptoms or pulmonary hypertension are usually tolerated well during pregnancy. Intracardiac shunts associated with pulmonary vascular hypertension are associated with a high maternal mortality during pregnancy, as a result of an increase in right-to-left shunting and worsening oxygen desaturation of the blood. In these women, pregnancy is contraindicated. If pregnancy should occur, a therapeutic abortion during the first trimester should be recommended. Women with uncorrected tetralogy of Fallot should undergo palliative or definitive repair before conception to improve maternal and fetal outcomes with pregnancy. Women with residual right ventricular outflow tract obstruction remain at high risk for right ventricular heart failure during pregnancy.

PROSTHETIC HEART VALVES

Most patients with a normally functioning prosthetic valve tolerate pregnancy without complications. However, in patients with mechanical valves, special attention to the choice and dose of anticoagulant therapy is necessary to avoid thromboembolic complications in the mother and teratogenic effects in the fetus. Women should start subcutaneous heparin before conception to avoid the potential teratogenic effects of warfarin during the first several months of critical fetal organ development. This therapy can be continued throughout pregnancy, or, alternatively, warfarin can be reinstituted late in the second trimester or during the third trimester. Heparin therapy, although reducing the risk of teratogenicity associated with warfarin use, is itself associated with a higher risk of maternal bleeding complications. Low-molecular-weight heparin may be an acceptable alternative; however, no firm data are available to support these recommendations. At the time of delivery, anticoagulation is interrupted to avoid bleeding complications. Antibiotic prophylaxis is generally not recommended at time of delivery.

HEART DISEASE ARISING DURING PREGNANCY

Cardiovascular disease can develop during pregnancy and may pose a significant risk to the mother and/or fetus. Hypertension is not an uncommon problem during pregnancy and is defined as a consistent increase in blood pressure of 30/15 mm Hg or as an absolute level greater than 140/90 mm Hg. The three major forms of hypertension that may develop during pregnancy include chronic hypertension, gestational hypertension, and toxemia. Toxemia is a form of hypertension that develops during the second half of pregnancy and is associated with proteinuria, edema, and, in severe forms, seizures. This problem is managed primarily by the obstetrician and is not discussed here. Gestational hypertension is an elevation in blood pressure that occurs late in the pregnancy, during delivery, or in the first postpartum days. This disease entity is not associated with proteinuria or edema and resolves within 2 weeks of delivery. Chronic hypertension is presumed to be present if an elevation in blood pressure is detected before the 20th week of pregnancy. No matter what the cause, fetal mortality correlates with the severity of the hypertension and begins to rise when the diastolic pressure exceeds 75 mm Hg during the second trimester and 85 mm Hg during the third trimester. Initial treatment includes a reduction in physical activity and salt restriction. If the blood pressure remains greater than 150/90 mm Hg, antihypertensive treatment should be instituted. Agents that have been safely used in pregnancy include hydralazine, α-methyldopa, clonidine, β blockers, and labetalol. Diuretics should be used with caution because of the increased risk of placental hypoperfusion.

Peripartum cardiomyopathy (PCM) is a form of dilated cardiomyopathy that may begin during the last trimester of pregnancy or within the first 6 months after delivery in a woman without prior heart disease or other definable cause for cardiac dysfunction. The true incidence of the disease is unknown, but it is estimated to affect one woman in 3000 to 4000 pregnancies. Although the cause of PCM is unknown, myocardial injury is thought to be immunologically mediated. Women usually present with symptoms and signs of congestive heart failure. Echocardiography is useful to assess chamber size and degree of ventricular dysfunction. The outcome with PCM is variable, with death or progressive heart failure occurring in approximately one third of affected women. The prognosis is particularly poor if symptoms developed before delivery. Despite this risk, many patients will have complete recovery of ventricular function, although recurrence, especially with subsequent pregnancies, can occur. Treatment is similar to that for congestive heart failure (see Chapter 6) and usually includes vasodilators, such as hydralazine, digoxin, and diuretics. Angiotensin-converting enzyme inhibitors have been associated with increased fetal wastage in pregnant animals and should be avoided. A thorough evaluation of cardiac function should be performed before subsequent pregnancies. If a woman decides to proceed with another pregnancy, she should be monitored regularly for signs of cardiac decompensation.

Approximately 50% of aortic dissections that occur in women younger than the age of 40 are associated with pregnancy. Although the cause of aortic dissection during pregnancy is unknown, it has been postulated that hemodynamic and hormonal changes associated with pregnancy may weaken the aortic wall. The highest incidence of dissection is during the third trimester, although it may occur any time during the pregnancy and early postpartum period. The presenting symptoms and diagnostic work-up are similar to those for the nonpregnant patient (see Chapter 13). Transesophageal echocardiography is highly sensitive and specific for the detection of aortic dissection and offers the advantage of not exposing the fetus to ionizing radiation. Management includes aggressive blood pressure control and β blocker therapy to reduce shear forces of the ejected blood. Recommendations for corrective surgery are similar to those for the nonpregnant patient and are discussed in Chapter 13.

REFERENCES

ACC/AHA Task Force Report: Guidelines for perioperative cardiovascular evaluation for noncardiac surgery. J Am Coll Cardiol 1996; 27:912–948.

Bhagwat AR, Engel PJ: Heart disease and pregnancy. Cardiol Clin 1995; 13:163–178.

Cardiac Transplantation 24th Bethesda Conference. J Am Coll Cardiol 1993; 22:1–64.

Mancini DM, Eisen H, Kussmaul W, et al: Value of peak exercise consumption for optimal timing of cardiac transplantation in ambulatory patients with heart failure. Circulation 1991; 83:778–786.

Salcedo EE, Cohen GI, White RD, Davison M: Cardiac tumors: Diagnosis and management. Curr Probl Cardiol 1992; 17:73–137.

Schick EC: Nonpenetrating cardiac trauma. Cardiol Clin 1995; 13:241–247.

13

VASCULAR DISEASES AND HYPERTENSION

Eric H. Awtry • *Joseph Loscalzo*

Diseases of the vasculature frequently coexist with diseases of the heart. Therefore, symptoms of vascular disease may be the first indication of the existence of an underlying cardiac condition, or the vascular disease may be asymptomatic in a patient with known cardiac disease. The range of vascular disease spans the spectrum from benign to life threatening and may be acute or chronic in presentation. In this chapter we review the diseases of the systemic vasculature, including aortic and peripheral vascular diseases, the diseases of the pulmonary vasculature, including pulmonary hypertension and thromboembolic disease, and the renovascular diseases and systemic hypertension.

Systemic Vascular Disease

PERIPHERAL ARTERIAL DISEASE

The most common etiology of chronic occlusive peripheral vascular disease (PVD) is atherosclerosis (Fig. 13–1). As the population ages, the incidence of PVD increases dramatically. It is estimated that 5% of people older than age 60 years have symptoms of PVD, and an additional 5% to 10% have asymptomatic disease. In addition, almost half of all patients with coronary artery disease (CAD) have some degree of PVD. The lower extremities are most commonly involved and, when symptomatic, manifest *claudication*. True claudication is an aching or cramping in the involved extremity that is exertionally related, is relieved by standing still, and occurs at a relatively constant walking distance. This must be distinguished from *pseudoclaudication*, which results from lumbar spinal stenosis, produces lower extremity discomfort on walking or standing, is not relieved by standing still, and requires a change in position (often hyperextension of the lumbar spine) for resolution. As PVD progresses, symptoms may occur at rest, often involve the toes, and are worse at night. Ischemic foot ulcers may also develop, frequently at the site of minor injury.

The examination of the patient with PVD may reveal smooth, shiny, hairless skin over the lower extremities; diminished or delayed distal pulses; and audible bruits over the involved arteries. The diagnosis of PVD is usually evident by symptoms and physical findings, although noninvasive testing (i.e., duplex ultrasonography) may help to quantify the extent of the disease. In normal persons, the systolic blood pressure in the leg is slightly higher than that in the arms (ankle-brachial index > 1.0). In patients with PVD, the ankle-brachial index decreases (especially if measured before and after exercise) and the magnitude of the decrease reflects the severity of PVD (Table 11–1). Contrast angiography or magnetic resonance angiography is rarely needed for diagnosis, although angiography is indicated for defining the vascular anatomy preoperatively.

Treatment of PVD is initially conservative unless resting ischemia or nonhealing ischemic ulcers are present. In patients with claudication, a regular walking regimen may increase the claudication distance by 100% to 400% over the course of several months. Pentoxifylline (400 mg three times daily) results in vasodilation, decreased platelet aggregation, and decreased blood viscosity and may also afford an improvement in symptoms. Cilostazol (100 mg twice daily) causes vasodilation and inhibits platelet aggregation and increases a patient's maximal walking distance by 28% to 100%. Similar medications have been associated with increased mortality in patients with congestive heart failure; thus, cilostazol should not be given to patients with heart failure. Smoking cessation, weight reduction, control of other modifiable cardiac risk factors, and avoidance of vasoconstricting medications are important interventions, and careful attention to foot care and avoidance of injury are of utmost importance. Indications for revascularization of the involved arteries include unacceptable or disabling symptoms, rest pain, ischemic ulceration, and gangrene. Percutaneous angioplasty with stent placement is a use-

145

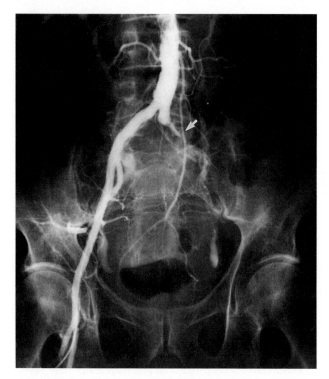

FIGURE 13–1 Arteriogram of the distal aorta and its bifurcation into the common iliac arteries in a patient with left lower extremity claudication. There is mild atherosclerotic disease of the distal aorta before its bifurcation. There is normal flow in the right iliac artery. The left iliac artery is totally occluded just distal to the aortic bifurcation *(arrow)*. The left leg was perfused through collateral arteries (not shown).

ful technique for treating disease of the iliac arteries but is less effective for more distal disease. Surgical revascularization offers excellent results for proximal (iliac and femoral arterial) disease but is less effective for more distal lesions. When a saphenous vein graft is used for these revascularization procedures, the postoperative use of ticlopidine, an inhibitor of platelet aggregation, improves long-term graft patency. Patients undergoing such surgical procedures require a complete cardiovascular evaluation; CAD frequently coexists with PVD (50% to 60% of patients with PVD have significant CAD) and results in a much higher perioperative risk of a cardiac complication.

The overall 5-year mortality rate in patients with claudication is approximately 30%, whereas the risk of limb amputation is 5%. This latter risk increases 4-fold in the presence of diabetes and more than 10-fold with concurrent use of tobacco products. Involvement of the upper extremities (most commonly the subclavian arteries) can occur with atherosclerotic disease; however, this feature, as well as the presence of PVD in a young patient and the sudden occurrence of limb ischemia in the absence of prior claudication, also raises the suspicion of less common vascular diseases (Table 13–2).

Thromboangiitis obliterans (Buerger's disease) is a disease of small arteries and veins of both the upper and lower extremities. It is most common in young males (< age 40) who are heavy smokers. Treatment is conservative, with particular emphasis on smoking cessation; the disease activity ceases with elimination of tobacco use.

Acute arterial occlusion is usually a dramatic event characterized by the sudden onset of pain, pallor, paresthesias, paralysis, and pulselessness of the involved extremity and may be the result of either thrombosis or embolism. Emboli usually originate from either the heart (i.e., atrial thrombus in the setting of atrial fibrillation, endocarditic vegetation, or intracardiac tumor) or areas of atherosclerotic disease in a proximal vessel. Many of these sources can be identified with transesophageal echocardiography (TEE). In rare cases, systemic emboli may result from venous thromboemboli that cross an atrial septal defect or patent foramen ovale to reach the systemic circulation (paradoxical embolus). Features suggesting an embolic cause of arterial occlusion include the presence of atrial fibrillation, endocarditis, recent myocardial infarction, and heart failure, whereas prior symptomatic PVD, active arteritis, hematologic disease, and trauma all suggest acute vascular thrombosis. Thromboembolectomy or thrombolysis may need to be considered if acute limb ischemia is present. Both of these therapeutic approaches offer similar rates of survival and limb salvage; thrombolysis decreases the need for surgery by approximately 50%, although it is associated with a higher frequency of hemorrhagic complications. After an embolic vascular event, the long-term use of oral anticoagulation may be warranted. Embolization of atheromatous debris from a diseased or aneurysmal aorta may occur spontaneously or after an intravascular procedure. The cholesterol emboli syndrome may result with manifestations that include livedo reticularis (cutaneous emboli), blue toe syndrome (digital emboli), hypertension and acute renal failure (renal emboli), and guaiac-positive stool (intestinal emboli). The peripheral blood smear often shows eosinophilia, and serum complement levels may be low. Anticoagulation may precipitate further embolic events and is relatively contraindicated. Surgical resection of the atheroembolic source is the optimal treatment.

Raynaud's phenomenon is a vasospastic disorder of the small arteries, primarily of the digits. It is usually induced by exposure to cold, resulting in intermittent pallor, cyanosis, and hyperemia, which produce the classic triphasic (white, blue, red) color changes in the involved digits. Primary Raynaud's phenomenon has no

TABLE 13–1 Noninvasive Assessment of the Severity of Lower Extremity Peripheral Vascular Disease

Extent of Disease	ABI at Rest	ABI After Exercise*
None or minimal	>1.0	No decrease
Mild	0.8–1.0	>0.5
Moderate	0.5–0.8	0.2–0.5
Severe	<0.5	<0.2

* Up to 5 minutes of exercise on a treadmill with a 10% grade at 1–2 mph.
ABI = systolic ankle:brachial pressure index.

identifiable underlying cause, is more common in younger women, is usually bilateral, and frequently involves the toes as well as the fingers. It is a benign condition that is usually controlled by avoidance of exposure to cold and occasionally by vasodilator therapy (calcium channel blockers or α-adrenergic blocking agents). Secondary Raynaud's phenomenon may accompany a variety of disorders, including systemic lupus erythematosus, progressive systemic sclerosis, and vasculitis. It is more common in older men, is frequently asymmetric, and involves mainly the hands. Ischemic complications are common. Therapy is directed at treatment of the underlying disorder.

ANEURYSMAL VASCULAR DISEASE

The term *aneurysm* refers to an abnormal, usually focal, dilatation of an artery (Fig. 13–2). Because most aneurysms are the result of atherosclerotic disease, they are more common in older men, and coronary and carotid vascular disease are frequent coexisting conditions. The incidence of aortic aneurysms increases with age, occurring in at least 3% of people older than 50. Hypertension, connective tissue disease, and a family history of aneurysmal disease are also risk factors for aneurysms. Aneurysms may occur at any point in the vascular tree from the aortic root to the distal peripheral vasculature, although they are most common in the abdominal aorta. Most aneurysms are asymptomatic and go undiagnosed; however, as they progressively enlarge, they may cause symptoms as a result of compression of surrounding structures, distal embolization of atherosclerotic debris or thrombus, or rupture.

The majority of abdominal aortic aneurysms are infrarenal in location. Suprarenal aneurysms can occur, usually as a result of extension of thoracic aneurysms. Abdominal aneurysms are frequently found on physical examination by detection of a pulsatile, expansile, some-

times tender, abdominal mass. In obese individuals even large aneurysms may be missed, whereas in thin patients, the normal aortic impulse may appear very prominent. Some patients with abdominal aneurysms describe a gnawing pain in the hypogastrium or lower back that may acutely worsen with expansion or impending rupture of the aneurysm. Acute rupture is a catastrophic event heralded by the triad of abdominal pain, hypotension, and a pulsatile abdominal mass.

Thoracic aortic aneurysms are also frequently atherosclerotic in origin, although ascending thoracic aortic aneurysms more commonly result from cystic medial necrosis, Marfan's syndrome (caused by an autosomal dominant mutation in the gene for fibrillin), aortic arteritis (see later discussion), or as a result of trauma. Most are asymptomatic, although aneurysms of the aortic root often distort the aortic valve and patients may present with symptoms of aortic insufficiency. A pulsatile mass may be felt in the suprasternal notch, although most thoracic aneurysms are first noted incidentally on chest radiography.

Iliac artery aneurysms are usually associated with abdominal aortic aneurysms, are occasionally noted on physical examination, and may result in ureteral obstruction, venous obstruction, and groin or perineal pain. Popliteal artery aneurysms are more common than femoral artery aneurysms; both are usually apparent on physical examination and are uncommon in women. Popliteal artery aneurysms are bilateral in more than half of cases and are frequently associated with other sites of aneurysm (usually of the abdominal aorta). These peripheral aneurysms may cause localized pain and frequently result in serious thromboembolic complications.

The diagnosis of aneurysmal disease of the abdominal aorta and peripheral vasculature can readily be made with ultrasonography. Thoracic aneurysms are well seen with TEE, and aneurysms at all levels are well visual-

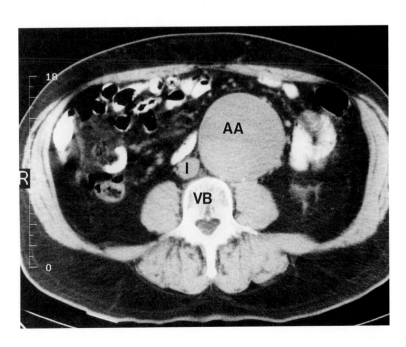

FIGURE 13–2 CT of the abdomen in a patient with a large aortic aneurysm (AA) measuring 8.5 cm in its greatest dimension. The normal-sized inferior vena cava (I) is labeled for comparison. VB = vertebral body.

TABLE 13-2 Peripheral Vascular Diseases

Disease	Pathology	Clinical Features	Physical Findings	Laboratory Findings	Treatment
Atherosclerotic occlusive peripheral vascular disease	Atherosclerotic narrowing of large and medium-sized arteries of lower extremities; segmental with skip areas; occasionally involves upper extremities	Male > female Common in diabetics Exertional leg pain relieved with rest (claudication); rest pain with severe disease Buttock claudication and impotence with aorto-iliac disease (Leriche's syndrome)	Decreased or absent lower extremity pulses Aortic, iliac, or femoral bruits Limb ischemia: cool, pale, cyanotic, shiny, hairless skin; ulcerations, gangrene	Decreased ankle:brachial index Arterial narrowing or obstruction on duplex exam or angiography	Intermittent claudication: Exercise as tolerated Stop smoking Avoid peripheral vaso-constricting drugs (e.g., β blockers) Meticulous skin and nail care Pentoxifylline, cilostazol Severe claudication or rest ischemia: Percutaneous angioplasty or surgical bypass; amputation if gangrene
Thromboangiitis obliterans (Buerger's disease)	Intimal proliferation and thrombi in small to medium-sized vessels with inflammatory infiltrates Segmental involvement of arteries and veins Upper and lower extremity involvement	Male > female Usually < age 30 Symptoms related to smoking Cool extremities Raynaud's phenomenon Distal limb claudication (instep or hand) Sudden onset limb pain	Cool extremities Digital ulcers Migratory thrombophlebitis	Characteristic findings on angiogram	Smoking cessation Sympathectomy to prevent vasospasm Amputation of gangrenous digits
Arterial embolism	May originate from the aorta or heart	Sudden onset of painful extremity (occasionally more gradual)	Cool, pale, painful extremity with absent pulses distal to embolus	Pathologic examination of embolus may reveal etiology	Heparin Embolectomy for larger vessels Chronic anticoagulation if source cannot be removed

Condition	Etiology/Pathology	Clinical Features	Physical Findings	Diagnosis	Treatment
Atheroembolism	Atheromatous debris ± thrombus, usually from aorta	Can be asymptomatic; May follow intravascular procedures; Digital (toe) ischemia common	Blue digits, livedo reticularis, renal insufficiency, guaiac + stool, abdominal petechiae	Eosinophilia, low complement levels; Skin or renal biopsy may reveal cholesterol emboli	Resection of source of debris, if possible; Heparin relatively contraindicated
Takayasu's arteritis	Probably immunologic; Intimal proliferation and fibrosis of the aortic wall; Involves the aortic arch and its branches; May involve renal arteries	Women > men; Systemic symptoms common (malaise, fever, weight loss)	Diminished or absent pulses; Hypertension and aortic insufficiency common	Elevated erythrocyte sedimentation rate; Characteristic pattern on arteriogram	Glucocorticoids reduce symptoms; Surgical or percutaneous revascularization for threatened vascular territories
Raynaud's phenomenon	Vasospasm of digital vessels precipitated by cold	Primary: female > male; age < 40; no underlying condition. Secondary: male > female; age > 40; multiple underlying conditions (arterial occlusive disease, connective tissue disease, neurologic disease, vasoconstricting drugs, cryoglobulinemia, cold agglutinins, post frostbite)	Triphasic color changes: white on exposure to cold, followed by blue (cyanosis), followed by red on rewarming (hyperemia); Normal pulses unless underlying arterial occlusive disease; Small areas of digital gangrene in severe cases, but amputation rare	Depends on underlying condition	Limitation of cold exposure; Treat underlying condition; Smoking cessation; Vasodilators; Regional sympathectomy in severe cases

ized with computed tomography (CT) or magnetic resonance imaging (MRI). Angiography is rarely needed for diagnosis.

The treatment of vascular aneurysms depends on their size and the presence of symptoms (Table 13–3). In general, all symptomatic aneurysms require surgical correction, unless other comorbidities preclude this approach. Aortic aneurysms tend to enlarge progressively, and the risk of rupture correlates with aneurysm size. In patients who are good surgical candidates, elective surgery should be considered for abdominal aortic aneurysms larger than 4 cm in diameter and (non-Marfan's) thoracic aortic aneurysms larger than 6 cm in diameter. With aneurysms smaller than this, serial imaging studies should be obtained every 3 to 6 months to identify enlarging lesions. Iliac artery aneurysms greater than 3 cm should be resected. Peripheral arterial aneurysms are associated with a high risk of thromboembolic complications, and, once diagnosed, surgical therapy is the treatment of choice. Nonsurgical repair of abdominal aortic aneurysms has been performed with percutaneously placed prosthetic grafts. These grafts are deployed intravascularly at the site of the aneurysm, are anchored to the nonaneurysmal proximal and distal aorta by expandable stents, and effectively isolate the aneurysm from the circulation. Early experience with this procedure has been promising.

A false (or pseudo) aneurysm is a localized tear in an arterial wall that allows blood to accumulate in the perivascular space. These most commonly result from trauma to a vessel, such as that occurring during catheterization of a femoral artery, although they may also occur after ulceration of an atherosclerotic plaque that then penetrates the vessel wall. Pseudoaneurysms are more prone to rupture than are true aneurysms. Ultrasonographically directed compression of a peripheral arterial pseudoaneurysm can sometimes be curative; however, surgical treatment is frequently necessary.

AORTIC DISSECTION

An aortic dissection is a tear in the aortic intima through which blood enters and subsequently dissects distally along the plane between the intima and media of the vessel, creating a true and false lumen in the aorta (Fig. 13–3). Hypertension and Marfan's syndrome

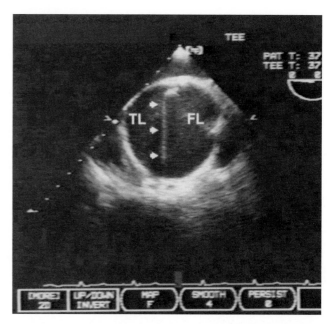

FIGURE 13-3 Transesophageal echocardiogram of the ascending aorta in a patient with Marfan's syndrome and severe chest pain. The aorta is dilated (5.5 cm), and a dissection flap is clearly seen *(arrows)* separating the true lumen (TL) from the false lumen (FL).

are the most common predisposing factors. Type A dissections originate in the ascending aorta, usually within a few centimeters of the aortic valve, and either extend around the aortic arch into the descending aorta (type I) or are limited to the ascending aorta (type II). Type B (or type III) dissections involve only the descending aorta and originate just distal to the origin of the left subclavian artery at the site of the ligamentum arteriosum. Patients with an acute aortic dissection usually present with sudden, severe chest pain, which may be "tearing" in quality. The pain may be substernal, classically radiating to the interscapular area. Proximal dissections may involve the aortic valve, resulting in acute aortic insufficiency; may dissect into a coronary artery (most commonly the right coronary artery), producing acute myocardial ischemia or infarction; and may rupture into the pericardial space, resulting in tamponade. As the dissection progresses distally, involvement of the subclavian, carotid, mesenteric, renal, and iliac arteries may result in pulse discrepancies or in cerebral, mesenteric, renal, or limb ischemia. The chest roentgenogram frequently demonstrates a widened mediastinum, although a normal mediastinal shadow does not exclude the diagnosis. The extent of dissection can be visualized with TEE, contrast CT, or MRI. In the hemodynamically unstable patient with suspected aortic dissection, TEE is the study of choice.

Once the diagnosis of aortic dissection is suspected, treatment should be instituted immediately. All patients should receive β-blocker therapy even if they are normotensive. Hypertensive patients should be treated with either intravenous nitroprusside or labetalol. Emergent surgery is indicated for patients with proximal (type A) dissection, whereas medical therapy is appropriate as

TABLE 13-3 Indications for Surgery in Aneurysmal Arterial Disease

Level of Disease	Surgical Indications
Thoracic aorta	Symptoms
	>6 cm in diameter or enlarging on serial exams
Abdominal aorta	Symptoms
	>4 cm in diameter or enlarging on serial exams
Iliac artery	Symptoms
	>3 cm in diameter
Femoral or popliteal	Always

initial therapy for patients with distal dissection. After surgery, all patients should remain on β-blocker therapy indefinitely, and repeated aortic imaging should be obtained at least yearly to evaluate for the development of progressive aortic dilatation or recurrent dissection. The percutaneous implantation of expandable endovascular stents offers a promising new option for the treatment of dissections of the abdominal aorta and peripheral vasculature. These stents may obliterate areas of the dissection, restore normal distal blood flow, and decrease the need for surgical intervention. As experience with these devices increases, they will likely play a greater role in the standard treatment of aneurysms and dissections.

OTHER ARTERIAL DISEASES

Inflammatory or infectious diseases may result in vascular disease. Aortic arteritis is an uncommon disorder in which the aorta and the origins of its major branches are involved with the inflammatory process. Giant cell arteritis is the classic example and may present as either Takayasu's arteritis in the young patient or temporal (cranial) arteritis in the older person. Takayasu's arteritis generally affects young women (most commonly Japanese women) and has a predilection for the aortic arch and the origins of the great vessels. Marked intimal proliferation and fibrosis occur in the aortic wall with resultant obliteration of the vessel lumen. It may involve the aortic root, resulting in aortic insufficiency. Aneurysm formation is uncommon. Treatment is with systemic corticosteroids, although surgery is occasionally required to bypass a threatened vascular bed. Giant cell arteritis affecting the extracranial branches of the carotid artery classically presents as temporal headaches and is referred to as *temporal arteritis*. It is almost exclusively a disease of people older than age 65; is slightly more common in women than in men; and, in addition to headaches, may be associated with temporal artery tenderness, visual loss, jaw claudication, weight loss, and fevers. The diagnosis is supported by a markedly elevated erythrocyte sedimentation rate (frequently >100 mm/hr), although definitive diagnosis is made with a temporal artery biopsy. Treatment requires the use of daily corticosteroids, which dramatically improve symptoms and prevent the ocular complications.

Bacterial infection of an aortic aneurysm is extremely rare; however, tertiary syphilis may produce an aortitis that, in contradistinction to atherosclerotic aortic disease, most commonly involves the ascending aorta. Aneurysmal dilation of the aortic root results, with variable amounts of aortic valve insufficiency and stenosis of the coronary artery ostia. It is a late complication of untreated syphilis, occurring 10 to 30 years after the index infection.

The most common congenital aortic disorder is coarctation (see later discussion). Congenital aneurysms of the sinuses of Valsalva can occur and may occasionally produce aortic valve dysfunction or occlusion of a coronary artery. These aneurysms may also rupture into the right cardiac chambers, producing a large left-to-right intracardiac shunt and a loud, continuous murmur. Infective endocarditis can be complicated by the development of an acquired sinus of Valsalva aneurysm.

Acute occlusion of the aorta may result from a large embolism that obstructs at the level of the aortic bifurcation (saddle embolus). In more rare cases, aortic occlusion occurs in the setting of thrombosis at the site of severe atherosclerotic disease. Aortic obstruction is usually characterized by the development of sudden, severe, bilateral lower extremity pain, paresthesias, and cyanosis. This must be distinguished from aortic dissection, and surgical removal of the clot with subsequent anticoagulation is mandatory. In rare cases, complete obstruction of the aorta may develop over time and is asymptomatic because of the development of collateral vessels.

Arteriovenous (AV) fistulas, abnormal connections between arteries and veins without intervening capillary systems, may be either congenital or acquired. Congenital AV fistulas are frequently multiple and small, and because the absolute amount of flow through any given AV fistula is low, they are often not associated with bruits or thrills. Nonetheless, because the sum of shunt flow across the multiple fistulas may be quite high, high-output heart failure can be a complication. Treatment is difficult, although single large fistulas may occasionally be resected. Acquired AV fistulas can occur after trauma to the vascular system, such as from a gunshot or stab wound, or after attempts at cannulating a vessel with a catheter during intravascular procedures. Frequently, AV fistulas are created surgically to facilitate hemodialysis. The augmented blood flow through these relatively large AV fistulas results in venous engorgement and warm skin overlying the fistula and produces a palpable thrill and an audible bruit detectable on examination. The AV fistula creates a low-resistance pathway for blood flow, resulting in a lower diastolic blood pressure and an increased pulse pressure. Larger AV fistulas may be associated with high-output heart failure. If the artery serving such an AV fistula is compressed, the shunt decreases and the patient's heart rate decreases (Nicaladoni-Branham sign). Acquired AV fistulas are best treated surgically.

CHRONIC VENOUS DISEASE

Varicose veins are caused by incompetent valves in the saphenous veins and may result from any condition that results in an increase in intra-abdominal pressure (e.g., pregnancy, ascites) or interferes with venous drainage from the lower extremities (e.g., intra-abdominal tumors, pelvic vein thrombosis). Varicosities may cause local discomfort, may be complicated by thrombosis (thrombophlebitis), and cause chronic edema. Treatment is initially conservative with compression stockings; sclerotherapy and surgical venous stripping are reserved for refractory cases. Chronic venous insufficiency may follow deep venous thrombophlebitis and results in chronic edema. Treatment also involves the use of support stockings and leg elevation. Leg ulcers commonly develop in the setting of venous stasis and require antibiotics and compressive bandages for optimal healing.

Edema caused by chronic venous disease or elevated venous pressure (e.g., right-sided heart failure, cirrhosis)

TABLE 13-4   Conditions Predisposing to Deep Venous Thrombosis

Venous Stasis
Congestive heart failure
Paralysis/cerebrovascular accident
Pregnancy
Major surgery
Immobility or prolonged bed rest
Polycythemia vera

Hypercoagulability
Acquired
Cancer, sepsis, pregnancy, oral contraceptives, lupus anticoagulant, nephrotic syndrome
Inherited
Deficiencies of antithrombin III, protein S, protein C, resistance to activated protein C (factor V Leiden), prothrombin gene mutation (20210A), dysfibrinogenemia, hyperhomocysteinemia

Vascular Injury
Trauma
Surgery
Central venous catheters
Certain chemotherapeutic agents

must be distinguished from that caused by ineffective lymphatic drainage (lymphedema). Venous disease produces pitting edema and an increased superficial venous pattern, involves the foot but not the toes, and is associated with relatively normal skin. Lymphedema is nonpitting, does not result in superficial venous prominence, involves the foot and the toes, and is associated with thickened skin. Lymphedema may be congenital (e.g., Milroy's disease), postinfectious, obstructive as a result of pelvic neoplasms, or iatrogenic after surgical removal of lymph nodes. Compression stocking use is the mainstay of therapy.

Venous Thromboembolic Disease

VENOUS THROMBOTIC DISEASE

Thrombosis of a vein is usually accompanied by inflammation of the wall of the involved vessel and is referred to as *thrombophlebitis*. Thrombophlebitis may involve the superficial or deep veins. Superficial thrombophlebitis produces a firm, tender cord at the site of the involved vein, and the warmth and erythema of the overlying skin may be difficult to distinguish from cellulitis. It may occur after minor trauma, especially in patients with varicose veins, or after placement of an intravenous catheter. A syndrome of migratory superficial thrombophlebitis may occur in patients with thromboangiitis obliterans and in patients with an occult malignancy (Trousseau's syndrome). Treatment with warm packs and anti-inflammatory agents and removal of indwelling catheters is usually effective. Thromboembolic events, in general, do not complicate superficial thrombophlebitis.

Deep venous thrombosis (DVT) most commonly affects the lower extremities, but it can also occur in veins of the pelvis and upper extremities. The triad of venous stasis, hypercoagulability, and venous injury (Virchow's triad) describes the main conditions that predispose to DVT (Table 13-4). The clinical diagnosis of DVT may be difficult. Classically, patients present with pain in the area of the involved vein and edema in the extremity distal to the thrombosis. However, almost half of patients with DVT are asymptomatic. DVT is frequently associated with embolic complications, and pulmonary emboli may be the initial presenting manifestation. The differential diagnosis of lower extremity DVT includes a ruptured Baker's cyst and trauma to the calf muscles. Because of the difficulty in diagnosing DVT clinically, specialized diagnostic tests are frequently required (Table 13-5).

The treatment of proximal (i.e., iliac and femoral) DVT is anticoagulation. It is not clear that distal (i.e., calf) DVT requires treatment, especially if there is no evidence of proximal propagation on serial ultrasound studies. Anticoagulation is initially accomplished with an intravenous bolus of heparin, followed by a continuous infusion to maintain the partial thromboplastin time 1.5 to 2 times the control value. Platelet counts must be monitored to identify the occasional patient who develops heparin-induced thrombocytopenia. Rapid achievement of therapeutic anticoagulation is imperative because failure to do so is associated with progression of thromboembolic disease. The use of weight-based dosing nomograms is useful to determine the appropriate heparin dose. Oral warfarin is started concurrently, and heparin is continued for 3 to 5 days until the warfarin reaches a therapeutic level. The goal is to maintain the international normalized ratio of the prothrombin time in the range of two to three times control. Warfarin is

TABLE 13-5   Diagnostic Tests for Deep Venous Thrombosis (DVT)

Method	Advantages	Disadvantages
Contrast venography	The "gold standard"; may differentiate new vs. old DVT	Invasive
Impedance plethysmography and Doppler ultrasonography (Duplex scan)	90–95% diagnostic accuracy for iliac and femoral DVTs Serial studies easily compared Noninvasive	Less accurate for DVTs below the knee

then continued for 3 to 6 months in patients no longer at risk for recurrent thrombosis, but it should be continued indefinitely in patients in whom the predisposing condition persists. Low-molecular-weight heparins (LMWHs) have been developed that can be administered subcutaneously and appear as effective as unfractionated heparin for initial treatment of DVT, with decreased risk of thrombocytopenia. In selected patients, treatment of acute DVT can be accomplished in the outpatient setting, with LMWHs continued until the international normalized ratio is in the therapeutic range. Warfarin is contraindicated during pregnancy, especially during the second trimester. In pregnant patients requiring anticoagulation, subcutaneous unfractionated or LMWHs may be used.

PULMONARY EMBOLISM

The lungs function as a filter for blood returning from the systemic circulation, and, therefore, material too large to pass through the pulmonary capillary system may become lodged in the pulmonary vasculature. Depending on the size and composition of the embolic material, these pulmonary emboli (PEs) may be asymptomatic or may result in profound abnormalities in gas exchange and hemodynamic collapse. The vast majority of PEs are the result of venous thromboemboli; however, other sources of embolic material must be considered in specific situations. Embolization of marrow fat (after major trauma or orthopedic surgery), amniotic fluid (during vaginal or caesarean delivery), or air (during placement of central venous catheters) may produce the adult respiratory distress syndrome. Sickled red blood cells or blood-borne parasites (e.g., schistosomes), as well as talc granules and cotton fibers unintentionally injected during intravenous drug use, may obstruct the pulmonary vasculature and produce progressive pulmonary hypertension.

Approximately 250,000 patients each year are hospitalized for pulmonary thromboembolism in the United States alone, and the 3-month mortality rate approaches 10% to 15%. The majority of pulmonary thromboemboli originate in the deep veins of the thigh, with less common sources including the veins of the upper extremities, pelvic veins, and right atrial mural thrombi. Predisposing factors for PE are similar to those for DVT, with stasis, hypercoagulability, and vessel trauma playing a central role. Increased age, smoking, and exogenous estrogen use also increase the risk of PE.

The presentation of an acute or chronic PE may be difficult to distinguish from that of other cardiopulmonary disorders; unless a high level of suspicion is maintained, the diagnosis is frequently missed. Historical features may be helpful, such as a prior history of DVT or PE, a family history of venous thrombosis, or a recent history of immobilization (e.g., recent surgery, prolonged car trips). The most frequent symptom is dyspnea (80%), with pleuritic chest pain and hemoptysis being less common (70% and 20% to 30%, respectively). Tachycardia and tachypnea are the most common physical findings; obvious thrombophlebitis, signs of acute pulmonary hypertension (e.g., loud P_2, right ventricular heave, bulging neck veins), and pleural rubs are less common. A low-grade fever is often present; however, high fever is unusual and suggests pneumonia rather than PE. Syncope and cyanosis are distinctly unusual and suggest a massive embolus. The vast majority of patients with an acute PE present with some combination of dyspnea, pleuritic chest pain, and tachypnea; patients with none of these findings are unlikely to have had an acute PE.

The most common finding on electrocardiogram is sinus tachycardia. Signs of acute right-sided heart strain, anterior T wave inversions, and pseudoinfarction patterns are also seen. The classic pattern of a deep S wave in lead I and a deep Q wave and T wave inversion in lead III ("S1-Q3-T3") is rare. Abnormal findings on chest radiography are common but nonspecific and include focal hypovascularity (Westermark's sign), a dilated right pulmonary artery (Palla's sign), and a wedge-shaped peripheral density above the diaphragm (Hampton's hump). Areas of atelectasis and small pleural effusions are common, but the radiograph is normal in up to 30% of patients with documented PE. Hypoxemia and hypocapnia are typical, and the extent of increase in the alveolar-arterial oxygen gradient correlates linearly with the severity of pulmonary embolus. However, a normal arterial blood gas finding occurs in 15% to 20% of patients with PE and, thus, cannot be used to exclude the diagnosis. Therefore, although features of the patient's history, physical examination, and routine diagnostic testing may suggest the diagnosis of pulmonary embolus, further specific testing is necessary for confirmation.

Because most PEs originate in the lower extremities, the finding of a DVT on bilateral venous duplex scanning can be used as a surrogate marker for PE. Unfortunately, as many as one third of patients with documented PE will have a negative lower extremity duplex examination for DVT, likely because either the clot has already embolized or it originated elsewhere. In patients with a DVT or PE, endogenous thrombolysis is activated, resulting in the breakdown of clot-bound fibrin. This process is clinically ineffective in removing most thromboemboli, but it results in the release of specific fibrin degradation products called D-dimers. These D-dimers are elevated in the blood of more than 90% of patients with a PE; however, they are also increased in patients with myocardial infarction, sepsis, pregnancy, or any systemic inflammatory disease, and, thus, high levels are not diagnostic of PE. A normal D-dimer level may, however, help to exclude the diagnosis. In patients in whom there is a low or moderate clinical suspicion for PE, a normal D-dimer level combined with a negative duplex scan can be used as reasonable evidence to exclude the diagnosis. Because of the false-negative rates of these studies, further diagnostic evaluation is warranted in patients in whom there is a high clinical suspicion.

Ventilation-perfusion scanning is commonly used to evaluate patients for pulmonary embolus. Radioactive tracers are inhaled and injected intravenously to visualize the areas of the lung that are ventilated and perfused, respectively. Normally, the ventilation and perfusion of a given lung segment are proportional. In the presence of a PE, perfusion to the lung is decreased but ventilation remains normal. A normal ventilation-perfusion scan excludes the diagnosis of PE with almost 100% accuracy. A "high-probability" ventilation-perfusion scan (a normal ventilation scan with a perfusion scan that demonstrates segmental or larger perfusion defects) is highly specific (>90%) for the presence of PE, especially if the clinical suspicion is high. "Intermediate-probability" ventilation-perfusion scans are nondiagnostic; and depending on the clinical suspicion, pulmonary embolus may be present in up to 40% of patients with these indeterminate scans. These patients, therefore, require further evaluation, usually with pulmonary angiography. Several alternatives to angiography have been proposed. In the stable patient, serial lower extremity duplex studies may be performed over a 10-day period. If no evidence of DVT develops, then treatment of PE is unnecessary because the treatment is aimed at preventing recurrent thrombus formation, not at treating the embolism. Ultrafast CT after intravenous contrast medium injection is highly sensitive and specific for the diagnosis of emboli in the proximal pulmonary arteries; more distal emboli cannot be reliably detected by this method. More recently, magnetic resonance pulmonary angiography has been shown to be quite sensitive and specific and may eventually substitute for conventional angiography. An approach to the patient with suspected PE is shown in Figure 13–4.

Echocardiography may be useful in patients with pulmonary emboli. Occasionally, thrombus can be identified in the right cardiac chambers or in the proximal pulmonary arteries. The extent of hemodynamic impairment of the right ventricle can be assessed, and other conditions that may mimic PE may be identified (e.g., right ventricular infarction, pericardial tamponade). Nonetheless, echocardiography plays a secondary role in the diagnosis of PE.

Treatment of PE is similar to that described earlier for DVT, with rapid institution of heparin followed by warfarin therapy. LMWHs have been shown to be as safe and effective as unfractionated heparin for the treatment of hemodynamically stable patients with PE. If the clinical suspicion of PE is high, anticoagulation should be started even before definitive diagnostic tests are performed. Heparin augments the action of endogenous antithrombin III, thereby preventing additional thrombus formation and allowing for endogenous thrombolysis to dissolve the embolism. The ideal duration of therapy is not clear in all patients, but 6 months of therapy appears to decrease the risk of recurrent PE compared with 6 weeks of therapy. As in DVTs, patients with persistent predisposing conditions warrant long-term or life-long anticoagulation.

Occasionally, alternative therapies are required (see Table 13–8), because anticoagulation either is contraindicated or is ineffective in treating or preventing recurrent emboli. In patients with massive pulmonary emboli, hemodynamic instability, or overt cardiogenic shock, thrombolytic therapy with streptokinase, urokinase, or tissue plasminogen activator hastens dissolution of the embolism and may decrease mortality. In hemodynamically stable patients with PEs, thrombolytic therapy has not been shown to decrease mortality, and the potential

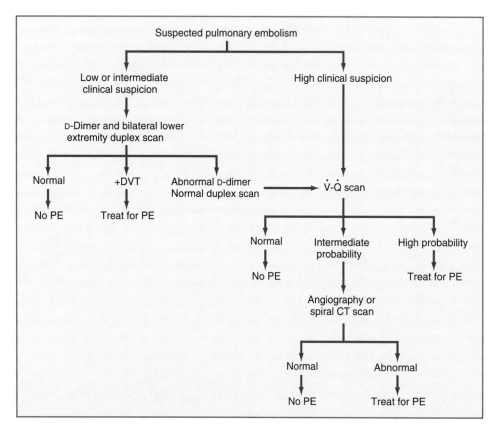

FIGURE 13–4 Diagnostic evaluation of suspected pulmonary embolism (PE).

benefits of more rapid thromboembolic resolution must be weighed against the increased risk of bleeding associated with this therapy. The routine use of thrombolytic therapy for PE is, therefore, not warranted. In unstable patients with contraindications to anticoagulation or thrombolysis, embolectomy by means of transvenous catheter techniques or open surgical procedures should be considered. Such therapy may result in dramatic improvement in the patient's condition, but it does not prevent recurrent thromboembolic events. In such cases, if the embolism is thought to have originated in the lower extremities, a filter can be placed in the inferior vena cava and is effective at reducing recurrent major emboli. Filters should also be considered in stable patients with contraindications to anticoagulation, and in patients who have recurrent PEs despite adequate anticoagulation. In this latter group of patients, anticoagulation should be continued because these filters can occasionally thrombose, resulting in chronic bilateral leg edema.

By far, the most effective treatment of thromboembolic disease is prevention. In patients at high risk for DVT or PE (e.g., patients in the intensive care unit, patients undergoing major surgery, patients with recent onset of paralysis), prophylactic therapy with subcutaneous unfractionated heparin (5000 units every 12 hours) or LMWHs (e.g., enoxaparin, 30 mg twice daily) significantly reduces the risk. In patients with contraindications to this therapy (e.g., after neurosurgery or with active bleeding), the use of pneumatic compression boots is an acceptable alternative.

Pulmonary Vascular Disease

PHYSIOLOGY OF PULMONARY HYPERTENSION

The pulmonary vasculature is a high-capacity, low-resistance system, and it functions under relatively low pressure (Table 13–6). The normal pulmonary arterial systolic and mean pressures are less than 30 mm Hg and less than 20 mm Hg, respectively. Diseases of this system impair gas exchange across the pulmonary alveoli and result in an increase in pulmonary arterial pressure with resultant detrimental effects on the function of the right ventricle. As a result of the extensive nature of the pulmonary capillary network and the distensibility of the pulmonary vasculature, the pulmonary system is able to

tolerate significant increases in blood flow with little or no rise in pulmonary pressure. Thus, pulmonary hypertension usually results from an increased pulmonary vascular resistance.

The pulmonary capillary system is uniquely arranged to maximize oxygen and carbon dioxide exchange across the alveolar-capillary membrane. Diseases associated with pulmonary hypertension are frequently complicated by impaired alveolar gas exchange with resultant hypoxemia, not as a direct result of the pulmonary vascular disease but, rather, as a result of the primary underlying lung disease. Pulmonary vascular occlusion and obliteration, which may be a secondary result of the pulmonary hypertension, may further decrease the diffusing capacity of the lungs and cause ventilation-perfusion mismatches, thus contributing to the hypoxemia.

Because of the low pressure of the normal pulmonary system, the right ventricle usually performs only minimal contractile work. Elevated pulmonary pressure is important mainly in regard to the effect it has on right ventricular function. When faced with an acute increase in pulmonary pressure, the right ventricle is able to generate a systolic pressure of up to 40 to 50 mm Hg without failing. More indolent development of pulmonary hypertension results in right ventricular hypertrophy and the ability of the right ventricle to generate pressures equal to or greater than systemic pressure. Acute or chronic pulmonary hypertension may lead to right ventricular failure; because of the interdependence of the right and left ventricles, the elevated pulmonary pressures can also affect left ventricular function. As the right ventricle dilates, the interventricular septum bows into the left ventricular cavity, thereby decreasing left ventricular stroke volume and compliance and producing left ventricular failure.

CAUSES OF PULMONARY HYPERTENSION

Table 13–7 reviews the causes of pulmonary hypertension, listed by pathophysiologic mechanism. Although increases in pulmonary blood flow are usually well tolerated, marked or prolonged increases in flow can result in pulmonary hypertension, as occurs in congenital heart diseases with left-to-right shunts. In pulmonary venous hypertension, the elevated pulmonary arterial pressure is secondary to elevated pulmonary venous pressure, most commonly as a result of left ventricular failure or mitral valve disease. Reactive pulmonary hypertension reflects arterial vasoconstriction, predominantly as a result of hypoxemia. Abnormalities of the pulmonary arteries or arterioles comprise a large group of disorders of which pulmonary thromboembolic disease and primary pulmonary hypertension (PPH) are the most important.

CLINICAL PRESENTATION

Irrespective of the etiology of pulmonary hypertension, the resultant hemodynamic effects and clinical signs and symptoms of chronically elevated pulmonary pressure are the same. In secondary pulmonary hypertension, however, the underlying condition frequently dominates the clinical picture.

TABLE 13–6   Values for Normal Adult Pulmonary Vascular Hemodynamics

Pulmonary artery pressure	
Systolic	15–30 mm Hg
Diastolic	3–12 mm Hg
Mean	<20 mm Hg
Pulmonary capillary wedge pressure	≤12 mm Hg
Pulmonary vascular resistance	30–120 dyne-cm/sec²

TABLE 13–7 **Causes of Pulmonary Hypertension**

Increased Pulmonary Flow

Atrial and ventricular septal defects
Patent ductus arteriosus
Peripheral arteriovenous shunts

Elevated Pulmonary Venous Pressure

Left ventricular failure
Mitral stenosis
Mitral regurgitation
Pulmonary venous thrombosis

Abnormalities of the Pulmonary Arteries or Arterioles

Pulmonary embolic disease
Parenchymal lung disease (e.g., fibrosis, COPD)
Pulmonary artery stenosis
Primary pulmonary hypertension
Toxic (e.g., *Crotalaria*, L-tryptophan, fenfluramine)
HIV associated
Vasculitides (e.g., systemic sclerosis, SLE)

Reactive Pulmonary Vasoconstriction

Hypoxia (e.g., high altitude)
Acidosis
Hypoventilation syndromes (e.g., sleep apnea, neuromuscular disorder)

COPD = chronic obstructive pulmonary disease; HIV = human immunodeficiency virus; SLE = systemic lupus erythematosus.

Exertional dyspnea and fatigue are early symptoms of pulmonary hypertension. As the disease progresses, angina-like chest pain is common and likely a result of right ventricular subendocardial ischemia. Presyncope or exertional syncope frequently occurs, presumably as a result of decreased left ventricular output. Hoarseness may occur as a result of compression of the left recurrent laryngeal nerve between the aorta and the dilated left pulmonary artery (Ortner's syndrome). Physical examination may disclose evidence of pulmonary hypertension (loud P_2, palpable pulmonary arterial impulse) or right ventricular pressure overload or overt failure (right ventricular heave, right-sided S_3, elevated jugular venous pressure, peripheral edema).

Laboratory evaluation may reveal evidence of the underlying disease. Hypoxemia is frequently present, although it is often only mild in patients with PPH. Chest radiography may demonstrate prominent central pulmonary arteries with a paucity of peripheral vessels ("vascular pruning") in patients with progressive pulmonary arteriopathy, as well as a dilated right atrium and ventricle. The electrocardiogram demonstrates right ventricular hypertrophy when the mean pulmonary arterial pressure exceeds 40 mm Hg, and evidence of right atrial enlargement is also common. Echocardiography provides important information regarding left and right ventricular size and function, can identify congenital or valvular disorders, and provides a means of estimating the pulmonary arterial pressure. The definitive diagnosis of pulmonary hypertension is made during right-sided heart catheterization with direct measurement of pulmonary arterial pressures.

PRIMARY PULMONARY HYPERTENSION

PPH is that which occurs in the absence of an identifiable cause. It is a relatively uncommon disorder characterized pathophysiologically by vasoconstriction, proliferation of vascular tissue, and in situ thrombosis. It may occur at almost any age, although most patients present in the third or fourth decade of life. In the adult population, more women than men are affected, but there appears to be no gender predilection in childhood. Familial cases have been described, leading to the suggestion of an inheritable predisposition. Most cases, however, are not familial, and so environmental factors likely play an important role. In support of this view, abnormalities identical to PPH have been described after exposure to such agents as L-tryptophan, crack cocaine, and anorexigenic drugs and in patients infected with the human immunodeficiency virus.

Vascular injury resulting in altered endothelial function with a resultant increase in vasomotor tone appears to play a central pathophysiologic role. This may be mediated by an increase in the endothelial production of vasoconstricting agents (thromboxane A_2, endothelin) or a decrease in vasodilating agents (prostacyclin, nitric oxide), abnormalities that have been described in patients with PPH. In addition, thromboxane A_2 promotes platelet aggregation, an effect that is opposed by nitric oxide and prostacyclin. An imbalance in these mediators could, therefore, result in a localized prothrombotic environment and account for the development of in situ pulmonary thrombosis seen in patients with PPH.

The prognosis of patients with PPH is poor and relates directly to the severity of the pulmonary hypertension and the level of impairment of right ventricular function. Overall mean survival is 2 to 3 years from the time of diagnosis.

TREATMENT OF PULMONARY HYPERTENSION

Because of the pathogenic role of pulmonary vascular thrombosis in patients with PPH, treatment with chronic anticoagulation is indicated and may offer a survival benefit. In patients whose pulmonary arterial pressures decrease acutely in response to a vasodilator challenge with adenosine or a calcium channel–blocking agent, long-term vasodilator therapy appears to be beneficial, at times with dramatic decreases in pulmonary pressures. Chronic vasodilator therapy can be achieved with oral calcium channel blockers (nifedipine, diltiazem), inhaled nitric oxide, or a continuous intravenous infusion of epoprostenol (prostacyclin). This last agent has been shown to decrease symptoms, increase exercise capacity, and decrease mortality in patients with PPH. In patients with progressive disease despite aggressive vasodilator therapy, lung transplantation or combined heart-lung transplantation has been performed.

The treatment of secondary pulmonary hypertension is directed at treating the underlying cause. Treatment of valvular heart disease, left ventricular failure, and intracardiac shunts may result in near normalization of the pulmonary pressures. Patients with these conditions, as well as patients with underlying lung diseases, often have resting or exercise-induced hypoxemia, and therapy with supplemental oxygen may decrease pulmonary pressure and improve right ventricular function by blunting the hypoxia-induced pulmonary vasoconstriction. Unfortunately, treatment aimed at decreasing pulmonary pressure with vasodilators has not been shown to be of benefit in secondary pulmonary hypertension. In patients with pulmonary embolic disease, most pulmonary emboli completely resolve over time, and chronic pulmonary hypertension develops in less than 2% of cases. The patients who do develop chronic pulmonary thromboembolic disease and subsequent right-sided heart failure may be candidates for surgical thromboendarterectomy by which the organized embolus is removed. The mortality of this procedure approaches 5% to 10%, but when the procedure is successful, pulmonary hypertension begins to resolve within the first postoperative months and the patient's quality of life significantly improves.

Hypertension

Hypertension is one of the greatest health problems facing industrialized nations and continues to be a major contributing factor in the development of, and death from CAD, stroke, heart failure, and renal failure. Because uncomplicated hypertension is an asymptomatic condition, many people are unaware that they have it. Campaigns by national medical organizations have raised public awareness, and the mass screening of patients has resulted in an increased recognition of the problem so that now only an estimated 30% of patients with hypertension are unaware of their diagnosis. This has contributed to significant decreases in the rates of death from stroke and CAD. Nonetheless, only 50% of patients with hypertension are on therapy, and only 30% have their blood pressure controlled to ideal levels. Because of the asymptomatic nature of this disease (at least until complications develop) and the frequent side effects associated with treatment, initiation of medical therapy and continued compliance with a treatment regimen is an ongoing challenge.

As currently defined, systemic hypertension is present in an adult (age ≥ 18) if the systolic blood pressure is greater than or equal to 140 mm Hg or the diastolic blood pressure is greater than or equal to 90 mm Hg. According to this definition, an estimated 50 million adult Americans have hypertension. This is a somewhat arbitrary definition in that it is not derived from any pathophysiologic data but, rather, from an analysis of the range of pressures in the population and the risks of associated morbidity and mortality. Nonetheless, the current definitions make clinical sense because the long-term risk of cardiovascular morbidity and mortality clearly rises in direct relation to increases in systemic blood pressure.

Hypertension can be further classified into various stages reflecting mild, moderate, or severe elevations in blood pressure (Table 13–8). When there is a discrep-

TABLE 13-8 Classification of Blood Pressure in Adults

Classification	Systolic BP		Diastolic BP
Normal	<130	and	<85
High-normal	130–139	or	85–89
Hypertensive			
Stage 1	140–159	or	90–99
Stage 2	160–179	or	100–109
Stage 3	≥180	or	≥110

BP = blood pressure (in mm Hg).

ancy between the classification of the systolic and diastolic blood pressures, the higher category should be used to classify the patient's hypertension. The diagnosis of hypertension is generally not based on a single elevated blood pressure measurement; rather, it reflects a pattern of elevated blood pressure, with abnormally high values obtained on at least three separate occasions. The normal blood pressure in children and pregnant women is slightly lower, although care must be taken in making the formal diagnosis of hypertension in children and adolescents because the blood pressure frequently normalizes in adulthood.

The incidence of hypertension increases with age and is more common in African-Americans than in whites. It is more common in younger men than in women, although this difference does not exist after the age of 55 and is reversed after the age of 75. Despite advances in the treatment of hypertension, much is still unknown regarding the etiology of the disease. In 90% to 95% of patients, no identifiable cause of the hypertension is found and the patients are said to have *primary* or *essential hypertension*. Familial patterns of primary hypertension are common and suggest that genetic factors are important. However, environmental factors, such as obesity, alcohol consumption, sedentary lifestyle, and salt intake, likely play a role. Proposed pathophysiologic mechanisms include excessive renal sodium retention, overactivity of the sympathetic nervous system, renin-angiotensin excess, hyperinsulinemia, and alterations in vascular endothelium. This last mechanism may result from a decrease in endothelium-derived vasorelaxing substances (e.g., nitric oxide) or an increase in endothelium-derived constricting factors (e.g., endothelin). Several of these factors may be present in a given individual and may mediate the hypertensive response through alterations in circulating blood volume, constriction of vascular smooth muscle, and/or vascular hypertrophy. In approximately 5% of hypertensive patients, the elevated blood pressure is the direct result of another disorder (Table 13–9).

EVALUATION OF THE HYPERTENSIVE PATIENT

The initial evaluation of a patient with hypertension should include a thorough history and physical examination and limited laboratory studies. The goals of this evaluation are to assess the patient for the presence and

TABLE 13–9 Secondary Causes of Hypertension

Renal

Renal parenchymal disease (glomerulonephritis, polycystic disease, diabetic nephropathy)

Renovascular disease (renal artery stenosis, fibromuscular dysplasia, vasculitis)

Endocrine

Hypo- or hyperthyroidism

Hyperparathyroidism

Adrenocorticoid excess (Cushing's syndrome, primary aldosteronism)

Pheochromocytoma

Exogenous hormones (oral contraceptives, estrogen replacement)

Neurologic Disorders

Brain tumors, sleep apnea, spinal cord injuries, lead poisoning, porphyria

Stress-Induced

Pain, anxiety, hypoglycemia, alcohol withdrawal, postoperative

Toxic/Pharmacologic

Alcohol and drug use, NSAIDs, ephedrine, corticosteroids, monoamine oxidase inhibitors

Miscellaneous

Aortic coarctation

Carcinoid syndrome

Pregnancy

NSAIDs = nonsteroidal anti-inflammatory drugs.

extent of hypertensive target organ damage, identify clinical factors that may influence the choice of therapy (e.g., renal failure, heart failure), determine the presence of other cardiovascular risk factors, and recognize the occasional patient with a secondary, and therefore potentially reversible, cause of hypertension. Hypertension itself is rarely symptomatic, although symptoms possibly attributable to the elevated blood pressure include headaches (usually occipital), blurred vision, fatigue, dizziness, epistaxis, dyspnea, and chest pain. In secondary hypertension, specific symptoms may develop that give clues to the underlying cause of the elevated blood pressure. Examples include weakness, polyuria, and muscle cramps caused by hypokalemia in primary hyperaldosteronism; weight gain and emotional lability in Cushing's syndrome; and headaches, palpitations, and hyperhidrosis in patients with pheochromocytoma. With chronic or severe hypertension, symptoms of organ damage may be present and include symptoms of congestive heart failure, CAD, cerebrovascular disease, uremia, and aortic dissection. Other historical features of importance include a history of alcohol use, prescription or nonprescription drug use (e.g., oral contraceptives, anabolic steroids), dietary sodium intake, and a family history of hypertension.

After confirming the presence of hypertension, the physical examination should focus on recognizing evidence of end-organ damage. The blood pressure and pulse should be checked in both arms and compared with the pressure in the legs to exclude the diagnosis of aortic coarctation. The fundoscopic examination should be carefully performed because it allows direct visual assessment of the extent of vascular injury and classification of the severity of hypertensive disease based on retinal changes (hypertensive retinopathy). "AV nicking" and "copper wire changes" in the arterioles characterize mild (grade I and II) retinopathy, whereas retinal hemorrhages and exudates (grade III) and papilledema (grade IV) reflect severe and potentially life-threatening disease. Evidence of left ventricular enlargement or failure should be noted. A thorough vascular examination should identify the presence of carotid or peripheral vascular disease, and abdominal bruits (reflecting possible renal artery stenosis) should be listened for carefully. A neurologic examination should be performed to search for evidence of prior strokes.

Initial laboratory screening should include serum electrolytes to identify potential metabolic disorders associated with secondary causes of hypertension. Measures of renal function (blood urea nitrogen and creatinine levels) and the urinalysis should be evaluated, because abnormalities in renal function may reflect either primary renal disease as a cause of the hypertension or secondary renal disease as a result of primary hypertension. Assessment of the serum glucose and fasting lipid levels are helpful in identifying other cardiovascular risk factors. An electrocardiogram should be obtained and evaluated for evidence of left ventricular hypertrophy or prior myocardial infarction. Echocardiography may be useful in selected patients to assess further the effects of hypertension on the heart.

Extreme elevations of blood pressure (>200 mm Hg systolic and/or >120 mm Hg diastolic) may occasionally be noted in asymptomatic patients. These patients are considered to have *accelerated hypertension* or *hypertensive urgency* and require the institution of antihypertensive therapy aimed at lowering the blood pressure over the course of several hours to several days. These elevated pressures, however, are often associated with symptoms of acute end-organ damage. Confusion, visual changes, seizures, headaches, and papilledema may occur as manifestations of hypertensive encephalopathy. Death may occur as a result of intracranial bleeding. Unstable angina, acute myocardial infarction, or left ventricular failure may be precipitated by profound hypertension. Hypertensive glomerulonephritis may result in proteinuria, hematuria, and acute renal failure. When these acute complications are present, patients are considered to have *malignant hypertension* or a *hypertensive emergency*. These patients require hospital admission and therapy aimed at immediate blood pressure reduction. Acute organ damage may resolve after aggressive treatment of the hypertension.

SECONDARY CAUSES OF HYPERTENSION

In approximately 5% of patients, a secondary cause of the hypertension can be found. Clinical features help to identify these patients, for whom a more extensive search for the etiology is warranted. Certain historical and physical examination findings (as described earlier) may point to a specific diagnosis. Patients with new-onset hypertension who are younger than the age of 30 or older than the age of 55 have a greater likelihood of having a reversible underlying cause. Patients with poorly controlled blood pressure, despite multiple anti-hypertensive medications, and those with previously well-controlled hypertension who develop a sudden increase in their blood pressure also require further evaluation. Table 13–9 lists the most frequently diagnosed secondary causes of hypertension. Several factors may contribute to failure of adequate blood pressure control despite a multidrug treatment regimen. Probably the most common reason for failure is medical noncompliance. Increased dietary sodium intake may aggravate hypertension, and a variety of drugs may interfere with the effectiveness of antihypertensive medications. These include oral contraceptive agents, corticosteroids, nonsteroidal anti-inflammatory drugs, and over-the-counter cold remedies containing ephedrine or sympathomimetics. These factors must be excluded before embarking on an extensive work-up for secondary causes of hypertension.

RENOVASCULAR HYPERTENSION

Renovascular hypertension accounts for 1% to 2% of cases of hypertension and is the most common secondary form of the disease. The pathophysiology of renovascular hypertension relates to a hemodynamically significant stenosis of the renal artery. The consequent decrease in renal blood flow stimulates an increase in renin release from the underperfused kidney and subsequently results in the increased production of angiotensin II. Angiotensin II is a potent vasoconstrictor and also stimulates the release of aldosterone from the adrenal gland, resulting in sodium and water retention and expansion of the intravascular volume. Both of these effects result in elevated blood pressure. The renal artery stenosis usually results from one of two processes: atherosclerotic renal artery disease or fibromuscular dysplasia. Atherosclerotic renal artery stenosis usually affects the proximal aspect of the renal artery and is most common in older men. Fibromuscular dysplasia results in fibrosis and aneurysm formation of the mid and distal renal arteries and is most common in younger women. Both these processes are bilateral in more than 50% of cases. Several clinical clues should raise the suspicion of renovascular hypertension. These include the sudden development of severe hypertension in a patient without a family history of hypertension, drug-resistant hypertension, the presence of diffuse atherosclerotic vascular disease or an abdominal bruit, and renal insufficiency in the setting of severe hypertension. Worsening of renal function after institution of an angiotensin-converting enzyme (ACE) inhibitor is also a common clue to the presence of bilateral renal artery stenosis.

The diagnosis can be made using functional or anatomic studies. Plasma renin activity can be measured, and, if low, essentially excludes the diagnosis. If renin activity is normal or high, documentation of an increase in activity after administration of an ACE inhibitor is

diagnostic. Nuclear renal scan performed before and after administration of ACE inhibitors also yields characteristic results. Ultrasonography may demonstrate a decreased size of the affected kidney. Definitive anatomic diagnosis is made by angiography, although advances in magnetic resonance angiography have made this a valuable noninvasive diagnostic technique. Treatment of renovascular hypertension involves eliminating the stenosis by surgical or percutaneous (balloon angioplasty) techniques.

ADRENAL CAUSES OF HYPERTENSION

Hyperaldosteronism

Primary hyperaldosteronism results from the autonomous production of aldosterone from the adrenal gland, independent of renin stimulation. It is a result of a unilateral adrenal adenoma (Conn's syndrome) in 54% of cases and bilateral adrenal hyperplasia in the majority of the rest. Hyperplasia is more common in men, and adenomas are more common in women. The increased aldosterone stimulates excessive renal sodium retention with resultant volume expansion and hypertension. The increased intravascular volume also augments renal perfusion, and renin secretion is thereby suppressed. Associated with the sodium retention is a loss of potassium and hydrogen ions, and, thus, these patients are hypokalemic and alkalotic. Patients are usually asymptomatic unless significant hypokalemia develops, in which case muscle cramps, palpitations, polyuria, and polydipsia are common.

This diagnosis should be considered in any patient with hypertension and either spontaneous hypokalemia or severe hypokalemia after treatment with diuretics. Measurement of plasma renin level is a useful screening test and should be low in patients with the disease. Urine aldosterone levels should be elevated, although a definitive diagnosis can be made by demonstrating an increased serum aldosterone level that does not suppress after saline-induced volume expansion. CT is useful in differentiating between adrenal adenomas and hyperplasia. This is an important distinction to make because it has important implications for therapy: patients with solitary adenomas are treated by resection of the tumor, which results in resolution of the hypertension approximately 50% of the time. Patients with adrenal hyperplasia are treated with the aldosterone antagonist spironolactone and, if necessary, additional diuretics.

Familial glucocorticoid-suppressible aldosteronism is an uncommon disorder causing hypertension in younger patients. It results from a mutation in the genes encoding for the enzymes aldosterone synthase and 11β-hydroxylase. This mutation places aldosterone synthesis under the control of adrenocorticotropic hormone (ACTH). The administration of dexamethasone suppresses ACTH and thereby ameliorates this syndrome by suppression of ACTH-induced aldosterone production. Most patients with Cushing's syndrome have hypertension, because of stimulation of mineralocorticoid receptors by the excess glucocorticoids. The diagnosis should be suspected in patients with truncal obesity,

TABLE 13–10   **Commonly Prescribed Oral Antihypertensive Medications**

Drug Class	Examples	Mechanism	Side Effects	Comments
Diuretics	Thiazide, furosemide	Inhibit tubular NaCl absorption	Hypokalemia, hyperuricemia, hyperglycemia	Thiazides ineffective when creatinine > 2.5 mg/dL
	Spironolactone	Aldosterone antagonist	Hyperkalemia, gynecomastia	Avoid with marked renal insufficiency
Adrenergic inhibitors				
Central α agonist	Clonidine, methyldopa	Decreases CNS sympathetic outflow	Drowsiness, fatigue, dry mouth, sexual dysfunction	Abruptly stopping clonidine may lead to rebound hypertension
Peripheral agents	Guanethidine, reserpine	Vasodilation	Orthostasis, sexual dysfunction	Use with caution in the elderly
β	Propranolol, atenolol, metoprolol	↓ Heart rate and contractility	Bradycardia, bronchospasm, fatigue, insomnia	Avoid in COPD, heart block
α₁	Prazocin, doxazocin, terazocin	Vasodilation	Orthostasis, "first-dose" hypotension, tachycardia	Tachyphylaxis to drug effect often noted
Combined α, β	Labetolol	↓ Heart rate and contractility; vasodilation	Bronchospasm, postural hypotension,	Avoid in COPD, heart block
Direct vasodilators	Hydralazine, minoxidil	Vasodilation	Tachycardia, fluid retention; lupus syndrome with hydralazine, hirsutism with minoxidil	Rarely first-line agents
Calcium channel blockers	Nifedipine, diltiazen, verapamil	Vasodilation	Tachycardia, fluid retention	Avoid in heart block, systolic failure
ACE inhibitors	Enalapril, captopril, fosinopril	Inhibits AII production	Angioedema, cough, hyperkalemia, rash	May worsen renal function, especially with RAS
Angiotensin receptor blockers	Losartan, valsartan	Inhibits binding of AII to its receptor	Hyperkalemia, rarely angioedema	May worsen renal function, especially with RAS

ACE = angiotensin-converting enzyme; AII = angiotensin II; CNS = central nervous system; COPD = chronic obstructive pulmonary disease; CRF = chronic renal failure; RAS = renal artery stenosis.

muscle weakness, and osteoporosis. The diagnosis can be confirmed by demonstrating an elevated urine cortisol level or an abnormal dexamethasone suppression test.

Pheochromocytoma

A pheochromocytoma is a rare catecholamine-producing tumor arising from the chromaffin cells of the neural crest. Approximately 85% of these tumors are located in the adrenal medulla, 10% of which are bilateral and 10% of which are malignant. The remaining 15% are extra-adrenal and may arise anywhere along the sympathetic chain. Multiple tumors are common in familial syndromes, especially the multiple endocrine neoplasia syndrome type 2, in which they occur in association with medullary carcinoma of the thyroid. Adrenal pheochromocytomas secrete predominantly epinephrine, resulting in mainly systolic hypertension caused by increased cardiac output, as well as tachycardia, hyperhidrosis, flushing, and apprehension. Extramedullary tumors secrete mainly norepinephrine, which produces systemic vasoconstriction, resulting in systolic and diastolic hypertension, but fewer associated symptoms. The secretion of catecholamines by these tumors is often episodic and results in wild fluctuations in blood pressure and sometimes dramatic paroxysms of adrenergic symptoms. Hypertensive crises and strokes may occur as a result of exceedingly high blood pressure.

The diagnosis is suggested by clinical symptoms. The complex of headaches, sweating episodes, and tachycardia in a hypertensive patient has a 91% sensitivity and 94% specificity. Laboratory confirmation of the diagnosis can be made by demonstrating elevated levels of serum or urine catecholamines or their metabolites (vanillylmandelic acid or metanephrines). The inability of clonidine to suppress the production of catecholamines in these patients also has diagnostic importance. Once diagnosed, the tumor can usually be localized by CT or MRI, although nuclear scanning with specific isotopes that localize to chromaffin tissue is occasionally needed to identify smaller tumors.

Treatment of these tumors is surgical resection. Patients must receive adequate β blockade, α blockade, and volume expansion before surgery to prevent the hemodynamic swings that can occur during manual manipulation of the tumor perioperatively. For unresectable tumors, chronic therapy with the α-adrenergic blocker phenoxybenzamine is usually effective.

TREATMENT OF HYPERTENSION

The goal of treating hypertension is to prevent the long-term morbidity and mortality associated with prolonged elevations in blood pressure. To this end, antihypertensive therapy should be instituted in patients with blood pressures in excess of 140/90 mm Hg. The method and aggressiveness of treatment depends on several factors, including the absolute level of blood pressure, the presence of end-organ damage, coexisting medical conditions, and overall cardiac risk.

In patients with mild or moderate hypertension without organ damage, it is reasonable to attempt a trial of nonpharmacologic therapy for 3 to 6 months. This therapy mainly consists of lifestyle modifications, including smoking cessation, weight reduction for overweight individuals, regular aerobic exercise, avoidance of alcohol, and restriction of dietary sodium intake (less than 6 g of sodium per day). These lifestyle changes may delay progression to sustained hypertension in patients with "high-normal" blood pressure, aid in control of established hypertension, decrease or eliminate the need for pharmacologic therapy, and reduce other cardiac risk factors. These measures should also be instituted in patients with more severe hypertension (>180/110 mm Hg), with multiple cardiac risk factors, or with evidence of end-organ damage; however, in these patients, pharmacologic therapy should be started concurrently.

Controlling hypertension with medications has clearly been shown to decrease cardiovascular morbidity and mortality, including the rate of stroke, myocardial infarction, heart failure, progressive renal disease, and all-cause mortality. Many antihypertensive agents are now available for the treatment of high blood pressure. The most commonly prescribed agents are listed in Table 13–10. The decision of which agent to use in a particular patient must take into account individual patient characteristics, comorbid conditions that may be affected by particular agents, possible interactions with other medications the patient is taking, as well as convenience of dosing and cost of therapy. Medications should be started at low doses and titrated to higher doses as needed. More than half of patients with mild to moderate hypertension can be controlled with a single antihypertensive medication. If the medication is ineffective at the maximal dose, a second agent should be added. In general, compliance is better with once daily medications.

The latest recommendation from the Joint National Committee on Detection, Evaluation, and Treatment of High Blood Pressure (JNC VI) is that β blockers and diuretics should remain the initial drugs of choice for the treatment of mild to moderate hypertension unless a contraindication to their use exists or there is a clear indication for another agent. This recommendation is based on randomized clinical trials that have demonstrated a decrease in morbidity and mortality with these

agents. A generalized approach to treatment of the hypertensive patient is shown in Figure 13–5.

The JNC does, however, recognize that certain medications have a real or theoretical advantage over β blockers or diuretics in certain situations or in certain populations (Table 13–11). An individualized approach to drug selection is, therefore, encouraged. For example, hypertension in African-Americans tends to respond better to treatment with diuretics or calcium channel blockers than with β blockers or ACE inhibitors. Patients with CAD should have their hypertension treated with β blockers, given the beneficial effects of these agents in this population. Similarly, patients with depressed left ventricular systolic function or overt heart failure are best managed with diuretics and ACE inhibitors. ACE inhibitors slow the progression of nephropathy in patients with diabetes and are the first-line agents in this setting. Sex and age do not appear to affect responsiveness to antihypertensives, although the start-

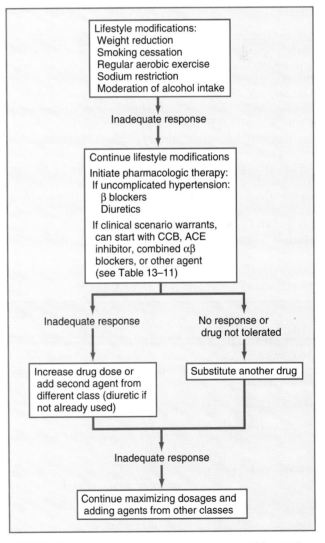

FIGURE 13–5 Hypertension treatment algorithm. ACE = angiotensin-converting enzyme inhibitor; CCB = calcium channel blocker.

TABLE 13–11 Preferred and/or Problematic Antihypertensive Agents in Selected Conditions

Condition	Preferred Drugs	Problematic Drugs
Diabetes	ACE inhibitors, CCB	β blockers, high-dose diuretics
Systolic heart failure	ACE inhibitors, diuretics	β blockers (except carvedilol), CCB (except amlodipine, felodipine)
Diastolic heart failure	ACE inhibitor, β blocker, CCB	Diuretics
Angina	β blockers, CCB	Short-acting dihydropyridine CCB (e.g., nifedipine)
Myocardial infarction	β blockers, ACE inhibitors (with systolic dysfunction)	Short-acting dihydropyridine CCB (e.g., nifedipine)
Pregnancy	Methyldopa; β blockers (in late pregnancy), hydralazine	ACE inhibitors, All receptor blockers
Obstructive lung disease	ACE inhibitors	β blockers, combined $\alpha\beta$ blockers
Renal insufficiency	Diuretics; ACE inhibitor (if creatinine <3 mg/dL)	ACE inhibitors, All receptor blockers, potassium-sparing agents

ACE = angiotensin-converting enzyme; CCB = calcium channel blocker; AII = angiotensin II.

ing dosages of medications should be lower in the elderly population. Antihypertensive medications may aggravate certain coexisting medical conditions and must be used with caution in specific settings. For instance, β blockers may induce bronchospasm in patients with lung disease, ACE inhibitors and diuretics may worsen renal insufficiency, and β blockers and calcium channel blockers may acutely worsen heart failure or conduction system disease.

Severe hypertension requires more aggressive therapy to prevent or limit organ damage. Hypertensive urgencies, without evidence of new or progressive end-organ damage, can usually be treated with oral doses of relatively fast-acting medications (e.g., β blockers, calcium channel blockers, or ACE inhibitors) with the aim of decreasing the blood pressure over the course of several hours to several days. Hypertensive emergencies require intravenous medications (e.g., nitroprusside, labetalol) to decrease the pressure over several minutes to an hour (Table 13–12). Such therapy should be given in an intensive care setting with close monitoring of the blood pressure and end-organ function. A precipitous drop in the blood pressure should be avoided because this may precipitate or exacerbate cerebral, renal, or myocardial ischemia. Establishing normal blood pressure is not the initial aim. A reasonable goal is to decrease the mean arterial pressure by 25% in the first 6 hours and then to levels less than 160/100 mm Hg over the next 6 hours. Once the pressure is adequately controlled, oral medications should be initiated and intravenous medications

TABLE 13–12 Parenteral Drugs for Hypertensive Emergencies

Drug	Advantages	Clinical Indications	Side Effects
Vasodilators			
Nitroprusside	Rapid onset, allows effective titration, no sedation	Most hypertensive emergencies	Thiocyanate toxicity with prolonged use; nausea
Nitroglycerin	Rapid onset	Hypertension with myocardial ischemia	Headache; tolerance with prolonged use
Enalaprilat	Longer duration of action	Hypertension with acute heart failure	Hyperkalemia; acute renal insufficiency
Hydralazine	Intramuscular preparation available	Eclampsia	Reflex tachycardia, angina
Adrenergic Inhibitors			
Labetolol	Prolonged duration of action	Most hypertensive emergencies except acute heart failure	Bronchspasm; bradyarrhythmias, worsened heart failure; vomiting
Esmolol	Short duration of action	Aortic dissection; perioperative	Hypotension; bronchospasm; bradyarrhythmias, worsened heart failure;
Phentolamine	Effective α blockade	Pheochromocytoma	Tachycardia; flushing; headache

weaned. The blood pressure can then be brought to ideal levels with titration of oral therapy.

REFERENCES

Calhoun A, Oparil S: Treatment of hypertensive crisis. N Engl J Med 1990; 323:1177.

Cigarroa JE, Isselbacher EM, DeSanctis RW, Eagle KA: Diagnostic imaging in the evaluation of suspected aortic dissection. N Engl J Med 1993; 328:35.

Dustan HP: Renal artery disease and hypertension. Med Clin North Am 1997; 81:1199.

Ginsberg JS: Drug therapy: Management of venous thromboembolism. N Engl J Med 1996; 335:1816.

Goldhaber SZ: Pulmonary embolism. N Engl J Med 1998; 339:93.

Joint National Committee on Prevention, Detection, Evaluation, and Treatment of High Blood Pressure: The sixth report of the Joint National Committee on Prevention, Detection, Evaluation, and Treatment of High Blood Pressure. Arch Intern Med 1997; 157: 2413.

Kouchoukos NT, Dougenis D: Surgery of the thoracic aorta. N Engl J Med 1997; 336:1876–1888.

Rubin LJ: Primary pulmonary hypertension. N Engl J Med 1997; 336: 111.

Werbel SS, Ober KP: Pheochromocytoma: Update on diagnosis, localization and management. Med Clin North Am 1995; 79:131.

SECTION IV

Pulmonary and Critical Care Medicine

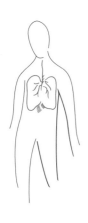

14

APPROACH TO THE PATIENT WITH RESPIRATORY DISEASE

Bonnie S. Slovis • Kenneth L. Brigham

Patients with respiratory disease present with various complaints that may be specific for their lung disease or may reflect diseases of other organ systems. For example, the most common symptoms of respiratory disease are dyspnea and cough. However, dyspnea is also a cardinal symptom of heart disease, and cough may be caused by gastroesophageal reflux or chronic sinusitis. An organized approach to the patient that starts with a careful history and a detailed physical examination focuses further diagnostic studies on the appropriate organ. Subsequent diagnostic testing and imaging, as indicated, usually lead to the correct diagnosis.

Common Presenting Complaints

Dyspnea (shortness of breath) is a common complaint of patients with pulmonary disease. Timing and acuity of onset, exacerbating and alleviating factors, and degree of functional impairment are key elements of the history. Associated symptoms such as cough, hemoptysis, chest pain, wheezing, orthopnea, and paroxysmal nocturnal dyspnea, as well as environmental triggers, should be elicited and are helpful in developing a differential diagnosis. If dyspnea is recent, of sudden onset, and accompanied by chest pain, diseases such as pneumothorax, pulmonary embolism, and pulmonary edema should come to mind. If the dyspnea is long-standing and is slowly progressive, chronic conditions such as chronic obstructive pulmonary disease, pulmonary fibrosis, and neuromuscular disease are in the differential diagnosis. In patients with chronic dyspnea, progression of the condition may be insidious and difficult to assess quanti-

tatively. Clinicians should ask patients how far they can walk on level ground without stopping, whether they can climb a flight of stairs without stopping, and what activities they did 1 year ago that they are unable to do now.

Dyspnea may be exertional or resting and episodic or continuous. Episodic dyspnea may have identified triggers, such as exertion, that suggest parenchymal lung disease or cardiac dysfunction, or it may be associated with environmental exposure, a feature that suggests asthma or hypersensitivity pneumonitis. Positional dyspnea is a useful symptom. Patients with severe obstructive lung disease, diaphragmatic paralysis, or neuromuscular weakness may have dyspnea immediately on lying down (orthopnea), because vital capacity is reduced when these patients are in the supine position. Paroxysmal nocturnal dyspnea is commonly associated with congestive heart failure. Paroxysmal nocturnal dyspnea occurs several hours after lying down because increased venous return to the heart results in mild pulmonary edema. Asthma also causes nocturnal dyspnea, in part because adrenal cortisol secretion is lowest at about 4:00 a.m. Exercise-induced asthma causes dyspnea out of proportion to the degree of exercise, with dyspnea often most severe in the 15 to 30 minutes after cessation of exercise. The absence of wheezing does not rule out asthma in any setting, and the presence of wheezing does not establish the diagnosis (i.e., asthma does not always cause wheezing, and not all patients who wheeze have asthma).

Cough is an often frustrating symptom for both the patient and the physician. The three most common causes of chronic cough are asthma, postnasal drip, and gastroesophageal reflux disease. Smokers with chronic cough may not volunteer the symptom because they believe that it is normal to cough and are unaware of the frequency and chronicity of their cough. Cough may be mild and infrequent, or it may be severe enough to induce emesis or syncope. Patients may have a dry cough or may produce sputum or blood (*hemoptysis*). A common cause of a dry, hacking cough is the use of angiotensin-converting enzyme inhibitors. The symptom may begin months or longer after initiation of the drug. Cough is much less common in patients taking angiotensin II receptor antagonists. *Bordetella pertussis* infection (whooping cough) and viral lower respiratory infections can produce a cough that may last for 3 months or longer. Patients with asthma often have cough, and on occasion it is their only symptom, a condition sometimes referred to as *cough-variant asthma*. Nocturnal cough should raise the suspicion of asthma or gastroesophageal reflux disease.

Sputum production is abnormal and should be characterized by quantity, color, presence or absence of blood, and timing. The physician should ask the patient to estimate the amount of sputum produced in 24 hours and should suggest ranges such as teaspoons, tablespoons, and fractions of a cup, because patients are often not accustomed to thinking in quantitative terms. *Chronic bronchitis* is defined as a persistent cough resulting in sputum production for more than 3 months in each of the last 3 years. Patients with chronic bronchitis usually produce more sputum in the morning, whereas patients with chronic aspiration may cough more after eating or drinking. Patients with asthma often have a productive cough resulting from excess mucus production. Yellow or gray sputum may indicate a bacterial infection but not necessarily because the color is a result of cellular debris, predominantly white cells, present in any inflammatory process. Patients with asthma who describe sputum with brown plugs or casts of the small bronchi may have allergic bronchopulmonary aspergillosis.

Hemoptysis is a frightening symptom. The volume of blood may be scant or heavy enough that its effects may be life-threatening. The most common cause of hemoptysis in the United States is chronic bronchitis, but worldwide the most common cause is pulmonary tuberculosis, and the incidence of tuberculosis is increasing throughout the world. Most cases of hemoptysis are small in volume and are self-limited with treatment of the underlying process. Massive hemoptysis, defined as more than 500 mL of blood in 24 hours, is rare, but when it occurs it is a medical emergency because it may be fatal. When patients with massive hemoptysis die, it is usually of asphyxiation rather than exsanguination. Causes of massive hemoptysis include lung cancer, lung cavities containing mycetomas, cavitary tuberculosis, pulmonary hemorrhage syndromes, pulmonary arteriovenous malformations, and bronchiectasis. The physician should distinguish among hemoptysis, epistaxis, and hematemesis. Because many patients have trouble identifying the source of the bleeding, a careful upper airway physical examination is essential.

Chest pain attributable to the lungs usually results from pleural disease, pulmonary vascular disease, or musculoskeletal pain precipitated by coughing because the lung parenchyma has no pain fibers. Lung cancer, for example, does not cause pain until it invades the pleura, chest wall, vertebral bodies, or mediastinal structures. Disease or inflammation of the pleura causes pleuritic chest pain (hence the term) characterized as a sharp or stabbing pain on deep inspiration that occasionally can be positional. Pain from pulmonary emboli, infection, pneumothoraces, and collagen vascular disease is usually pleuritic. Patients with pulmonary hypertension often complain of dull anterior chest pain unrelated to respiration that may be caused by right ventricular strain and demand ischemia. Other noncardiac causes of chest pain include esophageal disease, herpetic neuralgia, and trauma. Many elderly patients or those with a history of systemic steroid use have thoracic pain resulting from vertebral compression or rib fractures. Adequate analgesia, including narcotics, is essential in the treatment of chest pain in patients with underlying lung disease, to prevent the reduction in vital capacity caused by splinting of the chest in reaction to the pain. Musculoskeletal chest pain should be a diagnosis of exclusion after one has ruled out serious causes. The pain is usually reproducible with palpation over the affected area.

An accurate history of tobacco use as well as other toxic and environmental exposures is essential in patients with respiratory complaints. Tobacco smoke is the most prevalent environmental toxin seen in lung disease. Patients may be anxious about other inhaled toxins or irritants and yet may continue to smoke without concern. It is the physician's duty to ask about tobacco use and to attempt to motivate the patient to quit smoking (most smokers report that no physician has ever told them that they should quit smoking). The patient's history of cigarette smoking is quantified as the number of packs smoked per day times the cumulative number of years of smoking (i.e., pack-years). The risk of lung disease in susceptible persons is related directly to total pack-years of exposure and inversely to the age at onset of smoking and, in the case of lung cancer, the interval since smoking cessation.

A history of exposure to other inhaled toxins, irritants, or allergens should be elicited. A careful occupational history often uncovers exposure to inorganic dust or fibers such as asbestos, silica, or coal dust. Organic dusts may cause hypersensitivity pneumonitis and interstitial lung disease. Solvents and corrosive gases are also causes of pulmonary symptoms. The presence of household pets should be documented. Cats are the most allergenic for asthma, and birds may cause hypersensitivity or fungal lung disease. A travel history is important in evaluating infectious causes of pulmonary disease. For example, histoplasmosis is common in the Ohio and Mississippi River valleys, and coccidioidomycosis is found in the desert Southwest. Travel to developing countries increases the risk of exposure to tuberculosis. A family history is important in assessing the risk of genetic lung diseases such as cystic fibrosis and α_1-antitrypsin deficiency as well as the susceptibility to asthma or lung cancer.

Physical Examination

The first steps in the physical examination of the patient with pulmonary disease are observation and inspection, which must be done when the patient's chest is bare. The physician should watch the patient breathe and should note the effort required for breathing. An increased respiratory rate, use of accessory muscles of respiration, pursed-lip breathing, and paradoxical abdominal movement all indicate increased work of breathing. The patient's inability to speak in full sentences indicates severe airway obstruction. The physician should listen for cough and should note the strength of the cough, because this may signal respiratory muscle weakness or severe obstructive lung disease. The patient's rib cage should expand symmetrically with inspiration. The shape of the thoracic cage should be noted. Increased anteroposterior diameter is seen in obstructive lung disease. Severe kyphoscoliosis, pectus excavatum, ankylosing spondylitis, and morbid obesity all can produce restrictive ventilatory disease as a consequence of distortion and restriction of the volume of the thoracic cavity.

Palpation of the chest is performed by first palpating the accessory muscles of respiration in the patient's neck: the scalene and sternocleidomastoid muscles. Hypertrophy and contraction indicate increased respiratory effort. The trachea should be palpated and should lie in the midline of the neck. Deviation of the trachea suggests a unilateral process. Neck masses should be noted. The physician should place both hands on the lower half of the patient's posterior thorax with thumbs touching and fingers spread and should keep the hands in place while the patient takes several deep inspirations. The physician's thumbs should separate slightly and the hands should move symmetrically apart during the patient's inspiration. *Fremitus* is a faint vibration felt best with the edge of the hand against the patient's chest wall while the patient speaks. Fremitus is increased in patients with underlying consolidation, and it is decreased over a pleural effusion. Next, the patient's chest should be percussed. The level of the diaphragms on each side should be noted, and then the percussion note should be compared on the two sides starting at the apex and moving down, including posterior, anterior, and lateral aspects. Dullness to percussion can be caused by a pleural effusion, consolidation, a mass or an elevated diaphragm; hyperresonance can be caused by a pneumothorax or by hyperinflation.

Auscultation of the lung is performed to evaluate the quality of the breath sounds and to detect the presence of extra (adventitious) sounds not heard in normal lungs. Normal breath sounds have two qualities, vesicular and bronchial. Bronchial breath sounds are heard over the central airways and are louder and coarser than vesicular breath sounds, which are heard at the periphery and the base of the lungs. Bronchovesicular sounds are a combination of the two and are heard over medium-sized airways. Bronchial sounds have a longer inhaled component, and vesicular sounds a much longer expiratory component and are much softer. Bronchial breath sounds and bronchovesicular breath sounds at the periphery of the lungs are abnormal and may be caused by underlying consolidation. In the presence of consolidation, the patient has increased transmission of vocal sounds, called *whispered pectoriloquy*, as well as *egophony*, in which the spoken letter "e" sounds like an "a" over the area of consolidation (and is sometimes compared to the bleating of a goat).

Abnormal or extra pulmonary sounds are crackles, wheezes, and rubs. Crackles can be coarse rattles called *rhonchi* or fine, Velcro-like sounds, sometimes called *rales.* Coarse crackles are often caused by mucus in the airways or by the opening of large and medium-sized airways. Fine crackles, produced on inspiration by the opening of collapsed alveoli, are most common at the bases and are heard in pulmonary edema and interstitial fibrosis, as well as in healthy elderly patients during deep inspiration. *Wheezing* is a higher-pitched sound and when heard locally suggests large airway obstruction. The wheezing of patients with asthma or congestive heart failure is lower in pitch and is heard diffusely over all lung fields. Localized wheezing can also be heard in conditions such as pulmonary embolism, obstruction of a bronchus by a tumor, and foreign body aspiration. A *rub* is a pleural sound caused by inflamed pleural surfaces rubbing together. It has been described as the sound of pieces of leather rubbing against each other. Rubs are often evanescent and depend on the amount of fluid in the pleural space. Often, pleuritic chest pain and a rub develop after large-volume thoracentesis. A crunching sound timed with the cardiac cy-

TABLE 14–1   Physical Examination of the Chest

Inspection

Observation: anxiety, distress, malnutrition, somnolence
Chest wall shape, deformity
Respiratory rate, depth, pattern
Paradoxical respiratory motion of chest and abdomen
Retractions
Use of accessory muscles
Pursed-lip breathing
Cyanosis

Palpation

Tracheal deviation
Chest expansion
Vocal fremitus
Lymphadenopathy
Subcutaneous emphysema

Percussion

Normal, dull, or hyperresonant

Auscultation

Breath sounds: normal vesicular over periphery and
    bronchial centrally
Pleural rub
Added sounds: wheezes, crackles
Stridor

TABLE 14–2 Physical Findings in Common Pulmonary Disorders

Disorder	Mediastinal Displacement	Chest Wall Movement	Vocal Fremitus	Percussion Note	Breath Sounds	Added Sounds	Voice Sounds
Pleural effusion	Heart displaced to opposite side	Reduced over affected area	Absent or markedly decreased	Dull	Absent over fluid; bronchial at upper border	Absent; pleural rub may be found above effusion	Absent over effusion; increased with egophony at upper border
Consolidation	None	Reduced over affected area	Increased or normal	Dull	Bronchial	Crackles	Increased with egobronchophony and whispered pectoriloquy
Pneumothorax	Tracheal deviation to opposite side if under tension	Decreased over affected area	Absent	Resonant	Absent or decreased	Absent	Absent
Atelectasis	Ipsilateral shift	Decreased over affected area	Variable	Dull	Absent or diminished	Crackles may be heard	Absent
Bronchospasm	None	Decreased symmetrically	Normal or decreased	Normal or decreased	Bronchovesicular	Wheeze	Normal or decreased
Interstitial fibrosis	None	Decreased symmetrically	Normal or increased	Normal	Bronchovesicular	End-inspiratory crackles unaffected by cough or posture	Normal

cle, called *Hamman's crunch,* is heard in patients with a pneumomediastinum. The complete absence of breath sounds on one side should cause the examiner to think of pneumothorax, hydrothorax, or hemothorax, obstruction of a mainstem bronchus, or surgical or congenital absence of the lung. The elements of the complete physical examination of the chest are included in Table 14–1. The physical findings associated with various pulmonary disorders are outlined in Table 14–2.

REFERENCES

MacNee W: Pathophysiology of cor pulmonale in chronic obstructive pulmonary disease: Part one. Am J Respir Crit Care Med 1994; 150: 833–852.

MacNee W: Pathophysiology of cor pulmonale in chronic obstructive pulmonary disease: Part two. Am J Respir Crit Care Med 1994; 150: 1158–1168.

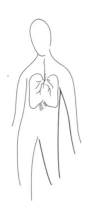

15

ANATOMIC AND PHYSIOLOGIC CONSIDERATIONS

Bonnie S. Slovis • Kenneth L. Brigham

The primary function of the lungs is gas exchange. The entire cardiac output goes through the lungs, where carbon dioxide is removed from blood and oxygen is absorbed. Gas exchange requires adequate cardiac output, alveolar ventilation, alveolar-capillary surface area, and regional matching of blood flow to ventilation. In the normal lung, alveolar-capillary surface can expand from 50 to 100 m² with the recruitment of closed capillaries and alveoli. Lung disease can compromise ventilation, pulmonary blood flow, or alveolar-capillary surface area and usually compromises the ability of the lung to match pulmonary blood flow with ventilation. All of these changes result in compromise of the lungs' ability to meet the body's demand for gas exchange.

Anatomy

THE AIRWAY

Inspired air travels through the nose and pharynx, where it is heated, humidified, and filtered of particles greater than 10 μm in diameter and soluble gases are removed. Entrance to the trachea is through the larynx, which is open during ventilation and closed and covered by the epiglottis during swallowing and Valsalva maneuvers.

The trachea, which is 10 to 12 mm in diameter, is held open by anterior, U-shaped, incomplete, cartilage rings. The trachea divides into the two mainstem bronchi at the level of the sternomanubrial junction. The right mainstem bronchus takes off at a less acute angle than the left, and therefore foreign bodies are more commonly aspirated into the right lung. The large airways, which are supported by circumferential cartilage rings, continue to branch with the cartilage disappearing in the smaller airways. These bronchial branches are

conducting airways and do not participate in gas exchange. At about the eighteenth branch the airways become respiratory bronchioles and contain increasing numbers of alveolar sacs. They continue to branch, becoming alveolar ducts, which ultimately terminate in alveoli (Fig. 15–1). Gas exchange takes place in the branches from the respiratory bronchioles to the alveoli, called the respiratory zone. After the tenth branch, the total cross-sectional area of the airways increases rapidly and resistance to air flow decreases. Air flow is laminar proximal to the respiratory zone, where turbulent flow begins and diffusion becomes the dominant mechanism of gas movement. The alveolar lining cells are predominantly flat, type I pneumocytes, which rest on a very thin basement membrane and allow rapid diffusion of gases to and from the adjacent capillary blood. Type II pneumocytes, about 5% of the alveolar lining cells, are round and secrete surfactant, a complex lipid-protein substance that coats the alveolar surface and decreases surface tension, thus stabilizing alveoli against collapse at low volumes. Type II cells are capable of regeneration and repair and are also the precursors of type I cells.

THE BLOOD VESSELS

The lungs have a dual circulation. The bronchial circulation originates from the aorta and, under systemic pressure, supplies nutrient flow to lung structures proximal to alveoli. One third of the venous outflow from the bronchial circulation returns through bronchial veins to the right side of the heart, similar to other organs perfused by systemic blood. The remainder of the bronchial circulation drains into the pulmonary veins, which empty into the left atrium, forming part of the normal anatomic right-to-left shunt.

The pulmonary circulation receives the entire output of the right cardiac ventricle, but it is a low resistance

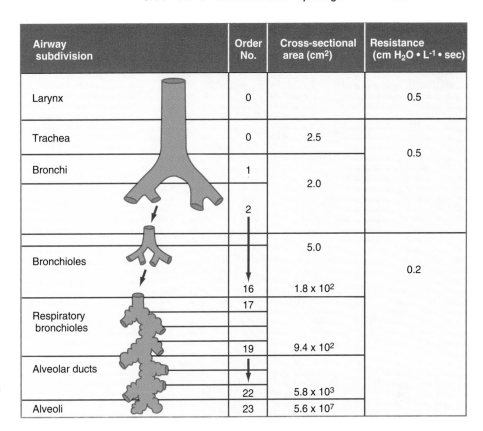

Airway subdivision	Order No.	Cross-sectional area (cm²)	Resistance (cm H₂O • L⁻¹ • sec)
Larynx	0		0.5
Trachea	0	2.5	
Bronchi	1	2.0	0.5
	2		
Bronchioles		5.0	
	16	1.8×10^2	0.2
Respiratory bronchioles	17		
	19	9.4×10^2	
Alveolar ducts			
	22	5.8×10^3	
Alveoli	23	5.6×10^7	

FIGURE 15–1 The subdivision of the airways and their nomenclature. The cross-sectional area increases dramatically toward the peripheral, small airways. (Adapted from Weibel ER: Morphometry of the Human Lung. Berlin: Springer, 1963.)

circuit (pulmonary artery pressure and pulmonary vascular resistance are about one tenth those of the systemic circulation). Pulmonary arteries are thin walled and have much less smooth muscle than systemic arteries. They accompany the bronchial tree to supply bronchopulmonary segments. At the level of the alveolar ducts the pulmonary arterioles terminate in a meshwork of capillaries, which form a sheet of blood surrounding the alveoli and create the large surface area necessary for gas exchange. Blood returns to the heart through pulmonary veins that course between lung lobules, coalesce into four main pulmonary veins, and empty into the left atrium.

Physiology

VENTILATION

Ventilation is the movement of air in and out of the lungs. The volume of air in the lungs is determined by the balance between the outward elastic force of the thoracic cage and the inward elastic recoil of the lungs. During inspiration, active contraction of the respiratory muscles increases intrathoracic volume and creates subatmospheric pressure in the pleural space and alveoli. Air enters the lung down the pressure gradient between atmospheric and intrathoracic pressure. Exhalation is passive in normal lungs and begins when inspiratory muscles relax; and then the intrinsic elastic recoil passively returns the lungs to their resting volume, where

alveolar pressure and ambient pressure are equal. With active contraction of expiratory muscles, alveolar pressure can be increased above ambient pressure, emptying additional volume from the lung. In disease states such as emphysema, when the elastic recoil of the lung is greatly diminished, active contraction of the expiratory muscles is required to empty enough air from the lungs to permit ventilation.

The primary respiratory muscle is the diaphragm. The so-called "accessory muscles of respiration"—the intercostal, sternocleidomastoid, scalene, and abdominal muscles—normally contribute little. At rest the diaphragm is dome shaped, curving into the thoracic cavity. During contraction it flattens, increasing the thoracic volume and distending the abdominal wall. If the lungs are hyperinflated because of trapped gas from emphysema or asthma (obstructive lung diseases), the diaphragm is flat or inverted at end expiration and its contraction will not produce an appreciable change in thoracic volume. In this situation the accessory muscles of respiration, the scalenes and sternocleidomastoids, contract and elevate the anterior chest wall. Although this increases intrathoracic volume, the increase is much less than that produced by the normal diaphragm so that effects on air movement are also much reduced. In addition to recruitment of accessory muscles during inspiration, with obstructive lung diseases expiration requires contraction of the abdominal muscles to exert pressure on the flattened diaphragm, which in turn increases intrathoracic pressure to force exhalation.

Respiratory muscles must overcome both elastic and resistive forces. The opposing elastic forces of the chest wall (outward force) and lungs (inward force) determine the resting lung volume at end passive expiration, which is called the functional residual capacity (FRC). The FRC should be less than 50% of the total amount of air that the lung can contain (total lung capacity [TLC]). Elasticity is usually measured as its inverse function, compliance. Compliance is the change in lung volume produced by a given change in transpulmonary pressure. In normal lungs at FRC, it takes about 1 cm H_2O pressure to inflate the lungs 200 mL. Compliance then would be 200 mL/cm H_2O. Compliance decreases in normal lungs as lung volume increases toward TLC. Compliance is decreased in diseases such as pulmonary fibrosis or pulmonary edema, which restrict lung volume expansion, and may be increased in emphysema because of the loss of elastic recoil (Fig. 15–2). When compliance is decreased, the work of breathing is increased, because of the increased pressure required to inflate the lungs. In diseases such as emphysema in which compliance is increased, the work of breathing is increased during inspiration as a result of the loss of mechanical advantage from hyperinflation and flattened diaphragms. It is also increased during expiration, because decreased lung elastic recoil requires active muscle contraction to empty the lungs in preparation for the next breath. In patients with severe lung disease, the work of breathing may be a major contributor to the resting metabolic rate. In extreme cases, this increase in energy expenditure can result in pulmonary cachexia. In people with

normal lungs, work of breathing uses only 4% to 5% of the total calories burned, but in severe lung disease up to 30% of the total-body oxygen consumption can be consumed by the work of breathing. Under these extreme circumstances, minute ventilation may decrease and arterial carbon dioxide ($PaCO_2$) increase as a homeostatic response of the body to decrease the energy cost of breathing.

Airway resistance (the ratio of transpulmonary pressure to air flow rate) is inversely related to the total cross-sectional area of the airways. Normal resistance is in the range of 1 to 2 cm H_2O/L/sec. Although the peripheral airways are narrow, their total cross-sectional area is large so that resistance to air flow at that level of the tracheobronchial tree is low. Airway resistance decreases as lung volume increases because of the tethering of airway walls to lung tissue, resulting in an increase in airway diameter as lung volume increases. Causes of increased airway resistance include airway obstruction resulting from an intrinsic or extrinsic mass or mucus plugging; airway smooth muscle contraction (bronchospasm); and the dynamic compression of a forced exhalation.

Because of the anatomy of the airways, not all air entering the lungs is in contact with gas-exchanging units. The portion of an inhaled breath that fills the respiratory zone is the alveolar volume (VA), and the portion remaining in the conducting airways is the dead space volume (VD). At end expiration, VD contains exhaled alveolar gas that has equilibrated with pulmonary capillary blood; thus, on the next breath the amount of fresh air reaching the alveoli is the VA minus the VD. The sum of alveolar and dead space ventilation with quiet breathing is the tidal volume (VT). The proportion of the VT that is VD varies with the tidal volume (although VD increases with larger inspirations because of traction on the bronchi, the increase is less than the increase in VA). Slow, deep breaths result in greater alveolar volume and therefore greater gas exchange than rapid shallow breaths at the same minute ventilation. Dead space in the seated position with quiet respiration is approximately 1 mL per pound of ideal body weight.

The distribution of ventilation in the lungs is unequal, with greater ventilation in the base and less at the apex in the upright position. The same is true for lung perfusion. This matching of ventilation and perfusion optimizes gas exchange. Ventilation is higher at the lung bases primarily because of greater negative pleural pressure at the apices, resulting in larger apical volumes at end expiration. During inspiration, the higher compliance of the lung at low volumes results in more air going to the bases.

CONTROL OF VENTILATION

Ventilation is the primary short-term homeostatic mechanism for maintaining normal blood pH. This is accomplished through elimination (increases pH) or retention (decreases pH) of CO_2. The PCO_2 in blood is inversely proportional to the minute ventilation and is the strongest factor controlling ventilation. The second strongest

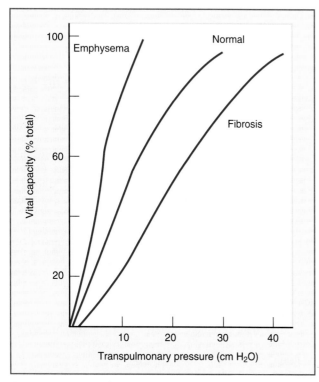

FIGURE 15–2 Compliance curves for normal subjects and patients with emphysema and pulmonary fibrosis. An elevation in the transpulmonary pressure required to achieve a given lung volume increases the work of breathing.

drive to ventilation is hypoxia. Maintaining pH and adequate oxygenation is accomplished through the respiratory control system, which consists of neurologic respiratory control centers, respiratory sensors, and respiratory effectors.

Respiratory Control Centers. Neuronal control of autonomic respiration resides in the brain stem, primarily the medullary reticular formation. The medulla receives input from the pons, which may modify or fine tune the rhythm of breathing. Voluntary ventilation originates in the cerebral cortex and can override autonomic ventilatory control.

Respiratory Effectors. The muscles of respiration include the diaphragm and accessory muscles, as previously discussed. For effective ventilation, these muscles must be coordinated by the respiratory control center through the phrenic, intercostal, cranial, and cervical nerves.

Respiratory Sensors. There are two types of respiratory receptors: chemoreceptors and mechanoreceptors. There are central and peripheral chemoreceptors, which detect changes in pH, P_{CO_2}, and P_{O_2}. Central chemoreceptors located in the medulla respond rapidly to changes in hydrogen ion concentration and P_{CO_2}. by stimulating or inhibiting ventilation to maintain blood pH within normal range. The peripheral chemoreceptors also respond to hydrogen ion concentration and Pa_{CO_2} but are most sensitive to changes in Pa_{O_2}. In contrast to the linear response of ventilation to Pa_{CO_2}, the response to changes in Pa_{O_2} are minimal until the Pa_{O_2} drops below 60 mm Hg. Below that level there is a steep relationship between Pa_{O_2} and ventilation, as illustrated in Figure 15–3. The Pa_{O_2} versus ventilation curve is a mirror image of the oxygen dissociation curve for hemoglobin. The lack of a significant ventilatory response to Pa_{O_2} above 60 mm Hg makes sense because changes in ventilation have very little impact on Pa_{O_2} unless the alveolar P_{CO_2} is elevated and levels of Pa_{O_2} above 60 mm Hg have minimal impact on total oxygen content of the blood.

Mechanoreceptors in the chest wall and airways modulate rate and depth of breathing in response to stretch. J receptors located in juxtacapillary regions in the lung periphery stimulate ventilation in response to pulmonary vascular engorgement. There are also airway irritant receptors that respond to physical and chemical stimuli.

PERFUSION

The pulmonary vascular bed receives the entire cardiac output from the right ventricle. The distribution of blood flow is not uniform throughout the lung and is dependent on several factors. Because the pulmonary circulation is a low pressure system it is affected by gravity, with the greatest blood flow going to the dependent portions of the lungs. The hydrostatic pressure increases from the top to the bottom of the lungs. Alveolar pressure, assuming open airways, is relatively constant throughout the lung. It is the relationship between

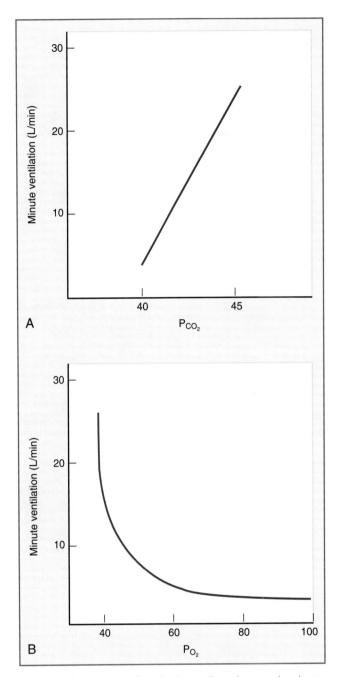

FIGURE 15–3 A rising P_{CO_2} leads to a linear increase in minute ventilation *(A)*. The ventilatory response to hypoxemia *(B)* is less sensitive and is clinically relevant only when the P_{O_2} has dropped significantly.

alveolar and pulmonary vascular pressure that largely determines blood flow in the normal lung.

In 1964, West devised a model of blood flow within the lungs that divides the lung into three zones, determined by the relationship between pulmonary vascular and alveolar pressures (Fig. 15–4). Zone 1 is defined as an area of the lungs in which alveolar pressure exceeds pulmonary artery pressure, thus inhibiting perfusion. Zone 1 conditions tend to occur in the most superior portions of the lungs in situations such as shock, in

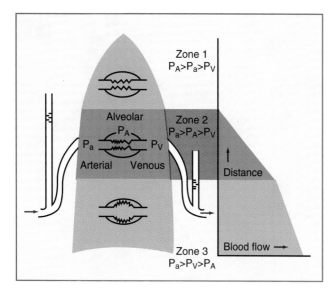

FIGURE 15–4   Zonal model of blood flow in the lung. Because of the interrelationship of vascular and alveolar pressures, the lung base receives the most flow (see text for explanation). (From West JB, Dollery CT, Naimark A: Distribution of blood flow in isolated lung: Relation to vascular and alveolar pressures. J Appl Physiol 1964; 19:713.)

which pulmonary artery pressure falls below alveolar pressure, or with positive pressure ventilation, in which the alveolar pressure rises above pulmonary artery pressure. This ventilated but unperfused area of the lung is called alveolar dead space and, depending on size, can markedly increase the minute ventilation required to remove CO_2 from the blood. Zone 2 conditions exist when pulmonary arterial pressure is higher than alveolar pressure but alveolar pressure is higher than pulmonary venous pressure. In zone 2, the hydrostatic pressure driving blood flow is the difference between pulmonary artery pressure and alveolar pressure. In zone 3, pulmonary venous pressure exceeds alveolar pressure and blood flow is determined by the arterial-venous pressure difference.

In states of increased oxygen demand, cardiac output rises but pulmonary vascular resistance actually falls because recruitment of previously unperfused vessels increases total vascular cross-sectional area. This allows blood flow to increase dramatically with relatively small increases in pulmonary artery pressure. The relationship between lung volume and pulmonary vascular resistance is complex. At low volumes, vascular resistance decreases with increasing volume, because of tethering of vessels to lung tissue; but at high lung volumes, resistance rises again, because of compression of capillaries by increasing alveolar volume.

Alveolar hypoxia causes local constriction of arterioles supplying the hypoxic area (hypoxic pulmonary vasoconstriction), which decreases blood flow to areas of low ventilation and thus helps to maintain ventilation-perfusion ($\dot{V}/\dot{Q}$) matching in a heterogeneously ventilated lung. In the case of generalized alveolar hypoxia, such as at altitude, global vasoconstriction results in pulmonary hypertension and can result in high altitude pulmonary

edema. Acidosis and increased sympathetic tone also cause lesser degrees of vasoconstriction, whereas mediators produced in the pulmonary vascular bed (e.g., nitric oxide and prostacyclin) can cause local vasodilation.

GAS TRANSFER

Oxygen and carbon dioxide are easily dissolved in plasma. Other atmospheric gases are much less soluble

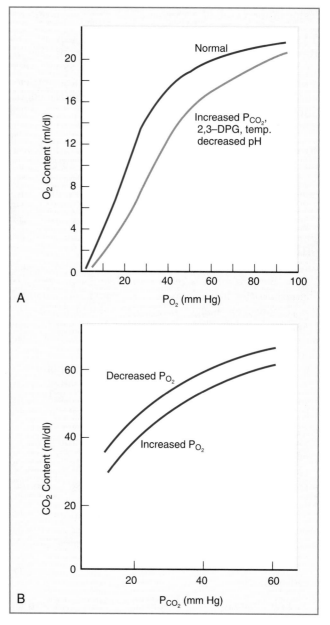

FIGURE 15–5   A, The oxyhemoglobin dissociation curve. The bulk of the O_2 is carried combined with hemoglobin. The various factors that decrease the hemoglobin O_2 affinity are shown. Opposite changes increase hemoglobin O_2 affinity, shifting the curve to the left. B, The CO_2 dissociation curve. It is more linear than the oxyhemoglobin curve throughout the physiologic range. Increased P_{O_2} shifts the curve to the right, which decreases CO_2 content for any given P_{CO_2} and thus facilitates CO_2 off-loading in the lungs. The shift to the left at a lower P_{O_2} facilitates CO_2 on-loading at the tissues. DPG = diphosphoglycerate.

and are not significantly exchanged across the alveolar-capillary interface. The solubility of O_2 and CO_2 allows complete equilibration between alveolar and plasma concentrations during each respiratory cycle. The majority of O_2 contained in the blood is bound to hemoglobin, with the remainder dissolved in plasma and creating the PaO_2. Each molecule of hemoglobin is capable of carrying four molecules of oxygen. Under normal conditions, at a PaO_2 of 150 mm Hg, hemoglobin is completely saturated, and further increases in PaO_2 have little effect on the oxygen content of blood. The oxygen-hemoglobin dissociation curve is a graph of the relationship between PaO_2 and hemoglobin saturation. Its shape reflects the cooperative binding of oxygen to hemoglobin (Fig. 15–5). Decreased blood pH, increased temperature, increased 2,3-diphosphoglycerate, and increased $PaCO_2$ all act to decrease the affinity of hemoglobin for oxygen, which facilitates unloading of oxygen into tissues. Carbon monoxide binds hemoglobin with 240 times greater affinity than does oxygen at the same sites and also induces cooperative binding. Binding of hemoglobin by carbon monoxide decreases the oxygen content of blood by decreasing the amount of oxygen bound to hemoglobin and simultaneously increasing the affinity of hemoglobin for oxygen by decreasing the release of oxygen into tissues.

Carbon dioxide is not cooperatively bound to hemoglobin, and thus the shape of the CO_2 dissociation is more linear than that of O_2 and affected predominantly by PaO_2. Higher PaO_2 shifts the curve to the right, facilitating unloading of CO_2 in the lungs; lower PaO_2 shifts the curve to the left, facilitating onloading of CO_2 in the tissues.

Abnormalities of Pulmonary Gas Exchange

Partial pressures of oxygen and carbon dioxide in arterial blood (arterial blood gas values) are determined by the degree of equilibration between the alveolar gas and capillary blood PO_2 and PCO_2. The degree of equilibration depends on four main factors. In order of importance, these factors are (1) matching of ventilation with perfusion, (2) ventilation, (3) shunt, and (4) diffusion.

VENTILATION/PERFUSION INEQUALITY (MISMATCH)

The lung is composed of units with varying ratios of ventilation to blood flow ($\dot{V}/\dot{Q}$). In normal lungs, the range of $\dot{V}/\dot{Q}$ ratios is narrow, from about 0.5 to 3.0. As lung disease develops, the range widens, so that $\dot{V}$ and $\dot{Q}$ are matched in fewer lung units ($\dot{V}/\dot{Q}$ mismatch). This mismatch without compensation will cause the PaO_2 to fall and the $PaCO_2$ to rise. In subjects with normal respiratory drive and ventilatory capacity, the increasing $PaCO_2$ triggers an increase in minute ventilation, which maintains $PaCO_2$ and pH within normal range but has very little effect on PaO_2. When the abil-

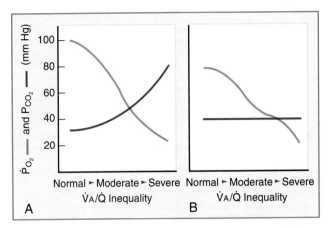

FIGURE 15–6 *A,* The effect of increasing ventilation-perfusion ($\dot{V}a/\dot{Q}$) inequality on arterial PO_2 and PCO_2 when cardiac output and minute ventilation are held constant. *B,* The change in gas tensions when ventilation is allowed to increase. Increased ventilation can maintain a normal PCO_2 but can only partially correct the hypoxemia. (Adapted from Dantzker DR: Gas exchange abnormalities. *In* Montenegro H [ed]: Chronic Obstructive Pulmonary Disease. New York: Churchill Livingstone, 1984, pp 141–160.)

ity to increase minute ventilation is exceeded, both hypoxemia and hypercarbia result (Fig. 15–6). $\dot{V}/\dot{Q}$ inequality is the primary cause of abnormal gas exchange in diseased lungs.

HYPOVENTILATION

Hypoventilation is defined as ventilation inadequate to keep arterial blood $PaCO_2$ from increasing above normal. In this situation, hypoxia occurs because increased CO_2 in alveoli displaces O_2. Alveolar PCO_2 is directly proportional to minute ventilation. The alveolar gas equation describes the reciprocal relationship between $PaCO_2$ and PaO_2:

$$PAO_2 = (PB - PH_2O)FIO_2 - PaCO_2/R$$

where PAO_2 is alveolar PO_2, PB is atmospheric pressure, PH_2O is the partial pressure of water vapor, FIO_2 is the fractional concentration of inspired O_2, and R is the respiratory exchange ratio. As minute ventilation falls, the $PaCO_2$ rises and the PAO_2 falls. Hypoventilation-induced hypoxia in patients breathing room air can be reversed by administration of supplemental O_2 (i.e., increased FIO_2).

SHUNT

Shunt is the portion of the blood that goes from the right side of the heart to the left without an opportunity for exchange of oxygen and carbon dioxide. Anatomic shunt occurs across intracardiac septal defects, across pulmonary arteriovenous malformations, and from the very small percentage of venous return from cardiac and bronchial circulations that empties directly into the left atrium. Physiologic shunt occurs when pulmonary capillary blood traverses unventilated lung units and is actu-

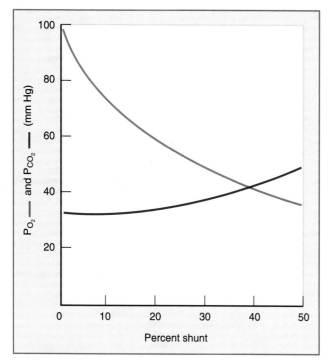

FIGURE 15-7 The effect of increasing shunt on the arterial P_{O_2} and P_{CO_2}. The minute ventilation has been held constant in this example. Under usual circumstances, the hypoxemia would lead to an increased minute ventilation and a fall in the P_{CO_2} as the shunt increases. (From Dantzker DR: Gas exchange abnormalities. *In* Montenegro H [ed]: Chronic Obstructive Pulmonary Disease. New York: Churchill Livingstone, 1984, pp 141–160.)

ally one extreme of $\dot{V}/\dot{Q}$ mismatch. Shunt is the most potent source of hypoxemia because the oxygen content of shunted blood cannot be affected by increases in the fraction of inspired oxygen. At values less than 50% of the cardiac output, shunt has very little effect on $PaCO_2$ (Fig. 15–7).

The fraction of blood shunted can be calculated only when the patient breathes 100% O_2 by the formula:

$$Qs/Qt = [Cc'O_2 - CaO_2]/[Cc'O_2 - C\bar{v}O_2]$$

where Qs = shunted blood flow, Qt = total blood flow, $Cc'O_2$ = end pulmonary capillary oxygen content, and $C\bar{v}O_2$ = mixed venous oxygen content.

DIFFUSION IMPAIRMENT

With normal cardiopulmonary function, blood spends an average of 0.75 second in the pulmonary capillaries at rest. During vigorous exercise, this time may be decreased to 0.25 second. Because it takes only 0.25 second for blood and alveolar oxygen to equilibrate across the thin alveolar capillary membrane, even under these conditions there is no fall in the end capillary oxygen concentration. If the diffusing distance is increased by alveolar capillary membrane thickening (so that more time is required for oxygen to equilibrate between alveolar gas and capillary blood), PaO_2 will first decrease

with exercise and only in extreme cases will resting PaO_2 be decreased. Hypoxemia is rarely caused solely by a diffusion impairment. The abnormalities in carbon monoxide diffusing capacity measured during pulmonary function testing reflect $\dot{V}/\dot{Q}$ matching far more often than diffusion impairment.

NONPULMONARY CAUSES OF HYPOXEMIA

The PaO_2 can be affected by the partial pressure of mixed systemic venous blood ($P\bar{v}O_2$) entering the lung circulation. $P\bar{v}O_2$ is decreased when the demand for oxygen in the tissues outstrips the supply. Inadequate cardiac output, low hemoglobin concentration, or low hemoglobin O_2 saturation all result in a low $P\bar{v}O_2$. The effect of decreased $P\bar{v}O_2$ on PaO_2 is usually only clinically significant in patients with underlying lung disease producing $\dot{V}/\dot{Q}$ mismatch or shunt (Fig. 15–8). Hypoxia caused by a combination of heart and lung disease should be understood and managed according to the contribution of each.

GROWTH AND AGING OF THE NORMAL LUNG

The lung grows by alveolar multiplication up to 8 years of age, after which it continues to grow until about age 20 by increasing alveolar diameter. Thereafter, both total alveolar surface area and elastic recoil decrease pro-

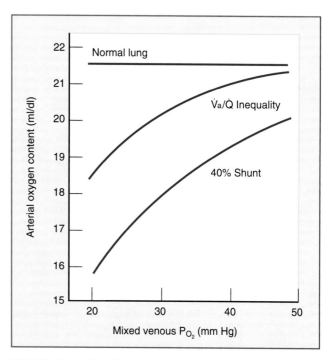

FIGURE 15-8 The effect of altering mixed venous P_{O_2} ($P\bar{v}O_2$) on the arterial oxygen content under three assumed conditions: a normal lung, severe ventilation-perfusion ($\dot{V}a/\dot{Q}$) inequality, and the presence of a 40% shunt. For each situation the patient is breathing 50% O_2 and the $P\bar{v}O_2$ is altered, keeping all other variables constant. (From Dantzker DR: Gas exchange in the adult respiratory distress syndrome. Clin Chest Med 1982; 3:57.)

gressively with age. By age 80, alveolar surface area is reduced by about 30%. Loss of elastic recoil results in less negative pleural pressure, which increases FRC. In addition, in older persons, small airways and alveoli in the lower lung zones tend to collapse during expiration, increasing V̇/Q̇, mismatch, which contributes to the progressive increase in the alveolar-arterial oxygen difference found in the normal lung with old age.

REFERENCES

Rubin LJ: Primary pulmonary hypertension. N Engl J Med 1997; 336: 111–117.

West JB: Pulmonary Pathology: The Essentials, 5th ed. Baltimore: Williams & Wilkins, 1998.

West JB: Respiratory Physiology: The Essentials, 5th ed. Baltimore: Williams & Wilkins, 1995.

West JB, Wagner PD: Pulmonary gas exchange. Am J Respir Crit Care Med 1988; 157:S82–S87.

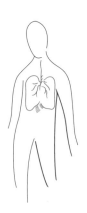

16

DIAGNOSTIC TECHNIQUES AND THEIR INDICATIONS

Bonnie S. Slovis • Kenneth L. Brigham

Imaging Procedures

Chest radiography is the most common and usually initial imaging procedure used to evaluate chest disease. The standard radiographic views are the posteroanterior and left lateral projections. These radiographs (called "plain films") can reveal abnormalities of bone, mediastinal structures, lung parenchyma, airways, and pleura. Both the presence and the absence of radiographic findings may be significant. The chest radiograph can conclusively eliminate some structural abnormalities from consideration and can demonstrate conclusively that abnormalities such as infiltrates, interstitial disease, vascular disease, masses, pleural effusions and thickening, cavitary lung disease, cardiac enlargement, and some airway diseases are present. The plain radiograph in combination with the history and physical examination is often sufficient to diagnose chest disease. In many circumstances, however, additional imaging techniques are necessary to define the disease process more clearly.

Computed tomography provides more information than the plain film by improving resolution, locating abnormalities in three dimensions, and, when studies are also done in the presence of intravascular contrast dye, distinguishing vascular from other structures. The spiral computed tomographic scan is an additional improvement in the technique; spiral computed tomography is faster, provides continuous sections through the chest, and permits the radiologist to define the thickness of the sections depending on the goal of the scan. Important uses of computed tomography are to evaluate pulmonary nodules and masses; to distinguish pleural thickening from pleural fluid; to estimate the size of the heart and the presence of pericardial fluid or thickening; to discriminate patterns of involvement in interstitial lung disease; to detect and define cavities; to identify intracavitary processes such as mycetomas or fluid; to quantify the extent and distribution of emphysema; to detect and measure mediastinal adenopathy and masses;

and, recently, to evaluate proximal clot in pulmonary arteries. Certain patterns of calcification of pulmonary nodules, such as eggshell or popcorn calcification, can rule out malignancy and the need for invasive diagnostic procedures.

Magnetic resonance imaging is not commonly used in the evaluation of pulmonary disease; however, there are special situations in which it can add important information. Magnetic resonance imaging is the imaging procedure of choice to evaluate neurologic and vertebral involvement in patients with superior sulcus tumors of the lung. It is also used to diagnose and evaluate vascular compromise in patients with mediastinal fibrosis, an uncommon but often fatal disease.

Positron emission tomography can aid in the diagnosis and staging of lung cancer. It detects masses greater than 1 cm in diameter and enlarged mediastinal nodes with considerable sensitivity. However, it does not distinguish between inflammation and malignancy. The availability of positron emission tomography is still limited, and its clinical utility is a topic of ongoing debate.

Pulmonary angiography is the gold standard for diagnosis of pulmonary emboli and arteriovenous malformations. Ultrasonography is useful for documenting and localizing fluid in the chest and to assist in diagnostic thoracocentesis if the effusion is small or loculated. Fluoroscopy is used to evaluate diaphragm function in patients with unexplained dyspnea. Ventilation/perfusion scanning is useful in the diagnosis of pulmonary embolism.

Evaluation of Lung Function

PULMONARY FUNCTION TESTING

Routine pulmonary function testing evaluates four areas of lung function: air flow (spirometry), lung volumes, gas exchange (diffusing capacity), and lung mechanics. Accu-

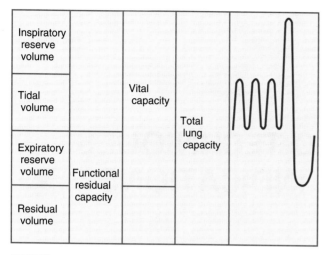

FIGURE 16-1 Lung volumes and capacities. Although vital capacity and its subdivision can be measured by spirometry, calculation of residual volume requires measurement of functional residual capacity by body plethysmography, helium dilution technique, or nitrogen washout.

capacity can be calculated by measuring dilution of an insoluble gas (usually helium or nitrogen) breathed by the patient in a closed circuit or from the pressure–volume relationship of gas measured in a whole-body plethysmograph. Although gas dilution techniques are easier and faster, their accuracy depends on uniform mixing of the indicator gas in the lungs. This does not occur in patients with severe obstructive lung disease, so that these techniques can greatly underestimate lung volume in patients with severe obstructive lung disease. Whole-body plethysmography, which measures a change in pressure with a change in volume, measures lung volumes more accurately in patients with obstructive lung disease, and also permits measurements of airway resistance, but the technique is cumbersome and time consuming.

Measurement of air flow is the most commonly performed pulmonary function test because of its value in the diagnosis and management of obstructive lung disease. Spirometry is used to measure air flow (Fig. 16–2). The patient breathes into an apparatus that measures inspiratory and expiratory flow rates with changing lung volumes and displays this information as a flow-volume loop the shape of which corresponds to certain lung function abnormalities (Fig. 16–3). Obstructive lung disease is diagnosed and evaluated by measuring the volume exhaled in 1 second with maximal effort starting from a full inspiration (forced expiratory volume in 1 second) and the forced vital capacity, which is the total amount of air the patient is able to exhale starting from a full inspiration. The ratio of forced expiratory volume in 1 second to forced vital capacity is the most useful expression of airway obstruction. In patients with obstructive lung disease, spirometry is often performed before and after administration of an inhaled bronchodilator as a measure of the reversibility of the obstruction. This test may also be a guide to therapy.

The gas exchange capacity of the lungs is measured

rate interpretation of pulmonary function tests requires appropriate reference standards. Variables that affect the standard values include age, sex, height, race, and hemoglobin concentration. The standard deviation of these variables and the day-to-day and test-to-test variation are considered when interpreting a given set of pulmonary function tests.

Pulmonary function testing divides the lung into four volumes and three capacities. Each capacity is the sum of two or more volumes (Fig. 16–1). All volumes except the residual volume can be measured directly by spirometry. Residual volume is calculated by measuring the functional residual capacity indirectly and subtracting the expiratory reserve volume. The functional residual

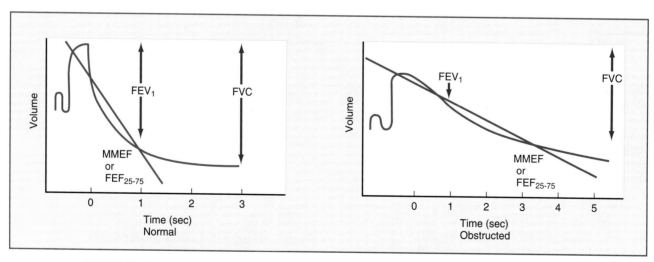

FIGURE 16-2 Spirometry in a normal subject and in a patient with obstructive lung disease. FEV_1 represents the forced expired volume in 1 second, and FVC represents the forced vital capacity. The slope of the line connecting the points at 25% and 75% of the FVC represents the forced expired flow, FEF_{25-75}, or maximum midexpiratory flow (MMEF). The FEF_{25-75} is less reproducible and less specific than the FEV_1.

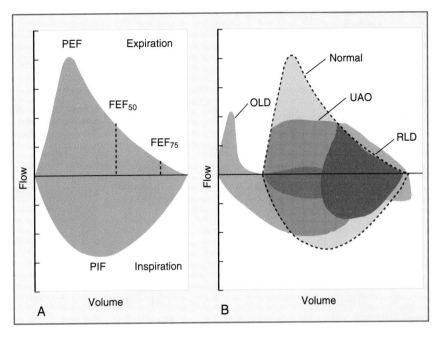

FIGURE 16–3 *A,* The maximum expired flow/volume curve in a normal subject. The peak expiratory flow (PEF) and forced expiratory flows at 50% and 75% of the exhaled vital capacity (FEF$_{50}$ and FEF$_{75}$) are indicated. PIF = Peak inspiratory flow. *B,* In obstructive lung disease (OLD), hyperinflation pushes the position of the curve to the left, and there is characteristic scalloping on expiration. In restrictive lung disease (RLD), lung volumes are reduced, but flow for any point in volume is normal. The flow/volume curve displays different patterns with various forms of upper airway obstruction (UAO), with reduction in respiratory flow if the obstruction is outside the thoracic cavity and, in addition, in expiratory flow if the obstruction is caused by a fixed deformity.

as the diffusing capacity for carbon monoxide. The patient takes a single breath of a gas mixture containing a low concentration of carbon monoxide and holds the breath for a fixed interval, and the amount of exhaled carbon monoxide is measured. The amount of unrecovered carbon monoxide is assumed to have diffused across the alveolar-capillary membrane and is therefore an expression of the gas exchange capacity of the lungs. The diffusing capacity for carbon monoxide is an integrated measure of the capacity of the lungs to take up and transport carbon monoxide (and by inference, oxygen), but an abnormal value does not define the nature of the gas exchange abnormality. Because hemoglobin is the sink for carbon monoxide, the hemoglobin concentration must be included in the interpretation of this test. Some causes of an abnormally low diffusing capacity of carbon monoxide are interstitial lung disease, emphysema, pneumonia, pulmonary vascular disease, and decreased cardiac output.

Maximum obtainable inspiratory and expiratory pressures are measured to evaluate respiratory muscle strength. In patients with neuromuscular disease and those with diaphragm dysfunction, this is a useful screening tool for assessing the degree of respiratory muscle weakness and for following the progression or resolution of the underlying process.

A diagnosis of reactive airways disease (asthma) in equivocal cases can be supported by measuring lung volumes and flow rates after inhalation of an aerosol of potentially provocative substances. These substances may be nonspecific bronchoconstrictor agents such as methacholine or may be specific agents to which the patient gives a history of sensitivity (e.g., cold air, organic and inorganic substances). Repeated measures after treatment with inhaled bronchodilator can demonstrate the degree of reversible obstruction, either at baseline or after bronchial provocation.

Cardiopulmonary exercise testing measures minute ventilation, respiratory rate, expired carbon dioxide, heart rate, electrocardiography, and pulse oximetry or arterial blood gases during graded exercise. The values are used to evaluate cardiac and pulmonary contributions to dyspnea and exercise limitation. The results can be used to differentiate between physiologic cardiac and pulmonary limitations and deconditioning.

Polysomnography is used to evaluate patients for sleep disturbances. Diagnoses are made from continuous recording of an electroencephalogram, an electrocardiogram, chest wall movement, a diaphragmatic electromyogram, pulse oximetry, and video-recorded observation performed while the subject sleeps. From such measurements it is possible to establish the presence of sleep-disordered breathing and to distinguish between central nervous system and peripheral causes of the disorder.

PULMONARY GAS EXCHANGE

The cornerstone in the evaluation of gas exchange is measurement of arterial blood gases. Arterial blood samples are analyzed for pH, the partial pressure of oxygen (PO$_2$), and the partial pressure of carbon dioxide (PCO$_2$). The percent hemoglobin saturation is routinely calculated from the PaO$_2$ and is an accurate estimate of PaO$_2$ except in the case of carbon monoxide poisoning. If carbon monoxide poisoning is suggested, saturation should be measured directly. The PaCO$_2$ reflects ventilation, and the PaO$_2$ reflects the adequacy of gas exchange. A calculation of the alveolar-arterial oxygen difference, sometimes called the A-a gradient, is used to evaluate the presence of decreased gas exchange as well as the severity of the impairment. To calculate the A-a gradient, subtract the measured PaO$_2$, drawn while the patient is breathing room air, from the calculated PaO$_2$. The normal A-a oxygen difference is about 10 mm Hg in young healthy individuals and increases with age and higher fraction of inspired oxygen. An abnormal A-a oxygen difference can be seen in patients with parenchymal lung disease, congestive heart failure, and pulmonary vascular disease, making it a sensitive but nonspecific test.

Arterial blood pH and PCO_2 and serum bicarbonate (HCO_3^-) are both used to calculate acid-base status using the Henderson-Hasselbalch equation:

$$pH = pK_a - log\ [HCO_3^-]/0.03\ PCO_2$$

Table 16–1 lists some additional equations, derived from this relationship, that help to interpret acid-base status. When an acid-base disorder is discovered, it is essential to determine whether the primary cause is respiratory or metabolic and to assess the degree of compensation that has occurred.

In patients who are hypoxemic, the measurement of the PaO_2 on room air compared with that measured while the patient is breathing 100% oxygen will distinguish between ventilation/perfusion mismatch and shunt as causes. In patients with ventilation/perfusion mismatch, the PaO_2 will rise significantly with increasing fraction of inspired oxygen. In patients with shunt the addition of supplemental oxygen has little impact on the PaO_2, because the blood is not coming in contact with ventilated alveoli. In reality, the majority of shunt is a very low ventilation/perfusion ratio (i.e., 0) and most severely hypoxemic patients will have some element of both. The more difficult it is to obtain an adequate PaO_2 with supplemental oxygen, the greater the contribution of shunt.

An elevated blood $PaCO_2$ (hypercapnia) means that alveolar ventilation is abnormally low. This may result from either too little movement of air or increased dead space. Sedative hypnotics, narcotics, and central nervous system disease are the primary causes of hypoventilation. In normal subjects, hypercapnia resulting from increased dead space can be overcome by increasing minute ventilation, but in patients with obstructive lung disease or respiratory muscle weakness the ventilatory limit may be reached before $PaCO_2$ becomes normal. Acute hypercapnia depresses the central nervous system (CO_2 narcosis), which can further depress ventilation. Mechanical ventilation is usually required for patients with acutely elevated $PaCO_2$ and resultant acidosis.

OXIMETRY

Oximetry is a reliable, noninvasive method for estimating arterial hemoglobin oxygen saturation. Oximetry devices rely on the different absorption spectra of oxyhemoglobin and deoxyhemoglobin to estimate the oxygen saturation. Sensors are usually placed on digits or ear lobes, which allow transmission of light from the source on one side of the tissue to the sensor on the other side. Accuracy of most of these devices is plus or minus 4% for saturations above 80%; they cannot be relied on below that level. Factors affecting the accuracy of oximetry readings are carboxyhemoglobin, methemoglobin, jaundice, and decreased local perfusion. Although useful in evaluating hemoglobin saturation, oximetry cannot be substituted for arterial blood gases in the evaluation of the A-a oxygen difference or the adequacy of ventilation.

REFERENCES

American Thoracic Society: Lung function testing: Selection of reference values and interpretive strategies. Am J Respir Crit Care Med 1991; 155:1201.

American Thoracic Society: Single-breath carbon monoxide diffusing capacity (transfer factor). Am J Respir Crit Care Med 1995; 152: 2158–2198.

Crapo RO: Pulmonary function testing. N Engl J Med 1994; 331:25–30.

TABLE 16–1   **Normal Values for Arterial Blood Gases**

$PO_2 = 104 - 0.27 \times age$
PCO_2: 36–44
pH: 7.35–7.45
Alveolar-arterial O_2 difference = $2.5 + 0.21 \times age$

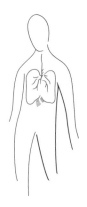

17

OBSTRUCTIVE LUNG DISEASE

Bonnie S. Slovis • Kenneth L. Brigham

Obstructive lung disease is a descriptive designation based on a physiologic abnormality: obstruction to the flow of air through the airways. Obstructive lung disease is characterized by decreased air flow rates during expiration, often accompanied by an elevated functional residual capacity resulting from trapped gas. The major disorders causing obstruction are asthma, bronchiectasis, emphysema, and chronic bronchitis. *Chronic obstructive pulmonary disease* (COPD) is the term applied to both emphysema and chronic bronchitis, diseases usually caused by cigarette smoking or other chronic irritant inhalation, although long-standing, poorly controlled asthma may also result in COPD. The clinical and laboratory classification of obstructive lung disease is presented in Table 17–1.

Pathophysiology of Air Flow Obstruction

The flow of air through the bronchial tree is directly proportional to the driving pressure and is inversely proportional to the resistance. Air flow to the lungs can be decreased by airway narrowing, which increases resistance, or by loss of elastic recoil of the lung, which decreases driving pressure. Most often, both these physiologic abnormalities are present.

Inflammation of the airways results in mucosal edema and increased mucus production, both of which narrow the airway. Persistent inflammation results in goblet cell hypertrophy, loss of ciliated epithelium (decreasing the ability to clear secretions), squamous metaplasia of airway epithelial cells, and peribronchiolar fibrosis. Inhaled tobacco smoke and other irritants, recurrent infection, and immunologic dysfunction characteristic of asthma are the most common causes of chronic airway inflammation in susceptible persons. Persistent or recurrent inflammation can destroy structural elements of the bronchial walls and can result in fixed bronchial dilatation and distortion *(bronchiectasis)*.

Contraction of smooth muscle narrows airways *(bronchoconstriction)* and increases resistance to air flow. Although bronchoconstriction is a normal response to inhalation of noxious stimuli, this constrictor response is exaggerated in some persons *(airway hyperreactivity)*. Conducting airways are surrounded by smooth muscle, which contains adrenergic and cholinergic receptors. Stimulation of β_2-adrenergic receptors by circulating catecholamines dilates airways, whereas stimulation of airway irritant receptors constricts airways through a cholinergic mechanism via the vagus nerve. The irritant bronchoconstricting pathways are normally present to protect against inhalation of noxious agents, but in pathologic states, these pathways may contribute to airway hyperreactivity. A host of other endogenous chemical mediators can affect airway tone (e.g., eicosanoids, histamine), but the roles of these mediators in the pathogenesis of airway hyperreactivity are not well defined.

Airway obstruction causes characteristic changes in lung volumes (Table 17–2). The residual volume and functional residual capacity are increased, whereas the total lung capacity is normal or increased. Vital capacity is reduced by the increase in the residual volume. Several factors contribute to the increase in functional residual capacity and residual volume in obstructive lung disease. Decreased lung elastic recoil increases the functional residual capacity because of reduced opposition to the outward force exerted by the chest wall. Loss of airway tone and decreased tethering by surrounding lung in COPD, as well as bronchoconstriction and mucus plugging in acute asthma, allow airways to collapse at higher lung volumes and trap excessive air. Finally, under demands for increased minute ventilation, the increased resistance to air flow may not allow the lungs to empty completely during the time available for expiration.

Three major consequences of these changes in lung volume are recognized. Breathing at higher lung volumes requires a higher change in pressure for the same change in lung volume (see Fig. 15–2), and this requirement increases the work of breathing. Second,

TABLE 17–1 Features of Obstructive Lung Diseases

Disorder	Clinical Features	Laboratory Findings
Chronic obstructive lung disease	Chronic progressive dyspnea	Decreased expiratory flow rates, hypoxia and hypercapnia in end-stage disease
Emphysema	Little or no sputum, cachexia—end stage	Hyperinflation, increased compliance, low DLCO, rarely α_1-antitrypsin deficiency
Chronic bronchitis	Sputum, history of smoking, industrial exposure	Nonspecific, rarely occurs in isolation without variable degree of emphysema
Asthma	Episodic dyspnea, cough, wheezing, with or without environmental triggers	Airway hyperreactivity, response to bronchodilators
Bronchiectasis	Usually large volume of sputum	Chest radiograph: dilated bronchi, thick-walled, tram track shadows, obstruction with or without restriction on pulmonary function tests
Immotile cilia syndrome	Situs inversus, dextrocardia, sinusitis, infertility	Abnormal dynenin in ciliated cells
Hypogammaglobulinemia		Decrease in one or more immunoglobulins
Cystic fibrosis	Sinusitis, bronchiectasis, meconium ileus, malabsorption, infertility	Increased sweat chloride, mutation in CFTR chloride channel, elevated fecal fat, abnormal nasal mucosal potential difference

larger lung volumes put the inspiratory muscles at a mechanical disadvantage. The diaphragm is flattened, thereby decreasing its ability to change intrathoracic volume, and all the inspiratory muscle fibers are shortened, thus decreasing the tension they are able to exert to effect changes in lung volume. The third consequence is beneficial. At larger lung volumes, the tethering of the narrowed and collapsing airways by the surrounding lung parenchyma reduces airway resistance and air trapping.

Obstructive lung disease results in abnormal gas exchange for several reasons. Destruction of alveoli decreases the gas exchange surface. This loss of surface area, coupled with bronchial obstruction and altered distribution of ventilated air, results in ventilation-perfusion mismatch, which may cause hypoxemia. Hyperinflation of the lungs creates or increases zone 1 conditions in which alveolar pressure exceeds pulmonary arterial pressure, a process that stops perfusion and creates a physiologic dead space. Because carbon dioxide diffuses more readily than oxygen, patients with obstructive lung disease can avoid hypercarbia by hyperventilating, even with substantial mismatching of ventilation and perfusion, but hyperventilation does not prevent hypoxemia.

TABLE 17–2 Abnormalities of Lung Volume

Lung Volume	Pulmonary Disorder	
	Obstructive Disease	Restrictive Disease
Vital capacity	D	D
Functional residual capacity	I	D
Residual volume	I	D
Total lung capacity	N or I	D

D = decreased; I = increased; N = normal.

Eventually, the metabolic costs of breathing become excessive, and respiratory muscles fatigue. Then chemoreceptors "reset," to allow $PaCO_2$ to rise, and ventilation becomes more efficient with a higher concentration of carbon dioxide eliminated at a lower minute ventilation and metabolic cost. Marked individual variation is seen in the degree of mechanical impairment and in the magnitude of increase in $PaCO_2$.

Asthma

Asthma, a chronic inflammatory disorder of the airways, affects 3% to 5% of the population in the United States and can be fatal. It is characterized by episodic airway narrowing, increased airway reactivity to a variety of stimuli, and pharmacologic or spontaneous reversibility. The inflammatory response involves mast cells, T lymphocytes, and eosinophils, which produce multiple soluble mediators (e.g., cytokines, leukotrienes, and bradykinins). An imbalance in proinflammatory versus inhibitory cytokines may be a fundamental part of the pathogenesis of asthma. The histologic findings in asthma are airway cellular infiltration, epithelial disruption, mucosal edema, and mucus plugging. The trigger or stimulus that provokes the inflammatory response may be exposure to extrinsic allergens or intrinsic host factors with no identifiable external cause. Even in people with no history of asthma, viral respiratory infection is occasionally associated with increased airway reactivity for several weeks to months after resolution of the infection; some of these persons develop chronic asthma. When a clear environmental trigger for asthmatic attacks can be identified, it can be avoided, or, in some cases, immunotherapy can desensitize the patient to the allergen. Some nonallergic factors that can precipitate or exacerbate asthma include postnasal drip, gastroesophageal reflux disease, exposure to cold, exercise, exposure to gases or fumes, emotional stress, hormones, and respiratory infections.

The diagnosis of asthma is based on clinical and laboratory data. The classic triad of symptoms is persistent wheeze, chronic episodic dyspnea, and chronic cough. Other associated symptoms are sputum production and chest pain or tightness. If hemoptysis is present, Churg-Strauss vasculitis, allergic bronchopulmonary aspergillosis, or bronchiectasis should be suspected as underlying causes. Patients may present with only one or a combination of the foregoing symptoms. Symptoms may be worse or only present at night.

Diagnostic testing can aid in confirming the diagnosis of asthma and in assessing the severity of an acute exacerbation and the reversibility of air flow obstruction (Table 17–3). Migratory infiltrates on serial chest radiographs, coupled with bronchospasm and expectoration, of mucus plugs suggest the diagnosis of allergic bronchopulmonary aspergillosis. Provocation testing with methacholine or histamine may detect bronchial hyperreactivity and can establish the diagnosis of asthma when results of routine pulmonary function tests are normal.

The management of asthma requires education and cooperation on the part of the patient. Simple, inexpensive peak expiratory flow meters can be used by the patient at home to monitor air flow obstruction. A diary should be maintained, and a clear plan should be in place for using the information to intervene early in exacerbations and to alter long-term therapy for optimal control of symptoms. The cornerstone of maintenance therapy is scheduled administration of inhaled corticosteroids. Long-acting and short-acting bronchodilators are added for additional symptomatic control as needed. Leukotriene inhibitors have been shown to be effective in maintenance therapy. Debate is ongoing about the relative efficacy of leukotriene antagonists versus inhaled corticosteroids as maintenance therapy. Theophylline preparations may have additional beneficial effects in some patients, but the narrow therapeutic window and modest efficacy of these preparations limit their value.

Acute severe asthma, or status asthmaticus, is an attack of severe bronchospasm that is unresponsive to routine therapy. Such attacks may be sudden (*hyperacute asthma*) and may be rapidly fatal, often before medical care can be obtained. In most cases, however, patients have a history of progressive dyspnea over hours to days, with increasing bronchodilator use. Patients with severe exacerbations may (1) have difficulty in talking, (2) use accessory muscles of inspiration, (3) have a pulsus paradoxus, (4) have orthopnea, (5) be diaphoretic, or (6) have mental status changes ranging from agitation to somnolence. In patients with these findings, treatment should be immediate and aggressive, with continuous monitoring of blood oxygen saturation by pulse oximetry, supplemented by arterial blood gas analysis to evaluate hypercarbia. Peak expiratory flow rates should be measured frequently to assess response to therapy. In patients who are unable to perform peak expiratory flow maneuvers and in those who have declining mental status or who appear to be worsening clinically, arterial blood gas analysis is essential. The arterial blood gas analysis in patients with mild attacks or early in the course of a severe attack shows hypoxemia (a widened alveolar-arterial oxygen gradient) and hyperventilation (a decreased $PaCO_2$). With increasing severity or respiratory muscle fatigue, the $PaCO_2$ returns to normal and ultimately begins to rise. A rising $PaCO_2$ in a patient with asthma is an ominous sign and may portend a medical emergency. These patients require continuous direct observation and monitoring, and many require mechanical ventilation.

TABLE 17–3 Diagnostic Studies in Asthma

Routine pulmonary function test	Decreased FEV_1; hyperinflation; improvement with bronchodilator
Special pulmonary function test	
Methacholine or cold-air challenge	Indicates the presence of nonspecific bronchial hyperreactivity; bronchoconstriction occurs at lower dose in asthma
Challenge with specific agents: occupational, drugs, etc.	Occasionally performed
Chest radiograph	Fleeting infiltrates and central bronchiectasis in ABPA
Skin tests	Demonstrate atopy; little value except prick test to *Aspergillus fumigatus* positive in ABPA
Blood tests	Eosinophils and IgE usually increased in atopy; levels may be very high in ABPA; *Aspergillus* precipitins increased in many but not all patients with ABPA

ABPA = allergic bronchopulmonary aspergillosis; FEV_1 = forced expiratory volume in 1 second.

Chronic Obstructive Pulmonary Disease

Patients with COPD have slowly progressive, irreversible airway obstruction. The course of the disease is punctuated by periodic exacerbations characterized by increased dyspnea, increased sputum production, a change in character of the sputum, and occasionally respiratory failure. Exacerbations may result from bacterial or viral respiratory infection, heart failure, poor patient compliance with prescribed therapy, or acute bronchospasm. Pulmonary emboli may be particularly difficult to diagnose in these patients because of their underlying lung disease and abnormal ventilation and perfusion patterns at baseline.

Because it is slowly progressive, COPD usually takes years to become clinically significant, so the diagnosis is usually made first in middle-aged and older persons. Dyspnea on exertion is the earliest symptom, but this symptom is often not seen until late in disease because patients gradually reduce their exercise level to match their respiratory capacity to avoid symptoms. Patients with chronic bronchitis have, by definition, a chronic productive cough. As the disease progresses, the physical examination may show increased anteroposterior chest diameter (indicating chronic lung overinflation), use of accessory muscles of respiration, peripheral cyanosis, and, on auscultation of the chest, decreased breath sounds, crackles, rhonchi, and wheezes.

In the early stages of COPD, pulmonary function testing is the most sensitive means of making the diagnosis. Although cigarette smoking is far and away the most frequent cause of COPD, less than one in five patients who smoke will develop the disease, and signs of air flow obstruction on pulmonary function tests, even in asymptomatic smokers, can identify susceptible patients. Early pulmonary function test findings are reduced flow rates at smaller lung volumes, followed by decreases in forced expiratory volume in 1 second (FEV_1) and forced vital capacity, with variable increases in residual volume and functional residual capacity and decreases in carbon monoxide diffusing capacity of the lungs. The pulmonary function testing patterns differ depending on whether the predominant disorder is chronic bronchitis or emphysema. Evidence of gas trapping and reduced diffusing capacity are hallmarks of emphysema, and these changes are less prominent in patients with chronic bronchitis. Because most patients have elements of both emphysema and chronic bronchitis, COPD is best viewed as a spectrum with emphysema and chronic bronchitis at either pole, but varying degrees of both disorders as the usual clinical picture. Patients with COPD generally have a weaker response to bronchodilators than do patients with asthma. Arterial blood gases usually show hypoxemia and, in more advanced cases, hypercarbia as well. Dyspnea is related to both hypoxemia and increased work of breathing in the presence of obstruction. Hypoxemia may worsen during exercise and sleep. Continued severe hypoxemia ($PaO_2 < 60$ mm Hg) may lead to secondary erythrocytosis. Pulmonary hypertension can result from a combination of loss of cross-sectional area of the pulmonary vascular bed, pulmonary vasoconstriction caused by alveolar hypoxia, and, in later stages of the disease, increased blood viscosity secondary to erythrocytosis. The increased afterload to the right ventricle produced by chronic pulmonary hypertension may lead to right ventricular failure (cor pulmonale), which may become the most difficult therapeutic problem.

Some precise definitions are useful in understanding COPD, as described in the following sections.

SMALL AIRWAY DISEASE

The earliest manifestation of COPD is in the peripheral airway. Pulmonary function tests first show decreased air flow at lower lung volumes even with a normal FEV_1. Anatomic abnormalities include inflammation of terminal and respiratory bronchioles, fibrosis of airway walls, goblet cell metaplasia, and occasionally areas of obliterative bronchiolitis.

EMPHYSEMA

Emphysema is abnormal enlargement of the air spaces as a result of progressive destruction of alveolar walls. In some patients, these abnormal air spaces coalesce to form giant, essentially nonfunctional air spaces (*bullae*) that compress surrounding areas of more normal lung. The degree of obstruction in patients with COPD correlates most closely with the severity of the emphysema.

The pathogenesis of emphysema is uncertain, although the most popular current theory is that repeated and prolonged inflammation releases proteolytic enzymes into the lungs in amounts too great to be neutralized by the endogenous antiproteases, a phenomenon termed a *protease-antiprotease imbalance*. The unopposed protease digests lung tissue and results in permanent destruction. This theory grew out of the discovery that an inherited defect in the gene encoding the principal endogenous antiprotease, α_1-antitrypsin, predisposes to the development of premature emphysema, especially in patients who smoke cigarettes. Cigarette smoking, the major cause of emphysema, increases the number of alveolar macrophages and neutrophils, enhances protease release from inflammatory cells, and impairs the activity of the antiproteases, a change that can produce a relative deficiency of antiprotease even in the presence of normal absolute amounts of α_1-antitrypsin.

Radiographic findings in emphysema reflect hyperinflation and loss of alveolar capillary surface area. Chest radiographs show lung hyperinflation, depressed diaphragm, increased anteroposterior chest diameter, and widened retrosternal air space. In addition, hyperlucent areas and attenuation of the vasculature may be evident. Enlarged pulmonary arteries indicate secondary pulmonary hypertension. Chest computed tomography is more sensitive than plain chest radiography in detecting emphysema and adds information about presence and location of bullae and the distribution of major anatomic abnormalities. This information is essential when patients are evaluated for bullectomy or lung reduction surgery.

CHRONIC BRONCHITIS

Chronic bronchitis is defined as a persistent cough resulting in sputum production for more than 3 months in each of the past 3 years. As with emphysema, cigarette smoking is the major cause, although exposure to other pollutants may play a role. Although cough and sputum production do not appear to affect the development of airway obstruction directly, patients with chronic bronchitis benefit from antibiotic therapy during exacerbations of their obstruction. The degree of air flow obstruction depends directly on the degree of coexisting emphysema and bronchospasm. No specific findings are noted on physical examination, chest radiography, or pulmonary function tests other than those associated with airway obstruction.

Bronchiectasis

Bronchiectasis, an abnormal and persistent dilation of the bronchi, results from destructive changes in the elastic and muscular layers of bronchial walls that may be diffuse or localized. Before the development of antibiotics and immunization against common childhood viral diseases, bronchiectasis usually began with a severe episode of necrotizing pneumonia during childhood, followed by a long, symptom-free interval and the appearance of clinical symptoms later in life. Currently, the common causes of bronchiectasis in developed nations are allergic bronchopulmonary aspergillosis, immunoglobulin deficiencies predisposing to chronic respiratory infections, abnormal airway clearance mechanisms, and, most commonly, cystic fibrosis (CF; see the following section of this chapter). Immotile cilia or Kartagener's syndrome is a rare inherited abnormality of ciliary microtubules that impairs airway clearance. The classic triad of Kartagener's syndrome is sinusitis, situs inversus, and infertility.

The diagnosis of bronchiectasis is made by a history of chronic cough, which may be dry or productive of large volumes of sputum. Patients who initially have dry bronchiectasis usually eventually produce sputum. Blood-streaked sputum is common in these patients, and massive hemoptysis occurs rarely. Auscultation of the lungs may show crackles over the affected lung segment, and occasionally digital clubbing is seen. Chest radiographs may be normal or may show mildly increased interstitial markings and linear atelectasis. The classic finding is parallel lines in peripheral lung fields described as "tram tracks," which represent thickened bronchial walls that do not taper from proximal to distal sites. The definitive diagnosis is made and the extent of disease is defined by high-resolution computed tomography. Pulmonary function testing shows variable degrees of obstruction.

Cystic Fibrosis

CF is an autosomal recessive genetic disorder that affects multiple organ systems (Table 17–4). It is the most common lethal genetic disorder in the white population, with a carrier frequency of about 1 in 25, affecting 1 in 3200 live births. The mutation occurs in a single gene that encodes the CF transmembrane conductance regulator (CFTR), a cyclic adenosine monophosphate–regulated chloride channel normally present in the apical surface of epithelial cells. Failure to produce the normal CFTR protein results in defective chloride transport and increased sodium reabsorption in airway and ductal epithelia and creates abnormally thick and viscous secretions in the respiratory, hepatobiliary, gastrointestinal, and reproductive tracts and in the pancreas. These abnormal secretions cause luminal obstruction and destruction of various exocrine ducts. The most common mutation, found in 65% of patients, is the ΔF508 mutation, which is a loss of the codon for

TABLE 17–4 Organ Involvement in Cystic Fibrosis

Pulmonary
Cough and sputum production
Recurrent pneumonias
Bronchial hyperreactivity
Hemoptysis
Pneumothorax
Marked digital clubbing
Cor pulmonale

Upper Respiratory Tract
Nasal polyps
Chronic sinusitis

Gastrointestinal
Meconium ileus in the neonate
Distal intestinal obstruction
Rectal prolapse
Hernias
Exocrine pancreatic dysfunction causing steatorrhea, malnutrition, and vitamin deficiency
Acute pancreatitis (rare)
Diabetes mellitus
Cirrhosis and portal hypertension
Salivary gland inflammation
Cholelithiasis

Genitourinary
Azoospermia
Decreased fertility rate in women
Nephrolithiasis

phenylalanine at the 508 position of the protein. To date, more than 700 mutations have been identified in the CFTR.

Although gastrointestinal manifestations of CF correlate with genotypes, the severity of CF lung disease, which accounts for 90% of deaths, does not. Ongoing research indicates that the genetic abnormality in CF results in a hyperinflammatory state in the lungs that precedes infection and is independent of mucus obstruction of airways. Other genetic and environmental factors undoubtedly contribute to the severity of lung disease in these patients.

In patients with CF, the upper and lower respiratory tract becomes colonized initially with *Staphylococcus aureus,* frequently followed by *Haemophilus influenzae* and, ultimately, *Pseudomonas aeruginosa.* Persistent inflammation and infection cause bronchial wall destruction and bronchiectasis. Mucus plugging of small airways produces postobstructive cystic dilations and parenchymal destruction. Progressive airway obstruction ensues, and most patients die of respiratory failure. Complications of CF lung disease are pneumothorax and hemoptysis. Hemoptysis is usually minor, although occasionally it can be massive and fatal.

The definitive diagnosis of CF is made by measuring the concentration of chloride in sweat. The diagnosis is considered definitive if the clinical picture is consistent with CF and if the sweat chloride concentration is greater than 60 mEq/L on each of two occasions. The diagnosis can be confirmed through genotyping. Genetic screening can detect 90% of carriers and is available to persons with a family history of CF. Although most patients are diagnosed in childhood, a few patients with milder disease are not diagnosed until adulthood. With improvements in diagnosis and management, the median survival of patients with CF has increased from 14 years in 1969 to 30 years in 1995. Investigators have estimated that by the end of the first decade of the twenty-first century, more than 50% of patients with CF will be more than 18 years old, a situation that will make CF predominately an adult disease. The diagnosis of CF should be considered and the appropriate tests performed in any patient with unexplained chronic sinus disease, bronchiectasis, or malabsorption resulting from exocrine pancreatic insufficiency.

The core treatment of CF is aggressive airway hygiene, nutritional support including pancreatic enzyme replacement, antibiotics, bronchodilators, and aerosolized recombinant human DNase, which decreases sputum viscosity by digesting inflammatory cell DNA. The use of inhaled antibiotics has increased since clinical studies found that inhaled tobramycin, at a dose of 300 mg bid during every other month, slows the rate of decline in pulmonary function. Research on the characterization and role of inflammatory mediators in CF, newly discovered endogenous antimicrobial peptides, and other genetic and environmental contributions to the disease are expanding the therapeutic options. The ultimate therapy for patients with end-stage lung disease is bilateral lung transplantation. Some centers are using two living donors, each of whom donates one lobe, for selected patients who are not expected to survive the wait until lung transplantation.

The finding that CF is a consequence of a defect in a single identified gene makes gene therapy a theoretic possibility for cure of the disease. Although attempts to develop the necessary technology are under way and some preliminary studies have been done in patients with CF, several obstacles to clinical application of this novel therapy remain. As yet, no delivery system for the normal gene exists that is proved safe and capable of delivering the gene to a sufficient number of airway cells and to achieve sufficient magnitude and duration of expression of the normal gene to be therapeutic. In addition, many of the alterations in the lungs of patients with CF lung disease probably are irreversible, even if the basic defect could be corrected.

Treatment

No curative therapies are available for COPD; therapy is aimed at controlling symptoms and avoiding harmful environments. Increased understanding of the pathogenesis of inflammation has led to development of leukotriene antagonists for treatment of asthma, and many new anti-inflammatory agents that could prove effective are under development. Gene therapy is on the horizon for genetic diseases such as CF and α_1-antitrypsin deficiency. In addition, the extension of gene therapy to the treatment of acquired diseases will be a major therapeutic advance during the first decade of the twenty-first century.

PHARMACOLOGIC THERAPY

Drugs used in the treatment of obstructive lung disease are categorized in four major groups: bronchodilators, anti-inflammatory drugs, antibiotics, and mucolytics (Table 17–5). The first two categories merit special comment here.

Bronchodilators

Sympathomimetics (β_2-adrenoreceptor agonists) are the most potent bronchodilators, although the anticholinergic drug ipratropium bromide may be superior in COPD. In practice, a combination of the two agents is probably best, except in young patients with pure asthma. Controversy exists over the role of anticholinergics added to β agonists in acute exacerbations of asthma. Albuterol is the most commonly used β agonist; its bronchodilator effect is rapid in onset and is relatively short lived. The long-acting β agonist salmeterol can be taken twice daily and is effective for maintenance therapy; it also has anti-inflammatory activity that may contribute to its efficacy. Bronchodilator aerosols can be delivered either by a metered-dose inhaler or a nebulizer. The metered-dose inhaler offers advantages of portability and ease of administration and convenience, and, when it is used correctly with a spacer, it is essentially as effective as nebulizers in delivering the drug. Nebulization has no advantage over the use of metered-dose inhalers, in the long-term management of obstructive lung disease.

Methylxanthines such as theophylline are weak systemic sympathomimetic agents with a narrow therapeutic window, and they are not first-line drugs in treatment of obstructive lung disease. Theophylline preparations may provide some additional bronchodilation in patients with COPD or asthma who do not respond adequately to inhaled β agonists. When these preparations are used, blood concentrations should be

TABLE 17–5   Pharmacologic Therapy for Airway Obstruction

Sympathomimetics
β_2-specific agents: metaproterenol, terbutaline, albuterol
Epinephrine
Methylxanthines
Theophylline
Aminophylline
Anticholinergics
Atropine
Ipratropium bromide
Anti-inflammatory Drugs
Corticosteroids
Cromolyn sodium

maintained in the lower end of the therapeutic range (between 8 and 12 μg/mL). Toxicity is common at concentrations higher than 20 μg/mL. The metabolism of theophylline is decreased by many commonly used drugs, and toxic serum concentrations of theophylline can be reached quickly when these other drugs are given unless the theophylline dose is adjusted appropriately. Toxic effects of theophylline are gastrointestinal, cardiac, and neurologic. Severe theophylline toxicity requires charcoal hemoperfusion and is frequently fatal.

Anti-Inflammatory Drugs

Inhaled corticosteroids are the first line anti-inflammatory therapeutic agents in patients with asthma who require more than occasional use of β agonists. Orally administered corticosteroids are necessary intermittently in patients with severe asthma or during moderate to severe exacerbations. Oral and intravenous routes of steroid administration are equally effective in patients who can take oral medications. Long-term systemic administration of corticosteroids should be avoided unless it is absolutely necessary. This is rarely the case in patients who are managed aggressively and for whom regimens of other medications are optimal. Adverse effects of long-term systemic steroids include weight gain, osteoporosis, hyperglycemia, immune suppression, adrenal suppression, systemic hypertension, Cushing's syndrome, myopathy, and psychologic disturbances. Long-term high-dose inhaled corticosteroids may have some mild systemic effects and may increase the risk of cataracts. As a general rule, patients should be maintained on the lowest long-term dose of inhaled steroid that controls their symptoms, with transient dose increases during exacerbations.

The oral leukotriene antagonists have been shown to be effective substitutes for inhaled corticosteroids in controlled clinical studies. Some studies have associated long-term use of leukotriene antagonists and the subsequent development of Churg-Strauss disease, but whether this association is an effect of leukotriene antagonists or whether withdrawal of corticosteroids unmasks underlying disease is unclear.

Inhaled sodium cromolyn and nedocromil are presumed to act by stabilizing mast cell membranes and thus by preventing release of inflammatory mediators from those cells. These are useful maintenance drugs in pediatric asthma and in occasional adults with atopy or a strong allergic component. They are not useful in acute exacerbations of asthma.

Algorithms for short-term and long-term therapy of asthma and COPD are outlined in Figure 17–1. Patient education, development and use of an action plan, and continuous rather than episodic care by a physician are keys to the control of these diseases.

OXYGEN THERAPY

Oxygen therapy is frequently necessary in acute exacerbations of obstructive lung disease. In patients who chronically hypoventilate (and thus have an elevated $PaCO_2$), elevating the inspired oxygen content may cause

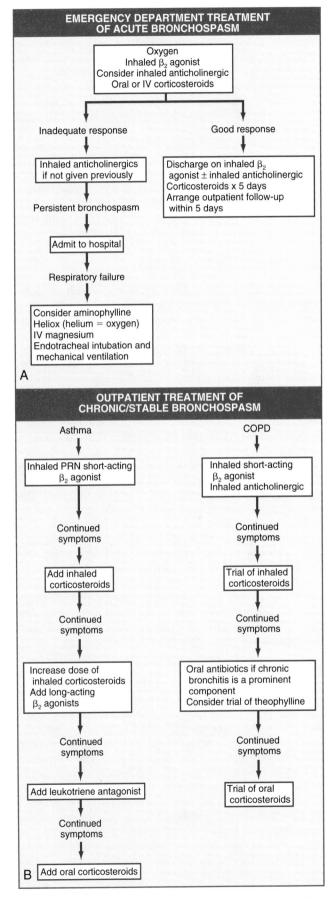

FIGURE 17–1 Algorithms for treatment of bronchospasm in the Emergency Department (*A*) and in outpatients with stable disease (*B*).

acutely worse hypercarbia. Supplemental oxygen probably has two effects that contribute to this response—a decrease in hypoxic ventilatory drive and a worsening ventilation-perfusion mismatch resulting from alveolar oxygen-mediated vasodilation in poorly ventilated lung units. Nonetheless, arterial oxygen must be maintained in a range compatible with life even at the expense of precipitating respiratory failure requiring mechanical ventilation.

Patients with persistent arterial oxygen saturations of less than 90%, PaO_2 lower than 55 mm Hg at rest, or oxygen saturations lower than 60% if cor pulmonale or erythrocytosis is present benefit from long-term continuous (24 hours/day) oxygen therapy. Long-term oxygen therapy is the only treatment that has been shown to prolong survival in patients with COPD.

ANTIBIOTICS AND VACCINES

Exacerbations of airway obstruction may result from viral or bacterial infection. The most common bacterial pathogens in COPD are *Streptococcus pneumoniae, H. influenzae,* and *Moraxella catarrhalis.* Management of acute exacerbations should include empiric antibiotics. In some patients with chronic bronchitis or bronchiectasis and frequent exacerbations, alternating use of different antibiotics may decrease the frequency and severity of exacerbations. In patients with CF, long-term, continuous, oral antibiotic administration has not been shown to be effective. However, inhaled high-dose tobramycin on alternating months and treatment of exacerbations with intravenous antibiotics, including double *Pseudomonas* coverage if the patient is colonized with that organism, slow the rate of decline in lung function. The use of home intravenous antibiotic therapy in adults with CF is increasing.

Immunization with influenza vaccines directed at specific epidemic strains is the single most effective intervention for reducing morbidity and mortality from obstructive lung disease. The efficacy of pneumococcal vaccine in elderly patients and in those with underlying lung disease has not been demonstrated, but the concept of immunization of these patients is rational, and the approach is generally recommended.

SMOKING CESSATION

Patients with COPD must be counseled about the importance of stopping smoking. Susceptible smokers have an increased rate of decline in FEV_1 of about 80 mL/year, in comparison with 30 mL/year in nonsusceptible smokers and nonsmokers (Fig. 17–2). The physician and other health care practitioners have the responsibility to counsel patients against tobacco use and to assist in patients' efforts to quit. Nicotine replacement with gum or transdermal patches, bupropion (an antidepressant that acts by inhibiting reuptake of serotonin at nerve endings), behavior modification, and long-term physician and group support increase the success of cessation attempts. Most patients who are successful at smoking cessation have had at least one prior failed attempt; this finding should encourage physicians to

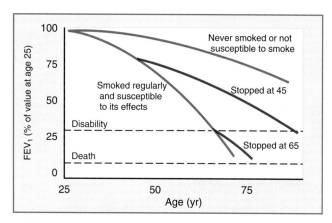

FIGURE 17–2 Pattern of decline in forced expiratory volume in 1 second (FEV_1), with risk of morbidity and mortality from respiratory disease in a susceptible smoker in comparison with a normal subject or a nonsusceptible smoker. Although cessation of smoking does not replenish the lung function already lost in a susceptible smoker, it decreases the rate of further decline. (Adapted from Fletcher C, Peto R: The natural history of chronic airflow obstruction. BMJ 1977; 1:1645.)

continue to counsel patients against smoking at every opportunity.

AIRWAY CLEARANCE TECHNIQUES

Multiple airway clearance techniques exist to aid clearing of airway secretions. In patients with CF, regular airway clearance, with or without DNase administration, decreases the rate of decline in pulmonary function. The optimal technique for airway clearance has not been clearly determined; however, percussion and postural drainage, flutter valves, and high-frequency oscillation vests are all effective, and the choice depends on cost and patient preference. No clear evidence indicates that these techniques are efficacious in treatment of chronic bronchitis or other causes of bronchiectasis, but when excessive thick airway secretions are a problem, some attempt to enhance airway clearance seems appropriate.

PULMONARY REHABILITATION PROGRAMS

Patients with pulmonary disease of sufficient severity to compromise normal activities of daily living commonly demonstrate improved quality of life and less subjective dyspnea when they are enrolled in a comprehensive, high-quality pulmonary rehabilitation program, even though pulmonary rehabilitation has not been shown to improve objective measures of pulmonary function, to affect the rate of decline in lung function, or to improve survival. An important part of rehabilitation in these patients is nutritional assessment and careful attention to maintaining adequate nutrition because malnutrition and cachexia are common in later stages of the disease and result in decreased respiratory muscle strength and compromised immune function.

SURGICAL THERAPY

Bullectomy, lung volume reduction surgery, and lung transplantation are all potentially effective surgical options for selected patients with end-stage COPD. Bullectomy is an established surgical procedure for patients with giant bullae that are compressing surrounding, less diseased lung. Although long-term experience is limited, lung volume reduction in patients with emphysema and severe air trapping can improve symptoms and pulmonary function in the short term in carefully selected patients. The best candidates are those with predominantly upper lobe disease, without an asthmatic or bronchitic component and without other major underlying diseases. Single or bilateral lung transplantation is an option for patients with end-stage obstruction. Patients with CF require bilateral lung transplantation because of the chronic necrotizing infection of their native lungs. Chronic rejection, viral infections, and late occurrence of obliterative bronchiolitis remain significant problems of lung transplantation, but the procedure clearly can improve the quality of life and can extend productive life in properly selected candidates.

REFERENCES

Standards for the diagnosis of care of patients with chronic obstructive pulmonary disease: American Thoracic Society. Am J Respir Crit Care Med 1995; 152(Suppl):S77–S121.

Barnes PJ: Inhaled glucocorticoids for asthma. N Engl J Med 1995; 332:868–875.

Drazen JM, Israel E, O'Byrne PM: Treatment of asthma with drugs modifying the leukotriene pathway. N Engl J Med 1999; 340:197–206.

Nelson HS: Beta-adrenergic bronchodilators. N Engl J Med 1995; 333:499–506.

Ramsey BW: Management of pulmonary disease in patients with cystic fibrosis [published erratum appears in N Engl J Med 1996; 335:1167]. N Engl J Med 1996; 335:179–188.

Wagner PD, Pauwels RA: National Asthma Education and Prevention Program: Highlights of the Expert Panel Report II: Guidelines for the Diagnosis and Management of Asthma [NIH Publication No. 97-4051]. Bethesda, MD: National Heart Lung and Blood Institute, 1997.

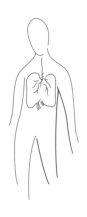

18

INTERSTITIAL AND INFILTRATIVE LUNG DISEASE

Bonnie S. Slovis • Kenneth L. Brigham

Interstitial lung disease (ILD) is the term used to describe a group of diseases characterized by diffuse lung injury and inflammation that frequently progresses to irreversible fibrosis and severely compromised gas exchange. These diseases may be classified according to the predominant location of the inflammation as bronchiolitis, alveolitis, vasculitis, or any combination of the three. As is common practice, the designation ILD is used here to describe these diseases regardless of whether the primary pathologic lesion originates in the interstitium or elsewhere in lung parenchyma. Unfortunately, the origin of many of these diseases is unknown, and treatment is not always effective, so progression of irreversible pulmonary fibrosis is frequently fatal.

Pathophysiology and Clinical Manifestations

The histologic features of ILD depend on the cause of the disease, and a definitive diagnosis can only be established by pathologic examination of lung tissue. ILDs are grouped by origin, when known, and by pathologic manifestations (Table 18–1). Known causes include pneumoconiosis, hypersensitivity pneumonitis, certain drugs, and toxic gas inhalation (see Chapter 22). Other diseases with characteristic pathologic features include sarcoidosis, collagen vascular disease, pulmonary vasculitis, alveolar hemorrhage, bronchiolitis obliterans with organizing pneumonia, and some rare but clinically important diseases such as eosinophilic granuloma (part of the spectrum of histiocytosis X) and lymphangioleiomyomatosis. Idiopathic pulmonary fibrosis, a disease of unknown origin, can be classified into types using pathologic criteria. A few cases cluster in families, a feature that suggests a genetic predisposition.

A careful and detailed history of the type and degree of environmental exposures, of the timing of symptoms

relative to exposures, occupations, and drug use, and of the symptoms of collagen vascular disease is essential in patients suspected of having ILD. Findings on physical examination depend on the degree of pathologic and physiologic abnormalities as well as on the underlying disease; typical findings include tachypnea, fine inspiratory crackles, and clubbing. Patients with sarcoidosis may have skin lesions, lacrimal and salivary gland enlargement, cranial nerve abnormalities, or hepatomegaly from involvement of the liver by infiltrating granulomas. Arthritis, alopecia, rash, or other evidence of rheumatologic disease is commonly apparent when ILD is caused by those diseases.

Most patients who present with ILD have cough and dyspnea. Characteristic abnormalities on pulmonary function tests include decreased total lung capacity (restriction) and decreased diffusing capacity. As the disease progresses, these abnormalities become more severe. Depending on the cause of the disorder, some patients may have evidence of air flow obstruction as well. With progressive fibrosis, the patient has loss of alveolar and pulmonary capillary bed surface area, ventilation-perfusion mismatch, and hypoxia. Early in the course of the disease, hypoxia occurs only with exercise, but as the disease progresses, hypoxia is present at rest, and these patients eventually require supplemental oxygen. Tachypnea is common and hypercapnia is uncommon in ILD.

The presence of ILD may be established clinically with the appropriate history, physical findings, and laboratory data; however, in most cases, pathologic examination of biopsy tissue is required for a definitive diagnosis. In some diseases such as sarcoidosis, transbronchial biopsy may provide sufficient tissue for diagnosis, but other diseases require thoracoscopic or open-lung biopsy. Idiopathic pulmonary fibrosis is a diagnosis of exclusion. Because this disease usually does not respond well to therapy, surgical lung biopsy is usually performed to rule out treatable disorders. Biopsy is most

TABLE 18-1 **Manifestations of Interstitial Lung Disease**

Disease	Physical Examination	Radiographs	Laboratory	Histology
Pneumonconioses Coal worker's Asbestos Silica Beryllium	Variable: Normal Crackles Clubbing	Diffuse reticulonodular infiltrates Large nodules Eggshell calcification of hilar nodes Pleural plaques	Nonspecific except beryllium: lymphocyte transformation test Obstructive and/or restrictive PFTs	Fibrosis Coal: anthracotic pigment Silicas: inflammation, birefringent crystals, alveolar proteinosis Asbestos: mesothelioma
Hypersensitivity pneumonitis	Fever Cough Crackles	Waxing and waning reticulonodular infiltrates Fibrosis	Serum precipitans to specific proteins Obstructive and/or restrictive PFTs	Obliterative bronchiolitis without granulomas Desquamative interstitial pneumonitis and diffuse alveolar damage
IPF DIP/RBILD	Variable: Normal Crackles Clubbing	Normal to end-stage honeycombing Abnormalities usually diffuse	Nonspecific Restrictive PFTs	Diffuse or patchy, intra-alveolar macrophages
UIP AIP NSIP				Patchy, fibroblasts, fibrosis Uniform, fibroblasts, no fibrosis Patchy or diffuse, prominent interstitial inflammation, fibrosis
Collagen vascular	Findings of collagen vascular disease Crackles Pleural rub	Pleural effusions Diffuse interstitial infiltrates Nodular infiltrates Occasional cavities	Serologies for specific disease Occasionally obstructive, usually restrictive PFTs	Interstitial inflammation Vasculitis Bronchiolar obstruction Organizing pneumonia Fibrosis
Drug-induced	Fever Crackles Pleural rub	Fibrosis Migratory infiltrates Diffuse interstitial infiltrates Pulmonary edema	Restrictive PFTs Anti-RNP antibodies	Alveolar macrophages with lamellar bodies in amiodarone Interstitial inflammation Fibrosis Eosinophilic infiltration
Sarcoid	Fever Malaise Weight loss Erythema nodosum Lupus pernio and skin plaques Salivary and lacrimal gland enlargement Iritis, uveitis, chorioretinitis, keratoconjunctivitis Cranial nerve palsies Arthritis Occasional rales or wheezes	Reticulonodular infiltrates Nodules Hilar adenopathy Mediastinal adenopathy Fibrosis	Lymphocytic bronchoalveolar lavage T8>T4 subsets Obstructive and/or restrictive PFTs Elevated transaminases with liver involvement Occasional hypercalcemia	Noncaseating granuloma with giant cells and negative acid-fast bacilli and fungal stains Fibrosis
Radiation	Crackles Fever	Focal interstitial infiltrates corresponding to radiation port Occasional diffuse infiltrates Fibrosis	None	Acute: endothelial and alveolar lining cell damage Chronic: fibrosis
Eosinophilic granuloma	None to cough Dyspnea Chest pain Fatigue Weight loss Occasionally fever	Spontaneous pneumothorax Nodules Reticulonodular infiltrates Middle and upper lobe predominance Honeycombing Sparing of costophrenic angle Cysts and nodules on HRCT	Normal lung volumes with decreased DLCO	OKT-6 (CD1) and S-100 positive immunostaining Few eosinophils Peribronchilolar inflammation Macrophages filling lumen of bronchioles and intraluminal fibrosis

Table continued on following page

TABLE 18-1 **Manifestations of Interstitial Lung Disease** *Continued*

Disease	Physical Examination	Radiographs	Laboratory	Histology
Lymphangio-leiomyomatosis	Dyspnea Cough Chest pain Decreased breath sounds or rales Hemoptysis Ascites	Spontaneous pneumo-thorax Pleural effusions Reticulonodular infiltrate Miliary pattern Honeycombing Hyperinflation Diffuse, small thin-walled systs on HRCT	Obstructive and/or restrictive PFTs Chylous pleural effusions Chylous ascites	HMB-45 positive immunostaining Atypical smooth muscle cell proliferation around broncho-vascular bundles
Bronchiolitis obliterans with organizing pneumonia	Fever Chills Malaise Fatigue Cough Dyspnea on exertion Weight loss	Peripheral patchy infiltrates, occasionally migratory CT scan: patchy consolidation, ground-glass opacities, small nodules	Restrictive and, in smokers, occasionally obstructive PFTs	Patchy peribronchiolar distribution Foamy macrophages in alveolar spaces Intraluminal buds of granulation tissue

CT = computed tomography; HRCT = high-resolution computed tomography; PFTs = pulmonary function tests.

informative early in disease, before end-stage fibrosis develops. In patients with severe radiographic fibrosis and pulmonary function test abnormalities, the disease may be sufficiently advanced to make surgical biopsy of no value.

TABLE 18-2 **Clinical Manifestations of Sarcoidosis**

Organ Systems	
Pulmonary	Dyspnea, cough, wheezing, hemoptysis, laryngeal, and endobronchial lesions
Dermatologic	Erythema nodosum, papules, plaques
Ocular	Uveitis, chorioretinitis, keratoconjunctivitis, lacrimal gland enlargement, optic neuritis
Neurologic	Cranial nerve palsy, headache, diabetes insipidus, mass lesions, seizures, meningitis, encephalitis
Rheumatologic	Arthralgias, arthropathy, myopathy
Gastrointestinal	Elevated transaminases, abdominal pain, jaundice
Cardiologic	Arrhythmias, conduction abnormalities, congestive heart failure
Hematologic	Lymphadenopathy (especially hilar), hypersplenism
Endocrine	Hypercalcemia, hypercalciuria, epididymitis, parotitis
Renal	Renal failure, renal calculi
Syndromes	
Löfgren's syndrome	Fever, arthralgias, bilateral hilar adenopathy, erythema nodosum
Heerfordt's syndrome (uveoparotid fever)	Fever, swelling of parotid gland and uveal tracts, cranial nerve VII palsy

SARCOIDOSIS

Sarcoidosis is a well-characterized systemic disease, the origin of which remains elusive despite years of intense research. It is characterized pathologically by noncaseating epithelioid granulomas that contain giant cells. As a systemic disease, it may affect any organ system (Table 18–2), but it commonly affects the lungs and lymph nodes. Skin manifestations are common, and patients with hilar adenopathy and erythema nodosum alone usually have less severe disease than those with parenchymal lung involvement and other extrapulmonary manifestations. Sarcoidosis occurs most commonly in adults 20 to 40 years old and is slightly more common in women than in men. In the United States, African-Americans are more commonly affected, but the disease is also prevalent in Scandinavian countries. Infectious, allergic, and environmental exposures have all been proposed as triggers of the disease in patients with a genetic susceptibility, but neither genetic factors nor specific triggers have been established.

Sarcoidosis has distinct immunologic features. Circulating CD4+ lymphocytes are decreased, and CD4+ cells obtained from bronchoalveolar lavage are increased. Findings include variable cutaneous anergy, increased concentrations of interleukin-1 and tumor necrosis factor in bronchoalveolar lavage fluid, decreased numbers of circulating B lymphocytes, and increased serum concentrations of polyclonal immunoglobulins. All these findings indicate activation of the immune system.

Symptoms of sarcoidosis reflect the organ systems involved. The most common presenting complaints are cough and dyspnea. Fatigue and low-grade fever are less common, but even high fevers can occur on occasion. Skin manifestations include erythema nodosum, plaques, nodules, and lupus pernio. Ocular symptoms are also common. The triad of uveitis, parotitis, and facial nerve palsy, called *uveoparotid fever*, is known as Heerfordt's

TABLE 18-3 Radiographic Staging of Sarcoidosis

Stage	Radiographic Findings
0	Normal radiograph
1	Adenopathy without parenchymal abnormality
2A	Adenopathy and parenchymal disease
2B	Parenchymal disease without adenopathy
3	Fibrosis and honeycombing

syndrome. Löfgren's syndrome is the constellation of erythema nodosum, arthralgias, and hilar adenopathy. Both syndromes are associated with better outcomes than are other clinical presentations of sarcoidosis. Liver granulomas are common but infrequently cause clinically significant liver disease. Less common but serious complications of sarcoidosis include cardiac and neurologic involvement. Hypercalcuria and hypercalcemia are thought to be due to increased intestinal absorption and increased conversion of vitamin D to its active form in sarcoid granulomas.

The diagnosis of sarcoidosis is made by the combination of clinical and histologic data. The presence of noncaseating granuloma, in the absence of positive stains or culture for infectious origin, supports the diagnosis. Transbronchial biopsy specimens are positive in 50% to 60% of patients with normal parenchyma on chest radiographs and in 85% to 90% of those with parenchymal abnormalities. Lymph node biopsies are performed if results of transbronchial biopsy are negative or if lymphoma is high on the list of differential diagnosis. A radiographic staging system for sarcoidosis has been created, but it does not correlate well with the clinical course of the disease (Table 18-3).

Although systemic administration of corticosteroids is accepted therapy for sarcoidosis, such therapy has not been proven to affect long-term prognosis. Roughly one third of patients with sarcoidosis have a spontaneous remission within 3 years of onset, one third remain stable, and one third have progression of their disease,

with about 10% progressing to severe pulmonary fibrosis. Treatment with corticosteroids is frequently withheld because the adverse side effects of prolonged steroid therapy can be worse than the effects of the disease. In patients who are asymptomatic and who have mild radiographic or pulmonary function abnormalities, close follow-up with repeat radiographs and pulmonary function testing is warranted. Indications for the use of corticosteroids are listed in Table 18-4. Other immunosuppressant agents are also used, and although they are associated with fewer side effects, they are also less efficacious. These agents, in combination with low-dose corticosteroids, are sometimes used for maintenance therapy to permit administration of lower doses of corticosteroids.

HYPERSENSITIVITY PNEUMONITIS

Hypersensitivity pneumonitis, or extrinsic allergic alveolitis, is an immunologically mediated disease that results from repeated inhalation and sensitization to certain organic dusts (Table 18-5). Acute, subacute, and chronic forms of the disease may occur, depending on the intensity and duration of exposure to the offending agent. In the acute form, intense exposure to the antigen is followed after 4 to 6 hours by cough, dyspnea, fever, chills, and malaise lasting for 18 to 24 hours. Subacute manifestations differ only in the severity of symptoms and have a more insidious onset. The chronic form of the disease results in progressive fibrosis and restrictive lung disease. The disease should be diagnosed early, to prevent exposure to the offending agent and to halt the progression of lung damage. Diffuse crackles are the predominant physical finding. Chest radiographic findings are variable and nonspecific. Hypersensitivity pneumonitis is in the differential diagnosis of any patient with restrictive lung disease, but this diagnosis should be highly suspected in patients with respiratory symptoms that worsen in certain environments, such as on returning to work after a weekend or vacation.

A presumptive diagnosis of extrinsic allergic alveolitis can be made on clinical grounds in the appropriate

TABLE 18-4 Indications for Use of Corticosteroids in Sarcoidosis

Disorder	Treatment
Iridocyclitis	Corticosteroid eye drops Local subconjunctival deposit of cortisone
Posterior uveitis	Oral prednisone
Pulmonary involvement	Steroids rarely recommended for stage I; usually employed if infiltrate remains static or worsens over 3-month period or the patient is symptomatic
Upper airway obstruction	Rare indication for intravenous steroids
Lupus pernio	Oral prednisone shrinks the disfiguring lesions
Hypercalcemia	Responds well to corticosteroids
Cardiac involvement	Corticosteroids usually recommended if patient has arrhythmias or conduction disturbances
CNS involvement	Response is best in patients with acute symptoms
Lacrimal/salivary gland involvement	Corticosteroids recommended for disordered function, *not* gland swelling
Bone cysts	Corticosteroids recommended if symptomatic

CNS = central nervous system.

TABLE 18-5 Hypersensitivity Pneumonitis

Antigen	Source	Disease Examples
Thermophilic bacteria	Moldy hay, sugar cane, compost	Farmer's lung, bagassosis, mushroom worker's disease
Other bacteria	Contaminated water, wood dust, fertilizer, paprika dust	Humidifier, detergent worker's, and familial hypersensitivity pneumonitis
Fungi	Moldy cork, contaminated wood dust, barley, maple logs	Suberosis, sequoiosis, and maple bark strippers, malt workers, and paprika splitter's lung
Animal protein	Bird droppings, animal urine, bovine and porcine pituitary powder	Pigeon breeder's lung, duck fever, turkey handler's disease, pituitary snuff taker's disease, laboratory worker's hypersensitivity pneumonitis
Chemically altered human proteins (albumin and others)	Toluene diisocyanate Trimellitic anhydride Diphenylmethane diisocyanate	Hypersensitivity pneumonitis
Phthalic anhydride	Heated epoxy resin	Epoxy resin lung

setting. Most patients with hypersensitivity pneumonitis have precipitating antibodies to the offending antigen, but serum precipitins also develop in 40% to 50% of asymptomatic persons with the same exposure. On occasion, environmental or laboratory challenge with the suspected antigen is repeated in specialized settings.

Effective treatment requires eliminating exposure to the offending antigen. Systemic corticosteroids can relieve symptoms in the acute phase. Although the efficacy of these agents in the chronic form of the disease is less clear, a trial of corticosteroids is usually given.

DRUG-INDUCED INTERSTITIAL LUNG DISEASE

Several drugs that can cause diffuse ILD either by direct injury of the lungs or by triggering a hypersensitivity response are listed in Table 18–6. Bleomycin causes dose-related cytotoxicity, which occurs in most patients who receive a cumulative dose of more than 450 U. The risk of bleomycin toxicity is increased in patients receiving radiation therapy, and high inspired oxygen concentrations can precipitate lung toxicity in patients previously treated with bleomycin, sometimes months after the previous dose. Other chemotherapeutic agents such as methotrexate are thought to produce hypersensitivity pneumonitis, although rechallenge with methotrexate after the pneumonitis has resolved may not provoke a recurrence.

Nitrofurantoin can produce hypersensitivity pneumonitis that may progress to chronic fibrosis if the reaction is not recognized and the drug is not discontinued. The antiarrhythmic drug amiodarone causes acute and chronic alveolar and interstitial disease. Amiodarone pulmonary toxicity is more common in patients taking 400 mg/day or more, although lower doses may also be toxic. Many drugs can cause a drug-induced lupus syndrome with pleural effusions and interstitial and alveolar infiltrates; the classic example is procainamide.

COLLAGEN VASCULAR DISEASE

Most collagen vascular diseases can involve the lungs. Well-described pulmonary manifestations occur in rheumatoid arthritis, systemic lupus erythematosus (SLE), and scleroderma, but pulmonary involvement may also occur in mixed connective tissue disease, Sjögren's disease, polymyositis, and dermatomyositis. Rheumatoid arthritis most commonly causes pleural effusions, but diffuse ILD, pulmonary hypertension, and pulmonary nodules are also seen. Pleural effusions and pneumonitis may occur in patients with SLE, Sjögren's disease, polymyositis, and dermatomyositis. Pulmonary hypertension is associated with scleroderma and SLE. Scleroderma also causes pneumonitis and pulmonary fibrosis. Patients receive supportive care, and, in addition, lung manifestations of these diseases are treated as part of the underlying disease. Although pulmonary fibrosis in these diseases is irreversible, studies using prostacyclin in pulmonary hypertension associated with collagen vascular diseases have been promising.

PULMONARY VASCULITIS

Vasculitides that involve the lung include granulomatous vasculitis, such as Wegener's granulomatosis, allergic granulomatosis and angiitis (Churg-Strauss syndrome), and an angiocentric T-cell lymphoma called lymphomatoid granulomatosis. Wegener's granulomatosis is characterized by alveolar hemorrhage, pulmonary infiltrates, lung nodules that may cavitate, and sinus involvement; eye, skin, and nervous system lesions may also occur. Classically, Wegener's granulomatosis is accompanied by glomerulonephritis, but a limited form involves the respiratory tract alone. Serologic testing is positive for the cytoplasmic antineutrophilic cytoplasmic antibody in 90% of patients, but it is not specific. A definitive diagnosis requires adequate tissue biopsy of either lung or kidney. A rapid diagnosis is essential because the disease is often fatal without therapy and usually responds to high-dose corticosteroids and cyclophosphamide. The granulomas in allergic granulomatosis and angiitis are eosinophilic, and the disease is accompanied by severe asthma and peripheral eosinophilia. Most patients with this disease respond well to corticosteroids. Pulmonary vasculitis and alveolar hemorrhage may be caused by any of the collagen vascular diseases that involve the

TABLE 18–6   Common Drug-Induced Lung Disease

Drug	Dose Relation	Manifestation
Chemotherapeutic		
Bleomycin	Acute/chronic, >450 U increased risk	Pneumonitis, fibrosis, BOOP
Busulfan	Chronic	Fibrosis, alveolar proteinosis
Cyclophosphamide	Chronic	Fibrosis, BOOP
Cytosine arabinoside	Acute	Pulmonary edema, ARDS
Methotrexate	Acute/chronic	Hypersensitivity pneumonitis, resolves with discontinuation, BOOP
Mitomycin C	Acute/delayed	Pneumonitis, ARDS, BOOP hemolytic uremic syndrome
Antimicrobial		
Nitrofurantoin	Acute/chronic	Acute pneumonitis, fibrosis
Sulfasalazine	Acute/chronic	Pulmonary infiltrate with eosinophilia/BOOP
Cardiovascular		
Amiodarone	Acute/chronic, >400 mg/day	Pneumonitis, fibrosis
Flecainide	Acute	ARDS, LIP
Tocainide	Weeks/months	Pneumonitis
Procainamide	Subacute/chronic	Drug-induced systemic lupus erythematosus, pleural effusions, infiltrates
Anti-inflammatory		
Aspirin	Acute	Pulmonary edema, bronchospasm
Illicit		
Opiates	Acute	Pulmonary edema
Cocaine	Acute	Pulmonary edema, diffuse alveolar damage, pulmonary hemorrhage, BOOP
Talc (in IV and inhaled illicit drugs)	Acute/chronic	Granulomatous interstitial fibrosis, granulomatous pulmonary artery occlusion, particulate embolization
Tocolytics		
Terbutaline, albuterol, ritodrine	Acute	Pulmonary edema

ARDS = acute respiratory distress syndrome; BOOP = bronchiolitis obliterans with organizing pneumonia; LIP = lymphoid interstitial pneumonia.

lungs, most commonly SLE. Hypersensitivity vasculitis occasionally involves pulmonary vessels.

DIFFUSE ALVEOLAR HEMORRHAGE

Diffuse alveolar hemorrhage may occur with or without the histologic finding of inflammation at the capillary level (pulmonary capillaritis). Some well-known causes of alveolar capillaritis include the systemic vasculitides, collagen vascular diseases, antiglomerular basement membrane antibody syndrome (Goodpasture's syndrome), and Henoch-Schönlein purpura. Both Goodpasture's syndrome and SLE can cause alveolar hemorrhage with or without associated capillaritis.

Goodpasture's syndrome is diffuse alveolar hemorrhage associated with glomerulonephritis caused by an antiglomerular basement membrane antibody that also has affinity for lung basement membrane components. The treatment of Goodpasture's syndrome is plasmapheresis and immunosuppression; untreated, the disease is fatal.

Idiopathic pulmonary hemorrhage or hemosiderosis is a diagnosis of exclusion. Patients with this syndrome have recurrent diffuse alveolar hemorrhage without associated renal or systemic disease. Histologically, the lungs show alveolar hemorrhage and hemosiderin accumulation without associated inflammation. Treatment includes supportive care, immunosuppression, and occasionally plasmapheresis, but response to therapy is variable. This syndrome is more common in children, who have a worse prognosis than do adults. The disease resolves in 25% of adults, but in the remaining 75% of cases, mean survival is 3 to 5 years from the time of diagnosis.

PULMONARY INFILTRATES WITH EOSINOPHILIA

Simple pulmonary eosinophilia (Löffler's syndrome) is usually a mild disease associated with transient or migratory pulmonary infiltrates and blood eosinophilia. The disease is usually caused by *Ascaris* infestation, but it is also seen in infestation with other parasites including *Entamoeba histolytica* and *Strongyloides stercoralis*. Tropical pulmonary eosinophilia is most common in Asia, Africa, and South America and is usually caused by *Wuchereria bancrofti*. Drug-induced eosinophilia, including pulmonary infiltrates, can be caused by a host of agents in common clinical use. Allergic bronchopulmonary aspergillosis is an allergic response to *Aspergillus* antigens in the lungs and does not require invasive *Aspergillus* infection. The clinical presentation includes asthma, migratory pulmonary infiltrates, peripheral eosinophilia, and, occasionally, bronchiectasis and expectoration of mucus plugs. Skin testing with *Aspergillus* antigen, elevated serum IgE, and *Aspergillus* precipitins in serum support the diagnosis. Symptoms respond to oral corticosteroids. Studies evaluating the effectiveness of treatment with itraconazole are under way. Chronic eosinophilic pneumonia is a disease of unknown origin that is associated with peripheral eosinophilia and pulmonary infiltrates. Predominant involvement of the lung periphery creates the classic radiographic finding described as a "photographic negative of pulmonary edema." The disease responds rapidly to oral corticosteroids, but relapse occurs if steroids are withdrawn too rapidly. Acute eosinophilic pneumonia is a similar illness, except the onset is more rapid and the initial pneumonia often progresses to involve most of the lung, to cause respiratory failure (acute respiratory distress syndrome). This disease responds rapidly to systemic corticosteroids, and relapse does not occur when these drugs are withdrawn.

IDIOPATHIC PULMONARY FIBROSIS

Idiopathic pulmonary fibrosis is a progressive ILD of unknown origin. The classification of this disease is based on histologic characteristics and has been revised. Giant cell pneumonitis and lymphoid interstitial pneumonitis have been removed from the prior classification because they are usually not idiopathic. The revised classification consists of four categories: (1) usual interstitial pneumonia, (2) desquamative interstitial pneumonia/respiratory bronchiolitis with ILD, (3) acute interstitial pneumonia (Hamman-Rich disease), and (4) nonspecific interstitial pneumonia. Subdividing idiopathic pulmonary fibrosis into these categories requires pathologic examination of an adequate sample of lung tissue, which can only be obtained by thoracoscopic or open-lung biopsy, and this method is also the most conclusive way to rule out other known causes of pulmonary fibrosis. Although the time course of idiopathic pulmonary fibrosis is variable, in most patients the disease progresses to end-stage fibrosis and death in spite of therapy. The exception is desquamative interstitial pneumonia, which usually resolves after treatment with systemic corticosteroids. For this reason, patients with idiopathic pulmonary fibrosis are usually treated with high-dose steroids and are monitored for clinical response.

RARE INTERSTITIAL LUNG DISEASES

Pulmonary eosinophilic granuloma is the pulmonary form of histiocytosis X, a disease characterized by proliferation of Langerhans' cells. The radiographic findings are diffuse, reticular, nodular, or reticulonodular infiltrates predominantly in the middle and upper lung fields. Unlike patients with most ILDs, patients with pulmonary eosinophilic granuloma have normal lung volumes. The disease is associated with smoking and has a highly variable course, frequently with spontaneous remission. Patients are at increased risk of spontaneous and often recurrent pneumothoraces.

Lymphangioleiomyomatosis is a disease of premenopausal women that is characterized by proliferation of smooth muscle in the walls of the pulmonary lymphatics and venules and causes obstruction and ILD. Lymphangioleiomyomatosis may produce chylous pleural effusions and alveolar hemorrhage and is a progressive, fatal disease. Because it occurs in premenopausal women and is accelerated during pregnancy, and because the pathologic cells resemble uterine muscle cells, hormonal manipulation has been used as therapy but without much success.

Pulmonary alveolar proteinosis is a disorder in which the alveoli fill with protein and phospholipid material similar to surfactant. The origin of pulmonary alveolar proteinosis is unknown, but it is thought to result from an unknown inhaled insult. In healthy lungs, surfactant is cleared by macrophages. Material like that found in pulmonary alveolar proteinosis is seen in the alveoli of patients with acute silicosis, a situation in which macrophage function is known to be inhibited. Investigators have postulated that the basic defect in pulmonary alveolar proteinosis is the inability of macrophages to clear surfactant. A genetically engineered mouse that does not express the gene that encodes granulocyte-monocyte colony-stimulating factor (GM-CSF) has been found to develop pulmonary alveolar proteinosis, and studies of therapy with this factor in patients with pulmonary alveolar proteinosis are currently under way. Traditionally, these patients have been treated by bilateral whole-lung lavage to "wash out" the abnormal material filling alveoli. This intervention dramatically improves oxygenation in the short term, but the course of the disease is variable. In some patients, the disease resolves after only one lavage, whereas in others, the disease progresses to severe fibrosis in spite of repeated lavage.

Bronchiolitis obliterans with organizing pneumonia is thought to be a response to lung injury resulting from infection, inhaled toxin, or autoimmune disease. The characteristic pathologic findings in this disease include filling of the lumen of distal bronchioles with inflammatory cells and fibrous tissue accompanied by an adjacent alveolitis. The disease is patchy, with the pathologic lesion and normal lung tissue often juxtaposed. Radiologically, bronchiolitis obliterans with organizing pneumonia may produce a single lesion suggesting neoplasm, a diffuse infiltrate, or scattered nodular infiltrates. The disease responds well to oral corticosteroids, and it usually does not cause permanent lung fibrosis.

REFERENCES

Katzenstein AL, Myers JL: Idiopathic pulmonary fibrosis: Clinical relevance of pathologic classification. Am J Respir Crit Care Med 1998; 157:1301–1315.

Raghu G: Interstitial lung disease: A diagnostic approach. Are CT scan and lung biopsy indicated in every patient? Am J Respir Crit Care Med 1995; 161:909.

Schwarz MI, King TE Jr: Interstitial Lung Disease, 2nd ed. Philadelphia: Mosby–Year Book, 1993.

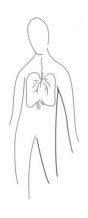

19

DISORDERS OF THE PLEURAL SPACE, MEDIASTINUM, AND CHEST WALL

Bonnie S. Slovis • Kenneth L. Brigham

Pleural Disease

PHYSIOLOGY OF THE PLEURAL SPACE

The *pleural spaces* are defined by the thin visceral pleura covering the lungs and the parietal pleura lining the chest wall, diaphragm, and mediastinum. The pleural spaces are potential spaces and normally contain only a thin film of fluid.

The elastic recoil of the lung exerts an inward force, and the chest wall exerts an outward force, so the net pressure in the pleural space when those forces are in balance (i.e., the lung is at functional residual capacity) is slightly less than atmospheric pressure. Fluid normally enters the space from the visceral pleura and is absorbed by the parietal pleura. Under normal conditions, the amount of fluid entering and exiting the pleural space is equal, so, despite a turnover of 5 to 10 L/day, fluid does not accumulate.

Fluid accumulates in the pleural space *(pleural effusion)* when the dynamics are altered by changes in hydrostatic or osmotic pressures, by increased permeability of pleural capillaries, or by lymphatic obstruction. Visceral pleural vessels are supplied from the pulmonary circulation, and parietal pleural vessels are part of the systemic circulation, so elevated pulmonary venous pressure increases the entry of fluid into the pleural space, and increased systemic venous pressure decreases absorption from the space. Pleural inflammation increases the permeability of pleural vessels and causes excessive fluid to enter the space for a given driving force. In addition, protein concentration in the fluid increases and creates an increased oncotic force with fluid accumula-

tion. Hypoalbuminemia decreases intravascular oncotic pressure and thus favors sequestration of fluid in extravascular spaces, including the pleural space. Because the lymphatic system is an important exit route for pleural fluid, central lymphatic obstruction or obstruction of channels at the pleural surface by tumor or exudate decreases pleural fluid absorption.

PLEURAL EFFUSIONS

Clinically, classification of pleural effusions on the basis of the characteristics of the fluid that reflect the underlying pathophysiologic features is useful. *Transudative effusions* result from increases in vascular hydrostatic pressure or decreases in plasma oncotic pressure. *Exudative effusions* result from increases in vascular permeability, from trauma, or, rarely, from abnormal communications between the pleural space and other structures such as the pancreas, esophagus, peritoneal space, or lung parenchyma (Table 19–1).

Patients with pleural effusions may present with dyspnea or chest pain, but they may be asymptomatic. The severity of symptoms depends on the underlying cause, size, and rate of accumulation of the effusion. Pleuritic chest pain is classically described as sharp and is exacerbated by coughing or deep breathing.

Physical signs of pleural effusion include dullness to percussion and decreased breath sounds over the effusion, decreased vocal fremitus, and bronchial breathing and egophony at the superior edge of the effusion resulting from lung compression. The sign of a pleural effusion on a chest radiograph taken with the patient in the upright position is apparent elevation of the hemidiaphragm caused by accumulation of fluid between the

TABLE 19–1 Pleural Effusions

Transudates

Congestive heart failure
Hypoalbuminemia
   Nephrotic syndrome
   Malnutrition
   Cirrhosis
Intra-abdominal fluid
   Ascites
   Peritoneal dialysis

Exudates

Infection
   Empyema
   Parapneumonic
Malignancy
   Primary lung cancer
   Lymphoma
   Metastatic cancer
Pulmonary embolism and infarction
Collagen vascular disease
   Systemic lupus erythematosus
   Rheumatoid arthritis
Intra-abdominal pathology
   Pancreatitis
   Subphrenic abscess
   Complication of abdominal surgery
   Meigs' syndrome
   Urinothorax
Trauma
   Hemothorax
   Chylothorax
   Ruptured esophagus
Miscellaneous
   Myxedema
   Uremia
   Asbestosis
   Lymphedema
   Drug-induced lupus
   Dressler's syndrome

From Light RW, Macgregor MI, Luchsinger PC, et al: Pleural effusions: The diagnostic separation of transudates and exudates. Ann Intern Med 1972; 77:507–513.

lung and the diaphragmatic surface. When the volume of fluid exceeds 250 mL, the costophrenic angle is blunted. Increasing amounts of fluid cause opacification of the lower thorax with a concave meniscus. Massive volumes of fluid may opacify the entire hemithorax and may compress the lung. These typical signs may not be present, and additional testing may be necessary to document and define the extent and location of pleural fluid. A lateral decubitus radiograph determines whether the effusion is free flowing, aids in estimating the volume, and possibly uncovers a subpulmonic effusion as the cause of an elevated hemidiaphragm. Ultrasonography and computed tomography of the chest are useful in evaluating loculated effusions, in patients who are unable to tolerate upright radiography, and in patients with coexisting parenchymal or pleural disease.

In any clinical situation in which pleural effusion is present and the cause is not known, thoracentesis and analysis of the fluid are essential. The gross appearance of the fluid is only helpful when the composition of the fluid is predominantly pus, chyle, or blood. If the fluid looks like blood, then the hematocrit will distinguish between hemothorax (bleeding into the pleural space) and hemorrhagic effusion.

Table 19–2 gives the laboratory criteria for classifying pleural effusions as transudate or exudate. Although not foolproof, these criteria are extremely helpful in limiting the differential diagnosis. Some characteristics of pleural fluid suggest specific diagnoses, such as the following: (1) a pH less than 7.0 suggests esophageal rupture or rheumatoid effusion; (2) glucose concentrations of less than 20 mg/dL are seen in rheumatoid arthritis and less commonly in malignant disease or infection; (3) bloody effusions occur in patients with malignant disease, trauma, pulmonary embolus, and collagen vascular disease; (4) frank pus defines an empyema, and organisms on Gram's stain or in culture define a pleural space infection; (5) eosinophils are found with blood or air in the pleural space; and (6) cytologic examination for malignant cells is positive in about 60% of malignant effusions on first thoracentesis, and positive results of cytologic examination rise to 80% if three separate samples are obtained. Gram's stain and routine bacterial and acid-fast cultures should always be performed, and fungal cultures should be added when fungal disease is suspected.

Transcutaneous needle biopsy of the parietal pleura can be performed as a bedside procedure, but this technique requires the presence of significant amounts of fluid, so the decision to perform this procedure should precede removal of most of the effusion by thoracentesis. Pleural biopsies are positive for acid-fast bacilli in more than 50% of tuberculous effusions, whereas fluid culture is positive in only 25%. Blind pleural biopsy can occasionally enable the clinician to make a diagnosis of malignancy when pleural fluid is negative. Visually directed thoracoscopic biopsy has the highest yield and should be performed if less invasive tests do not establish the cause of an exudative effusion. Exudative effusions may require chest tube drainage or serial thoracenteses to prevent loculation, draining cutaneous

TABLE 19–2 Differentiation of Exudative and Transudative Pleural Effusion

	Exudate	Transudate
Protein	>3 g/dL	<3 g/dL
Pleural/serum protein	>0.5	<0.5
LDH	2/3 upper limit of normal	2/3 upper limit of normal
Pleural/serum LDH	>0.6	<0.6

LDH = lactate dehydrogenase.
Adapted from Light RW, Macgregor MI, Luchsinger PC, et al: Pleural effusions: The diagnostic separation of transudates and exudates. Ann Intern Med 1972; 77:507–513.

fistulas *(empyema necessitans),* lung abscess, and bronchopleural fistula.

Treatment of pleural effusions depends on the cause and on the degree of impairment of lung function. When possible, the underlying cause of the effusion should be treated specifically. Transudative effusions seldom require drainage, and they will resolve without consequence if the underlying abnormality is corrected. Exudative effusions, on the other hand, may or may not require drainage. Removing the effusion by thoracentesis or by chest tube drainage may improve the patient's symptoms even when no improvements in lung function or gas exchange can be measured. Sterile parapneumonic effusions resolve with antibiotic therapy of the underlying pneumonia. *Empyemas,* defined as pus in the pleural space or exudative fluid with a positive Gram stain or culture, should be drained, usually by a large thoracostomy tube. Antibiotic therapy alone is rarely successful in resolving these effusions, and delay in drainage may result in significant residual pleural disease requiring thoracotomy and pleurectomy. The best palliative therapy of malignant effusions is treatment of the underlying malignant disease. Life expectancy of patients with malignant pleural effusions resulting from lung cancer is about 12 weeks. Serial thoracenteses have been discouraged because they cause protein wasting. Thoracostomy tube drainage and chemical pleurodesis may reduce the recurrence of malignant effusions, but these procedures are painful and require several days in the hospital. Outpatient continuous catheter drainage has been advocated for patients who have symptomatic improvement with large-volume thoracentesis and in whom the fluid reaccumulates rapidly.

PNEUMOTHORAX

Spontaneous pneumothorax is associated with Marfan's syndrome, but it is most commonly idiopathic and occurs in young people without any known predisposition. Classic symptoms are sudden onset of dyspnea and sharp chest pain. The diagnosis is made radiographically, and without either surgical or chemical pleurodesis, 50% of these pneumothoraces recur within 2 years.

Tension pneumothorax is the accumulation of air under positive pressure in the pleural space. Because tension pneumothorax can cause hemodynamic collapse, it is a medical emergency that requires immediate decompression. Treatment of a pneumothorax when tension is not present depends on the amount of air and on the underlying cardiorespiratory status of the patient, and it also depends on whether the patient is being ventilated mechanically. Every patient with a pneumothorax who is being mechanically ventilated requires a chest tube because of the risk of tension physiology in these patients. In the absence of mechanical ventilation, small pneumothoraces may resolve without intervention. Occasionally, needle drainage can be performed without reaccumulation, and in other situations, small-bore catheters placed percutaneously may suffice. In patients with recurrent pneumothoraces and in those with emphysema or pleural blebs, thoracoscopy or thoracotomy with oversewing of the blebs or wound of the pleural surface is required.

Mediastinal Disease

The *mediastinum* can be conveniently divided into three compartments based on the lateral chest radiograph (Fig. 19–1). The *anterior compartment* lies between the sternum and the heart shadow. It contains the thymus gland, the aortic arch, lymphatic tissue, and ectopic thyroid and parathyroid tissue. Masses in this compartment are most likely thymomas, ectopic or malignant thyroid or parathyroid glands, germ cell tumors, or lymphomas. The *middle mediastinum* contains the pericardial sac, the lung hila, and central and hilar lymph nodes. Masses in this compartment are commonly bronchogenic or pleuropericardial cysts, lymphomas, sarcoid, carcinomas, or granulomatous diseases, usually tuberculosis or histoplasmosis. *Mediastinal fibrosis* is a progressive accumulation of fibrous tissue in the mediastinum that encroaches on major airways and blood vessels and results in inexorably progressive airway or vascular obstruction and death. No effective therapy is available for this disease. The *posterior mediastinum* is the space just anterior to the vertebral bodies. It contains the descending aorta, the azygos venous system, the thoracic duct, lymph nodes, and the sympathetic nerve chain. Masses found in this compartment are neurogenic tumors (e.g., neurofibromas), lymphomas, esophageal tumors, and vascular aneurysms.

Chest Wall Disease

PHYSIOLOGY

Adequate ventilation depends on efficient movement of the chest wall and diaphragm in response to neural stimulation. Any disease that restricts chest wall movement or interferes with neuromuscular function may produce hypoventilation. In these diseases, the total lung capacity and vital capacity are decreased, but the residual volume is usually normal or even increased. Hypoventilation produces hypercapnea and progressive atelectasis. The decrease in vital capacity causes ventilation-perfusion inequality leading to hypoxemia.

SPECIFIC DISORDERS

Vertebral Disease

Scoliosis is an abnormal lateral curvature and decreased mobility of the vertebral column. *Kyphosis* is extreme flexion of the thoracic spine. Usually, these deformities coexist, and the resulting restriction of thoracic cavity volume may cause cardiorespiratory failure. Surgical correction of the deformity in adults does not improve respiratory function or the incidence of complications.

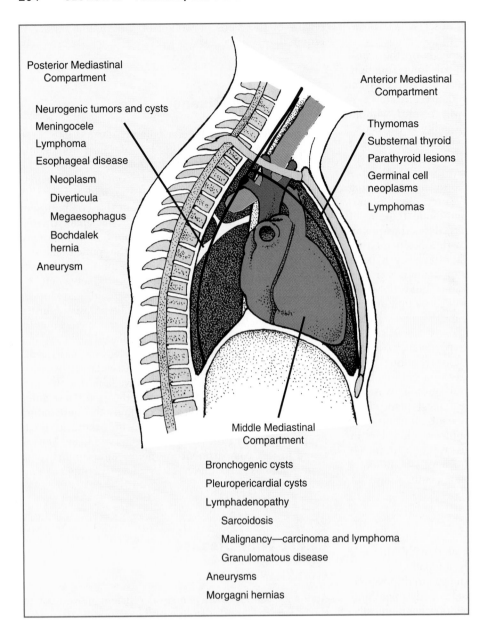

Posterior Mediastinal
Compartment

Neurogenic tumors and cysts
Meningocele
Lymphoma
Esophageal disease
   Neoplasm
   Diverticula
   Megaesophagus
   Bochdalek hernia
Aneurysm

Anterior Mediastinal
Compartment

Thymomas
Substernal thyroid
Parathyroid lesions
Germinal cell neoplasms
Lymphomas

Middle Mediastinal
Compartment

Bronchogenic cysts
Pleuropericardial cysts
Lymphadenopathy
   Sarcoidosis
   Malignancy—carcinoma and lymphoma
   Granulomatous disease
Aneurysms
Morgagni hernias

FIGURE 19–1 Masses of the mediastinum indicated by their anatomic location.

Obesity

Obesity causes a decrease in the expiratory reserve volume and decreased ventilation of basilar portions of the lungs and hypoxemia. The abnormalities are magnified when the patient is in the supine position and are frequently accompanied by disorders of ventilatory control and upper airway obstruction.

Diaphragmatic Paralysis

Unilateral diaphragmatic paralysis in the absence of other disease may affect pulmonary function minimally, and the patient may be without symptoms. Most patients retain 75% of normal vital capacity in spite of the loss of function of half the diaphragm. The supine position worsens symptoms by virtue of encroachment of abdominal contents on the thoracic cavity. Causes of

diaphragmatic paralysis include injury of the phrenic nerve by tumor invasion or compression, surgical injury, and herpes zoster or other viral neuropathy. The diagnosis of diaphragmatic paralysis is made by fluoroscopic observation of the diaphragm during a "sniff" maneuver; the affected diaphragm moves paradoxically. Definitive diagnosis is made from nerve conduction studies.

Bilateral diaphragmatic paralysis is rarely subtle. Patients are markedly dyspneic and have difficulty in sleeping in the recumbent position. Paradoxical inward motion of the abdominal wall during inspiration is a classic physical finding. Maximal inspiratory force is markedly decreased. Chest radiographs show decreased lung volumes, and this condition may occasionally be mistaken for pulmonary fibrosis because of crowding of the parenchyma and vasculature at the bases. Bilateral diaphragmatic paralysis is rarely idiopathic and usually is a manifestation of an acute or chronic generalized neuromuscular disease such as Guillain-Barré syndrome, muscular dystrophy, amyotrophic lateral sclerosis, or postpolio syndrome, a diagnosis that is frequently overlooked.

Treatment of the underlying disease rarely corrects the paralysis, so the focus must be on management of the progressive respiratory failure. Decisions to use supplemental oxygen, noninvasive positive pressure ventilation, or tracheostomy with long-term mechanical ventilation depend on the medical condition and on the patient's preference.

REFERENCES

MacNee W: Pleural Diseases, 3rd ed. Baltimore: Williams & Wilkins, 1996.

Sahn SA: The pleura. Am Rev Respir Dis 1998; 138:184.

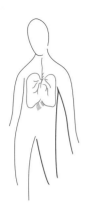

20

NEOPLASTIC DISEASES OF THE LUNG

Bonnie S. Slovis • Kenneth L. Brigham

Risk Factors

Lung cancer kills more than 120,000 Americans each year and is the leading cause of death in persons with cancer. Cigarette smoking is responsible for at least 90% of lung cancers and is the number one preventable cause of cardiopulmonary disease that results in death. The risk of lung cancer increases with dose and length of exposure to tobacco smoke and is greater in persons who begin smoking at an early age. There is also a small but significant increased risk for lung cancer in persons passively exposed to tobacco smoke. Heavy occupational asbestos exposure is the second most important cause of lung cancer, and when asbestos exposure is combined with cigarette smoking the risk is 50 times greater than in the nonsmoking, non–asbestos-exposed population.

Also related to lung cancer is exposure to uranium, arsenic, chromium, methylethers, polycyclic aromatic hydrocarbons, nickel, and possibly beryllium. Exposure to radon is associated with a dose-related increase in the risk of developing bronchogenic carcinoma. Chronic inflammatory (e.g., cystic fibrosis) and fibrosing (e.g., pulmonary fibrosis from any cause) lung diseases increase the risk for bronchogenic carcinoma, as does the acquired immunodeficiency syndrome, especially when coupled with smoking. Chronic immunosuppression after solid organ transplant places patients at risk for posttransplant lymphoproliferative disorders. This risk is associated with the degree of immunosuppression and the presence of Epstein-Barr virus infection.

Pathology

Approximately 5% of bronchogenic tumors are benign and are usually seen on routine chest radiographs. When there are symptoms, they are related to bronchial obstruction. Bronchial adenomas are the most common benign endobronchial tumor. Bronchial carcinoid tumors are usually low-grade malignancies, but they may have atypical histologic features and a more aggressive clinical course. The most common benign peripheral lung tumor is the pulmonary hamartoma, which has a characteristic "popcorn" pattern of calcification.

Primary malignant neoplasms in the lung are classified as small cell or non–small cell carcinomas. The non–small cell tumors are further divided into four histologic types—squamous cell carcinoma, adenocarcinoma, large cell or anaplastic carcinoma, and bronchoalveolar carcinoma, but these categories have little clinical significance because the treatment and prognosis are the same. Some non–small cell carcinomas are too poorly differentiated to be assigned a type or they have mixed histologic features. This may become a problem if the tumor has mixed small cell and non–small cell histology because the treatment of these cell types is different.

Primary neoplasms originating in organs other than the lungs commonly metastasize to lung parenchyma, endobronchial mucosa, chest wall, pleural space, or mediastinum. Uncommonly, primary tumors of breast, pancreas, or liver may invade the lungs by direct extension. Sarcomas as well as renal, colon, thyroid, and testicular malignancies reach the lungs by hematogenous spread. Adenocarcinomas of breast, prostate, stomach, ovary, and pancreas typically spread to the lungs by lymphangitic dissemination, appearing as an infiltrate or diffuse reticulonodular pattern on chest radiograph and causing dyspnea out of proportion to the radiographic appearance.

Clinical Presentation

The clinical presentation of patients with lung cancer depends on tumor location, tumor size, and whether there is metastatic spread or paraneoplastic manifestations. Most patients present with cough, hemoptysis, dyspnea, or postobstructive pneumonia. Chest pain usually signifies chest wall or neurologic invasion or malignant pleural or pericardial effusions. Bronchorrhea, the classic symptom for bronchoalveolar cell carcinoma, occurs in a minority of these patients. Pancoast's syndrome is the coexistence of pain, Horner's syndrome, and brachial nerve palsies, caused by superior sulcus tumors that invade the brachial plexus, the inferior cervical ganglion, and vertebral column. Superior vena cava syndrome results from obstruction of the superior vena cava by central upper lobe tumors, usually the small cell tumors. Symptoms include facial and upper extremity edema, dilatation of superficial veins over the upper part of the body, cerebral edema, and stridor. Partial obstruction of a bronchus by tumor may produce localized wheezing, whereas complete obstruction causes atelectasis or postobstructive pneumonia. Hoarseness may result from recurrent laryngeal nerve injury by a hilar mass or adenopathy, usually on the left side. Phrenic nerve involvement by tumor causes unilateral diaphragmatic paralysis. Direct or metastatic spread of the tumor to the pleura or pericardium causes malignant effusions and, rarely, cardiac tamponade.

Symptoms in patients with bronchogenic carcinoma frequently do not develop until the tumor metastasizes, most often to lymph nodes, adrenal glands, brain, liver, or bone. Bronchogenic carcinoma may produce a paraneoplastic syndrome resulting from ectopic production of hormones or induction of autoantibodies to neuronal antigens (Table 20–1).

Diagnosis and Evaluation

The history and physical examination, coupled with current and prior radiographic studies, are the first steps in the evaluation of lung cancer. A lesion that is radiographically stable for more than 2 years is assumed to be benign. Routine laboratory evaluation is not helpful in the diagnosis.

Because therapeutic options for lung cancer depend on histologic character of the tumor and clinical staging (Table 20–2), attempts to obtain tissue should start with the least invasive procedure and progress to more invasive methods until a tissue diagnosis is obtained. Cytologic examination of sputum in patients who have productive coughs, especially with hemoptysis and relatively central lesions, yields a noninvasive diagnosis in 40% to 50% of patients. Fiberoptic bronchoscopy can localize tumors and provide information about the degree of bronchial obstruction as well as provide biopsy material. Bronchoscopy establishes the diagnosis of about 90% of visible endobronchial lesions but only about 50% or fewer of peripheral lesions, depending on tumor size and location. Transthoracic needle aspiration of peripheral lesions that abut the pleura yields a diagnosis in about 80% of cases. A negative needle biopsy does not rule out malignancy, and therefore many clinicians advocate going directly to the more invasive thoracoscopic wedge resection. If that is done, a diagnosis can be made on frozen tissue sections; and, if the lesion is malignant, a complete lobectomy can be performed. For treatment of non–small cell tumors, some centers prefer giving neoadjuvant therapy before resection, in which case a tissue diagnosis is necessary before surgery.

Therapeutic options for lung cancer depend on tumor type, stage of disease, and performance status of the patient. Lung cancer staging was recently revised to better classify patients according to predicted outcome and the use of therapeutic interventions. Performance status at diagnosis is the strongest predictor of long-term survival. The best chance of curing a non–small cell lung cancer is complete surgical resection. Patients with stage I, II, or IIIA disease should have the tumor resected if they are otherwise operative candidates. Operability is determined by the patient's overall performance status as well as by specific cardiopulmonary functional status. Patients with significant cardiac disease may not be candidates. Preoperative pulmonary function testing has been used to exclude patients with a pre-

TABLE 20–1   Paraneoplastic Syndromes Associated with Bronchogenic Carcinoma

Syndrome	Cell Type	Mechanism
Hypertrophic pulmonary osteoarthropathy and clubbing	All except small cell	Unknown
Hyponatremia	Small cell most common, may be any type	Syndrome of inappropriate secretion of antidiuretic hormone (SIADH), ectopic antidiuretic hormone production by tumor
Hypercalcemia	Usually squamous cell	Bone metastases, osteoclast-activating factor, parathyroid hormone–like hormone, prostaglandins
Cushing's syndrome	Usually small cell	Ectopic ACTH production
Eaton-Lambert myasthenic syndrome	Usually small cell	Voltage-sensitive calcium channel antibodies in >75%; affect presynaptic neuronal calcium channel activity
Other neuromyopathic disorders	Small cell most common, may be any type	Anti-neuronal nuclear antibodies, also known as anti-Hu; others unknown
Thrombophlebitis	All types	Unknown

TABLE 20–2 **International Staging System for Lung Cancer, 1997 Revision**

Primary Tumor (T)

T1–Tumor ≤3 cm diameter without invasion more proximal than lobar bronchus
T2–Tumor >3 cm diameter *or*
  Tumor of any size with any of the following:
    Invades visceral pleura
    Atelectasis of less than entire lung
    Proximal extent at least 2 cm from carina
T3–Tumor of any size with any of following:
    Invasion of chest wall
    Involvement of diaphragm, mediastinal pleura, or pericardium
    Atelectasis involving entire lung
    Proximal extent within 2 cm of carina
T4–Tumor of any size with any of following:
    Invasion of mediastinum
    Invasion of heart or great vessels
    Invasion of trachea or esophagus
    Invasion of vertebral body or carina
    Presence of malignant pleural or pericardial effusion
    Satellite tumor nodule(s) within same lobe as primary tumor

Nodal Involvement (N)

N0–No regional node involvement
N1–Metastasis to ipsilateral hilar and/or ipsilateral peribronchial nodes
N2–Metastasis to ipsilateral mediastinal and/or subcarinal nodes
N3–Metastasis to contralateral mediastinal or hilar nodes *or* ipsilateral or contralateral scalene or
  supraclavicular nodes

Metastasis (M)

M0–Distant metastasis absent
M1–Distant metastasis present (includes metastatic tumor nodules in a different lobe from the
  primary tumor)

Stage Groupings of TNM Subsets

Stage IA	T1 N0 M0	Stage IIIA	T3 N1 M0
IB	T2 N0 M0		T1-3 N2 M0
Stage IIA	T1 N1 M0	Stage IIIB	Any T N3 M0
IIB	T2 N1 M0		T4 Any N M0
	T3 N0 M0	Stage IV	Any T Any N M1

Adapted from Mountain CF: Revisions in the international system for staging lung cancer. Chest 1997; 111:1710.

dicted postoperative FEV$_1$ of less than a liter. However, because resection offers the best chance at cure, more sophisticated estimates of the functional consequences of the proposed surgery are being done. These include using the percent predicted FEV$_1$ instead of the absolute value to estimate postoperative status and "split function studies" (separate ventilation of the two lungs using radionuclides) to accurately predict postoperative performance.

Resectability depends on the stage and location of the tumor. Tumors with endobronchial invasion within 2 cm of the carina are generally not resectable, although sleeve resection is occasionally performed. The patient receives no benefit from resection of tumors with direct invasion of great vessels or mediastinal structures or of those with contralateral lymph node involvement or when there are distant metastases. Staging is based on the computed tomographic scan of the chest and abdomen, followed by mediastinal lymph node biopsy in those patients with enlarged nodes. Bone scan, computed tomography of the head, and magnetic resonance imaging are not indicated in the absence of symptoms suggesting metastases.

Solitary Pulmonary Nodule

Although solitary pulmonary nodules are frequently benign, they may be malignant, and resection is usually required for diagnosis. Lesions may be considered benign without a tissue diagnosis if (1) there is radiographic documentation that the lesion has not increased in size over 2 years or (2) the tumor contains calcifications in a central, speckled, diffuse, laminar, or "popcorn" pattern. Lesions larger than 3 cm are called masses rather than nodules and are likely to be malignant. The practice of observing newly discovered noncalcified nodules without intervention by serial radiographs is not advised, because small lesions may metastasize or patients may be lost to follow up.

Treatment and Prognosis

Surgery is the therapy of choice for patients with non–small cell lung cancer who are operable candidates and have resectable lesions. Chest wall invasion or ipsilateral hilar and mediastinal nodal involvement does not preclude surgery. There is growing evidence to support neoadjuvant chemoradiation therapy in patients with stage II or IIIA disease. Radiation therapy may be curative in a small percentage of patients who are not operative candidates but does not spare pulmonary function any more than surgery does. Palliative radiation can relieve bronchial and superior vena cava obstruction, as well as provide symptomatic relief of brain and bone metastases.

Small cell lung cancer is staged and treated differently than non–small cell lung cancer. Small cell lung cancer is classified as "limited stage" if the tumor can be irradiated entirely within a single port. If that is not the case, the tumor is classified as "extensive stage." Usual therapy for limited stage disease is chemotherapy combined with irradiation. Small cell lung cancer is very chemosensitive, and most patients respond to therapy with clinical remission, although the length of the remission is variable and very rarely are patients cured. These tumors frequently metastasize to the brain, and prophy-

lactic cranial irradiation in patients with limited disease reduces the incidence of brain metastases but does not prolong survival. Patients with extensive-stage disease are usually treated with chemotherapy alone, which increases survival and decreases symptoms.

On average, only 14% of patients with lung cancer survive as long as 5 years after the time of diagnosis. Although the stage of the disease at the time of diagnosis predicts the response to therapy and survival, no screening strategy has been shown to be beneficial or cost effective. Even in clinical stage I disease, the 5-year survival rate is only 60%. This may relate in part to the fact that not all patients undergo surgical staging, but it also reflects the aggressive nature of this disease.

REFERENCES

Edell ES, Cortese DA, McDougall JC: Ancillary therapies in the management of lung cancer: Photodynamic therapy, laser therapy, and endobronchial prosthetic devices. Mayo Clin Proc 1993; 68:685–690.

Jett JR: Current treatment of unresectable lung cancer. Mayo Clin Proc 1993; 68:603–611.

Johnson BE, Johnson DH: Lung Cancer. New York: Wiley-Liss, 1995.

Karsell PR, McDougall JC: Diagnostic tests for lung cancer. Mayo Clin Proc 1993; 68:288–296.

Mountain CF, Dresler CM: Regional lymph node classification for lung cancer staging. Chest 1997; 111:1718–1723.

Patel AM, Davila DG, Peters SG: Paraneoplastic syndromes associated with lung cancer [see comments]. Mayo Clin Proc 1993; 68:278–287.

Patel AM, Peters SG: Clinical manifestations of lung cancer. Mayo Clin Proc 1993; 68:273–277.

21

DISORDERED BREATHING

Bonnie S. Slovis • Kenneth L. Brigham

Sleep Apnea Syndrome

During normal sleep, ventilation declines, arterial carbon dioxide increases, and pharyngeal muscles relax, resulting in narrowing of the upper airway, which adds a resistive load to the respiratory system. A normal sleep pattern consists of several stages occurring cyclically with typical electroencephalographic brain wave patterns that correspond to the sleep stage. One stage is rapid eye movement (REM) sleep, which coincides with dreaming and is characterized by rapid eye movements, generalized skeletal muscle atonia except for the diaphragm, and irregular respiration.

Apnea is defined as complete cessation of air flow for 10 or more seconds. *Hypopnea* is a significant decrease in air flow. Occasional apneas and hypopneas occur during normal sleep, and their frequency increases with age. In patients with sleep apnea syndrome, however, the apneas and hypopneas are increased in frequency and duration to a degree sufficient to fragment sleep and produce clinically significant hypoxia and hypercapnia. Sleep apnea may be obstructive, caused by upper airway obstruction, or central, caused by decreased central respiratory drive, or a mixture of the two patterns. Consequences of the sleep disturbance include excessive daytime somnolence, increased risk for vehicular accidents, irritability, headache, hypertension, and an increase in sudden death probably due to cardiac arrhythmias.

Obstructive sleep apnea is estimated to occur in 4% of middle-aged and older men and is less common in women. The primary risk factors for obstructive sleep apnea are obesity and abnormal upper airway anatomy produced by enlarged tonsils, macroglossia, a long soft palate and uvula, or micrognathia. In those situations, even the normal upper airway muscle relaxation that occurs during sleep may allow complete occlusion of the airway and complete cessation of air flow. After variable periods of airway occlusion, the patient arouses, reestablishes muscle tone, and opens the airway. This cycle may be repeated hundreds of times a night, resulting in multiple episodes of hypoxemia and hypercapnia and marked disruption of the normal sleep pattern. During airway occlusion, there is an increase in sympathetic tone, producing vasoconstriction and hypertension. Hypoxemia can cause bradycardia and cardiac arrhythmias. There is an increased incidence of stroke and coronary artery disease in patients with obstructive sleep apnea, but a causal relationship is difficult to establish because of shared risk factors.

The diagnosis of sleep apnea should be considered when patients complain of daytime hypersomnolence that interferes with daily activities, especially when accompanied by complaints of loud snoring and gasping by the sleeping partner. Patients are usually, but not invariably, obese. On physical examination, a small pharyngeal opening or redundant or increased soft tissue is usually seen. Patients may be hypertensive and in extreme cases have evidence of right-sided heart failure. In patients who are morbidly obese, sleep apnea is often accompanied by the obesity hypoventilation syndrome, characterized by daytime hypoxemia and hypercarbia. Establishing a diagnosis of sleep apnea requires polysomnography. While the patient sleeps during the night, continuous recordings are made of electroencephalographic and electrocardiographic tracings. Air flow; respiratory, eye, chin, and limb muscle movement; and oxygen saturation are monitored and recorded. From these data, a score is derived that defines whether clinically significant sleep apnea is present. If the pattern is one of obstructive apnea, patients are usually fitted with a continuous positive airway pressure mask. Maintaining positive airway pressure at the end of expiration keeps the upper airway open and prevents collapse. The amount of positive pressure can be titrated to the lowest level that prevents the apneic episodes and clinical symptoms. Although highly effective, the devices are cumbersome and often uncomfortable, and long-term patient compliance remains low.

All sedatives depress ventilatory drive to some degree, and patients with sleep apnea should be counseled against their use. When patients are obese, significant weight loss can eliminate or reduce the severity of sleep apnea. Hypothyroidism, acromegaly, and amyloidosis are

210

rare causes of sleep apnea that should be ruled out. Surgery to remove obstructing tonsils, adenoids, or polyps or uvulopalatopharyngoplasty in patients with specific anatomic abnormalities and mild obstruction is sometimes useful. A permanent tracheostomy is a last resort but is highly effective therapy.

Other Breathing Disorders

Apnea or hypopnea resulting from decreased central respiratory drive may be a consequence of central nervous system injury or may be idiopathic (Ondine's curse). Affected patients may hypoventilate even when awake, although they are capable of completely normal voluntary breaths; during sleep, frequent apnea is the rule. Central apnea is usually due to some structural abnormality of the brain stem, which may be discovered only at autopsy.

In patients with obstructive lung disease, increased work of breathing eventually makes it impossible to maintain sufficient ventilation to keep arterial blood gases normal. When that occurs, the patient hypoventilates chronically, causing $PaCO_2$ to increase; the kidneys respond by retaining enough bicarbonate to keep arterial blood pH normal. These patients appear to have normal ventilatory drive but lack the ability to increase minute ventilation to meet increased metabolic demand.

Lower brain stem and upper pontine lesions may cause *central hyperventilation*. However, hyperventilation seldom occurs in the absence of other physiologic or chemical abnormalities. Hepatic cirrhosis, pregnancy, pain, and extreme anxiety are all causes of central hyperventilation. *Apneustic breathing* consists of sustained inspiratory pauses, as a result of damage to the midpons, most commonly due to a basilar artery infarct. *Biot's* or *ataxic breathing*, a haphazard random pattern of deep and shallow breaths, is caused by disruption of the respiratory rhythm generator in the medulla.

Cheyne-Stokes respiration is the regular cycling of crescendo-decrescendo tidal volumes separated by apneic or hypopneic pauses. These patients usually have generalized central nervous system disease or congestive heart failure. Heart failure affects respiratory patterns because the resulting prolonged circulatory times cause a delay between changes in blood gases at the tissue level and the arrival of the respiratory stimulus at the brain stem chemoreceptors. This delay means that the ventilatory response is out of sync with tissue needs, which sets up a cycle of gradually increasing ventilation to the point of overcompensation followed by gradually decreasing ventilation to apnea and then repetition of the cycle.

REFERENCES

Bella I, Chad DA: Neuromuscular disorders and acute respiratory failure. Neurol Clin 1998; 16:391–417.

Johnson DC, Kazemi H: Central control of ventilation in neuromuscular disease. Clin Chest Med 1994; 15:604–617.

Rochester DF, Esau SA: Assessment of ventilatory function in patients with neuromuscular disease. Clin Chest Med 1994; 15:751–763.

Strollo FJ, Rogers RM: Current concepts: Obstructive sleep apnea. N Engl J Med 1996; 334:99–104.

Thorsteinsson G: Management of postpolio syndrome. Mayo Clin Proc 1997; 72:627–638.

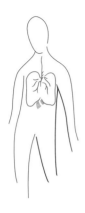

22

ENVIRONMENTAL AND OCCUPATIONAL INJURY

Bonnie S. Slovis • Kenneth L. Brigham

Exposure to certain respirable substances may produce lung injury. The degree of injury depends on the size of the particles, the noxiousness of the material inhaled, and the dose and duration of exposure. The pneumoconioses are lung diseases caused by inhalation of inorganic dusts. Inhalational lung injury may also be caused by toxic fumes, gases, and heavy metals. The inhalation of organic dust may cause a hypersensitivity pneumonitis, which is covered in Chapter 18.

Pneumoconioses

The four major pneumoconioses result from inhalation of asbestos, coal dust, silica, or beryllium (see Table 18–1). *Asbestos* is the most important because of the frequency of exposure and severity of disease. Disease is related to the intensity and duration of exposure as well as to the fiber type. Manifestations of asbestosis range from benign pleural effusions and pleural thickening to progressive pulmonary fibrosis and increased risk of lung cancer and mesothelioma. The risk of lung cancer is six times greater in persons with significant asbestos exposure and 59-fold higher in smokers with similar exposure. The time between asbestos exposure and the development of malignancy is long, usually from 20 to 40 years. Asbestos-related lung fibrosis also progresses slowly and continues to progress after exposure ceases. The asbestos fibers are not easily cleared from the lung and continue to stimulate ongoing inflammation and fibrosis. The fibers appear on histologic examination as "asbestos bodies." They are also called *ferruginous bodies* because of the accumulation of iron and protein on their surface over time.

Silicosis resulting from significant silica exposure is less common but produces an intense inflammatory response and progressive massive fibrosis. Latency from exposure to disease can be as short as 5 years, with intense exposure, or as long as 20 years. Acute silicosis may develop in months and has the clinical features of an acute infectious pneumonia. The pathology, however, will show refractile particles and alveolar proteinosis. Classic radiographic findings are coalescent upper lobe nodules and eggshell calcification of hilar nodes. The disease predisposes to infection with mycobacteria.

Coal workers' pneumoconiosis is the result of a long and intense inhalation of coal dust. Coal dust alone does not cause any significant inflammation or physiologic abnormalities in most people exposed. Simultaneous exposure to silica is largely responsible for significant fibrosis, and radon exposure increases the risk of lung cancer. Concurrent cigarette smoking increases the risk of symptomatic disease. The chest radiograph when abnormal has a reticulonodular pattern. Pneumoconioses are graded on the basis of the number, distribution, size, and shape of these fine nodules by specially trained radiologists.

Berylliosis occurs in an acute and chronic form. Acutely, beryllium causes an intense inflammatory reaction resembling a chemical pneumonitis. The chronic form is a granulomatous disease, primarily affecting the lung. The clinical features of the chronic form are similar to sarcoid, and the diagnosis is made by history of exposure, histologic examination, and laboratory confirmation through a lymphocyte transformation test, available at specialized centers.

Air Pollution

Sulfur oxides, ozone, and nitrogen dioxide are increasing in concentration in the atmosphere, especially in industrial areas. The pulmonary effects of the gases are varied but include bronchoconstriction and exacerbations of asthma, bronchitis, and chronic obstructive pulmonary disease. Elevated household levels of radon gas have raised concerns about carcinogenesis. Miners exposed to high levels have been documented to have a higher risk of lung cancer, but the evidence for household air exposure has been difficult to confirm and define.

Noxious Gases and Fumes

The inhalation of certain gases and fumes may cause asphyxia or cellular and metabolic injury (Table 22–1). Inhalation of concentrated gases normally found in the atmosphere, such as carbon dioxide, nitrogen, or methane, causes asphyxia by replacement of alveolar oxygen, but these gases are not directly toxic. Carbon monoxide (CO) poisoning is a common and frequently unsuspected cause of inhalational injury and results in tissue hypoxia by competitively displacing oxygen from hemoglobin. Affinity of CO for the hemoglobin oxygen-binding sites is approximately 250 times greater than that of oxygen. The correlation between CO levels and symptoms is weak, but generally patients with levels greater than 30% are symptomatic. Much lower levels may cause neuropsychiatric symptoms and myocardial ischemia in persons with underlying coronary artery disease. The neuropsychiatric symptoms range from mild confusion or fatigue, usually accompanied by headache and nausea, to profound coma and death. Long-term neurologic sequelae are common and unpredictable. The diagnosis of CO poisoning is made on clinical grounds and supported by laboratory data. A history of other family members with the same symptoms, symptoms occurring in a closed automobile, or an exposure to kerosene heaters or charcoal fires in closed spaces should prompt further evaluation. Laboratory evaluation requires an arterial blood gas with a measured, not calculated hemoglobin oxygen saturation. A CO level should be measured in patients with a measured oxygen saturation (SaO_2) lower than the calculated SaO_2 obtained from the oxygen tension (PaO_2). Be aware that victims of CO poisoning may have very low CO levels if sufficient time has elapsed since exposure. Nonetheless, it is important to take an in-depth history to prevent further exposure.

Treatment of patients with elevated CO levels is with 100% inspired oxygen, which lowers the elimination half-life from approximately 3 hours to 1.5 hours or less. There is great individual variation in the rate of CO elimination. Treatment with hyperbaric oxygen decreases the elimination half-life to less than 30 minutes, but studies of the clinical utility of this therapy are conflicting.

Inhalation of caustic substances such as ammonia, chlorine, and hydrogen fluoride causes acute symptoms of eye and upper airway inflammation. Pain, lacrimation, rhinorrhea, and upper airway symptoms cause the individual to flee the environment, preventing further exposure and injury. Lower airway injury is usually not severe unless the exposure is massive or the victim is trapped. Subsequent reactive airways disease may occur and last months.

Inhalation of nitrogen dioxide, also known as silo filler's disease, occurs in farmers working in silos where fermentation of grain produces large quantities of the gas. It does not cause immediate discomfort. Initial symptoms are cough and dyspnea, followed by pulmonary edema if exposure continues. Most patients recover without sequelae; however, a small minority may develop bronchiolitis obliterans with obstructing pneumonia.

Metal fume fever is a flulike illness caused by inhalation of metal oxides generated by welding. There are no long-term sequelae. Inhalation of platinum, formalin, and isocyanates may precipitate asthma. Acute pneumonitis can occur with high-intensity inhalation of cadmium and mercury vapors.

Smoke Inhalation

There are several mechanisms of injury resulting from smoke inhalation. Direct thermal injury is usually confined to the upper airways, but it may produce injury to the lower airways if there is sufficient steam due to the high thermal content of water. Laryngeal edema may lead to obstruction and must be anticipated to avoid

TABLE 22–1 Toxic Gases and Fumes

Injury	Agent	Occupational Exposure
Simple asphyxia	Carbon dioxide	Mining, foundries
	Nitrogen	Mining, diving
	Methane	Mining
Cellular hypoxia/oxygen transport	Carbon monoxide	Mining, combustion in closed spaces Smoke inhalation
	Cyanide	Petroleum refining
	Hydrogen sulfide	
Direct tissue injury	Ammonia	Fertilizer, cleaning agents
	Chlorine	Bleaches, swimming pools
	Nitrogen dioxide	Farming, fertilizer, combustion in closed spaces
	Phosgene	Welding, paint removal
	Cadmium, mercury	Welding

emergent intubation of a difficult airway. Anoxia from consumption of oxygen by the fire as well as cytotoxic injury from gases such as carbon monoxide, cyanide, and oxidants liberated during combustion occur. Cyanide poisoning disrupts the cytochrome oxygen transport chain, uncoupling oxygen from energy production. Treatment with 100% oxygen and sodium thiosulfate is safe and effective if administered early. Most hospitals have cyanide kits available with instructions for administration. The combustion of natural and synthetic polymers often produces aldehydes such as formaldehyde, acetaldehyde, and acrolein that cause irritant injury. Of these chemicals, acrolein, liberated during the combustion of acrylic and natural polymers, has the highest irritant potential.

The treatment of all persons suspected of having significant smoke inhalation is supportive, with close attention paid to the airway. The administration of 100% oxygen, cardiac and hemodynamic monitoring, direct laryngoscopy followed by early intubation for signs of laryngeal edema, arterial blood gas analysis, and measurement of CO and cyanide levels should be routine in any patient with significant exposure. Supportive care for adult respiratory distress syndrome from smoke inhalation is the same as for all other causes of this syndrome. Long-term complications for patients who survive are uncommon but may include tracheal stenosis, bronchiolitis obliterans, and persistent reactive airways disease. There is no evidence that corticosteroids improve outcome, and they are not recommended.

High-Altitude Injury

The acute ascent to high altitude may produce the acute mountain sickness syndrome of cerebral and pulmonary edema. The hypoxia of altitude may increase vascular permeability and result in edema. In the lungs, the alveolar hypoxia causes pulmonary vasoconstriction and elevated pulmonary artery pressures, which increase right ventricular afterload. The therapy is descent. Treatment with supplemental oxygen and corticosteroids is helpful in severe cases.

Drowning and Near-Drowning

Submersion in water beyond the ability to hold one's breath results in aspiration of variable amounts of water. Some victims develop laryngeal edema after very small volume aspirations, and lung injury may be caused by respiratory efforts against a closed larynx. This may produce high-negative intrapulmonary pressures and hydrostatic pulmonary edema. In other cases, large amounts of water may be aspirated. The distinction between freshwater and saltwater drowning is minor. The primary effects are dilution of surfactant and hypoxic organ injury. Restoration of ventilation and circulation must be accomplished as soon as possible, and attempts to evacuate water from the lungs are futile and waste valuable time. The baroreflex of bradycardia and shunting of blood to vital organs during submersion, accompanied by the decreased metabolism induced by hypothermia, increases survival even after prolonged resuscitation efforts. Resuscitation efforts should not be terminated until the patient is normothermic.

REFERENCES

Ernst A, Zibrak JD: Carbon monoxide poisoning. N Engl J Med 1998; 339:1603–1608.

Fraser RG, Pare JAP, Pare PD, et al: Pleuropulmonary disease caused by inhalation of inorganic dust (pneumoconiosis). *In* Fraser RG, Fraser RS, Genereuz GP (eds): Diagnosis of Diseases of the Chest, 3rd ed. Philadelphia: WB Saunders, 1990, pp 2346–2486.

Hall AH, Rumack BH: Clinical toxicology of cyanide. Ann Emerg Med 1986; 15:1067–1074.

Haponik EF, Crapo RO, Herndon DN, et al: Smoke inhalation. Am Rev Respir Dis 1988; 138:1060–1063.

Mossman BT, Churg A: Mechanisms in the pathogenesis of asbestosis and silicosis. Am J Respir Crit Care Med 1998; 157:1666–1680.

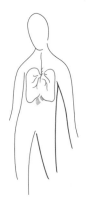

23

ESSENTIALS OF PULMONARY CRITICAL CARE MEDICINE

Bonnie S. Slovis • Kenneth L. Brigham

The medical intensive care unit is a specialized unit for patients who have suffered or are at high risk for cardiovascular or respiratory collapse. Services unique to this setting are invasive or continuous monitoring, mechanical ventilation for respiratory support, and hemodynamic support with vasoactive and inotropic drugs. Although physicians caring for patients in this setting must have expertise in the management of critical illness affecting all organ systems, this chapter focuses on the diagnosis and treatment of respiratory and circulatory collapse, mechanical ventilation, and the multiple organ dysfunction syndrome.

Shock

Shock is the profound and widespread failure of adequate tissue perfusion that leads to cell injury and death. Classically, shock has been divided into four etiologic categories: (1) hypovolemic, (2) cardiogenic, (3) obstructive, and (4) distributive. The classic hemodynamic variables for each category are outlined in Table 23–1.

Hypotension and tachycardia are characteristic of shock from any cause. Depending on the degree and duration of shock, the patient may have abnormal mental status and decreased urine output. It is often difficult to determine the cause of shock immediately, and in some patients there is more than a single cause. Treatment of shock should be directed at the underlying etiology, but the mere presence of the clinical syndrome is a medical emergency and requires immediate intervention, often before the cause is clear. Initially, resuscitation is attempted by expanding intravascular volume with vigorous administration of intravenous fluids. If volume expansion does not restore blood pressure, vasopressor drugs are given.

Invention of the percutaneous flow-directed pulmo-

nary artery catheter by Swan and Ganz made continuous measurements of pulmonary artery and left atrial pressure and frequent measurements of cardiac output feasible. These measurements have been in widespread use in caring for patients in shock since the technology was introduced. However, some authorities have questioned the utility and safety of the pulmonary artery catheter from the beginning of its use, and a report of a meta-analysis of published studies suggests that the pulmonary artery catheter may do more harm than good. A large, multicenter, randomized, prospective trial is being planned to answer this question. In the meantime, monitoring in most medical intensive care units is commonly done by placement of the pulmonary artery catheter, but detailed discussion of technique of insertion, interpretation of the data, and management based on those data is beyond the scope of this chapter.

Hypovolemic shock may be related to dehydration or hemorrhage. Patients are typically cool and clammy, because of peripheral vasoconstriction in response to decreased circulating volume. Neck veins are flat, urine output is decreased, and there may be altered mental status. The metabolic demand is usually unchanged, but the maximal oxygen consumption is decreased because decreased cardiac output and tissue perfusion make the oxygen consumption supply limited.

In *cardiogenic shock,* signs of left-sided heart failure are usually present unless the cause is a right ventricular infarct. Jugular and peripheral veins are distended, and the skin is cold and clammy from peripheral vasoconstriction in response to an inadequate cardiac output. Left ventricular preload is increased because of the decreased left ventricular ejection fraction. Elevated left atrial pressure results in increased pulmonary capillary pressure so that hydrostatic pulmonary edema is common. Cardiac output is low, myocardial oxygen consumption is decreased, and the arteriovenous oxygen content difference is increased because the low flow state results in increased extraction of oxygen at the

TABLE 23-1   Hemodynamic Variables in the Four Types of Shock

Type of Shock	Pulmonary Wedge Pressure (PCWP)	Cardiac Index (CI)	Systemic Vascular Resistance Index (SVRI)
Hypovolemic	Low	Low	High
Cardiogenic	High	Low	High
Extracardiac obstructive	Normal or low (high in tamponade)	Low	High
Distributive	Normal or low	High (rarely low)	Low

Adapted from Parrillo JE, Ayres SM (eds): Major Issues in Critical Care Medicine. Baltimore: Williams & Wilkins, 1984.

tissue level. The most common cause of cardiogenic shock is myocardial ischemia with or without infarction. Other causes include acute valvular dysfunction, myocarditis, cardiomyopathies, traumatic myocardial contusion, and persistent bradycardia or tachycardia.

Obstructive shock results from significant obstruction to blood flow within the cardiovascular circuit. Examples include massive pulmonary emboli, like the classic "saddle embolus" lodged at the bifurcation of the right and left pulmonary arteries, and acute pulmonary hypertension associated with illicit intravenous drug use. In both of these situations there is obstruction of flow from the right to the left side of the heart. Pericardial tamponade and constrictive pericarditis impair diastolic filling of the right ventricle. Tension pneumothorax and intrathoracic tumors exert pressure on the great veins in the thorax and thus impair venous return, and aortic dissection may obstruct left ventricular outflow. Findings common to all causes of obstructive shock are hypotension, decreased cardiac output, decreased myocardial oxygen consumption, and increased arteriovenous oxygen difference. Other findings depend on the site of the obstruction. Obstruction to left ventricular outflow mimics cardiogenic shock whereas obstruction to right ventricular filling or outflow mimics right-sided heart failure.

Distributive shock results from systemic vasodilation so profound that even a normally functioning heart cannot increase cardiac output enough to maintain blood pressure. Causes include sepsis, anaphylaxis, spinal injury, and adrenal insufficiency. In contrast to other forms of shock, peripheral vasodilation results in warm and well-perfused extremities, low systemic vascular resistance, and high cardiac output.

Acute Respiratory Failure

The two major functions of respiration are to add oxygen to and remove carbon dioxide from the blood. Acute respiratory failure is the relatively sudden decline in either or both of these functions. If an acute insult is of sufficient magnitude, acute respiratory failure may occur even though lung function before the insult was normal. If chronic compensated respiratory failure is present because of pre-existing lung disease, even a

minimal insult may lead to acute or chronic respiratory failure. All causes of respiratory failure result in hypoxemia. The causes of hypoxemia can be divided into four classes: (1) ventilation/perfusion mismatch, (2) alveolar hypoventilation, (3) right-to-left shunt, and (4) decreased inspired oxygen tension (e.g., at high altitude or in fires where oxygen is rapidly consumed).

Elevated arterial carbon dioxide tension is, by definition, due to alveolar hypoventilation. Hypercapnia is commonly present in patients with severe obstructive lung disease, neuromuscular weakness, or a depressed central nervous system. In patients with normal lungs, hypoventilation can cause hypoxemia owing to lowering of alveolar oxygen tension (PAO_2) by displacement of oxygen by the increased carbon dioxide. Hypoxemia in this situation is easily reversed by increasing the concentration of oxygen in the air being breathed in all but the most extreme cases of hypoventilation. In this situation, when the patient is receiving supplemental oxygen, direct measurement of arterial oxygen tension (PaO_2), arterial carbon dioxide tension (PCO_2), and pH is the only way to determine the degree of respiratory failure. Most patients with ventilatory failure also have significant underlying lung disease, creating hypoxic as well as hypercapnic respiratory failure.

Oxygen Therapy

Hypoxia is treated with supplemental oxygen. Hypercapnia is treated with assisted or complete support of ventilation, until the underlying cause of the respiratory failure can be corrected. Severe hypoxemia is immediately life threatening, so that ensuring an arterial blood oxygen saturation greater than 88% is urgent and essential. If hypoxemia is due to ventilation/perfusion mismatch, it is easily corrected with relatively small increases in oxygen content of inspired air (FIO_2). Hypoxemia due to anatomic or physiologic shunt is refractory to increases in FIO_2. Hypoxemia that is not adequately corrected by increasing FIO_2 requires that the patient be ventilated mechanically. Mechanical ventilation can deliver higher concentrations of oxygen to the lungs than can be achieved by less invasive means and also permits the use of positive end-expiratory pressure (PEEP), which improves ventilation/perfusion matching. FIO_2 should be increased cautiously in patients with hypoxemia in the presence of hypercapnia because the increase in oxygen may depress hypoxic ventilatory drive and increase physiologic shunt, both of which could worsen respiratory failure. The goal is to use the lowest FIO_2 necessary to maintain an arterial oxygen saturation of 88% to 90%.

These patients often require mechanical ventilation to ensure adequate oxygenation and ventilation. Noninvasive positive-pressure masks have been shown to be effective in some patients who are cooperative and alert. If mechanical ventilation is not elected in this setting, close monitoring of arterial blood gas determinations is essential so that mechanical ventilation can be instigated at the first sign of worsening clinical status. When mechanical ventilation is begun, the target effect on arterial blood gases is not normalization of arterial carbon dioxide tension ($PaCO_2$) but maintenance of arterial pH of 7.32 to 7.38. Acute normalization of $PaCO_2$ in patients with chronic hypercapnia will result in a profound alkalosis because of renal metabolic compensation for the previous elevation of CO_2. If patients on mechanical ventilation are mildly hyperventilated over time, their kidneys will compensate by wasting bicarbonate, which will make it more difficult to discontinue mechanical ventilation because of uncompensated respiratory acidosis.

Mechanical Ventilation

Mechanical ventilation in the acute setting is accomplished by using a mechanical device to deliver positive inspiratory pressure through an endotracheal or tracheostomy tube. Modern mechanical ventilators permit control of numerous variables related to ventilation. The respiratory cycle is divided into an inspiratory and an expiratory phase. The duty cycle is the time required for a full respiratory cycle (i.e., the sum of the inspiratory cycle and the expiratory cycle). During inspiration, the inhaled gas is delivered at a controllable flow rate under positive pressure. The machine may be set so that inspiration stops either when a preset volume is delivered (volume cycled) or when a preset pressure is reached (pressure cycled). In volume-cycled ventilation, the inspiratory time is determined by the set tidal volume and the flow rate so that peak airway pressure may vary from breath to breath. If the inspiratory time takes up too much of the duty cycle, the time available for passive exhalation will decrease and may not allow complete emptying of the previous tidal volume; if this occurs over several breaths, end-expiratory pressure increases and the lungs overdistend (a condition referred to as "auto-peep"). Possible complications of volume-cycled ventilation are overdistention of the lungs, barotrauma, and air trapping. In pressure-cycled ventilation the inspiratory time and tidal volume may vary from breath to breath. The biggest drawback of pressure-cycled ventilation is the inability to guarantee the desired minute ventilation. Ventilators contain alarms for maximum airway pressure and minimum minute ventila-

tion that can be set to alert medical intensive care unit staff before serious complications develop.

After the variables affecting the respiratory cycle are set to achieve the therapeutic goal, a mode of ventilation can be selected to further enhance ventilatory efficiency. The most common volume-cycled modes are *assist-control* and *synchronized intermittent mandatory ventilation.* Both of these modes can be used with PEEP, and synchronized intermittent mandatory ventilation can also include *pressure support ventilation* (PSV).

The assist-control ventilatory mode delivers a guaranteed set number of breaths per minute at a set tidal volume. Any spontaneous breaths initiated by the patient over the set rate will trigger the ventilator to deliver the set tidal volume as well. The synchronized intermittent mandatory ventilation mode delivers a guaranteed set number of breaths per minute synchronized with the patient's efforts, at a set tidal volume, but the volume of any breaths initiated by the patient over the set rate is determined by the patient's effort.

When PEEP is used, the ventilator ensures positive pressure at the end of expiration, preventing the collapse of alveoli that might otherwise close. Over time, closed alveoli may be recruited to participate in gas exchange. The effect is to improve ventilation/perfusion mismatch and thus improve oxygenation. As lungs become less compliant due to hydrostatic pulmonary edema or adult respiratory distress syndrome, increasing levels of PEEP are required to have the same effect. As PEEP is set beyond 10 cm H_2O, the resulting increase in intrathoracic pressure may decrease venous return and cardiac output. High levels of PEEP may also increase zone 1 lung, and therefore increase dead space ventilation. Nonetheless, higher levels are often required to maintain adequate oxygenation, and the best level of PEEP is highly individual and may be difficult to determine.

Continuous positive airway pressure is similar to PEEP except that the patient is breathing spontaneously. It is achieved by using a device that supplies a constant flow of gas that exceeds the patient's peak inspiratory flow demands and thus keeps airway pressure above atmospheric. This mode of ventilation is frequently used as a trial in the course of removing patients from mechanical ventilation, to ensure the patient can support spontaneous ventilation and survive extubation. Noninvasive continuous positive airway pressure can be applied through a nasal mask, and on occasion this approach obviates the need for endotracheal intubation.

PSV can be used alone or in support of the spontaneous breaths of patients being mechanically ventilated in the SIMV mode. As the patient inhales, the ventilator automatically provides an inspiratory flow rate sufficient to achieve a preset inspiratory pressure. Because PSV supports only spontaneous non–volume-cycled breaths, it has no role in the assist-control mode. Some physicians use PSV alone or with SIMV as a mode of weaning from mechanical ventilation. The difference between PSV and pressure-controlled (cycled) ventilation is that in PSV the patient must initiate each breath and in pressure-controlled ventilation a demand rate is set.

Barotrauma is a significant complication of mechanical ventilation. In patients with severe air flow obstruction, air trapping and lung overdistention may lead to rupture of the alveolar sacs, producing a pneumothorax that may rapidly progress to a tension pneumothorax as the ventilator continues to deliver air under positive pressure. In patients with stiff lungs who require high pressures to accomplish adequate ventilation, pneumomediastinum, subcutaneous emphysema, or pneumothorax may result from dissection of air along bronchovesicular planes. All patients on mechanical ventilation who develop a pneumothorax require placement of a chest tube.

Complications of Endotracheal Intubation and Mechanical Ventilation

Complications of endotracheal intubation fall generally into two groups: (1) those that occur when the endotracheal tube is placed and (2) those that result from prolonged intubation. Complications occurring at the time the tube is placed include tooth avulsion, pharyngeal injury, esophageal intubation, aspiration, right mainstem bronchus intubation, and laryngeal spasm. Transnasal intubation carries the risk of turbinate injury and epistaxis. Complications of prolonged intubation include nose and lip ulcers and necrosis, laryngeal dysfunction, tracheal stenosis, and, with nasotracheal intubation, sinusitis. Patients who require mechanical ventilation for more than 21 days should be evaluated for tracheostomy.

Pneumonia acquired in the medical intensive care unit (nosocomial pneumonia) is a frequent complication of endotracheal intubation and prolonged mechanical ventilation. Two avoidable risk factors are supine posture and extubation with reintubation. In patients whose hemodynamics will allow, the head of the bed should be kept elevated at 30 degrees with close supervision to avoid unplanned extubation. The most common organism causing pneumonia during mechanical ventilation in the first 4 days of hospitalization is *Staphylococcus aureus*, but as duration of hospitalization and mechanical ventilation increases, both upper and lower airways become colonized with gram-negative organisms and these become the most frequent organisms causing nosocomial pneumonia.

Systemic Inflammatory Response Syndrome, Sepsis, Multiple Organ Dysfunction Syndrome, and Adult Respiratory Distress Syndrome

The *systemic inflammatory response syndrome (SIRS)* is a constellation of clinical signs and symptoms resulting from the host response to various insults. When caused by infection, SIRS is called sepsis. The diagnosis of SIRS requires at least two of the following: temperature greater than 38°C or less than 36°C, tachycardia greater than 90 beats/min, tachypnea greater than 20 breaths/min or $PaCO_2$ less than 32 mm Hg, and white blood cell count greater than 12,000/μL or less than 4,000/μL. This systemic response to inflammation may result in dysfunction of multiple organs (usually lung, liver, kidneys, cardiovascular system, or central nervous system), and this clinical situation is called multiple organ dysfunction syndrome or multiple organ system failure. Mortality of patients with SIRS increases with the number of organs failing, from a low of 30% to 40% for two failing organs to greater than 90% with five or more failing organs.

Lung dysfunction occurs often and early in SIRS and is termed the *adult respiratory distress syndrome*. The usual criteria defining this syndrome are PaO_2 to FIO_2 of 200 or less (commonly called the P/F ratio) and bilateral pulmonary infiltrates evident on the chest radiograph in the absence of volume overload. If a pulmonary artery catheter is in place, the pulmonary artery wedge pressure must be less than or equal to 18 mm Hg. There is no specific therapy for the adult respiratory distress syndrome that has been shown to be efficacious; thus, treatment is supportive. Mechanical ventilation is the principal form of supportive therapy in these patients. Because patients with adult respiratory distress syndrome are often difficult to ventilate and oxygenate, multiple ventilatory strategies have evolved with little more than anecdotal information about effects on the course of the disease. A major exception is a recent large multicenter controlled trial that showed a 30% lower mortality in patients with adult respiratory distress syndrome who were ventilated using low tidal volumes than in patients who were ventilated with high tidal volumes. On the basis of that study, it now appears that patients with adult respiratory distress syndrome should be mechanically ventilated with low tidal volumes (approximately 6 mL/kg ideal body weight). It is possible to ventilate the lungs with liquid perfluorocarbons, which have a very high capacity for dissolving oxygen and distribute evenly in even injured lungs. Partial liquid ventilation with these chemicals is being evaluated as a method of treating patients who cannot be adequately oxygenated despite use of the optimal available ventilatory strategies. Extracorporeal membrane oxygenation and jet ventilation have been successfully used in infants but have not proved beneficial in adults.

Cytokines are endogenously produced inflammatory mediators that appear to be important in the pathogenesis of SIRS. In sepsis, tumor necrosis factor and interleukin-1 are produced early. Interleukin-8, a powerful neutrophil chemotaxin, is produced later and plays a major role in perpetuating tissue inflammation. Interleukin-6 is produced later in the course of sepsis and has both proinflammatory and anti-inflammatory effects. Interleukin-10 is anti-inflammatory. Some studies indicate that the balance between proinflammatory and anti-inflammatory cytokines is important in determining outcomes in patients with SIRS. Treatments directed at blocking the production or action of inflammatory cytokines or administering or enhancing the production of anti-inflammatory cytokines are being studied in clinical trials. Multiple prostanoids, biologically active metabolites of arachidonic acid, are produced in the setting of SIRS and may be involved in the pathogenesis. These include the potent pulmonary vasoconstrictor thromboxane A_2, the potent pulmonary vasodilator prostacyclin, and prostaglandin E_2, which has anti-inflammatory effects. Precise roles for these mediators in the pathophysiology of SIRS are not yet defined.

Patients with SIRS, multiple organ dysfunction syndrome, adult respiratory distress syndrome, or sepsis are severely ill and often require prolonged aggressive supportive therapy as well as intense therapy aimed at the underlying causes of organ failure. This may require weeks to months in the medical intensive care unit, but patients who survive usually recover normal function of their failing organs.

REFERENCES

Esteban A, Alia I, Tobin MJ, et al, and the Spanish Lung Failure Collaborative: Effect of spontaneous breathing trial duration on outcome of attempts to discontinue mechanical ventilation. Am J Respir Crit Care Med 1999; 159:512–518.

Leung P, Jubran A, Tobin MJ: Comparison of assisted ventilator modes on triggering, patient effort, and dyspnea. Am J Respir Crit Care Med 1997; 155:1940–1948.

Manthous CA, Schmidt GA, Hall JB: Liberation from mechanical ventilation: A decade of progress [see comments]. Chest 1998; 114:886–901.

Swan HJ, Forrester JS, Diamond G, et al: Hemodynamic spectrum of myocardial infarction and cardiogenic shock: A conceptual model. Circulation 1972; 45:1097–1110.

Wheeler AP, Bernard GR: Current concepts: Treating patients with severe sepsis. N Engl J Med 1999; 130:207–214.

SECTION V

Renal Disease

ELEMENTS OF RENAL STRUCTURE AND FUNCTION

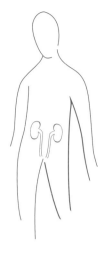

Dinesh K. Chatoth

Elements of Renal Structure

GROSS ANATOMY

The human kidneys are a pair of bean-shaped organs situated in the retroperitoneal space, positioned on either side of the vertebral column at the level of the lower thoracic and upper lumbar vertebrae. The right kidney is slightly lower than the left kidney because of the location of the liver. Each adult kidney weighs about 120 to 170 g and measures about 12 × 6 × 3 cm. The renal hilum is a slitlike opening in the medial concave margin of the kidney that allows the passage of the renal artery and vein, the nerve plexus, lymphatics, and the renal pelvis into the sinus of the kidney.

A coronal section of the kidney shows two distinct regions (Fig. 24–1A). The pale outer region is called the cortex and is about 1 cm in thickness. The dark inner region is the medulla and contains 6 to 15 (average, 8) conical structures called pyramids. The base of each pyramid is situated at the corticomedullary junction, and the apex extends into the hilum of the kidney as the papilla. The renal cortex caps around the base of each renal pyramid and extends in between the pyramids as the renal columns of Bertin.

The upper expanded section of the urinary tract is called the renal pelvis. In humans, the renal pelvis extends outward to form three major calyces, each of which branches into eight or more minor calyces. The funnel-shaped minor calyx extends toward the pyramid and encompasses each papilla, thereby draining the urine formed by the pyramidal unit. Urine from several minor calyces drains into a major calyx and subsequently into the renal pelvis. The ureters originate from the lower end of the renal pelvis and descend toward the bladder. Urine from the renal pelvis passes to the bladder through the ureters.

RENAL BLOOD SUPPLY

Blood is delivered to each kidney from a main renal artery branching from the aorta at the level of the first lumbar vertebra (see Fig. 24–1B). The renal artery enters the hilum and usually divides into two main segmental branches, which are further subdivided into several lobar arteries supplying the upper, middle, and lower regions of the kidney. These vessels branch further as they enter the renal parenchyma and create interlobar arteries that course toward the renal cortex along the lateral margin of the medullary pyramids. At the corticomedullary junction, these smaller arteries provide perpendicular branches that continue in an archlike manner, appropriately named the *arcuate arteries*. Interlobular arteries arise from the arcuate arteries and branch radially within the cortex. The glomerular capillaries receive blood through afferent arterioles that originate from these terminal interlobular arteries. The efferent arteriole leaves the glomerular capillary bed and supplies a network of vessels that surround the tubular structures. The efferent arterioles of the juxtamedullary glomeruli form hairpin loops called vasa recta that extend deep into the medulla.

The peritubular capillary networks drain into venules. Interlobular, arcuate, and lobular veins accompany the corresponding arteries and provide the venous drainage of the kidney. They drain into the renal vein, which ultimately drains into the inferior vena cava.

INNERVATION OF THE KIDNEY

Kidneys are richly innervated by the autonomic nervous system. Sympathetic nerve endings are present in all segments of renal vasculature, tubules, and the juxtaglomerular apparatus. Stimulation of the renal sympathetic nerves enhances the release of renin from the juxtaglomerular cells, thereby increasing angiotensin and aldo-

223

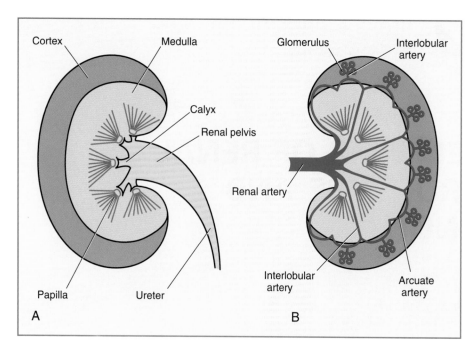

FIGURE 24–1   Basic renal structure. *A,* Urinary collecting structures; *B,* the arterial supply.

sterone production. The sympathetic nervous system may not play a major role in day-to-day regulation of glomerular filtration rate, but it becomes important in pathologic states.

THE NEPHRON

Histologically, the kidney is composed of a basic structural and functional unit known as the nephron (Fig. 24–2). Each human kidney contains approximately 1 million nephrons, and each nephron is composed of two major components: a filtering element that consists of an enclosed capillary network (the renal, or malpighian, corpuscle) and its attached tubule. The tubule contains several distinct anatomic and functional segments. They include the proximal tubule, the loop of Henle (composed of the straight portion of the proximal tubule, the thin descending limb, and the thick ascending limb), the distal tubule, and the connecting segment. They drain into the collecting duct system that contains the cortical collecting duct and the outer and inner medullary collecting segments. Whereas embryologically the collecting duct system is different from the nephron, functionally they are intimately related to the nephron segments.

Nephrons are mainly classified into two types on the basis of whether they possess a short or a long loop of Henle. The short-looped nephrons usually originate from the superficial and midcortical regions, and their loops of Henle bend within the outer medulla. In contrast, the long-looped nephrons originate from the juxtamedullary (corticomedullary) region, and their loops of Henle extend into the inner medulla.

The Renal Corpuscle (Glomerulus)

The glomerulus (Fig. 24–3) is a unique network of capillaries suspended between the afferent and efferent

arterioles enclosed within an epithelial structure (Bowman's capsule). The capillaries are arranged into lobular structures called glomerular tufts and are lined by a thin layer of endothelial cells. The central region of the glomerulus consists of mesangial cells along with surrounding mesangial matrix. Other components of the glomerulus include the glomerular basement membrane and

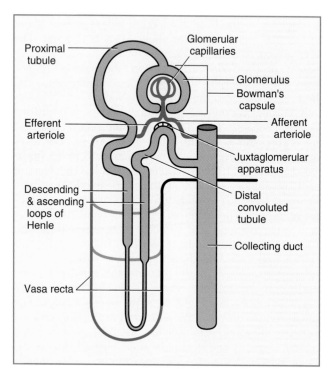

FIGURE 24–2   The nephron, with the basic vascular structures. The glomerular capillaries are supplied by the afferent arterioles and drain into the efferent arterioles. Blood then flows through the vasa recta and is returned to the venous circulation.

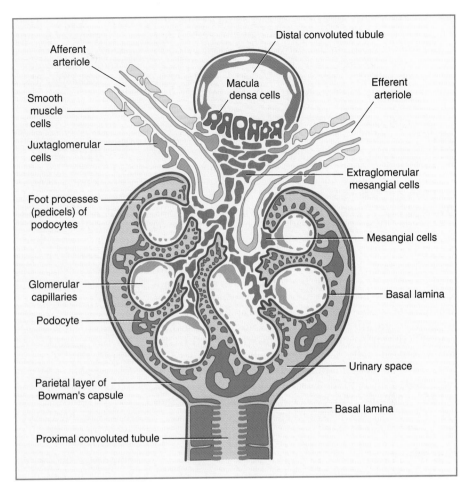

FIGURE 24–3 Schematic diagram of a renal glomerulus and the structures associated at the vascular pole *(top)* and urinary pole *(bottom)* (not drawn to scale). Mesangial cells are associated with the capillary endothelium and the glomerular basement membrane. The macula densa cells of the distal tubule are shown intimately associated with the juxtaglomerular cells of the afferent arteriole and the extraglomerular mesangial cells. (Modified from Kriz W, Sakai T: Morphological aspects of glomerular function. *In* Davison AM [ed]: Nephrology: Proceedings of the Tenth International Congress of Nephrology. London: Bailliére-Tindall, 1987; with permission.)

visceral and parietal epithelial cells. The afferent and efferent arterioles enter and leave the glomerulus at the vascular pole, and Bowman's capsule continues as the proximal tubule at the urinary pole.

Endothelial Cells. A thin layer of fenestrated endothelial cells lines the glomerular capillary lumen. The endothelial cells form the initial defense that impedes the passage of blood constituents from the capillary lumen to the urinary space. Furthermore, the endothelial surface is negatively charged and contributes to the charge selective properties of the filtration barrier. The glomerular endothelial cells also play an important role in glomerular pathophysiology.

Glomerular Basement Membrane. The glomerular basement membrane is a layer of hydrated gel composed of glycoproteins containing interwoven collagen fibers (type IV and type V collagen). It is made up of a central dense layer, called the *lamina densa*, and two outer layers, called the *lamina rara interna* and the *lamina rara externa*. The glomerular basement membrane acts as the principal barrier to the filtration of plasma proteins, and in humans its thickness ranges from 315 to 373 nm.

The glomerular epithelial cells and mesangial cells are important in maintaining the integrity of the glomerular basement membrane. The basement membrane functions as a filtration barrier because of the pore size and negative charge, so that for a given molecular size, negatively charged particles are filtered less easily than positively charged particles. Although the largest pores in the glomerular basement membrane are 80 Å in diameter, albumin, which is 60 Å, is not filtered because of the negative surface charge.

Epithelial Cells. The visceral epithelial cells, or podocytes, are the largest cells in the glomerulus. They extend foot processes that lie in direct contact with the lamina rara externa of the basement membrane. The gap between the adjacent foot processes is known as the filtration slit. The podocytes have a negative surface charge because of the presence of sialoproteins, and thus they contribute to the filtration barrier. Furthermore, they play a significant role in the synthesis and maintenance of the glomerular basement membrane. The parietal epithelial cells form the outer wall of the Bowman's capsule and are continuous with the parietal epithelial cells at the vascular pole. There is evidence to suggest that glomerular epithelial cells may be the major sites of injury in various noninflammatory glomerulopathies.

Mesangium. The glomerular tufts are suspended within the urinary space of Bowman's capsule on a lattice known as the mesangium. Mesangial cells are enclosed by a matrix of homogeneous fibrillary material containing mucopolysaccharides and glycoprotein. There is no basement membrane between the capillary endothelium and mesangial cells (see Fig. 24–3). This arrangement provides easy entry of plasma products, as well as allowing for interaction with the inflammatory cells.

Mesangial cells have actin-myosin elements in their cytoplasm, which accounts for their well-established contractile properties. Mesangial cell contraction alters the surface area for filtration, which may lead to a decrease in the glomerular filtration rate. Furthermore, receptors for various vasoconstrictor hormones such as antidiuretic hormone (ADH) and angiotensin II are present on these cells. In addition to the effects on renal blood flow, these hormones alter the glomerular filtration rate through mesangial cell contraction. Another important function of mesangial cells is the production and remodeling of the extracellular matrix composed of collagen and glycoproteins, which provides structural support to the glomerular capillary loops. In response to growth factors such as transforming growth factor (TGF) and platelet-derived growth factor (PDGF), the mesangial cells secrete extracellular matrix. This process results in glomerular basement membrane thickening and is an important factor in the pathogenesis of various glomerular diseases, especially diabetes. Mesangial cells also exhibit some phagocytic properties.

The Tubule

The glomerular capsule funnels ultrafiltrate into the renal tubules. The proximal tubule begins at the urinary pole of the glomerulus and consists of two segments. The initial segment, the proximal convoluted tubule, is located in the cortex. The second segment, the straight portion of the proximal tubule, is located in the medullary ray and enters the medulla to deliver fluid to the loop of Henle. The thin descending limb of the loop of Henle forms a hairpin turn in the medulla and returns toward the cortex, forming the distal tubule. The distal tubule consists of two segments: the thick ascending limb of the loop of Henle and the distal convoluted tubule. The distal tubule leads to the connecting segment, which marks the transition between distal tubule and the collecting segment. The collecting segment comprises the cortical collecting duct and the outer and inner medullary collecting ducts. They terminate as the papillary collecting duct or the ducts of Bellini that empty into the renal pelvis at the tips of the renal papillae.

Juxtaglomerular Apparatus. The structural arrangement of the nephron allows the distal tubule to come into close approximation with the vascular pole of the parent glomerulus. This distinct region of the distal tubule, known as the *macula densa*, contains distal tubular cells that are taller and more numerous than those in other parts of the tubule. The vascular component consists of the terminal portion of the afferent arteriole and the initial portion of the efferent arteriole. The macula densa and the vascular component, together with the extraglomerular mesangial cells, create a specialized structure known as the juxtaglomerular apparatus. This structure is the site of renin formation and is important in coordinating the function of the glomerulus and tubule.

Elements of Renal Physiology

The kidney contributes to body fluid homeostasis by excreting excess solute and water in the urine. The first step in the formation of urine by the kidney requires the production of an ultrafiltrate of plasma at the glomerulus. This fluid, which is relatively free of cellular elements and proteins, flows through the various tubular segments, which absorb solutes and water.

RENAL BLOOD FLOW

Approximately one fifth of the cardiac output is received by the kidneys, which translates to a renal blood flow (RBF) rate of approximately 1200 mL/min and a renal plasma flow (RPF) rate of about 600 mL/min. The blood supply to the kidney is not proportional to its oxygen consumption. For instance, the medulla has a relatively high oxygen consumption rate in comparison with the cortex, but it receives only 15% of the renal blood flow. The RBF is modulated by several circulatory hormones and autocrine factors such as thromboxanes, endothelin, and angiotensin.

GLOMERULAR FILTRATION RATE

In a healthy adult, the glomerular filtration rate (GFR) is approximately 120 mL/min. The filtration fraction is the percentage of renal plasma flow that is filtered, and it is mathematically expressed as the ratio of GFR to RPF. The normal filtration fraction is 0.2, or 20%. Glomerular filtration is a net result of an outwardly directed net pressure that moves fluid across the semipermeable capillary wall. The hydrostatic pressure and plasma oncotic pressure gradients govern this transfer of fluid across the capillary wall, which is expressed by the Starling equation:

$$GFR = Kf(P - \Pi)$$

where GFR is the rate of fluid transfer between the glomerular capillaries and Bowman's space, Kf is the permeability of the glomerular capillary bed, P is the difference in hydrostatic pressure between the glomerular capillaries and Bowman's space, and Π is the difference in oncotic pressure between the glomerular capillary and Bowman's space. The oncotic pressure in Bowman's space is negligible because of the absence of proteins and therefore equals the colloid oncotic pressure in the glomerular capillary.

A normal GFR of 120 mL/min translates to a glomerular ultrafiltrate of 180 L/day. Of this, about 178.5 L of fluid is reabsorbed daily after filtration, and alterations in renal perfusion pressure could significantly affect the net volume of urine produced. However, as described later, there exist regulatory mechanisms in the kidney that prevent major alterations in salt and fluid balance. These regulatory mechanisms operate at the level of glomerular filtration and tubular reabsorption. These mechanisms remain operative in an isolated kidney that is devoid of any contact with the circulatory factors or renal nerves, which indicates that these adaptations are intrinsic to the kidney.

Autoregulation of RBF and GFR

The RBF and GFR are maintained at constant levels over a wide range of arterial pressures between 70 and 180 mm Hg. This phenomenon, in which the GFR is constant in the presence of perturbations that otherwise would result in alteration of GFR, is referred to as *renal autoregulation*. The following mechanisms are operative in regulating GFR and RPF:

1. Myogenic mechanism, which is an inherent property of smooth muscle cells. Alterations in the renal perfusion pressure result in pressure-mediated release of vasoactive factors from the arteriolar endothelium, thus maintaining a constant glomerular perfusion pressure. In other words, a rise in renal perfusion pressure results in stretching of the afferent arteriolar smooth muscle cells, which triggers afferent arteriolar constriction and prevents the transmission of the high capillary pressure to the glomerular capillaries.
2. Tubuloglomerular feedback, which is a fundamental property of the kidney whereby changes in sodium delivery to the macula densa control afferent arteriolar tone. An increase in arterial pressure leads to an initial increase in GFR that subsequently results in increased sodium chloride delivery to the macula densa of the distal tubule. The macula densa senses this and sends a signal to the afferent arteriole, which results in vasoconstriction. The opposite response occurs when the GFR is decreased.

Glomerulotubular Balance

This mechanism operates at the level of the proximal tubules, whereby the fractional rate of proximal tubular sodium reabsorption remains constant despite variations in GFR. This balance is modulated by alterations in the effective circulating volume. In empirical terms, this modulation includes down-setting and up-setting of the glomerulotubular balance in the volume-expanded and volume-depleted states, respectively. These alterations occur independently of changes in GFR.

THE PROXIMAL TUBULE

The primary function of the proximal tubule is the bulk isosmotic reabsorption of the glomerular ultrafiltrate.

Sodium is the most abundant cation in the glomerular filtrate, and therefore it is not surprising that most of the transport processes in the proximal tubule involve sodium transport (Fig. 24–4).

The majority of sodium reabsorption in the proximal tubule involves active transport mechanisms. The Na^+,K^+-ATPase transporter, by pumping sodium from the tubular cell across the basolateral membrane, generates an electrochemical gradient for movement of sodium across the luminal membrane. In general, the transport of sodium across the luminal membrane occurs by combined processes involving other solutes. A countertransport mechanism involving hydrogen ions (H^+) results in the reclamation of most of the filtered bicarbonate. The absorption of glucose and amino acids involves cotransport with sodium. Phosphate is substantially reclaimed in this segment by a mechanism coupled to active sodium absorption. Calcium reabsorption in the proximal tubule also parallels the reabsorption of sodium. Other electrolytes are absorbed in the proximal tubule by mechanisms unrelated to sodium transport. Furthermore, the bulk of the filtered potassium is reabsorbed in this segment.

In the straight portion of the proximal tubule, organic acids such as uric acid and drugs such penicillin are secreted. Most diuretics are also secreted in this neph-

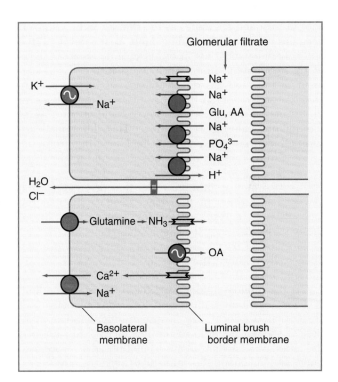

FIGURE 24–4 The major transport processes of the proximal tubular cells. Sodium can be reabsorbed alone; in cotransport with amino acids (AA), glucose (Glu), or anionic compounds such as phosphate (PO_4^{3-}); or by antitransport with hydrogen ions. The proximal nephron is also responsible for reabsorption of calcium, secretion of organic acids (OA), and formation of ammonia, which is important for the secretion of hydrogen ions in the distal nephron. Water and chloride absorption occurs primarily through paracellular pathways.

ron segment. This process is important for the efficacy of these compounds because their activity is mediated through an effect on luminal solute transport mechanisms. Furthermore, ammonia synthesis, an important step in renal acid excretion, also occurs in the proximal tubule.

The removal of solutes, principally sodium salts, from the glomerular filtrate creates an osmotic gradient for water movement from the proximal tubular lumen to the peritubular space. This slight osmotic gradient is adequate to account for proximal isotonic water absorption, because permeability of water is relatively high.

The physical forces surrounding the tubule also govern the solute and water reabsorption in proximal tubules. For example, a high peritubular capillary hydrostatic pressure impairs water and sodium reabsorption from the proximal tubule, and a high colloid oncotic pressure in the peritubular capillary favors the absorption of water and electrolytes from the proximal tubule. The primary determinant of peritubular capillary oncotic pressure is the filtration fraction, and the glomerular capillary hydrostatic pressure determines the hydrostatic pressure in the peritubular capillary.

THE LOOP OF HENLE

The loop of Henle begins at the corticomedullary junction as the thin descending limb and then makes a hairpin turn and continues as the thin ascending limb. It becomes the thick ascending limb at the level of the outer medulla and ends in the macula densa at the level of the glomerulus from which it originated. Each segment of the loop has different permeability for sodium chloride and water, so that about 15% of the volume of the isosmotic ultrafiltrate is absorbed and about 25% of the sodium chloride is absorbed. This differential absorption converts the isotonic fluid entering from the proximal tubule into a dilute fluid delivered to the distal tubule (Fig. 24–5).

Passive water absorption in the thin descending limb and salt absorption in the thin ascending limb of the loop occur as a result of the selective permeability of these segments. The thick ascending limb absorbs sodium chloride by an active, energy-dependent process. Specifically, luminal transport involves an Na$^+$/K$^+$/2 Cl$^-$ cotransporter. Because this segment is impermeable to water, the luminal fluid leaving the thick ascending limb is made hypotonic with regard to plasma by active salt absorption, a critical step in urinary dilution. The addition of sodium chloride to the medullary interstitium is the primary step that allows a multiplicative process to build and maintain the interstitial hypertonicity necessary to absorb water from thin descending limbs and from collecting ducts during antidiuresis.

The hairpin arrangement and countercurrent flow of the loop minimize the work needed to maintain a papillary osmolality of 1200 mOsm/kg H$_2$O, in comparison with the 300 mOsm/kg H$_2$O osmolality of the cortex. A similar organization of the vasa recta allows the sodium chloride absorbed from the loop of Henle and urea absorbed from the papillary collecting duct to be trapped within the interstitium at increasing concentra-

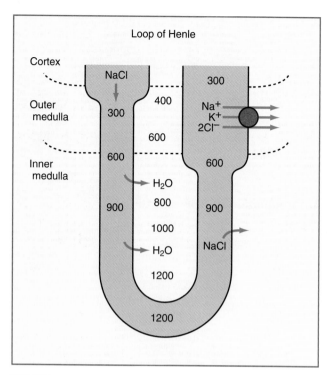

FIGURE 24–5 The loop of Henle is responsible for additional absorption of filtrate. Water is absorbed in the solute-impermeable descending limb. The concentrated medullary interstitium, established by solute transport at the water-impermeable ascending limb, drives water absorption from the descending limb. The hyperosmolar interstitium also provides the driving force for urinary concentration at the collecting duct. The relative osmolarity of the tubular fluid and interstitium is demonstrated by the numerals.

tions. The integrity of these anatomic relationships is essential to the concentrating ability of the kidney.

A significant portion of calcium reabsorption occurs within the loop of Henle. Calcium absorption in the medullary portion of the thick ascending limb varies with the magnitude of the positive luminal transepithelial voltage that accompanies active salt absorption and is not influenced by parathyroid hormone (PTH). In contrast, PTH stimulates the rate of calcium absorption in the cortical thick ascending limb without altering sodium absorption. The thick ascending limb of the loop of Henle is also the major site of magnesium reabsorption.

THE DISTAL NEPHRON

The distal convoluted tubule is a water-impermeable segment of the nephron that continues the dilution of luminal fluid through active sodium chloride absorption. Sodium absorption in the distal nephron occurs primarily by a thiazide diuretic–sensitive, chloride-coupled transport process. The cortical collecting duct reabsorbs sodium by a mineralocorticoid-sensitive process. In states of volume depletion and maximal aldosterone production, the urine can be rendered virtually free of sodium. Because the cortical interstitium remains isotonic to plasma, salt absorption from these segments affects urinary dilution but not urinary concentration.

Potassium secretion begins in the distal convoluted tubule and continues along the collecting ducts. Virtually all of the filtered potassium is reabsorbed in proximal nephron segments, and the potassium that appears in the urine is mostly a result of secretion by the distal nephron segments. Potassium secretion proceeds by diffusion of the intracellular cation down both concentration and electrical gradients into the tubular lumen. The *principal cell* in the collecting duct is the major site of potassium secretion (Fig. 24–6). The basolateral Na^+,K^+-ATPase establishes the concentration gradient by maintaining a high intracellular potassium concentration. The potassium is then secreted into the tubular lumen down its concentration gradient through a potassium channel. Although some potassium may leak back across the basolateral membrane, two factors favor the movement of potassium into the luminal fluid. First, the concentration of potassium in the luminal fluid is low; enhanced distal tubular flow thus results in the maintenance of low intraluminal potassium concentrations and stimulates potassium secretion. Second, the principal cells also have a sodium channel on the apical side, which results in sodium reabsorption from the tubular lumen. This results in a negative electrical potential in the tubular lumen that favors the movement of potassium from the cell into the tubular lumen. Aldo-

sterone stimulates potassium secretion by enhancing the activity of the basolateral Na^+,K^+-ATPase transporter and by increasing the permeability of the luminal cell membrane to sodium.

Proton secretion in the distal nephron allows absorption of any bicarbonate present in these segments, thereby completing reclamation of filtered bicarbonate. The major contribution of the distal nephron to acid-base homeostasis, however, is new bicarbonate generation, mediated by proton secretion into tubular fluid by a proton ATPase. The secreted H^+ can be either buffered by phosphate or excreted as ammonium ions. The secretory process in the collecting duct generates an intraluminal free H^+ concentration 1000 times greater than the free H^+ concentration in blood. The secretory process allows for the generation of bicarbonate within the cell, which is transported into the blood to replenish bicarbonate consumed during buffering of nonvolatile acids. The quantity of new bicarbonate added to body fluids is equal to the daily H^+ generation from dietary protein and is approximately 1 mEq/kg of body weight daily. The same factors that determine the rate of distal potassium secretion—namely, the luminal delivery of sodium and the presence of aldosterone—also promote secretion of H^+ in the distal tubule.

The collecting ducts (cortical, medullary, and papillary) are the primary sites of ADH action. They are minimally permeable to water in the absence of ADH and, in that circumstance, can deliver the hypotonic (50 to 100 mOsm/kg of H_2O) fluid issuing from the distal convoluted tubule unchanged into the urine. When ADH is present, water passes across the tubule wall readily, and the luminal fluid tonicity approaches that of the interstitium at any level. Maximal urinary concentrating ability thus depends on the availability of ADH plus the degree of the medullary hypertonicity generated from thick ascending limb sodium chloride absorption and trapping of salt and urea. Intrinsic renal prostaglandins impair distal water reabsorption through several mechanisms, including blockade of ADH action in the collecting duct. Thus, nonsteroidal anti-inflammatory drugs, by blocking prostaglandins, may impair renal free water excretion.

RENAL HOMEOSTATIC FUNCTIONS
(Table 24–1)

Regulation of Water, Acid-Base, and Electrolyte Balance

The kidney is responsible for eliminating any excess fluid and solute that are ingested. The most commonly encountered abnormalities in fluid and electrolyte balance are referable to sodium, potassium, water, and acid-base physiology. The renal contribution to these abnormalities is discussed in detail in Chapter 26.

The kidney also plays a major role in the balance of other electrolytes. Calcium reabsorption from the glomerular ultrafiltrate helps to regulate body calcium balance. The bulk of filtered calcium (approximately 60%) is reabsorbed in the proximal tubule, along with sodium. Factors that alter fractional proximal tubular reabsorp-

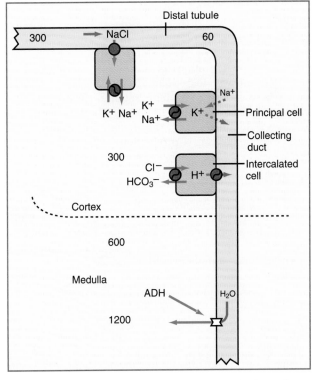

FIGURE 24–6 The distal nephron is responsible for fine adjustment of the final urinary constituents. Solute absorption in the water-impermeable cortical segments results in dilute urine. Cortical collecting segments provide secretion of potassium and hydrogen ions. The medullary collecting duct is the site of urinary concentration as water is absorbed across a membrane made permeable by antidiuretic hormone (ADH) down a concentration gradient into the hypertonic interstitial compartment.

TABLE 24–1   Renal Homeostatic Functions

Function	Mechanism	Affected Elements
Waste excretion	Glomerular filtration	Urea, creatinine
	Tubular secretion	Urate, lactate, drugs (diuretics)
	Tubular catabolism	Pituitary hormones, insulin
Electrolyte balance	Tubular NaCl absorption	Volume status, osmolar balance
	Tubular K^+ secretion	Potassium concentration
	Tubular H^+ secretion	Acid-base balance
	Tubular water absorption	Osmolar balance
	Tubular Ca, Phos, Mg transport	Ca, Phos, Mg homeostasis
Hormonal regulation	Erythropoietin production	Red blood cell mass
	Vitamin D activation	Calcium homeostasis
Blood pressure regulation	Altered sodium excretion	Extracellular volume
	Renin production	Vascular resistance
Glucose homeostasis	Gluconeogenesis	Glucose supply (maintained) in prolonged starvation

Ca = calcium; Mg = magnesium; NaCl = sodium chloride; Phos = phosphate.

tion greatly influence calcium excretion. PTH, through its action in the cortical thick ascending limb and the distal convoluted tubule, enhances calcium reabsorption.

In hypocalcemic conditions, the serum PTH is increased, and the renal conservation of filtered calcium is maximized. Concomitantly, when the serum calcium concentration is elevated, PTH is suppressed and renal tubular calcium absorption is decreased. Unfortunately, the symptoms of hypercalcemia often lead to volume depletion, which stimulates sodium and calcium conservation by the nephron. Hypercalcemia also leads to a decrease in the GFR, further limiting the urinary excretion of calcium.

Magnesium is absorbed in the proximal tubule at a lower rate than is sodium. The majority of magnesium absorption occurs in the loop of Henle. Decreases in fractional proximal tubular absorption (caused by extracellular fluid expansion) and decreases in sodium chloride absorption in the loop of Henle (caused by diuretics) increase the excretion of magnesium. Renal loss of magnesium is a common cause of hypomagnesemia, and hypermagnesemia is almost always the result of a severely diminished GFR.

Waste Excretion

The kidney is responsible for elimination of nitrogenous products of protein catabolism. This is accomplished primarily by filtration at the glomerulus. Because homeostatic requirements necessitate the maintenance of low concentrations of these compounds, large volumes of ultrafiltrate formation are necessary for excretion of the absolute quantity of material. The normal daily GFR of 180 L makes such mass elimination possible.

A second mechanism of solute entry into the urine is tubular secretion. Organic acids (such as urate and lactate) and organic bases (such as creatinine) are excreted in this manner. The secretory process is the major route of elimination for substances that are protein-bound. A large number of drugs, including antibiotics and diuretics, are excreted through this mechanism.

The kidney contributes to the metabolic degradation of a number of peptide hormones, including most pituitary hormones, glucagon, and insulin. This is accomplished by filtration of these substances at the glomerulus and catabolism by the renal tubular cells. Decreased renal catabolism of insulin in diabetics with renal insufficiency may be manifested as a prolongation of the effect of exogenous insulin.

Regulation of Blood Pressure

It has been proposed that the kidney plays a major role in the genesis of hypertension. In certain forms of essential hypertension, the primary defect may be impaired sodium excretion by the kidney, which leads to expanded intravascular volume. Natriuretic factors released in response to sodium retention cause vasoconstriction and promote hypertension. The blood pressure is further modulated by the release of renin, which results in angiotensin II production.

Renal Hormonal Regulation

The kidney is the major site of *erythropoietin* production. This hormone is a highly glycosylated, 39,000-d protein. It is produced in the renal cortex, either by peritubular capillary cells or peritubular fibroblasts. Erythropoietin stimulates red blood cell production by its effect on the bone marrow. Erythropoietin production increases in states of decreased tissue oxygen delivery. This may occur as a result of chronic hypoxemia, as seen in persons living at high altitudes or in patients with lung disease, or as a result of decreased oxygen-carrying capacity of blood, as seen in anemic individuals.

The kidney contributes to calcium homeostasis not only by directly regulating excretion but also by affecting hormonal production. *Vitamin D* requires two in vivo hydroxylations to become the potent hormone that regulates intestinal calcium absorption. After hydroxylation in the liver at the 25 position of the molecule, renal proximal tubular cells add a second hydroxyl ion at the 1 or 24 position. This hydroxylation step is controlled and stimulated by PTH and low phosphate.

As noted previously, the juxtaglomerular cells produce and secrete *renin*. Renin promotes the formation of angiotensin II, a potent vasoconstrictor that is a stimulus to aldosterone secretion. Aldosterone stimulates renal sodium absorption and excretion of potassium and hydrogen ions.

Glucose Homeostasis

The kidney participates in the regulation of plasma glucose by its ability to synthesize glucose by the gluconeogenetic pathway. Lactate, pyruvate, and amino acids are used by the kidney for gluconeogenesis. This function becomes important in prolonged starvation states, in which up to 40% of plasma glucose is contributed by the kidney. In addition to decreased clearance and degradation of insulin, absence of this gluconeogenetic pathway in patients with severe renal dysfunction may contribute to hypoglycemia.

REFERENCES

Guyton AC, Hall JE: Urine formation by the kidney: Glomerular filtration, renal blood flow, and their control. *In* Guyton AC, Hall JE (eds): Textbook of Medical Physiology, 9th ed. Philadelphia: WB Saunders, 1996, pp 315–330.

Tisher CC: Structure and function of the kidneys. *In* Goldman L, Bennett JC (eds): Cecil Textbook of Medicine, 21st ed. Philadelphia: WB Saunders, 2000, pp 532–539.

Tisher CC, Madsen KM: Anatomy of the kidney. *In* Brenner BM, Rector FC Jr (eds): The Kidney, 4th ed. Philadelphia: WB Saunders, 1991, pp 3–75.

25

APPROACH TO THE PATIENT WITH RENAL DISEASE

Yousri M. H. Barri • Sudhir V. Shah

Assessment of the Patient with Renal Disease

RENAL FUNCTION TESTS

An approximate assessment of glomerular filtration rate (GFR) is most easily obtained by measuring the concentration of creatinine and blood urea nitrogen. Creatinine is a metabolite of creatine, a major muscle constituent. In a given individual, the daily rate of production of creatinine is constant and is determined by the mass of skeletal muscle. Creatinine is eliminated almost entirely by glomerular filtration, and its concentration in the serum has been used as a marker of renal function. The "normal" range for serum creatinine concentration is 0.8 to 1.3 mg/dL in men and 0.6 to 1.1 mg/dL in women. The serum creatinine value is lower in women because of less muscle mass, which leads to a lower rate of creatinine production. However, a value in this range does not necessarily imply normal renal function. For example, in a patient whose creatinine increases from 0.6 to 1.2 mg/dL, a 50% decrease in GFR has occurred, despite creatinine remaining in the "normal" range. Certain drugs such as cimetidine, trimethoprim, triamterene, and amiloride may interfere with creatinine excretion and cause a false elevation in the serum creatinine value. A more accurate assessment of renal function is obtained by determining the creatinine clearance. However, once the relation between the serum creatinine and the creatinine clearance is established for a given patient, the serum creatinine can be followed as a reliable indicator of GFR, provided there is no significant change in muscle mass.

The blood urea nitrogen concentration is often used in conjunction with the serum creatinine concentration as a measure of renal function. Urea is the major end product of protein metabolism, and its production reflects the dietary intake of protein as well as the protein catabolic rate. Urea is excreted by glomerular filtration, but a significant amount of urea is reabsorbed along the tubule, particularly in sodium-avid states such as volume depletion. Consequently, the blood urea nitrogen value may vary in relation to the extracellular fluid volume, whereas the serum creatinine concentration is less dependent on volume status. The usual ratio of urea nitrogen to creatinine concentration in the serum is 10:1. This ratio is increased in a number of clinical settings (Table 25–1).

Determination of the clearance of endogenous creatinine is a convenient test and provides a reasonable estimate of the GFR. Two major errors limit the accuracy of creatinine clearance: increasing creatinine secretion and incomplete urine collection. Approximately 10% of creatinine is excreted by the process of tubular secretion. Therefore, creatinine clearance overestimates the true GFR, particularly in azotemic patients. The creatinine clearance (C_{cr}) is calculated as shown in Table 25–2. The daily excretion of creatinine in the urine is relatively constant and averages 20 to 25 mg/kg/day in men and 15 to 20 mg/kg/day in women. If in a 24-hour urine collection the creatinine excretion deviates significantly from these values, the urine collection may be incomplete. A simpler approach is the Cockroft-Gault formula in which the serum creatinine concentration is used along with age, sex, and weight to estimate the GFR (Table 25–3). Averaged creatinine and urea clearance is an alternative in patients with moderate renal failure (creatinine level, >2.5 mg/dL). The clearance of creatinine overestimates the GFR, whereas urea clearance underestimates the GFR and results in a more reliable estimation of renal function.

Renal tubular function is evaluated by tests that examine the ability of the kidney to maintain salt and water balance as well as acid-base homeostasis. Maximal urinary concentrating ability can be assessed by the wa-

TABLE 25–1   Factors Affecting Blood Urea Nitrogen Level Independent of Renal Function

Disproportionate Increase in Blood Urea Nitrogen
Volume depletion "prerenal azotemia"
Gastrointestinal hemorrhage
Corticosteroid or cytotoxic agents
High-protein diet
Obstructive uropathy
Sepsis
Catabolic states tissue breakdown

Disproportionate Decrease in Blood Urea Nitrogen
Low-protein diet
Liver disease

ter deprivation test. In the polyuric patient suspected of having a defect in urinary concentrating ability, the administration of 5 units of aqueous vasopressin once the urinary osmolality reaches a steady state distinguishes patients with either central or nephrogenic diabetes insipidus. Patients with central diabetes insipidus develop a doubling of the urinary osmolality with aqueous vasopressin. In contrast, individuals with nephrogenic diabetes insipidus do not respond with further increase in urinary concentration.

The fractional excretion of various solutes in the urine provides useful information about the tubular handling of a solute relative to its GFR. The fractional excretion of sodium (Fe_{Na}) is the fraction of sodium filtered at the glomerulus, which is ultimately excreted in the urine (Table 25–4). Determination of the Fe_{Na} is most useful in the differential diagnosis of acute oliguric renal failure. Note that the Fe_{Na} can be calculated on a spot specimen because the volume terms in the numerator and denominator cancel each other. A value for Fe_{Na} less than 1% suggests prerenal failure such as volume depletion, whereas a value greater than 1% is consistent with parenchymal renal disease such as acute tubular necrosis or interstitial nephritis. The Fe_{Na} may, however, be less than 1% in patients with acute glomerular disease or radiocontrast-induced acute renal failure. In patients with persistent vomiting, volume depletion may be associated with high Fe_{Na} because of metabolic alkalosis leading to increased urinary sodium. However, the urinary chloride concentration typically is low and is a better index of volume depletion.

Acidification of the urine is an important tubular

TABLE 25–2   Calculation of the Creatinine Clearance

$C_{cr} = U_{cr} \times V/P_{cr}$
where C_{cr} = clearance of creatinine (mL/min)
        U_{cr} = urine creatinine (mg/dL)
        V = volume of urine (mL/min) (for 24-hr volume: divide by 1440)
        P_{cr} = plasma creatinine (mg/dL)
Normal range: 95 to 105 mL/min/1.75 m²

TABLE 25–3   Cockroft-Gault Formula to Calculate Creatinine Clearance (C_{cr})

$$C_{cr} = \frac{(140 - \text{age in years}) \times (\text{lean body weight in kg})}{S_{cr} \text{ in mg/dL} \times 72}$$
For women multiply final value by 0.85

S_{cr} = serum creatinine.

function that can be assessed by the measurement of the urine pH. In the presence of systemic acidosis (arterial pH, <7.3), the urine pH should be less than 5.3. Failure to acidify urine in the presence of systemic acidosis suggests distal renal tubular acidosis.

A normal individual excretes less than 150 mg/day of protein. The glomerular basement membrane serves as an effective barrier to the passage of high-molecular-weight proteins such as albumin, and the renal tubules have the capacity to reabsorb the small amount of protein that is filtered. Abnormal proteinuria may occur as a transient phenomenon in individuals with febrile illnesses or congestive heart failure or after vigorous exercise. Orthostatic proteinuria is a benign condition that is confirmed by the absence of proteinuria in overnight urine collection while the patient is supine. Persistent proteinuria almost always indicates renal disease. On all timed urine samples for protein, a simultaneous determination of urine creatinine is useful as a means of assessing the accuracy of urine collection. Patients who excrete more than 3.5 g of protein have, with rare exceptions, glomerular disease. Less than 3.5 g of urinary protein can be found in patients with glomerular and tubular diseases. Microalbuminuria of 30 to 300 mg/24 hr is associated with progression of renal disease and with higher cardiovascular morbidity and mortality in patients with diabetes and hypertension.

URINALYSIS

Urinalysis is a simple, noninvasive, and inexpensive means of detecting renal disease. A clean-catch voided urine specimen should be examined promptly by both chemical and microscopic means.

Normal urine color ranges from almost colorless to deep yellow, depending on the concentration of the urochrome pigment. Abnormal urine colors may be a sign of disease or may indicate the presence of a pigment,

TABLE 25–4   Calculation of the Fractional Excretion of Sodium

Fractional excretion of sodium (Fe_{Na}) = fraction of sodium filtered at the glomerulus that is ultimately excreted in the urine
Fe_{Na} = clearance of sodium/clearance of creatinine
$Fe_{Na} = U_{Na} V \div P_{Na}/U_{cr} \div VP_{cr} = U_{Na}/P_{Na}(P_{cr}/U_{cr})$
where P_{Na} = plasma sodium (mEq/L)
P_{cr} = plasma creatinine (mg/dL)
U_{Na} = urine sodium (mEq/L)
U_{cr} = urine creatinine (mg/dL)

drug, or dye. The presence of red blood cells or myoglobin often results in red or smoke-colored urine. Cloudiness of the urine may occur when a high concentration of white blood cells is present (pyuria) or when amorphous phosphates precipitate in alkaline urine.

A chemical assessment of the urine is performed with the "dipstick," a plastic strip impregnated with various reagents that detect the pH, protein, hemoglobin, glucose, and ketones in the urine. These assays are semiquantitative and are graded on the basis of color changes in the various reagent strips. The dipstick method for the detection of urinary protein is sensitive for albumin but does not detect immunoglobulins or tubular proteins (Tamm-Horsfall mucoprotein). The disadvantage of the dipstick method is its failure to detect Bence Jones proteins. The urine sulfosalicylic acid test is an alternate test that detects all urinary proteins by a process of precipitation. A very concentrated urine may show trace to 1+ protein (10 to 30 mg/dL) in a normal individual. The finding of blood in the urine is abnormal and generally indicates the presence of intact red blood cells. Blood detected by a dipstick that cannot be accounted for by red blood cells in the urine sediment is due to either hemoglobin or myoglobin.

Microscopic examination of the urine sediment is used to detect cellular elements, casts, crystals, and microorganisms (Table 25–5). *Microscopic hematuria* is defined as more than two red blood cells per high-power field on a centrifuged urine specimen in the absence of contamination by menstrual blood. Red cells of glomerular origin tend to be dysmorphic and have many sizes and shapes, whereas nonglomerular red cells are uniform in size and shape. The presence of red cell casts confirms the nephronic origin of hematuria. *Pyuria* is defined as the presence of more than four white blood cells per high-power field. The presence of pyuria suggests urinary tract infection or inflammation. Sterile pyuria (negative culture in the presence of pyuria) suggests the diagnosis of prostatitis, chronic urethritis, renal tuberculosis, renal stones, or papillary necrosis. Documentation of eosinophiluria by Wright's or Hansel's stain is suggestive of interstitial nephritis. Renal tubular epithelial cells are large, with prominent nuclei, and are often seen in acute tubular necrosis, glomerulonephritis, or pyelonephritis. Epithelial cells are commonly found in the urinary sediment and may derive from any site along the urinary tract from the renal pelvis to the urethra. Renal tubular cells that contain absorbed lipids are termed *oval fat bodies*. Free fat droplets composed primarily of cholesterol esters may also be observed in the urine, usually in association with heavy proteinuria.

Urinary casts are cylindric structures derived from the intratubular precipitation of Tamm-Horsfall protein. The presence of red or white blood cells in the casts provides presumptive evidence of inflammatory parenchymal renal disease. *Red blood cell casts* most frequently indicate the presence of a proliferative glomerular lesion but may also be seen in patients with acute interstitial nephritis. *Renal tubular cell casts* (often with dirty brown, coarse granular casts) in a patient with acute renal failure help to make the diagnosis of acute tubular necrosis. The presence of *leukocyte casts* in a patient with urinary tract infection indicates a diagnosis of pyelonephritis rather than a lower urinary tract infection. Leukocyte casts may also be seen in interstitial nephritis and, less commonly, in glomerulonephritis.

In the absence of specific symptoms, crystals of calcium oxalate (envelope shaped) and uric acid (rhomboid) often identified in acidic urine are of little clinical significance. The presence of cystine crystals (benzene ring shaped) in the urine indicates the rare disease cystinuria. Triple phosphate crystals ("coffin-lid" shaped) may be identified in alkaline urine. Bacteria in the urine are almost always recognized in a centrifuged specimen but do not necessarily imply significant bacteriuria. The presence of bacteria in an unspun specimen, however, is significant and provides presumptive evidence for a urinary tract infection.

TABLE 25–5 **Microscopic Examination of the Urine**

Finding	Associations
Casts	
Red blood cell	Glomerulonephritis, vasculitis
White blood cell	Interstitial nephritis, pyelonephritis
Epithelial cell	Acute tubular necrosis, interstitial nephritis, glomerulonephritis
Granular	Renal parenchymal disease (nonspecific)
Waxy, broad	Advanced renal failure
Hyaline	Normal finding in concentrated urine
Fatty	Heavy proteinuria
Cells	
Red blood cell	Urinary tract infection, urinary tract inflammation
White blood cell	Urinary tract infection, urinary tract inflammation
Eosinophil	Acute interstitial nephritis
(Squamous) epithelial cell	Contaminants
Crystals	
Uric acid	Acid urine, acute uric acid nephropathy, hyperuricosuria
Calcium phosphate	Alkaline urine
Calcium oxalate	Acid urine, hyperoxaluria, ethylene glycol poisoning
Cystine	Cystinuria
Sulfur	Sulfa-containing antibiotics

The Major Renal Syndromes

A patient with renal disease may present with hematuria, proteinuria, nocturia, polyuria, or edema. Often, however, the symptoms are nonspecific, and it is not unusual for a patient to present with moderate-to-severe renal insufficiency already present. Although the division of clinical manifestations into separate clinical syndromes is arbitrary and overlap exists, classification of the expression of renal injury into common themes serves a useful purpose, namely, consideration of specific clinicopathologic entities (Table 25–6).

The *acute nephritic syndrome* is a clinical syndrome characterized by relatively abrupt onset of renal dysfunction accompanied by hematuria that is nephronic in origin. The presence of red blood cell casts and dysmorphic erythrocytes in the urine sediment, as well as significant degrees of proteinuria, is highly suggestive of the nephronic origin of the hematuria. Sodium avidity in the acute nephritic syndrome is considerably greater than what would be expected from decreased GFR. Plasma albumin is generally normal, so that a significant fraction of the retained sodium remains intravascular and may explain the presence of hypertension, plasma volume dilution, circulatory overload, and congestive heart failure.

Although acute poststreptococcal glomerulonephritis is the prototype for the acute nephritic syndrome, other infections may also lead to this syndrome. This syndrome may also be due to primary glomerular diseases, such as mesangioproliferative glomerulonephritis, and multisystem diseases, such as systemic lupus erythematosus, Henoch-Schönlein syndrome, and essential mixed cryoglobulinemia.

The *nephrotic syndrome* is characterized by increased glomerular permeability, manifested by proteinuria in excess of 3.5 g/day/1.73 m² body surface area. There is a variable tendency toward edema, hypoalbuminemia, and hyperlipidemia.

An important step in classifying and therefore determining the type of glomerular involvement is the urinalysis. On the basis of the urinalysis, a patient with massive proteinuria may be classified as having a nephrotic or a nephritic form. Patients with a nephrotic form, in addition to proteinuria, may demonstrate oval fat bodies, coarse granular casts, and occasional cellular elements, but the lack of "active" sediment is characteristic. The differential diagnosis includes glomerular diseases such as minimal change disease, membranous nephropathy,

diabetic nephropathy, and amyloidosis. In patients with the nephrotic syndrome and an active urinary sediment that has glomerular hematuria (by virtue of dysmorphic red blood cells and/or red blood cell casts) along with moderate to heavy proteinuria (nephrotic/nephritic syndromes), membranoproliferative nephritis, systemic lupus erythematosus, postinfectious glomerulonephritis, and mixed essential cryoglobulinemia are the most likely diagnostic considerations.

The term *rapidly progressive renal failure* is applied to patients who have a rapid deterioration in renal function over weeks to months. This contrasts to patients with *acute renal failure*, who have an abrupt decline in renal function over several days, and to patients with *chronic renal failure*, who have a decline in renal function over years. The differential diagnosis of a patient who presents with rapidly progressive renal failure is shown in Table 25–7. One of the important but uncommon causes of rapidly progressive renal failure is rapidly progressive glomerulonephritis. This is a clinical syndrome of rapid and progressive decline in renal function (usually at least a 50% decline in GFR over 3 months) associated with extensive glomerular crescent formation (usually more than 50%) as the principal histologic finding on renal biopsy. Dysmorphic erythrocytes, red blood cell casts, and moderate proteinuria are characteristic in rapidly progressive glomerulonephritis, as in other nephritic syndromes.

Acute renal failure is a syndrome that can be broadly defined as an abrupt decline in renal function sufficient to result in azotemia over days to a few weeks. Acute renal failure can result from a decrease in renal blood flow (prerenal azotemia), intrinsic parenchymal disease (renal azotemia), or obstruction to urine flow (postrenal azotemia). The general approach for evaluating acute renal failure is detailed in Chapter 30.

Tubulointerstitial nephropathy designates a group of clinical disorders that principally affect the renal tubules and interstitium, with relative sparing of the glomeruli and renal vasculature. In the majority of cases it is

TABLE 25–6   Major Renal Syndromes

Syndrome	Definition	Example
Acute nephritic syndrome	Abrupt onset of renal insufficiency accompanied by hematuria that is glomerular or tubular in origin	Poststreptococcal glomerulonephritis
Nephrotic syndrome	Increased glomerular permeability manifested by massive proteinuria (>3.5 g/day/1.73 m²)/edema and hypoalbuminuria	
With "bland" urine sediment (pure nephrotic)	Oval fat bodies, coarse granular casts	Minimal change disease
Asymptomatic urinary abnormalities	Isolated proteinuria (<2.0 g/day/1.73 m²) or hematuria (with or without proteinuria)	IgA nephropathy
Tubulointerstitial nephropathy	Renal insufficiency associated with non–nephrotic-range proteinuria and functional tubular defects	Analgesic nephropathy
Acute renal failure	An abrupt decline in renal function sufficient to result in retention of nitrogenous waste (e.g., blood urea nitrogen and creatinine)	Acute tubular necrosis
Rapidly progressive renal failure	Rapid deterioration of renal function over a period of weeks to months	Rapidly progressive glomerulonephritis
Tubular defects	Isolated or multiple tubular transport defects	Renal tubular acidosis

TABLE 25–7   Causes of Rapidly Progressive Renal Failure

Obstructive uropathy
Malignant hypertension
Rapidly progressive glomerulonephritis
Thrombotic thrombocytopenic purpura/hemolytic-uremic syndrome
Atheromatous embolic disease
Bilateral renal artery stenosis
Scleroderma crisis
Multiple myeloma

possible to classify the disease into acute interstitial nephritis or chronic interstitial nephropathy on the basis of the rate of progression of renal dysfunction. Chronic tubulointerstitial nephropathy is characterized by renal insufficiency, non–nephrotic-range proteinuria, and tubular damage disproportionately severe relative to the degree of azotemia. Thus, patients with chronic tubulointerstitial disease often have modest degrees of sodium wasting, hyperkalemia, and a normal anion gap metabolic acidosis even when renal dysfunction is modest. Acute interstitial nephritis, often caused by a drug, is characterized by sudden onset of clinical signs of renal dysfunction associated with a prominent inflammatory cell infiltrate within the renal interstitium and is often important in the differential diagnosis of patients with acute renal failure.

Radiologic Imaging of the Urinary Tract

The plain film of the abdomen or the kidney/ureter/bladder view is a simple way to determine renal size and shape. Renal ultrasonography is a more reliable test to determine kidney size, and the kidney/ureter/bladder film is rarely used for this purpose. Radiopaque renal calculi composed of calcium, magnesium ammonium phosphate (struvite), or cystine are often apparent in a plain film of the abdomen.

Renal ultrasonography is a noninvasive method of obtaining an anatomic image of the kidney and the collecting system. This technique is particularly useful for the detection of renal masses, cysts, and dilatation of the collecting system (hydronephrosis). Renal ultrasonography may serve as the primary imaging procedure for patients with unexplained renal failure to assess renal size and determine whether a patient has obstructive uropathy. The absence of evidence of hydronephrosis on an ultrasonogram does not rule out obstructive uropathy, particularly in the presence of acute obstruction, volume depletion, or retroperitoneal fibrosis. In a patient with advanced renal failure, the presence of bilaterally small kidneys implies a chronic, irreversible process whereas the presence of normal-sized kidneys indicates acute renal failure or chronic renal failure due

to diseases such as diabetes, amyloid, or multiple myeloma. Duplex ultrasonography in which B-mode ultrasonography has been combined with pulsed Doppler imaging may be useful in detecting disease of the major renal arteries or veins. Simple cysts are easily identified by ultrasound. However, complex cysts or solid lesions require further investigation by computed tomography or magnetic resonance imaging. Discrepancy in kidney size by more than 1.5 cm may suggest renovascular disease. Ultrasonography is used routinely to guide kidney biopsy, to introduce nephrostomy tubes, or to drain fluid collection around the kidney.

Intravenous pyelography involves the intravenous administration of iodinated radiographic contrast medium that is excreted through the kidney by glomerular filtration. The contrast medium concentrates in the renal tubules and produces a nephrogram image within the first few minutes after injection. As the medium passes into the collecting system, the calyces, renal pelvis, ureters, and bladder are visualized. The advantages of intravenous pyelography over ultrasonography include a low false-positive rate, the ability to identify the site and cause of obstruction, and the detection of papillary necrosis or caliceal blunting. The disadvantage of intravenous pyelography is the requirement for radiocontrast, which can induce nephrotoxicity, particularly in patients with renal insufficiency, volume depletion, diabetes, or multiple myeloma.

Retrograde pyelography is performed by injection of radiocontrast material directly into the ureters at the time of cystoscopy. This technique is useful in the definition of obstructing lesions within the ureter or renal pelvis, particularly in the setting of a nonvisualizing kidney on intravenous pyelography. Ureteric stones can be removed during this procedure using a special basket.

Computed tomography of the kidney is useful to define further abnormalities seen on ultrasonography or intravenous pyelography. The studies are usually done with instillation of a contrast medium, except when investigating renal calculi or hemorrhage when contrast medium is not required. Computed tomography is most helpful to evaluate renal masses, complex cysts, perinephric pathology, and vascular pathology such as renal vein thrombosis. In selected cases, it is used to guide kidney biopsy, biopsy from renal masses, or fluid collection such as perinephric abscess.

Magnetic resonance imaging uses high magnetic fields and radiofrequencies to construct images. The method avoids the use of ionizing radiation and the administration of contrast material. Magnetic resonance imaging is most helpful in delineating complex renal masses, staging renal tumors and detecting invasion of renal veins, and diagnosing renovascular disease and as an alternative to computed tomography in patients with renal failure to avoid use of a radiocontrast agent. Technical improvement in magnetic resonance angiography has enhanced the detection of renal artery stenosis and the identification of its hemodynamic significance. Magnetic resonance imaging should be avoided in patients with claustrophobia and implanted ferromagnetic devices such as pacemakers.

The *radioisotopic renal scan* provides important non-invasive information about renal blood flow. The test involves the intravenous administration of radiolabeled compounds that are excreted by the kidney. An external scintillation camera provides an image of the kidneys and calculates the rate of uptake and excretion of the labeled compound. Technetium-99m diethylenetriamine-pentaacetic acid (DTPA) and technetium-labeled mercaptoacetyl triglycine are two compounds used to assess renal vascular perfusion qualitatively. Renal scans are useful in assessing renal perfusion and outflow tract integrity. The indications for radioisotope scans include (1) assessment of renal function by calculation of GFR and effective renal plasma flow, (2) measurement of split renal function to determine if one kidney is non-functioning, (3) assessment of the hemodynamic significance of renal artery stenosis by a renal scan after captopril therapy, and (4) evaluation for obstructive uropathy by renal scan after furosemide therapy in the presence of a dilated collecting system.

Renal arteriography involves the direct injection of radiographic contrast medium into the aorta and renal arteries and is used to assess renal vasculature. It is particularly useful in the evaluation of patients with suspected renal artery stenosis or thrombosis and in those with a renal mass. Patients with unexplained hematuria or with a suggested vascular malformation should have a renal arteriogram. A renal arteriogram is an important part of the work-up of living kidney donors. Patients with suspected polyarteritis nodosa may require selective renal arteriography to detect microaneurysms. Renal arteriography is generally limited to situations in which a strong clinical indication exists and the patient is considered a candidate for surgical intervention. Renal vein catheterization is used to confirm the diagnosis of renal vein thrombosis or to obtain blood samples from the renal vein, particularly when renovascular hypertension is suspected. Although renal vein thrombosis can be diagnosed by computed tomography or magnetic resonance imaging, renal venography may be required when the diagnosis is in doubt.

TABLE 25–8   Indications for Kidney Biopsy

Nephrotic syndrome
Persistent proteinuria particularly with abnormal sediment or abnormal renal function
Hematuria associated with abnormal urine sediment or proteinuria
Unexplained hematuria after exclusion of lower urinary tract causes
Systemic disorders with kidney involvement (e.g., systemic lupus erythematosus, Henoch-Schönlein purpura)
Acute renal failure
   Atypical features
   Failure to recover in 6 weeks
Rapidly progressive renal failure
Renal allograft dysfunction

Renal Biopsy

Most renal biopsies are performed when a glomerular lesion is suspected and less commonly in patients with unexplained acute renal failure. Table 25–8 lists the indications for kidney biopsy. The percutaneous biopsy is the most commonly used technique and is a relatively safe procedure. Potential complications of a closed renal biopsy include hematuria, renal hematoma, vascular laceration with the development of arteriovenous fistula, and the inadvertent biopsy of liver, spleen, or bowel. Percutaneous kidney biopsy is contraindicated in solitary or ectopic kidneys (except kidney transplants), horseshoe kidney, uncontrolled bleeding disorders, uncontrolled hypertension, renal infection, renal neoplasm, and uncooperative patients.

REFERENCE

Kokko JP: Approach to the patient with renal disease. *In* Goldman L, Bennett JC (eds): Cecil Textbook of Medicine, 21st ed. Philadelphia: WB Saunders, 2000, pp 526–532.

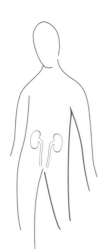

26

FLUID AND ELECTROLYTE DISORDERS

Thomas E. Andreoli • Sameh R. Abul-Ezz

The concentrations of fluid and electrolytes in the cells and fluid compartments of the body are remarkably constant despite a widely varying intake. This equilibrium is maintained by fluid and solute shifts across the cells of the body through well-defined mechanisms and by the capacity of the kidney to regulate the urinary excretion of water, electrolytes, and solutes in response to the needs of the body. In health, the solute content of body water is maintained between 285 and 295 mOsm/kg of water. Tight regulation of body water and solute concentrations is made possible by the remarkable ability of the kidney to regulate urine volume from 500 mL to 24 L per 24-hour period. The ability of the kidney to carry out its functions is intrinsically tied to the thirst-neuro-hypophysial-renal axis.

Volume Disorders

Water is the most abundant molecular component of living matter and constitutes approximately 60% of total-body weight in humans (Fig. 26–1). Total-body water is inversely proportional to the amount of body fat, which varies with age, sex, and nutritional status. Approximately two thirds of the total-body water is in the intracellular compartment. Three fourths of the extracellular water is in the interstitial space, and one fourth is in the plasma. Potassium and magnesium constitute the major cations of the intracellular space, whereas sodium is the major cation of the extracellular space. Phosphate and protein are the major anions of the intracellular space, whereas chloride and bicarbonate are the major anions of extracellular space. The cell membrane represents the barrier between the intracellular and extracellular fluid compartments. Because membranes are relatively permeable to water, the movement of fluid across the cell membrane is determined by the osmotic gradient. Thus, except for transient changes, the intracellular and extracellular fluid compartments are in *osmotic equilibrium.*

The transfer of fluid between the vascular and interstitial compartments occurs across the capillary wall and is governed by the balance between hydrostatic pressure gradients and plasma oncotic pressure gradients, as related in the *Starling equation:*

$$J_v = [K_f(P_C - P_I) - \sigma(COP_P - COP_I)]$$

where J_v is the rate of fluid transfer between vascular and interstitial compartments, K_f is the water permeability of the capillary bed, P_C and P_I are average hydrostatic pressures in the capillary and interstitium, respectively, and COP_P and COP_I are the colloid osmotic pressures in the plasma and interstitial fluid, respectively. Thus, an increase in the driving force for fluid movement into the interstitial compartment may result from a decrease in the colloid oncotic pressure of plasma, as may occur in hypoalbuminemia, and/or an increase in the capillary hydrostatic pressure.

NORMAL VOLUME HOMEOSTASIS

Protection of extracellular fluid volume is a fundamental characteristic of fluid and electrolyte homeostasis. The homeostatic mechanisms sense changes in the *effective circulating volume* (ECV). ECV is difficult to define because it is not a measurable and distinct body fluid compartment. ECV relates to the "fullness" and pressure within the arterial tree. Because only 15% of total blood volume is in the arterial compartment, arterial blood volume can be decreased in relation to the holding capacity of the arterial tree. In most circumstances, ECV correlates with the total extracellular fluid volume, except in certain disorders in which ECV is decreased in the presence of an increased total extracellular fluid volume (Table 26–1). In these disorders, the ECV is decreased as a result of either decreased cardiac output or arterial vasodilatation, which decreases fullness and pressure in the arterial circulation.

The afferent mechanisms sense alterations in the

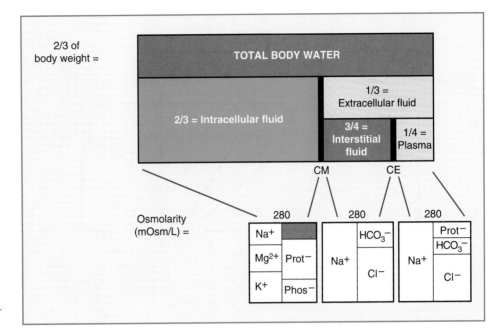

FIGURE 26–1 Composition of body fluid compartments. The compartments are anatomically defined by the cell membrane (CM) and capillary endothelium (CE). The osmolar concentration among compartments is equivalent despite wide variation in cation and anion composition.

ECV and activate a series of effectors that create an *integrated volume response* (Fig. 26–2). Two cardinal mechanisms protect the extracellular fluid volume: alterations in systemic hemodynamics and alterations in the external sodium and water balance. Hemodynamic alterations occur within minutes of a perceived volume reduction and are characterized by tachycardia, increased peripheral resistance from arterial vasoconstriction, and decreased venous capacitance from venoconstriction. Renal conservation of salt and water lags behind by 12 to 24 hours and involves release of various hormones (see Fig. 26–2). Stimulation of the extrarenal baroreceptors also results in the release of antidiuretic hormone (ADH), which promotes water retention in the kidney. Vasoconstrictive factors, such as endothelins, produced and released by vascular endothelial cells, also play a role in modulating systemic hemodynamics. Alterations in the glomerular hemodynamics, through changes in the peritubular Starling forces, directly modulate sodium and water reabsorption in the proximal tubules. Furthermore, vasodilator prostaglandins, such as prostaglandin E_2, maintain the glomerular filtration rate (GFR) by enhancing the renal blood flow in states associated with ECV depletion.

In response to volume expansion, the renal excretion of salt and water is increased because of the suppression of the aforementioned pathways. The release of atrial natriuretic peptide is a major factor promoting natriuresis in volume expanded states. Atrial natriuretic peptide is released from the atrial myocytes in response to atrial stretch associated with volume expansion. It promotes natriuresis through direct effects on the filtration fraction and collecting duct sodium reabsorption and has an indirect inhibitory effect on the renin-angiotensin system.

Because the afferent sensors respond to ECV rather than to the total extracellular fluid volume, in disease states such as congestive heart failure and hepatic cirrhosis, continued activation of the integrated volume response occurs and thus promotes further salt and water retention.

VOLUME DEPLETION

Disorders of extracellular volume result from alterations in sodium balance. The causes of true volume depletion—that is, decreased ECV and total extracellular fluid volume—are illustrated in Table 26–2. The clinical findings in states of true volume depletion are secondary to an underfilling of the arterial tree and to the renal and hemodynamic responses to this underfilling. Mild volume depletion may be associated with orthostatic dizziness and tachycardia. As the intracellular compartment becomes further depleted, recumbent tachycardia becomes evident, and urine output diminishes. Patients with severe volume depletion may present with vasoconstriction, hypotension, mental obtundation, cool extremities, and negligible urine output. Many of these clinical features can be explained on the basis of effects of vasoconstrictor hormones, such as catecholamine and angiotensin II, that are released in response to hypovolemia.

Volume depletion can occur in the absence of classic

TABLE 26–1   Disorders Characterized by Decreased Effective Circulating Volume with Increased Total Extracellular Fluid Volume

Congestive heart failure
Liver disease
Sepsis
Nephrotic syndrome (minority)
Pregnancy
Anaphylaxis

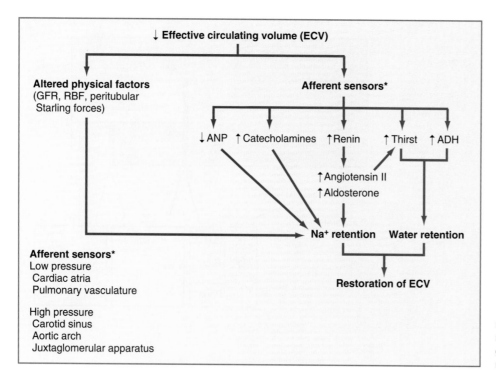

FIGURE 26–2   Volume repletion reaction. ADH = antidiuretic hormone; ANP = atriopeptin; GFR = glomerular filtration rate; RBF = renal blood flow.

clinical findings. States of volume depletion in patients receiving cardiovascular drugs and excess renal sodium loss from intrinsic renal disease or diuretics are examples of clinical circumstances in which an assessment of the state of hydration may be difficult. An appropriate clinical history is always mandatory. If doubt exists about the state of hydration, particularly if the patient appears to be critically ill, measurement of the pulmonary capillary wedge pressure by means of right-sided heart catheterization permits assessment of the intravascular volume status.

The absolute quantity and the rate of fluid replacement depend on the severity of volume depletion, which is estimated by the clinical presentation. If fluid repletion is to involve parenteral infusions, one should consider the distribution of the infused fluid. Solutions containing 0.9% sodium chloride and colloid solutions, which are retained in the extracellular space, are the preferred parenteral solutions for the treatment of hypovolemia. In contrast, only one third of infused 5% glucose (D_5W) remains in the extracellular compartment.

VOLUME EXCESS

Volume expansion occurs when salt and water intake exceeds renal and extrarenal losses. The causes are listed in Table 26–3. The underlying disturbance common to these disorders is sodium and water retention by the kidney. The sodium and water retention may be primary, from an increased ECV, or secondary, in response to a decreased ECV. The net result of renal

---

TABLE 26-2   Causes of Volume Depletion

Gastrointestinal losses
   Upper: bleeding, nasogastric suction, vomiting
   Lower: bleeding, diarrhea, enteric or pancreatic fistula, tube drainage
Renal losses
   Salt and water: diuretics, osmotic diuresis, postobstructive diuresis, acute tubular necrosis (recovery phase), salt-losing nephropathy, adrenal insufficiency, renal tubular acidosis
   Water loss: diabetes insipidus
Skin and respiratory losses
   Sweat, burns, insensible losses
Sequestration without external fluid loss
   Intestinal obstruction, peritonitis, pancreatitis, rhabdomyolysis, internal bleeding

---

TABLE 26-3   Causes of Volume Excess

Primary Renal Sodium Retention (Increased Effective Circulating Volume)
Acute renal failure
Acute glomerulonephritis
Severe chronic renal failure
Nephrotic syndrome
Primary hyperaldosteronism
Cushing's syndrome
Liver disease

Secondary Renal Sodium Retention (Decreased Effective Circulating Volume)
Heart failure
Liver disease
Nephrotic syndrome (minimal change disease)
Pregnancy

sodium and water retention is an alteration of Starling forces that leads to increased capillary hydrostatic pressure and favors fluid shifts from the intravascular to interstitial space. Most patients with nephrotic syndrome have an increased ECV volume resulting from primary renal sodium retention, whereas in a subgroup of patients with nephrotic syndrome with minimal pathologic change, secondary renal sodium retention is due to a decreased ECV. In advanced liver disease, the ECV is decreased because of arterial underfilling from vasodilatation that results in secondary renal sodium retention. However, in early liver disease, the volume excess may result from primary renal sodium retention. Severe hypoalbuminemia associated with liver disease, nephrotic syndrome, or severe malnutrition may overwhelm the local capillary homeostatic mechanisms and may lead to edema formation.

The mainstay in treating volume excess is dietary sodium restriction in combination with diuretics (Table 26–4). Diuretics enhance natriuresis by inhibiting the reabsorption of sodium at various sites along the nephron. The cardinal example of a proximal tubular diuretic is acetazolamide, a *carbonic anhydrase inhibitor,* which blocks proximal reabsorption of sodium bicarbonate. Consequently, prolonged use of acetazolamide may lead to hyperchloremic acidosis. Metolazone, a congener of the thiazide class of diuretics, in addition to blocking sodium reabsorption in the distal tubule, exerts its natriuretic effect in the proximal tubule. Because the proximal tubule is the major site for phosphate reabsorption, profound phosphaturia may accompany the use of metolazone. *Loop diuretics* such as furosemide and bumetanide inhibit the coupled entry of sodium, chloride, and potassium across the apical membranes in the thick ascending limb of the loop of Henle. *Thiazide diuretics* inhibit coupled entry of sodium and chloride across the apical membrane of the distal tubule. The loop diuretics promote calcium excretion, and the thiazide diuretics decrease calcium excretion. Thus, the former are useful in the management of hypercalcemia, whereas the latter are useful in preventing calcium stone formation. Spironolactone, an *aldosterone antagonist,* decreases sodium reabsorption in the cortical collecting duct. Primary *sodium channel blockers,* such as amiloride, also block sodium reabsorption in the cortical collecting duct by an aldosterone-independent mechanism. The last two groups of diuretics do not cause hypokalemia, which is a common complication associated with the use of other diuretics. In states of severe sodium retention and edema formation, such as severe congestive heart failure and nephrotic syndrome, a combination of diuretics working at different sites in the nephron may be more effective than the use of a single class of diuretics. Moreover, potassium and magnesium deficits can be minimized by using potassium-sparing diuretics in combination with a potassium-wasting diuretic. In patients with cirrhosis and ascites, abdominal paracentesis has been used as a good therapeutic alternative to diuretics.

Osmolality Disorders

Body fluid osmolality, the ratio of solute to water in all fluid compartments, is maintained within an extremely narrow range. Because water moves freely across most cell membranes, changes in the extracellular fluid osmolality cause reciprocal changes in the intracellular volume. The extracellular fluid osmolality can be approximated by calculating the serum osmolality based upon the major solutes in that compartment:

$$\text{Calculated osmolality} = 2[Na^+] + [\text{glucose}]/18 + [\text{BUN}]/2.8$$

where the glucose and blood urea nitrogen (BUN) concentrations are expressed as milligrams per deciliters, and the serum sodium concentration is expressed as milliequivalents per liter.

Measured osmolality usually equals the calculated osmolality. However, in the presence of osmotically active substances, such as ethanol, methanol, or ethylene glycol, the measured osmolality is higher than the calculated osmolality. Under these circumstances, the *osmolar gap* (measured calculated osmolality) provides a clue to the presence of toxins and gives an estimated concen-

TABLE 26–4 **Characteristics of Commonly Used Diuretics**

Agent	Site	Primary Effect	Secondary Effect
Carbonic anhydrase inhibitors (acetazolamide)	Proximal tubule	Blocking of Na^+/H^+ exchange	K^+, HCO_3^- loss
Loop diuretics (furosemide, bumetanide, ethacrynic acid)	Thick ascending limb of loop of Henle	↓ $Na^+/K^+/2Cl^-$ transport	K^+ loss ↑ H^+ secretion ↑ Ca^{2+} excretion
Thiazide diuretics			
Thiazides	Distal convoluted tubule	↓ NaCl cotransport	K^+ loss, ↑ H^+ secretion ↓ Ca^{2+} excretion
Metolazone	Distal tubule, proximal tubule	↓ NaCl reabsorption	
Aldosterone antagonists (spironolactone)	Cortical collecting duct	↓ Na reabsorption	↓ K^+ loss ↓ H^+ secretion
Primary sodium channel blockers (triamterene, amiloride)	Cortical collecting duct	↓ Na reabsorption	↓ K^+ loss ↓ H^+ secretion

tration of these solutes. Calculated or measured osmolality differs from the *effective osmolality* (2[Na$^+$]). Because urea freely distributes across cell membranes, it does not contribute to the effective osmolality. Alterations in the plasma sodium concentration almost always reflect changes in water balance. Because sodium is the major cation in the extracellular fluid, disorders of osmolality are generally reflected by an abnormal sodium concentration in the extracellular fluid.

Regulation of osmolality involves alteration in renal water excretion, and the sodium excretion is not affected by osmoregulatory factors unless concomitant ECV depletion exists. Extracellular fluid osmolality is regulated by dual pathways in the *water repletion reaction* (Fig. 26–3). Osmoreceptor cells in the central nervous system that are located in the wall of the third ventricle sense minor changes in the osmolality of blood in the internal carotid circulation. Neuronal signals from osmoreceptors stimulate the release of ADH from the posterior pituitary gland and simultaneously stimulate the sensation of thirst. ADH causes renal water conservation by increasing water permeability and water reabsorption in the collecting ducts. Thirst leads to an increase in water intake. When the extracellular fluid volume is reduced by about 10%, water repletion is activated as a means of replenishing extracellular fluid volume irrespective of osmolality. In this case, baroreceptors in the venous and arterial circulation stimulate ADH release through neuronal pathways. This *nonosmotic* stimulation of ADH release occurs independently of osmoreceptor function. Water repletion activates mechanisms that counterregulate water conservation. Suppression of thirst and inhibition of ADH release lead to decreased water intake and increased renal water excretion.

Hyponatremia

PATHOPHYSIOLOGY

A diagnostic approach to hyponatremia is outlined in Figure 26–4. The causes of hyponatremia show that it can be associated with normal, high, or low total-body sodium content. In some hyponatremic disorders, the serum osmolality is elevated; thus, the intracellular water content is not increased, and no risk of brain edema exists. Hyperglycemia and the use of hypertonic mannitol may result in hyponatremia because of water shift from the intracellular to extracellular space. Hyponatremia associated with normal serum osmolality may be seen in patients with extreme hyperlipidemia and hyperproteinemia, resulting from methodologic errors in techniques to measure serum electrolyte concentration. The increasing use of ion-selective electrodes for these measurements is making these causes of "pseudohyponatremia" uncommon. Hyponatremia may also be seen in patients who undergo transurethral resection of the prostate or hysteroscopy because of the absorption of large amounts of hypo-osmolar glycine or sorbitol irrigating solutions.

Most hyponatremic disorders are associated with hypo-osmolality. In principle, hypo-osmolality can result from an increase in water intake and/or a decrease in renal water excretion. Under normal circumstances, the kidneys can excrete 16 to 20 L of water per day. Water excretion may be impaired secondary to a reduced GFR rate, impaired sodium chloride reabsorption in the renal diluting segments of the distal nephron, or failure to suppress ADH secretion in response to hypertonicity (syndrome of inappropriate ADH [SIADH]). Thus, for a

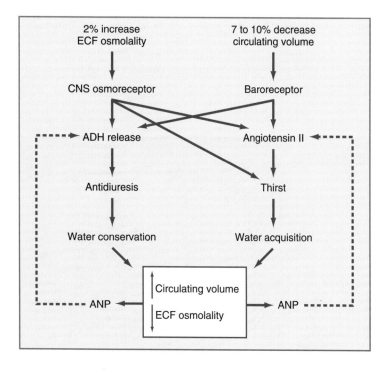

FIGURE 26–3 Water regulatory mechanisms. Alterations in extracellular fluid osmolality or volume stimulate *(solid lines)* thirst and release of antidiuretic hormone (ADH). The net result is a positive water balance. Counterregulation is provided by the inhibitory effects *(dashed lines)* of atriopeptins (ANP). CNS = central nervous system; ECF = extracellular fluid.

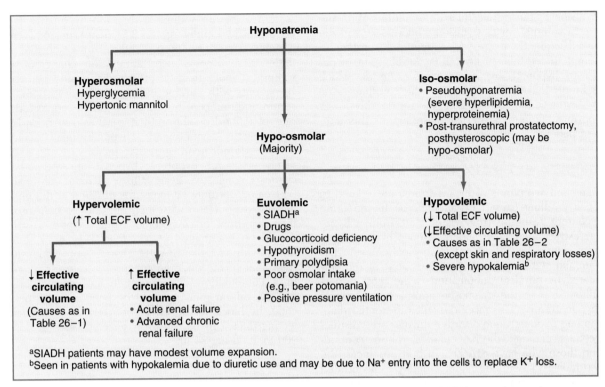

FIGURE 26-4   Diagnostic approach to hyponatremia. ECF = extracellular fluid; SIADH = syndrome of inappropriate antidiuretic hormone.

patient to develop hyponatremia solely as a result of excess water intake is unusual.

In *primary polydipsia*, the hyponatremia is caused by large water intake in the presence of impaired water excretion. Hyponatremia may also occur with modestly increased water intake in the presence of impaired GFR or decreased solute intake. In patients with decreased GFR, renal water excretion is impaired because of decreased delivery of filtrate to the distal nephron. Patients with chronic starvation or beer potomania have deficient oral intake of solutes. Because renal water excretion depends on osmolar intake, these patients may develop hyponatremia at a modestly increased level of water intake.

More commonly, hyponatremia occurs as a result of the inability to dilute urine maximally because of reduction in the rate of salt absorption by the diluting segment, sustained nonosmotic release of ADH, or a combination of these two factors. In the disorders associated with decreased ECV, nonosmotic ADH release occurs and promotes water retention by the kidney. In addition, these patients have enhanced proximal sodium chloride reabsorption with diminished distal delivery. These disorders may be associated with signs of either volume expansion or volume depletion.

SIADH is the prototype of the primary release of ADH or ADH-like substances. It occurs most often in association with pathologic processes of the central nervous system or pulmonary system. Many medications can enhance the release of ADH or can potentiate its effect (Table 26–5). The circulating ADH allows excessive water absorption in the collecting duct with a mod-

TABLE 26-5   Causes of Syndrome of Inappropriate Antidiuretic Hormone

Central Nervous System Disorders

Trauma
Infection
Tumors
Porphyria

Pulmonary Disorders

Tuberculosis
Pneumonia
Positive pressure ventilation

Neoplasia

Carcinoma: bronchogenic, pancreatic, ureteral, prostatic, bladder
Lymphoma and leukemia
Thymoma and mesothelioma

Drugs

Increased ADH release
    Chlorpropamide
    Clofibrate
    Carbamazepine
    Vincristine
Potentiated ADH action
    Chlorpropamide
    Cyclophosphamide
    Nonsteroidal anti-inflammatory agents

ADH = antidiuretic hormone.
Modified from Andreoli TE: Disorders of fluid volume, electrolyte, and acid-base balance. *In* Wyngaarden JB, Smith LH Jr, Bennett JC (eds): Cecil Textbook of Medicine, 19th ed. Philadelphia: WB Saunders, 1992, p 509.

est expansion of the extracellular fluid volume. With the increase in volume, renal perfusion is increased, and the kidney subsequently decreases sodium reabsorption in an attempt to reestablish euvolemia. A subgroup of patients with hyponatremia has a *reset osmostat,* which means simply that these patients are able to dilute urine but at serum sodium levels that are appreciably lower than normal. Treatment of hyponatremia in this subgroup of patients is difficult.

DIAGNOSIS AND TREATMENT

The signs and symptoms of hyponatremia are related to brain cell swelling caused by an increase in the brain water content resulting from water shift from a hypoosmolar extracellular environment. Hence hyponatremic disorders should be considered in any patient who has acute mental status changes. An assessment of the volume status by physical examination is the most important initial step in the diagnostic approach to patients with hyponatremia. The most difficult differential diagnosis among hyponatremic disorders involves the distinction between patients who have modest volume contraction and those who have SIADH. In both instances, the urine osmolality may be inappropriately concentrated relative to the serum osmolality. When the volume depletion is secondary to extrarenal losses, the urine sodium concentration is negligible, whereas it is usually higher than 30 mEq/L in patients with SIADH. High BUN and serum uric acid levels suggest hypovolemia. When hyponatremia is associated with a low BUN and uric acid level, SIADH is the most likely diagnosis.

Baseline data should include body weight, serum electrolytes, serum osmolality, urine electrolytes, and urine osmolality; frequent measurement of serum and urine electrolytes, intake, and urine output should be performed during the treatment of hyponatremia. As a general rule, the administration of solutions with a tonicity ($[Na^+] + [K^+]$) greater than that of urine sodium and potassium concentration raises serum sodium concentrations. The treatment should depend on the underlying clinical disease and volume status of the patient. Sodium and water intake should be restricted in the volume-expanded patient. In patients with decreased ECV and hypovolemia, treatment should include isotonic sodium chloride.

In patients with SIADH, restriction of water intake is the mainstay of therapy. Demeclocycline is also useful in the treatment of this syndrome. Hypertonic saline, often in combination with furosemide, should be reserved solely for the treatment of acute symptomatic hyponatremia with circulatory collapse.

When hyponatremia occurs acutely (<48 hours), cerebral edema can ensue. The typical presentation is with headache, nausea, vomiting, weakness, incoordination with falls, delirium, and seizures. Patients with hyponatremia that develops over days to weeks present with fever or no neurologic signs and symptoms. Caution should be taken when hyponatremia is corrected to avoid central pontine myelinolysis from the overzealous correction of low serum sodium concentrations.

The rate of correction of serum sodium depends on the symptoms and duration of hyponatremia. The correction of serum sodium with acute hyponatremia may be achieved rapidly up to 2.5 mEq/L/hr until central nervous system symptoms and seizures subside. Even under these circumstances, an absolute change of serum sodium of more than 20 mEq/L/day should be avoided. In patients with chronic hyponatremia (>48 hours), the serum sodium concentration should be corrected at a rate of 0.5 mEq/L/hr until it reaches 120 mEq/L. Patients with asymptomatic hyponatremia (acute or chronic) do not need aggressive therapy.

Hypervolemic hypotonic hyponatremia secondary to cirrhosis, congestive heart failure, or renal failure should be treated not only by measures directed at the underlying disease but also with loop diuretics to help promote the excretion of hypotonic urine. Water restriction should be maintained at less than 1 L/24 hr. For patients with chronic SIADH that is not responsive to treatment of the underlying cause, free water restriction or a combination of furosemide and normal or high dietary sodium intake should be beneficial. Demeclocycline, by blocking the effect of ADH on the renal collecting duct, can be useful in selected cases at doses of 900 to 1200 mg/24 hr.

Hypernatremia

PATHOPHYSIOLOGY

In most cases, hypernatremia is caused by excess water loss, rather than by sodium gain. Hypertonicity of the plasma is a powerful stimulus for thirst. Patients unable to sense thirst owing to diseases of the brain or patients who are physically unable to obtain water may develop hypernatremia. Most hypernatremic patients, however, manifest a primary defect in urinary concentrating ability along with insufficient administration of free water (Fig. 26–5).

Water can be lost in the urine, in excess of electrolytes, in conditions characterized by the presence of large quantities of osmotically active solutes in the filtrate. This type of *osmotic diuresis* can occur in patients with hyperglycemia, after the infusion of mannitol, or in patients excreting excessive amounts of amino acids or urea. The last situation occurs in patients receiving high-protein tube feedings or total parenteral nutrition.

Diabetes insipidus is a disorder in which the collecting tubule is impermeable to water. Patients may have a central defect in the release of ADH or a defect in renal responsiveness to the hormone (nephrogenic). This is covered in greater detail in Chapter 64.

In hypernatremia caused by osmotic diuresis, urine osmolality may be higher than serum osmolality because of the presence of solutes, such as glucose, mannitol, or urea in the urine. In these patients, the urine osmolality caused by the presence of electrolytes ($2 \times [Na^+ + K^+]$) is lower than the effective plasma osmolality ($2 \times [Na^+]$).

TREATMENT

Hypernatremia that is associated with hypovolemia implies a sodium deficit in addition to the water deficit

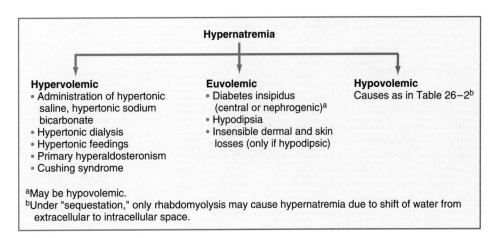

FIGURE 26-5 Diagnostic approach to hypernatremia.

and may require isotonic saline infusion. In other patients, hypotonic intravenous solutions (D_5W, half-normal saline, quarter-normal saline) should be administered to correct hypernatremia. The water content of these fluids varies according to the electrolyte concentration. For example, 1 L of D_5W essentially equals 1 L of free water, because all glucose is eventually metabolized. However, 1 L of half-normal saline or quarter-normal saline contains 500 or 750 mL, respectively, of free water. In addition, if other solutes, such as potassium or magnesium, are added to the intravenous fluids, their contribution to the tonicity of the administered fluid should be taken into account. Administration of solutions that are hypotonic relative to the urine corrects hypernatremia.

The serum sodium concentration can be used as a guide to the replacement of free water by the following formula:

Water deficit
$$= 0.6 \times \text{body weight (kg)} \times [1 - (140/Na^+)]$$

where Na^+ = plasma sodium and body weight (kg) = estimated body weight when hydrated.

The treatment of patients with central diabetes insipidus is discussed in Chapter 64.

As is the case in hyponatremic patients, the rate of correction of hypernatremia is important. In chronic hypernatremia (>36 to 48 hours), the brain generates compounds that raise the intracellular osmolality and thereby minimize cell shrinkage. Thus, rapid correction of plasma osmolality may lead to a shift of water to the relatively hypertonic intracellular compartment and may result in brain edema. As a general rule, hypernatremia should be corrected over 48 hours at a rate not exceeding 0.5 mEq/L/hr, or 12 mEq/L/day.

Disturbances in Potassium Balance

The human body contains approximately 3500 mEq of potassium. With a normal concentration of 3.5 to 5.0 mEq/L, the ECF contains approximately 70 mEq of potassium, or only 2% of total-body stores. In response to a dietary potassium load, rapid removal of potassium from the extracellular space is necessary to prevent life-threatening hyperkalemia. For example, in the absence of a homeostatic mechanism, if a person ingests 50 mEq of dietary potassium in a single meal (the average daily American diet contains 100 to 120 mEq potassium per day), the serum potassium could rise to 7 mEq/L (assuming an extracellular volume of 14 L with a baseline serum potassium of 4 mEq/L). Thus, the initial adaptation to a potassium load is the rapid redistribution of potassium from the extracellular space to the intracellular space. Various hormones including insulin, aldosterone, and catecholamines cause movement of potassium into cells. The acid-base status of the patient is another determinant of the serum potassium concentration, presumably because of an exchange of potassium for hydrogen across the cells. The greatest effect on the serum potassium concentration is associated with metabolic acidosis involving mineral acids. The cellular permeability to the anions of the mineral acids is low, so hydrogen moves relatively unaccompanied into the cell. By contrast, metabolic acidosis caused by organic acids, such as lactic acid and keto acids, does not cause hyperkalemia. The anions of these acids are relatively permeable and accompany hydrogen into the cell. This situation diminishes the electrochemical gradient favoring potassium efflux.

Although these mechanisms affect the distribution of potassium between the fluid compartments, other mechanisms are necessary to maintain overall potassium balance. People ingest approximately 100 mEq potassium daily, the bulk of which is eliminated by the kidney. The basic mechanism in the distal tubular secretion is the movement of intracellular potassium from the principal cell into the tubular lumen down an electrochemical gradient. Factors that enhance this gradient promote potassium secretion. These factors include the rate of distal tubular flow, the distal delivery of sodium, the presence of poorly reabsorbable anions in the tubular fluid, and stimulation by aldosterone.

The ratio of extracellular to intracellular potassium establishes the resting membrane potential of the cell. Hence, hyperkalemia or hypokalemia is associated with alteration of the resting membrane potential, which accounts for most of the symptoms and findings in these disorders.

DIAGNOSTIC APPROACH

A careful history with emphasis on the patient's diet and use of medications and laxatives should be obtained. Spurious hyperkalemia and hypokalemia must be excluded. In addition to serum electrolytes and magnesium, urine electrolytes and urine osmolality should be obtained. The next step should be to determine whether abnormal renal potassium handling is involved in the genesis of the disorder. This may be determined by measuring the 24-hour urine potassium excretion. In extrarenal hyperkalemia, renal potassium excretion should be more than 200 mEq/day, and if hypokalemia is caused by extrarenal losses, the renal potassium excretion should be less than 20 mEq/day. An alternative method to estimate distal tubule potassium secretion, the major determinant of final urine potassium, is *TTKG (transtubular potassium gradient)*. This is expressed as

TTKG

$$= \text{urine K} \times \text{serum osm./urine osm.} \times \text{serum K}$$

In hyperkalemia, the appropriate renal response is reflected in a TTKG ranging from more than 8 to 10, and in hypokalemia with appropriate renal potassium conservation, TTKG is generally less than 2. Any deviation from these values suggests that renal defect in potassium handling is contributing to the potassium disorder. This formula is not useful in conditions in which urine is hypo-osmolar to plasma.

HYPERKALEMIA

The ratio of intracellular to extracellular potassium concentration is the major determinant of the resting potential of the cell membrane. As the extracellular potassium concentration increases, the cell membrane is partially depolarized, the sodium permeability is diminished, and the ability to generate action potentials is decreased. In muscle tissue, this change accounts for muscle weakness and paralysis. In the heart, hyperkalemia is manifest as changes in the electrocardiogram. These changes include peaked T waves, decreased amplitude or the absence of P waves, wide QRS complexes, sinus bradycardia, and conduction defects.

A pathophysiologic approach to the causes of hyperkalemia is outlined in Figure 26–6. Vigorous phlebotomy techniques can result in lysis of red blood cells, a process that releases intracellular potassium into the serum sample. Thrombocytosis ($>1 \times 10^6/\mu L$) and leukocytosis ($>60,000/\mu L$) may also be associated with "spurious hyperkalemia." These disorders can be diagnosed rapidly by determining the plasma and serum concentrations of potassium. True hyperkalemia is present if these values differ by ≤ 0.2 mEq/L.

Chronic renal insufficiency does not cause hyperkalemia unless it is advanced, with a GFR ranging from less than 10 to 15 mL/min. Thus, hyperkalemia in chronic renal insufficiency is usually caused by a distal tubular defect in potassium secretion rather than by the impaired GFR, as shown in Figure 26–6. Failure to increase plasma aldosterone by the administration of corticotropin or furosemide confirms the diagnosis of *hyporeninemic hypoaldosteronism*. Prostaglandin defi-

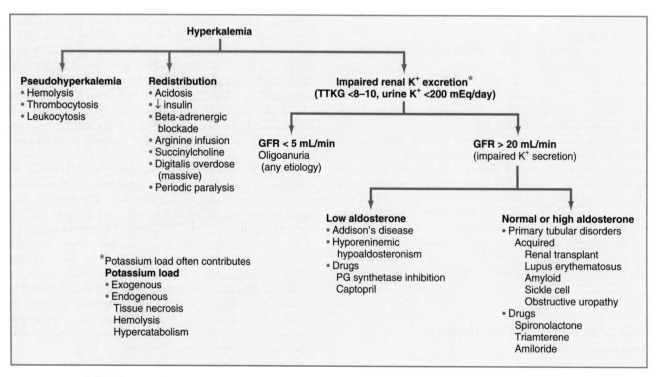

FIGURE 26–6 Diagnostic approach to hyperkalemia. GFR = glomerular filtration rate; PG = prostaglandin; TTKG = transtubular potassium gradient.

ciency may play a role in the pathogenesis of this disorder. Determination of the urine potassium in response to a single dose of an oral mineralocorticoid (such as 9α-fludrocortisone) may help to differentiate hypoaldosteronism from aldosterone resistance. In aldosterone resistance, no increase in urine potassium excretion occurs in response to the mineralocorticoid.

Treatment of hyperkalemia depends on the urgency of clinical findings. If cardiac standstill is imminent, the most rapid method of reversing the effects of hyperkalemia is to reestablish the normal membrane potential. Calcium antagonizes the membrane effects of hyperkalemia and can provide rapid protection of the cardiac conduction system. This protection, however, is short-lived and must be accompanied by other therapies to decrease the extracellular potassium concentration. The distribution of potassium into the intracellular compartment by administration of sodium bicarbonate, β_2-adrenergic agonists, or insulin rapidly decreases the serum concentration of potassium. The ultimate goal of the treatment is the net removal of potassium from the body. Exchange resins, such as sodium polystyrene sulfonate, can enhance the potassium excretion from the gastrointestinal tract. Attempts can be made to enhance renal excretion by improving the distal delivery of sodium with sodium bicarbonate and administration of loop diuretics. Finally, dialysis can be used to remove excess extracellular potassium. For long-term management of patients with an aldosterone deficiency, an oral preparation of a mineralocorticoid can be used. The clinician should identify and discontinue any offending drug that may contribute to the patient's hyperkalemia.

HYPOKALEMIA

Because potassium is the most abundant intracellular cation, its deficiency results in a wide variety of defects. For example, rhabdomyolysis and adynamic ileus have been associated with hypokalemia. Chronic hypokalemia stimulates thirst and may cause nephrogenic diabetes insipidus. However, the most prominent abnormalities relate to the cardiovascular system. Typically, hypokalemia is associated with flattening of the T waves and development of U waves. The most urgent abnormality is an association with arrhythmias, particularly in patients receiving digitalis. Hypokalemia, through stimulation of renal ammonia synthesis, may worsen hepatic encephalopathy in patients with hepatic cirrhosis.

A diagnostic approach to hypokalemia is outlined in Figure 26–7. As in hyperkalemia, spurious hypokalemia can also occur with leukocytosis (>60,000 cells/μL) resulting from active uptake of potassium by white cells from the serum. True hypokalemia is caused by redistribution, extrarenal potassium loss, poor intake, or renal potassium losses. Because only 2% of total-body potassium is distributed in the extracellular compartment, serum potassium measurements may not accurately reflect the total-body stores. In fact, hypokalemia can occur in

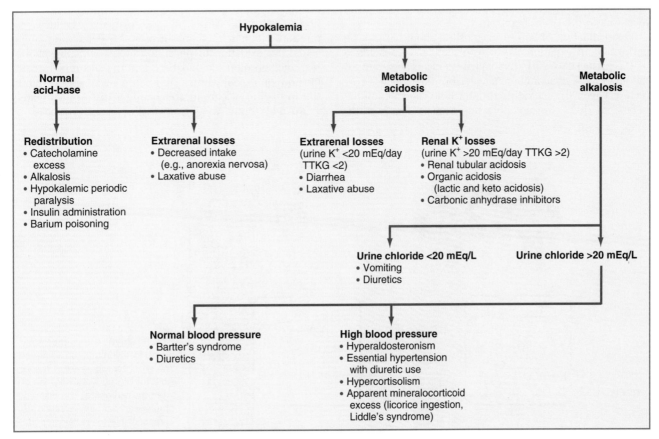

FIGURE 26–7 Diagnostic approach to hypokalemia. TTKG = transtubular potassium gradient.

the presence of normal total-body potassium stores. This occurs when potassium shifts from the extracellular space to the intracellular space. Excess circulating catecholamines, insulin administration, and alkalosis are the major causes of redistribution of potassium from the extracellular space to the intracellular space. Redistribution hypokalemia is particularly important in the clinical setting of myocardial infarction and exacerbation of chronic obstructive pulmonary disease. These patients are especially prone to arrhythmias, because excess catecholamines (in response to stress, inhaled β_2-agonists) cause potassium shifts in the setting of total-body potassium depletion from frequent diuretic usage.

In patients with hypokalemia, the acid-base status, the presence or absence of hypertension, and measurement of urinary chloride and potassium are helpful in narrowing the diagnostic possibilities. In patients with diuretic abuse (usually patients with eating disorders), the urine sodium and chloride concentrations are high in the presence of metabolic alkalosis, a profile similar to that of *Bartter's syndrome*, which is a rare defect of primary renal tubular sodium chloride reabsorption. In this setting, a urine screen for diuretics may be necessary to make the diagnosis. In comparison, patients with surreptitious vomiting have a low urinary chloride concentration. Patients who abuse laxatives have low urine sodium and chloride concentrations, with metabolic acidosis or normal acid-base status. Glycyrrhizic acid, the active ingredient in licorice, blocks 11β-dehydrogenase, an enzyme that normally protects the mineralocorticoid receptor from the glucocorticoids, and this change results in unregulated activation of the mineralocorticoid receptors in the distal nephron.

Determination of serum magnesium should always be performed in a patient with hypokalemia. Hypokalemia that is associated with hypomagnesemia is resistant to therapy unless concomitant magnesium deficiency is corrected. Given the factors that determine transmembrane potassium shifts, the net potassium deficit may be diffi-

cult to calculate. An estimate for a 70-kg man based on the serum concentration is 100 to 200 mEq deficit in total-body potassium when the serum concentration decreases from 4 to 3 mEq/L. At less than 3 mEq/L, every 1 mEq/L decrease in the serum concentration of potassium reflects an additional 200 to 400 mEq deficit in total-body potassium. Hypokalemia should be treated with oral potassium supplementation. Intravenous potassium administration should only be used in urgent situations such as in patients with arrhythmias, digitalis toxicity, and intolerance to oral formulations in patients with adynamic ileus. The rate of intravenous potassium administration generally should not exceed 10 mEq/hr, and, only under electrocardiographic monitoring, the potassium administration rate can be increased up to 20 mEq/hr. Hypokalemia associated with long-term diuretic therapy may be treated with the addition of a potassium-sparing diuretic.

Disturbances in Acid-Base Balance

Most metabolic processes occurring in the body result in the production of acid. The largest source of endogenous acid production is from the catabolism of glucose and fatty acids to carbon dioxide and water or, effectively, carbonic acid. The amount of volatile acid production is about 22,000 mEq of hydrogen daily and is effectively eliminated by the lungs. Pulmonary ventilation excretes the carbon dioxide formed by cellular respiration. Cellular metabolism of sulfur-containing amino acids, the oxidation of phosphoproteins and phospholipids, nucleoprotein degradation, and the incomplete combustion of carbohydrates and fatty acids also result in the formation of certain nonvolatile acids. Approximately 1 mEq/kg body weight of hydrogen is produced by

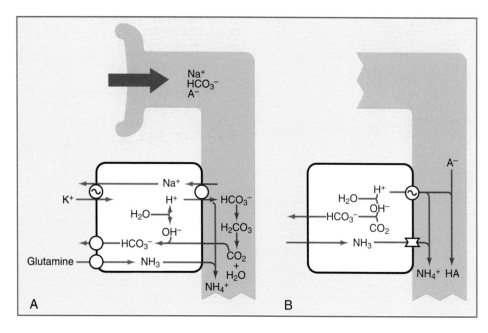

FIGURE 26-8 Renal mechanisms for hydrogen ion secretion. The proximal tubule *(A)* is responsible for the bulk reabsorption of filtered bicarbonate. The distal nephron hydrogen ion secretion *(B)* is responsible for reclaiming additional bicarbonate as well as for titrating inorganic anions (A−).

these processes daily. The primary factors regulating alteration in the rate of minute ventilation are subtle changes in cerebrospinal fluid pH or arterial pH.

The normal concentration of hydrogen in arterial blood is 40 mEq/L, equating to a pH of 7.40. This concentration is maintained relatively constant despite variations in the endogenous and exogenous acid input. An acid load is acutely neutralized by circulating and intracellular buffers. The capacity of these buffering systems is limited, however, and would be quickly depleted by normal endogenous acid production. Mechanisms for excreting acid must therefore be effective to maintain acid-base homeostasis. Nonvolatile acid excretion is effected through the kidneys.

RENAL HYDROGEN ION EXCRETION

The kidney contributes to acid-base homeostasis by the reclamation of 4500 mEq of bicarbonate filtered at the glomerulus daily and by the generation of new bicarbonate that replenishes the body buffer stores. These functions are accomplished by the secretion of hydrogen by various nephron segments (Fig. 26–8). The bulk of filtered bicarbonate is reabsorbed in the proximal tubule. In contrast to the distal tubule, the proximal tubule is a high-capacity bicarbonate reabsorption system resulting from the presence of carbonic anhydrase in the luminal membrane. Carbonic anhydrase in the luminal membrane rapidly catalyzes the dehydration of carbonic acid to carbon dioxide and water and thus maintains the gradient for hydrogen secretion in the proximal tubule. The distal tubule lacks a luminal carbonic anhydrase and has only a cytoplasmic carbonic anhydrase, which limits its capacity to reclaim bicarbonate. The rate of proximal bicarbonate reabsorption is increased by the following: volume depletion; an elevation in the pressure of carbon dioxide (PCO_2), as seen in chronic respiratory acidosis; and hypokalemia. Conversely, volume expansion or the reduction of the PCO_2 lowers the proximal tubular resorptive rate for bicarbonate.

The distal tubule is responsible for reclaiming the remainder of the filtered bicarbonate. This segment must also eliminate hydrogen quantitatively equivalent to the nonvolatile acid production. Hydrogen excretion is accomplished by secretion into the tubular fluid. The inorganic bases of nonvolatile acid production, such as phosphates, are filtered at the glomerulus and are poorly reabsorbed by the nephron. These "fixed" bases, as well as ammonia produced by proximal tubular cells, can effectively trap the secreted hydrogen in the tubular fluid for elimination in the urine. Aldosterone and the PCO_2 affect the distal secretion of hydrogen.

ASSESSMENT OF ACID-BASE STATUS

The initial step in evaluating acid-base problems is to obtain an arterial blood gas measurement and serum electrolyte concentrations (Fig. 26–9). The arterial blood gas measures the pH, oxygen pressure (PO_2), and PCO_2. The bicarbonate concentration is then calculated using the Henderson-Hasselbalch equation, which re-

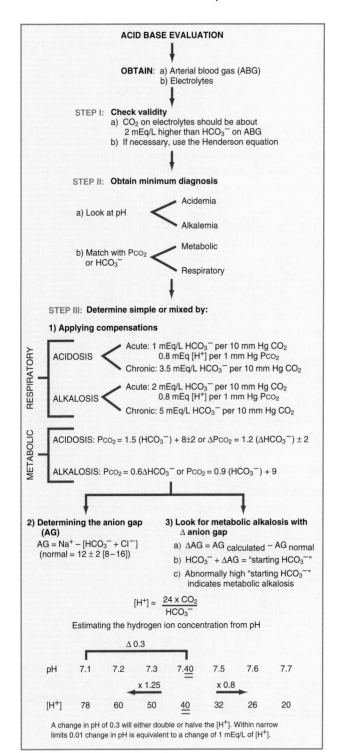

FIGURE 26–9 Scheme for assessing acid-base homeostasis.

lates the pH directly to the bicarbonate concentration and inversely to the PCO_2. Because little soluble carbon dioxide is present in serum, the total carbon dioxide obtained with the serum electrolytes is effectively a measure of the serum bicarbonate concentration. This measured value should differ from that calculated on a concomitant blood gas determination by no more than 2 mEq/L. The validity of the blood gas determination can be estimated further by applying the bicarbonate concentration and the measured PCO_2 to the Henderson-Hasselbalch equation:

$$[H^+] = 24 \times PCO_2/[HCO_3^-]$$

Based on the pH, PCO_2, and serum bicarbonate, a minimum diagnosis should be established, as shown in Figure 26–9. Next, a measurement of the compensatory response and the anion gap should be performed. If the compensation of a primary acid-base defect is inappropriate, then a mixed acid-base disorder is considered. The presence of a normal serum pH in combination with abnormal PCO_2 and serum bicarbonate values provides another clue to a mixed acid-base disorder. The anion gap (see Fig. 26–9) is useful in the diagnostic approach to metabolic acidosis. When an organic acid (such as lactic acid) is added to the extracellular fluid compartment, the bicarbonate concentration falls as the acid is buffered. The anion gap increases as the organic base is accumulated. Quantitatively, the increase in anion gap should be equivalent to the decrease in bicarbonate concentration. Thus, by adding the difference between the calculated and normal anion gap to the prevailing bicarbonate concentration, an estimate of the "starting" bicarbonate concentration can be made. An abnormally elevated initial bicarbonate concentration indicates concomitant metabolic alkalosis.

METABOLIC ACIDOSIS

Metabolic acidosis is characterized by a decrease in the serum bicarbonate concentration. This decrease occurs either by excretion of bicarbonate-containing fluids or by utilization of bicarbonate as a buffer of acids. In the latter instance, the nature of the base may affect the electrolyte composition. Thus, considering metabolic acidosis by means of the anion gap is convenient (Table 26–6).

Metabolic acidoses have a normal anion gap whenever net bicarbonate losses are abnormally large. This condition may occur because the kidneys fail to reabsorb or regenerate bicarbonate, extrarenal losses of bicarbonate occur, or excessive amounts of substances yielding hydrochloric acid have been administered. Thus, gastrointestinal bicarbonate loss and renal tubular acidosis (RTA) are the major causes of normal anion gap acidosis.

The urinary anion gap is defined as follows:

Urinary anion gap
$$= \text{unmeasured anions} - \text{unmeasured cations}$$
$$= [Na^+ + K^+] - Cl^-$$

This equation is useful in evaluating patients with acidosis characterized by a normal anion gap. The test provides an approximate index of urinary ammonia excretion, as measured by a negative urinary anion gap. Thus, a normal renal response would be a negative urinary anion gap, generally in the range of 30 to 50 mEq/L. In such an instance, the acidosis is probably

TABLE 26–6   Causes of Metabolic Acidosis

Normal Anion Gap
Bicarbonate losses
    Extrarenal
        Small bowel drainage
        Diarrhea
    Renal
        Proximal renal tubular acidosis
        Carbonic anhydrase inhibitors
        Primary hyperparathyroidism
Failure of bicarbonate regeneration
Distal renal tubular acidosis
Aldosterone deficiency
    Addison's disease
    Hyporeninemic hypoaldosteronism
Aldosterone insensitivity
    Interstitial renal disease
    Aldosterone antagonists
Ureteroileostomy (ileal bladder)
Acidifying salts
    Ammonium chloride
    Lysine or arginine hydrochloride
Diabetes mellitus (recovery phase)

Wide Anion Gap
Reduced excretion of acids
    Renal failure
Overproduction of acids
    Ketoacidosis
        Diabetic
        Alcoholic
        Starvation
    Lactic acidosis
    Toxin ingestion
        Methanol
        Ethylene glycol
        Salicylates
        Paraldehyde
        Isopropyl alcohol

Modified from Andreoli TE: Disorders of fluid volume, electrolyte, and acid-base balance. *In* Wyngaarden JB, Smith LH Jr, Bennett JC (eds): Cecil Textbook of Medicine, 19th ed. Philadelphia: WB Saunders, 1992, p 523.

caused by gastrointestinal losses, rather than by a renal lesion.

A classification scheme and diagnostic features of the RTA syndromes are outlined in Table 26–7. In proximal RTA, the primary defect is an impairment of bicarbonate reabsorption in the proximal tubule, and it may be associated with defective phosphate, glucose, urate, and amino acid reabsorption. Type I distal RTA is characterized by the inability to acidify urine maximally. Patients with type IV distal RTA have impaired urinary acidification because of hypoaldosteronism. A large subset of these patients has diabetes mellitus.

The causes of acidosis characterized by a wide anion gap are listed in Table 26–6. In *renal failure*, inorganic compounds such as phosphates and sulfates are the major contributors to the increased anion gap. Organic compounds also accumulate in patients with diminished renal function. *Ketoacidosis* results from accelerated lipolysis and ketogenesis, caused by a relative insulin defi-

TABLE 26-7 **Characteristics of Renal Tubular Acidosis (RTA) Syndromes**

Condition	Urine pH*	Serum Potassium
Type I distal RTA†	>5.5	Normal or ↓
Proximal RTA (type II)	<5.5	↓
Type IV distal RTA (hyporeninemic hypoaldosteronism)	<5.5	↑
Voltage-dependent RTA‡	>5.5	↑

* Urine pH assessed during acidemia.
† May be seen with amphotericin use.
‡ Described in patients with obstructive uropathy.

ciency. This disorder can occur in patients with diabetes who have an absolute deficiency of insulin production. Alcoholic ketoacidosis and starvation ketoacidosis result from the suppression of endogenous insulin secretion caused by inadequate carbohydrate ingestion. In addition, in alcoholic ketoacidosis, insulin resistance contributes to ketone formation. The syndrome of *lactic acidosis* results from impaired cellular respiration. Lactate is produced from the reduction of pyruvate in muscle, red blood cells, and other tissues as a consequence of anaerobic glycolysis. In situations of diminished oxidative metabolism, excess lactic acid is produced. This anaerobic state also favors a shift of keto acids to the reduced form, β-hydroxybutyrate. The nitroprusside reaction, which is catalyzed by the keto acids acetoacetate and acetone, is thus nonreactive in the setting of lactic acidosis. Lactic acidosis occurs most commonly in disorders characterized by inadequate oxygen delivery to tissues, such as shock, septicemia, and profound hypoxemia. Certain toxins may also sufficiently alter mitochondrial function and may establish an effective anaerobic state. Some of these toxins may undergo metabolism into organic acids that can contribute to the generation of acidosis characterized by a large anion gap. Methanol is metabolized by alcohol dehydrogenase to formic acid. Ethylene glycol is metabolized to glycolic and oxalic acids. Salicylates are themselves acidic compounds and can cause acidosis characterized by a wide anion gap.

The treatment of metabolic acidosis depends on the underlying cause and the severity of the manifestations. The rapid administration of parenteral sodium bicarbonate is generally indicated when the pH is less than 7.1, and hemodynamic instability is evident. Oral bicarbonate supplementation may be sufficient if the acidosis is caused by gastrointestinal bicarbonate loss or RTA.

Although bicarbonate supplementation is beneficial in patients with proximal RTA, a normal serum bicarbonate concentration is difficult to achieve. This problem is a result of bicarbonaturia, which accompanies the rise in serum bicarbonate. In contrast, in type I distal RTA, adequate bicarbonate supplementation may correct the acidosis completely. Furthermore, the treatment of acidosis also corrects hypercalciuria and nephrocalcinosis, which are commonly seen in type I distal RTA. Therapy of type IV distal RTA involves correction of hyperkalemia and bicarbonate supplementation.

The treatment of organic acidosis should be directed at the underlying disorder. If the generation of the organic acid can be interrupted, the organic base pair may be metabolized, effectively regenerating bicarbonate. The acidemia of diabetic ketoacidosis, for example, can be effectively treated by administration of insulin, thereby inhibiting further ketogenesis. In lactic acidosis, therapy should be directed toward improving tissue perfusion. In alcoholic and starvation ketoacidosis, administration of dextrose-containing intravenous fluids corrects the acidosis.

METABOLIC ALKALOSIS

The administration of base or the effective removal of hydrogen increases the bicarbonate concentration of the extracellular fluid. Normally, an elevation of the serum bicarbonate concentration is corrected by excretion of the excess bicarbonate. The maintenance of *metabolic alkalosis*, therefore, implies a defect in the renal mechanism regulating bicarbonate excretion, mainly the proximal tubular bicarbonate absorption. Elevation of the PCO_2, hypokalemia, or volume depletion increases the proximal tubular bicarbonate absorption and can sustain metabolic alkalosis.

The most common cause of metabolic alkalosis is gastric loss of hydrochloric acid by vomiting or mechanical drainage. Diuretic (thiazide and loop) use is commonly associated with metabolic alkalosis. Volume depletion associated with vomiting and diuretic use enhances proximal bicarbonate reabsorption. Volume depletion also leads to aldosterone secretion, which stimulates distal tubular hydrogen secretion. Potassium secretion is likewise stimulated. Endogenous or exogenous mineralocorticoid excess (see Fig. 26–7) is another important cause of metabolic alkalosis. In all these disorders, concomitant hypokalemia promotes the maintenance of metabolic alkalosis.

The renal compensation for sustained hypercapnia results in an increase in the serum bicarbonate concentration. If the ventilatory rate acutely increases, the PCO_2 will fall rapidly but the bicarbonate concentration will remain transiently elevated, with consequent posthypercapnic alkalosis. Furthermore, the elevated PCO_2 stimulates proximal tubular bicarbonate absorption. As noted before, administration of bicarbonate in a setting of organic acidosis may result in alkalosis when the organic anion is metabolized. Excessive alkali ingestion (e.g., milk-alkali syndrome) is an uncommon cause of metabolic alkalosis. It results from impaired renal bicarbonate excretion caused by renal failure in the setting of excess alkali intake.

The determination of urinary chloride concentrations is helpful in formulating a rational approach to the diagnosis and treatment of metabolic alkalosis (see Fig. 26–7). Volume expansion with sodium chloride is the mainstay of therapy in patients with vomiting-induced, diuretic-induced, and posthypercapnic metabolic alkalosis (*chloride-responsive alkalosis*). Potassium and chloride repletion also aids in therapy. However, volume expansion may be harmful in diuretic-induced alkalosis associated with congestive heart failure. The use of carbonic anhydrase inhibitors may be beneficial in this setting. Metabolic alkalosis associated with primary mineralocorticoid excess, Bartter's syndrome, and milk-alkali syndrome is unresponsive to volume expansion (*chloride-resistant alkalosis*). Treatment of the underlying cause is the mainstay of therapy in primary mineralocorticoid excess states. In Bartter's syndrome, potassium chloride supplements and potassium-sparing diuretics are required.

RESPIRATORY ACIDOSIS

Respiratory acidosis occurs with any impairment in the rate of alveolar ventilation. Acute respiratory acidosis occurs with a sudden depression of the medullary respiratory center (narcotic overdose), with paralysis of the respiratory muscles, and with airway obstruction. Chronic respiratory acidosis generally occurs in patients with chronic airway disease (emphysema), with extreme kyphoscoliosis, and with extreme obesity (pickwickian syndrome).

The serum bicarbonate concentration is increased, the magnitude of which depends on the acuity and the severity of the respiratory disorder. Acute increases in the PCO_2 result in somnolence, confusion, and, ultimately, carbon dioxide narcosis. Asterixis may be present. Because carbon dioxide is a cerebral vasodilator, the blood vessels in the optic fundi are often dilated, engorged, and tortuous. Frank papilledema may be present in patients with severe hypercapnic states.

The only practical therapy of acute respiratory acidosis involves treatment of the underlying disorder and ventilatory support. In patients with chronic hypercapnia who develop an acute increase in the PCO_2, attention should be directed toward identifying factors that may have aggravated the chronic disorder. Alkalinizing salts should be avoided in patients with chronic respiratory acidosis.

RESPIRATORY ALKALOSIS

Respiratory alkalosis occurs when hyperventilation reduces the arterial PCO_2 and consequently increases the arterial pH. Acute respiratory alkalosis is most commonly a result of the hyperventilation syndrome. It may also occur in damage to the respiratory centers, in acute salicylism, in fever and septic states, and in association with various pulmonary processes (pneumonia, pulmonary emboli, or congestive heart failure). The disorder may be produced iatrogenically by injudicious mechanical ventilatory support. Chronic hyperventilation occurs in the acclimatization response to high altitudes (a low ambient oxygen tension), in advanced liver disease, and in pregnancy.

Acute hyperventilation is characterized by lightheadedness, paresthesias, circumoral numbness, and tingling of the extremities. Tetany occurs in severe cases. When anxiety provokes hyperventilation, air rebreathing with a paper bag generally terminates the acute attack.

REFERENCES

Andreoli TE: Disorders of fluid volume, electrolyte, and acid-base balance. *In* Wyngaarden JB, Smith LH Jr, Bennett JC (eds): Cecil Textbook of Medicine, 19th ed. Philadelphia: WB Saunders, 1992, pp 499–528.
Coher JJ, Kassierer JP (eds): Acid-Base. Boston: Little, Brown, 1982.
Narins RG (ed): Maxwell and Kleeman's Clinical Disorders of Fluid and Electrolyte Metabolism, 5th ed. New York: McGraw-Hill, 1994.

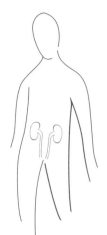

27

GLOMERULAR DISEASES

Sudhir V. Shah

The Glomerulus

The glomerulus consists of a capillary bed that receives blood from the afferent arteriole and is drained by the efferent arteriole. It contains four different cell types: the glomerular (visceral) epithelial cell (podocyte), the endothelial cell, the mesangial cell, and the parietal epithelial cell (Fig. 27–1). The podocyte supports the delicate glomerular basement membrane (GBM) by means of an extensive trabecular network. The mesangium provides a skeletal framework for the entire capillary network and, owing to its contractile capability, can control blood flow along the glomerular capillaries in response to a host of mediators. The endothelial cells line the capillary lumen, and the parietal epithelial cells cover Bowman's capsule.

Mechanisms of Glomerular Injury

Both humoral and cell-mediated immune mechanisms play a major role in glomerular injury and consist primarily of two types (Fig. 27–2). Occasionally, antibodies to the GBM develop, resulting in a glomerulonephritis (GN) characterized by linear deposition of IgG along the capillary walls. Much more frequently, discrete deposition of granular deposits of immunoglobulins and complement is seen. These immunoglobulins, together with their respective circulating antigens, may be deposited in the GBM. Alternatively, antigens may localize individually to the GBM and in situ activation of antigen-antibody complexes may occur. In both instances, the antigen-antibody complex localization in the GBM initiates the cascade of glomerular injury. Such deposits may be seen in the mesangium, along the subendothelial surface of the GBM, or within the outer region of the capillary wall in the subepithelial space.

Other glomerular diseases occur in which immunologic mechanisms are thought to play a role but no deposits are detectable. Minimal change nephrotic syndrome, now thought to be a disorder of the glomerular epithelial cell, may be due to non–complement-fixing antiglomerular epithelial cell antibodies. Idiopathic crescentic GN (anti-GBM antibodies are absent) is possibly mediated by mononuclear cell–mediated immune reactions, induction of endothelial leukocyte adhesion molecules on endothelium, or antineutrophil cytoplasmic antibody (ANCA)–mediated local neutrophil activation.

Neutrophil infiltration in response to immune complex-complement interaction, endothelial leukocyte adhesion molecule induction, or the presence of ANCA can lead to glomerular injury through the release of proteolytic enzymes and/or reactive oxygen metabolites. Other circulating cells have been suggested to play a role in glomerular injury. Platelets may be important in various forms of glomerular injury and are particularly important in mesangial proliferative lesions. Macrophages in concert with activated lymphocytes are likely important in antibody-independent, cell-mediated glomerular injury. The glomerular cells themselves may be activated to produce oxidants and/or proteases with subsequent damage to either the GBM or the mesangium. Finally, in other disorders such as diabetes or amyloidosis, the glomerular injury may be secondary to metabolic imbalances.

Clinical Manifestations of Glomerular Disease

The initial manifestations of glomerular disease are often nonspecific (hypertension, edema, malaise) or urinary abnormalities (proteinuria, hematuria). Altered glomerular function, either proteinuria consequent to changes in GBM permeability or decreased glomerular filtration rate (GFR) secondary to abnormal ultrafiltration, characterizes glomerular disease.

The glomerular capillaries provide a filtration barrier that prevents the passage of proteins into the urine on the basis of protein size, shape, and electrical charge. Normally, less than 50 mg of protein is excreted in the

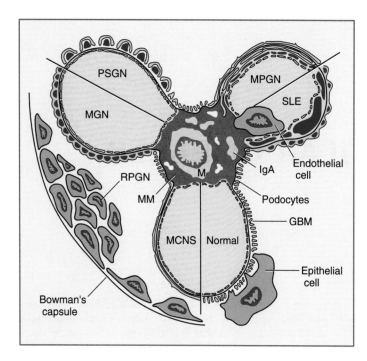

FIGURE 27–1 Schematic drawing of a glomerulus illustrating the normal features as well as several diseases. GBM = glomerular basement membrane; IgA = immunoglobulin A deposits in IgA nephropathy; M = mesangial cell; MCNS = minimal change nephrotic syndrome; MGN = membranous glomerulopathy; MM = mesangial matrix; MPGN = membranoproliferative glomerulopathy; PSGN = poststreptococcal glomerulonephritis; RPGN = rapidly progressive glomerulonephritis; SLE = systemic lupus erythematosus.

urine per day. Nephrotic-range proteinuria (>3.5 g/day in adults) represents diffuse glomerular injury with loss of the net negative charge on the capillary wall and/or structural defects in the filtration barrier. The presence of either red blood cell casts or dysmorphic red blood cells in the urine characterizes nephronal bleeding indicative of either proliferative GN or acute interstitial nephritis. Dysmorphic red blood cells are best seen using phase-contrast microscopy and consist of red blood cells of varying size, shape, and hemoglobin content.

Renal salt retention is a common feature of glomerular disease and may lead to edema, volume overload, congestive heart failure, and hypertension. Although the mechanisms responsible for reduced salt excretion are poorly understood, sodium acquisitiveness is considerably greater than that expected solely from the reduction in GFR.

The renal function in glomerular disease depends on the type and varies from normal renal function (e.g., minimal change disease) to relentless progressive end-stage renal disease (e.g., rapidly progressive glomerulonephritis [RPGN]).

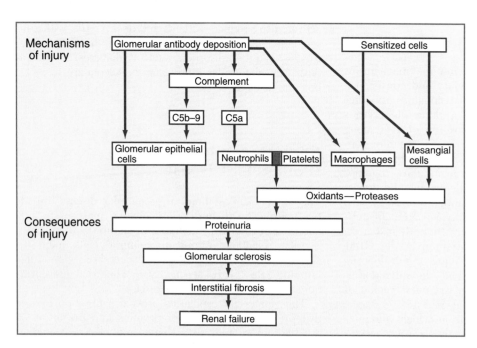

FIGURE 27–2 Schematic depiction of the mechanisms that mediate glomerular injury *(top)* and the consequences of those processes *(bottom)* leading to renal failure. (From Shah SV: Mechanisms of glomerular injury. Semin Nephrol 1991; 11:320–331.)

TABLE 27-1 Characteristics of Glomerular Syndromes

Syndrome	Features
Acute nephritic syndrome	Nephronal hematuria (RBC casts and/or dysmorphic RBCs) temporally associated with acute renal failure
Rapidly progressive glomerulonephritis	Nephronal hematuria (RBC casts and/or dysmorphic RBCs) with renal failure developing over weeks to months and diffuse glomerular crescent formation
Nephrotic syndrome	Massive proteinuria (>3.5 g/day/1.73 m^2) with variable edema, hypoalbuminemia, hyperlipidemia, and hyperlipiduria
With "bland" sediment	"Pure" nephrotic syndrome
With "active" sediment	"Mixed" nephrotic/nephritic syndrome
Asymptomatic urinary abnormalities	Isolated proteinuria (usually <2.0 g/day/1.73 m^2) or hematuria (with or without proteinuria)

RBC = red blood cell.

Approach to the Patient with Glomerular Disease

Glomerular diseases have been classified in numerous ways. Here they are organized and discussed as they relate to the four major glomerular syndromes: acute nephritic syndrome, RPGN, nephrotic syndrome (with either "bland" or "active" urine sediment), and asymptomatic urinary abnormalities (Table 27-1). The diagnosis of glomerular diseases is based on pathologic features related to glomerular alterations. Definitions of some of the more commonly used terms are given in Table 27-2.

Acute Nephritic Syndrome

Acute nephritic syndrome is characterized by the abrupt onset (days) of hematuria with red blood cell casts or dysmorphic red blood cells and proteinuria (usually non–nephrotic-range), temporally associated with impairment of renal function. The manifestation of altered renal function may be oliguria, with impairment of renal function as measured by a rise in blood urea nitrogen and creatinine, or retention of salt and water, resulting in the development of hypertension. Acute nephritic syndrome is most commonly due to proliferative GN, of which poststreptococcal glomerulonephritis (PSGN) is a prototype, and less commonly from acute interstitial nephritis. Table 27-3 lists the diseases commonly associated with this condition. The measurement of complement levels is useful in narrowing down the diagnostic possibilities.

PSGN occurs as a postinfectious complication of nephritogenic strains of group A β-hemolytic streptococcal infection. Pharyngitis (strep throat) is a common antecedent infection in northern states, but PSGN occurs in fewer than 5% of those infected, usually within a 7- to 28-day latent period. Streptococcal pyoderma more commonly occurs in the southern United States and may also lead to PSGN in as many as 50% of infected individuals. PSGN is the hallmark disease for the acute nephritic syndrome and is typically seen in children aged 3 to 12, although it can occur in adults. Both sexes are equally affected with PSGN, which occurs more

TABLE 27-2 Pathologic Features of Glomerular Disease

Type of Disease	Feature
Focal	Some (but not all) glomeruli contain the lesion.
Diffuse (global)	Most glomeruli ($>75\%$) contain the lesion.
Segmental	Only a part of the glomerulus is affected by the lesion (most focal lesions are also segmental, e.g., focal segmental glomerulosclerosis).
Proliferation	An increase in cell number due to hyperplasia of one or more of the resident glomerular cells with or without inflammatory cell infiltration
Membrane alterations	Capillary wall thickening due to deposition of immune deposits or alterations in basement membrane
Crescent formation	Epithelial cell proliferation and mononuclear cell infiltration in Bowman's space

TABLE 27–3   Differential Diagnosis of Acute Nephritic Syndrome

Low Serum Complement Level	Normal Serum Complement Level
Acute postinfectious glomerulonephritis	IgA nephropathy
Membranoproliferative glomerulonephritis	Idiopathic rapidly progressive glomerulo-nephritis
Type I	Anti–glomerular basement membrane disease
Type II	Polyarteritis nodosa
Systemic lupus erythematosus	Wegener's granulomatosis
Subacute bacterial endocarditis	Henoch-Schönlein purpura
Visceral abscess "shunt" nephritis	Goodpasture's syndrome
Cryoglobulinemia	

frequently in the summer and autumn in North America. The patient presents with typical acute nephritic syndrome associated with malaise, cola-colored urine, mild hypertension, periorbital edema, and non–nephrotic-range proteinuria.

Laboratory findings include red blood cells and red blood cell casts, white blood cells, and proteinuria on urinalysis; antibodies to streptococcal antigens; a low serum complement (usually returning to normal at 6 to 12 weeks); and azotemia. Histologically, PSGN is a diffuse proliferative (mesangial and endothelial cells) and exudative (neutrophils and monocytes) GN with coarsely granular capillary loop deposits of IgG and C3 and subepithelial electron-dense humplike deposits by electron microscopy (Fig. 27–3).

The differential diagnosis is that of an acute GN with hypocomplementemia and includes other forms of postinfectious GN (e.g., bacterial endocarditis, shunt nephritis), systemic lupus erythematosus (SLE), and membranoproliferative GN. The diagnosis can usually be based on the typical renal presentation following a streptococcal infection, hypocomplementemia, and serologic evidence. Because the diagnosis is most often straightforward, a renal biopsy is indicated only if the disease follows an atypical course in children. Most adults with acute nephritic syndrome require a kidney biopsy to establish the diagnosis.

There is no specific therapy for PSGN, although antibiotics should be administered if cultures are positive for *Streptococcus*. Salt restriction and, in some cases, diuretics and antihypertensive agents may be required to manage sodium retention (manifested by hypertension, edema, congestive heart failure, and other signs). Complete recovery occurs in at least 90% to 95% of all patients. However, proteinuria and/or hematuria may continue for 1 to 2 years in some patients, but progression to chronic renal failure is exceedingly rare, typically occurring only in older adults who contract the disease. Less than 5% of patients have oliguria for more than 7 to 9 days, and the prognosis in these patients is less favorable.

Nonstreptococcal postinfectious GN may occur after bacterial infections (e.g., staphylococcal, pneumococcal), viral infections (e.g., mumps, hepatitis B, varicella, coxsackievirus infection, infectious mononucleosis), protozoal infection (e.g., malaria, toxoplasmosis), and a host of others (e.g., schistosomiasis, syphilis). The clinical and histologic manifestations may vary somewhat, depending on the infecting agent. Still, most have features similar to those of PSGN and an equally good prognosis if the underlying infection is eradicated.

GN associated with infective endocarditis usually manifests as a mild form of the acute nephritic syndrome (hematuria and proteinuria with a mild decrease in renal function). Endocarditis is now more common in prosthetic valves and in patients with intravenous drug abuse rather than patients with rheumatic heart disease. *Staphylococcus aureus* is the most common organism, although a variety of gram-positive and gram-negative organisms may be involved. In patients with infected ventriculoatrial shunts (shunt nephritis) the most common organism is *Staphylococcus epidermidis*. Shunt nephritis usually manifests as hematuria and proteinuria with nephritic-range proteinuria in about one fourth of the patients. As in other forms of postinfectious GN, cryoglobulins, rheumatoid factor, and low levels of complement are generally present. Light microscopy shows mesangioproliferative GN. Elimination of infection with appropriate antibiotic therapy may result in a return of renal function to normal.

GN associated with visceral abscess has been reported in patients with pulmonary, hepatic, and retroperitoneal abscesses. These patients develop the acute nephritic syndrome with a mesangioproliferative GN, often with complement deposition by immunofluores-

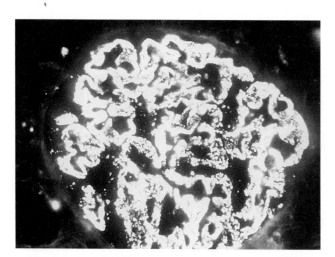

FIGURE 27–3   Immunofluorescence demonstrating coarsely granular capillary loop deposits of IgG.

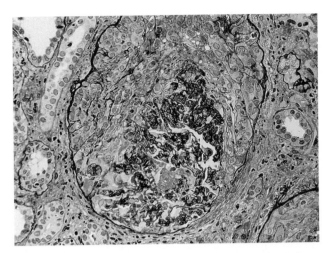

FIGURE 27–4 Glomerulus demonstrating crescent formation.

TABLE 27–4 Types of Rapidly Progressive Glomerulonephritis (RPGN)

Anti–Glomerular Basement Membrane Antibody-Mediated RPGN (Linear Immunofluorescent Pattern)

Idiopathic anti–glomerular basement membrane antibody-mediated RPGN

Goodpasture's syndrome

Associated with other primary glomerular diseases
   Membranous glomerulopathy

Immune Complex–Mediated RPGN (Granular Immunofluorescent Pattern)

Idiopathic immune complex–mediated RPGN

Associated with other primary glomerular diseases
   Membranoproliferative glomerulopathy (type II > type I)
   IgA nephropathy

Associated with secondary glomerular diseases
   Postinfectious glomerulonephritides
   Systemic lupus erythematosus
   Mixed essential cryoglobulinemia
   Henoch-Schönlein purpura

Non–Immune-Mediated RPGN (Negative Immunofluorescent Pattern)

Idiopathic pauci-immune RPGN (ANCA-associated)

Vasculitides including Wegener's and microscopic polyarteritis

ANCA = antineutrophil cytoplasmic antibody.

cence. The complement levels are usually not modestly depressed in about half the patients, and rheumatoid factor is usually negative. Successful antibiotic therapy results in recovery of renal function in only 50% of patients.

SLE, Henoch-Schönlein purpura, and mixed essential cryoglobulinemia may present as acute GN, but more typically they are associated with other glomerular syndromes and are therefore discussed later.

Rapidly Progressive Glomerulonephritis

Rapidly progressive glomerulonephritis (RPGN) is a syndrome characterized by nephronal hematuria (red blood cell casts and/or dysmorphic red blood cells) with renal failure developing over weeks to months and diffuse glomerular crescent formation evident on renal biopsy (Fig. 27–4). Classification is complicated by the fact that RPGN can occur with immune deposits (either anti-GBM or immune complex type) or without immune deposits. In addition, it can be an idiopathic primary glomerular disease or can be superimposed on other glomerular diseases either primary or secondary. The classification scheme used here is based on the immunofluorescence information obtained from renal biopsy (Table 27–4).

Anti-GBM GN, characterized by linear capillary loop staining with IgG and C3 (Fig. 27–5) and extensive crescent formation, accounts for 10% to 20% of all cases of RPGN, although overall it accounts for less than 5% of all forms of GN. About two thirds of these patients have Goodpasture's syndrome with associated pulmonary hemorrhage. The remainder have an idiopathic form of anti-GBM GN. The pathogenesis of anti-GBM antibody disease appears to be linked to the development of autoimmunity to the noncollagenous domain of the $\alpha 3$ chain of type IV collagen (NCI$\alpha 3$ IV), and there is a strong association with human leukocyte antigen HLA-DR2. Goodpasture's syndrome affects young men six times more frequently than women and usually presents as hemoptysis and dyspnea. Idiopathic anti-GBM GN is seen in older patients (older than 50 years) and affects both sexes equally. Anti-GBM antibodies are present in serum (detectable using indirect immunofluorescence on normal kidney); serum C3 is normal. Therapy consists of high-dose oral prednisone, cytotoxic agents such as cyclophosphamide, and plasma exchange. A high index of suspicion resulting in earlier diagnosis and vigorous treatment has increased survival to more than 50%, as opposed to 10% to 15% a decade ago.

Immune complex RPGN is almost always associated

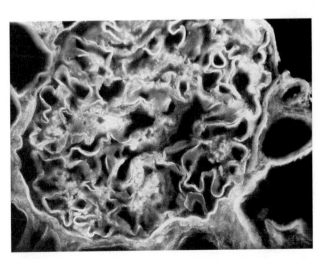

FIGURE 27–5 Immunofluorescence demonstrating a linear pattern of IgG.

with another underlying disease, and the correct diagnosis can usually be made by seeking the other clinical and laboratory features of these conditions (see Table 27–4). About 30% of all cases of RPGN are of this type (granular deposits of immunoglobulins and complement).

Non–immune-mediated RPGN (also called pauci-immune GN) is found in about 50% of patients with crescentic GN and is seen in association with one of the systemic vasculitides such as polyarteritis nodosa or Wegener's granulomatosis or as an idiopathic form that is thought to represent a vasculitis limited to the glomerular capillaries. The idiopathic form is usually found in patients in their 50s or 60s. A helpful diagnostic feature is the presence of ANCA, which is found in approximately 80% of patients with pauci-immune GN. When ANCA is detected by indirect immunofluorescence, two major patterns are observed: cytoplasmic staining (C-ANCA) and perinuclear staining (P-ANCA). P-ANCA is most common in pauci-immune necrotizing and crescentic GN and in patients with microscopic polyarteritis nodosa. Patients with sinus involvement (Wegener's granulomatosis) commonly have C-ANCA, although there is a great deal of overlap. Because of the success in treatment of Wegener's granulomatosis with cytotoxic agents such as cyclophosphamide and corticosteroids, patients with ANCA-positive pauci-immune GN receive a similar type of treatment, although the duration of treatment with cyclophosphamide has not been resolved.

Nephrotic Syndrome

The nephrotic syndrome is characterized by the presence of proteinuria, hypoalbuminemia, edema, hyperlipiduria, and hyperlipidemia. However, the finding of proteinuria of more than 3.5 g/24 hr/1.73 m², so-called nephrotic-range proteinuria, is sufficient for the designation of nephrotic syndrome. Table 27–5 includes the renal lesions commonly associated with the nephrotic syndrome. They are divided into diseases with or without red blood cell casts ("bland" or "active" urine sediment). Each of these entities may occur as a primary renal lesion or as a secondary component of a systemic disease.

NEPHROTIC SYNDROME WITH "BLAND" URINE SEDIMENT

Minimal Change Nephrotic Syndrome

Minimal change nephrotic syndrome (MCNS) is also known as nil lesion or lipoid nephrosis; more than 85% to 90% of all children with nephrotic syndrome have this condition. It almost always presents as insidious or sudden onset of the nephrotic syndrome in children aged 2 to 8 years with a male-to-female ratio of 2:1. In adults, MCNS accounts for about 20%, with a more equal male-to-female ratio. As children approach teenage years and early adulthood, the incidence of MCNS

TABLE 27–5 Glomerulopathies Associated with Nephrotic Syndrome

Nephrotic–Range Proteinuria with "Bland" Urine Sediment (Pure Nephrotic)
Primary glomerular disease
Minimal change nephrotic syndrome (nil lesion, lipoid nephrosis)
Membranous glomerulopathy
Focal glomerulosclerosis
Secondary glomerular disease
Diabetic nephropathy (Kimmelstiel-Wilson glomerulosclerosis)
Amyloidosis
Nephrotic-Range Proteinuria with "Active" Urine Sediment ("Mixed," Nephrotic/Nephritic)
Primary glomerular disease
Membranoproliferative glomerulopathy, types I, II, III
Secondary glomerular disease
Membranoproliferative glomerulopathy
Systemic lupus erythematosus
Henoch-Schönlein purpura
Mixed essential cryoglobulinemia

as a cause of nephrotic syndrome diminishes. In adult patients the association of MCNS with the use of non-steroidal anti-inflammatory agents and Hodgkin's disease must be kept in mind.

Laboratory features include those of the typical nephrotic syndrome with bland urinary sediment, normal renal function (unless there is severe volume contraction), and normal complement levels. Histologically, light microscopy is normal (hence the term *nil lesion*) and no immunoglobulins or complement deposition is seen. Electron microscopy reveals effacement (fusion) of the foot processes, which is the result of the proteinuria (see Fig. 27–1).

MCNS, especially in children, is extremely responsive to treatment with corticosteroids. Patients are given a trial of 60 mg/m²/day in children and about 2 mg/kg/day in adults. At 4 weeks, alternate-day therapy with 35 mg/m² in children and 0.9 mg/kg in adults is begun and continued for 4 to 8 more weeks, with a tapering regimen given over the next 4 to 6 months. Eighty-five to 90% of all patients with MCNS respond to this protocol (usually by the fourth week in children and the eighth week in adults). Adults older than 40 may require 16 to 20 weeks of corticosteroid therapy before a complete remission occurs.

After a remission, about 70% of patients have one or more episodes of relapse. The remainder become frequent relapsers (more than twice a year) or corticosteroid dependent. These patients may benefit from adjunctive therapy with cytotoxic alkylating agents such as chlorambucil (0.1 to 0.2 mg/kg/day) or cyclophosphamide (2.0 mg/kg/day) for 12 weeks. However, there are significant risks associated with the use of these agents, including gonadal failure and carcinogenesis, particularly with long-term use or in combination with corticosteroids. Recent studies indicate that cyclosporine therapy

TABLE 27-6   Features of Focal Segmental Glomerulosclerosis

Nephrotic-range proteinuria with "bland" urinary sediment
Focal, segmental collapse of capillary loops and mesangial
  sclerosis with hyaline droplets
Etiology
  Idiopathic
    "Collapsing" glomerulonephritis
  Secondary
    Heroin
    Acquired immunodeficiency syndrome (AIDS)
    Reflux nephropathy

is of value in selected patients and may induce remissions more often in corticosteroid-dependent patients and less often in corticosteroid-resistant patients.

About three fourths of individuals are disease free at 10 years, with a 10-year survival rate of 95%. Patients show an increased risk of infection (particularly pneumococcus and *Haemophilus* infection) and thrombosis of renal and peripheral veins. The development of chronic renal failure due to MCNS is essentially nonexistent. Patients failing to respond to corticosteroids are generally found to have another glomerulopathy, most often focal glomerulosclerosis (FGS).

Focal Glomerulosclerosis

FGS accounts for 10% to 15% of children and 15% to 20% of adults with idiopathic nephrotic syndrome (Table 27–6). Although heavy proteinuria and edema are usually present at onset, some patients have asymptomatic proteinuria and hematuria. Hypertension, azotemia, and microscopic hematuria are commonly found at the time of diagnosis. Serum complement levels are normal. Recently, a glomerular permeability factor present in the blood has been implicated in the proteinuria in patients with FGS.

Light microscopy shows focal and segmental collapse of capillary loops and mesangial sclerosis sometimes associated with hyalin insudation at the edge of the sclerotic focus. Proliferation or infiltration is absent. Focal mild tubular dropout with interstitial fibrosis is often present. Patchy deposition of IgM, C3, and occasionally other immunoreactants is seen in the segmental sclerotic foci. Electron-dense deposits are typically absent by electron microscopy. Patients with acquired immunodeficiency syndrome–related FGS often show numerous tubuloreticular structures within the endothelial cytoplasm—collections of microtubules that apparently form in response to elevated serum levels of interferon. Such structures are also very common in biopsies of patients with SLE.

Approximately one third of patients respond to corticosteroid therapy with a lasting remission and good long-term renal function. But most (60% to 70%), particularly those with persistent nephrotic syndrome, progress to chronic renal failure (55% by 10 years). The remainder follow a long-term course with relapses and remissions and late onset of renal failure. Recurrence of FGS in transplants occurs in as many as 40% of patients.

Heroin users and patients with the acquired immunodeficiency syndrome may develop the nephrotic syndrome and the histologic lesion of FGS. These patients typically follow a much more rapid downhill course, often with progression to end-stage renal failure in less than 1 year. A variant of FGS known as "collapsing glomerulopathy" is a distinct entity characterized by black racial predominance, massive proteinuria, relatively rapidly progressive renal insufficiency, and distinctive pathologic findings. Although collapsing glomerulopathy resembles human immunodeficiency virus nephropathy both pathologically and clinically, it differs clinically by having no evidence for associated human immunodeficiency virus infection and differs pathologically by lacking endothelial or tubuloreticular inclusions.

Membranous Glomerulopathy

Membranous glomerulopathy (Table 27–7) accounts for 25% to 30% of nephrotic syndrome in adults, with peaks between ages of 30 to 40 and 50 to 60 years. Microscopic hematuria is present in about 50% of the patients. Spontaneous complete remissions occur in about 20% of patients, with another 20% to 25% experiencing a partial remission with non–nephrotic-range proteinuria. These patients may maintain a stable GFR for decades. Of the remaining 50%, about half progress to end-stage renal failure by 5 to 10 years.

Treatment of membranous nephropathy is controversial. At this time, it is reasonable to suggest or recommend that patients with a favorable long-term prognosis (e.g., children, adults with non–nephrotic-range proteinuria) need not receive specific treatment. Similarly, adult patients, particularly women younger than 40 years old with nephrotic syndrome but with normal renal function and modest degree of proteinuria (<9 g/day), could be managed conservatively, without corticosteriods or cytotoxic agents, and observed for either spontaneous remission or progression. In these patients it may be appropriate to use angiotensin-converting enzyme inhibitors, which have been shown to reduce proteinuria in

TABLE 27-7   Features of Membranous Glomerulopathy

Nephrotic-range proteinuria with "bland" urinary sediment
Glomerular basement membrane thickening with "spike"
  formation, granular deposits of IgG and complement, and
  subepithelial electron-dense deposits
Etiology
  Idiopathic
  Secondary
    Infections: hepatitis B, syphilis
    Neoplasms: carcinoma of the lung, stomach, breast
    Drugs: gold, D-penicillamine, captopril
    Collagen vascular diseases: systemic lupus erythematosus, mixed connective tissue disease

about a third of patients. Patients with persisting severe proteinuria (>9 g/day), particularly men older than 40 years, with symptomatic nephrotic syndrome or progressive renal failure may be best treated by a combination of cytotoxic drugs, such as oral methylprednisone and chlorambucil used sequentially over a 6-month period. This treatment may improve the likelihood of remission and decrease the incidence of chronic renal failure.

Diabetic Nephropathy

Diabetic nephropathy is the single most important cause of end-stage renal disease in the United States, with diabetic patients accounting for approximately 40% of all patients enrolled in the end-stage renal disease program. The cumulative incidence of nephropathy is 30% to 50% in type 1 diabetes and about 20% in type 2 diabetes, although certain populations of patients with type 2 diabetes (e.g., Pima Indians) have a higher incidence of nephropathy. More than half of patients with ESRD secondary to diabetes have type 2 diabetes. Currently available data strongly support the concept that diabetic nephropathy is a direct result of the metabolic derangements seen in diabetics and that normalization of carbohydrate metabolism would be protective against the development of renal disease. In early diabetes, some of the biochemical alterations can lead to hyperfiltration, with the GFR elevated above normal by 20% to 30%.

Diabetic nephropathy is a clinical syndrome characterized by persistent albuminuria (>300 mg/24 hr), a relentless decline in GFR, and raised arterial blood pressure. Nephropathy is rare during the first 5 years of diabetes, after which the incidence increases until it reaches a peak at approximately 15 to 20 years of diabetes. Several studies have suggested that microalbuminuria, being defined as a urinary albumin excretion rate greater than 30 mg/24 hr (20 μg/min) and less than or equal to 300 mg/24 hr (200 μg/min), strongly predicts the development of diabetic nephropathy in both types of diabetes. Excessive cardiovascular mortality has been associated with microalbuminuria. One to 5 years after the onset of microalbuminuria, proteinuria increases and can be detected by protein dipstick measurement on routine urinalysis. This increment in proteinuria is associated with a significant risk for the development or worsening of existing hypertension and progressive decline in renal function. Once proteinuria is established, renal function declines, with 50% of patients reaching end-stage renal disease in 7 to 10 years after the onset of proteinuria. The rate at which patients with proteinuria progress is highly variable, but if the nephropathy is untreated, the GFR may decrease at an average rate of 1 mL/min/mo. A high percentage of patients with type 2 diabetes (in contrast to type 1 diabetes) have modest proteinuria and hypertension when initially seen, indicating that other diseases may be responsible for the renal damage. Diabetic retinopathy is found in more than 90% of patients with type 1 diabetes; nearly one third of the patients with type 2 diabetes diabetic nephropathy have no evidence of retinopathy. Regardless, the absence of retinopathy and/or renal insufficiency without proteinuria, presence of red blood cell casts,

and low levels of complement should lead to a search for other causes of renal disease.

Kimmelstiel-Wilson nodular glomerulosclerosis, although the classic diabetic glomerular lesion, is found in only 15% to 20% of patients with diabetic nephropathy. It consists of a nodular increase in hyaline material that massively expands the mesangial areas surrounded by dilated and uniformly thickened capillary loops. The nodular foci have a focal and segmental distribution. The more common lesion is that of diffuse glomerulosclerosis, a uniform increase in hyaline material within the mesangial areas associated with capillary loop changes described previously. Hyaline arteriolosclerosis involving both the afferent and efferent arterioles, as well as tubulointerstitial atrophy and fibrosis, accompanies both the nodular and the diffuse forms of diabetic glomerulosclerosis. The insudative lesions—capsular drops and fibrin caps—consist of small, eosinophilic droplets on the parietal side of Bowman's capsule or the inner surface of a capillary loop, respectively. The presence of linear deposition of IgG along the capillary walls, as well as focal, segmental deposition of IgM and C3, is nonspecific and is thought to represent passive trapping.

The major therapeutic interventions in diabetic nephropathy include vigorous control of blood sugar, antihypertensive treatment, and restriction of dietary proteins. Strict control of blood glucose prevents diabetic microangiopathic lesions in experimental animals, and evidence is accumulating that euglycemia in humans with early diabetes has similar effects. Meticulous control of hypertension slows the rate of decline in GFR. In addition, angiotensin-converting enzyme inhibitors appear to have a more marked antiproteinuric effect than other antihypertensive agents. Thus, the current practice is to use angiotensin-converting enzyme inhibitors in patients with either incipient or overt diabetic nephropathy. Their use has also been recommended in patients who have microalbuminuria, even in the face of normal blood pressure. There is suggestive evidence that in patients with diabetic nephropathy, protein restriction reduces the progression of kidney disease.

Dysproteinemias and Amyloidosis

The most common histologic diagnosis, found in 80% of patients with myeloma, is cast nephropathy or myeloma kidney. Light-chain deposition disease, occurring in 5% to 10%, and amyloidosis, occurring in 10%, can present as the nephrotic syndrome, which is present in up to 25% of the cases.

Patients with *cast nephropathy* usually present with proteinuria and renal insufficiency. Renal failure can evolve rapidly despite stable paraprotein production and excretion. The typical light microscopic findings include large refractile tubular casts surrounded by multinucleated giant cells located in the distal and collecting tubules. The casts are composed of light chains and Tamm-Horsfall protein and are strongly eosinophilic and periodic acid–Schiff positive.

Light chain deposition disease is a monoclonal gammopathy characterized by deposition of light chains in the kidney and other vital organs (liver, heart, peripheral nerves). This disorder predominantly affects men, with a sex ratio of 2:1 to 4:1 and an age range between 35 and 75 years. The primary renal presentation is impairment, evident by an elevated serum creatinine level and proteinuria, with nephrotic-range proteinuria being detected in 25%. Extrarenal manifestation of light chain deposition may be noted at presentation with abnormal results of liver function tests.

The characteristic light microscopic findings vary from normal glomeruli to degrees of mesangial expansion along with thickened tubular basement membranes outlined by continuous deposits. One third of the biopsy cases have a pattern of nodular glomerulosclerosis similar to Kimmelstiel-Wilson glomerulopathy seen with diabetic nephropathy. Immunofluorescence shows deposits composed of monoclonal light chains (usually kappa type).

Systemic *amyloidosis* is classified into four types according to the chemical composition of fibrillar deposits, which correspond to clinical patterns termed *primary, secondary, hereditary,* and *dialysis associated.* The most common form in the United States is primary or AL, which is a plasma cell dyscrasia. Secondary amyloidosis, which develops after chronic inflammatory or infectious disease, has deposits composed of AA proteins. There are several autosomal dominant hereditary forms, of which the most well known is familial amyloidotic polyneuropathy. The fourth form occurs in chronic hemodialysis patients, and the amyloid fibril is a β_2-microglobulin. Up to 80% of patients with AL or AA forms of amyloidosis have renal involvement. Nephrotic syndrome is the initial feature in 75% of patients with secondary amyloidosis and in approximately 25% of patients with primary amyloidosis and is a rare complication of familial amyloidosis. Renal insufficiency is present in approximately 50% at diagnosis, and the most common cause of death is cardiac failure with a median survival of 4 months. Diagnosis is often not suspected on clinical grounds and is made when a patient undergoes renal biopsy for nephrotic syndrome (Fig. 27–6).

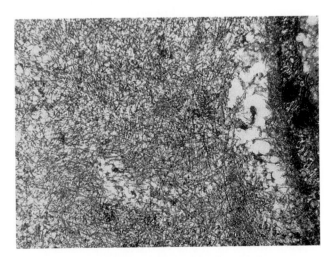

FIGURE 27–6 Electron micrograph demonstrating the non-branching fibrils characteristic of amyloidosis.

There are no reliable biochemical tests for diagnosis, and definitive diagnosis must be made by tissue biopsy. Most patients with primary amyloidosis and 65% of patients with secondary amyloidosis have a positive abdominal fat aspirate. It is positive in only a minority of patients with dialysis-associated amyloidosis. Even when amyloid is known to be present, a kidney biopsy may be necessary to make a definitive diagnosis and to rule out other diseases. By light microscopy, the deposits are extracellular, eosinophilic, and metachromatic. The amyloid proteins are Congo-red positive, show apple-green birefringence under polarized light, and are fibrillar by electron microscopy. Figure 27–6 shows the typical Congo-red staining and electron microscopic findings of AL amyloidosis. There are no specific treatments for amyloidosis. In patients with primary amyloidosis, colchicine, melphalan, and prednisone have been used. Colchicine is the drug of choice in patients with amyloidosis secondary to familial Mediterranean fever.

NEPHROTIC SYNDROME WITH "ACTIVE" URINE SEDIMENT

Many patients present with pure nephrotic syndrome. However, a variety of patients with glomerular diseases present with a "mixed" pattern of nephrotic/nephritic syndrome, including the various forms of membranoproliferative glomerulopathy as well as SLE, Henoch-Schönlein purpura, and mixed essential cryoglobulinemia.

Types of Membranoproliferative Glomerulopathy

Membranoproliferative glomerulopathy (MPGN) may be idiopathic or associated with a number of other diseases. An important recent recognition is the association with hepatitis C, which may account for 10% to 20% of adult MPGN (see later). Idiopathic MPGN is a disease of young persons, with most cases diagnosed in those between the ages of 5 and 30 years. Overall, MPGN accounts for 10% to 15% of all cases of idiopathic nephrotic syndrome. The clinical manifestations are variable, with around 50% presenting with nephrotic syndrome, 25% to 30% with asymptomatic proteinuria, and 15% to 20% with acute nephritic syndrome. Regardless of the major pattern, concurrent hematuria and proteinuria are almost always present. Serum C3 levels are depressed in more than 70% of patients at disease onset. The presence of C3 nephritic factor is most likely an associated event rather than a cause of MPGN, and its presence does not appear to alter the prognosis. Thus, MPGN must be differentiated from other forms of GN showing hypocomplementemia (Table 27–8).

MPGN is characterized overall by thickening of capillary loops and mesangial hypercellularity, often with lobular accentuation. Several subtypes exist. Type I MPGN has subendothelial deposits with mesangial interposition producing capillary loop splitting (see Fig. 27–1). Type II (dense deposit disease [DDD]) has characteristic broad, very electron-dense deposits widening the GBM. Immunofluorescence examination of both types I and II

TABLE 27–8 Features of Membranoproliferative Glomerulopathy

Nephrotic-range proteinuria with "active" urinary sediment
Idiopathic
Type I: Mesangial hypercellularity and capillary loop "splitting"
Type II: Mesangial hypercellularity with glomerular basement membrane "dense deposits"
Type III: Morphologic variants
Type I changes plus subepithelial deposits
Changes intermediate between type I and type II
Associated with other diseases (secondary)
Hepatitis C and B
Systemic lupus erythematosus
Essential mixed cryoglobulinemia
Sickle cell disease
Partial lipodystrophy (type II)

cells shows extensive granular C3 deposition in the capillary loops, usually with absence of immunoglobulins. There are several different morphologic variants with features similar to either type I or II MPGN that have been reported as type III MPGN.

MPGN is a slow but progressive disease, with approximately 30% of patients in chronic renal failure at the end of 10 years. Poor prognostic indicators include the presence of nephrotic syndrome or azotemia at the time of diagnosis. Spontaneous remission of proteinuria occasionally occurs but does not usually affect the long-term outcome. There is currently no consensus on any given therapeutic regimen that is both safe and effective in MPGN, although a combination of corticosteroid and cytotoxic drug therapy or antiplatelet agents have been used.

Type II MPGN recurs in virtually 100% of renal transplants, but recurrence is far less common in type I MPGN (about 25%). However, recurrence does not interfere with long-term graft survival.

Essential Mixed Cryoglobulinemia

Mixed cryoglobulins composed of monoclonal IgM rheumatoid factor and polyclonal IgG are characteristic of a disorder called essential mixed cryoglobulinemia. It occurs usually in middle age, affecting women slightly more than men, and presents as purpura, fever, Raynaud's phenomenon, arthralgias, and weakness. Renal manifestations are seen in 40% to 50% of patients and vary from proteinuria and/or hematuria to acute nephritic syndrome. Many patients are hypocomplementemic with a decrease in early complement components such as C4 and normal levels of C3. Thus, the presence of palpable purpura in a patient with proteinuria and hematuria with high titers of rheumatoid factor with or without low levels of C4 is highly suggestive of the diagnosis of essential mixed cryoglobulinemia. The glomeruli show a diffuse proliferative GN with intraluminal hyaline thrombi. IgG, IgM, and C3 are usually present in subendothelial areas and the mesangium.

About 50% of patients with essential mixed IgG-IgM cryoglobulinemia have underlying chronic hepatitis C virus infection. Anti–hepatitis C viral antibody, hepatitis C viral core antigens, and hepatitis C RNA can be found in the cryoglobulins and in the renal deposits of patients with hepatitis C virus infection associated with mixed cryoglobulinemia. All patients should be screened for the presence of hepatitis C; and in those patients who demonstrate the presence of hepatitis C, interferon alfa therapy should be considered. Patients with renal insufficiency or acute nephritic syndrome usually progress to end-stage renal failure. However, the overall survival rate in patients with renal manifestations is about 75%. Plasmapheresis to decrease the circulating cryoprecipitates may improve the prognosis of patients with severe renal disease. Although treatment with interferon alfa appears to cause improvement, relapses are common after stopping treatment.

Systemic Lupus Erythematosus Glomerulonephritis

SLE is primarily a disease of young women, although it may occur in both sexes at any age. It accounts for 5% to 10% of patients with nephrotic syndrome, and it can be the presenting manifestation of a patient with SLE without any other systemic manifestations. It should be suspected in any individual, especially a young woman, who presents with proteinuria accompanied by hematuria, especially when accompanied by low levels of complement. Diagnosis rests on serologic evidence of antinuclear antibody production in the presence of inflammation of multiple organs. Clinical evidence of renal disease is present in as many as 85% to 90% of SLE patients, varying from minimal changes to nephritic and/or nephrotic syndrome. Virtually all patients are found to have renal injury if a kidney biopsy is performed. The nephrotic syndrome with a "nephritic" sediment is most common, and 10% to 15% of patients also have azotemia. Serum complement levels are usually low during periods of active renal disease. A small number of patients present with RPGN. Renal function deteriorates over a matter of weeks, and numerous cellular crescents are seen on renal biopsy.

The clinical presentation and the severity of renal disease correlate with the underlying histopathology, best classified using the World Health Organization scheme (Table 27–9). Essentially, these categories can be grouped as proliferative (types II, III, IV) or membranous (type V) glomerulopathies, with greater proliferation (type IV) associated with poorer prognosis. Multiple immunoglobulins and various components of complement are almost invariably present within the glomeruli and may involve all levels of the GBM as well as the mesangium (Fig. 27–7; see also Fig. 27–1). It has been suggested that the presence and amount of subendothelial deposits seen by electron microscopy are good predictors of progression.

The treatment of lupus nephritis is controversial, but patients with class I and II disease do not need any treatment directed at the renal lesions. Therapy should

TABLE 27-9 Histologic Class, Clinical Presentation, and Prognosis in Systemic Lupus Erythematosus Nephritis

Histologic Type	WHO Class	Frequency (%)*	Proteinuria (%)	Nephrotic Syndrome (%)†	Azotemia (%)‡
Normal	I	<5			
Mesangial	II	15	70	0	~10
Focal proliferative	III	20	100	15	20
Diffuse prolifera-tive	IV	50	100	~90	75
Membranous	V	15	100	~90	20

* Percent of patients with systemic lupus erythematosus who show this lesion on biopsy.
† Proteinuria exceeding 3.0 g/24 hr.
‡ Serum creatinine exceeding 1.2 mg/dL or blood urea nitrogen exceeding 25 mg/dL.
Adapted from Couser WG: Glomerular disorders. *In* Wyngaarden JB, Smith LH Jr, Bennett JC (eds): Cecil Textbook of Medicine, 19th ed. Philadelphia: WB Saunders, 1992, p 566.

be dictated by the extrarenal manifestations. Patients with definite but mild to moderate renal disease accompanied by focal glomerular lesions detected by light microscopy may be managed by the lowest possible dose of corticosteroids and observed carefully for the development of more diffuse renal disease. Several long-range studies of patients with diffuse proliferative GN (class IV) and severe focal proliferative GN have suggested that the addition of cytotoxic drugs to a regimen of prednisone may offer benefit in these patients with SLE by providing a better preservation of renal function. The outlook for patients even with class IV lupus nephritis has improved enormously over the past decade, with survival as high as 90% at 10 years.

Patients with SLE tolerate dialysis about as well as patients with non-SLE renal failure. Indeed, for reasons that are not yet understood, patients with SLE who are placed on chronic dialysis often note dramatic amelioration of other manifestations of SLE. Renal transplantation is also well tolerated, with recurrence of SLE GN being relatively rare.

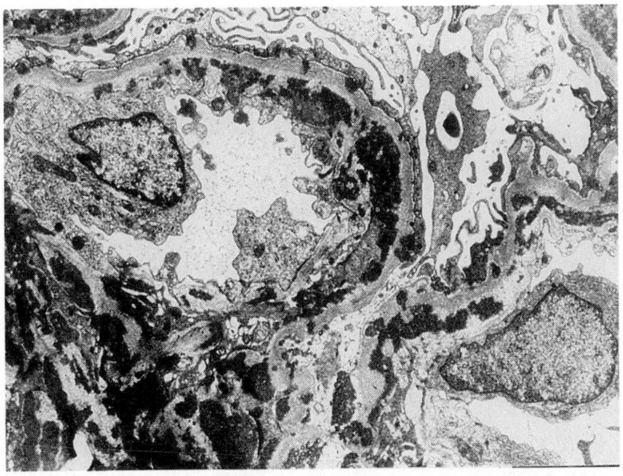

Henoch-Schönlein Purpura

Henoch-Schönlein purpura is seen most often in children (boys more than girls) and is characterized by purpuric lesions on the buttocks and legs, episodic abdominal pain, arthralgias, fever, malaise, and proteinuria (often nephrotic range) with hematuria and red blood cell casts. Serum C3 levels are typically normal.

The glomeruli show varying degrees of mesangial hypercellularity and crescent formation, with the prognosis declining as the proliferation increases. Uncommonly, exuberant crescent formation occurs associated with a rapid progression to renal failure. IgA and C3 staining of the mesangium is prominent with numerous mesangial electron-dense deposits seen by electron microscopy. Immunofluorescence examination of lesions or of unaffected skin shows IgA and C3 within dermal capillaries.

Henoch-Schönlein purpura tends toward a benign, self-limited course of remission and relapse, usually disappearing after a few months to years. More than half of the patients recover completely from their renal injury, but about 10% progress to end-stage renal disease. Persistent nephrotic syndrome, acute nephritic syndrome at onset, and older age suggest a poor prognosis. Therapy is unproven for the renal manifestations of Henoch-Schönlein purpura, although patients with extensive crescent formation should be managed aggressively. Recurrence is uncommon in renal transplants.

FIGURE 27-7 Electron micrograph from a patient with SLE with (a) massive subendothelial deposits, (b) a few subepithelial deposits, and (c) mesangial deposits.

Asymptomatic Urinary Abnormalities

A variety of renal lesions may present as either isolated proteinuria or hematuria, with or without proteinuria

TABLE 27–10 **Asymptomatic Urinary Abnormalities**

Isolated Proteinuria
Proteinuria without hematuria
Postural proteinuria

Isolated Hematuria (with or Without Proteinuria)
IgA nephropathy (Berger's disease)
Hereditary nephritis
   Alport's syndrome
    Thin basement membrane disease
Benign recurrent hematuria

(Table 27–10). Isolated proteinuria without hematuria is usually an incidental finding in an asymptomatic patient. These patients generally excrete less than 2 g of protein per day with a bland urine sediment and have normal renal function. About 60% of these patients have so-called postural proteinuria, with absence of proteinuria while lying flat and return of proteinuria on standing. The long-term outcome of isolated proteinuria (postural or nonpostural) is excellent, with the majority of patients showing steady decline in protein excretion. However, in some patients, this condition represents a very early manifestation of a more serious glomerular disease such as membranous glomerulopathy, IgA nephropathy, focal glomerulosclerosis, diabetic nephropathy, or amyloidosis. Finally, it should be noted that mild proteinuria may accompany a febrile illness, congestive heart failure, or infectious diseases.

Hematuria with or without proteinuria in an otherwise asymptomatic patient may represent the fortuitous early discovery of another glomerular disease such as SLE, Henoch-Schönlein purpura, postinfectious GN, or idiopathic hypercalciuria in children. However, asymptomatic hematuria is also the primary presenting manifestation of a number of specific glomerular diseases discussed next.

IG

IgA nephropathy, characterized by mesangial IgA deposits (Fig. 27–8), is the final diagnosis in as many as 50% of patients with asymptomatic hematuria. It is the most common cause of primary glomerular disease worldwide. The typical presentation is gross hematuria after a viral illness, with men affected two to three times more frequently than women and whites much more commonly affected than blacks. Most other patients present with asymptomatic hematuria discovered on an incidental examination, accompanied by mild to moderate proteinuria. Most patients are between the ages of 15 and 35. Microscopic hematuria usually remains after the gross hematuria resolves. Mild proteinuria of less than 1 g/day is common, but nephrotic-range proteinuria may be seen in as many as 10% of patients. Serum complement is normal.

Light microscopic changes vary from normal glomeruli (grade I), through mesangial hypercellularity (grade II), to a mixed group of abnormalities, including seg-

mental sclerosis, crescent formation, tubular atrophy, and interstitial fibrosis (grade III). Mesangial deposits of IgA, even in glomeruli unaffected when judged by light microscopy, are characteristic of this disease (see Fig. 27–1); some patients also have IgG and C3 deposition.

Progressive renal insufficiency develops in 20% to 30% of patients after 20 years. Some have a more rapid progression, with renal failure in as little as 4 years. Poor prognostic indicators include nephrotic-range proteinuria, hypertension, and the higher-grade renal biopsy changes. No effective therapy is currently available. Mesangial IgA deposits recur frequently in renal transplants but with minimal long-term effects on function.

HEREDITARY NEPHRITIS (ALPORT'S SYNDROME)

Hereditary nephritis usually presents in childhood with recurrent gross hematuria, with or without vague lower back or abdominal pain. Mild proteinuria is often present, but nephrotic syndrome is rare. Sensorineural deafness is present in about 50% of the patients. Family history may show any of a number of different patterns, although 80% of pedigrees show some X-linkage and over half of these result from a mutation of *COL4A5*, the gene located at Xq22 that codes for the α5 chain of type IV collagen. Boys are usually more affected than girls and often develop renal failure by age 30. Light microscopy reveals nonspecific interstitial foam cells, and immunofluorescence is negative for immunoglobulins and complement. The diagnostic ultrastructural abnormalities include alternating areas of thinned and thickened capillary loops with lamination and splitting of the GBM.

No effective treatment is currently available. It has been shown that the GBM in patients with Alport's syndrome does not react with anti-GBM antibody, implying a lack of certain GBM antigens. Therefore, although Alport's syndrome does not recur in renal transplants, allografts may develop anti-GBM antibody GN,

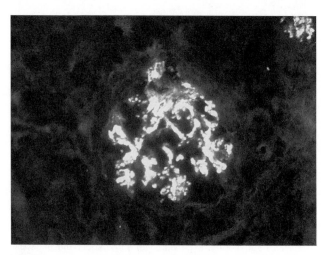

FIGURE 27–8 Immunofluorescence demonstrating the mesangial distribution of IgA.

owing to the presence of GBM antigens for which the recipient lacks immune "tolerance."

THIN BASEMENT MEMBRANE DISEASE

Thin basement membrane disease is an autosomal dominant basement membrane glomerulopathy, with some cases resulting from mutation of *COL4A4* gene at 2q35-q37 location. The disease usually presents as microscopic hematuria without proteinuria in an otherwise asymptomatic young adult. Light and immunofluorescence examinations are normal, whereas ultrastructural examination demonstrates the markedly thinned GBM. Prognosis is excellent, although a few patients with progressive renal failure have been reported.

BENIGN RECURRENT HEMATURIA

The majority of these patients are young adults found to have microscopic hematuria on routine examination or with gross hematuria associated with a febrile illness, exercise, or immunization. The common causes of hematuria are depicted in Table 27–11. Hypercalciuria is a common cause of macroscopic and microscopic hematuria in children. Recent studies indicate that adults have similar consequences from hypercalciuria and/or hyperuricosuria. Benign recurrent hematuria is diagnosed in patients with asymptomatic hematuria when the other possibilities are excluded. Renal biopsy is normal in most, but focal or diffuse mesangial proliferation may be shown. Immunofluorescence is sometimes negative but may show mesangial deposits of IgM or IgG with C3 or C3 alone. Ultrastructural studies are equally variable, with many reports of normal glomeruli, although electron-dense deposits have been seen in GBM and/or mesangium in some patients. Overall the prognosis is excellent, with as many as 50% in complete remission at 5 years and only a few with declining renal function.

TABLE 27–11 **Common Causes of Hematuria by Age and Sex**

Age 0–20 yr
Glomerulonephritis
Urinary tract infection
Congenital urinary tract anomalies
Age 20–40 yr
Urinary tract infection (females > males)
Calculi
Bladder cancer
Age 40–60 yr
Urinary tract infection (females > males)
Bladder cancer
Calculi
Age ≥ 60 yr (men)
Benign prostatic hypertrophy
Bladder cancer
Urinary tract infection
Age ≥ 60 yr (women)
Urinary tract infection
Bladder cancer

From Koenig KG, Bolton WK: Clinical evaluation and management of hematuria and proteinuria. *In* Neilson EG, Couser WG (eds): Immunologic Renal Diseases. Philadelphia: Lippincott–Raven, 1997, p 809.

REFERENCES

Glassock RJ, Cohen AH, Adler SG: Primary glomerular diseases. *In* Brenner BM (ed): The Kidney, 5th ed. Philadelphia: WB Saunders, 1996, pp 1392–1497.

Glassock RJ, Cohen AH, Adler SG: Secondary glomerular diseases. *In* Brenner BM (ed): The Kidney, 5th ed. Philadelphia: WB Saunders, 1996, pp 1498–1596.

Hricik DE, Chung-Park M, Sedor JR: Glomerulonephritis. N Engl J Med 1998; 339:888–899.

Neilson EG, Couser WG (eds): Immunologic Renal Diseases. Philadelphia: Lippincott–Raven, 1997.

Shah SV (ed): Mechanisms of glomerular injury. Semin Nephrol 1991; 11:253–372.

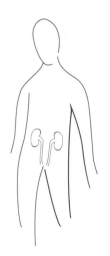

28

MAJOR NONGLOMERULAR DISORDERS

Dinesh K. Chatoth

Tubulointerstitial Nephropathy

Tubulointerstitial nephropathy encompasses a group of clinical disorders that affect principally the renal tubules and interstitium, with relative sparing of the glomeruli and renal vasculature. Most cases of tubulointerstitial nephropathy can be classified into two types on the basis of morphologic changes, as well as on the basis of the rate of deterioration in renal function: *Acute interstitial nephritis* causes a rapid (days to weeks) decline in renal function and is characterized histologically by an acute inflammatory infiltrate. *Chronic interstitial nephropathy* causes a slowly progressive (years) deterioration in renal function and is characterized histologically by predominantly interstitial scarring and fibrosis, with a variable but less impressive amount of monocytic infiltration.

ACUTE INTERSTITIAL NEPHRITIS

Acute interstitial nephritis (AIN) is a clinicopathologic syndrome that is characterized by the sudden onset of clinical signs of renal dysfunction associated with a prominent inflammatory cell infiltrate within the renal interstitium. It is an important cause of acute renal failure (ARF) and may account for 10 to 20% of all cases of ARF.

Etiology

The most common causes of AIN are listed in Table 28–1. The best documented cases of AIN have resulted from complications of therapy with a wide variety of drugs, especially antibiotics and nonsteroidal anti-inflammatory drugs. Septicemia from any cause can also result in AIN, and certain infectious agents such as leptospirosis, legionnaires' disease, and mononucleosis appear to have a particular tendency to cause AIN.

Acute pyelonephritis can be classified histologically as a form of AIN. In contrast to the allergic form of AIN, acute pyelonephritis is associated with direct bacterial invasion of the renal medulla. The clinical manifestations are predominantly those of infection, fever, chills, and flank pain, and acute pyelonephritis only rarely causes ARF.

Severe glomerulonephritis, although sometimes accompanied by an interstitial inflammatory infiltrate, is generally excluded from classifications of AIN. In some patients, such as those with systemic lupus erythematosus, interstitial inflammation may be out of proportion to the degree of glomerular injury, and interstitial nephritis is the predominant finding.

Clinical Features

The major clinical manifestation of AIN is the development of acute renal insufficiency. Many patients develop a systemic manifestation of hypersensitivity reaction with some combination of fever, skin rash, peripheral eosinophilia, and arthralgias. The absence of any or all of these features is common and therefore does not preclude the diagnosis of AIN. Hypertension and edema, important features of acute glomerulonephritis, are uncommon in AIN.

Signs of renal inflammation often accompany acute interstitial nephritis, and urinary abnormalities often provide the first clue to the diagnosis of AIN in a patient with ARF. Hematuria (sometimes macroscopic), sterile pyuria, and leukocyte casts are common findings in AIN, especially secondary to drugs. Eosinophiluria is highly suggestive of AIN but is not often observed. Furthermore, Hansel's stain of the urine is necessary to

TABLE 28-1   Causes of Acute Interstitial Nephritis

Drugs

Antimicrobial drugs
Penicillins (especially methicillin)
Rifampin
Sulfonamides
Ciprofloxacin
Cephalosporins
Nonsteroidal anti-inflammatory drugs
Allopurinol
Sulfonamide diuretics

Systemic Infections

Legionnaires' disease
Leptospirosis
Streptococcal infections
Cytomegalovirus infection
Infectious mononucleosis

Primary Renal Infections

Acute bacterial pyelonephritis

Immune Disorders

Acute allograft rejection
Systemic lupus erythematosus
Sjögren's syndrome

demonstrate eosinophils. Red blood cell (RBC) casts have been found on rare occasions to be associated with AIN and may make the presentation indistinguishable from that of glomerulonephritis. Mild to moderate proteinuria (usually <1 g/day) is present in the majority of patients. Electrolyte abnormalities associated with AIN include hyperkalemia, renal tubular acidosis, and renal sodium wasting.

Discontinuing use of the offending drug is the primary treatment of drug-induced AIN. In situations in which antibiotics are used to treat underlying infection, another appropriate drug can be substituted. In most cases, this usually results in restoration of renal function within several weeks. A short course of high-dose corticosteroids (e.g., prednisone, 1 mg/kg/day for 1 to 2 weeks) may accelerate recovery, but the added risk in patients with underlying infections must be weighed against possible benefits, especially because the latter have not been established unambiguously. Definitive diagnosis of AIN can be made only by renal biopsy, which may be indicated if the diagnosis of ARF is uncertain.

CHRONIC TUBULOINTERSTITIAL NEPHROPATHY

Chronic tubulointerstitial nephropathy is a clinicopathologic entity characterized clinically by slowly progressive renal insufficiency, non-nephrotic–range proteinuria, and functional tubular defects. Pathologically, it is characterized by interstitial fibrosis with atrophy and loss of renal tubules. Chronic interstitial nephropathy is an important cause of chronic renal failure and appears to be responsible for 15% to 30% of all cases of end-stage renal disease (ESRD).

Diagnosis and Clinical Features

Chronic tubulointerstitial nephropathy is characterized by an interstitial mononuclear cell infiltrate along with fibrosis and tubular atrophy. These tubular defects are disproportionately severe in relation to the degree of azotemia. Furthermore, this disease is characterized by the absence of renal manifestations (RBC casts or the nephrotic syndrome) that are usually associated with glomerular disease (Table 28–2). Most patients with chronic interstitial nephropathy have little or no clinical evidence of active renal inflammation. The urinalysis may show modest pyuria and minimal hematuria and in some cases shows WBC casts and occasional granular casts. Proteinuria levels are usually less than 1 g/day.

Certain causes of chronic interstitial nephritis tend to damage a specific segment of the nephron and thereby alter only the tubular functions that are normally ascribed to that segment. Conditions such as multiple myeloma or heavy metal toxicity, which affect primarily proximal tubule structures, may manifest with proximal renal tubular acidosis (RTA), glycosuria, aminoaciduria, and uricosuria. Distal RTA, salt wasting, and hyperkalemia are seen in patients with isolated distal tubular damage, as may occur with chronic obstruction or amyloidosis. Alternatively, patients with analgesic nephropathy, sickle cell disease, or polycystic kidney disease may present with polyuria that is caused by a urinary concentrating defect secondary to medullary involvement.

Specific Causes of Chronic Tubulointerstitial Nephropathy (Table 28–3)

Urinary Tract Obstruction. Urinary tract obstruction is the most important cause of chronic tubulointerstitial nephropathy and is discussed later in this chapter.

TABLE 28-2   Clinical Findings That Suggest Chronic Tubulointerstitial Disease

Hyperchloremic metabolic acidosis (out of proportion to the degree of renal insufficiency)
Hyperkalemia (out of proportion to the degree of renal insufficiency)
Reduced maximal urinary concentrating ability (polyuria, nocturia)
Partial or complete Fanconi's syndrome
    Phosphaturia
    Bicarbonaturia
    Aminoaciduria
    Uricosuria
    Glycosuria
Urinalysis
    May be normal but may contain cellular elements; absence of RBC casts
    Modest proteinuria (<2.0 g/day); absence of nephrotic-range proteinuria

RBC = red blood cell.

TABLE 28-3 Conditions Associated with Chronic Tubulointerstitial Nephropathy

Urinary Tract Obstruction
Drugs
Analgesics/NSAIDs
Nitrosourea
Cisplatin
Cyclosporine
Tacrolimus
Lithium
Vascular Diseases
Nephrosclerosis
Atheroembolic disease
Heavy Metals
Lead
Cadmium
Metabolic Disorders
Hyperuricemia/hyperuricosuria
Hypercalcemia/hypercalciuria
Hyperoxaluria
Potassium depletion
Cystinosis
Hereditary Diseases
Medullary cystic disease
Hereditary nephritis
Polycystic kidney disease
Sickle hemoglobinopathies
Malignancies and Granulomatous Diseases
Multiple myeloma
Sarcoidosis
Tuberculosis
Wegener's granulomatosis
Immunologic Diseases
Systemic lupus erythematosus
Sjögren's syndrome
Cryoglobulinemia
Goodpasture's syndrome
Vasculitis
Amyloidosis
Renal allograft rejection
Other Diseases
Balkan nephropathy
Radiation nephritis
Chinese herb nephropathy

NSAID = nonsteroidal anti-inflammatory drug.

Chronic Pyelonephritis and Reflux Nephropathy. The term *chronic pyelonephritis* was previously used to describe what is currently known as chronic tubulointerstitial nephropathy. The term *chronic pyelonephritis* is now reserved specifically for radiologic findings that demonstrate deformity of the pelvis and calyces that are typically most pronounced in the upper and lower poles. It is now generally accepted that bacteriuria alone is unlikely to result in chronic renal injury. The lesion of chronic pyelonephritis results from vesicoureteral reflux or urinary tract infection in association with obstruction. The development of nephrotic-range pro-

teinuria is usually due to focal segmental sclerosis seen in association with reflux and carries a poor prognosis.

Drugs

Analgesic Nephropathy. Excessive consumption of certain analgesic agents such as phenacetin or acetaminophen (phenacetin is largely converted to acetaminophen), usually in combination with aspirin, may result in chronic interstitial nephritis. Analgesic nephropathy occurs more frequently in women who have ingested large quantities (cumulative ingestion, >3 kg) of antipyretic-analgesic mixtures. Patients frequently do not report taking analgesics, so when the diagnosis is suspected, the possibility of analgesic nephropathy should be vigorously investigated. Emotional stress, neuropsychiatric disturbances, and gastrointestinal disturbances are commonly associated with analgesic nephropathy. Anemia is present in most patients and is frequently more severe than can be attributed to the degree of renal insufficiency; this is because of associated gastrointestinal blood loss that is commonly seen in this condition. Sloughing of a necrotic papilla into the urinary tract may be associated with gross hematuria, flank pain (ureteral colic), passage of tissue in the urine, and an abrupt decline in renal function.

A variety of findings on intravenous urography or retrograde pyelography, including calyceal filling defects resulting from the presence of a sloughed papilla (ring sign), may suggest the diagnosis. Demonstration of papillary necrosis in the absence of other common causes (e.g., diabetes mellitus, urinary tract obstruction, infection, or sickle cell disease) suggests analgesic nephropathy. Patients with analgesic nephropathy are at increased risk for development of transitional cell carcinoma of the urinary tract, particularly of the renal pelvis. The appearance of hematuria should lead to prompt evaluation to rule out a uroepithelial neoplasm. With cessation of analgesic use, renal function generally stabilizes.

Cytotoxic and Immunosuppressive Agents. Several agents such as cyclosporine, tacrolimus, cisplatin, and nitrosoureas, which are more often associated with ARF, may also sometimes cause chronic tubulointerstitial nephropathy.

Vascular Diseases

Hypertensive Nephrosclerosis. The pathologic hallmark of benign nephrosclerosis is an arteriolopathy that is most pronounced in the interlobular and afferent arterioles. Interstitial and glomerular changes appear to result from the subsequent ischemia. Tubular atrophy and interstitial scarring may precede signs of glomerular injury in arteriolar nephrosclerosis.

Radiation Nephritis. Clinically evident renal injury is uncommon with less than 1000 to 2000 cGy but develops in approximately 50% of patients receiving higher doses. In the early stage of radiation nephritis, tubular necrosis, medial and intimal thickening of the small renal arteries, and damage to the glomerular endothelium are present. Later, glomerulosclerosis, collagenous thickening of the small renal arteries, and interstitial fibrosis are prominent. Evidence of renal damage occurs several months to years after renal irradiation. Manifestations range from mild proteinuria, urinary concentrating defects, and benign hypertension with a reduced glomerular filtration rate, to malignant hypertension with end-stage renal failure (ESRF).

Heavy Metals

Lead. Although occupational lead exposure has declined since the 1960s, environmental exposure to lead aerosols has remained relatively high. Lead exposure sometimes occurs as a result of contaminated drinking water (from lead pipes/soldered joints) or from consumption of "moonshine" whiskey. Lead accumulates in tubule cells and causes a predominantly proximal tubular injury, which may lead to glycosuria, aminoaciduria, and chronic interstitial disease. The clinical triad of hypertension, gout ("saturnine" gout), and renal insufficiency in a patient suggests the possibility of lead nephropathy. Disodium ethylenediaminetetraacetic acid, a chelator of lead, may be used to test for a lead burden as well as to treat some cases of lead nephropathy.

Metabolic Abnormalities. Although prolonged hyperuricemia is associated with renal dysfunction, the role of chronic hyperuricemia in producing renal insufficiency is not entirely clear. It has been suggested that the nephropathy seen in association with saturnine gout may actually be secondary to chronic lead exposure, on the basis of the greater mobilization of lead after administration of ethylenediaminetetraacetic acid in these patients. Furthermore, hypertension that is a feature of lead nephropathy often accompanies primary or secondary hyperuricemia.

Primary hyperoxaluria, enteric hyperoxaluria, and cystinosis are inherited diseases that may lead to chronic interstitial nephritis and subsequent ESRF. Hypokalemia and hypercalcemia can also cause chronic tubular injury, leading to nephrogenic diabetes insipidus. Chronic hypercalcemia may result in nephrocalcinosis and chronic interstitial nephritis with reduced glomerular filtration rate that may be only slowly and incompletely reversible.

Malignancies. Renal involvement is common in patients with multiple myeloma; progressive renal insufficiency is seen in more than two thirds of these patients. The so-called myeloma kidney (cast nephropathy) is characterized by laminated refractile tubular casts (surrounded by inflammatory cells and multinucleated giant cells) and by tubular atrophy and interstitial fibrosis. In patients with kappa light chain disease, Fanconi's syndrome may precede the diagnosis of myeloma or the onset of renal insufficiency by many months. Furthermore, in 5% to 15% of cases of myeloma, nephrotic syndrome develops as a result of glomerular lesions (amyloidosis).

In patients with lymphomas and leukemias, particularly acute lymphoblastic leukemia, neoplastic cells may infiltrate the renal interstitium and cause renal enlargement. However, renal function is rarely compromised in such situations.

Immune Disorders. A variety of immune disorders may be associated with both acute and chronic interstitial nephritis, including several types of glomerulonephritis, chronic renal transplant rejection, and systemic lupus erythematosus. Renal involvement in Sjögren's syndrome is usually in the form of chronic interstitial nephritis. The most common functional abnormalities are distal hypokalemic RTA and urinary concentrating defects.

Cystic Diseases of the Kidney

Renal cystic diseases are characterized by epithelium-lined cavities filled with fluid or semisolid debris within the kidneys. Certain clinical settings suggest specific cystic disorders (Table 28–4). An abdominal mass in a neonate or older infant suggests the possibility of either autosomal dominant polycystic kidney disease (ADPKD) or autosomal recessive polycystic kidney disease (ARPKD). Renal failure in adolescence suggests ARPKD or medullary cystic disease. The finding of a solitary cyst in a healthy 50-year-old person is suggestive of a simple cyst. A history of renal disease in a family raises the possibility of ADPKD, ARPKD, or medullary cystic disease. Recurrent renal stones can occur in patients with ADPKD or medullary sponge kidney. The onset of hematuria in a patient undergoing chronic hemodialysis may indicate the possibility of acquired cystic disease.

SIMPLE CYSTS

Simple renal cysts increase in frequency with age, being present in up to 50% of the population over 50 years of age. Simple cysts are most often asymptomatic and are usually incidental findings during imaging studies. Renal ultrasonography, together with computed tomography (CT), permits accurate differentiation of benign from malignant lesions in most instances.

POLYCYSTIC KIDNEY DISEASE

Polycystic kidney diseases (PKDs) include ADPKD, usually referred to as adult PKD, and ARPKD, often referred to as infantile or childhood PKD. ARPKD occurs in association with congenital hepatic fibrosis and causes death from renal failure during the first year of life.

AUTOSOMAL DOMINANT POLYCYSTIC KIDNEY DISEASE

Autosomal dominant PKD is the most common hereditary renal disease in the United States and affects more than 500,000 people. The clinical disorder can be caused by at least three different genes. The most common type, ADPKD1, is carried on the short arm of chromosome 16, and the ADPKD2 gene is carried on chromosome 4. The location of the ADPKD3 gene has not yet been determined.

Clinical manifestations of ADPKD rarely occur before the age of 20 to 25 years. Therefore, many affected people of childbearing age pass the genetic trait on to offspring while they are still asymptomatic and thus un-

TABLE 28–4 Characteristics of Renal Cystic Disorders

Feature	Simple Cysts	ADPKD	ARPKD	ACKD	MCD	MSK
Inheritance pattern	None	Autosomal dominant	Autosomal recessive	None	Often present, variable pattern	None
Incidence or prevalence	Common, increasing with age	1/200–1/1000	Rare	40% in dialysis patients	Rare	Common
Age at onset	Adulthood	Usually adulthood	Neonatal period, childhood	Late adulthood	Adolescence, early adulthood	Adulthood
Presenting symptoms	Incidental finding	Pain, hematuria, infection, family screening	Abdominal mass, renal failure, failure to thrive	Hematuria	Polyuria, polydipsia, enuresis, renal failure, failure to thrive	Incidental, urinary tract infections, hematuria, renal calculi
Hematuria	Occurs	Common	Occurs	Occurs	Rare	Common
Recurrent infections	Rare	Common	Occurs	No	Rare	Common
Renal calculi	No	Common	No	No	No	Common
Hypertension	Rare	Common	Common	Present from underlying disease	Rare	No
Method of diagnosis	Ultrasonography	Ultrasonography, gene linkage analysis	Ultrasonography	CT scan	None reliable	Excretory urogram
Renal size	Normal	Normal to very large	Large initially	Small to normal, occasionally large	Small	Normal

ACKD = acquired cystic kidney disease; ADPKD = autosomal dominant polycystic kidney disease; ARPKD = autosomal recessive polycystic kidney disease; CT = computed tomography; MCD = medullary cystic disease; MSK = medullary sponge kidney.
From Gabow PA: Cystic diseases of the kidney. *In* Wyngaarden JB; Smith LH Jr, Bennett JC (eds): Cecil Textbook of Medicine, 19th ed. Philadelphia: WB Saunders, 1992, p 609.

aware that they have the disease. Patients usually present either for screening because of a family history of the disease or for evaluation of symptoms. Acute abdominal flank pain and back pain along with hematuria are the most common clinical manifestations. Nonspecific, dull lumbar pain is a frequent symptom and usually occurs when the kidneys are sufficiently enlarged to be palpable on examination of the abdomen. Sharp, localized pain may result from cyst rupture or infection or from passage of a renal calculus. Microhematuria is frequently the initial sign of PKD; gross hematuria may also occur.

Hypertension, the most common cardiovascular manifestation of ADPKD, occurs in about 60% of patients before the onset of renal insufficiency. Nocturia resulting from a urinary concentrating defect is often present at the time of diagnosis, and most patients show impaired salt conservation on restricted salt intake. Urinary tract infection and pyelonephritis are common complications. Up to one third of patients with PKD have multiple, asymptomatic hepatic cysts; about 10% of patients have cerebral aneurysms; and about 25% of patients have mitral valve prolapse. Diverticulosis has also been commonly associated with ADPKD.

The natural history of renal functional impairment with ADPKD is variable. The disease progresses to ESRF in almost 50% of patients by age 60. Some of the conditions associated with poor prognosis in ADPKD include presence of the ADPKD1 gene, male sex, black race, hypertension, clinical presentation at an earlier age, and episodes of gross hematuria.

The diagnosis of PKD is made on the basis of radiographic evidence of multiple cysts distributed throughout the renal parenchyma, in association with renal enlargement, increased cortical thickness, and elongation and splaying of the renal calyces. The demonstration of the characteristic bilateral renal cystic involvement is best accomplished by renal ultrasonography. In adults, CT scan with contrast medium occasionally reveals more cystic involvement than is apparent by ultrasonography. Imaging studies that show only a few cysts require differentiation of early ADPKD from multiple simple cysts. The presence of extrarenal involvement, particularly hepatic cysts, lends support to the diagnosis of ADPKD. The information on gene location now permits identification of presymptomatic carriers of ADPKD1 through gene linkage analysis. Because gene linkage is expensive, requires the cooperation of other family members, and supplies no anatomic information, it is probably best reserved for patients with nondiagnostic imaging studies.

The treatment for patients with ADPKD is aimed at preventing complications of the disease and preserving renal function. Patients and family members should be educated about the inheritance and manifestations of the disease. Screening of all patients with ADPKD for cerebral aneurysms is not cost effective. However, screening is recommended in patients with strong family history of aneurysmal hemorrhages and for individuals with certain occupations (e.g., pilots). Therapy for PKD is directed toward control of hypertension and toward prevention and early treatment of urinary tract infections. ESRF is managed by either dialysis or transplan-

tation. Bilateral nephrectomy may be required before transplantation in patients with inordinately large kidneys or those with a history of frequent or persistent urinary tract infection.

ACQUIRED CYSTIC KIDNEY DISEASE

Acquired cystic kidney disease refers to the development of cysts in patients with chronic renal failure or ESRD who are undergoing dialysis. On occasion, carcinomas may complicate this disorder. Although the diagnosis can be established with ultrasonography, CT scan is the diagnostic method of choice in acquired cystic kidney disease because the kidneys and cysts are often small.

MEDULLARY CYSTIC DISORDERS

Medullary cystic disease is part of a group of congenital tubulointerstitial nephropathies known as juvenile nephronophthisis–medullary cystic disease complex. It occurs as a rare, autosomal dominant disease, sometimes accompanied by eye deformities. Anemia and prolonged childhood enuresis that is caused by a urinary concentrating defect are early indications of the renal disease. Other associated clinical features include short stature and failure to thrive. Neither radiography nor renal biopsy has a high rate of success in demonstrating the small medullary cysts because they are about 1 to 2 mm in diameter. Medullary cystic disease regularly results in ESRF during adolescence or early adulthood.

Medullary sponge kidney is a more common, benign disorder that is often detected incidentally on abdominal radiographs. Medullary sponge kidney is relatively common and often manifests as a result of passage of a renal calculus. It is estimated that about 10% of patients who present with renal stones may have medullary sponge kidney. Nephrocalcinosis occurs in about half the patients and accounts for identification of asymptomatic patients on routine abdominal radiography. The diagnosis is made on intravenous pyelography (IVP) by the characteristic radial pattern ("bouquet of flowers" or "bunch of grapes") of contrast-filled medullary cysts. Treatment for urinary tract infection and renal calculus formation is indicated. Renal failure is not a feature of this condition.

Urinary Tract Obstruction

Obstruction to urine flow may occur at any point from the renal pelvis to the urethral meatus. The several causes of urinary tract obstruction are classified in Table 28–5. The age and sex of the patient influence the likelihood of a given pairing of etiology and site of urinary obstruction. Unilateral ureteral obstruction usually causes no detectable change in urinary flow or total renal function. Azotemia or renal failure occurs only if the drainage of both kidneys is significantly compromised. Total urinary tract obstruction is an important cause of ESRF.

TABLE 28-5   Causes of Urinary Tract Obstruction

Congenital Urinary Tract Malformation
Meatal stenosis
Ureterocele
Posterior urethral valves
Intraluminal Obstruction
Calculi
Blood clots
Sloughed papillary tissue
Extrinsic Compression
Pelvic tumors
Prostatic hypertrophy
Retroperitoneal fibrosis
Acquired Anomalies
Urethral strictures
Neurogenic bladder
Intratubular precipitates

A change in urinary habits is often the presenting sign of urinary tract obstruction. Complete obstruction is the most common cause of true anuria. However, polyuria, especially nocturia, is not uncommon in partial obstruction and may occur as a consequence of defective urinary concentration.

Urinary tract obstruction as a cause of renal failure must be sought in any patient who presents with renal failure of unknown etiology, especially in the absence of proteinuria. In addition, total anuria in a setting of acute renal failure or widely varying urine output is highly suggestive of urinary tract destruction. Renal sonography is the preferred means of diagnosing urinary tract obstruction and depends on identification of hydronephrosis. Dilation of the urinary tract may not be evident within the first 24 hours of obstruction or in some severely dehydrated patients. In these situations, an IVP showing a prolonged nephrogram phase with delayed filling can provide valuable diagnostic information. A 24- or 48-hour film may show contrast medium concentrated either in dilated calyces or in the renal pelvis. Retrograde examination of the ureters is rarely necessary for making the diagnosis but may be necessary for defining the anatomy of the obstruction before surgical intervention.

Management of urinary tract obstruction is directed toward identification of the site and cause of obstruction and relief of the obstruction, usually through surgical intervention. Elimination of obstruction is at times associated with a *postobstructive diuresis,* which is caused partially by a solute diuresis from salt and urea retained during obstruction and partially by the renal concentrating defect. In some cases, definitive relief of obstruction is not possible, and urinary diversion may be required. This may be as simple as an indwelling urethral catheter or more complex, such as an ileal conduit. In all cases, control of urinary tract infection is of paramount concern. Urinary tract infection in an obstructed kidney constitutes a urologic emergency and necessitates prompt relief of the obstruction.

Nephrolithiasis

Nephrolithiasis is a common cause of morbidity in the United States. The peak incidence is in the age group of 20 to 45 years, with a predilection for men (the incidence is five times higher in men than in women). The incidence of nephrolithiasis is higher in developed countries, mainly because of high intake of animal protein coupled with a low-fiber diet.

Depending on stone composition, five types of renal calculi are recognized (Table 28–6). Calcium stones are the most common, accounting for 75% of all stone. The majority of these are calcium oxalate stones, which contribute to more than 50% of all diagnosed renal calculi. Calcium phosphate stones require an alkaline pH for their precipitation and therefore are less common except in patients with RTA, primary hyperparathyroidism, or milk alkali syndrome.

Patients with nephrolithiasis usually have hematuria (both gross and microscopic) and sudden onset of excruciating colicky pain located in the flank and radiating to the groin on the same side. Nephrolithiasis may sometimes be associated with polyuria, dysuria, vomiting, and ileus. Initial evaluation of the patient with nephrolithiasis should include past history of hematuria or passing a stone, urinary infections, family history, and a detailed dietary analysis. Initial screening should include measurements of electrolytes, creatinine, serum calcium, phosphate, and uric acid. Management of patients with nephrolithiasis requires identification of the specific type of stone. Urinalysis is helpful in determining the pH, identifying hematuria, ruling out infection, and, most important, identifying the type of crystals. An IVP with tomographic cuts can identify many of the stone types. Uric acid stones are easily identifiable because they are the only radiolucent stones. Cystine stones are less radiopaque and may assume the calyceal shape. Also, triple phosphate stones have a staghorn appearance and can be easily identified radiologically. The most reliable method of identifying stones is crystallographic study when the stone is identified through straining of urine.

Forty percent of patients with a first episode of nephrolithiasis have a second episode within 2 to 3 years, and 75% have a recurrence in 7 to 10 years. After 20 years of follow-up, less than 10% of the patients remain stone free. On the basis of these figures, all patients with a first episode of nephrolithiasis should be advised to consume approximately 3 L of fluid per day to maintain at least 2 L of urinary volume per day. Eight to 10 ounces should be consumed during the night, because this is the period of maximum urinary concentration. Restricting intake of animal protein and reducing daily salt intake are the two dietary modifications that have been shown to lower the risk of recurrent nephrolithiasis. Accordingly, patients should be advised to restrict their intake of protein to 1 to 1.5 g/kg

TABLE 28-6 Frequency Distribution, Risk Factors, and Radiologic Appearance of Renal Calculi

Type of Stone	Percentage of All Stones	Risk Factors	Radiologic Appearance
Calcium oxalate/phosphate	75	Hypercalciuria (40%–50%) Hypocitraturia (20%–40%) Hyperuricosuria (15%–25%) Hyperoxaluria (<5%) Decreased urine volume (5%–10%)	Opaque, round, multiple calculi
Magnesium-ammonium-phosphate (triple phosphate/struvite)	10–15	Anatomic urologic abnormality Infection with urease-producing organism Hypercalciuria Hyperuricosuria	Opaque, staghorn
Uric acid	10–15	Hyperuricosuria Urine pH <5.0 Decreased urine volume	Radiolucent
Cystine	1	Hypercystinuria Decreased urine volume	Radiopaque, may be staghorn

and to use salt in moderation. A comprehensive metabolic work-up may be initiated 6 to 8 weeks after passage of the first stone, especially in patients with high occupational or dietary risk of recurrence. This should include two 24-hour urine collections for volume, pH, creatinine, urea, sodium, calcium, phosphate, urate, oxalate, and citrate excretion, together with serum parathyroid hormone determination (Fig. 28–1).

The majority of renal stones (about 90%) are passed spontaneously. The probability of passing a stone depends on the size (especially the width), as well as on its anatomic location. Ureteral stones that are less than 4 mm in width usually pass within a year. Stones that are wider than 8 mm are very unlikely to pass. Symptoms of obstruction, pain, and fever may necessitate surgical intervention. Extracorporeal shock wave lithotripsy treatment is more beneficial in patients with renal pelvic or upper ureteral stones. Ureteroscopy with basket retrieval or ultrasonic lithotripsy may be more successful in patients with lower ureteral stones.

CALCIUM STONES

As mentioned previously, calcium stones can be made up of either calcium oxalate or calcium phosphate. Only a minority of patients with calcium stones have identifiable systemic disease such as hyperparathyroidism, sarcoidosis, hypervitaminosis D, RTA, or gastrointestinal disease responsible for hyperoxaluria. About 50% of patients have hypercalciuria in the absence of any of the diseases described here along with normal serum calcium and parathyroid hormone levels.

Several risk factors are identified in patients with calcium stones. Hypercalciuria can result from hypercalcemia secondary to primary hyperparathyroidism, sarcoidosis, malignancy, and immobilization. It can sometimes also result from familial hypercalciuric syndromes.

RTA, volume overload, and loop diuretics can also increase calcium concentration in the urine. In 90% of patients with hypercalciuria, the condition is idiopathic. In these patients, the presence of hypercalciuric levels of more than 4 mg/kg per 24 hours in the absence of the causes described here is usual. Hypercalciuria tends to be familial, with hyperabsorption at the gut, normal or low serum parathyroid hormone levels, increased 1,25-vitamin D levels, and mild hypophosphatemia.

Other risk factors for calcium stones include low urinary volume and increased intake of animal protein. Epidemiologic studies have shown that urine volumes of less than 1100 mL/day are significantly associated with increased risk of calcium stones. Increased intake of animal protein leads to increased acid load that results in increased urinary calcium excretion. The high protein intake also increases urinary calcium excretion by increasing the glomerular filtration rate.

Hyperuricosuria is a risk factor because urate crystals increase the precipitability of calcium oxalate and calcium phosphate. Hypocitraturia is a well-known risk factor for calcium stones, inasmuch as citrate in urine binds calcium and prevents its precipitation. Normally, citrate is reabsorbed in the proximal tubule, and this reabsorption is enhanced in the presence of acidosis. Accordingly, conditions such as distal RTA, renal failure, severe hypokalemia, chronic diarrheal states, or treatment with acetazolamide can result in hypocitraturia and increase risk for calcium stones. A proportion of patients with hypocitraturia have none of the risk factors described here and are said to have idiopathic hypocitraturia.

Oxalate is a byproduct of normal metabolism. Increased excretion of oxalates occurs in primary hyperoxaluria as a result of an enzymatic defect. More commonly, hyperoxaluria is a result of increased gastrointestinal absorption in patients with small bowel dys-

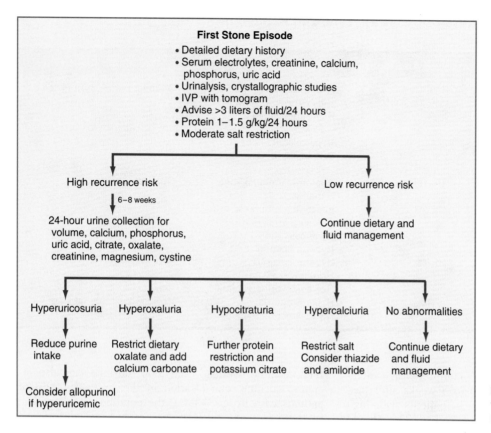

First Stone Episode
- Detailed dietary history
- Serum electrolytes, creatinine, calcium, phosphorus, uric acid
- Urinalysis, crystallographic studies
- IVP with tomogram
- Advise >3 liters of fluid/24 hours
- Protein 1–1.5 g/kg/24 hours
- Moderate salt restriction

High recurrence risk

6–8 weeks

24-hour urine collection for volume, calcium, phosphorus, uric acid, citrate, oxalate, creatinine, magnesium, cystine

Low recurrence risk

Continue dietary and fluid management

Hyperuricosuria	Hyperoxaluria	Hypocitraturia	Hypercalciuria	No abnormalities
Reduce purine intake	Restrict dietary oxalate and add calcium carbonate	Further protein restriction and potassium citrate	Restrict salt Consider thiazide and amiloride	Continue dietary and fluid management
Consider allopurinol if hyperuricemic				

FIGURE 28–1 Management protocol for patients with idiopathic nephrolithiasis.

function, such as inflammatory bowel disease. Increased gastrointestinal absorption of oxalates can also be seen with intestinal malabsorption syndromes as well as with diets high in oxalates (found in tea, colas, citrus juices, spinach, and peanuts).

Medical management of patients with calcium stones depends on identification of a metabolic disorder contributing to the stone formation. Hypercalciuria can be managed by reducing dietary sodium and protein intake, consuming a high-fiber diet, and increasing fluid intake. Thiazides, by virtue of increasing distal renal tubular calcium reabsorption, can also help in the management of hypercalciuria. Hyperoxaluria can be managed by reducing the intake of dietary oxalates. Magnesium-containing supplements are also helpful by reducing the gastrointestinal oxalate load by binding intestinal oxalate. Enteric hyperoxaluria can also be managed by dietary calcium supplements. Hypocitraturia is effectively treated by controlling the underlying condition as well as by treatment with potassium citrate.

Calcium stones 4 to 7 mm in diameter have a 50% chance of passing spontaneously. Surgical intervention is indicated when a stone is unlikely to pass spontaneously or when serial studies show loss of renal function or increasing hydronephrosis, when there is infection, and when there is intractable pain.

URIC ACID STONES

Uric acid stones are caused by the precipitation of uric acid in the urine. The main risk factors are dehydration, persistently acidic urine, hyperuricosuria resulting from overproduction of uric acid, or increased secretion associated with RTA. Ten to 15 percent of patients have elevated serum uric acid levels, whereas 80% of those forming uric acid stones have no definable abnormality of either serum uric acid or urinary uric acid excretion. More than 75% of patients with recurrent uric acid stones have hyperacidic urine, which accelerates the precipitation of uric acid.

The mainstay of treatment of uric acid stones is to increase volume and alkalinize the urine in an effort to reduce precipitation of uric acid. Alkalinization of urine (with a urinary pH goal of 6.5 to 7) can be achieved during the day with oral sodium bicarbonate. To achieve alkalinization at night when the urine is most acidic, acetazolamide may be used in an evening dose. In a very small number of patients with hyperuricosuria, allopurinol may be indicated. The majority of uric acid stones dissolve with effective urinary alkalinization within a few weeks. Patients in whom such treatment fails can be treated with extracorporeal shock wave lithotripsy.

MAGNESIUM-AMMONIUM-PHOSPHATE (STRUVITE) STONES

Patients with struvite stones usually have a past medical history of several intractable urinary tract infections treated with multiple courses of antibiotics. Infection with urease-producing organisms (*Proteus* and *Providencia* species) results in formation of ammonium. Ammonium raises the urine pH, making the urine alkaline, which in turn precipitates struvite and apatite. Ammonium phosphate traps calcium and magnesium, which results in magnesium ammonium phosphate stones. Radiologically, triple phosphate stones appear as radiopaque stones, usually filling the collecting system of the involved kidney. Although infection is an important factor in producing triple phosphate stones, there is often a nidus responsible for initiation of infection. Forty percent of patients with struvite stones have hypercalciuria, and approximately 15% have hyperuricosuria. Patients with metabolic abnormalities resulting in either hypercalciuria or hyperuricosuria should be managed in the same way as patients with calcium or uric acid stones. Management of patients with triple phosphate stones should focus on treating risk factors and on evaluation for anatomic abnormalities. The goal of treatment is to eradicate infection, which is difficult to achieve. Percutaneous nephrolithotomy is currently the primary surgical intervention of choice.

CYSTINE STONES

Cystine crystals are hexagonal in shape and, when present in urine, indicate the presence of excess cystine excretion that leads to the formation of cystine stones. The normal solubility of cystine is 240 to 400 mg/L, and patients with cystine stones have an excretion rate of about 480 to 3600 mg per 24 hours. Solubility of cystine in the urine can be achieved by maintaining high urine output as well as by alkalinizing the urine. The goal is to ensure a urine output of 3 to 4 L per day and achieve a urine pH of about 7.0. Drugs such as penicillamine or tiopronin can be added to the therapeutic armamentarium in patients who experience failure of fluid management and urine alkalinization. Cystine stones are refractory to extracorporeal shock wave lithotripsy; therefore, ultrasonic lithotripsy may be indicated in the management of patients in whom medical treatment fails.

Renal Neoplasia

RENAL CELL CARCINOMA

Renal cell carcinoma is the most frequent malignant renal neoplasm and accounts for about 2% of all cancer deaths in both sexes. It has an increased predilection for men, with a male-to-female ratio of about 2:1. The incidence of this malignancy peaks between the ages of 50 and 70 years. The term *hypernephroma* originated from the gross appearance of these tumors, which, because of their high lipid content, resemble adrenal tissue. Some cases of renal cell carcinoma are associated with an abnormality in chromosome 3. Von Hippel–Lindau disease is associated with renal cell carcinoma and is also characterized by an abnormality in chromosome 3. Other features of von Hippel–Lindau disease include spinal and cerebellar hemangioblastomas, renal and pancreatic cysts, retinal angiomas, and pheochromocytomas.

Renal cell carcinoma originates from the proximal tubular elements. The tumors usually have three cell types: clear cells, granular cells, and spindle cells. The spindle cell type has extensive nuclear anaplasia and confers a poor prognosis. The tumors are highly vascular, supplied by vessels with thin, amuscular walls. Extension of the tumor into normal renal veins and even into the inferior vena cava is not uncommon. Metastatic spread is chiefly via vascular routes, and the lungs, bone, and liver are the most frequent sites of metastasis. The tumors often undergo cystic internal degeneration, thus mimicking benign renal cysts. Calcification within a renal mass, the result of internal necrosis, is a significant radiographic indicator of malignancy.

The classic clinical manifestation of renal cell carcinoma—a triad of hematuria, flank pain, and palpable flank mass—is seen in only about 10% of affected patients. However, any one of these features is present in more than half of all patients as an initial manifestation of the tumor. These tumors are commonly diagnosed as incidental findings during radiodiagnostic procedures. Renal cell carcinoma is notable for the large number of systemic, extrarenal manifestations of the tumor (Table 28–7). Fever is present in about 20% of cases, and an elevated erythrocyte sedimentation rate is present in about 50% of the patients. Anemia is present in about one third of patients, and polycythemia secondary to increased erythropoietin is a striking finding in some cases. Reversible hepatic dysfunction has been found, as has peripheral neuropathy. Ectopic hormone syndromes associated with renal cell carcinoma include hypercalcemia from osteoclast-stimulating factors and Cushing's syndrome from tumor production of an adrenocorticotropic hormone (ACTH)–like factor. Hypercalcemia in renal cell carcinoma is frequently associated with bone metastasis of the tumor.

Treatment of renal cell carcinoma requires surgical excision of the tumor, usually by radical nephrectomy. A small, localized tumor may be removed by hemine-

TABLE 28-7 Manifestations of Renal Cell Carcinoma: Approximate Incidence at Presentation

Manifestation	Percentage of Total
Local	
Hematuria	60
Abdominal mass	45
Pain	40
Classic triad: hematuria, mass, pain	10
Systemic	
Common	
Weight loss	30
Anemia	20
Fever	10
Uncommon	
Erythrocytosis	<5
Leukemoid reaction	<5
Varicocele	<5
Hepatopathy	<5
Hypercalcemia	<5
Cushing syndrome	<5
Galactorrhea	<5

phrectomy, or even ex vivo dissection, when preservation of renal functional mass is critical. The tumors respond poorly to radiation and chemotherapy. Vena caval angiography may be valuable preoperatively to ascertain the presence of venous tumor thrombus. Survival is related to cellular morphology, local extension, and distant metastases; the 10-year survival rate ranges from about 10% to 50% on the basis of these factors.

RENAL ONCOCYTOMA

Renal oncocytomas account for approximately 5% of all renal neoplasms. They are benign tumors and originate primarily from the distal collecting tubular elements. It is very difficult to differentiate oncocytomas from renal cell carcinomas. Moreover, oncocytomas may coexist with renal call carcinomas in some situations. Therefore, radical nephrectomy is the treatment of choice for renal oncocytomas.

OTHER RENAL TUMORS

Renal angiomyolipomas are hamartomas, and more than half of these tumors are found in patients with tuberous sclerosis. They are usually multiple tumors that frequently involve both kidneys. Angiomyolipomas are highly vascular fatty tumors that can mimic renal cell carcinomas in both manifestation and angiographic appearance. CT scan is diagnostic in most situations because of the fat content of the tumor. However, surgical exploration may be necessary for differentiating angiomyolipoma from renal cell carcinoma in patients without tuberous sclerosis, especially if CT scan results are equivocal.

Renal sarcomas constitute fewer than 5% of all renal malignant neoplasms. The most common type of renal sarcoma is leiomyosarcoma. The treatment is usually radical nephrectomy.

Metastatic tumors are common in the kidney because of the rich vascularity. These tumors are often asymptomatic and are incidental findings during radioimaging studies or autopsy.

WORK-UP OF RENAL MASS

The evaluation of a patient with a renal mass should proceed according to the schema given in Figure 28–2.

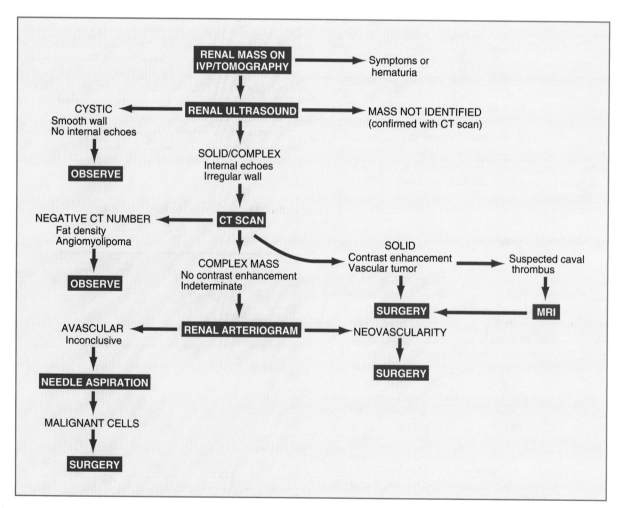

FIGURE 28–2 Schema for the evaluation of a patient with a renal mass. (Adapted from Williams RD: Tumors of the kidney, ureter, and bladder. *In* Wyngaarden JB, Smith JL Jr, Bennett JC [eds]: Cecil Textbook of Medicine, 19th ed. Philadelphia: WB Saunders, 1992, p 615.)

This plan attempts to differentiate benign cystic lesions from solid masses and to identify malignant characteristics in solid renal masses. Multiple modalities exist for the accurate diagnosis of renal masses, and because of their sensitivity, an increasing number of incidental renal masses are being identified in asymptomatic patients. A systematic algorithmic approach should determine the types of more than 90% of renal masses before management.

When a renal mass is demonstrated by IVP with or without nephrotomography, renal ultrasonography is necessary to determine more accurately whether the mass is cystic or solid. About two thirds of renal masses fulfill all ultrasonographic criteria for a simple cyst, and no further work-up is required. When a mass is suspected on IVP but is not confirmed on ultrasonography (15% of cases), renal CT scanning is required, particularly in symptomatic patients.

If the mass on ultrasonography is solid or complex (20% of cases), a renal CT scan (both with and without intravenous injection of iodine contrast), which has replaced renal arteriography, is the next diagnostic step. CT is as accurate as, and obviates the potential morbidity of, angiography in defining renal masses. In addition, CT can usually give sufficient local staging information to allow definitive surgical management. When contrast enhancement on CT is coupled with areas of a negative CT number (relative tissue density in Hounsfield units) that are typical of fat, a diagnosis of angiomyolipoma is appropriate, and no further work-up is required. In indeterminate cases, arteriography or needle aspiration cytologic study or both may be needed to further define the diagnosis; however, in these unusual cases, final definition is likely to require surgery.

REFERENCES

Eknoyan G: Tubulointerstitial diseases and toxic nephropathies. *In* Goldman L, Bennett JC (eds): Cecil Textbook of Medicine, 21st ed. Philadelphia: WB Saunders, 2000, pp 594–600.

Fick GM, Gabow PA: Hereditary and acquired cystic disease of the kidney. Kidney Int 1994; 46:951–964.

Hruska K: Renal calculi (nephrolithiasis). *In* Goldman L, Bennett JC (eds): Cecil Textbook of Medicine, 21st ed. Philadelphia: WB Saunders, 2000, pp 622–627.

Kelly CJ, Neilson EG: Tubulointerstitial diseases. *In* Brenner BM (ed): The Kidney, 5th ed. Philadelphia: WB Saunders, 1995, pp 1655–1679.

Shapiro CL, Garnick MB, Kantoff PW: Tumors of the kidney, ureter, and bladder. *In* Goldman L, Bennett JC (eds): Cecil Textbook of Medicine, 21st ed. Philadelphia: WB Saunders, 2000, pp 631–635.

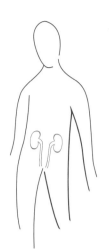

29

VASCULAR DISORDERS OF THE KIDNEY

Yousri M. H. Barri

In this chapter a wide spectrum of diseases are covered that have the common theme of affecting the renal vasculature. These include diseases that affect larger vessels (e.g., renal artery occlusion) and more recently recognized ischemic nephropathy as well as atheroembolic disease, which involves the smaller vessels. Also discussed are malignant hypertension and scleroderma, which have common histologic patterns, and thrombotic microangiopathy.

Renal Arterial Occlusion

Partial renal artery occlusion may be caused by arteriosclerotic disease or fibromuscular dysplasia, which may lead to renovascular hypertension or ischemic nephropathy as a result of progressive atherosclerotic arterial stenosis. Renal artery occlusion may also occur as a result of thrombotic or embolic phenomena. Thrombosis may result from blunt trauma or dissection of the renal artery or may complicate procedures such as renal angioplasty, stent placement, or surgical procedures. Inflammatory conditions such as Takayasu's syndrome, systemic vasculitis, and thromboangiitis obliterans may also be associated with renal arterial thrombosis. However, embolization is more common than thrombosis, and in 90% of the cases it originates from the heart. The causes of embolic disease of cardiac origin include atrial fibrillation, valvular heart disease, bacterial or nonbacterial endocarditis, and atrial myxoma.

Clinical symptoms associated with occlusion of a primary or secondary branch of the renal artery depend on the presence of collateral circulation. Acute renal infarction is associated with lumbar or flank pain, abdominal pain, nausea, vomiting, and fever. If infarction occurs, leukocytosis will develop and levels of serum enzymes such as serum aspartate aminotransferase, lactate dehydrogenase, and alkaline phosphatase will be elevated. Microscopic hematuria may also be seen. Significant renal dysfunction may be associated with bilateral renal infarction or infarction of a solitary kidney. It is frequently associated with acute onset of hypertension owing to the activation of the renin-angiotensin system.

Radiologic evaluation is necessary to establish the diagnosis of renal vascular occlusive disease. Radionuclide imaging with technetium-DTPA (diethylenetriamine pentaacetic acid) or DMSA (dimercaptosuccinic acid) will show nonprofusion of the kidney. Enhanced computed tomography or magnetic resonance angiography and duplex Doppler studies have shown improved diagnostic accuracy. However, the diagnosis is more reliably established by renal arteriography.

The goal of management is to restore blood flow to the ischemic kidney promptly to avoid irreversible damage. Therefore, rapid diagnosis and localization of the thrombus is critical. Traumatic renal artery thrombosis can lead to irreversible renal damage unless surgical thrombectomy is performed within 4 to 6 hours. In acute atheroembolic disease, early diagnosis and revascularization within hours has the highest success in preserving renal function. In contrast, in chronic ischemic renal disease and in the presence of collateral circulation the return of renal function may occur even when diagnosis and treatment are delayed. Return of renal function has been documented after surgical treatment for up to 6 weeks after thrombosis. Therapeutic options include anticoagulation, intravenous or intra-arterial thrombolytic therapy, percutaneous angioplasty, clot extraction by a percutaneous catheter, and surgical thrombectomy.

Ischemic Renal Disease

Renal artery stenosis is now recognized as an important cause of renal insufficiency and end-stage renal disease. Ischemic nephropathy is defined as chronic renal impairment secondary to hemodynamically significant renal artery stenosis. The most common cause of vascular disease is bilateral atherosclerotic renal artery stenosis.

Approximately 15% of patients with end-stage renal disease who are older than age 50 years have ischemic renal disease. The incidence of renal vascular disease is even higher, 30% to 40%, in patients with evidence of coronary, cerebral, or peripheral vascular disease.

The diagnosis of atherosclerotic ischemic nephropathy should be considered in patients with significant risk factors (Table 29–1). The urinalysis is usually benign, with few cells and mild to moderate proteinuria. These patients may have nephrotic-range proteinuria, although this is unusual. The natural history of atherosclerotic renal vascular disease is that of progression. Angiographic progression of renal artery stenosis has been documented in 40% to 50% of patients over a period of 2 to 5 years. With progression, atherosclerotic renal vascular disease can lead to end-stage renal disease. Many patients who were classified as having hypertensive nephrosclerosis may have had progressive renal vascular ischemic nephropathy. Ischemic nephropathy as the cause of renal insufficiency is probably underestimated.

The diagnosis of ischemic nephropathy depends on the finding of significant renal artery stenosis and proving that these lesions are the cause of renal impairment. Currently, there are no tests that have been shown to be predictive of improvement in renal function after correction of renal artery stenosis. Furthermore, tests used for the diagnosis of renovascular hypertension, such as angiotensin-converting enzyme inhibitor renography, is not reliable in patients with renal dysfunction. Discrepancy in renal size on ultrasound is an important clue for considering the diagnosis. Duplex Doppler ultrasonography is a good screening test, but it is highly operator dependent, may be technically difficult, and is time consuming. Magnetic resonance angiography appears to be an effective noninvasive test to detect the stenosis of proximal renal blood vessels. However, it is unreliable in the diagnosis of renal artery branch stenosis. The gold standard test for the diagnosis of ischemic nephropathy is renal arteriography. However, the risks of arteriography include contrast medium–induced acute renal failure, atheroembolic renal disease, and irreversible loss of renal function. These patients usually have underlying renal insufficiency and are at an increased risk for contrast medium–induced acute renal failure, which may be prevented by hydration, use of nonionic contrast, or CO_2 angiography. The recommended approach in these patients is to proceed to renal arteriography in patients with multiple risk factors for ischemic nephropathy. However, in patients with equivocal risk factors, initial noninvasive tests such as duplex Doppler ultrasonography or magnetic resonance angiography before proceeding to angiography is the best approach.

Treatment options for these patients include percutaneous angioplasty, surgical revascularization, and medical therapy. Medical therapy does not reliably prevent disease progression and is associated with a higher mortality that has been observed even after initiation of dialysis. However, medical therapy with appropriate antihypertensive agents may be the only available option in patients who are unlikely to tolerate invasive procedures. There is an increased risk of acute renal failure with the use of angiotensin-converting enzyme inhibitors in these patients. Either percutaneous angioplasty or surgical revascularization can restore renal function lost as a result of renal artery stenosis. The selection of either procedure will be dependent on individual patients. Percutaneous angioplasty is the treatment of choice in patients at high surgical risks. However, surgical revascularization may be the best option in patients with bilateral high-grade osteal renal artery stenosis that is not amenable to angioplasty. Surgical revascularization has been documented to improve renal function in patients with ischemic nephropathy. In addition, surgical revascularization has a higher technical success rate and a lower rate of recurrence when compared with percutaneous angioplasty.

Arterioles and Microvasculature

The processes that involve the smaller vessels of the kidney are usually diffuse and involve both kidneys. Most of the diseases of renal arterioles are associated with systemic involvement of other organ systems. Clinically, arteriolar diseases are usually associated with hypertension as a result of the activation of the renin-angiotensin system. Renal insufficiency may be of acute onset but more commonly is progressive over weeks to months.

Atheroembolic Diseases of the Kidney

Atheroembolic renal disease is a progressive disorder presenting with worsening renal insufficiency as a result of embolic obstruction of small and medium-sized renal blood vessels by atheromatous emboli. It usually occurs in patients with widespread atheromatous disease, either spontaneously or more commonly after renal artery manipulation or surgery, or after procedures such as angiography or percutaneous angioplasty. Atheroembolic disease may also occur after treatment with anticoagulants or thrombolytic therapy, which may interfere with the healing of ulcerated plaques (Table 29–2).

TABLE 29–1 Risk Factors Associated with Ischemic Nephropathy

Severe or refractory hypertension
Hypertensive crisis
Asymmetry of renal size
Flash pulmonary edema with normal left ventricular function
Age >50 years
Rise in serum creatinine level with angiotensin-converting enzyme inhibitors
History of smoking
Presence of atherosclerosis elsewhere (e.g., coronary arteries)

TABLE 29-2 Risk Factors for Atheroembolic Renal Disease

Angiography or angioplasty (aortic, coronary, renal)
Surgical procedures with manipulation of the aorta and/or renal arteries
Anticoagulation or thrombolytic therapy
Spontaneous in patients with severe atherosclerotic disease

The most common clinical problem is acute, subacute, or chronic renal dysfunction. Labile hypertension may occur secondary to renal ischemia and activation of the renin-angiotensin system. Renal insufficiency may be nonoliguric and is usually progressive. Evidence of cholesterol embolization in the retina, muscles, or skin manifested as livedo reticularis may be helpful in making the diagnosis. Atheroembolic disease may also involve other organs, leading to cerebrovascular disease, acute pancreatitis, ischemic bowel, or peripheral gangrene.

The urinalysis is typically benign with few cells, and proteinuria is usually mild. Eosinophilia, eosinophiluria, leukocytosis, and hypocomplementemia may be seen during the active phase of the disease. These findings indicate immunologic activation of the surface of the exposed atheroemboli. The diagnosis of renal atheroemboli should be considered when acute renal failure develops after aortic or renal artery manipulation. The presence of extrarenal atheroemboli such as cyanosis, gangrenous lesions on the toes, and/or livedo reticularis in the legs further supports the diagnosis. Pathologic examination of the kidney shows the presence of cholesterol clefts surrounded by tissue reaction in small to medium-sized renal arteries. There is no effective treatment for this disorder. Avoiding angiographic and surgical procedures in patients with diffuse atherosclerosis may help to prevent this disease. Anticoagulants and thrombolytic agents may worsen atheroembolic process and are to be avoided. Peritoneal dialysis is preferred in patients who develop end-stage renal disease to avoid heparin use with hemodialysis. The prognosis is generally poor and is dependent on the extent of organ involvement and the degree of embolization.

Chronic Hypertensive Nephrosclerosis

This disorder is described as a slow process of intrarenal vascular sclerosis and ischemic changes associated with chronic hypertension. When advanced, these changes can lead to end-stage renal disease. Risk factors for this disorder include race (African-American), marked elevation in blood pressure, and underlying chronic renal disease. Patients usually have long-standing hypertension (>10 years), and a slowly progressive rise in serum creatinine value. Urinalysis findings are usually benign, the sediment revealing few cells, and proteinuria is usually mild, less than 1.5 g/24 hr.

The diagnosis of chronic hypertensive nephrosclerosis is based on clinical presentation in the setting of long-standing hypertension. Typically, patients have a normal urine sediment, non-nephrotic range proteinuria, and small kidneys on ultrasound examination. Kidney biopsy is rarely necessary for diagnosis. Progression of renal failure is related to the degree of blood pressure control. Accelerated hypertension may worsen the rate of progression of renal disease. The primary goal of therapy is to control the blood pressure. The outcome of these patients depends on blood pressure control, compliance with medications, and regular follow-up. In some patients, worsening renal function occurs despite apparently good blood pressure control. It is possible that genetic factors are important in some of these patients. Survival of patients with chronic nephrosclerosis is lower than patients with primary glomerular disease.

Malignant Nephrosclerosis

Malignant nephrosclerosis describes renal vascular changes associated with accelerated hypertension leading to renal ischemia and acute renal failure. The rise in arteriolar and capillary pressure leads to disruption of the vascular endothelium, resulting in the characteristic fibrinoid necrosis. The plasma renin-angiotensin system is activated and may contribute to the development of fibrinoid necrosis.

Patients usually present with extreme elevations in diastolic blood pressure (>120 mm Hg). Hypertensive encephalopathy often occurs concurrently. Proteinuria and hematuria occur in association with acute renal failure. Renal biopsy shows fibrinoid necrosis of the arterioles and produces a histologic picture similar to microangiopathy seen in hemolytic-uremic syndrome. The initial goal of therapy is to lower rapidly the diastolic blood pressure to 100 to 110 mm Hg within 6 hours. It is advisable not to lower blood pressure initially by more than 25% of the initial blood pressure. More aggressive blood pressure control is unnecessary and may lead to ischemic events as a result of decreased perfusion. More gradual lowering of the diastolic blood pressure to 80 to 90 mm/Hg can be achieved over weeks. Renal function commonly deteriorates further during the initial phase of blood pressure control but recovers as the vascular lesions heal and autoregulation of blood flow is re-established. If the vascular injury is severe, the healing may occur as normal blood pressure is maintained. Most patients with accelerated hypertension will have moderate to severe chronic and acute vascular damage and are at increased risk for coronary, cerebrovascular, and renal disease. Patients who develop renal insufficiency tend to have a lower survival rate.

Scleroderma

Scleroderma is a progressive connective tissue disorder associated with proliferation of connective tissue, thickening of vascular walls, and vascular lumen narrowing. The typical manifestations associated with renal involvement include internal proliferation, medial thickening, and increased collagen deposition in the small renal arteries. Approximately 50% of patients may have signs of renal involvement such as mild proteinuria, abnormal serum creatinine level, and associated systemic hypertension. Risk factors associated with renal disease caused by scleroderma include rapidly progressive diffuse skin involvement, cooler months, and race (African-American). Scleroderma renal crisis occurs in 10% to 15% of patients and is characterized by acute renal failure accompanied by an abrupt onset of severe hypertension. Other findings with renal crisis include microangiopathy, volume overload, visual symptoms, and hypertensive encephalopathy. The renin-angiotensin system is activated and may contribute to the development or worsening of renal crisis. The diagnosis of scleroderma renal crisis requires the presence of other features of scleroderma. In rare instances, patients with scleroderma may present with renal crisis. Therapy should be started before the occurrence of irreversible changes. Blood pressure control is the primary goal to slow progression of renal failure. Angiotensin-converting enzyme inhibitors are the drugs of choice and lead to improvement of blood pressure control in the majority of patients. In comparison with other antihypertensive agents, angiotensin-converting enzyme inhibitors have been associated with better preservation of renal function. With adequate blood pressure control and use of angiotensin-converting enzyme inhibitors, some patients may regain sufficient renal function to discontinue dialysis.

Hemolytic-Uremic Syndrome and Thrombotic Thrombocytopenic Purpura

Hemolytic-uremic syndrome (HUS) and thrombotic thrombocytopenic purpura (TTP) are characterized by thrombotic microangiopathy and thrombocytopenia. The clinical features of and therapy for these disorders are similar, although some differences exist (Table 29–3). Renal involvement is more common in HUS and is characterized by fibrin thrombi in the glomerular capillary loops. The arterioles may also show thrombi with fibrinoid necrosis.

HUS is more common in children after nonspecific diarrheal illness. Verotoxin-producing *Escherichia coli* (O157:H7) have been associated with hemorrhagic colitis and HUS. HUS may be associated with renal failure, thrombocytopenia, and microangiopathic hemolytic anemia. Similar features are observed with TTP, and mental status change and neurologic symptoms are observed more frequently with TTP. Both disorders may be associated with malignancy, oral contraceptives, antineoplastic agents, infections, and autoimmune diseases. The clinical course of renal involvement may be acute or rapidly progressive renal failure. The rate of spontaneous recovery of HUS is high in children, and only sup-

TABLE 29–3 Comparison Between Hemolytic-Uremic Syndrome and Thrombotic Thrombocytopenic Purpura

Feature	Hemolytic-Uremic Syndrome	Thrombotic Thrombocytopenic Purpura
Neurologic manifestations	Rare	Common
Thrombocytopenia	Moderate	Severe
Renal failure	Common	Occasionally
Diarrhea and colitis	Common	Rare
Multiorgan involvement	Unusual	Common
Recurrence	Rare	Common
Mortality	Low	High

portive therapy may be required. The prognosis in adults is less favorable, and additional therapy is usually necessary. Plasma exchange is the most effective modality, with a good response in up to 90% of cases. It has a greater efficacy compared with fresh plasma infusion. Therefore, plasma exchange should be initiated as soon as the diagnosis is made. In patients with TTP, plasma exchange daily for 1 week, then on alternate days until remission is achieved, is recommended as initial therapy. Vincristine is of value in patients who do not respond to plasma exchange. Corticosteroids are usually given in combination with other therapies, and it is difficult to evaluate their efficacy. Splenectomy is reserved for patients with TTP resistant to therapy.

Antiphospholipid Syndrome and the Kidney

Patients with the antiphospholipid syndrome may develop venous or arterial thrombosis, thrombocytopenia, and recurrent fetal loss. This disorder may be associated with systemic disorders such as systemic lupus erythematosus or other autoimmune diseases, certain infections, and drugs, or it may occur alone as a primary disease. It is associated with a false-positive result of a Venereal Disease Research Laboratory (VDRL) test, lupus anticoagulants, or anticardiolipin antibodies. Patients on dialysis or renal transplant patients have an increased risk of thrombosis. Renal involvement is associated with vascular occlusive disease affecting renal blood vessels, ranging from the main renal artery to glomerular capillaries. The findings of glomerular microthrombi similar to those seen in HUS have been seen.

Some patients have mild proteinuria with normal renal function, whereas others develop acute or rapidly progressive renal failure associated with proteinuria and an active urinary sediment. Large renal artery thrombosis with renal infarction may be associated with flank pain, hematuria, and worsening renal function. Renal vein thrombosis may be silent and asymptomatic or acute and associated with flank pain and acute renal dysfunction.

Antiphospholipid antibodies may occur in patients treated with hemodialysis or after renal transplantation. Increased incidence of thrombotic events has been reported in hemodialysis patients. Treatment with warfarin can be successful in reducing the incidence of clotting of an arteriovenous graft. Antiphospholipid antibodies are associated with an increased incidence of renal allograft thrombosis and loss. Treatment with anticoagulants may prevent recurrence of thrombosis and loss of the renal allograft. Treatment of antiphospholipid syndrome is the same independent of the presence of renal involvement. A patient with thrombotic microangiopathy or thrombosis of a small or larger artery requires anticoagulation to prevent vascular injury. High-intensity anticoagulation with warfarin (international normalized ratio > 3) markedly reduces the incidence of new thrombotic events in these patients. Immunosuppressive agents are not successful in the treatment of this syndrome.

Renal Vein Thrombosis

The incidence of renal vein thrombosis may be as high as 30% in patients with nephrotic syndrome, especially those with membranous nephropathy. However, renal vein thrombosis can also occur in association with other hypercoagulable states, volume depletion and hemoconcentration, extrinsic compression, renal cell carcinoma, sickle cell disease, papillary necrosis, and sepsis (Table 29–4). In nephrotic syndrome, antithrombin III levels are decreased and protein C and S levels may be altered and contribute to the hypercoagulable state.

Patients with acute renal vein thrombosis present with nausea, vomiting, flank pain, microscopic or gross hematuria, and marked elevation of plasma lactate dehydrogenase level. A rise in serum creatinine value and increased renal size may also be noted. These patients benefit from thrombolytic therapy followed by anticoagulation. Patients with chronic renal vein thrombosis, however, may have nonspecific findings such as worsening proteinuria or evidence of renal tubular dysfunction.

The gold standard for the diagnosis of renal vein

TABLE 29-4   Conditions That Predispose to Renal Vein Thrombosis

Hypercoagulable States
Nephrotic syndrome
Oral contraceptives and pregnancy
Protein S or C deficiency
Antiphospholipid syndrome
Systemic lupus erythematosus

Extracellular Fluid Depletion
Extrinsic Compression of the Renal Vein
Lymph node enlargement
Tumors
Retroperitoneal fibrosis
Aortic aneurysm

Other Disorders
Renal cell carcinoma
Trauma or surgery
Sickle cell disease
Renal papillary necrosis

thrombosis is selective renal venography. Recently, computed tomography, magnetic resonance angiography, and ultrasonography have been found to be useful noninvasive screening tools, but they are less reliable than renal venography.

Treatment of established renal vein thrombosis consists of anticoagulation with heparin and then long-term anticoagulation with warfarin. Therapy usually continues for 1 year, or indefinitely in the case of recurrence or persistence of risk factors. Thrombolytic therapy is considered in patients with acute renal vein thrombosis accompanied by acute renal failure. Rarely, surgical thrombectomy may be required in patients who fail to respond to anticoagulant therapy.

REFERENCES

DuBose TD: Vascular disorders of the kidney. *In* Goldman L, Bennett JC (eds): Cecil Textbook of Medicine, 21st ed. Philadelphia: WB Saunders, 2000, pp 617–620.
Freedman BI, Iskandar SS, Appel RG: The link between hypertension and nephrosclerosis. Am J Kidney Dis 1995; 25:207.
Greco BA, Breyer JA: Atherosclerotic ischemic renal disease. Am J Kidney Dis 1997; 29:167.

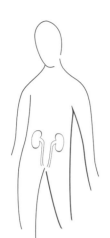

30

ACUTE RENAL FAILURE

Sudhir V. Shah

Definition and Etiology

Acute renal failure (ARF) is a syndrome that can be broadly defined as an abrupt decrease in renal function sufficient to result in retention of nitrogenous waste (blood urea nitrogen [BUN] and creatinine) in the body. ARF can result from a decrease of renal blood flow (*prerenal azotemia*), intrinsic renal parenchymal diseases (*renal azotemia*), or obstruction of urine flow (*postrenal azotemia*) (Fig. 30–1).

The most common intrinsic renal disease that leads to ARF is an entity referred to as *acute tubular necrosis* (ATN), which is a clinical syndrome characterized by an abrupt and sustained decline in glomerular filtration rate occurring within minutes to days in response to an acute ischemic or nephrotoxic insult. The clinical recognition of ATN is largely predicated on exclusion of prerenal and postrenal causes of sudden azotemia, followed by exclusion of other causes of intrinsic ARF (glomerulonephritis, acute interstitial nephritis, vasculitis). One must exclude carefully the other defined renal syndromes before concluding that ATN is present. Although the name *acute tubular necrosis* is not an entirely valid histologic description of this syndrome, the term is ingrained in clinical medicine and is therefore used in this chapter.

Differential Diagnosis and Diagnostic Evaluation of the Patient

ACUTE AZOTEMIA DURING HOSPITALIZATION

Despite the exhaustive list of conditions that can cause acute azotemia in hospitalized patients, a careful history and physical examination and simple laboratory tests often suffice for diagnosis. In hospitalized adults, prerenal azotemia is the single most common cause of acute azotemia, and ATN is the most common intrinsic renal disease that leads to ARF. Thus, the most important differential diagnosis is between prerenal azotemia (e.g., volume depletion) and ATN (secondary to ischemia or nephrotoxins). In the elderly male patient, bladder outlet obstruction must also be excluded. In addition, depending on the clinical setting, other diagnoses to be considered are acute interstitial nephritis (secondary to antibiotics), atheromatous emboli (from prior aortic surgery and/or aortogram), ureteral obstruction (pelvic or colon surgery), or intrarenal obstruction (acute uric acid nephropathy).

CHART REVIEW, HISTORY, AND PHYSICAL EXAMINATION

Determination of the cause of ARF depends on a systematic approach, as depicted in Table 30–1. The difficulty in arriving at a correct diagnosis in a hospitalized patient is not the failure to identify a possible cause of the ARF; the problem is often just the opposite, in that several causes of ARF may be possible. The correct diagnosis depends on careful analysis of available data concerning the patient with ARF and on examination of the sequence of deterioration in renal function in relation to chronology of the potential causes of ARF. The correct diagnosis also requires a knowledge of the natural history of the different causes of ARF. Some of the important data that should be sought from the patient's chart review are presented in Table 30–2.

Reduced body weight, postural changes in blood pressure and pulse, and decreased jugular venous pulse all suggest a reduction in extracellular fluid volume. Prerenal azotemia may also develop in states in which extracellular fluids are expanded (cardiac failure, cirrhosis, nephrotic syndrome) but the "effective" blood volume is decreased. Careful abdominal examination may show a distended, tender bladder that indicates lower urinary tract obstruction. When lower urinary tract obstruction is suspected as a cause of acute azotemia, examination of the prostate and a sterile "in-and-out" diagnostic postvoid bladder catheterization should be performed as a part of the physical examination. The urine volume

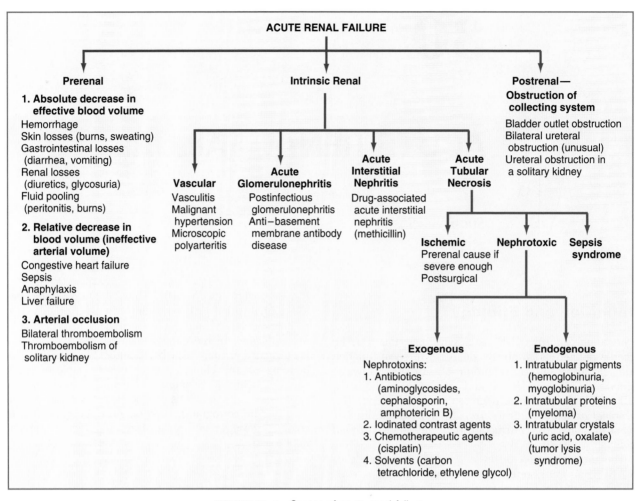

FIGURE 30–1 Causes of acute renal failure.

should be recorded and a specimen saved for studies described later.

Additional findings that may be helpful are the occurrence of fever and rash in some patients with acute interstitial nephritis. A history of recent aortic catheterization and the finding of livedo reticularis are diagnostic clues for cholesterol or atheromatous emboli.

TABLE 30–1   Diagnostic Approach to Acute Renal Failure

1. Record review (see Table 30–2); special attention to evidence of recent reduction in GFR and sequence of events leading to deterioration of renal function to determine possible causative factors
2. Physical examination, including evaluation of hemodynamic status
3. Urinalysis, including careful sediment examination
4. Determination of urinary indices
5. Bladder catheterization
6. Fluid diuretic challenge
7. Radiologic studies, particular procedure dictated by clinical setting, e.g., ultrasonography to look for obstruction
8. Renal biopsy

GFR = glomerular filtration rate.

Differentiating prerenal azotemia from ATN may be difficult, partly because evaluation of volume status in a critically ill patient is not easy, and any cause of prerenal azotemia, if severe enough, may lead to ATN. Evaluation of the urine volume and urine sediment and of certain urinary indices is particularly helpful in making the correct diagnosis.

URINE VOLUME

The urine volume is often less than 400 mL/day in oliguric ATN. Normal urine output does not exclude the diagnosis of ATN because many patients with ATN have urine outputs as high as 1.5 to 2.0 L/day. This nonoliguric ATN is frequently associated with nephrotoxic antibiotic-induced ARF. On the other hand, anuria (no urine output) should suggest a diagnosis other than ATN, the most important being obstruction. Widely varying daily urine outputs also suggest obstruction.

URINE SEDIMENT

In prerenal failure, a moderate number of hyaline and finely granular casts may be seen, but coarsely granular and cellular casts are infrequent. In ATN, the sediment

TABLE 30-2   **Record Review in a Hospitalized Patient Who Develops Acute Renal Failure**

Record Finding	Comments
Prior renal function	Determination whether the azotemia is acute; patients with prior renal insufficiency particularly susceptible to ARF, secondary to contrast dyes
Presence of infection	Sepsis a possible cause of ARF, even in the absence of hypotension
Nephrotoxic agents	Aminoglycosides (e.g., gentamicin) important cause of ATN in hospitalized patients, typically nonoliguric ATN during first 2 wks of therapy; antibiotics possible cause of acute interstitial nephritis; cytotoxic drugs (e.g., cisplatin) possible cause of ARF
Contrast studies including oral cholecystography, intravenous pyelography, angiography	Important cause of ATN in hospitalized patients; typically causes oliguric ATN within 24–48 hr after study
Episodes of hypotension	Suggestion of prerenal azotemia or ischemic ATN
History of blood transfusions	Incompatible blood transfusion an unusual cause of ATN
Review of chart for history of loss or sequestration of extracellular fluid volume, intake-output, and serial weights	Important clues to the possibility of prerenal azotemia
Type of surgery	Patients who have had cardiac or vascular surgery or with obstructive jaundice particularly susceptible to ATN
Type of anesthesia	Methoxyflurane and the related less toxic enflurane causes of nonoliguric ATN
Amount of blood loss during surgery and whether associated with hypotension	Suggestion of prerenal azotemia or ischemic ATN

ARF = acute renal failure; ATN = acute tubular necrosis.

is usually quite characteristic: "dirty" brown granular casts and renal tubular epithelial cells, free and in casts, are the most striking elements and are present in 70 to 80% of patients with ATN. A benign sediment containing few formed elements should alert the physician to the possibility that obstruction is present. In ARF associated with intratubular oxalate (e.g., methoxyflurane anesthesia) or uric acid deposition (associated with acute hyperuricemia after chemotherapy of neoplastic disease), the sediment contains abundant oxalate or uric acid crystals.

"URINARY INDICES"

An important series of diagnostic tests relates to an assessment of renal tubular function. The most widely used and convenient tests are measurements of sodium and creatinine simultaneously obtained from plasma and urine serum samples to calculate the fractional excretion of sodium. The rationale for the use of these indices is as follows: the ratio of urine to plasma creatinine (U/P_{Cr}) provides an index of the fraction of filtered water excreted. If one assumes that all the creatinine filtered at the glomerulus is excreted into the urine and that relatively little is added by secretion (an oversimplification but an acceptable one), then any increment in the concentration of creatinine in urine over that in plasma must result from the removal of water.

In prerenal azotemia, owing to the reduction in the amount of glomerular filtrate entering each nephron and to an added stimulus to salt and water retention, U/P_{Cr} typically is considerably greater than it is in ATN, and urinary sodium concentrations characteristically are low (Table 30–3). In contrast, in the ATN variety of ARF,

the nephrons excrete a large fraction of their filtered sodium and water, and the results are a lower U/P_{Cr} and a higher fractional excretion of sodium. Interpretations of these tests, however, must be made in conjunction with other assessments of the patient because clinically important exceptions to these generalizations exist. For example, certain types of ATN, such as radiographic dye–induced renal injury, may manifest with all the clinical characteristics of ATN but with a fractional excretion of sodium of less than 1%.

INDICATIONS FOR OTHER DIAGNOSTIC TESTS AND RENAL BIOPSY

If the diagnosis of prerenal azotemia or ATN is reasonably certain and the clinical setting does not require the

TABLE 30-3   **Urinary Diagnostic Indices**

Index	Prerenal Azotemia	Acute Tubular Necrosis
Urine sodium (U_{Na})(mEq/L)	<20	>40
Urine creatinine (U_{Cr})(mg/dL)/ P_{Cr} mg/dL	>40	<20
Urine osmolarity (U_{OSM})(mOsm/kg H_2O)	>500	<350
Renal failure index (RFI) RFI = $U_{Na}U_{Cr}/P_{Cr}$	<1	>1
Fractional excretion of filtered sodium (FeNa) FeNa = $U_{Na}P_{Cr}/P_{Na}U_{Cr}$ (100)	<1	>1

P_{Cr} = plasma creatinine; P_{Na} = plasma sodium.

exclusion of other causes of acute azotemia, generally no further diagnostic evaluation is necessary. Further diagnostic evaluation is indicated in the following situations: (1) when the diagnosis is uncertain, especially if the clinical setting suggests other possibilities (obstruction, vascular accident); (2) when clinical findings make the diagnosis of prerenal azotemia or ATN unlikely (anuria); and/or (3) when oliguria persists beyond 4 weeks.

Sonography provides a noninvasive method of determining the presence or absence of dilatation of the collecting system. It is, therefore, an important and safe screening test to rule out obstruction. Radionuclide methods are available to assess renal blood flow and excretory (secretory) function. Blood flow studies can easily discriminate between the presence and absence of renal blood flow and the symmetry of flow to the two kidneys, but these studies are less accurate in quantitating absolute rates of flow. Renal biopsy is rarely required for ARF occurring in the hospital setting, in contrast to ARF occurring outside the hospital, for which renal biopsy is often indicated.

APPROACH TO THE PATIENT WITH RENAL FAILURE

Azotemia first discovered outside the hospital may be either chronic or acute in origin. Useful points in deciding whether renal failure is acute or chronic are summarized in Table 30–4. Most patients who have advanced azotemia have chronic renal failure. Before a detailed evaluation is carried out, one should give priority to identifying complications of renal failure that may be lethal unless they are treated promptly. Some of these complications, such as marked fluid overload and pericardial tamponade, may be detected on clinical examination. However, life-threatening complications such as severe hyperkalemia or extreme metabolic acidosis require laboratory evaluation.

Even before the nature of the underlying disease causing azotemia is known, a decision to initiate dialysis has to be made. Dialysis should be instituted promptly in patients with severe hyperkalemia, acidosis, marked fluid overload, or uremic manifestations. Many uremic manifestations are nonspecific. However, a pericardial rub and neurologic manifestations such as asterixis are indications for prompt dialysis.

LABORATORY EVALUATION

In hospitalized adults in whom the diagnoses of prerenal and postrenal azotemia have been excluded, ARF is usually caused by ATN. By contrast, in an outpatient setting in which prerenal and postrenal causes have been excluded, ARF is more often caused by other renal parenchymal diseases. Examination of the urine for blood and protein and of the urine sediment can give valuable information that often helps to narrow considerably the diagnostic possibilities and to suggest further appropriate laboratory evaluation.

The presence of 3+ to 4+ protein, 2+ to 3+ blood, and an active sediment with red blood cells (RBCs) and RBC casts is characteristic of proliferative glomerulonephritis. A history of an underlying disease such as systemic lupus erythematosus, complement levels, antinuclear factor, and kidney biopsy (if the kidney size is normal) generally helps to clarify the diagnosis.

The presence of only a few RBCs in the urine sediment with a strongly heme-positive urine or a heme-positive supernatant (with the RBCs removed by centrifugation) most commonly results from myoglobinuria or hemoglobinuria. Patients with rhabdomyolysis have a marked increase in the muscle enzymes such as creatinine phosphokinase. The urine sediment in patients with myoglobinuria may show RBCs, pigmented casts, granular casts, and numerous uric acid crystals.

Kidney size gives important clues about whether the renal failure is acute or chronic and whether obstruction is present. Renal ultrasonography is the initial procedure of choice because it is noninvasive and reliable. The finding of normal-sized kidneys in a patient with advanced azotemia generally suggests that the patient has acute rather than chronic renal failure; however, several important causes of chronic renal failure, including diabetes mellitus, multiple myeloma, and amyloidosis, may be associated with normal-sized kidneys. The renal ultrasound examination is also helpful in (1) making a diagnosis of polycystic kidney disease; (2) determining whether one or two kidneys are present; and (3) localizing the kidney for renal biopsy.

Normal kidney size in a patient with renal failure is often an indication for renal biopsy. Before a renal biopsy is carried out, the patient's blood pressure must be controlled, bleeding and coagulation parameters must be checked, and the presence of two kidneys must be confirmed.

TABLE 30–4   Useful Features That Suggest Acute or Chronic Renal Failure

Feature	Acute Renal Failure	Chronic Renal Failure
Previous history	Normal renal function	Prior history of elevated blood urea nitrogen or creatinine
Kidney size	Normal	Small, with exception of multiple myeloma, diabetes, amyloid, polycystic kidney disease
Bone film	No evidence of renal osteodystrophy	Possible evidence of renal osteodystrophy
Hemoglobin/hematocrit	Anemia possible, but normal hemoglobin level in a patient with advanced azotemia presumptive evidence of acute renal failure	Anemia common

Clinical Presentation, Complications, and Management of Acute Tubular Necrosis

ARF results in signs and symptoms that reflect loss of the regulatory, excretory, and endocrine functions of the kidney. The loss of excretory ability of the kidney is expressed by a rise in the plasma concentration of specific substances normally excreted by the kidney. The most widely monitored indices are the concentrations of BUN and creatinine in the serum. In patients without other complications, the BUN rises by about 10 to 20 mg/dL/day, and the bicarbonate level falls to a steady-state level of 17 to 18 mEq/L. The serum potassium level need not rise appreciably, except in the presence of a hypercatabolic state, gastrointestinal bleeding, or extensive tissue trauma.

Because ATN is inherently a catabolic disorder, patients with ATN generally lose about 0.5 lb per day. Further weight loss can be minimized by providing adequate calories (1800 to 2500 kcal) and about 40 g of protein per day. The use of hyperalimentation with 50% dextrose and essential amino acids has had little effect on minimizing mortality and morbidity in patients with ATN, except in patients who also have significant burns.

Hyperkalemia is a life-threatening complication of ARF and often necessitates urgent intervention. The electromechanical effects of hyperkalemia on the heart are potentiated by hypocalcemia, acidosis, and hyponatremia. Thus, the electrocardiogram, which measures the summation of these effects, is a better guide to therapy than a single potassium determination. The cardiac effects of hyperkalemia are primarily referable to blunting of the magnitude of the action potential in response to a depolarizing stimulus. The sequential electrocardiographic changes observed in hyperkalemia are peaked T waves, prolongation of the PR interval, widening of the QRS complex, and a sine wave pattern, and these changes are mandatory indications for prompt treatment. The most common biochemical abnormality responsible for death in patients with ATN is hyperkalemia.

Moderate acidosis is generally well tolerated and does not need treatment unless it is used as an adjunct to controlling hyperkalemia or when plasma bicarbonate levels fall to less than 15 mEq/L. Hyperkalemia and acidosis not easily controlled by medical therapy are indications for initiating dialysis.

In most patients, hypocalcemia is asymptomatic and does not require treatment. Phosphate-binding gels may be used in patients with significant hyperphosphatemia. Anemia regularly develops in patients with ATN and does not require treatment unless it is symptomatic or contributes to heart failure.

In a well-managed patient (with use of early dialysis), many of the uremic manifestations outlined in Table 30–5 either do not develop or are minimal. However, infection remains the main cause of death despite vigorous dialysis. Thus, meticulous aseptic care of intravenous catheters and wounds and avoidance of the use of indwelling urinary catheters are important in the management of such patients.

The indications for initiating dialysis are severe hyperkalemia and/or acidosis not easily controlled by medical treatment or fluid overload. In the absence of any of the foregoing conditions, most nephrologists advocate dialysis when the BUN reaches about 100 mg/dL because the goal of modern therapy is to avoid the occur-

TABLE 30–5   Major Complications of Acute Renal Failure

Impairment of fluid and electrolyte excretion	
Water	Hyponatremia
Sodium chloride	Volume expansion
	Congestive heart failure
Potassium	Hyperkalemia
	Arrhythmias
Hydrogen	Acidosis
Phosphate	Hyperphosphatemia
	Hypocalcemia
	Metastatic calcifications
Magnesium	Hypermagnesemia
Uric acid	Hyperuricemia
Retention of urea and other solutes	Uremia
	Cardiac: pericarditis
	Neurologic: asterixis, confusion, somnolence, coma, seizures
	Hematologic: anemia, coagulopathy, bleeding diathesis
	Infection
	Gastrointestinal: nausea, vomiting, gastritis, bleeding
	Skin: pruritus
	Glucose intolerance
Synthetic impairment	
1,25-Dihydroxyvitamin D_3	Hypocalcemia
Erythropoietin	Anemia
Impaired drug metabolism and excretion	Drug toxicity, decreased diuretic effectiveness

rence of uremic symptoms. Therefore, the patient is dialyzed as frequently as necessary to keep the BUN at <100 mg/dL. When this approach is used, most patients do not develop uremic symptoms, the diet and fluid intake can be liberalized, and the overall management of the patient is easier. Finally, the clinician must review carefully the indications for and the doses of all drugs administered to patients with ATN. Monitoring of blood concentrations of drugs is an important adjunct to effective treatment.

OUTCOME AND PROGNOSIS

The oliguric phase of ATN typically lasts for 1 to 2 weeks and is followed by the diuretic phase. About one fourth to one third of the deaths occur in the diuretic phase. This finding is not surprising because with the availability of dialysis, the most important determinant of the outcome is not the uremia itself but rather the underlying disease that causes the ATN.

As noted previously, infection continues to be the most important cause of death in patients with ATN. In modern acute care hospitals, the outcome of patients who develop ATN is highly variable, and, depending on the nature of the underlying disease, mortality rates may be in excess of 50%. In patients who survive the acute episode, renal function returns essentially to normal, with the only residual findings being a modest reduction in glomerular filtration rate and an inability to concentrate and acidify urine maximally.

PREVENTION

The first principle of good management is prophylaxis. This requires recognition of the clinical settings in which ATN normally occurs (e.g., in patients undergoing cardiac or aortic surgery) and recognition of patients particularly susceptible to ATN. Useful measures include correcting fluid deficiencies before surgical procedures and keeping patients who are particularly at risk adequately hydrated before radiocontrast studies. Nephrotoxic drugs should be used only when essential and then only with careful monitoring of the patient. Finally, pretreatment with allopurinol before chemotherapy of massive tumors diminishes uric acid excretion.

PATHOGENESIS OF ACUTE TUBULAR NECROSIS

Although an initial decrease in renal blood flow appears to be a requisite for the development of ischemic ATN, blood flow returns nearly to normal within 24 to 48 hours after the initial insult. Despite adequate renal blood flow, tubular dysfunction persists, and the glomerular filtration rate remains depressed. Leakage of glomerular ultrafiltrate from the tubular lumen into the renal interstitium across the damaged renal tubular cells, obstruction to flow resulting from debris or crystals in the lumen of the tubules, and a decrease in the glomerular capillary ultrafiltration coefficient (K_f) have

all been proposed to play a pathophysiologic role in sustaining the clinical picture of ATN.

Various biochemical changes have been implicated in cell injury in ARF. These changes include mitochondrial dysfunction, ATP depletion, phospholipid degradation, elevation in cytosolic free calcium, decrease in Na^+,K^+-ATPase activity, alterations in substrate metabolism, lysosomal changes, and the production of oxygen free radicals. Which changes are causative and which may simply be by-products of advanced cell injury are not yet clear.

Despite the common use of the term *acute tubular necrosis*, necrosis of the tubules is seen infrequently in either ischemic or nephrotoxic ARF. In addition, although two kinds of cell death, *apoptosis* and *necrosis*, are recognized, one of the major advances in our understanding of cell death has been the recognition that the pathways traditionally associated with apoptosis may be critical in the form of cell injury associated with necrosis. Thus, evidence indicates that apoptotic mechanisms, including endonuclease activation, are important in renal tubular injury and that certain mediators (oxidants, caspases, and ceramide) regulate this process. The pathway that is followed by the cell depends on both the nature and the severity of insults. Integral to the path that is followed is thought to be the expression of many genes involved in cell cycle regulation as well as a group of genes that are proinflammatory and chemotactic. The cascades that lead to the apoptotic or necrotic mode of cell death probably are activated almost simultaneously and may share some common pathways.

Specific Causes of Acute Renal Failure

EXOGENOUS NEPHROTOXINS

Radiographic Contrast Agents

Radiocontrast-induced ARF is one of the most common causes of nephrotoxic ARF. Nonionic agents do not appear to be any less nephrotoxic than ionic ones. The most important risk factor is preexisting renal insufficiency, although dehydration and concomitant exposure to other nephrotoxins are also important. High-risk patients should be kept well hydrated by administration of half-normal saline (0.45%) at the rate of 1 mL/kg/hour for 8 to 12 hours before and after the procedure.

Aminoglycosides

The most important manifestation of aminoglycoside (tobramycin, gentamicin, amikacin) nephrotoxicity is ARF, which occurs in about 10% of patients receiving these drugs. Maintaining blood levels in the therapeutic range reduces but does not eliminate the risk of nephrotoxicity. ARF is usually mild and nonoliguric and is manifested by a rise in the serum creatinine level after about a week of therapy with one of the aminoglycosides. The prognosis for recovery of renal function after several days is excellent, although some patients may need dialysis support before recovery.

Nonsteroidal Anti-Inflammatory Drugs

Nonsteroidal anti-inflammatory drugs (NSAIDs) have several acute renal effects. NSAIDs are potent inhibitors of prostaglandin synthesis, a property that contributes to their nephrotoxic potential in certain high-risk patients in whom renal vasodilatation depends on prostaglandins. The most frequent pattern of injury related to NSAIDs is prerenal azotemia, particularly in patients who either are volume contracted or have a reduced effective circulating volume. Susceptible persons include those with congestive heart failure, cirrhosis, chronic renal disease, and volume depletion. Hyperchloremic metabolic acidosis, often associated with hyperkalemia, has also been recognized as an effect of the NSAIDs, particularly in persons with preexisting chronic interstitial renal disease. Hyporeninemic hypoaldosteronism occurs in these persons in states of renal prostaglandin inhibition. Finally, NSAIDs have been associated with the development of acute interstitial nephritis, often associated with renal insufficiency and nephrotic-range proteinuria. This complication appears to be an idiosyncratic reaction to propionic acid derivatives such as ibuprofen, naproxen, and fenprofen. In contrast to acute interstitial nephritis associated with other drugs, the incidence of hypersensitivity symptoms and eosinophilia is low. Discontinuation of the offending agent usually results in resolution of this disorder.

Cisplatin

Renal injury is a well-recognized and dose-dependent complication of cisplatin use in the management of many carcinomas. Hypomagnesemia resulting from renal losses of magnesium may be severe and can occur in as many as 50% of patients. Patients should be well hydrated before they receive cisplatin, and known nephrotoxins should be avoided whenever possible. The usual lesion is that of ATN, but with severe damage or recurrent administration of the drug, chronic interstitial disease may ensue.

Ethylene Glycol Toxicity

Ingestion of ethylene glycol, usually in the form of antifreeze, produces a characteristic syndrome of a severe anion gap metabolic acidosis and a large osmolal gap. ARF generally manifests after 48 to 72 hours. Patients are disoriented and agitated initially, and they progress to central nervous system depression, stupor, and coma. Cardiovascular collapse and death then follow.

Angiotensin-Converting Enzyme Inhibitors

ARF associated with angiotensin-converting enzyme inhibitors is thought to be hemodynamic in origin from loss of autoregulation of renal blood flow and glomerular filtration rate and has been typically reported when these drugs are given to patients with bilateral renal artery stenosis or with moderately advanced azotemia. Allergic acute interstitial nephritis similar to that observed with antibiotic administration has also been reported.

ENDOGENOUS NEPHROTOXINS

Rhabdomyolysis

Since the first description of the causative association between rhabdomyolysis and ARF in persons with crush injuries during World War II, the spectrum of causes of rhabdomyolysis, myoglobinuria, and renal failure has broadened. The most frequent causes are (in order) alcoholism, muscle compression, seizures, metabolic derangements, drugs, and infections. Muscle pain and dark brown orthotoluidine-positive urine without RBCs are important diagnostic clues, but the diagnosis must be confirmed by elevations of creatine phosphokinase and myoglobin. About one third of patients with rhabdomyolysis develop ARF, frequently associated with hyperkalemia, hyperuricemia, hyperphosphatemia, early hypocalcemia, and a reduced ratio of BUN to creatinine because of excessive creatinine release from muscle. Late hypercalcemia is also a typical feature of the disease.

Hyperuricemic Acute Renal Failure

ARF may occur in patients with "high turnover" malignant diseases (acute lymphoblastic leukemia and poorly differentiated lymphomas) who either spontaneously or, more frequently, after cytotoxic therapy release massive amounts of purine uric acid precursors. This process leads to uric acid precipitation in the renal tubules. During massive cell lysis, phosphate and potassium are also released in large amounts, with resulting hyperphosphatemia and hyperkalemia. The peak uric acid level is often >20 mg/dL, and a ratio of urinary uric acid to creatinine concentrations greater than 1:1 suggests the diagnosis of acute uric acid nephropathy. Prevention of ARF includes establishing a urinary output of 3 L or more per 24 hours and treatment with allopurinol before cytotoxic therapy is instituted.

Hepatorenal Syndrome

The *hepatorenal syndrome* is defined as kidney failure in patients with severely compromised liver function in the absence of clinical, laboratory, or anatomic evidence of other known causes of renal failure. It closely resembles prerenal failure, except it does not respond to conventional volume replacement. In the United States and Europe, most cases of hepatorenal syndrome occur in patients with advanced alcoholic cirrhosis. Hepatorenal syndrome may begin insidiously over a period of weeks to months, or it may appear suddenly and may cause severe azotemia within days. The common precipitating causes are deterioration of liver function, sepsis, use of nephrotoxic antibiotics or NSAIDs, overzealous use of diuretics, diarrhea, and gastrointestinal bleeding. The disorder can, however, occur without any apparent precipitating cause. The hallmark of hepatorenal syndrome is oliguria with urine osmolality two to three times the concentration of plasma, as well as urine that is virtually sodium free, similar to that of patients with prerenal azotemia.

The initial step in management is to search diligently for and to treat correctable causes of azotemia. An important step in the management of these patients is to exclude reversible prerenal azotemia. Because hepatorenal syndrome and prerenal azotemia have similar urinary diagnostic indices, one must often use a functional maneuver, such as the administration of volume expanders, to differentiate between these two entities. Once a diagnosis of hepatorenal syndrome is established, no specific treatment exists, and management is conservative. The prognosis is poor.

Acute Renal Failure Related to Pregnancy

ARF of pregnancy, a rare disorder in industrialized nations, occurs in fewer than 1 in 10,000 deliveries. In the first trimester, septic abortion accounts for the majority of patients with ARF. Although many organisms have been implicated, *Clostridium welchii,* which produces a toxin causing hemolysis and renal failure, accounts for a disproportionate number of cases. In late pregnancy, renal insufficiency manifested by a mild increase in serum creatinine, which returns to normal after delivery, is often a feature of preeclampsia. ATN is an uncommon complication of preeclampsia and occurs in about 1% to 2% of cases; however, it does occur in a larger percentage, in approximately 5% of patients with hemolysis, elevated liver enzymes, and low platelets (HELLP syndrome). Abruptio placentae can also cause ATN, but it is also the most common cause of renal cortical necrosis.

Postpartum ARF, also known as *postpartum hemolytic uremic syndrome,* is characterized by hypertension and microangiopathic hemolytic anemia, and it occurs anywhere from 1 to 2 days to several months after delivery, most commonly 2 to 5 weeks post partum. Glomerular lesions resemble those found in adult hemolytic uremic syndrome, with fibrin deposition, thickened capillary walls, and subendothelial swelling with large granular subendothelial deposits. Overall, prognosis is poor, with a chance of recovery of renal function in only a minority of patients.

REFERENCES

Chapman AB, Schrier RW: Acute renal failure in pregnancy. *In* Jacobson HR, Striker GE, Klahr S (eds): The Principles and Practice of Nephrology, 2nd ed. St. Louis: Mosby–Year Book, 1995, pp 445–453.

Lazarus JM, Brenner BM: Acute Renal Failure, 3rd ed. New York: Churchill Livingstone, 1993.

Safirstein R: Pathophysiology of acute renal failure. *In* Greenberg A (ed): Primer on Kidney Diseases, 2nd ed. San Diego: Academic Press, 1998, pp 247–253.

Shah SV: Acute renal failure. *In* Jacobson HR, Striker GE, Klahr S (eds): The Principles and Practice of Nephrology, 2nd ed. St. Louis: Mosby–Year Book, 1995, pp 544–594.

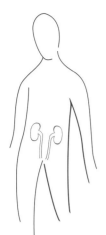

31

CHRONIC RENAL FAILURE

Mary Jo Shaver

Chronic renal failure is defined as progressive and irreversible loss of renal function. The most common causes of renal insufficiency ultimately leading to end-stage renal disease (ESRD) are listed in Table 31–1. Loss of 75% of glomerular filtration rate (GFR) does not usually result in pronounced symptoms because the remaining glomeruli adapt with hyperfiltration, and the surviving tubules adjust by maintaining adequate acid-base, fluid, and electrolyte balance. For example, the doubling of serum creatinine from 0.7 to 1.4 mg/dL signifies a loss of approximately 50% of the GFR and emphasizes the importance of early recognition and intervention at this stage. Serum creatinine, creatinine clearance, and the reciprocal of the serum creatinine plotted against time are commonly used for diagnosing and monitoring renal dysfunction. These techniques are limited in their accuracy and may be affected by drugs or other illnesses, but are the only practical and cost-effective means of monitoring patients with chronic renal insufficiency.

When patients have an elevated serum creatinine, acute renal failure must be differentiated from chronic renal failure, as discussed in Chapter 30. Every attempt should be made to arrive at the specific cause of chronic renal failure. One of the most important pieces of data is prior laboratory measurements of the serum creatinine concentration. Renal biopsy is the most specific tool to reach a definitive diagnosis. This allows treatment of the underlying cause, assessment of the prognosis, and determination of suitability for kidney transplantation. If the biopsy is not performed because of small kidney size, diagnosis is made based on present, past, and family history, serologic evaluation, examination of the urine sediment, and ultrasound evaluation. Although most chronic kidney diseases are associated with a progressive decrease in kidney size, a few systemic diseases are characterized by normal kidney size despite advanced renal failure. These diseases include diabetes mellitus, multiple myeloma, polycystic kidney disease, nephropathy related to acquired immunodeficiency syndrome, and amyloidosis.

Adaptation to Nephron Loss

To ensure adequate solute, water, and acid-base balance, the surviving nephrons in the diseased kidney must adjust by increasing their filtration and excretion rates. Without such adjustments, patients with chronic renal failure are vulnerable to edema formation and severe volume overload, hyperkalemia, hyponatremia, and azotemia. Thus, during progressive renal disease, sodium balance is maintained by increasing fractional excretion of sodium by the nephrons. Acid excretion is usually maintained until the late stages of chronic renal failure, when the GFR falls to less than 15 mL/min. Initially, increased tubular ammonia synthesis provides an adequate buffer for hydrogen in the distal nephron. Later, a significant decrease in distal bicarbonate regeneration results in hyperchloremic metabolic acidosis. Further loss of nephronal mass leads to retention of organic ions such as sulfates and results in anion gap metabolic acidosis and titration of bone bicarbonate stores.

Once renal insufficiency is established, the tendency is for renal disease to progress regardless of the initial insult. Glomerular sclerosis ensues, most likely the result of glomerular hyperfiltration and/or hypertension. Compensatory glomerular hypertrophy is invariably associated with tubular hypertrophy in the remaining nephrons. Tubular hypertrophy is associated with increased energy expenditure, a metabolic event related to generation of reactive oxygen metabolites. Reactive oxygen metabolites have been proposed as a mechanism of tubulointerstitial damage in animal models. In addition, hyperlipidemia is believed to play a role in progressive renal insufficiency through mesangial proliferation and sclerosis.

Although this adaptive mechanism can be beneficial in maintaining fluid, electrolyte, and acid-base balance, the long-term consequence is perpetuation of tubulointerstitial damage. Interventions that reduce intraglomerular pressure such as protein restriction and the use of

TABLE 31–1 Percentage of Distribution of Incidence of End-Stage Renal Disease by Primary Diagnosis, 1992–1996

Primary Cause	Incidence (%)
Diabetes	39.2
Hypertension/large-vessel disease	28.2
Glomerulonephritis	11.0
Cystic/hereditary/congenital disease	3.5
Interstitial nephritis/pyelonephritis	4.4
Obstruction	2.0
Miscellaneous and origin uncertain	9.0

angiotensin-converting enzyme inhibitors have been shown to help attenuate progression of renal disease. Figure 31–1 illustrates different pathways through which these maladaptive mechanisms can result in progression of renal insufficiency and, ultimately, ESRD.

Conservative Management

Conservative management of chronic renal failure should include (1) measures to slow progression, (2) identification of potentially reversible causes of renal failure when unexpected declines in renal function occur, (3) identification and treatment of complications of chronic renal failure, and (4) preparation of patients emotionally for the problems associated with ESRD.

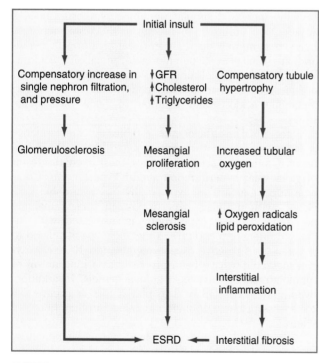

FIGURE 31–1 Factors responsible for the progression of renal disease. ESRD = end-stage renal disease; GFR = glomerular filtration rate.

MANAGEMENT OF HYPERTENSION

Several controlled trials have conclusively confirmed that aggressive management of hypertension attenuates the rate of progression of renal failure. Significant benefit has been shown in patients with diabetic nephropathy, as well as in patients with other chronic renal diseases. In addition, studies demonstrate the nephroprotective effect of angiotensin-converting enzyme inhibitors above and beyond control of hypertension alone in patients with nephropathy and type 1 diabetes mellitus. In addition, the use of nondihydropyridine calcium channel blockers (verapamil, diltiazem) may be beneficial by blocking the deleterious effect of angiotensin II on the progression of renal insufficiency. Thus, it may be helpful to combine angiotensin-converting enzyme inhibitors and calcium channel blockers in patients who require more than one drug for control of hypertension.

DIET

In the past, dietary protein restriction was advocated to reduce uremic symptoms. More recently, animal and human studies have shown that dietary protein restriction tends to slow the rate of progression of renal insufficiency. Although the evidence from human studies is less certain, strong evidence of the beneficial effect of dietary protein restriction has been provided by several animal studies. The National Study of Dietary Modification in Renal Disease suggests a beneficial effect of protein restriction to 0.6 g/kg/day in patients with a GFR of less than 25 mL/min/1.73 m². At present, advising aggressive dietary management in patients with renal insufficiency, with proper restriction of sodium, potassium, phosphorus, and protein intake, seems prudent. Sodium should be restricted, especially in hypertensive and edematous patients. Malnutrition at the initiation of dialysis is a strong predictor of increased mortality. Therefore, a protein-restricted diet must be approached with great surveillance and caution, and all efforts must be made to deliver adequate calories of more than 35 kcal/kg/day.

The most common dyslipidemia in chronic renal failure is hypertriglyceridemia, which occurs in 30% to 70% of patients. Hypercholesterolemia occurs in only 20% of patients who do not have nephrosis. The treatment of choice in patients in whom dietary management fails or in those at high risk or with known cardiovascular disease is hydroxymethylglutaryl–coenzyme A reductase inhibitors.

MANAGEMENT OF REVERSIBLE CAUSES OF ACUTE DETERIORATION IN RENAL FUNCTION

The rate of decline in GFR for individual patients is log linear. Accordingly, plotting 1 over the serum creatinine against time usually predicts the rate at which a specific patient will reach ESRD, as shown in Figure 31–2. When such a patient suddenly shows acceleration of renal failure, the differential diagnosis for such acceleration should be considered, as presented in Table 31–2.

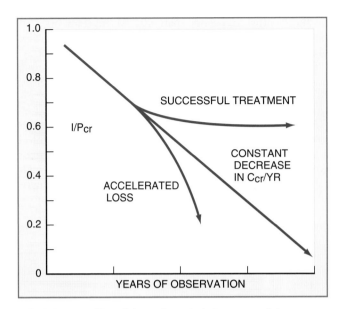

FIGURE 31–2   Use of the reciprocal of plasma creatinine concentration, $1/P_{cr}$, to follow the progress of glomerular disease in a patient. (From Sullivan LP, Grantham JJ: Physiology of the Kidney, 2nd ed. Philadelphia: Lea & Febiger, 1982.)

Patients with chronic renal impairment are more susceptible to factors leading to acute renal failure, and these entities should be investigated aggressively.

AVOIDING TOXIC DRUG EFFECTS

Many drugs that are excreted by the kidney should be avoided or adjusted in patients with renal insufficiency, as shown in Table 31–3. In hospitalized patients, aminoglycosides are one of the most common offenders. Patients with chronic renal insufficiency are at increased risk, and dose adjustments should be made based on the GFR. By inhibiting vasodilatory prostaglandins, nonsteroidal anti-inflammatory drugs can decrease GFR as well as cause acute interstitial nephritis and acute renal failure. Radiocontrast agents are another common cause of acute or acute on chronic renal failure in hospitalized patients. Risk factors for contrast induced acute renal failure include volume depletion and preexisting renal insufficiency. Patients at high risk of contrast-induced acute renal failure should receive intravenous fluid hydration with 5% dextrose in normal saline 8 to 10 hours before and after the procedure.

Clinical Manifestations

GENERAL FEATURES OF THE UREMIC SYNDROME

Patients with renal insufficiency usually become symptomatic when the GFR is less than 10 mL/min. Patients with diabetes and renal insufficiency usually have symptoms at lesser degrees of renal impairment. *Uremia* is a syndrome that affects every organ system. The uremic

TABLE 31–2   **Reversible Causes of Acute Deterioration in Renal Function**

Decreased renal perfusion
  Intravascular volume depletion
  Heart failure
  Third spacing
Obstruction
Infection
  Urinary tract infection
  Sepsis
Nephrotoxins
  Endogenous: myoglobulin, hemoglobin, uric acid, calcium, phosphorus
  Exogenous: contrast media, drugs
Poorly controlled hypertension: malignant or accelerated hypertension

syndrome is likely the consequence of a combination of factors including retained molecules, deficiencies of important hormones, and metabolic factors, rather than the effect of a single uremic toxin (Fig. 31–3). Urea, in addition to being the most commonly used measure of renal failure and adequacy of dialysis, can cause symptoms of fatigue, nausea, vomiting, and headaches. Its breakdown product (cyanate) can result in carbamylation of lipoproteins and peptides, with adverse effects leading to multiple organ dysfunctions.

Guanidines, by-products of exogenous or endogenous protein metabolism, are increased in renal failure. They can inhibit α_1-hydroxylase activity within the kidney and can lead to deficient calcitriol production and secondary hyperparathyroidism. High parathyroid hormone levels have been implicated in various manifestations of ure-

TABLE 31–3   **Drug Dosage in Chronic Renal Failure**

Major Dosage Reduction	Minor or No Reduction	Avoid Usage
Antibiotics		
Aminoglycosides	Erythromycin	NSAIDs
Penicillin	Nafcillin	Nitrofurantoin
Cephalosporins	Clindamycin	Nalidixic acid
Sulfonamides	Chloramphenicol	Tetracycline
Vancomycin	Isoniazid/rifampin	
Quinolones	Amphotericin B	
Fluconazole	Aztreonam/tazo-	
Acyclovir/ganci-	bactam	
clovir	Doxycycline	
Foscarnet		
Imipenem		
Others		
Digoxin	Antihypertensives	Aspirin
Procainamide	Benzodiazepines	Sulfonylureas
H_2 antagonists	Quinidine	Lithium carbonate
Meperidine	Lidocaine	Acetazolamide
Codeine	Spironolactone	
Propoxyphene	Triamterene	

NSAIDs = nonsteroidal anti-inflammatory drugs.

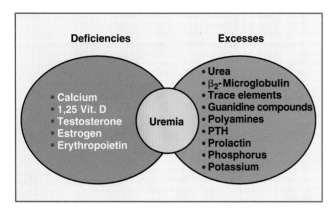

FIGURE 31–3   Etiologic factors of uremia. PTH = parathyroid hormone.

mia, especially in cardiomyopathy and metastatic calcifications. β_2-Microglobulin accumulation in patients with renal failure has been associated with neuropathy, carpal tunnel syndrome, and amyloid infiltration of the joints.

SPECIFIC MANIFESTATIONS OF UREMIA

Major manifestations of uremia are shown in Figure 31–4.

Cardiovascular Effects

Mortality from cardiovascular disease in renal failure patients is three and a half times that of an age-matched population. Heart disease accounts for more than 50%

of the deaths in uremic patients. More than 60% of patients who start undergoing dialysis have echocardiographic manifestations of left ventricular hypertrophy, dilation, and systolic or diastolic dysfunction. Anemia and hypertension, commonly seen in patients before they begin dialysis, contribute to left ventricular hypertrophy and congestive heart failure. Secondary hyperparathyroidism can lead to metastatic calcification in the myocardium, cardiac valves, and arteries. Accelerated atherogenesis is responsible for the high prevalence of coronary artery disease in this population and the high rate of recurrent coronary artery stenosis after angioplasty. Pericarditis can occur in uremic patients before they start dialysis and in patients who are already undergoing dialysis. Initiation of dialysis or intensifying dialytic therapy usually results in resolution of pericarditis in patients who are receiving inadequate dialysis. Pericarditis occurring in the setting of adequate dialysis may not respond to a further increase in dialysis therapy and may require surgical drainage or the use of nonsteroidal anti-inflammatory agents.

Gastrointestinal Disease

Gastrointestinal disturbances are among the earliest and most common signs of the uremic syndrome. Patients with renal failure usually describe a metallic taste and loss of appetite. Later, they experience anorexia, nausea, vomiting, and weight loss, which improve after dialysis is initiated. Several pathologic processes can lead to gastrointestinal bleeding. Among these, gastritis, peptic ulceration, and arteriovenous malformations are the most common.

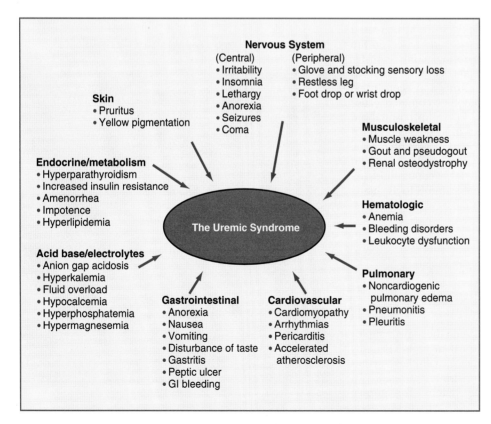

FIGURE 31–4   Diagrammatic summary of the major manifestations of the uremic syndrome. GI = gastrointestinal.

Neurologic Manifestations

Central nervous system manifestations are frequent and occur early, often with subtle changes in cognitive function, memory, and disturbances in sleep. Lethargy, irritability, frank encephalopathy, asterixis, and seizures are late manifestations of uremia and are usually avoided by early initiation of dialysis. Peripheral neurologic manifestations appear as symmetric sensory neuropathy in a glove-and-stocking distribution. Peripheral motor impairment can result in restless legs and foot or wrist drop. Clinically, these patients have decreased distal tendon reflexes and loss of vibratory perception. After the initiation of dialysis, they exhibit amelioration of impaired mentation, generalized weakness, and peripheral neuropathy.

Musculoskeletal Manifestations

Alterations in calcium and phosphate homeostasis and renal osteodystrophy are common manifestations of ESRD. Hyperparathyroidism and disturbance of vitamin D metabolism are commonly found. Hypocalcemia and secondary hyperparathyroidism are the result of phosphate retention and the lack of α_1-hydroxylase activity in the failing kidney, with consequent deficiency of the most active form of vitamin D. Over time, the adaptive parathyroid hypertrophy becomes maladaptive and leads to bone disease and tissue calcinosis. Calcium and phosphate homeostasis in the setting of renal failure is demonstrated in Figure 31–5. Control of hyperparathyroidism with phosphate binders, calcium supplementation, and 1,25(OH)$_2$-vitamin D, together with dialysis therapy, is now achievable. This aggressive management approach has resulted in a significant reduction in renal osteodystrophy in patients who are undergoing dialysis.

Hematologic Effects

Erythropoietin, a hormone produced by the kidney that regulates the production of erythrocytes by the bone marrow, becomes progressively deficient as renal mass declines. This is one of the most common causes of anemia in chronic renal failure, after iron deficiency. Routine administration of erythropoietin to patients with ESRD results in correction of anemia, improved quality of life, and decreased dependence on blood transfusions. Bleeding disorders, primarily from defects in platelet adherence and aggregation, are common in patients with uremia. Uremic bleeding can be generally controlled with cryoprecipitate, 1-deamino-(8-D-arginine)-vasopressin, conjugated estrogens, and dialysis.

Endocrine Abnormalities

Alterations in thyroid function testing may contribute to the difficulty of diagnosing thyroid disease in the uremic patient. Common laboratory findings may include an increased triiodothyronine resin uptake, a low triiodothyronine level resulting from the impaired conversion of thyroxine to triiodothyronine peripherally, and normal thyroxine levels. Thyroid-stimulating hormone levels are usually normal. On occasion, the use of a thyrotropin-

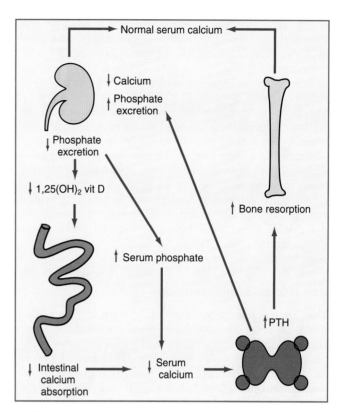

FIGURE 31–5   Calcium and phosphate homeostasis in the setting of renal failure. The decreased excretion of phosphate initiates the cycle directed at normalization of the serum calcium concentration. PTH = parathyroid hormone.

releasing hormone stimulation test may be needed for diagnosis of thyroid disorders in uremia. Interestingly, goiter is present in up to one third of patients with chronic renal failure.

A deranged pituitary gonadal axis can result in sexual dysfunction manifested by impotence, decreased libido, amenorrhea, sterility, and uterine bleeding. Hyperprolactinemia may be responsible for some of these abnormalities of the pituitary gonadal axis. Patients have decreased plasma levels of testosterone, estrogen, and progesterone, with normal or increased levels of follicle-stimulating hormone and luteinizing hormones. Pregnancy is uncommon in female patients who have a GFR of <30 mL/min.

Immunologic Function

Defects occur in both humoral and cellular immune systems in patients with ESRD. These patients are generally immunosuppressed and are susceptible to bacterial, fungal, and microbacterial infections.

Metabolic Disorders

As renal function diminishes, many diabetic patients have a decrease in their insulin requirements. This change is partly a result of the increased half-life of exogenously administered insulin secondary to decreased insulin clearance. At the same time, increased peripheral insulin resistance in uremic patients has been recognized. Insulin resistance occurs secondary to tissue insensitivity to insulin, as well as metabolic acidosis and hyperparathyroidism, which impairs insulin release and secretion.

Lipid abnormalities are common findings in the early course of renal failure. They are most consistent with type IV hyperlipoproteinemia, with a marked increase in plasma triglycerides and less of an increase in total cholesterol. The activity of lipoprotein lipase is decreased in uremia with a reduction in the conversion of very-low-density lipoprotein to low-density lipoprotein and thus hypertriglyceridemia. These abnormalities of lipid metabolism are considered contributors to accelerated atherosclerosis in patients with renal failure, in addition to the role of these substances in mesangial proliferation and progressive renal failure.

Dermatologic Manifestations

The uremic hue, a yellowish skin color, is likely the result of retained liposoluble pigments, such as lipochromes and carotenoids. Pruritus is a common complaint of patients with renal failure. It usually responds to dialysis, control of hyperparathyroidism, improved calcium and phosphate balance, and, occasionally, ultraviolet rays. Calciphylaxis is rare in patients with well-managed renal failure. It results from painful skin calcification in patients with a serum calcium × phosphate product that exceeds 70 mg/dL in the presence of severe hyperparathyroidism. Nail findings include the half-and-half nail, characterized by red, pink, or brownish discoloration of the distal nail bed, pale nails, and splinter hemorrhages.

Treatment of End-Stage Renal Failure

A plan for a modality of renal replacement therapy should be discussed with the patient early in the course of renal failure and before the appearance of uremic symptoms. The current criteria for initiation of dialysis are GFR 15 mL/min or less for patients with diabetes and 10 mL/min or less for patients without diabetes. Creatinine clearance overestimates GFR in advanced renal failure because of tubular secretion of creatinine. A more accurate estimation of the GFR can be calculated from the average of the creatinine and urea clearances. Patients with volume overload resistant to diuretics, metabolic acidosis, pericarditis, persistent hyperkalemia, intractable gastrointestinal symptoms, or encephalopathy should be started on dialysis even though their creatinine clearance may exceed the previously set criteria. The choice of renal replacement therapy largely depends on the patient's physical and sociodemographic characteristics. Most patients are started either on hemodialysis or on peritoneal dialysis. Renal transplantation is encouraged because of a better quality of life and a greater chance for rehabilitation.

HEMODIALYSIS

By the mid-1990s, 283,932 patients had been treated for ESRD, and 73,091 new patients had been started on treatment for ESRD. Hemodialysis continues to be the most common modality of renal replacement therapy for patients in the United States, although the trend is toward the initiation of more patients on peritoneal dialysis. As illustrated in Figure 31–6, blood obtained through a temporary or permanent vascular access that ensures blood flows of 300 mL/min or more is pumped through a large number of capillaries manufactured from semisynthetic membranes. Moving in the opposite direction is a dialysate solution that contains sodium chloride, bicarbonate, and varying concentrations of potassium. Diffusion through the membrane allows low-molecular-weight substances such as urea to leave the blood and to move to the dialysate according to the concentration gradient. Similarly, bicarbonate, which is usually at a concentration of 35 mEq/L, diffuses to the plasma. Removal of excess water is achieved by ultrafiltration, which depends on the hydrostatic pressure across the membrane. The average patient undergoing hemodialysis requires 3.5 to 4.0 hours of dialysis three times a week to achieve creatinine clearance of more than 140 L/week.

PERITONEAL DIALYSIS

In this modality of renal replacement therapy, the peritoneum acts as a semipermeable membrane similar to a hemodialysis filter. This technique has several advantages because it allows independence from the long time spent in dialysis units, it does not require stringent dietary restrictions as in hemodialysis, and rehabilitation rates are better than those observed in hemodialysis, with more patients returning to full-time employment. Residual renal function is maintained for a longer period, for instance 1 to 2 years, while the patient is undergoing peritoneal dialysis, thus improving morbidity and mortality. In continuous ambulatory peritoneal dialysis, dialysate of 2.0- to 3.0-L volumes is left in the peritoneal cavity for varying amounts of time to be exchanged four to six times daily. In continuous cyclic peritoneal dialysis, the patient is connected to a machine referred to as a *cycler* that allows inflow of smaller volumes of dialysate with shorter dwell time through the night, so the patient is free of dialysis during the day. Several modifications in this regimen can be made to fit the specific patient to achieve adequate clearance. The rate of removal of various solutes depends on the concentration gradient, surface area, and permeability of the peritoneal membrane to the solute. Smaller molecules move across the peritoneal membrane with ease and are influenced by dialysate flow rates or ultrafiltration rates. Ultrafiltration is achieved through increasing dextrose concentration in the dialysate. In spite of lower weekly creatinine clearance values in patients undergoing peritoneal dialysis, residual renal function is preserved longer, and the survival of these patients matches that of patients undergoing hemodialysis.

The two major drawbacks of peritoneal dialysis are

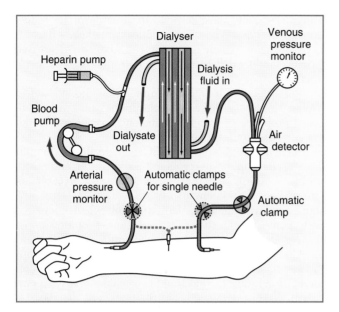

FIGURE 31–6 Essential components of a dialysis delivery system that, together with the dialyzer, make up an "artificial kidney." In isolated ultrafiltration, no dialysis fluid is used (bypass mode). Also shown is the apparatus for using a single needle for inflow and outflow of blood from the patient. (From Keshaviah PR, Shaldon S. *In* Drukker W, Parsons FM, Maher JF [eds]: Replacement of Renal Function by Dialysis, 3rd ed. Boston: Martinus Nijhoff Publishers, 1988. Reprinted by permission of Kluwer Academic Publishers.)

infection of the percutaneous catheter placed into the peritoneal cavity and difficulty in achieving adequate clearance in patients with large body mass. Peritonitis in patients undergoing peritoneal dialysis can be treated with intraperitoneal antibiotics. Catheter removal is indicated in some cases of peritonitis, for instance, bacterial peritonitis not responding to antibiotics and fungal peritonitis.

KIDNEY TRANSPLANTATION

Renal transplantation is one of several modalities for renal replacement therapy, with hemodialysis or peritoneal dialysis often required before, during, or after transplantation. Successful renal transplantation is probably the most satisfactory treatment for ESRD. When cyclosporine became available in 1983, the success rate improved significantly, with an 85% to 90% 1-year-graft survival, compared with 65% with azathioprine and steroids. A decrease in the incidence of acute rejection has been seen secondary to the introduction of newer immunosuppressive agents that include mycophenolate mofetil, tacrolimus, and daclizumab. This advance has been associated with some improvement in short-term allograft survival. The current 1-year graft survival for cadaveric renal transplantation is ≥90%.

Cadaver Versus Living Donor Kidney Transplantation

Advantages and disadvantages of cadaver versus living, related or unrelated, kidney donor transplantation are listed in Table 31–4. Living related-donor organs are involved in about 25% of all kidney transplantations. Because the cadaver donor organ supply fails to meet the demand, the pressure for living kidney donation has increased. Unrelated donors with a stable and close emotional relationship with the recipient, such as a spouse, have been considered appropriate donors in many transplant centers. Survival of grafts from these unrelated donors is better than survival of grafts from cadavers, despite less histocompatibility matching of human leukocyte antigen (HLA). Living or cadaver donation should only be performed between ABO blood group–compatible donors. A major advantage of a living donor-related transplant is histocompatibility matching. Figure 31–7 is a representation of the inheritance pattern of HLA within a family. HLA-identical matches

TABLE 31–4 **Comparison of Donor Sources for Kidney Transplantation**

Advantages	Disadvantages
Living Donor	
Better tissue match with less likelihood of rejection	Small potential risk of operation to donor
Smaller doses of drugs for immunosuppression	Requirement of willing, medically suitable family member or other person
Waiting time for transplant reduced	
Sequelae of long-term dialysis avoided	
Elective surgical procedure	
Better early graft function with shorter hospitalization	
Better short-term and long-term success	
Cadaver Donor	
Availability to any recipient	Tissue match not as similar
Availability of other organs for combined transplants (i.e., kidney-pancreas transplant)	Waiting time variable
Availability of vascular conduits for complex vascular reconstruction	Operation performed urgently
	Early graft function possibly compromised
	Short-term and long-term success not as good as from living donor

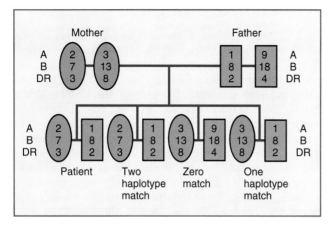

FIGURE 31-7 Diagrammatic representation of inheritance of human leukocyte antigen (HLA) tissue types in a family with four siblings.

consistently demonstrate superior graft survival and less chance for rejection than either one-haplo or cadaveric renal transplants. From 1993 to 1996, the increase in living donor-unrelated transplant donations was 46.6%, and the increase in living donor-related transplant donation was 5.4%, as compared with only a 1.6% increase in cadaveric kidney donation.

Immunosuppressant Drug Therapy

Prophylaxis against and treatment of graft rejection are at the heart of the success of kidney transplantation. Since the 1960s, the immunosuppressive protocols for renal transplantation have undergone remarkable evolution. All the protocols for immunosuppression aim at disruption of the lymphocyte cell cycle. Azathioprine and steroids, with or without antilymphocyte preparations, were the mainstay of clinical immunosuppression in the 1960s and 1970s. Since the introduction of cyclosporine in the early 1980s, the number of drugs capable of suppressing the immune system has increased steadily. These agents, by virtue of their specific mode of action, have succeeded in preventing most patients from having early and irreversible graft rejections without severe toxic effects. The mechanism of action of some of the most commonly used immunosuppressants is illustrated in Figure 31-8.

The addition of *cyclosporine* to immunosuppressive protocols in the early 1980s favorably affected graft survival, with a 20% increase in cadaveric kidney survival in the first year. The newer microemulsion preparations of cyclosporine result in more predictable levels and less dependence on bile for absorption. The hepatic cytochrome oxidase P-450 system is essential for cyclosporine metabolism, and several drugs can induce or inhibit this system and thus may cause significant changes in cyclosporine levels.

Cyclosporine exerts its specific immunosuppressive activity by inhibition of immunocompetent lymphocytes in the G_0 and G_1 phases of the cell cycle. Some of the most important side effects of cyclosporine are listed in

Table 31-5, and most respond to an appropriate reduction in the dose. The most significant of these effects is nephrotoxicity, which is usually secondary to decreased glomerular blood flow and, again, responds to dose reduction.

Tacrolimus has a mechanism of action and side effect profile similar to those of cyclosporine, but with additional problems of hyperglycemia and an increased tendency toward neurotoxicity.

Mycophenolate mofetil (CellCept) specifically inhibits T- and B-lymphocyte proliferation by interfering with purine synthesis and thus DNA synthesis. Mycophenolate mofetil has been associated with a 60% to 70% reduction in acute transplant rejection when compared with conventional therapies and thus promotes long-term graft survival. Mycophenolate mofetil is replacing azathioprine either as initial immunosuppressive therapy in combination with steroids and cyclosporine or after an acute episode of rejection. The major toxicity, occurring in 30% of patients, is gastric distress or diarrhea.

Acute Rejection

T lymphocytes survey the human body and are capable of recognizing foreign antigens when these antigens are presented in association with HLA antigens, especially class 2 histocompatibility antigens. When the recipient's T-helper cells identify foreign HLA class 2 antigens presented by dendritic or other antigen-presenting cells in the transplanted kidney, lymphocyte activation results. Activated cytotoxic lymphocytes invade the tubular interstitial region of the transplanted kidney, with resulting

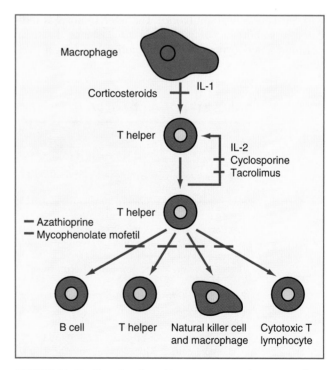

FIGURE 31-8 Site of action of immunosuppressive agents. IL = interleukin.

TABLE 31-5 **Side Effects of Commonly Used Immunosuppressive Drugs**

Effect	Corticosteroids	Azathioprine	Cyclosporine	Mycophenolate Mofetil
Renal	Fluid retention		Preglomerular vaso-constriction Striped interstitial fibrosis Hyperkalemia	
Cardiovascular	Hypertension	Hypertension		
Hematologic	Bone marrow suppression	Macrocytosis	Hemolytic uremic syndrome	Leukopenia Anemia
Neurologic	Proximal muscle weakness Mood changes Depression		Tremor Seizures	
Gastrointestinal	Gastritis	Acute pancreatitis	Cholestasis	Vomiting Diarrhea Abdominal pain
Metabolic	Glucose intolerance Dislipidemia		Dislipidemia Decreased glucose tolerance	
Dermatologic	Acne Easy bruisability	Hair loss	Hypertrichosis Brittle fingernails	
Miscellaneous	Osteoporosis Aseptic necrosis Obesity Accelerated cataract formation		Gingival hypertrophy	

tubulitis and deterioration in renal function. Clinically, acute rejection is detected by graft tenderness, rise in serum creatinine levels, oliguria, and sometimes fever. Frequent monitoring of renal function has allowed early detection of acute rejection based on rising serum creatinine before any clinical signs or symptoms become manifest. The incidence of acute rejection is highest between the second and twelfth weeks after transplantation. Severe forms of acute rejection, carrying a poor prognosis, involve the intrarenal arteries and lead to vasculitis. This type of rejection is usually resistant to steroids, thus necessitating antilymphocyte therapy. *Hyperacute rejection,* occurring in the first few hours after renal transplantation and resulting from preformed anti-

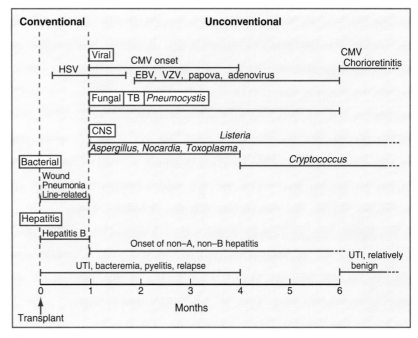

FIGURE 31-9 Timetable for the occurrence of infection in the renal transplant recipient. Exceptions to this timetable should initiate a search for an unusual hazard. CMV = cytomegalovirus; CNS = central nervous system; EBV = Epstein-Barr virus; HSV = herpes simplex virus; TB = tuberculosis; UTI = urinary tract infection; VZV = varicella-zoster virus. (From Rubin RH, Wolfson JS, Cosimi AB, et al: Infection in the renal transplant recipient. Am J Med 1981; 70:405–411. Copyright 1981 by Excerpta Medica, Inc.)

bodies to the donor kidney, may lead to loss of the allograft.

Post-Transplant Infection

Infection is second only to vascular disease as the leading cause of mortality in kidney transplant recipients. In addition to common community-acquired bacterial and viral infections, kidney transplant recipients are also susceptible to numerous viral, fungal, and other opportunistic infections, which normally do not cause severe illness in the immunocompetent host. Fortunately, the timetable of these infections is predictable, and an educated guess based on the time of infection after transplantation, together with the specific set of syndromes associated with each infection, can help early recognition and prompt treatment of these infections. Figure 31–9 shows the temporal relationship between renal transplantation and these infections.

Post-Transplant Malignant Disease

Immunosuppression increases the risk of developing malignant disease. Skin cancer has the highest incidence in transplant recipients as compared with all other types of malignancy. Sun exposure is the most significant risk factor, and skin protection provides excellent primary prevention. With continuous surveillance and aggressive management, metastasis from skin cancers is rare.

Transplant recipients are also at high risk of developing Kaposi's sarcoma and post-transplant lymphoproliferative disease, a rare occurrence in the immunocompetent host. Cancer surveillance should be an essential part of post-transplant follow-up. Transplant recipients should be educated to recognize and report early changes in bowel habits, respiratory symptoms, hematuria, musculoskeletal symptoms, skin changes, or weight changes.

REFERENCES

Dubrow A, Levin NW: Chronic renal failure. *In* Jacobson HR, Striker GE, Klahr S (eds): The Principles and Practice of Nephrology, 2nd ed. St. Louis: Mosby–Year Book, 1995, pp 596–620.

England BK, Mitch WE: Mechanisms of progression of renal insufficiency. *In* Massry SG, Glassock RJ (eds): Massry and Glassock's Textbook of Nephrology, 3rd ed, vol 2. Baltimore: Williams & Wilkins, 1995, pp 1261–1269.

Levey AS, Adler S, Caggiula AW, et al: Effects of dietary protein restriction on the progression of advanced renal disease in the modification of diet in renal disease study. Am J Kidney Dis 1996; 27: 652–663.

Rahman M, Smith MC: Chronic renal insufficiency. Arch Intern Med 1998; 158:1743–1752.

Rubin RH: Infection in the organ transplant recipient. *In* Rubin RH, Young LS (eds): Clinical Approach to Infection in the Compromised Host, 3rd ed. New York: Plenum, 1994, pp 629–705.

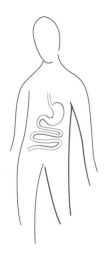

SECTION VI

Gastrointestinal Disease

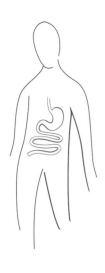

32

COMMON CLINICAL MANIFESTATIONS OF GASTROINTESTINAL DISEASE

A. Abdominal Pain

Edgar Achkar

Abdominal pain is a frequent manifestation of intra-abdominal disease. It is difficult to gauge pain origin and severity because it is subjective by nature and because it is affected by emotional as well as physical factors.

Abdominal pain may be acute or chronic. Acute pain occurs suddenly and suggests serious physiologic alterations. On the other hand, chronic pain may be present for several months and, although it does not mandate immediate attention, it may lead to lengthy investigation.

Appropriate evaluation of abdominal pain requires a knowledge of pain mechanisms, close attention to history and physical examination findings, and recognition of important accompanying symptoms.

Physiology

Abdominal pain may be classified as somatic or visceral. Somatic pain originates from the abdominal wall and parietal peritoneum, whereas visceral pain originates in internal organs and from the visceral peritoneum. Abdominal pain results from stimulation of receptors specific for thermal, mechanical, or chemical stimuli. Once these receptors are excited, pain impulses travel through sympathetic fibers. There are two types of nerve fibers that carry pain: A fibers, which have rapid conduction, and C fibers, which have slow conduction. Most visceral fibers are of the C type, and the pain resulting from their stimulation tends to be dull. In contrast, fibers originating from the parietal peritoneum and abdominal wall are of both the A and C types, and the pain tends to be sharp and more distinctly localized.

Abdominal viscera are not sensitive to cutting, tearing, burning, or crushing. However, visceral pain results from stretching of the wall of hollow organs or the capsule of solid organs as well as by inflammation or ischemia.

Causes of Abdominal Pain

Multiple intra-abdominal and extra-abdominal disorders produce abdominal pain. It is helpful to distinguish acute from chronic abdominal pain. The approach varies with each specific cause but acute abdominal pain demands quick intervention.

The major causes of abdominal pain are listed in Table 32–1.

Clinical Features

HISTORY

The differential diagnosis of abdominal pain, whether acute or chronic, requires careful history taking with regard to pain characteristics, location and radiation, timing, and the presence of any other accompanying symptoms.

TABLE 32–1 Major Causes of Abdominal Pain

Acute
Inflammation
  Appendicitis
  Cholecystitis
  Pancreatitis
  Diverticulitis
Perforation
Obstruction
Vascular causes
  Acute ischemia
  Ruptured aneurysm

Chronic
Inflammation
  Peptic ulcer
  Esophagitis
  Inflammatory bowel disease
  Chronic pancreatitis
Vascular causes
  Chronic ischemia
Metabolic causes
  Diabetes
  Porphyria
Functional causes
  Dyspepsia
  Irritable bowel syndrome
Abdominal wall pain
  Neurogenic
  Musculoskeletal
Chronic benign abdominal pain syndrome

Pain location often indicates the organ responsible for the problem. For instance, epigastric pain is usually typical of peptic ulcer or dyspepsia, whereas right upper quadrant pain is more typical of cholecystitis. However, pain may start in one location and settle in another. For instance, in acute appendicitis, it is not unusual for pain to start in the epigastrium before settling in the right lower quadrant. Similarly, pain of acute cholecystitis initially may be localized in the epigastric area.

In acute cases, abdominal pain tends to be sharp and severe. The pain of a perforated viscus is intense, and the pain from a dissecting aneurysm may be crushing. On the other hand, pain from irritable bowel or dyspepsia is constant and dull, and the pain of chronic peptic ulcer is described as gnawing or hunger pain. The pattern of pain relief is helpful for some conditions but rarely for acute cases. For instance, pain of dyspepsia may respond to antacids and the pain of irritable bowel may be relieved by defecation. However, the classic relief of pain from duodenal ulcer with food is not universal, and basing the diagnosis of peptic ulcer on history is not reliable.

The physician should also inquire about whether pain is steady or intermittent and whether it occurs at night. For nocturnal pain, a distinction should be made between pain that awakens the patient from pain that is felt when the patient wakes up for other reasons.

Table 32–2 outlines characteristics, location, and radiation of pain for a few common acute and chronic abdominal conditions.

PHYSICAL EXAMINATION

Examination of the abdomen may provide invaluable clues to the diagnosis. A patient writhing in bed and unable to find a comfortable position may be suffering from obstruction. On the other hand, a patient lying with the lower extremities flexed and avoiding any motion may be suffering from peritonitis. Abdominal distention indicates obstruction or ascites. Visual inspection for visible peristalsis is helpful for the diagnosis of small bowel obstruction, but this sign is present only in the early stages.

The abdomen should be palpated gently, starting in an area away from the area of pain. The physician looks for areas of localized tenderness and rebound but also for masses and enlarged organs. Pain upon percussion of the abdomen indicates peritoneal reaction.

A rectal examination is important for identifying a rectal tumor in the case of colon obstruction or tenderness high in the rectum in acute appendicitis. Pelvic

TABLE 32–2 Characteristics of Various Types of Abdominal Pain

Condition	Type	Location	Radiation
Acute Abdominal Pain			
Appendicitis	Crampy, steady	Periumbilical, RLQ	Back
Cholecystitis	Colicky, steady	Epigastric, RUQ	Right scapula
Pancreatitis	Steady	Epigastric, periumbilical	Back
Perforation	Sudden, severe	Epigastric	Entire abdomen
Obstruction	Crampy	Periumbilical	Back
Infarction	Severe, diffuse	Periumbilical	Entire abdomen
Chronic Abdominal Pain			
Esophagitis	Burning	Substernal	Left arm, back
Peptic ulcer	Gnawing	Epigastric	Back
Dyspepsia	Bloating, dull	Epigastric	None
IBS	Crampy	LLQ, RLQ	None

IBS = irritable bowel syndrome; LLQ = left lower quadrant; RLQ = right lower quadrant; RUQ = right upper quadrant.

examination should be performed in women to rule out pelvic inflammatory disease.

The Acute Abdomen

The acute abdomen is a challenging condition in medical practice. The first question to be answered is whether immediate surgery is needed. Therefore, a quick evaluation is necessary in order not to delay intervention in patients who need it. It is preferable to obtain early surgical consultation even in doubtful cases rather than waiting for confirmation of the diagnosis by laboratory or radiologic studies.

The acute abdomen is caused by sudden inflammation, perforation, obstruction, or infarction of various intra-abdominal organs. However, some intrathoracic conditions such as pneumonia, nephrolithiasis, and some metabolic disorders may cause acute abdominal pain.

It is possible that the acute abdomen, in its early stages, reveals very few findings. It is also important to be aware that patients with benign chronic conditions may come to the emergency department with severe pain that is in contrast with a lack of any physical findings.

The importance of a detailed history and careful physical examination has already been mentioned. With the acute abdomen, it is important to inquire about past medical history, particularly previous abdominal surgery. Indeed, a patient with sudden crampy pain and abdominal distention may have intestinal obstruction caused by adhesions. It is also important to perform an entire examination of the patient, looking for jaundice, skin lesions, or evidence of chronic liver disease.

There may be no need for extensive laboratory testing. However, a complete blood cell count with differential, a urinalysis, and measurements of serum amylase, lipase, bilirubin, and electrolytes are necessary. An elevated white blood cell count indicates inflammatory disease, and extremely high values are quite typical of acute intestinal ischemia. An elevated serum amylase concentration usually indicates acute pancreatitis, but a perforated ulcer or mesenteric thrombosis may also lead to high amylase values.

Radiographic examination is an important part of the work-up of the patient with acute abdomen. An abdominal film is important in revealing the intra-abdominal gas pattern, and an upright film that includes the diaphragm is very important in identifying intra-abdominal air. If an upright film cannot be obtained, a left lateral decubitus film may be sufficient. Examination with radiopaque medium should be used cautiously, particularly if surgery is being planned. The use of ultrasonography or biliary scintigraphy for acute cholecystitis and a computed tomographic (CT) scan for the diagnosis of abscess or diverticulitis may be indicated, but CT scan is not necessary when the diagnosis of acute pancreatitis has already been established.

Chronic Abdominal Pain

Chronic abdominal pain does not impose the urgency that acute abdominal pain does. However, the challenge

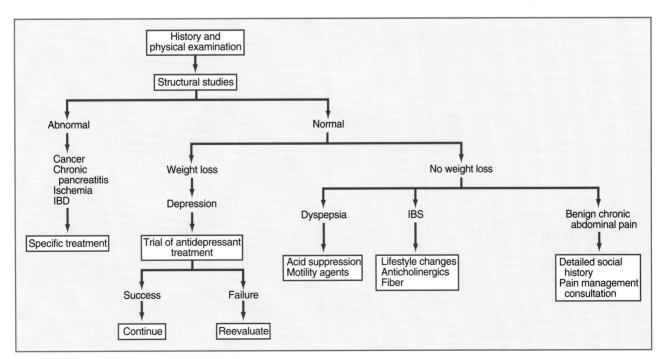

FIGURE 32-1 Approach to the patient with chronic abdominal pain. IBD = inflammatory bowel disease; IBS = irritable bowel syndrome.

for the physician is to differentiate organic pain resulting from a specific pathologic process from functional chronic pain. The location and characteristics of pain, as already discussed, serve as important guides, as do other accompanying symptoms. The presence of postprandial nausea and vomiting suggests chronic peptic ulcer, disorders of gastric emptying, or outlet obstruction. The documentation of weight loss dictates the search for an organic cause. If anorexia accompanies weight loss, cancer must be ruled out, particularly in elderly patients. If no cancer can be found and if all objective tests are normal, the possibility of a chronic depressive state must be entertained.

The most frequent causes of chronic abdominal pain are functional. The distinction between dyspepsia and irritable bowel syndrome is sometimes unclear. However, dyspepsia is characterized by chronic intermittent epigastric discomfort with or without heartburn and with or without nausea. Irritable bowel syndrome is a very common disorder. It is estimated that 15% of Americans suffer from it on a regular basis and that 40 to 50% of referrals to gastroenterologists are related to irritable bowel. The syndrome manifests itself by abdominal distention, flatulence, and disordered bowel function. The abdominal pain of irritable bowel syndrome tends to be in the left lower quadrant but can be located elsewhere or be more generalized. Weight loss and other serious symptoms are usually absent. In spite of a tendency for constipation or diarrhea, rectal bleeding is not reported. A limited work-up to rule out colonic obstruction and, in some cases, inflammatory bowel disease is generally sufficient. Patients are reassured, counseled, and treated with anticholinergic agents and bowel softeners.

The more challenging clinical problem is the one of benign chronic abdominal pain syndrome. This term describes a condition in which the pain has been present for months or years. The patient is likely to be a woman who has undergone numerous examinations and diagnostic studies with negative findings and, in many cases, surgical operations without any relief. Lengthy or repeated diagnostic work-ups are counterproductive and only convince the patient that one more test is what is needed to determine the source of the pain. The physician must establish that organic disease is not present. The physician must also realize that the pain is real: that the patients are not malingerers in spite of the fact that the pain does not fit any familiar pattern. Depression may be the result rather than the cause of the pain.

Chronic abdominal pain is a clinical situation requiring as much tact, diplomacy, and compassion as scientific knowledge. An effort should be made to inquire about social factors, including history of physical and sexual abuse, particularly in women. Psychiatric evaluation may be necessary, but the suggestion for such a consultation will be interpreted by the patient as a belief from the physician that the "pain is in my head." A referral to a competent pain management specialist is helpful in a certain number of cases. This approach offers the possibility of providing relief with nerve blocks when the pain is localized or the use of other pain-relieving devices. If this fails, referral to a psychologist or psychiatrist may be more acceptable to the patient.

For a practical approach to chronic abdominal pain, see the algorithm in Figure 32–1.

REFERENCES

Drossman DA, Leserman J, Nachman G, et al: Sexual and physical abuse in women with functional or organic gastrointestinal disorders. Ann Intern Med 1990; 113:822–828.

Grundfest-Broniatowski S: Abdominal pain. *In* Achkar E, Farmer RG, Fleshler B [eds]: Clinical Gastroenterology, 2nd ed. Philadelphia: Lea & Febiger, 1992, pp 39–46.

Yamada T: Approach to the patient with acute abdomen. *In* Yamada T [ed]: Handbook of Gastroenterology. Philadelphia: Lippincott-Raven, 1998, pp 59–67.

....

B. Gastrointestinal Hemorrhage

Gregory Zuccaro, Jr.

....

Acute Gastrointestinal Hemorrhage

PRESENTATION OF GASTROINTESTINAL BLEEDING

Patients generally present with overt evidence of acute gastrointestinal (GI) blood loss, including lightheadedness, postural changes in blood pressure or pulse or both, and anemia. The characteristics of this bleeding may help localize the source of bleeding to the upper or lower GI tract. Acute bleeding may present as one of the following:

Hematemesis. It is extremely likely that the patient presenting with vomiting of bright red blood or of material that looks like coffee grounds has a source of bleeding proximal to the ligament of Treitz.

Melena. Black, tarry, usually foul-smelling stools are most often a manifestation of upper GI bleeding; however, a small bowel or proximal colonic source of bleeding may on occasion lead to melanic stools.

Hematochezia. Passage of red blood or maroon stools per rectum frequently indicates a lower GI source of bleeding. However, in cases of rapid upper GI bleeding, especially from a duodenal ulcer, patients may present with hematochezia rather than melena.

ETIOLOGY OF GASTROINTESTINAL BLEEDING

Common sources of acute gastrointestinal hemorrhage are listed in Table 32–3. The astute clinician always considers the most likely diagnosis as the evaluation is planned. For example, there would be some similarities and some important differences in the evaluation of hematochezia in a 20-year-old patient in comparison with an 80-year-old patient. In both patients, the possibility of upper GI bleeding must be considered.

However, once it is established that bleeding originates from the lower GI tract, a colonic source may be sought in the 80-year-old patient (the bleeding source is most likely a diverticulum, angioectasia, or cancer),

whereas a small bowel source might be sought in the 20-year-old (Meckel's diverticulum is most likely).

APPROACH TO THE PATIENT WITH ACUTE GASTROINTESTINAL BLEEDING (Fig. 32–2)

Assessment of Vital Signs/Resuscitation

This is the first priority in the evaluation and therapy for the patient with acute GI hemorrhage. Vital signs with postural changes should be recorded immediately. If the systolic blood pressure drops more than 10 mm Hg and/or the pulse increases more than 10 beats per minute as the patient changes positions from supine to standing, it is likely the patient has lost at least 800 mL (15%) of circulating blood volume. Hypotension, tachycardia, tachypnea, and mental status changes in the setting of acute GI hemorrhage suggest at least a 1500-mL (30%) loss of circulating blood volume.

The goal of resuscitation is to restore the normal circulatory volume. Initially, large-bore intravenous catheters are used to administer isotonic solutions (lactated

TABLE 32–3   Common Sources of Acute Gastrointestinal Hemorrhage

Source	Associated Clinical Factors	Treatment
Upper Gastrointestinal Tract		
Esophagitis	Heartburn, regurgitation, dysphagia	Medication,* antireflux surgery
Esophageal cancer	Progressive dysphagia, weight loss	Chemoradiotherapy, surgery
Gastritis/gastric or duodenal ulcer	Use of aspirin/NSAIDs	Withdrawal agent
	Abdominal pain/dyspepsia	Medication†
	Nausea/vomiting	Endoscopic therapy to arrest bleeding
	Helicobacter pylori infection	
Esophageal varices	History of CLD	Variceal banding, TIPS, or decompressive surgery
	Stigmata of CLD on physical examination	
Mallory-Weiss tear	History of vomiting before hematemesis	None (usually self-limited)
Lower Gastrointestinal Tract		
Diverticulum	Painless hematochezia	Supportive (usually self-limited)
Angioectasia	Painless hematochezia	Endoscopic therapy
	Often in ascending colon	Surgery if extensive
	?Association with aortic valvular disease	
Colon cancer	Change in bowel habits/weight loss	Surgery
Ischemic colitis	Typically elderly patients	Supportive (usually self-limited)
	May have other vascular disease	
	May present with abdominal pain	
Meckel's diverticulum	Young patient with painless hematochezia	Surgery
	Located 60 cm proximal to ileocecal valve	
Hemorrhoids	Not typically associated with hemodynamic instability	Surgery

* Proton pump inhibitors or histamine-2 antagonists.
† Proton pump inhibitors or histamine-2 antagonists in the absence of *H. pylori* infection; various combinations of antibiotics, proton pump inhibitors, and bismuth products in the presence of *H. pylori* infection.
CLD = chronic liver disease; NSAIDs = nonsteroidal anti-inflammatory drugs; TIPS = transjugular intrahepatic shunt.

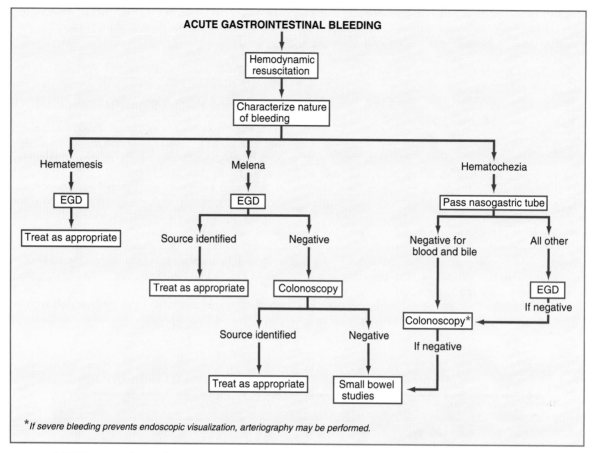

FIGURE 32-2 Approach to the patient with acute gastrointestinal bleeding. EGD = esophagogastroduodenoscopy; GI = gastrointestinal; NG = nasogastric.

Ringer's solution, 0.9% NaCl). The amount of blood products to be transfused must be individualized. Transfusions of packed red blood cells are provided to prevent complications (e.g., angina, congestive heart failure, stroke) of acute blood loss. Therefore, the need for blood transfusion depends on the multiple factors, including the patient's age, overall health, and response of vital signs to initial resuscitation. In view of the risks of blood transfusion, it is not appropriate to simply transfuse until an arbitrary hemoglobin/hematocrit level is reached.

Initial Evaluation

As the patient is resuscitated, the clinician must ascertain certain key historical points:

1. The nature of bleeding: melena, hematemesis, hematochezia.
2. The duration of GI bleeding (because this helps dictate the necessary pace of the evaluation to determine the bleeding source).
3. The presence or absence of abdominal pain; for example, hematochezia caused by bleeding diverticula or angioectasia is typically painless, but when caused by ischemia, it may be accompanied by abdominal pain.
4. Other associated symptoms, including fever, urgency/tenesmus, recent change in bowel habits, weight loss.
5. Current/recent medication use, particularly nonsteroidal anti-inflammatory drugs (NSAIDs) or aspirin (which may predispose to ulcer disease or bleeding gastritis), anticoagulants, and alcohol use.
6. Medication allergies.
7. Relevant past medical and surgical history, including history of prior bleeding, prior abdominal surgery, history of radiation therapy, and history of major organ disease (including cardiopulmonary, hepatic, or renal disease).
8. Angina, dyspnea, postural symptoms, or palpitations since the onset of bleeding episode.

The physical examination must include assessment of vital signs, cardiac and pulmonary examination, abdominal examination, and digital rectal examination. The initial laboratory examination should include complete blood cell count and measurements of serum electrolytes, blood urea nitrogen, and creatinine.

The initial disposition of the patient must also be considered. Patients over the age of 60, those with severe blood loss, and those with significant comorbid illness are at the greatest risk of complications of GI hemorrhage and are best managed in an intensive care setting until stabilized.

Identification of the Bleeding Source

In the majority of cases, acute GI hemorrhage resolves spontaneously. Nevertheless, it is prudent to localize the bleeding source, because proper identification allows for direct treatment in cases in which bleeding does not spontaneously resolve and allows for identification of the patient at risk for further bleeding. For example, in the patient with a bleeding duodenal ulcer, there are various stigmata of hemorrhage that may be identified within the ulcer crater during endoscopy. These include active bleeding, a pigmented protuberance (artery visible within the ulcer crater), and clot over the ulcer. The patient with a "clean base," in which there are no such stigmata, has an excellent prognosis for cessation of bleeding. The patient with an actively bleeding ulcer or visible artery without active bleeding is extremely likely (>50% chance) to have continued bleeding. Plans for disposition and length of hospital stay may be based in part on these endoscopic findings. Furthermore, the site of bleeding may be injected with vasoconstrictors or sclerosants or may be cauterized at the time of endoscopy, all of which decrease the need for transfusion, the need for surgery, and length of hospital stay.

An approach to the patient with acute GI bleeding is outlined in Figure 32–2. Historical points and objective findings often enable localization of the bleeding site to the upper GI tract (proximal to the ligament of Treitz) or to the lower GI tract (distal to that point). For the patient with melena or hematemesis, the upper GI tract should be examined first. Patients with hematochezia more commonly have lower GI bleeding, but when the pace of bleeding is brisk, an upper GI tract lesion may manifest with hematochezia. Placement of a nasogastric tube with aspiration of contents is a reasonable first step. The absence of blood does not by itself rule out the presence of an upper GI source, because blood from a duodenal bulb ulcer may not flow back into the stomach and allow for sampling by the nasogastric tube. Only when copious bile, and no blood, is aspirated should the clinician conclude that the source of bleeding is from the lower GI tract. In any other nasogastric finding, an upper endoscopy should be the initial step in the evaluation. Once the lower GI tract has been identified as the source of bleeding, sigmoidoscopy or colonoscopy is the test of choice. In cases of lower GI bleeding in which the pace of bleeding is so brisk as to preclude endoscopic visualization of the colon and rectum, visceral arteriography may be performed. There is no role for barium studies in the evaluation of acute GI hemorrhage.

Chronic Gastrointestinal Hemorrhage

This condition may manifest as self-limited, recurrent episodes of melena or hematochezia, usually not with the degree of hemodynamic compromise discussed earlier. Patients may also have no overt evidence of blood loss, but rather may have persistent anemia and stools consistently positive for occult blood.

The evaluation of this condition differs from that of acute GI hemorrhage. Obviously, the pace of the evaluation is less urgent. Furthermore, the likely causes for this bleeding differ from those of acute GI bleeding. Patients with this condition usually have undergone upper endoscopy and colonoscopy at least once, with no source of chronic bleeding identified. Therefore, the bleeding either must have an upper GI tract or colonic source that is difficult to identify and was overlooked at the previous examination or emanates from the small intestine. The small intestine is a difficult area to examine in this regard because of its length and configuration. In general, the small intestine is evaluated radiographically. The patient may ingest barium, which is followed through the length of the small intestine. To distend the small bowel and give greater mucosal detail, an enteroclysis tube may be placed with its distal tip near the ligament of Treitz, allowing more forceful administration of barium and air. Endoscopic evaluation may be attempted with instruments with long insertion tubes (enteroscopy), but in general, this examination is limited to the proximal to mid-jejunum. For the patient with persistent blood loss, no source of bleeding in the upper GI tract or colon as determined by endoscopy, and negative findings on radiologic studies, the entire small intestine may be examined at laparotomy with endoscopy in the operative suite.

REFERENCES

Kollef MH, Canfield DA, Zuckerman GA: Triage considerations for patients with acute gastrointestinal hemorrhage admitted to a medical intensive care unit. Crit Care Med 1995; 23:1048–1054.

Luk GD, Bynum TE, Hendrix TR: Gastric aspiration in localization of gastrointestinal hemorrhage. JAMA 1979; 241:576–578.

Rossini FP, Ferrari A, Spandre M, et al: Emergency colonoscopy. World J Surg 1989; 13:190–192.

Zuccaro G: Bleeding peptic ulcer: Pathogenesis and endoscopic therapy. Gastrointest Endosc Clin North Am 1993; 22(4):747–750.

Zuccaro G: Management of the adult patient with acute lower gastrointestinal bleeding. Am J Gastroenterol 1998; 93:1202–1208.

C. Malabsorption

Edy E. Soffer

The main purpose of the GI tract is to digest and absorb major nutrients (fat, carbohydrates, and protein), essential micronutrients (vitamins and trace elements), water, and electrolytes. Digestion involves both mechanical and biochemical breakdown of the food. The former is achieved by mastication and gastric trituration, and the latter is achieved by a complex enzymatic process that depends on gastric, pancreatic, and biliary secretions and is completed by enzymes located at the brush border of enterocytes. The final products are then absorbed through the intestinal brush border. Controlled release of food from the stomach, normal progression through the intestine, and adequate intestinal surface area are important factors.

Most food components can be absorbed throughout the length of the small intestine, but some can be absorbed only at specific segments (e.g., vitamin B_{12} and bile acids can be absorbed only in the terminal ileum). The primary absorptive function of the colon is the salvage of water and electrolytes. This section discusses normal assimilation of major nutrients and the approach to patients with maldigestion or malabsorption.

Digestion and Absorption of Fat

Dietary fat is composed predominantly of triglycerides with long-chain fatty acids (16- and 18-carbon–length chain). In animal fat, fatty acids are mostly saturated (i.e., have only single bonds in the carbon chain), whereas those of vegetable origin are mostly polyunsaturated (i.e., have more than one double bond in the carbon chain). Because fats are insoluble in water, their digestion requires a number of phases. In the gastric and intestinal lumen, fat is first physically released and broken down into emulsion particles (i.e., fat globules dispersed in the aqueous phase). Bile salts and pancreatic colipase on the surface of these particles result in release of fatty acids, leaving a 2-monoglyceride. The formation of mixed micelles with bile salts allows these hydrophobic lipolytic products to cross the unstirred water layer that overlies the cellular epithelium. Once within the cell, most of these products are resynthesized into triglycerides and, together with cholesterol and phospholipids, are packaged into chylomicrons and very-low-density lipoproteins (VLDL) and exported into the lymphatic channels. Bile salts remain in the lumen, are recycled into new micelles, and are finally reabsorbed in the terminal ileum. Most dietary lipids are absorbed in the jejunum, together with fat-soluble vitamins (A, D, E, K).

Digestion and Absorption of Carbohydrates

The bulk of dietary carbohydrates consists of starch, a glucose polymer, and the disaccharides sucrose and lactose, but only monosaccharides can be absorbed. Salivary and pancreatic amylases release oligosaccharides from starch, and final hydrolysis to glucose monomers takes place at the brush border. The disaccharides are hydrolyzed at the brush border by sucrase and lactase. Glucose and galactose are actively transported in conjunction with sodium, whereas fructose absorption occurs by facilitated diffusion.

Digestion and Absorption of Proteins

Dietary proteins are the major source for amino acids. Digestion starts in the stomach by pepsins secreted by the gastric mucosa, but most of the hydrolysis is accomplished by pancreatic enzymes in the proximal small bowel. Pancreatic proteases, trypsin, elastase, chymotrypsin, and carboxypeptidase are secreted by the pancreas as inactive proenzymes. Enterokinase, secreted from intestinal brush border by bile acids, converts trypsinogen to its active form, trypsin. Trypsin in turn converts the other proenzymes to their active forms. The products of luminal digestion consist of amino acids and short peptides. Both amino acids and dipeptides or tripeptides, the results of brush border digestion by peptidases, can be transferred across the intestinal cell membranes. The transfer of most amino acids is sodium dependent. Most of the absorption process takes place in the proximal small bowel.

Mechanisms of Malabsorption

The term *maldigestion* refers to defective hydrolysis of nutrients, whereas *malabsorption* refers to impaired mucosal absorption. In clinical practice, however, *malabsorption* refers to all aspects of impaired assimilation of nutrients. Malabsorption can involve multiple nutrients or be more selective. As a consequence, the clinical manifestations are highly variable.

The full process of absorption consists of a *luminal phase,* in which various nutrients are hydrolyzed and solubilized; a *mucosal phase,* in which further breakdown takes place at the cell membrane, followed by transfer into the cell; and finally a *transport phase,* in which nutrients are removed to the vascular or lymphatic circulation. Impairment of one or more of these phases can result in malabsorption (Table 32–4).

LUMINAL PHASE

Digestion is accomplished for the most part by pancreatic enzymes, particularly lipase, colipase, and trypsin. As a consequence, chronic pancreatitis can result in malabsorption, particularly that of fat and protein. Deficiency in bile salts can lead to fat malabsorption and can be the result of cholestatic liver states that impair the secretion of bile into the lumen, bacterial overgrowth that causes bile salt deconjugation, or ileal disease or resection that impairs reabsorption.

MUCOSAL PHASE

Mucosal impairment is the more common cause of malabsorption. It can occur because of diffuse small intestinal disease, such as that seen in celiac sprue or Crohn's disease, or a decreased amount of otherwise normal surface area after surgical resection or small bowel infarction. Selective defects in an otherwise normal intestine results in specific entities such as lactase deficiency, abetalipoproteinemia, or cystinuria.

TRANSPORT PHASE

After absorption, nutrients leave the cells through the vascular or lymphatic circulation. Consequently, mesenteric vascular disease, primary lymphangiectasia, or lymphatic obstruction secondary to infiltrative diseases can result in malabsorption.

Multiple Mechanisms

Certain disorders can impair the absorptive process at various stages. Patients with subtotal gastrectomy can have a modest degree of malabsorption. This is caused by impaired mixing of food with bile and pancreatic enzymes as a result of anatomic changes and impaired gastric emptying. Because food bypasses the duodenum, release of secretin and cholecystokinin is decreased, and bacterial overgrowth may occur in the blind loop. Likewise, in diabetes mellitus, abnormal gastric and intestinal motility and bacterial overgrowth may be compounded by pancreatic exocrine insufficiency.

Clinical Manifestations of Malabsorption

The clinical manifestations of malabsorption are usually nonspecific. Bloating, fatigue, a change in bowel habits,

TABLE 32-4   Pathophysiologic Mechanisms in Malabsorption

Luminal Phase	Mucosal Phase	Transport Phase
Reduced Nutrient Availability	Extensive mucosal loss (resection or infarction)	Vascular conditions (vasculitis; atheroma)
Cofactor deficiency (pernicious anemia; gastric surgery)	Diffuse mucosal disease (celiac sprue; Crohn's disease; irradiation; infection; infiltrations; drugs: alcohol, colchicin, neomycin, iron salts)	Lymphatic conditions (lymphangiectasia; irradiation; nodal tumor, cavitation, or infiltrations)
Nutrient consumption (bacterial overgrowth)	Brush border hydrolase deficiency (lactase deficiency)	
Impaired Fat Solubilization	Transport defects (Hartnup's cystinuria; vitamin B_{12} and folate uptake)	
Reduced bile salt synthesis (hepatocellular disease)	Epithelial processing ($\alpha\beta$-lipoproteinemia)	
Impaired bile salt secretion (chronic cholestasis)		
Bile salt inactivation (bacterial overgrowth)		
Impaired CCK release (mucosal disease)		
Increased bile salt losses (terminal ileal disease or resection)		
Defective Nutrient Hydrolysis		
Lipase inactivation (ZE syndrome)		
Enzyme deficiency (pancreatic insufficiency or cancer)		
Improper mixing or rapid transit (resection; bypass; hyperthyroidism)		

Adapted from Riley SA, Marsh MN: Maldigestion and malabsorption. *In* Feldman M, Scharschmidt BF, Sleisenger MH (eds): Sleisenger and Fordtran's Gastrointestinal and Liver Disease: Pathophysiology/Diagnosis/Management, 6th ed. Philadelphia: WB Saunders, 1998, pp 1501–1522.
CCK = cholecystokinin; ZE = Zollinger-Ellison.

and some weight loss may occur in the early course of the syndrome. At later stages, symptoms and signs related to nutrient deficiency are observed. Wasting may be accompanied by edema, which results from protein malabsorption. Anemia, resulting from iron and vitamin deficiency, contributes to fatigue. Bleeding tendencies such as ecchymoses result from vitamin K deficiency. Bulky, oily stool, the hallmark of steatorrhea, is the result of fat malabsorption, whereas abdominal distention and watery diarrhea are the result of carbohydrate malabsorption, specifically that of disaccharidases.

Signs associated with malabsorption are presented in Table 32–5.

Tests for Malabsorption

Blood tests for measurement of albumin, carotene, cholesterol, calcium, and folic acid levels and of prothrombin time are usually performed when malabsorption is suspected. The tests are helpful in assessing the severity

TABLE 32–5   Signs Associated with Malabsorption Syndromes

Gastrointestinal Signs	
Mass	Crohn's disease, lymphoma, tuberculosis, glands
Distention	Intestinal obstruction, gas, ascites, pseudocyst (pancreatic), motility disorder
Steatorrheic stool	Mucosal disease, bacterial overgrowth, pancreatic insufficiency, infective/inflammatory, drug-induced
Extraintestinal Signs	
Skin	
Nonspecific	Pigmentation, thinning, inelasticity, reduced subcutaneous fat
Specific	Blisters (dermatitis herpetiformis), erythema nodosum (Crohn's disease), petechiae (vitamin K deficiency), edema (hypoproteinemia)
Hair	
Alopecia	Gluten sensitivity
Loss or thinning	Generalized inanition, hypothyroidism, gluten sensitivity
Eyes	
Conjunctivitis, episcleritis	Crohn's disease, Behçet's disease
Paleness	Severe anemia
Mouth	
Aphthous ulcers	Crohn's disease, gluten sensitivity, Behçet's disease
Glossitis	Deficiencies of vitamin B_{12}, iron, folate and niacin
Angular cheilosis	Deficiencies of vitamin B_{12}, iron, folate, B complex
Dental hypoplasia (pitting/dystrophy)	Gluten sensitivity
Hands	
Raynaud's phenomenon	Scleroderma
Finger clubbing	Crohn's disease, lymphoma
Koilonychia	Iron deficiency
Leukonychia	Inanition
Musculoskeletal	
Mono/polyarthropathy	Crohn's disease, gluten sensitivity, Whipple's disease, Behçet's disease
Back pain (osteomalacia/osteoporosis/sacroiliitis)	Crohn's disease, malnutrition, gluten sensitivity
Muscle weakness (low K, magnesium, vitamin D, generalized inanition)	Diffuse mucosal disease, bacterial overgrowth, lymphoma
Nervous system	
Peripheral neuropathy (weakness, paresthesias, numbness)	Vitamin B_{12} deficiency
Cerebral (seizures, dementia, intracerebral calcification, meningitis, pseudotumor, cranial nerve palsies)	Whipple's disease, gluten sensitivity, diffuse lymphoma

From Riley SA, Marsh MN: Maldigestion and malabsorption. *In* Feldman M, Scharschmidt BF, Sleisenger MH (eds): Sleisenger and Fordtran's Gastrointestinal and Liver Diseases: Pathophysiology/Diagnosis/Management, 6th ed. Philadelphia: WB Saunders, 1998, pp 1501–1522.

of malabsorption but do not aid in the differential diagnosis. Many other tests are available in diagnosing malabsorption. Those that are more clinically useful are discussed.

FECAL FAT ANALYSIS

The simplest method of detecting stool fat is to assess a Sudan stain on a stool smear. It has a limited sensitivity because of its affinity for dietary triglyceride and its lipolytic products only, but the test has the advantage of simplicity and low cost. A more sensitive test for steatorrhea is the quantitative measurement of fat in the stool. Stool is collected for three consecutive days while the patient is on a diet containing 80 to 100 g of fat per day, and the specimen is analyzed for fat content. Normal fat excretion should not exceed 6 g/day. The test is cumbersome and does not identify the cause of fat malabsorption, but it gives an accurate quantification of stool fat excretion.

TESTS OF PANCREATIC EXOCRINE FUNCTION

Intubation studies of the duodenum near the ampulla of Vater are the best index of pancreatic function. After stimulation of the pancreas, duodenal contents are aspirated and analyzed for bicarbonate and enzyme output. However, these tests are invasive and time consuming and therefore are not suitable for screening. The measurement of pancreatic enzymes in the blood (trypsinogen) or in the stool (chymotrypsin or elastase) is a simple and helpful diagnostic tool in the diagnosis of moderate to severe pancreatitis. Pancreatic calcifications seen on abdominal films or CT scan indicate the presence of chronic pancreatitis. Abnormal ductal anatomy can be demonstrated by an endoscopic retrograde cholangiopancreatography (ERCP), but this test is invasive and has adverse side effects.

SMALL INTESTINAL BIOPSY

Small intestinal mucosal biopsy is a key diagnostic test for diseases that affect the cellular phase of absorption. In some diseases, the histologic features are diagnostic; in others, the findings are suggestive (Table 32–6). Endoscopic biopsies from the duodenum have mostly replaced jejunal biopsies obtained by specially designed peroral capsules. A number of biopsies should be taken from the distal duodenum to increase the diagnostic yield.

D-XYLOSE TEST

D-xylose is a 5-carbon monosaccharide that, when given in a large dose, can cross the intestinal mucosa largely by passive diffusion. In this test, a patient ingests 25 g of D-xylose and urine is collected for the next 5 hours. Healthy subjects excrete more than 4.5 g of D-xylose in 5 hours. The test reflects the permeability and surface area of the mucosa and serves as an indicator of mucosal integrity. Abnormally low false-positive results may occur in the presence of poor renal function, large

TABLE 32–6   Utility of Small Bowel Biopsy Specimens in Malabsorption

Often Diagnostic
Whipple's disease
Amyloidosis
Eosinophilic enteritis
Lymphangiectasia
Primary intestinal lymphoma
Giardiasis
Abetalipoproteinemia
Agammaglobulinemia
Mastocytosis
Abnormal But Not Diagnostic
Celiac sprue
Systemic sclerosis
Radiation enteritis
Bacterial overgrowth syndrome
Tropical sprue
Crohn's disease

amounts of edema, or ascites. Abnormal results can also be seen in the presence of bacterial overgrowth but may be normalized after treatment with antibiotics.

RADIOGRAPHIC STUDIES

Barium studies of the small bowel in malabsorption usually yield nonspecific findings. However, they are helpful in the presence of distinct anatomic changes such as small bowel diverticulosis, lymphoma, Crohn's disease, strictures, or enteric fistulas.

SCHILLING TEST

Absorption of vitamin B_{12} requires several steps. First, it binds to salivary R protein. In the duodenum, pancreatic proteases hydrolyze the R protein, allowing the vitamin to bind with intrinsic factor secreted by gastric parietal cells. The vitamin B_{12}–intrinsic factor complex is then absorbed by specific receptors found on enterocytes in the distal ileum. Consequently, malabsorption of vitamin B_{12} can occur because of lack of intrinsic factor (pernicious anemia or gastric resection), pancreatic insufficiency, bacterial overgrowth, or ileal resection or disease. The Schilling test helps identify the cause of vitamin B_{12} deficiency. The test consists of several phases: In phase 1, after the injection of 1 mg of vitamin B_{12} to saturate hepatic storage, the patient ingests radiolabeled vitamin, and urine is collected for measurement of radioactivity. In phase 2, if malabsorption is diagnosed, the test is repeated while the patient is given vitamin B_{12} and intrinsic factor; if malabsorption is corrected, pernicious anemia is diagnosed. In phase 3, if malabsorption is still present, and if the test result remains abnormal in spite of treatment with antibiotics, an ileal disease is diagnosed.

BREATH TESTS

These tests rely on the principle that bacterial degradation of luminal compounds causes the release of gases that can be measured in the breath. In the case of disaccharidase deficiency, oral ingestion of specific carbohydrates (such as lactose) results in colonic fermentation, as a result of malabsorption in the small bowel, with increased hydrogen in the breath. In the presence of bacterial overgrowth, orally ingested glucose ferments in the small bowel (instead of being absorbed), which results in increased breath hydrogen. The measurement of radioactive carbon (carbon 14 [^{14}C]) in the breath has been used in tests devised to measure malabsorption of fat or bile acids and for measurement of bacterial overgrowth (^{14}C-xylose). The radioactive tests are cumbersome, and their usefulness in clinical practice is limited.

Approach to the Patient with Suspected Malabsorption

Because of the large number of available diagnostic tests, a rational use of these tests is necessary in evaluating the patient with suspected malabsorption (Fig. 32–3). The best screening test for steatorrhea is the 72-hour fecal fat analysis; however, the test is cumbersome and the stool collection is difficult to obtain in practice. Alternatively, test selection may depend on the clinical presentation. The presence of cholestatic hepatobiliary disease is usually quite obvious clinically. When weight loss, nutritional deficiencies, and diarrhea are present, a qualitative stool analysis may be performed to establish steatorrhea. The absence of a history of excessive alcohol intake, previous episodes of pancreatitis, or abdominal pain makes the presence of chronic pancreatitis unlikely. A urinary D-xylose test or a small bowel biopsy can then be performed to determine whether mucosal disease is present. If results of these tests are normal, enzyme tests and abdominal films can be obtained next to assess for pancreatic disease. If test results are non-revealing or if the D-xylose test result is abnormal in the presence of a normal mucosal biopsy, a hydrogen breath test and small bowel films can be obtained to assess for bacterial overgrowth. When abdominal pain suggestive of pancreatic origin is present, imaging tests such as ultrasonography, CT scan of the abdomen, and ERCP may be performed first to rule out chronic pancreatitis or pancreatic cancer. When diarrhea is associated with cramps and flatulence with minimal or no weight loss and no nutritional deficiencies, the possibility of carbohydrate malabsorption, particularly lactose intolerance, should be investigated. Empirical treatment with pancreatic enzyme supplementation and antibiotics for suspected bacterial overgrowth or infection with *Giardia lamblia* is occasionally given when the etiology remains unclear.

Treatment

The treatment of malabsorption depends on the underlying condition. It consists of dietary manipulations for celiac sprue, antibiotic therapy for bacterial overgrowth,

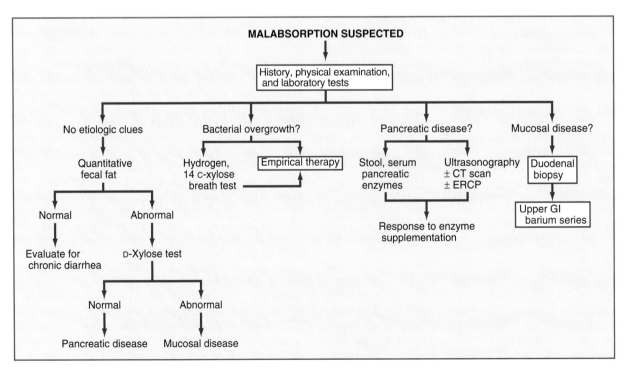

FIGURE 32–3 Approach to the patient with suspected malabsorption. CT = computed tomography; ERCP = endoscopic retrograde cholangiopancreatography; GI = gastrointestinal. (Adapted from Riley SA, Marsh MN: Maldigestion and malabsorption. *In* Feldman M, Scharschmidt BF, Sleisenger MH [eds]: Sleisenger and Fordtran's Gastrointestinal and Liver Diseases: Pathophysiology/Diagnosis/Management, 6th ed. Philadelphia: WB Saunders, 1998, pp 1501–1522.)

enzyme supplementation for pancreatic insufficiency, surgery for small bowel obstruction, or parenteral nutrition when treatment options have failed to maintain an adequate nutritional status. These treatment modalities are discussed in the sections devoted to the corresponding diseases.

ASSOCIATED DISORDERS

Malabsorption can be caused by a large number of disorders, some of them listed in Table 32–4. Two of these disorders, celiac sprue and bacterial overgrowth, are discussed in this section.

Celiac Sprue (Nontropical Sprue, Gluten-Sensitive Enteropathy)

Celiac disease is characterized by intestinal mucosal injury resulting from immunologic intolerance to gluten in persons genetically predisposed to this condition. The prevalence of the disease among relatives of patients with celiac sprue is approximately 10%. There is a strong association of celiac sprue with human leukocyte antigen (HLA) class II molecules, particularly HLA-DQ2 and HLA-DQ8. The disease is induced by exposure to storage proteins found in grain plants such as wheat (which contains gliadin), barley, rye, oats, and their products. The exposure initiates a cellular immune response that results in mucosal damage, particularly in the proximal intestine. Results of investigations suggest that an enzyme, tissue transglutaminase, may be the autoantigen of celiac sprue.

Clinical Presentation. Celiac disease can manifest with the classic constellation of symptoms and signs of a malabsorption syndrome. Not uncommonly, the manifestation may be atypical with nonspecific GI symptoms such as bloating, chronic diarrhea without steatorrhea, flatulence, lactose intolerance, or deficiencies of a single micronutrient, as in iron deficiency anemia. Non-GI complaints such as depression, fatigue, arthralgias, osteoporosis, or osteomalacia may predominate. A number of diseases, including dermatitis herpetiformis, type I diabetes mellitus, autoimmune thyroid disease, and selective IgA deficiency, are associated with a higher incidence of celiac disease.

Diagnosis. Although celiac disease is part of the differential diagnosis of every malabsorptive syndrome, a high index of suspicion should be kept in mind for patients with atypical manifestations. Intestinal biopsy is the most valuable test in establishing the diagnosis of celiac sprue. There is a spectrum of pathologic changes ranging from normal villous architecture with an increase in mucosal lymphocytes and plasma cells (the infiltrative lesion) to partial or total villous atrophy. Although abnormal findings in intestinal biopsy are not specific, they are highly suggestive, particularly because most other conditions that can mimic celiac disease (such as Crohn's disease, lymphoma, tropical sprue, graft-vs.-host disease, or immune deficiency) may be distinguished on clinical grounds. A clinical response to a gluten-free diet, in the presence of abnormal biopsy, establishes the diagnosis and precludes the need, in adults, to document healing by repeated biopsies. Serologic blood tests (gliadin; endomysial and reticulin antibodies) are helpful in screening of patients with atypical symptoms or asymptomatic relatives of patients with celiac sprue.

Treatment. Strict, lifelong adherence to a gluten-free diet is the only treatment for celiac disease. Specific nutritional supplementation should be provided to correct deficiencies, particularly those of iron, vitamins, and calcium. A clinical response may be seen within a few weeks. Patients should be monitored to ensure adequate response and proper adherence to the diet. The long-term prognosis is excellent in patients who adhere to the diet, although there may be a slight increase in the incidence of malignancies, particularly lymphoma.

Bacterial Overgrowth Syndrome

The proximal small bowel normally contains only a small number of bacteria, fewer than 1000 per milliliter of fluid, with no anaerobic *Bacteroides* organisms and few coliforms. Overgrowth of bacteria can result in diarrhea and malabsorption by a number of mechanisms: (1) deconjugation of bile salts, which leads to impaired micelle formation and fat malabsorption; (2) patchy injury to enterocytes on the intestinal mucosal surface; (3) direct use of nutrients, such as uptake of vitamin B_{12} by gram-negative organisms; and (4) secretion of water and electrolytes by products of bacterial metabolism such as hydroxylated bile acids and organic acids.

Conditions Associated with Bacterial Overgrowth. The most important factor maintaining the relative sterility of the upper gut is normal motor function, other factors being gastric acid and intestinal immunoglobulins. As a consequence, conditions that impair these functions can result in bacterial overgrowth. GI stasis can be caused by motility disorder (scleroderma, intestinal pseudo-obstruction, diabetes) or anatomic impairment (blind loops, obstruction, diverticulosis). Achlorhydria, pancreatic insufficiency and immunodeficiency syndromes are also associated with bacterial overgrowth.

Diagnosis. Direct culture of jejunal aspirate is the most definitive diagnostic test, but it is invasive and uncomfortable. The ^{14}C-xylose breath test is the most appropriate test, whereas the glucose breath hydrogen is the simplest, although not as sensitive or specific. Empirical therapeutic trial with antibiotics is an acceptable alternative to diagnostic testing.

Treatment. When appropriate, specific therapy, such as surgery for intestinal obstruction, should be provided. More commonly, patients are treated with antibiotics, the most appropriate being those effective against aerobic and anaerobic enteric organisms. Tetracycline, trimethoprim-sulfamethoxazole, or metronidazole in combination with cephalosporin is a suitable agent. A single course of therapy for 7 to 10 days may be therapeutic for months. In other patients, intermittent therapy (one week of every four) or even continuous therapy for a month or two may be needed.

REFERENCES

Corrao G, Corazza GR, Andreani ML, et al: Serological screening of coeliac disease: Choosing the optimal procedure according to various prevalence values. Gut 1994; 35:771.

Dietrich W, Ebnis T, Bauer M, et al: Identification of tissue transglutaminase as the autoantigen of celiac disease. Nat Med 1997; 3:797.

Kerlin P, Wong L: Breath hydrogen testing in bacterial overgrowth of the small intestine. Gastroenterology 1988; 95:982.

Riley SA, Marsh MN: Maldigestion and malabsorption. *In* Feldman M, Scharschmidt BF, Sleisenger MH (eds): Sleisenger and Fordtran's Gastrointestinal and Liver Diseases: Pathophysiology/Diagnosis/Management, 6th ed. Philadelphia: WB Saunders, 1998, pp 1501–1522.

D. Diarrhea

Edy E. Soffer

Definition

Diarrhea is defined as an increase in stool weight (>200 g/day). Clinically, it is commonly reported as decreased stool consistency, although the term is also used to describe increased frequency, urgency, and fecal incontinence. This section discusses the physiology of water and solute transport across the intestine and the pathophysiology and management of diarrhea.

Normal Physiology

Approximately 8 to 9 L of fluid enter the intestine daily: 1 to 2 L consists of food and liquid intake, and the rest is derived from endogenous sources such as salivary, gastric, pancreatic, biliary, and intestinal secretions. After small bowel absorption, only 1 to 2 L are presented to the colon; most of this amount is absorbed as it passes through the colon, leaving a stool output of up to 100 to 200 g/day.

The small intestine and the colon vary in their handling of ions. However, they share two principles: Ions are absorbed by specific mechanisms that are energy dependent, whereas water moves passively along osmotic gradients. Epithelial cells share some common properties: membrane polarity with apical (luminal) and basolateral (serosal) sides; joining of cells by tight junctions; a sodium pump located on the basolateral membrane; and an electrochemical profile characterized by an intracellular Na^+ concentration that is low and voltage that is negative in comparison to the extracellular milieu, resulting in an electrochemical gradient. Movement of ions across the epithelium can be either passive, along electrochemical and concentration gradients, or active, against such gradients, which requires energy expenditure. Active transport of ions is always through the cells (transcellular). Because of the lipid composition of cell membranes, movement of ions is controlled by specialized membrane proteins termed *channels, carriers,* and *pumps.*

Pumps are carriers capable of transporting ions and solutes against an electrochemical gradient and require

energy expenditure. The most important intestinal epithelial pump is the Na^+,K^+-ATPase pump, which moves Na^+ out of the cell, across the basolateral membrane, and against both concentration and electrochemical gradients. By extruding three Na^+ ions for every two K^+ ions that enter the cell, this pump maintains the electronegativity of the cell and its low Na^+ concentration, which drive sodium and water absorption (Fig. 32–4).

Fluid secretion in the small bowel and the colon depends on electrogenic chloride secretion. This entails basolateral entry and apical exit of chloride. Chloride accumulates in the cell above its electrochemical equilibrium and exits the cell through specific channels into the lumen. One of those channels, activated by cyclic

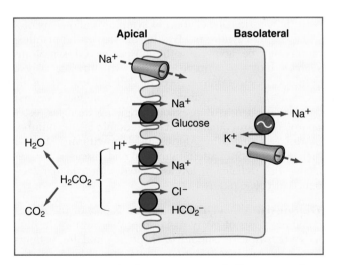

FIGURE 32–4 Apical sodium transporters. Sodium crosses the apical membrane of the epithelial cell, down an electrochemical gradient. The mechanism for this may be (1) an ion-specific channel that can be blocked by amiloride; (2) a carrier that couples the movement of sodium and nutrients, such as glucose; or (3) a carrier that allows electroneutral entry of sodium in exchange for intracellular hydrogen (antiport carrier). The common exit pathway across the basolateral membrane is the sodium pump. (From Selin JH: Intestinal electrolyte absorption and secretion. *In* Feldman M, Scharschmidt BF, Sleisenger MH [eds]: Sleisenger and Fordtran's Gastrointestinal and Liver Diseases: Pathophysiology/Diagnosis/Management, 6th ed. Philadelphia: WB Saunders, 1998, pp 1451–1471.)

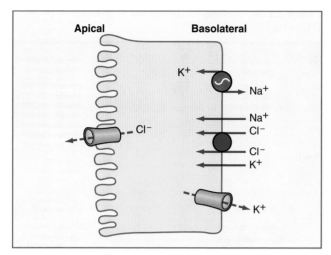

Apical   **Basolateral**

FIGURE 32–5   Chloride secretion. Discrete basolateral entry steps and apical exit steps are integral to chloride secretion. A carrier couples the movement of sodium, potassium, and chloride in a 1:1:2 stoichiometry and permits chloride to accumulate in the cell above its electrochemical equilibrium. Chloride exits the cell across the apical membrane by means of a chloride channel. The sodium and potassium that entered with the chloride are recycled by, respectively, the sodium pump and a basolateral potassium channel. (From Selin JH: Intestinal electrolyte absorption and secretion. *In* Feldman M, Scharschmidt BF, Sleisenger MH [eds]: Sleisenger and Fordtran's Gastrointestinal and Liver Diseases: Pathophysiology/Diagnosis/Management, 6th ed. Philadelphia: WB Saunders, 1998, pp 1451–1471.)

adenosine monophosphate (cAMP), has been identified as the defective gene product in cystic fibrosis. It is called *cystic fibrosis transmembrane regulator* (CFTR) and is the chloride channel activated by several media-

tors implicated in secretory diarrhea. The process of chloride secretion is shown in Figure 32–5.

Although the small bowel and the colon share many basic mechanisms with regard to ion transport, differences exist. Thus, the composition of electrolytes in the small bowel fluid that enters the colon is comparable with that of plasma, whereas fecal fluid contains twice as much potassium as sodium.

Pathophysiology

A number of mechanisms can cause diarrhea, and they are listed in Table 32–7. However, most diarrheal states are caused by either inadequate absorption of ions, solutes, and water or by increased secretion of electrolytes that results in water accumulation in the lumen.

SECRETORY DIARRHEA

Secretory diarrhea is caused by abnormal ion transport across intestinal epithelial cells, which results in decreased absorption, increased secretion, or both. It is typically caused by abnormal mediators, such as enteric hormones, bacterial enterotoxins, or laxatives that affect intracellular levels of cAMP, cyclic guanosine monophosphate (cGMP), calcium, and/or protein kinase. These in turn cause a decrease in sodium chloride absorption or an increase in chloride secretion; the end result is increased water accumulation in the gut lumen. A classic example of secretory diarrhea is cholera. A toxin produced by the organism binds to membrane receptors on enterocytes, resulting in activation of guanine-nucleotide binding protein (G-protein) causing in-

TABLE 32–7   **Classification of Diarrhea**

Type	Mechanism	Examples	Characteristics
Secretory	Increased secretion and/or decreased absorption of Na^+ and Cl^-	Cholera Vasoactive intestinal peptide–secreting tumor Bile salt enteropathy Fatty acid-induced diarrhea	Large volume, watery diarrhea. No gas or pus No solute gap Little or no response to fasting
Osmotic	Nonabsorbable molecules in gut lumen	Lactose intolerance (lactase deficiency) Generalized malabsorption (particularly carbohydrates) Mg^{2+}-containing laxatives	Watery stool, no blood or pus Improves with fasting Stool may contain fat globules or meat fibers and may have an increased solute gap
Inflammatory	Destruction of mucosa Impaired absorption Outpouring of blood, mucus	Ulcerative colitis Shigellosis Amebiasis	Small frequent stools with blood and pus Fever
Decreased absorptive surface	Impaired reabsorption of electrolytes and/or nutrients	Bowel resection Enteric fistula	Variable
Motility disorder	Increased motility with decreased time for absorption of electrolytes and/or nutrients Decreased motility with bacterial overgrowth	Hyperthyroidism Irritable bowel syndrome Scleroderma Diabetic diarrhea	Variable Malabsorption

creased cAMP production. The increased concentration of cAMP inhibits the Na^+/Cl^- cotransport mechanism, blocking NaCl absorption, and at the same time induces chloride secretion by activating the Cl^- channel. These events can result in massive diarrhea, without evidence of cell injury, as shown by the ability of the cell to absorb Na^+ if coupled to nutrients (Na^+-glucose, Na^+-amino acids). This is why cholera and other forms of secretory diarrhea can be treated with oral solutions containing sodium and glucose.

Some of the causes of secretory diarrhea are listed in Table 32–8. In diseases such as celiac disease or any malabsorptive syndrome, secretory and osmotic mechanisms coexist. For instance, fatty acids can inhibit fluid from both the small intestine and the colon, whereas bile acids can interfere with absorption of water and electrolytes or induce their secretion in the colon. Clinically, secretory diarrhea has two characteristics: (1) Diarrhea persists during fasting, and (2) the stool osmotic gap is small (<50 mOsm) because the product $2(Na^+ + K^+)$ accounts for most of stool osmolality. Although these features are present in cases of pure secretory diarrhea, they may be absent when different mechanisms coexist. For instance, secretory diarrhea related to malabsorption of fatty acids may be substantially reduced during fasting, but the stool osmotic gap may reflect the osmotic component of unabsorbed carbohydrates and the secretory effects of fatty acids.

OSMOTIC DIARRHEA

Osmotic diarrhea is caused by the presence in the lumen of poorly absorbed, osmotically active solutes. Because water movement is passive, governed by osmotic gradient across mucosal membranes, water content in the lumen is increased. Some causes of osmotic diarrhea are presented in Table 32–9. There are two important clinical features of osmotic diarrhea: First, diarrhea stops when patients fast (thus avoiding both malabsorption of nutrients and the ingestion of poorly absorbed solutes). Second, stool analysis shows the presence of an

TABLE 32–8   Some Causes of Secretory Diarrhea

Infections
Bacterial toxins (enterotoxigenic *Escherichia coli*)
Stimulant Laxatives
Ricinoleic acid (castor oil), senna (Senekot), bisacodyl (Dulcolax)
Bile Acid and Fatty Acid Malabsorption
Intestinal Resection
Neuroendocrine Tumors
Zollinger-Ellison syndrome (gastrin)
Carcinoid syndrome (serotonin, substance P, prostaglandins)
Medullary carcinoma of the thyroid (calcitonin, prostaglandins)
Pancreatic cholera syndrome (vasoactive intestinal peptide)

TABLE 32–9   Some Causes of Osmotic Diarrhea

Laxatives Containing Poorly Absorbed Anion
Sodium phosphate (Phospho-soda)
Laxatives Containing Poorly Absorbed Cation
Magnesium hydroxide (Philips Milk of Magnesia), magnesium citrate (Citrate of Magnesia)
Disaccharidase Deficiency
Lactose intolerance
Poorly Absorbed Carbohydrate
Lactulose, sorbitol ("sugar free" gum), mannitol, congenital glucose-galactose or fructose malabsorption
General Malabsorption Syndromes

osmotic gap; the product $2(Na^+ + K^+)$ (to account for the anions) is less than 290 mOsm/kg, which is the normal osmolality of secreted fecal fluid. The osmotic gap is caused by the presence in stool of osmotically active, unabsorbed agents.

ABNORMAL INTESTINAL MOTILITY

Abnormal motility can cause diarrhea by two mechanisms:

1. Enhanced motility, resulting in rapid gut transit and decreased contact time between luminal contents and absorptive epithelial cells. This mechanism may contribute to the diarrhea seen in conditions such as the carcinoid syndrome, hyperthyroidism, diabetes, or the irritable bowel syndrome and that seen after gastrectomy and after vagotomy.
2. Slow motility, caused by diseases such as scleroderma or diabetes, may result in bacterial overgrowth, which can cause diarrhea and steatorrhea by deconjugation of bile acids.

EXUDATION

Inflammatory or infectious conditions that result in damage to the intestinal mucosa can cause diarrhea by a number of mechanisms. There is loss of blood, mucous proteins, and serum proteins; the extent of loss depends on the degree of injury. However, mucosal damage can interfere with absorption, induce secretion, and affect motility, all of which contribute to diarrhea.

Evaluation of Diarrhea

HISTORY AND PHYSICAL EXAMINATION

A careful interview can yield valuable clues that aid in choosing the most appropriate and cost-effective investigations. Of particular usefulness is the duration of diarrhea; acute diarrheas are usually infectious in origin and for the most part resolve with or without intervention. Chronic diarrhea, defined as lasting more than 4 weeks, is unlikely to be infectious. The presence of blood is also a useful clue; it suggests inflammation, ischemia, infections by invasive organisms, or neoplasms. Large-volume diarrhea suggests small bowel or proximal colonic disease, whereas small, frequent stools associated with urgency suggest left-sided colon or rectal disease. All current and recent medications (specifically new medications, antibiotics, and antacids) and alcohol intake should be reviewed. Nutritional supplements should be reviewed; they include the intake of "sugar-free" foods (containing nonabsorbed carbohydrates), fat substitutes, milk products, shellfish, and heavy intake of fruits, fruit juices, and caffeine. The social history should include travel, source of drinking water (treated city water or well water), rural conditions with consumption of raw milk, exposure to farm animals that may spread *Salmonella* or *Brucella*, and sexual practices. Familial occurrence of celiac disease, inflammatory bowel disease, or multiple endocrine neoplasia syndromes should be checked as well. Physical examination in acute diarrhea is helpful in determining severity of disease and hydration status. It is less helpful in chronic diarrhea, although findings such as oral ulcers and pyoderma gangrenosum suggest inflammatory bowel disease, dermatitis herpetiformis is associated with celiac disease, and lymphadenopathy is associated with lymphoma.

Further evaluation by laboratory tests and the appropriate selection of tests depend to a great extent on the duration and severity of diarrhea and the presence of blood, overt or occult, in the stool.

Acute Diarrhea

Acute diarrhea is defined as lasting less than 4 weeks and is commonly caused by infectious organisms or toxins. It is usually self-limited and, in the absence of blood in the stool, usually remains undiagnosed. If a patient is seen early in the course of illness and has no systemic symptoms or blood in the stool, and if diarrhea is mild, observation and follow-up are the most appropriate courses of action. Otherwise, and particularly in the presence of blood, stool should be sent for evaluation of infectious organisms, and treatment should be instituted when appropriate. If organisms are not identified, sigmoidoscopy should be performed and biopsies obtained. Performance of further investigations depends on the results of sigmoidoscopy (for instance, if inflammatory bowel disease is suspected), severity of diarrhea, the immune status of the host, and the presence of systemic toxicity. A general algorithm for the evaluation of acute diarrhea is shown in Figure 32–6.

Chronic Diarrhea

Clinicians have multiple tests at their disposal when evaluating a patient with chronic diarrhea, and proper judgment should be used in choosing the most appropriate ones. Duration of diarrhea, evidence of systemic involvement, nutritional deficiencies and previous investigations should guide the evaluation of the patient. In contrast to acute diarrhea, infectious etiology is uncommon with chronic diarrhea. Weight loss and evidence of nutritional deficiencies suggest malabsorption caused by a pathologic process in the small bowel or pancreas, the latter implicated by a history of excessive alcohol intake or abdominal pain. Chronic bloody diarrhea suggests inflammatory bowel disease, particularly ulcerative colitis. Chronic diarrhea with no evidence of nutritional or metabolic deficiency suggests lactose intolerance (common); irritable bowel syndrome, particularly when associated with abdominal pain (common); microscopic colitis (particularly in elderly women); fecal incontinence; or surreptitious laxative abuse. Colon cancer should always be ruled out. Large-volume diarrhea, in the absence of nutritional deficiencies, with features of a secretory process usually prompts a search for hormone-producing tumors, but they are rarely found. Therapy is directed toward the underlying etiology when possible. When no specific therapy is available (as in microscopic colitis) or no cause is found, it is appropriate to give empirical therapy (such as antibiotics for possible bacterial overgrowth or *Giardia* infection, or cholestyramine

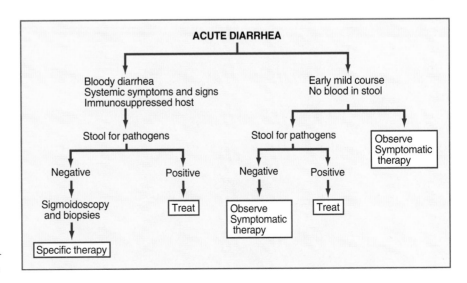

FIGURE 32–6 Algorithm for the evaluation of the patient with acute diarrhea.

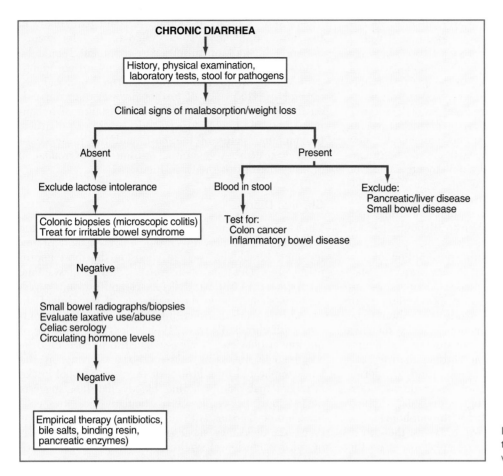

FIGURE 32–7   Algorithm for the evaluation of the patient with chronic diarrhea.

for bile acid malabsorption) or nonspecific therapy with constipating agents such as loperamide, diphenoxylate, and, in more severe cases, codeine, paregoric, or a trial of long-acting somatostatin analogue. A general algorithm for the approach to chronic diarrhea is illustrated in Figure 32–7.

REFERENCES

Afzalpurkar RG, Schiller LR, Little KH, et al: The self-limited nature of chronic idiopathic diarrhea. N Engl J Med 1992; 327:1849.

Donowitz M, Freddy T, Saidi R: Evaluation of patients with chronic diarrhea. N Engl J Med 1995; 332:725.

Eherer AJ, Fordtran JS: Fecal osmotic gap and pH in experimental diarrhea of various causes. Gastroenterology 1992; 103:545.

Fine KD: Diarrhea. *In* Feldman M, Scharschmidt BF, Sleisenger MH (eds): Sleisenger and Fordtran's Gastrointestinal and Liver Diseases: Pathophysiology/Diagnosis/Management, 6th ed. Philadelphia: WB Saunders, 1998, pp 128–152.

Selin JH: Intestinal electrolyte absorption and secretion. *In* Feldman M, Scharschmidt BF, Sleisenger MH (eds): Sleisenger and Fordtran's Gastrointestinal and Liver Diseases: Pathophysiology/Diagnosis/Management, 6th ed. Philadelphia: WB Saunders, 1998, pp 1451–1471.

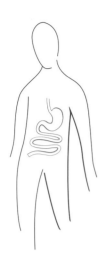

33

ENDOSCOPIC AND RADIOGRAPHIC PROCEDURES IN GASTROENTEROLOGY

John J. Vargo II

Historically, visualization of the gastrointestinal tract was limited to plain radiographs, barium contrast studies, and use of rigid endoscopic instruments with limited depth of insertion and no therapeutic capabilities. Technologic advances now allow the clinician to investigate both the hollow and solid components of the gastrointestinal tract in multiple ways. Each radiographic and endoscopic procedure has its own defined set of indications, advantages, and shortcomings (Table 33–1). The clinician must be attuned to the most appropriate diagnostic test to use in various clinical settings and understand that some tests also carry with them the possibility of therapeutic intervention. This chapter provides a brief review of the endoscopic and radiographic procedures currently available and their optimal uses.

Gastrointestinal Endoscopy

Endoscopes used today are flexible instruments that permit visualization of the gastrointestinal mucosa. Examination of the mucosa can be optimized through the insufflation of air and irrigation of the field with water. A variety of instruments can be passed through the endoscope for mucosal biopsies, removal or ablation of lesions, and control of hemorrhage. Endoscopy has several advantages over routine barium contrast studies, including (1) the ability to detect subtle mucosal lesions, (2) the ability to perform mucosal biopsies and cytology brushings, and (3) the ability to perform therapy at the time of diagnosis, such as controlling bleeding, dilating strictures, and removing polyps. Disadvantages of endoscopy include its invasiveness and expense, the inability

to detect motility disorders and subtle esophageal rings, and the potential for morbidity and mortality, although death is extremely rare (<1 death per 10,000 upper endoscopic procedures).

Esophagogastroduodenoscopy and Enteroscopy

Esophagogastroduodenoscopy visualizes the upper gastrointestinal tract to the second portion of the duodenum. It is the procedure of choice for the diagnosis and treatment of upper gastrointestinal bleeding. Other indications include the diagnosis of ulcers, esophagitis, or cancer; foreign body removal; the evaluation of dyspepsia refractory to medical management; the investigation of lesions identified on upper gastrointestinal series; and screening for precancerous conditions, such as Barrett's esophagus.

Enteroscopes are specialized endoscopes that can examine variable lengths of the small bowel beyond the reach of the upper endoscope. Push enteroscopes permit mucosal biopsies and treatment of lesions but do not visualize the entire small bowel. Passive enteroscopes are much longer than push enteroscopes and are propelled through the small bowel by means of peristalsis acting on an inflated balloon at the tip, thus allowing for deeper insertion into the small bowel. The passive instrument, however, does not have mucosal biopsy or treatment capabilities. Indications for enteroscopy include the evaluation and treatment of obscure gastrointestinal bleeding and the evaluation of abnormalities identified on small bowel radiographs.

TABLE 33–1 Endoscopic and Radiographic Procedures

Procedure	Advantages	Disadvantages
Plain film of the abdomen	Identifies intraluminal, intramural, intraperitoneal gas, and calcifications	Few specific features
Barium swallow	Demonstrates luminal narrowing, mass lesions, and motility disorders	Misses some superficial mucosal lesions
Double contrast examination of the upper gastrointestinal tract (UGI series)	Demonstrates ulcers and tumors	Misses some superficial lesions; no biopsy capability
Small bowel series	Evaluates transit time, luminal narrowing, and mass lesions Easier to perform than enteroclysis	May miss subtle or distal lesions
Enteroclysis	High fidelity examination of small bowel mucosa	Requires tube placement
Double contrast barium enema	Demonstrates polyps, masses, strictures, diverticulosis; reflux into terminal ileum helpful to rule out Crohn's disease	Can be uncomfortable Unable to differentiate retained stool from small polyps
Visceral angiography	Demonstration and treatment of bleeding lesions Demonstration of vascularity of mass lesions	Invasive Large contrast load Bleeding lesions visualized only if blood loss exceeds 0.5 mL/min
Ultrasonography	Portable, no radiation exposure Excellent for the evaluation of the biliary tree, gallbladder, and cystic lesions Real-time imaging, biopsy capability	Air interface leads to suboptimal images
Computed tomography	Visualizes hollow and solid organs, including retroperitoneal structures and vasculature Biopsy capability	Expensive Radiation exposure Contrast load
Magnetic resonance imaging	Excellent anatomic definition Useful for characterizing hepatic lesions Magnetic resonance cholangiopancreatography allows for noninvasive imaging of biliary tree and main pancreatic duct	Expensive Patient must be cooperative
Percutaneous transhepatic cholangiography (PTC)	Allows visualization of biliary tree Capability for tissue sampling and bile duct decompression	Invasive Success lower with nondilated ducts
^{99m}Tc-HIDA liver scan	Best test for cystic duct obstruction	Poor anatomic definition Will not visualize if bilirubin >6 mg/dL
^{99m}Tc-RBC scan	Approximate location of intermittently bleeding site	Poor anatomic definition
Esophagogastroduodenoscopy	Direct visualization of upper gastrointestinal tract Biopsy and therapeutic capability	Expensive Invasive May miss motility disorder
Flexible sigmoidoscopy (to 60 cm)	Direct visualization of rectum, sigmoid colon, and descending colon Permits biopsy	May miss compressive lesions No visualization of proximal colon
Colonoscopy	Direct visualization of the colonic and ileal mucosa Permits biopsy, polyp removal, and treatment of some bleeding lesions	Expensive Invasive
Endoscopic retrograde cholangiopancreatography (ERCP)	Permits direct access to bile and pancreatic ducts for removal of stones, tissue sampling, and treatment of strictures	Requires high level of skill
Endoscopic ultrasonography (EUS)	Differentiates between intramural and extramural lesions Test of choice for determining local staging of gastrointestinal malignancies Tissue sampling of lymph nodes and pancreas	Requires high level of skill

Endoscopic Retrograde Cholangiopancreatography

Endoscopic retrograde cholangiopancreatography (ERCP) is a highly technical procedure that uses a duodenoscope designed to visualize the papilla of Vater and allow for selective cannulation of the bile and pancreatic ducts. The subsequent injection of contrast medium into the ducts coupled with fluoroscopy allows the ductal anatomy to be defined. Indications for this procedure include the evaluation and treatment of obstructive jaundice, acute recurrent pancreatitis, and chronic pancreatitis. In specialized centers, manometry of the sphincter of Oddi located within the ampulla is performed in patients with recurrent biliary type pain without gallstones or idiopathic recurrent acute pancreatitis.

In most therapeutic ERCP cases, a sphincterotomy is performed. This involves an electrocautery incision of the ampulla of Vater with a special catheter, thereby allowing for the removal of bile duct stones, cytology brushing and biopsy of suspicious lesions, and placement of bile and pancreatic duct stents. When performed by an experienced endoscopist, sphincterotomy has a morbidity of 5% (bleeding, pancreatitis) and a mortality of 0.5%.

Endoscopic Ultrasonography

Endoscopic ultrasonography (EUS) is usually performed with a specially adapted endoscope with an ultrasound probe at its tip. As opposed to conventional endoscopy, which visualizes the surface or mucosa of the gastrointestinal tract, EUS allows the examiner to see the components of the hollow viscus wall (mucosa, submucosa, muscularis propria, and serosa) as well as anatomic structures outside the gut wall (e.g., masses, lymph nodes). EUS is the examination of choice for determining whether a lesion originates within or outside the gut wall and for the staging of esophageal, gastric, pancreatic, and rectal cancers. EUS is as accurate as ERCP for the diagnosis of common bile duct stones without the risk of pancreatitis. The advent of EUS-guided fine-needle aspiration has further increased our ability to define malignant masses or lymph nodes.

Sigmoidoscopy and Colonoscopy

Sigmoidoscopy is performed using a 30-cm or, more commonly, a 60-cm instrument. Indications include acute bloody diarrhea, chronic diarrhea, the evaluation of distal colorectal disease, and screening for colon polyps and cancer. Preparation for a flexible sigmoidoscopy involves enemas, but sedation is not required.

Colonoscopy allows for the entire colon and, in most cases, the terminal ileum to be visualized. In contrast to flexible sigmoidoscopy, the preparation is more extensive, with osmotically active agents used to cleanse the entire colon. Intravenous sedation is usually administered. The perforation rate for diagnostic colonoscopy is 0.05%, which increases to 0.5% with polypectomy. Colonoscopy is done in patients with lower gastrointestinal bleeding, suspected colon cancer, as a followup to abnormalities identified on barium enema, to diagnose the presence and extent of inflammatory bowel disease, and in the surveillance follow-up of ulcerative colitis patients for cancer or of patients with previously documented colon cancer or polyps for recurrent disease. Important therapeutic applications of colonoscopy include the removal of colonic polyps, the ablation of lesions such as vascular ectasia, and the control of lower gastrointestinal bleeding.

Radiographic Procedures

PLAIN RADIOGRAPHS AND BARIUM CONTRAST STUDIES

Plain radiographs of the abdomen, consisting of the upright, supine, and left lateral decubitus views, are inexpensive and easy to obtain. The information gained is most helpful in the patient with acute abdominal pain or in the perioperative period. The presence of a pneumoperitoneum, dilated loops of bowel with air fluid levels, and displacement of normal loops of bowel can be indicative of perforation, obstruction, or organ enlargement, respectively. Plain abdominal radiographs are useful in detecting calcifications associated with such diseases as chronic pancreatitis, cholelithiasis, and nephrolithiasis.

Barium studies are obtained using water-soluble agents (Hypaque, Gastrografin) or different concentrations of barium. Water-soluble agents are helpful in the identification of perforations, and they result in less tissue reaction with the peritoneum than barium. Water-soluble contrast agents can also identify colonic obstructing lesions because the retention of barium can be problematic when surgery is indicated. Barium is the agent of choice in patients suspected of having aspiration or a tracheoesophageal fistula because it is associated with less pulmonary toxicity. Single-contrast studies involve the administration of a barium bolus and can detect luminal narrowing, obstruction, or large lesions. The double-contrast technique involves the administration of a small amount of high-density barium followed by the instillation of air or gas-forming agents. The fine coating of the hollow viscus produces a higher fidelity study that is more sensitive for the detection of smaller mucosal lesions.

Cine-esophagography involves the dynamic assessment of the swallowing function and esophageal motility. This test is useful for detecting abnormalities in the pharyngeal phase of swallowing, documenting aspiration risk, assessing the adequacy of esophageal peristalsis, and identifying esophageal motility disorders. Single-contrast esophageal studies can detect extrinsic compression on the esophagus by an enlarged thyroid, left atrium, or mediastinal tumor. It is also useful for detecting esophageal masses, tumors, or strictures. The use of a barium impregnated marshmallow or tablet can demonstrate more subtle strictures and rings. Double-contrast esophagography is more sensitive for the detection of mucosal lesions such as erosions, ulcers, webs, and rings.

A single-contrast upper gastrointestinal barium study is useful for detecting gastric ulcers, luminal narrowing, and disordered motility characterized by poor gastric emptying. A double-contrast study allows for the identification of more subtle lesions, such as gastric erosions and abnormalities at anastomotic sites, and can be helpful in assessing thickened gastric or duodenal folds. Upper endoscopy with biopsy is more sensitive than barium studies in determining whether a gastric ulcer is benign or malignant.

A small bowel series can be useful in the evaluation of malabsorption, occult blood loss, gross mucosal lesions, and luminal narrowing and to rule out small bowel Crohn's disease. A small bowel enema or enteroclysis involves placing a tube past the ligament of Treitz and injecting small amounts of high-density barium followed by methylcellulose. This leads to a more sensitive test that is able to detect subtle mucosal abnormalities as well as a Meckel diverticulum.

Single- and air-contrast barium enemas are useful in the detection of colonic luminal narrowing, diverticulosis, and large masses. The double-contrast examination allows for the identification of small mucosal lesions, such as polyps. Colonoscopy more reliably identifies mucosal abnormalities and allows for tissue biopsy and polyp removal. In general, colonoscopy should be favored over a barium enema for the evaluation of fecal occult blood, colonic polyps, chronic diarrhea, and possible inflammatory bowel disease, owing to its ability to provide tissue sampling.

ULTRASONOGRAPHY

Ultrasonography utilizes high-frequency sound waves to examine solid and fluid-filled organs noninvasively. This modality has a 98% accuracy for detecting gallstones and is useful in assessing biliary dilation and focal or infiltrative processes of the liver (e.g., fatty liver, cysts, tumors) and can help in examining retroperitoneal organs, such as the pancreas. Real-time examination allows for fine-needle aspiration or core biopsies of suspicious lesions and color Doppler assessment of vasculature to determine vessel patency. The portability and lack of radiation exposure are other important advantages with ultrasonography. The presence of air within the gut degrades the ultrasound image. This is an important shortcoming of the procedure, which can particularly affect visualization of the pancreas and other retroperitoneal organs.

COMPUTED TOMOGRAPHY

Computed tomography (CT) utilizes computer-aided reconstruction of multiple radiographic images to render composite views based on tissue density. It has many applications, including the evaluation of parenchymal abnormalities (e.g., mass lesions, cysts, abscesses, calcifications). CT is particularly useful in demonstrating thickening of the small and large bowel, which can be seen in ischemia and inflammatory bowel disease, diverticulitis, and vascular abnormalities such as thrombosis and portal hypertension. In the emergent setting, CT is invaluable in assessing the type and extent of abdominal trauma. As with ultrasonography, CT can be used to perform biopsies or drain fluid collections. Newer uses for CT involve computer-aided reconstruction of vasculature, which may replace visceral angiography in the future.

MAGNETIC RESONANCE IMAGING

The role of magnetic resonance imaging of the abdomen continues to evolve. It may be superior to dynamic CT in the detection of liver lesions, such as metastases and hemangiomas. By utilizing various contrast agents, such as superparamagnetic iron oxide taken up by Kupffer cells and protein bound chelates of gadolinium taken up by hepatocytes, magnetic resonance imaging can characterize various liver lesions, including focal nodular hyperplasia, hepatocellular carcinoma, adenoma, and regenerative nodules. Magnetic resonance cholangiopancreatography serves as a noninvasive alternative to ERCP in the diagnosis of common bile duct stones, bile duct strictures, chronic pancreatitis, and congenital abnormalities of the pancreas such as pancreas divisum.

VISCERAL ANGIOGRAPHY

Angiography is a specialized, invasive technique that visualizes the vascular architecture of an organ. Typically, a percutaneous approach with the Seldinger technique is employed in which a catheter is threaded into the desired artery or vein and contrast medium is injected. This procedure is usually reserved for the evaluation of acute massive gastrointestinal bleeding, particularly of the small and large bowel, that cannot be visualized endoscopically. Once a bleeding site is identified, pharmacotherapy with vasoconstrictors such as vasopressin or embolization with coils or Gelfoam can be delivered through the angiography catheter. Other indications for angiography include placement of transjugular intrahepatic portosystemic shunts in cirrhotic patients with intractable variceal bleeding or refractory ascites and chemoembolization of malignant hepatic lesions. In the future, carbon dioxide digital subtraction angiography and the noninvasive modalities of CT and magnetic resonance angiography may replace standard angiography for most diagnostic procedures.

RADIONUCLIDE IMAGING

Technetium-99m sulfur colloid (^{99m}Tc)–labeled red blood cells can be used to localize the approximate source of gastrointestinal hemorrhage. This technique detects bleeding rates as low as 0.5 mL/min. Drawbacks include the time necessary to tag the erythrocytes with the radiopharmaceutical and the inaccuracy in defining the exact anatomic site of bleeding. Radionuclide imaging (biliary scintigraphy) of the biliary tree by derivatives of ^{99m}Tc-labeled N-substituted iminodiacetic acid (e.g., ^{99m}Tc-HIDA) provides functional and morphologic information about the hepatic parenchyma, the extrahepatic biliary tree, and excretion into the small bowel. Biliary scintigraphy is highly sensitive for diagnosing acute cholecystitis, suggested by persistent nonvisualization of the gallbladder due to cystic duct obstruction by a gallstone. A liver spleen scan utilizing ^{99m}Tc-sulfur colloid has largely been supplanted by other imaging modalities, such as ultrasonography and CT. The agent ^{99m}Tc-pertechnetate has a high affinity for gastric mucosa and can be useful in the localization of Meckel's diverticulum.

Radiolabeled foods are used to calculate the gastric emptying of solids and liquids in disorders such as diabetic gastroparesis.

OTHER METHODS OF BILIARY TREE VISUALIZATION

Percutaneous transhepatic cholangiography involves the direct puncture of the intrahepatic bile ducts using a fine-gauge needle followed by opacification of the biliary tree with contrast medium. In expert hands, this procedure has a 98% success rate. Technical success is reduced with nondilated duct systems. The major indication for percutaneous transhepatic cholangiography is to define the level and cause for obstruction in jaundiced patients with dilated bile ducts on ultrasonography. Serious complications occur in 3% of patients and include sepsis, biliary peritonitis, and bleeding. The choice between percutaneous transhepatic cholangiography and ERCP depends on several variables, including institutional expertise and postsurgical anatomy. Oral cholecystography was used for many years to detect gallstones, but it has been supplanted by ultrasonography.

REFERENCES

Feldman M, Scharschmidt BF, Sleisenger MH (eds): Sleisenger and Fordtran's Gastrointestinal and Liver Disease: Pathophysiology/Diagnosis/Management, 6th ed. Philadelphia: WB Saunders, 1998.

Sutton D (ed): A Textbook of Radiology and Imaging, 6th ed. New York: Churchill Livingstone, 1998.

34

DISEASES OF THE ESOPHAGUS

Joel E. Richter

Although the esophagus appears to be a simple organ, esophageal diseases are common and range from trivial complaints of heartburn to major clinical problems of aspiration, obstruction, and hemorrhage. This chapter briefly outlines normal esophageal function and describes a group of unique symptoms characteristic of esophageal disorders. The major benign categories of esophageal diseases, gastroesophageal reflux disease (GERD), and motility disorders are discussed, followed by a brief review of other common esophageal diseases.

Normal Esophageal Physiology

The esophagus is a hollow tube bordered at each end by high-pressure valves, or *sphincters*. The esophagus serves a single but important function: conveying solids and liquids from the mouth to the stomach. The upper esophageal sphincter (UES) prevents aspiration and swallowing of excessive amounts of air, and the lower esophageal sphincter (LES) prevents the movement of gastric contents in the opposite direction (i.e., *gastroesophageal reflux*). Swallowing is a complex and well-coordinated motor activity that involves many muscle groups and five cranial nerves (V, VII, IX, X, and XII). Swallowing can be divided into three stages: the oral stage, which is voluntary, and the pharyngeal and esophageal stages, which are involuntary. The oral stage involves chewing food and forming it into an oral bolus while propelling it by the tongue into the posterior pharynx. In the pharyngeal stage, food is passed from the pharynx across the UES into the proximal esophagus. This entire process occurs in about 1 second and involves five important steps: (1) the soft palate is elevated and retracted to prevent nasopharyngeal regurgitation; (2) the vocal cords are closed, and the epiglottis swings backward to close the larynx and to prevent aspiration; (3) the UES relaxes; (4) the larynx is pulled upward, thereby stretching the opening of the esophagus and UES; and (5) contractions of the pharyngeal

muscles provide a driving force to propel food into the esophagus. In the esophageal stage, ingested food is transported from the UES to the stomach while the LES is relaxed. This transport is accomplished primarily by an orderly wave initiated by swallowing and progressing along the esophagus (*primary peristalsis*). After the food bolus passes, the LES reestablishes a tonic contraction that prevents regurgitation of gastric contents.

Clinical Symptoms of Esophageal Disease

Dysphagia is the sensation that food is hindered ("sticking") in its normal passage from the mouth to the stomach. Dysphagia is divided into two distinct syndromes (Fig. 34–1): that resulting from abnormalities affecting the pharynx and UES (*oropharyngeal dysphagia*) and that caused by any of a variety of disorders affecting the esophagus itself (*esophageal dysphagia*). Oropharyngeal dysphagia is usually described as the inability to initiate the act of swallowing. It is a "transfer" problem of impaired ability to move food from the mouth into the upper esophagus. Esophageal dysphagia results from difficulty in transporting food down the esophagus and may be caused by motility disorders or mechanical obstructing lesions. Patients most often report that their food hangs up somewhere behind the sternum. If this symptom is localized to the lower part of the sternum, then the lesion is most likely in the distal esophagus, although the patient may also refer the feeling of blockage to the lower part of the neck. To classify the symptom of esophageal dysphagia, three questions are crucial: (1) What type of food causes symptoms? (2) Is the dysphagia intermittent or progressive? and (3) Does the patient have heartburn? An algorithm for approaching patients with dysphagia is shown in Figure 34–1.

Heartburn (pyrosis), the most common of all esophageal symptoms, results from the reflux of gastric contents into the stomach. It is usually described as a burn-

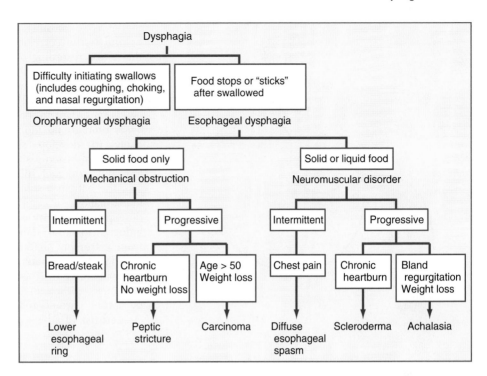

FIGURE 34-1 Algorithm for the differential diagnosis of dysphagia.

ing pain that radiates up behind the sternum. It has many synonyms, including "indigestion," "acid regurgitation," "sour stomach," and "bitter belching." Heartburn is predictably aggravated by several factors, including certain foods (fatty foods, chocolate, or spicy products), the act of bending over or lying down, alcohol (especially red wines), caffeine, smoking, and emotions. Heartburn is usually relieved, albeit only transiently, by ingesting antacids, baking soda, or milk. Heartburn may be accompanied by regurgitation or water brash. *Regurgitation* is the flow into the mouth of a sour or bitter fluid that comes from the stomach and often occurs at night or when bending over. *Water brash* describes the sudden filling of the mouth with clear, slightly salty fluid. This fluid is not regurgitated material, but rather it consists of secretions from the salivary glands as part of a protective, vagally mediated reflex from the distal esophagus.

Odynophagia, or pain on swallowing, is usually associated with caustic ingestion, pill-induced esophagitis, infectious esophagitis caused by viral or fungal agents, and, rarely, severe GERD.

Severe substernal chest pain that is often indistinguishable from angina pectoris may be esophageal in origin. Although this pain was once commonly thought to be secondary to spasms of the esophagus, later studies have suggested that gastroesophageal reflux is more likely the cause.

Gastroesophageal Reflux Disease

GERD refers to a spectrum of clinical manifestations resulting from reflux of stomach and duodenal contents into the esophagus. Many otherwise healthy individuals

have occasional heartburn or regurgitation. However, this condition becomes a disease when the symptoms are severe and frequent or when associated esophageal mucosal damage occurs.

ETIOLOGY AND PATHOGENESIS

The common denominator for gastroesophageal reflux is the creation of a common cavity phenomenon representing equalization of intragastric and esophageal pressures. The LES is the major barrier against GERD, with a secondary component from the crural diaphragm during inspiration. Acid refluxing into the esophagus is normally cleared by a two-step process: peristaltic motor contractions rapidly clear fluid volume from the esophagus, and residual acid is neutralized by swallowed saliva. Patients with symptomatic GERD usually exhibit one or more of the following (Fig. 34–2): decreased or absent tone in the LES, inappropriate relaxation of the LES unassociated with swallowing, and decreased acid clearance resulting from impaired peristalsis. Other factors such as abnormal saliva production, excessive acid production, delayed gastric emptying, and reflux of bile salts and pancreatic enzymes may be implicated in some patients. Patients with moderate to severe GERD have a sliding hiatal hernia that interferes with normal esophageal clearance by acting as a fluid trap.

CLINICAL MANIFESTATIONS

Heartburn, ranging in degree from mild to severe, is the most common symptom of GERD, and associated complaints include dysphagia, odynophagia, regurgitation, water brash, and belching. Dysphagia for solids is usually secondary to a peptic stricture. Other causes may include esophageal inflammation alone, peristaltic

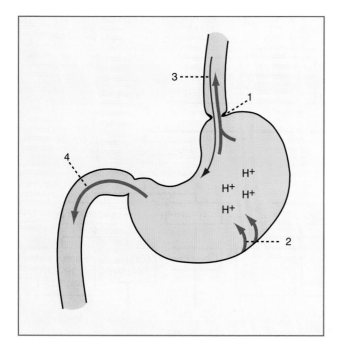

FIGURE 34–2 Pathogenesis of gastroesophageal reflux disease: *1,* impaired lower esophageal sphincter—low pressures or frequent transient lower esophageal sphincter relaxation; *2,* hypersecretion of acid; *3,* decreased acid clearance resulting from impaired peristalsis or abnormal saliva production; *4,* delayed gastric emptying or duodenogastric reflux of bile salts and pancreatic enzymes.

dysfunction seen with severe esophagitis, and esophageal cancer arising from Barrett's esophagus. GERD may present in patients whose symptoms are not immediately referable to the gastrointestinal tract, including patients with chest pain, respiratory disorders, and ear, nose, and throat problems. Respiratory complaints include chronic cough, recurrent aspiration, and asthma. Associated complaints related to the ear, nose, and throat include hoarseness, sore throat, throat clearing, and a full sensation in the neck (*globus sensation*).

DIAGNOSIS

The diagnosis of GERD is best made by the patient's history. Objective tests are useful to quantify the severity of disease and to address three questions: (1) Does reflux exist? (2) Is acid reflux responsible for the patient's symptoms? and (3) Has reflux led to esophageal damage? Reflux may be demonstrated during a barium swallow or by radionuclide scintigraphy after placing technetium-99m sulfur colloid in the patient's stomach. Esophageal manometry is useful for demonstrating abnormal peristalsis and poor LES tone, but it does not show reflux. The most sensitive and physiologic test for the presence of acid reflux is *prolonged esophageal pH monitoring*. This is done by placing a pH probe in the distal esophagus and monitoring acid exposure in an ambulatory state in the patient's home or work environment. The presence of reflux does not necessarily mean

that it is responsible for the patient's symptoms. Most helpful is the correlation of a patient's symptoms with the actual recording of acid reflux episodes during prolonged esophageal pH monitoring. Finally, symptoms resulting from acid reflux do not always correlate with the extent of damage to the esophageal mucosa. This damage is important to identify because patients with esophagitis tend to be more difficult to treat and are more likely to develop severe esophageal complications. Esophageal strictures can be assessed by barium swallow, but to detect subtle narrowings, one may need to give the patient a solid bolus challenge such as a tablet, marshmallow, or even an aggravating food product. Endoscopy with biopsy is the most sensitive test for reflux-induced mucosal damage. Endoscopic changes range from extremely shallow linear erosions associated with friability to confluent ulcerations to complete mucosal denudation. A few patients exhibit *Barrett's epithelium,* columnar epithelium in the esophagus that is produced by severe chronic reflux and is associated with an increased risk of adenocarcinoma.

TREATMENT AND PROGNOSIS

GERD is a chronic problem that may wax and wane in intensity, and relapses are common. In patients without esophagitis, the therapeutic goal is simply to relieve the acid-related symptoms. In patients with esophagitis, the

TABLE 34–1 Treatment of Gastroesophageal Reflux Disease

Simple (Lifestyle) Measures
Elevation of the head of the bed
Avoidance of food or liquids 2–3 hr before bedtime
Avoidance of fatty or spicy foods
Avoidance of cigarettes, alcohol
Weight loss
Liquid antacid (aluminum hydroxide–magnesium hydroxide) 30 mL 30 min after meals and at bedtime *or* over-the-counter H_2-receptor blockers

Persistent Symptoms
Without esophagitis
  Alginic acid antacids (Gaviscon), 10 mL 30 min after meals and at bedtime
  Promotility drugs
    Cisapride, 10 mg qid
    Metoclopramide, 10 mg qid
  H_2-receptor blockers
    Cimetidine, 400 mg bid
    Ranitidine, 150 mg bid
    Famotidine, 20 mg bid
    Nizatidine, 150 mg bid
With esophagitis
  H_2-receptor blockers—regular or double dose depending on severity
  H_2-receptor blocker and promotility agent
  Proton pump inhibitor
    Omeprazole, 20 mg every morning
    Lansoprazole, 30 mg every morning
Antireflux surgery

ultimate goal is to heal or to minimize the esophagitis while attempting to prevent further complications. As shown in Table 34–1, lifestyle modifications remain the cornerstone of effective antireflux treatment and may be curative in patients with mild symptoms. Patients with more severe symptoms who do not have esophagitis generally respond to alginic acid, promotility drugs, or histamine (H_2)–receptor blockers. Promotility drugs, such as cisapride, act by increasing LES pressure, improving esophageal contractions, and increasing gastric emptying when emptying is delayed. H_2-receptor blockers act solely by decreasing acid secretion. Patients with mild esophagitis generally need an H_2-receptor blocker, usually in a twice-daily dose, to heal their mucosal injury. Patients with more severe esophagitis or intractable symptoms need a proton pump inhibitor to control their disease by turning off acid secretion. Long-term therapy is necessary in patients with severe reflux symptoms and in those with more severe grades of esophagitis. Surgical management is reserved for those younger and healthier patients who require constant high-dose and powerful medications to control their reflux disease. Several procedures are available, but all generally consist of returning the hiatal hernia and esophageal gastric junction into the abdomen and restoring LES function by wrapping the lower esophagus with a cuff of gastric fundal muscle.

Motility Disorders of the Oropharynx and Esophagus

OROPHARYNGEAL DISORDERS

Definition and Pathogenesis

Oropharyngeal motility problems may arise from dysfunction of the UES (Zenker's diverticulum or cricopharyngeal bar), neurologic disorders (stroke, multiple sclerosis, amyotrophic lateral sclerosis, brain tumors), skeletal muscle disorders (muscular dystrophies, myasthenia gravis, metabolic myopathy), or local structural lesions (cancer, thyromegaly, cervical spurs). This dysfunction is a common problem in the elderly population, is frequently associated with a poor prognosis, and is related to a high incidence of aspiration pneumonia.

Clinical Manifestations

Symptoms may occur gradually, or they may have a rapid onset. Patients present with a variety of complaints, including sticking of food in the throat, difficulty in initiating a swallow, nasal regurgitation, coughing when swallowing, and dysarthria, or these patients may have nasal speech because of associated muscle weakness.

Diagnosis

The clinical history is often characteristic, and associated neurologic and muscular abnormalities discovered on physical examination help in making a correct diagnosis.

Rapid-sequence cine-esophagography is required to assess adequately the abnormalities occurring in swallowing; esophageal manometry and endoscopy have only ancillary diagnostic roles.

Treatment and Prognosis

Treatment consists of correcting recognizable reversible causes, including Parkinson's disease, myasthenia gravis, hyperthyroidism or hypothyroidism, and polymyositis. Unfortunately, most cases are not amenable to medical or surgical therapy. Some cases may improve or may resolve with time. For example, many patients with oropharyngeal dysphagia secondary to strokes improve over a 6-month period. Other patients require retraining and use of various swallowing maneuvers and techniques to achieve an adequate and safe swallow. This rehabilitation is managed by a therapist specializing in swallowing techniques who uses cine-esophagography with various types of foods to help plan and evaluate therapy. Rare patients may be helped by a cricopharyngeal myotomy, which cuts the UES.

ESOPHAGEAL DISORDERS

Definition and Pathogenesis

Motility disorders of the esophageal body arise from diseases of smooth muscle (e.g., scleroderma) or the intrinsic nervous system (e.g., achalasia, Chagas' disease). In achalasia, loss of the ganglion cells in Auerbach's plexus leads to increased tone and impaired relaxation of the LES, which are also associated with absent peristalsis. The cause of the other motility disorders, such as diffuse esophageal spasm and its variants, is uncertain.

Clinical Manifestations

The three most common causes of motility disorders are achalasia, scleroderma, and diffuse esophageal spasm, each of which exhibits a unique pattern of symptoms (Table 34–2).

Diagnoses

The clinical history is often suggestive, and cine-esophagography (Fig. 34–3) combined with esophageal manometry (see Table 34–2) confirms the diagnosis in most patients. An infiltrating carcinoma of the gastric cardia can mimic achalasia; thus, endoscopy with biopsy is needed.

Treatment and Prognosis

Achalasia usually responds to brisk dilatation of the LES with a pneumatic bag, a procedure that ruptures some of the sphincter muscle fibers or a surgical myotomy (the Heller procedure). Therapy for scleroderma includes aggressive treatment of GERD because more

TABLE 34–2 **Esophageal Motor Disorders**

	Achalasia	Scleroderma	Diffuse Esophageal Spasm
Symptoms	Dysphagia Regurgitation of nonacidic material	Gastroesophageal reflux disease Dysphagia	Substernal chest pain (angina-like) Dysphagia with pain
X-ray appearance	Dilated, fluid-filled esophagus Distal "bird beak" stricture	Aperistaltic esophagus Free reflux Peptic stricture	Simultaneous noncoordinated contractions
Manometric findings			
Lower esophageal sphincter	High resting pressure Incomplete or abnormal relaxation with swallow	Low resting pressure	Normal pressure
Body	Low-amplitude, simultaneous contractions after swallow	Low-amplitude peristaltic contractions or no peristalsis	Some peristalsis Diffuse and simultaneous nonperistaltic contractions, occasionally high amplitude

than half these patients have esophagitis. Patients with diffuse esophageal spasm and its variants may respond to nitroglycerin and anticholinergic agents or calcium channel blocking drugs, although results are often disappointing. Occasionally, these patients, especially if they have severe dysphagia and weight loss, may improve with pneumatic dilatation or a long esophageal myotomy.

Other Esophageal Disorders

RINGS AND WEBS

These lesions may occur in the proximal or distal (Schatzki's ring) esophagus. The cause is uncertain, but

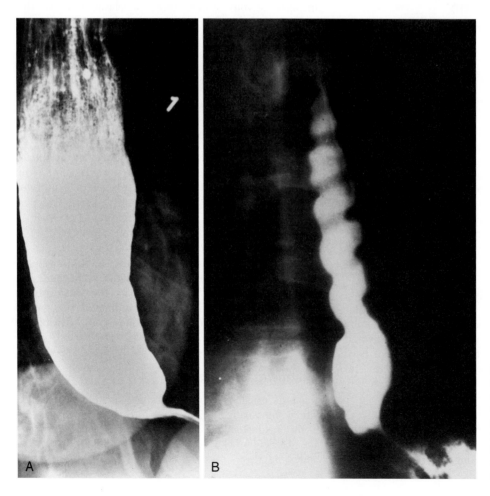

FIGURE 34–3 Radiologic appearance of achalasia *(A)* and diffuse esophageal spasm *(B)*. In achalasia, the esophageal body is dilated and terminates in a narrowed segment or "bird beak." The appearance of numerous simultaneous contractions is typical of diffuse esophageal spasm.

they may be congenital or secondary to GERD. Many rings and webs are asymptomatic; however, dysphagia is the rule if the luminal diameter is less than 13 mm, but it is unlikely if the ring diameter is more than 20 mm. Patients complain of intermittent dysphagia when they eat solid foods such as bread and steak. Rings and webs can easily be disrupted mechanically with peroral dilators.

PILL ESOPHAGITIS

More than half the cases of pill-induced esophagitis result from tetracycline and its derivatives, particularly doxycycline. Other commonly prescribed medications that cause esophageal injury include slow-release potassium chloride, iron sulfate, quinidine, aldrononates, and nonsteroidal anti-inflammatory drugs. A common factor is a history of improper pill ingestion, including taking the pills with too little water or no fluids or taking them just before bedtime and lying down. Patients usually present with odynophagia and dysphagia. A careful history can make the diagnosis, and endoscopic examination confirms the presence of mucosal erosions or ulcerations. Symptoms usually resolve when the drug is stopped. These patients need to be educated about the proper techniques for ingesting medications.

INFECTION

The most common infections causing esophagitis are fungal (*Candida*) and viral (herpes, cytomegalovirus). These infections usually occur in patients with acquired immunodeficiency syndrome or in patients who are receiving immunosuppressant therapy. However, these infections also occur in patients with less severe immune defects (patients with diabetes, malnourished elderly persons, postoperative patients, and those treated with antibiotics and steroids), and occasionally these infections occur in otherwise healthy persons. Severe odynophagia and dysphagia are the common symptoms of mucosal inflammation and ulceration. Diagnosis is best made by endoscopic visualization with biopsies and brushings.

REFERENCES

Castell DO, Donner MW: Evaluation of dysphagia: A careful history is crucial. Dysphagia 1987; 2:65.

DeVault KR, Castell DO: Guidelines for the diagnosis and treatment of gastroesophageal reflux disease. Arch Intern Med 1995; 115: 2165–2173.

Richter JE: Motility disorders of the esophagus. *In* Yamada T ed): Textbook of Gastroenterology. Philadelphia: JB Lippincott, 1996.

Richter JE: Disorders of esophageal function. *In* McCallum RW, Phillips SF, Reynolds JC (eds): Gastrointestinal Motility Disorders for the Clinician: A Practical Guide for Patient Care. New York: Academy Professional Information Services, 1998.

Wilcox CM, Karowe MW: Esophageal infections: Etiology, diagnosis, and management. Gastroenterology 1994; 2:188.

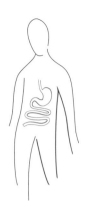

35

DISEASES OF THE STOMACH AND DUODENUM

Gary W. Falk

The stomach acts as a reservoir for ingested foods and initiates the process of digestion. A wide variety of disorders affect the stomach and duodenum, the most important being peptic ulcer disease and its sequelae. This chapter reviews the normal physiology of the stomach and duodenum as well as many of the disorders that involve these two organs.

Gastroduodenal Anatomy

The stomach is a J-shaped dilation of the alimentary tract bounded proximally by the lower esophageal sphincter and distally by the pyloric sphincter. The stomach is divided into four regions (Fig. 35–1). The cardia is a poorly defined transition from the esophagogastric junction to the fundus. The fundus projects up above the cardia and is continuous with the body (corpus), which is characterized by longitudinal folds known as rugae. The antrum is the distalmost part of the stomach commencing at the incisura angularis and continuing on to the pylorus, a circular muscle region joining the stomach to the duodenum.

The stomach is lined by a mucosa of columnar cells underneath which is a submucosa of connective tissue. Beneath that are inner oblique, middle circular, and outer longitudinal smooth muscle layers that are covered by serosa. The anterior and posterior trunks of the vagus nerve provide parasympathetic innervation, whereas sympathetic nerves originating from the celiac ganglia travel in concert with blood vessels supplying the stomach.

The stomach is characterized microscopically by mucus-containing columnar surface cells and invaginated pits for gastric glands that vary in the different regions of the stomach. The oxyntic, or acid-producing, region of the stomach is found in the fundus and body, where gastric glands contain characteristic parietal cells, which secrete both acid and intrinsic factor. These glands also contain zymogen-rich chief cells, which synthesize pepsinogen, and enterochromaffin-like endocrine cells, which secrete histamine. Antral glands have different endocrine cells: gastrin-secreting G cells and somatostatin-secreting D cells, which are often in close proximity to the G cells.

The duodenum, the first part of the small intestine, forms a C-shaped loop around the head of the pancreas and is bounded by the pylorus proximally and the jejunum distally (see Fig. 35–1). The first part of the duodenum is the duodenal bulb, which is characterized by a featureless surface, whereas the remainder of the duodenum has characteristic circular folds that increase the surface area available for digestion. The duodenum is divided into a mucosa, submucosa, muscularis, and serosa much like the stomach and is innervated in a similar fashion. The mucosa consists of columnar cells with a villiform appearance, underneath which are submucosal Brunner's glands that secrete bicarbonate-rich secretions needed to commence the neutralization of gastric acid.

Gastroduodenal Mucosal Secretion and Protective Factors

The stomach secretes water, electrolytes, enzymes, and glycoproteins to assist in a variety of physiologic functions. It begins the digestion of proteins and triglycerides, begins the complex process of vitamin B_{12} absorption, and inhibits the entry of microorganisms. Acid secretion occurs in the parietal cells located in the oxyntic glands of the fundus and body of the stomach (Fig. 35–2). These cells may be stimulated to secrete acid by three different pathways. The neurocrine pathway in-

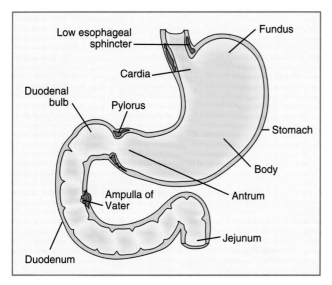

FIGURE 35–1 Anatomic regions of the stomach and duodenum.

for potassium ions. Prostaglandins and somatostatin inhibit parietal cell function by binding to receptors that act through inhibitory G proteins (G_i) to inhibit adenylate cyclase. Somatostatin also inhibits gastrin release. Acid is necessary to convert pepsinogen, secreted from gastric chief cells, into pepsin, a proteolytic enzyme that is inactive at a pH greater than 4. Parietal cells also secrete intrinsic factor, a glycoprotein important in vitamin B_{12} absorption.

Under normal circumstances, gastroduodenal surface epithelial cells resist injury by several protective mechanisms. First, these cells secrete mucins, phospholipids, and bicarbonate to create a pH gradient in the mucus layer between the acidic gastric lumen and the cell surface. Second, the surface cells resist back-diffusion of acid by intrinsic mechanisms of cellular integrity. Finally, prostaglandins enhance mucosal protection by increasing mucus secretion, increasing bicarbonate production, maintaining mucosal blood flow, and enhancing the resistance of epithelial cells to injury.

volves the vagal release of acetylcholine, the paracrine pathway is mediated by the release of histamine from mast cells and enterochromaffin-like cells in the stomach, and the endocrine pathway is mediated by the release of gastrin from antral G cells. Each of these transmitters has a specific receptor located on the basolateral surface of the parietal cell. Stimulation of these receptors leads to activation of intracellular second messenger systems: gastrin and acetylcholine promote the accumulation of intracellular calcium, whereas histamine causes a stimulatory G protein (G_s) to activate adenylate cyclase, which in turn generates cyclic adenosine monophosphate. These intracellular messengers then activate protein kinases, which activate the proton pump, the H^+,K^+-ATPase enzyme, located at the apical surface of the parietal cell to secrete hydrogen ions in exchange

Gastroduodenal Motor Physiology

Based on electrophysiologic and functional characteristics, the stomach can be divided into two functional compartments. The proximal stomach, consisting of the fundus and proximal third of the body, acts as a reservoir for incoming gastric contents, whereas the distal stomach grinds, mixes, and sieves food. The smooth muscle of the proximal stomach has a characteristic tonic contraction. This allows for gastric accommodation, a process by which the fundus relaxes in response to incoming food and fluid with little increase in intragastric pressure. This unique property is destroyed by prox-

FIGURE 35–2 Schematic representation of acid secretion by the parietal cell. Each transmitter has a specific receptor located on the basolateral surface of the parietal cell. Stimulation of these receptors leads to activation of intracellular second messenger systems: gastrin and acetylcholine promote the accumulation of intracellular calcium whereas histamine causes a stimulatory G protein (G_s) to activate adenylate cyclase, which, in turn, generates cyclic adenosine monophosphate (cAMP). These intracellular messengers then activate protein kinases, which activate the proton pump, the H^+,K^+-ATPase enzyme, located at the apical surface of the parietal cell to secrete hydrogen ions (H^+) in exchange for potassium ions (K^+). Prostaglandins and somatostatin inhibit parietal cell function by binding to receptors that act through inhibitory G proteins (G_i) to inhibit adenylate cyclase. Long arrows indicate sites of action of various drugs that inhibit acid secretion. ECL = enterochromaffin-like endocrine cells.

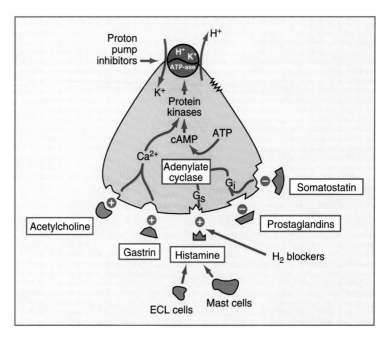

imal or truncal vagotomy. In contrast, the distal stomach is characterized by regular three cycle per minute fluctuations of transmembrane potential originating from the pacemaker region in the midportion of the greater curvature of the stomach, which then propagate circumferentially and distally toward the pylorus. Unlike the heart, electrical activity in the stomach is propagated myogenically; there is no anatomically specialized pacemaker zone or conduction fibers.

Motor events in the stomach and duodenum are very different in the fasted and fed states. During fasting, motor activity of the stomach is characterized by a pattern of cyclic changes known as the migrating motor complex (MMC) that typically occurs every 90 to 120 minutes. The MMC begins in the stomach and migrates down the length of the small bowel. Immediately after eating a meal, the motor activity of the stomach and small intestine changes from a fasted to a fed pattern. This is characterized by irregular contractile activity that lasts for a variable period of time depending on the contents of the meal.

Gastric emptying of a mixed solid liquid meal involves an interplay between fundic relaxation, antral contractions, pyloric resistance, and duodenal contractions as well as the composition and volume of the meal. Liquids empty the stomach first in a "decanting" process, which decreases the volume in the stomach. The solid part of the meal is then propelled forward by gastric contractions toward the antrum, where high-amplitude contractions triturate solids until they are reduced in size to 1 mm or less before being emptied through the pylorus. Regulatory defects of the gastrointestinal tract may occur at the level of the smooth muscle contractile apparatus, the myenteric plexus, or the extrinsic nervous system.

Gastritis

CLINICAL PRESENTATION

Gastritis represents a nonspecific inflammation of the stomach. Clinically, the three most common and important causes of gastritis are infection with the bacteria *Helicobacter pylori*, ingestion of nonsteroidal anti-inflammatory drugs (NSAIDs), and stress-related mucosal changes.

Helicobacter pylori

H. pylori is a gram-negative, curved, flagellated rod found only in gastric epithelium or in gastric metaplastic epithelium. *H. pylori* clearly causes histologic gastritis and is found in 80% to 95% of patients with duodenal ulcers and 70% to 90% of patients with gastric ulcers. However, only a minority of patients with *H. pylori* gastritis develop peptic ulcer disease or gastric cancer. There is a clear age-related prevalence of *H. pylori* infection in healthy subjects, increasing from 10% in those younger than age 30 to 60% in subjects older than age 60 in the Western world. The majority are infected early in life, although the mode of transmission remains unknown. *H. pylori* colonization is more common in blacks, individuals in lower socioeconomic classes, and inhabitants of custodial institutions. In the developing world, infection is far more common, with over 80% of the population infected by age 20. Infection with *H. pylori* typically is lifelong unless treated.

H. pylori is a noninvasive organism that colonizes the mucus layer overlying gastric epithelium. Factors important in the organism's ability to colonize the stomach include its flagellae, which facilitate locomotion, ability to adhere to the mucus layer, and production of urease. Urease increases juxtamucosal pH, creating a more hospitable microclimate than that of the acidic stomach. Colonization causes acute and chronic inflammation consisting of neutrophils, plasma cells, T cells, and macrophages accompanied by varying degrees of epithelial cell injury, all of which resolve after treatment.

The ultimate clinical outcome of infection depends on a complex interplay between virulence factors of the organism, the host response, environmental factors, and age at the time of infection. It is now clear that there are many different strains of *H. pylori* with different virulence factors. Two such virulence factors are the *vacA* and *cagA* genes. The *vacA* gene encodes a vacuolating cytotoxin that directly damages epithelial cells and is more common in patients with peptic ulcer disease. There is a strong association between production of the vacuolating cytotoxin and presence of the *cagA* gene, both of which are more common in patients with peptic ulcer disease. The most common endpoint of *H. pylori* infection is chronic superficial gastritis, which may persist for years. Duodenal and gastric ulcers develop in the minority of infected patients. Atrophic gastritis is another end result of infection that may increase the risk of gastric cancer. Finally, the mucosal lymphocytic response to *H. pylori* infection may lead to a monoclonal B cell proliferation in mucosa-associated lymphoid tissue (MALT) lymphoma.

Nonsteroidal Anti-inflammatory Drugs

The NSAIDs are among the most widely used classes of drugs. There is a clear relationship between ingestion of NSAIDs and injury to the gastrointestinal tract. Two types of mucosal injury are caused by NSAIDs. The first form develops after acute ingestion and is related to direct topical injury to mucosal cells. Acute ingestion of aspirin enhances mucosal permeability by lowering the mucosal potential difference and enhancing back-diffusion of hydrogen ions. Hyperemia, subepithelial hemorrhage, and superficial erosions are seen endoscopically, although these lesions are typically asymptomatic. Microscopically, there is a "reactive" pattern of injury characterized by little or no increase in inflammatory cells. With longer term NSAID use, these lesions disappear and frank ulceration may develop. Chronic NSAID ingestion results in inhibition of gastroduodenal mucosal prostaglandin synthesis caused by inhibition of the enzyme cyclooxygenase, and hence a decrease in mucus and bicarbonate production and mucosal blood flow.

Stress-Related Gastric Mucosal Damage

Whereas mucosal damage develops in the majority of critically ill patients, there is a low incidence of clinically significant upper gastrointestinal bleeding. The etiology of stress-related mucosal injury is multifactorial. Mucosal ischemia caused by decreased blood flow (from shock, hypotension, or catecholamine release) impairs mucosal resistance to acid back-diffusion. Hyperemia of the mucosa evolves into erosions and then frank ulceration in the stomach and duodenum, which may go on to bleed.

TREATMENT

A variety of prophylactic treatment strategies are effective in preventing upper gastrointestinal bleeding in critically ill patients although there is no proof that prophylaxis decreases mortality. Antacids administered every 2 hours neutralize gastric acid but are inconvenient to use because of increased nursing time and diarrhea. Sucralfate at a dose of 1 g every 6 hours is also effective but requires placement of a nasogastric tube. H_2-receptor antagonists given as either a continuous infusion or by bolus injection every 12 hours in the case of more potent agents such as famotidine or ranitidine are safe, convenient, and should be titrated to an intragastric pH of greater than 4 to minimize the activity of pepsin. Studies now show that administration of H_2-receptor antagonists does not increase the risk of pneumonia in these patients.

Studies suggest that routine prophylaxis is no longer indicated in all critically ill patients. Coagulopathy and respiratory failure requiring mechanical ventilation for 48 hours are clear risk factors for clinically significant bleeding in the intensive care unit. Other patients who need prophylaxis include those with central nervous system trauma, burns, organ transplantation, a history of peptic ulcer disease with or without bleeding, multiorgan failure, trauma, and major surgery.

OTHER CAUSES OF GASTRITIS

There are a wide variety of other causes of gastritis. Atrophic gastritis is characterized by a variable loss of gastric glands accompanied by varying degrees of intestinal metaplasia. Multifocal gastric atrophy is associated with chronic *H. pylori* infection and is especially common in populations at increased risk for adenocarcinoma of the stomach. Atrophy of the oxyntic mucosa may also be encountered in the elderly and is accompanied by achlorhydria or hypochlorhydria. Gastric atrophy may also be encountered in patients with pernicious anemia, which is characterized by malabsorption of vitamin B_{12}, absolute achlorhydria, and megaloblastic anemia. Atrophy in these patients is autoimmune in etiology, with antibodies to intrinsic factor. A variety of uncommon disorders may cause gastritis. Lymphocytic gastritis is characterized by a mononuclear infiltration of T cells, often in association with celiac disease, collagenous/lymphocytic colitis, and Ménétrier's disease. Eosinophilic gastritis is characterized by an eosinophilic infiltration of any of the layers of the stomach, especially in the an-

trum. Ménétrier's disease is characterized by giant gastric folds in the fundus and the body of the stomach, with a histologic appearance of increased mucosal thickness, glandular atrophy, and an increase in the size of the gastric pits. A variety of infections may involve the stomach in addition to *H. pylori*. These are typically seen in immunocompromised patients in the setting of human immunodeficiency virus infection, chemotherapy, or organ transplantation. Some of the more important infections include tuberculosis, syphilis, and cytomegalovirus infection, although many other fungal and parasitic infections are possible. Systemic diseases such as sarcoid and Crohn's disease may also involve the stomach. Both will have characteristic granulomas histologically.

Peptic Ulcer Disease

Peptic ulcer disease (gastric ulcer and duodenal ulcer) is a common clinical problem. The lifetime prevalence of peptic ulcer disease is 5% to 10%. The most important risk factors are infection with *H. pylori*, NSAID ingestion, and the unopposed hypergastrinemia of Zollinger-Ellison syndrome. A number of "myth" factors are clearly not associated with the development of ulcers: stress, personality, occupation, alcohol consumption, and diet.

PATHOPHYSIOLOGY

Peptic ulcer disease was once thought of simply as a problem of hypersecretion of acid and pepsin. However, it is now clear that an ulcer is the end result of an imbalance between aggressive and defensive factors in the gastroduodenal mucosa. *H. pylori*, NSAIDs, and acid secretory abnormalities are the major factors that disrupt this equilibrium. Whereas acid peptic injury is necessary for ulcers to form, acid secretion is normal in almost all patients with gastric ulcers and increased in approximately one third of patients with duodenal ulcers. Zollinger-Ellison syndrome accounts for 0.1% of patients who present with peptic ulcer disease. A defect in bicarbonate production, and hence acid neutralization in the duodenal bulb, is also seen in patients with duodenal ulcer disease. This abnormality resolves with eradication of *H. pylori* if it is present.

Duodenal and gastric ulcers develop in a minority of patients infected with *H. pylori*. Acute infection results in short-lived acid hyposecretion that then resolves despite persistence of the organism. Chronic infection increases the basal gastrin, the gastrin response to a meal, basal acid output, and gastrin-stimulated acid output. Regulation of antral G cells may be altered by abnormalities in the ability of adjacent somatostatin-producing D cells to shut down gastrin release. All of these abnormalities resolve after eradication of the organism. Gastric ulcers may develop in the setting of intense gastritis associated with certain strains of *H. pylori* (Fig. 35–3A). The development of duodenal ulcers is more complex and probably involves enhanced gastric acid secretion caused by dysregulation of somatostatin and gastrin: gas-

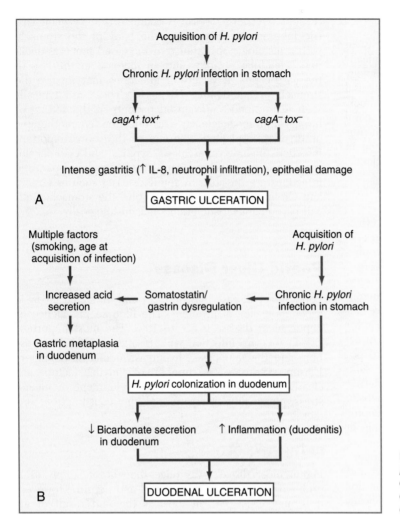

FIGURE 35–3 Mechanisms by which *Helicobacter pylori* may cause gastric ulcers *(A)* and duodenal ulcers *(B)*. (From Peek RM, Blaser MJ: Pathophysiology of *Helicobacter pylori*-induced gastritis and peptic ulcer disease. Am J Med 1997; 102:200–207.)

trin release is increased, whereas the inhibitory influence of somatostatin is diminished. This results in duodenal gastric metaplasia and subsequent *H. pylori* colonization and inflammation in the duodenum (see Fig. 35–3*B*). Duodenal bicarbonate production is also inhibited by *H. pylori* infection.

NSAIDs clearly predispose patients to ulcers, both duodenal and gastric, as well as to complications of ulcer disease, including hemorrhage, perforation, and obstruction. The risk for gastric ulcers is somewhat greater than that for duodenal ulcers. It is estimated that symptomatic ulceration occurs in 2% to 4% of patients treated with NSAIDs for 1 year. Many more individuals will develop asymptomatic ulcers of uncertain significance. NSAID-induced ulceration occurs with all NSAIDs, except for the newer cyclooxygenase-2 selective agents such as celecoxib (Celebrex), regardless of enteric coating or delivery as a prodrug formulation. The risk of NSAID-induced ulceration and complications is dose related and increases with age older than 60, concurrent corticosteroid use, increasing duration and dose of therapy, anticoagulant therapy, and a history of prior ulcer disease.

CLINICAL PRESENTATION

Dyspepsia, the classic symptom of peptic ulcer disease, is defined as a pain centered in the upper abdomen or discomfort characterized by fullness, bloating, distention, or nausea. Symptoms may be chronic, recurrent, or of new onset. Dyspepsia is a common clinical problem and may be seen in 25% to 40% of adults. Only 15% to 25% of patients with dyspepsia are found to have a gastric or duodenal ulcer. Other causes of dyspepsia include gastroesophageal reflux disease, gastric cancer, and gastroparesis. Up to 60% of patients have no definite diagnosis and are classified as having functional dyspepsia, a condition most likely related to an abnormal perception of events in the stomach caused by afferent visceral hypersensitivity.

DIAGNOSTIC APPROACH

There are four possible diagnostic approaches to the patient with dyspepsia: (1) a short trial of empirical antisecretory therapy; (2) immediate endoscopy; (3) noninvasive testing for *H. pylori infection* followed by antibiotic treatment of positive patients; and (4) empirical antibiotic therapy for *H. pylori* without testing for *H. pylori* infection (Fig. 35–4). There are no randomized controlled clinical trials that allow the physician to make evidence-based decisions in the *H. pylori* era.

Immediate endoscopic evaluation without a trial of empirical therapy is indicated for individuals with obvious systemic symptoms such as weight loss, bleeding, nausea, and vomiting as well as in individuals with new-onset dyspepsia older than age 45 to 50 years in whom gastric neoplasia is a consideration. If a gastric ulcer is found at endoscopy, multiple biopsies and brush cytology are required to exclude a malignancy. Endoscopy is also indicated in patients who fail to respond to the empirical therapy. There is no longer any role for barium radiography in the evaluation of dyspepsia, because of its poor sensitivity and specificity. Initial noninvasive testing for *H. pylori* followed by antimicrobial therapy

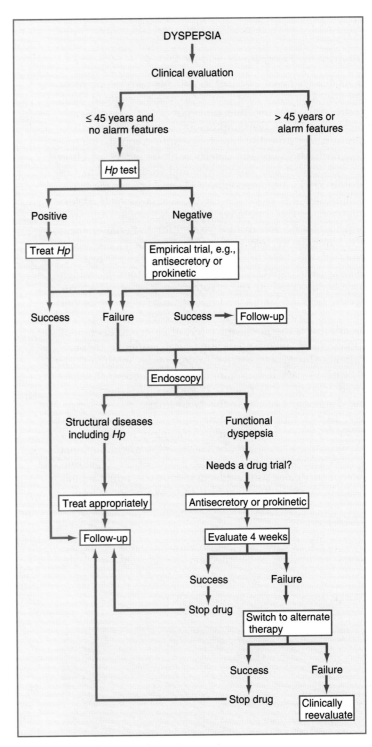

FIGURE 35–4 Diagnostic approach to patients presenting with uninvestigated dyspepsia. Alarm features include weight loss, vomiting, dysphagia, evidence of anemia, gastrointestinal bleeding, or an abdominal mass or lymphadenopathy. *Hp* = *H. pylori.* (Modified from American Gastroenterological Association medical position statement: Evaluation of dyspepsia. Gastroenterology 1998; 114:579–581.)

in patients with positive features is a cost-effective approach for patients younger than age 45 years with uncomplicated dyspepsia. The rationale for this is that ulcer disease, if present, will heal and future ulcer diathesis is eliminated. However, a decision to treat empirically patients with dyspepsia with antibiotics for presumed *H. pylori* infection without proof of infection is not supported by any model and should never be done. Indiscriminate use of antimicrobial therapy may also be associated with illnesses related to alteration of normal human flora, increased resistance of *H. pylori* and other bacteria that are not a target of therapy, and a host of adverse effects such as *Clostridium difficile* colitis.

Diagnostic Tests for *H. pylori*

H. pylori testing is essential in patients with peptic ulcer disease. A negative test will focus the subsequent diagnostic evaluation on other causes of peptic ulcer disease, such as NSAID consumption or gastrinoma. Furthermore, a negative test precludes antimicrobial therapy. Diagnostic tests for the detection of *H. pylori* infection are subdivided into noninvasive and invasive techniques (Table 35–1). Immunoglobulin G serologic testing is the noninvasive test of choice for the diagnosis of *H. pylori* infection in the untreated patient. Serologic tests may remain positive for up to 3 years after bacterial eradication, limiting its role in the documentation of eradication. In the ^{13}C- or ^{14}C-labeled urea breath test, *H. pylori* urease splits off labeled carbon dioxide, which may be detected in the breath of a patient. The urea breath tests are more accurate than serologic tests but more expensive and less widely available. The urea breath test is the noninvasive test of choice to document successful *H. pylori* eradication after antibiotic therapy. Patients should not receive proton pump inhibitors for at least 14 days before administration of breath tests to avoid false-negative results. If endoscopy is performed, the diagnosis is made by the rapid urease test or histology. In the rapid urease test, mucosal biopsies are directly inoculated into a urea-containing media with a pH-sensitive indicator that changes color when ammonia is metabolized from urea by the urease of the organism. Recent treatment with antibiotics or proton pump inhibitors will decrease the yield of both of these biopsy tests.

TREATMENT

Cost precludes routine post-treatment testing in all patients. Instead, cure of infection should only be sought

TABLE 35–1   Diagnostic Tests for *Helicobacter pylori*

Invasive (endoscopic biopsy required)

Rapid urease test
Histology
Culture

Noninvasive

Serology
Urea breath test (^{13}C or ^{14}C)

in selected patients: complicated peptic ulcer disease (i.e., bleeding, perforation or obstruction), MALT lymphoma, or after resection of early gastric cancer. Because antibiotic treatment suppresses the organism even if it is not eradicated, confirmation of cure should only be done 4 weeks after completion of therapy.

Initial Treatment of Peptic Ulcer Disease

A number of excellent treatment options are available for the healing of peptic ulcers. Antacids are highly effective agents for healing ulcers and controlling symptoms. However, from a practical perspective, the inconvenient dosing frequency and adverse effects of therapy limit the use of antacids to symptom control only. Antacids neutralize acid that is already secreted. This increases intragastric pH, which also inactivates pepsin. The greatest buffering capacity is achieved when antacids are given 1 hour after eating.

H_2-receptor antagonists remain a mainstay of ulcer therapy. Acid secretion is decreased by competitively and selectively inhibiting the H_2 receptor of the parietal cell. There are four different H_2-receptor antagonists: cimetidine, ranitidine, famotidine, and nizatidine. All of these compounds act by the same mechanism but have different relative potencies for inhibiting gastric acid secretion; cimetidine is the least potent, whereas famotidine is the most potent. As a consequence of inhibiting gastric acid secretion, gastric pH rises and pepsin activity decreases. This class of drugs is uniformly safe and well tolerated, although the risk of adverse effects is slightly increased with cimetidine because of binding to cytochrome P-450 and hence increased drug interactions. H_2-receptor antagonists heal 90% to 95% of duodenal ulcers and 88% of gastric ulcers at 8 weeks. Given as a single full dose at bedtime, each of the available compounds (cimetidine, 800 mg; ranitidine, 300 mg; famotidine, 40 mg; and nizatidine, 300 mg) has a comparable efficacy for ulcer healing.

The proton pump inhibitors omeprazole and lansoprazole are substituted benzimidazoles that bind irreversibly to the H^+,K^+-ATPase enzyme of the gastric parietal cell, thereby blocking the final step of gastric acid secretion in response to any type of stimulation, resulting in long-lasting inhibition of gastric acid secretion. For gastric secretory activity to be restored, new enzyme needs to be resynthesized, which normally takes 2 to 5 days. The proton pump inhibitors are remarkably well tolerated. Adverse effects are uncommon and are typically no more common than those experienced with placebo. The proton pump inhibitors achieve duodenal ulcer healing rates at 4 weeks that typically are noted at 8 weeks with H_2-receptor antagonists. Omeprazole, 20 mg once daily, and lansoprazole, 15 mg daily, result in healing rates of 90% to 100% at 4 weeks. In addition to accelerating duodenal ulcer healing, the proton pump inhibitors typically relieve symptoms more rapidly than H_2-receptor antagonists. In contrast to the dramatic acceleration of healing of duodenal ulcers with proton pump inhibitors, gastric ulcer healing is essentially comparable to that from H_2-receptor antagonists at 8 weeks. Furthermore, doubling of the dosage used for duodenal ulcer therapy (omeprazole, 40 mg daily; lansoprazole, 30 mg daily) is required to achieve comparable healing rates, which results in higher costs to the patient.

Sucralfate is a complex salt of sucrose sulfate and aluminum hydroxide that is as effective as H_2-receptor antagonists in the treatment of duodenal ulcer disease. It is insoluble in water; and in the acid milieu of the stomach, sucralfate is broken down into sucrose sulfate and an aluminum salt. There, it becomes a gel-like substance that binds to both defective and normal mucosa in the stomach and the duodenum. Sucralfate has little or no effect on acid secretion and acts through several different mucosal protective mechanisms. It binds to mucosal surfaces and acts as a physical barrier to the diffusion of acid, pepsin, and bile acids. Sucralfate is as effective as H_2-receptor antagonists in the treatment of duodenal ulcer disease. The drug is well tolerated with few adverse effects. The evidence for efficacy in gastric ulcer disease is less compelling. The correct dose is 1 g four times a day, which makes it less convenient than other agents for treating peptic ulcer disease.

Treatment of *H. pylori* Infection

Eradication of *H. pylori* accelerates the rate of duodenal and gastric ulcer healing to approximate that of omeprazole at 4 weeks. Eradication of *H. pylori* essentially cures both duodenal and gastric ulcers and should be attempted in all patients with current or past documented peptic ulcer disease and evidence of infection.

However, treatment of *H. pylori* infection is confusing and rapidly evolving. Despite in vitro sensitivity to a variety of antibiotics, in vivo activity of these same drugs against *H. pylori* is disappointing. As such, eradication of the organism is difficult. Combinations of two antibiotics plus either a proton pump inhibitor or ranitidine bismuth are used to maximize the chance of eradication. Current treatment regimens for *H. pylori* are shown in Table 35–2. Factors such as compliance and antibiotic resistance, especially to clarithromycin and metronidazole, influence treatment efficacy. Compliance is essential for treatment success, and all of these regimens offer simpler dosing than earlier options. Nevertheless, antibiotic resistance remains a problem in the treatment of *H. pylori*. Resistance to metronidazole is approximately 50% and that to clarithromycin is 10%.

Treatment and Prophylaxis of NSAID-Induced Ulceration

For patients who develop ulcers while ingesting NSAIDs, therapy should be stopped, if possible, and the patient placed on conventional doses of H_2-receptor antagonists or proton pump inhibitors. *H. pylori* should be sought and treated if present. For patients who need continued NSAID therapy, the dosage should be reduced as much as possible. Small ulcers (5 mm or less) in the stomach or duodenum will heal with co-administration of H_2-receptor antagonists, whereas larger ulcers require co-administration of a proton pump inhibitor for healing.

Given the fact that prophylactic medications are ex-

TABLE 35-2   14-Day Treatment Regimens for *Helicobacter pylori* Infection

Regimen	Wholesale Cost ($)	Efficacy
Bismuth subsalicylate, 524 mg qid Metronidazole, 250 mg qid Tetracycline 500 mg qid	30	90%
Bismuth subsalicylate, 524 mg qid Metronidazole, 250 mg qid Tetracycline, 500 mg qid Omeprazole, 20 mg bid	137	95%
Ranitidine bismuth, 400 mg bid Amoxicillin, 1 g bid Clarithromycin, 500 mg bid	136	90%
Ranitidine bismuth, 400 mg bid Metronidazole, 500 mg bid Clarithromycin, 500 mg bid	124	90%
Omeprazole, 20 mg bid, or lansoprazole, 30 mg bid Metronidazole, 500 mg bid Clarithromycin, 500 mg bid	172–180	90%
Omeprazole, 20 mg bid, or lansoprazole, 30 mg bid Amoxicillin, 1 g bid Clarithromycin, 500 mg bid	184–192	90%

pensive and NSAID use is common, ulcer prophylaxis should be considered only in high-risk individuals: age older than 60 years, history of prior peptic ulcer disease or ulcer hemorrhage, co-administration of anticoagulants or corticosteroids, and high dose of NSAIDS (Table 35–3). Misoprostol is a prostaglandin E_1 analogue that is effective for the prophylaxis of NSAID-induced ulcers in patients and decreases the incidence of serious gastrointestinal complications such as bleeding, perforation, and gastric outlet obstruction. It acts by prostaglandin-dependent pathways to decrease gastric acid secretion and enhance mucosal defenses. Lower doses of misoprostol

TABLE 35-3   Strategy for Prophylaxis of NSAID-Induced Ulcers

Discontinue NSAIDs.
If NSAIDs are necessary, use lowest dose possible.
Consider prophylactic therapy for at-risk populations:
    Age >60
    Underlying cardiovascular disease
    Prior peptic ulcer disease
    Prior peptic ulcer bleeding
    Concurrent use of corticosteroids
    Concurrent use of anticoagulants
    High NSAID dosage
If prophylaxis is indicated, use:
    Omeprazole, 20 mg/day
    Misoprostol, 200 μg bid to qid
    Famotidine, 40 mg bid

(200 μg bid or tid) are just as effective as four times a day dosing for prevention of duodenal and gastric ulcers. Adverse effects with misoprostol are diarrhea and abdominal cramps, especially in patients treated with full doses (200 μg qid). Data suggest that omeprazole at a dose of 20 mg daily is more effective than either H$_2$-receptor antagonists or misoprostol for the prophylaxis of NSAID ulcers. Furthermore, omeprazole is typically better tolerated than misoprostol. High-dose famotidine, 40 mg twice daily, is more effective than placebo in preventing both duodenal and gastric ulcers in patients receiving long-term NSAID therapy. Conventional doses of famotidine and the other H$_2$-receptor antagonists are effective for the prophylaxis of duodenal ulcers but not gastric ulcers.

The frequency of both *H. pylori* infection and NSAID ingestion increases with age. It is unclear if eradication of *H. pylori* results in a decrease in the frequency of NSAID-induced peptic ulcers. Nevertheless, patients with a history of prior peptic ulcer disease or its complications should be tested and treated for *H. pylori*, if present, before beginning NSAID therapy.

Maintenance Therapy

Maintenance therapy with a chronic low dose (half strength) of any of the H$_2$ blockers is now an obsolete concept. Maintenance therapy is now indicated only for patients with *H. pylori*–positive peptic ulcer disease if eradication is unsuccessful.

Surgery

Once central to the management of peptic ulcer disease, surgery now has a negligible role in the management of uncomplicated peptic ulcer disease, with the recognition that ulcers can be cured by elimination of *H. pylori* and NSAIDs. However, complications of peptic ulcer disease have not decreased and surgery continues to play an important role in the management of complications. Some of the different surgical approaches are shown in Figure 35–5.

COMPLICATIONS

Bleeding Peptic Ulcers

Peptic ulcer disease is the most common cause of upper gastrointestinal bleeding, which occurs in 15% to 20% of patients. Although bleeding ceases spontaneously in 80%, the mortality of bleeding ulcers is 6% to 7%. The major risk factor for bleeding ulcers is consumption of NSAIDs. Patients with bleeding ulcers present with he-

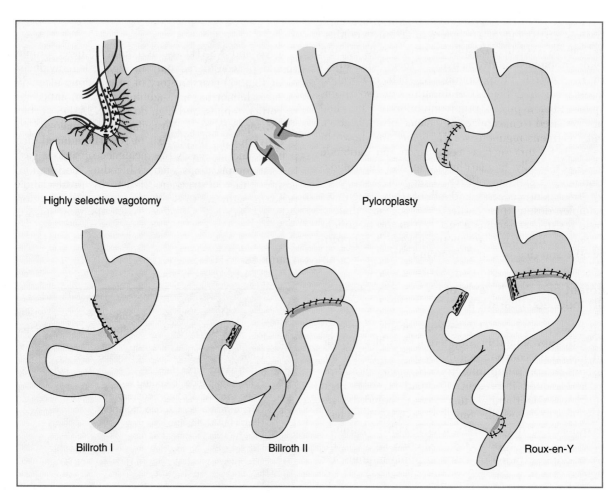

Highly selective vagotomy

Pyloroplasty

Billroth I

Billroth II

Roux-en-Y

FIGURE 35–5 Operations for peptic ulcer disease.

matemesis, melena, or hematochezia, often without antecedent pain. Predictors for an adverse outcome include hemodynamic instability at presentation, bright red blood per rectum and through the nasogastric tube, age older than 60, ongoing transfusion requirements, and increasing number of underlying medical illnesses. All patients with upper gastrointestinal bleeding should undergo early upper endoscopy, which allows for both therapeutic intervention and the determination of other predictors for rebleeding. Rebleeding rates are approximately 5% for clean based ulcers, 10% for ulcers with flat spots, 22% for adherent clots, 43% for nonbleeding visible vessels, and 55% for active oozing or spurting from an ulcer. Patients with large ulcers, greater than 1 to 2 cm, also have higher rebleeding rates and mortality. Endoscopic therapy with techniques such as bipolar or thermal coagulation or injection with epinephrine clearly improves the outcome in patients with bleeding ulcers by decreasing mortality, length of hospital stay, number of blood transfusions, and need for emergency surgery.

Because most bleeding recurs within 3 days of initial presentation, patients with active bleeding or stigmata of hemorrhage such as pigmented spots in an ulcer crater or clot can be discharged within 3 days if they are stable. Given the excellent prognosis for patients with clean based ulcers, discharge within 24 hours of presentation is also reasonable. Approximately 20% of patients rebleed after endoscopic therapy, of whom 50% can be successfully re-treated. The remainder are then candidates for surgical intervention; or if the surgical risk is deemed too high, they can be treated angiographically with either intra-arterial vasopressin or embolization techniques. Surgery generally involves control of the bleeding vessel. The role of definitive ulcer surgery in this setting is less certain at present. After initial therapy of bleeding ulcers is completed, the ulcer should be healed with antisecretory therapy as described earlier.

Gastric Outlet Obstruction

Gastric outlet obstruction is typically caused by either pyloric channel or duodenal ulceration and may be seen in the setting of acute ulceration, where edema, spasm, or inflammation causes gastric outlet obstruction, or as a sequelae of chronic ulceration with scarring and fibrosis. Patients present with symptoms of early satiety, bloating, nausea, vomiting, and weight loss. Endoscopy is the diagnostic test of choice for gastric outlet obstruction; it should only be performed after adequate gastric decompression and lavage of retained gastric contents. Malignancy may now account for 50% of cases of gastric outlet obstruction and should be excluded with adequate biopsy and cytology samples. Treatment of gastric outlet obstruction is aimed at correcting any underlying electrolyte abnormalities resulting from persistent vomiting, in conjunction with nasogastric decompression for 3 to 5 days. During that time, H_2-receptor antagonists should be administered parenterally as well. Adequacy of response may be assessed empirically with a trial of refeeding. In those patients who respond, the underlying cause of ulcer disease should be treated (*H. pylori* and/or NSAIDs) appropriately in conjunction with continued antisecretory therapy. For patients failing to respond, treatment options include endoscopic balloon dilation or surgery.

Perforation

Peptic ulcer perforation occurs when an ulcer penetrates through the full thickness of the stomach or duodenum. This then leads to peritonitis, which, if untreated, results in sepsis and death. Perforation can occur with either duodenal or gastric ulcers but is a far less common complication than bleeding. Patients present with the sudden onset of severe abdominal pain beginning in the epigastrium and radiating throughout the entire abdomen. Physical examination demonstrates peritoneal findings, including abdominal pain, rebound tenderness, and boardlike rigidity. The clinical suspicion of perforation may be confirmed in most cases by demonstrating pneumoperitoneum with either an upright chest radiograph or upright and supine abdominal radiographs. In less clear-cut cases, computed tomography or a water-soluble upper gastrointestinal contrast study may be helpful. Perforation mandates surgical intervention. A perforated duodenal ulcer is typically repaired with an omental patch, whereas a perforated gastric ulcer necessitates either an omental patch or resection.

Zollinger-Ellison Syndrome

Zollinger-Ellison syndrome is characterized by marked hypersecretion of acid caused by high circulating levels of gastrin caused by the presence of a gastrin-secreting tumor. It accounts for less than 1% of patients with peptic ulcer disease. Approximately 75% of gastrinomas are sporadic, whereas the other 25% are associated with type I multiple endocrine neoplasia syndrome (MEN-I). MEN-I is an autosomal dominant condition with a locus on chromosome 11, which may allow for genetic testing in the future. It is typically associated with hyperparathyroidism and pituitary tumors.

Zollinger-Ellison syndrome should be suspected in patients with recurrent peptic ulcer disease in the absence of *H. pylori* infection or NSAID consumption. Up to 50% of patients may have diarrhea, whereas others may also have symptoms of gastroesophageal reflux and its complications. The diagnosis of Zollinger-Ellison syndrome is made when there is a high fasting gastrin concentration of more than 1000 pg/mL in the setting of gastric acid hypersecretion (>15 mEq/hr if the patient has not undergone gastric surgery; >5 mEq/hr if the patient has had prior gastric surgery). However, gastrinomas are a relatively uncommon cause of hypergastrinemia. The most common causes of hypergastrinemia are *H. pylori* infection or hypochlorhydria related to either decreased intraluminal acid in the setting of atrophic gastritis or antisecretory therapy. Other causes of hypergastrinemia include retained gastric antrum (after ulcer surgery), idiopathic G cell hyperfunction, chronic gastric outlet obstruction, and chronic renal failure. Therefore, acid hypersecretion, as documented by gastric acid analysis, is necessary for the diagnosis of

Zollinger-Ellison syndrome. The secretin stimulation test has limited value, because it yields false-negative and false-positive results in up to 10% of cases. The single best imaging test for gastrinomas is somatostatin receptor scintigraphy, which is superior to ultrasonography, computed tomography, magnetic resonance imaging, and angiography for tumor localization. Endoscopic ultrasonography is also superior to conventional imaging techniques. Should either of these studies be negative in the setting of a suspected gastrinoma, then magnetic resonance imaging is the best alternative imaging technique.

Surgical therapy is the preferred management of sporadic Zollinger-Ellison syndrome. The tumors are often found in the "gastrinoma triangle," demarcated by the common bile duct, the junction of the second and third portions of the duodenum, and the body of the pancreas. All patients with sporadic gastrinomas without evidence of liver metastases should be explored surgically with the intent of removal of local and regional disease. Multiple pancreatic or duodenal tumors are the classic finding in gastrinomas as part of the MEN-I syndrome, and the role of surgery in these patients is less clear-cut, although some recommend surgery if a lesion greater than 3 cm is identified with preoperative imaging techniques. Studies clearly show that surgical extirpation of these tumors decreases the chance of metastatic spread to the liver, which is the primary determinant of survival. Proton pump inhibitors are the agents of choice to control acid secretion in these patients. Omeprazole or lansoprazole should be begun at an initial dose of 60 mg daily, and the dose should then be titrated to a basal acid output of less than 10 mEq/hr, 24 hours after the last dose of the drug. If more than 120 mg of a proton pump inhibitor is required, then the dose should be split to twice daily. Chronic therapy with proton pump inhibitors uniformly results in continued inhibition of acid secretion, good symptom control, complete healing of any mucosal lesions, and lack of adverse effects. Treatment of Zollinger-Ellison syndrome with proton pump inhibitors does not result in further elevation of gastrin levels.

TABLE 35–4 Causes of Delayed Gastric Emptying

Mechanical Causes
Peptic ulcer disease, scarred pylorus
Malignancy: gastric cancer, gastric lymphoma, pancreatic cancer
Gastric surgery: vagotomy, gastric resection, roux-en-Y anastomosis
Crohn's disease

Endocrine and Metabolic
Diabetes mellitus
Hypothyroidism
Hypoadrenal states
Electrolyte abnormalities
Chronic renal failure

Medications
Anticholinergics
Opiates
Dopamine agonists
Tricyclic antidepressants

Abnormalities of Gastric Smooth Muscle
Scleroderma
Polymyositis/dermatomyositis
Amyloidosis
Pseudo-obstruction
Myotonic dystrophy

Neuropathy
Scleroderma
Amyloidosis
Pseudo-obstruction
Autonomic neuropathy

Central Nervous System or Psychiatric Disorders
Brain stem tumors
Spinal cord injury
Anorexia nervosa
Stress

Miscellaneous
Idiopathic gastroparesis
Gastroesophageal reflux disease
Nonulcer (functional) dyspepsia
Cancer cachexia or anorexia

Delayed Gastric Emptying

Typical symptoms of delayed gastric emptying include early satiety, bloating, epigastric fullness, nausea, and vomiting. Symptoms are worsened by eating, which may lead to anorexia, weight loss, and nutritional deficiencies. A wide range of clinical disorders are associated with impaired gastric emptying (Table 35–4). Diabetic gastroparesis is the most important of these disorders. It is typically seen in individuals with long-standing type I diabetes who have other complications, such as peripheral and autonomic neuropathy, nephropathy, and retinopathy. The cause of diabetic gastroparesis is unclear but is most likely related to neural injury. Idiopathic gastroparesis is another common cause of delayed gastric emptying, which generally occurs in otherwise

healthy women. The etiology is unknown, but it may be related to recent viral infection.

The diagnostic evaluation of delayed gastric emptying should first focus on excluding structural and metabolic abnormalities. Endoscopy is the best tool to exclude a structural abnormality. A small bowel follow-through may be warranted to exclude a small bowel lesion. Basic blood chemistries, blood cell counts, and thyroid studies should also be performed. Should these studies be negative, radionuclide scintigraphy using a mixed solid liquid meal can quantitate delayed gastric emptying. Assessment of solid emptying is more relevant clinically than liquid emptying. In especially difficult cases, gastrointestinal manometry and electrogastrography may help in the diagnosis.

Treatment of gastroparesis begins with seeking and

treating potentially correctable causes. For example, medications that slow gastric emptying should be avoided. Because liquids empty more easily than solids, and liquid emptying is often preserved in patients with gastroparesis, simple dietary modifications may be helpful in treatment. The diet should be modified to include blenderized foods and liquid supplements. High-fat foods should be avoided, since they inhibit gastric emptying under normal conditions, and high fiber foods are less likely to empty because of disruption of the migrating motor complex. Medical options are limited and involve the use of prokinetic drugs, which are agents that improve transit in the gastrointestinal tract.

Metoclopramide is a D_2-receptor antagonist that also facilitates the release of acetylcholine from cholinergic nerve terminals in the gut, thereby accelerating gastric emptying. The efficacy of metoclopramide is inconsistent, and long-term therapy is complicated by adverse effects and the development of tolerance. Adverse effects occur in up to 20% of patients and include drowsiness, anxiety, fatigue, insomnia, restlessness, agitation, extrapyramidal effects, galactorrhea, and menstrual irregularities. The typical dosage is 10 mg, 20 to 30 minutes before meals and at bedtime, although doses as high as 80 mg or as low as 20 mg may be used daily. Doses should be lowered for patients with renal failure. Although the pill form is usually used, the liquid preparation may allow for more reliable absorption in disorders of gastric emptying.

Cisapride increases gastric motor activity by facilitating the release of acetylcholine at the myenteric plexus. Cisapride is well tolerated because of the lack of extragastrointestinal actions. The most frequently reported side effects are headaches, cramping, and diarrhea. Ventricular tachycardia, ventricular fibrillation, torsades de pointes, and prolongation of the QT interval have been reported when cisapride is administered with other drugs that inhibit the cytochrome P-450 3A4 system. Drugs to be avoided during the use of cisapride include clarithromycin, ketoconazole, fluconazole, itraconazole, miconazole, and erythromycin. In addition, a 12-lead ECG should be obtained before cisapride therapy is initiated. If the QT interval is more than 450 msec, cisapride should not be used. It is also contraindicated in patients with electrolyte disorders. Cisapride consistently accelerates gastric emptying in patients with gastroparesis of various causes. Cisapride is available in pill and suspension formulations; the suspension may be more useful in gastroparesis. The typical dose is 10 to 20 mg, 15 to 20 minutes before meals and at bedtime. No dosage modification is necessary in renal failure.

Erythromycin is a macrolide antibiotic that stimulates smooth muscle motilin receptors located at all levels of the gastrointestinal tract. The prokinetic effect of erythromycin is related to its ability to mimic the effect of the gastrointestinal peptide motilin to stimulate smooth muscle contraction. This accounts for the acceleration of solid and liquid gastric emptying caused by erythromycin. The role of erythromycin as a prokinetic agent is fairly limited. It may have beneficial effects in diabetic gastroparesis, postvagotomy gastric stasis, and roux-en-Y

syndrome. It is most useful when given acutely at an intravenous dose of 1 to 3 mg/kg every 8 hours. Erythromycin may dramatically improve gastric emptying in patients with severe diabetic gastroparesis when given in this fashion. Long-term use of the drug at a dose of 250 to 500 mg orally every 8 hours in patients with gastric stasis is of limited efficacy, owing either to tachyphylaxis or to side effects, especially cramping and increased nausea and vomiting.

In patients refractory to these measures, surgical placement of a jejunal tube may be necessary, with or without a venting gastrostomy. Total parenteral nutrition is rarely indicated. Surgical gastrectomy should only be considered in patients with postsurgical gastric stasis. Gastric pacemakers may be an option in the future.

Rapid Gastric Emptying

Rapid gastric emptying is much less of a clinical problem than delayed gastric emptying. Its major clinical significance is in the dumping syndrome. This is seen after peptic ulcer disease surgery, which disrupts the normal reservoir, grinding, and sieving properties of the stomach. These disruptions lead to accelerated emptying of hypertonic boluses of nutrient material into the small intestine, resulting in secretion of large amounts of fluid into the small intestine, splanchnic vasodilation, and release of vasoactive peptides. Early dumping symptoms, occurring approximately 30 minutes after a meal, are characterized by epigastric fullness and pain, nausea, vomiting, early satiety, and vasomotor features such as flushing, palpitations, and diaphoresis. Later symptoms, such as diaphoresis, tremulousness, and weakness, occur approximately 2 hours after a meal and may be caused by hypoglycemia from oversecretion of insulin. Treatment of dumping syndrome involves dietary manipulation to decrease the volume and osmotic load emptied into the intestine. Frequent small feedings of low-carbohydrate meals, separation of fluid and solid intake, and avoidance of hypertonic fluids and lactose are usually helpful. Should these measures fail, administration of octreotide at a dose of 25 to 50 μg subcutaneously 30 minutes before meals may be helpful. Octreotide acts by slowing gastric emptying and intestinal transit as well as by inhibiting the release of insulin. Surgical procedures to slow gastric emptying have limited success.

REFERENCES

American Gastroenterological Association medical position statement: Evaluation of dyspepsia. Gastroenterology 1998; 114:579–581.

Howden CW, Hunt RH: Guidelines for the management of *Helicobacter pylori* infection. Am J Gastroenterol 1998; 93:2330–2338.

Laine L, Peterson WL: Bleeding peptic ulcer. N Engl J Med 1994; 331:717–727.

Lanza FL: A guideline for the treatment and prevention of NSAID-induced ulcers. Am J Gastroenterol 1998; 93:2037–2046.

Peek RM, Blaser MJ: Pathophysiology of *Helicobacter pylori*--induced gastritis and peptic ulcer disease. Am J Med 1997; 102:200–207.

Soll AH: Medical treatment of peptic ulcer disease: Practice guidelines. JAMA 1996; 275:622–629.

Talley NJ, Silverstein MD, Agreus L, et al: AGA technical review: Evaluation of dyspepsia. Gastroenterology 1998; 114:582–595.

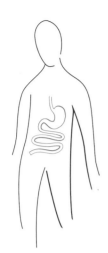

36

INFLAMMATORY BOWEL DISEASE

Aaron Brzezinski

The term *inflammatory bowel disease* (IBD) refers mainly to two idiopathic diseases of the gastrointestinal system that are characterized by acute and chronic inflammation: ulcerative colitis and Crohn's disease. *Ulcerative colitis* is characterized by inflammatory changes involving the colonic mucosa and submucosa in a continuous fashion, starting at the rectum and extending proximally. Depending on the extent of the disease, ulcerative colitis can be divided into proctitis (rectum only), proctosigmoiditis, left-sided colitis (extending to the splenic flexure), or universal colitis (pancolitis). Such classification is important for therapeutic and prognostic reasons. *Crohn's disease,* on the other hand, can involve any segment of the gastrointestinal system, usually in a discontinuous fashion *(skip lesions),* and the inflammation is frequently transmural.

Etiology

The immune system has separate compartments, including the systemic compartment, represented by the peripheral blood lymphocytes, and the gastrointestinal mucosa, in which numerous intraepithelial lymphocytes and lamina propria lymphocytes are found. Patients with IBD have an abnormality in the expression and activation in the gastrointestinal mucosal compartment.

The gastrointestinal system is normally in a "controlled state of inflammation." To regulate immune and inflammatory functions, constant cell-to-cell communication is mediated through cytokines. *Cytokines* are small peptides that regulate immune function and include interleukins (IL), interferons, monokines, and lymphokines. Some cytokines are primarily proinflammatory (tumor necrosis factor-α, IL-1), whereas others have immunoregulatory or anti-inflammatory actions (IL-2, IL-4, IL-10, transforming growth factor-β). In a simplistic way, homeostasis is disrupted in patients with IBD because of overexpression of proinflammatory cytokines, underexpression of regulatory or anti-inflammatory cytokines, or both.

Evidence also suggests that genetic factors play a role in IBD, and the disease is most likely polygenic. First-degree relatives of patients with ulcerative colitis or Crohn's disease have a 10- to 15-fold increased risk of developing IBD, usually with the same disease as the patient. Furthermore, about 10% of patients with IBD have a first-degree relative with the disease. Infectious agents have been implicated, but none have fulfilled Koch's criteria. Environmental factors are suspected because the disease is more common in industrialized countries, and the frequency is increasing in countries that are becoming industrialized. However, to date, the only environmental factor clearly associated with IBD is cigarette smoking. Cigarette smoking seems to be protective for ulcerative colitis; some patients develop symptoms when they stop smoking cigarettes, whereas smokers with Crohn's disease have more aggressive disease than do nonsmokers with Crohn's disease.

Incidence and Epidemiology

Whereas the incidence of ulcerative colitis has remained stable, the incidence of Crohn's disease is increasing worldwide. Both diseases are more common in the northern parts of the Western world, among whites, and particularly in Ashkenazi Jews living in Europe or North America. However, both diseases can occur in any ethnic group. The incidence of both diseases is between 5 and 15 new cases per 100,000 population, with the prevalence between 50 and 100 per 100,000 population. IBD affects both sexes equally and has a bimodal age of presentation. The most common age of presentation is between the second and fourth decades of life, followed by a second smaller peak after the sixth decade of life.

Ulcerative Colitis: Clinical Features

Patients with ulcerative colitis usually present with bloody diarrhea, which has a chronic intermittent course, with episodes of remissions and exacerbations. The symptoms, severity, and prognosis of the disease are often determined by the extent of the disease. At presentation, nearly 50% of patients have proctitis or proctosigmoiditis; however, after 13 years, the disease extends to involve the entire colon in more than 30% of patients. Patients with proctitis have urgency and frequent trips to the toilet to pass small amounts of mucus and blood. Patients with more extensive disease have bloody diarrhea, predefecational cramps, and, if they have severe or fulminant disease, signs and symptoms of dehydration, abdominal pain, and fever. Not infrequently, patients present with extraintestinal manifestations such as erythema nodosum, arthritis, or pyoderma gangrenosum before they develop intestinal symptoms.

Crohn's Disease: Clinical Features

Crohn's disease is a heterogeneous disease with the clinical manifestations depending on the site of involvement and the behavior of disease. Patients can have mostly *inflammatory* symptoms, characterized by abdominal pain in the right lower quadrant, fever, weight loss, and a palpable inflammatory mass. They may have *obstructive* symptoms, characterized by postprandial abdominal pain, bloating, nausea, and vomiting; or they may have *fistulous* disease, characterized by enterovaginal fistula, enterocutaneous fistulas, or other internal fistula or abscess. However, the three patterns of disease can occur in the same patient. Not infrequently, patients present with perianal disease including anal fissures, abscess, fistula, or skin tags. These manifestations should not be confused with "hemorrhoids." The most common site of involvement is ileocolonic disease; such patients usually have inflammatory disease that, over time, becomes stricturing disease. Patients with disease confined to the colon have nonbloody diarrhea, abdominal pain, fever, and weight loss. Patients with gastroduodenal Crohn's disease have dyspeptic symptoms, whereas patients with jejunoileal disease have obstruction or symptoms related to fistulae.

Extraintestinal Manifestations

IBD is a systemic disease that affects primarily the gastrointestinal system and has numerous extraintestinal manifestations, including musculoskeletal, skin, hepatic, ocular, renal, and other features. The most frequent musculoskeletal complication is seronegative "arthritis." This pauciarticular, asymmetric, nondeforming arthritis involves large joints more commonly. It occurs in 15% to 45% of patients with colonic disease, either Crohn's disease or ulcerative colitis. The other major musculoskeletal manifestations are sacroiliitis and ankylosing spondylitis, which are axial arthropathies. These disorders are more common in patients with ulcerative colitis, have a close association with the histocompatibility antigen HLA-B27, and run a course independent of disease activity. To date, more than 40 skin manifestations of IBD have been described; the 3 most commonly seen are aphthous ulcerations of the oral mucosa, erythema nodosum, and pyoderma gangrenosum. *Erythema nodosum* occurs in 15% of patients with Crohn's disease and in 4% of patients with ulcerative colitis. It is characterized by red, tender subcutaneous nodules, usually on the anterior tibial surface. *Pyoderma gangrenosum* does not have a clear association with disease activity. It occurs in ~2% of patients with IBD, and it usually presents at sites of trauma. It usually occurs over the shins or on the face and is characterized by large ulcers of the skin, with a necrotic center and an advancing border that is undermined or rolled.

Ocular manifestations occur in approximately 6% of patients with IBD. The most common manifestation is *episcleritis,* which occurs more commonly in patients with Crohn's colitis. A less frequent, but more serious manifestation is *uveitis,* which usually presents with a sudden-onset headache and blurred vision and is an ophthalmologic emergency. Hematologic features are multiple. Some are complications of the intestinal disease such as iron deficiency anemia or vitamin B_{12} malabsorption, whereas others are extraintestinal manifestations such as a hypercoagulable state leading to venous and arterial thrombosis that can have fatal complications.

Hepatic complications occur in approximately 5% of patients with IBD. The most common finding is asymptomatic elevation of hepatic transaminases with fatty infiltration of the liver, either resulting from nutritional factors or secondary to medications used to treat IBD. A more significant hepatobiliary complication is *primary sclerosing cholangitis,* which is characterized by progressive inflammation of the intrahepatic and extrahepatic biliary tree, leading to strictures, with sepsis, cirrhosis, and cholangiocarcinoma as possible complications. Primary sclerosing cholangitis occurs more commonly in patients with ulcerative colitis than in those with Crohn's disease, and it follows a course that is independent of disease activity.

Other Complications

Patients with Crohn's disease can develop multiple metabolic abnormalities. They have increased absorption of oxalate that leads to kidney stones and a disrupted enterohepatic circulation with increased frequency of gallstones. Metabolic bone disease is a complication of IBD, either because of vitamin D malabsorption or as a side effect of steroid use. Other rare complications include acute pancreatitis, pleuropericarditis, fibrosing alveolitis, bronchiolitis obliterans, clubbing, hypertrophic osteoarthropathy, and amyloidosis.

Colon Cancer

The risk of colon cancer is increased in patients with IBD, particularly in those with ulcerative colitis. The risk is related to the extent and duration of disease, and it is increased in patients with primary sclerosing cholangitis. In patients with pancolitis, the risk increases after 10 years and is estimated to increase by 0.5% to 1% per year, to reach an absolute risk of 30% after 35 years of disease. Patients with extensive Crohn's colitis and those with left-sided ulcerative colitis also have an increased risk of colorectal cancer, but the risk is lower than in patients with ulcerative pancolitis. Proctitis is not associated with a cancer risk. Because of the evolution from diseased mucosa to dysplasia to cancer, different regimens with colonoscopy and multiple biopsies throughout the colon are recommended, and whenever dysplasia is found, colectomy is recommended.

Diagnosis

The diagnosis of IBD is based on clinical features, laboratory tests, and endoscopic and histologic features (Table 36–1). Laboratory tests are not specific and usually reflect inflammation and/or anemia. The only specific feature is perinuclear antineutrophil cytoplasmic antibody (pANCA), which is positive in up to 70% of patients with ulcerative colitis but rarely positive in patients with Crohn's disease. During colonoscopy in patients with ulcerative colitis, the mucosa has a granular appearance, decreased vessel markings and mucosal shine, and superficial ulcerations (Fig. 36–1), and in more severe cases, the mucosa is friable, with deeper ulcerations and an exudate. Patients with long-standing disease have "pseudopolyps." Histologically, crypt architecture is distorted, with crypt abscesses and inflammation consisting of plasma cells, neutrophils, lymphocytes, and eosinophils.

Stool cultures for ova and parasite identification and stool testing for *Clostridium difficile* toxin, are helpful,

because these infections can mimic IBD. In Crohn's disease, small bowel radiography remains the best study with which to investigate the jejunum and ileum. Involved areas have edema and thickening of the wall that lead to bowel loop separation and can also show ulcerations of the mucosa, fistulas, or strictures. A tight, long stricture in the terminal ileum is commonly called the "string sign" (Fig. 36–2). On endoscopic examination, the involved mucosa shows aphthoid ulcerations (Fig. 36–3), deep linear or stellate ulcers (Fig. 36–4), edema, erythema, exudate, and friability with intervening areas of normal mucosa *(skip lesions)*. Linear ulcers with segments of edematous or uninvolved mucosa lead to the characteristic pattern called "cobblestoning." Patients with a suspected abscess should have a computed tomographic examination before other radiologic or endoscopic studies are performed.

Differential Diagnosis

The differential diagnosis of IBD includes infectious colitis, ischemic colitis, radiation enteritis, enterocolitis induced by nonsteroidal anti-inflammatory drugs, diverticulitis, appendicitis, colon cancer, and lymphoma. Among the infectious causes, *Yersinia enterocolitica* infection can mimic Crohn's disease because the pathogen causes ileitis, mesenteric adenitis, fever, diarrhea, and abdominal pain in the right lower quadrant, all of which are features of Crohn's disease. Tuberculosis, strongyloidiasis, and amebiasis must be excluded in populations at high risk because these diseases can mimic IBD, and treatment with corticosteroids can lead to death.

Treatment

As part of the initial management of patients with IBD, the clinician must determine the extent and severity of the patient's disease. Patients with mild or moderate disease can be managed as outpatients, whereas patients with severe or fulminant disease require hospital admission and multidisciplinary management with a colorectal surgeon. Patients with severe disease are febrile, tachycardic, and anemic, and they have leukocytosis and ab-

TABLE 36–1   Differentiating Features

	Ulcerative Colitis	Crohn's Disease
Site of involvement	Rectum always, colon only	Any segment of the gastrointestinal tract
Pattern of involvement	Continuous	Skip
Diarrhea	Bloody	Usually nonbloody
Abdominal pain	In severe disease	Frequent
Perianal disease	No	In 30% of patients
Fistula	No	Yes
Endoscopic findings	Erythema, friable, superficial ulceration	Aphthoid ulcers, deep ulcers, skip lesions
Histologic features	Crypt abscess	Granulomas (~30%)

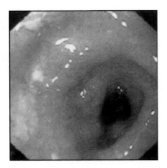

FIGURE 36-1   Ulcerative colitis.

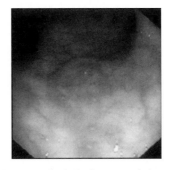

FIGURE 36-3   Crohn's disease: aphthous ulcers.

dominal pain. Because IBD is a chronic recurrent illness, treatment is divided first into management of the acute attack, next into treatment to induce remission, and finally into maintenance of remission.

NUTRITION

Nutritional support is an important aspect of supportive treatment in patients with IBD. However, as primary treatment it has a role only in small bowel Crohn's disease, because these patients may achieve remission when they are treated with total parenteral nutrition or elemental diets for prolonged periods (at least 4 weeks). Vitamins and minerals should be supplemented; patients with extensive ileal disease cannot absorb vitamin B_{12} orally, whereas patients taking corticosteroids require supplemental calcium and vitamin D. Patients with extensive small bowel involvement develop malabsorption of fat-soluble vitamins (A, D, E, and K), iron deficiency, folate deficiency, and, if diarrhea is significant, zinc deficiency.

ANTIDIARRHEAL MEDICATIONS

Antidiarrheal agents should be used cautiously during exacerbations because they can precipitate toxic colitis or megacolon. Their main role is in controlling postoperative diarrhea. When less than 100 cm of terminal ileum is resected, patients develop bile salt malabsorption, in which bile salts enter the colon and cause diarrhea. Bile salt resin binders such as cholestyramine antidiarrheal agents are effective treatment. When patients

have undergone more extensive resections, the bile salt pool is depleted, and fat malabsorption develops. These patients respond to a low-fat diet supplemented with medium-chain triglycerides and antidiarrheal agents.

ANTI-INFLAMMATORY MEDICATIONS

These groups are the 5-aminosalicylic acid compounds (5-ASA), not to be confused with acetylsalicylic acid (aspirin) or with nonsteroidal anti-inflammatory drugs and corticosteroids. 5-ASA medications need to contact the diseased mucosa because the effect is topical, not systemic. For this reason, different delivery systems exist (Table 36-2). The purpose of such delivery systems is to release the agent at the site of inflammation. These agents are indicated for the treatment of mild or moderate active disease. In patients with ulcerative colitis, these agents play a significant role in maintenance of remission. Patients with ulcerative colitis who do not take a 5-ASA compound have a 50% risk of recurrent attacks within 6 months of discontinuation, whereas in those who continue to take a 5-ASA agent, the risk of disease recurrence is less than 10% per year. In patients with Crohn's disease, high doses of 5-ASA may have a beneficial long-term effect in maintenance of remission, although this is a subject of debate. A clear dose-dependent response exists for 5-ASA medications, with higher doses more effective in inducing and maintaining remission. Patients who take sulfasalazine (metabolized to 5-ASA and sulfapyridine) need folic acid supplementation. Patients allergic to sulfa drugs can take oral 5-ASA preparations; however, allergic reactions to these com-

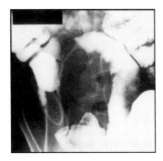

FIGURE 36-2   Crohn's disease: "string sign."

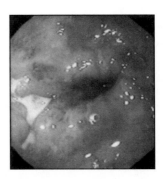

FIGURE 36-4   Crohn's disease: stellate ulcer.

TABLE 36-2 5-Aminosalicylic Acid Preparations, Common Uses, and Doses

	Site of Action	Active Disease	Maintenance of Remission
Diazo-Bond			
Sulfasalazine	Colon	4–6 g/day	2–4 g/day
Olsalazine	Colon	1–2 g/day	1 g/day
Resin-Coated			
Mesalamine (Asacol)	Colon	2.4–6.2 g/day	1.2–2.4 g/day
Time-Release			
Mesalamine (Pentasa)	Small bowel and colon	4 g/day	2–4 g/day
Topical			
Mesalamine (Rowasa supp)	Rectum	1 g/day	?
Mesalamine (Rowasa enema)	Rectum and sigmoid colon	4 g/day	?

pounds have also been described. Side effects requiring discontinuation of medication occur in ~30% of patients and include headaches, nausea, and skin reactions.

Reversible oligospermia occurs and is related to sulfapyridine, rather than to 5-ASA. Less frequent, but more serious side effects are pleuropericarditis, pancreatitis, agranulocytosis, interstitial nephritis, and hemolytic anemia.

Corticosteroids remain the most effective anti-inflammatory agents for inducing remission in patients with active IBD. They are indicated for moderate or severe disease and in patients in whom treatment with 5-ASA fails. Corticosteroids should be used only to induce remission, because they do not maintain remission and have significant long-term side effects. The most common agent used is prednisone, started in doses between 40 and 60 mg per day. Patients improve rapidly, and the medication is usually tapered down slowly, that is, 5 to 10 mg per week until discontinuation. Patients who do not improve after 1 week of oral treatment or those with more severe disease are best treated in the hospital with intravenous (IV) corticosteroids, that is, hydrocortisone, 300 mg IV per day, which can be given either by continuous infusion or in three divided doses.

ANTIBIOTICS

The main role for antibiotics is in patients with Crohn's disease who have colonic or perianal involvement. The two more commonly used antibiotics are metronidazole and ciprofloxacin. Metronidazole is prescribed at a dose of 20 mg/kg/day in three divided doses. Patients should be warned of potential side effects such as a disulfiram (Antabuse) effect and peripheral neuropathy. IV antibiotics are part of the initial treatment in patients with toxic or fulminant colitis.

IMMUNOSUPPRESSIVE AGENTS

Azathioprine (Imuran) and 6-mercaptopurine (6-MP) are used as steroid-sparing agents in patients with steroid-refractory disease, fistulous disease, or perianal dis-

ease. Other regimens include intramuscular methotrexate for active Crohn's disease and cyclosporine IV as "bridge" treatment for severe steroid-refractory ulcerative colitis. Given the potential for both short-term and long-term side effects, as well as the need for close follow-up, patients needing these medications are best managed by gastroenterologists.

BIOLOGIC MEDICATIONS

The newest drugs used for IBD are the "biologic agents." These are produced by molecular biology techniques and are designed to work at a specific site in the inflammatory cascade. The first agent approved by the United States Food and Drug Administration for treating patients with Crohn's disease is infliximab, a chimeric tumor necrosis factor-α antibody. It is indicated in patients with active Crohn's disease who are not responding to conventional medical treatment and who do not need immediate surgical treatment and in patients with enterocutaneous or perianal fistulas.

SURGICAL TREATMENT

When patients have a fulminant presentation, toxic colitis, symptomatic strictures, or severe disease that does not respond to medical treatment, they are best treated surgically. The other main indication for surgical treatment is dysplasia or cancer. For patients with ulcerative colitis, regardless of the extent of disease, the entire colon must be removed. Patients with Crohn's disease undergo segmental resections or stricturoplasty, and they also require surgical treatment for symptomatic fistulas and for abscess drainage. Crohn's disease is recurrent, and most patients require subsequent operations within 5 to 10 years.

REFERENCES

Hanauer SB: Inflammatory bowel disease. N Engl J Med 1996; 334: 841–848.

Pearson DC, May GR, Fick GH, et al: Azathioprine and 6-mercaptopurine in Crohn's disease: A meta-analysis. Ann Intern Med 1995; 122:132–142.

Sandborn WJ: A review of immune modulator therapy for inflammatory bowel disease. Am J Gastroenterol 1996; 91:423.

Sutherland LR, May GR, Shaffer EA: Sulfasalazine revisited: A meta-analysis of 5-aminisalicylic acid in the treatment of ulcerative colitis. Ann Intern Med 1993; 118:540–549.

Targan SR, Hanauer SB, van Deventer SJH, et al: A short-term study of chimeric monoclonal antibody cA2 to tumor necrosis alpha for Crohn's disease. N Engl J Med 1997; 337:1029–1035.

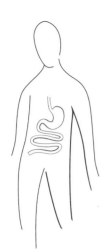

37

NEOPLASMS OF THE GASTROINTESTINAL TRACT

Carol A. Burke

Esophageal Carcinoma

Carcinoma of the esophagus is one of the most lethal of all cancers. The lack of early symptoms and serosal barrier, as well as the rich, bidirectional esophageal lymphatic flow, results in advanced disease by the time of diagnosis. Traditionally, squamous cell carcinoma (SCC) constituted 95% of all esophageal carcinomas. Since 1980, the incidence of adenocarcinoma of the esophagus has rapidly increased and represents up to 50% of newly diagnosed cases of esophageal carcinoma. The epidemiology of SCC differs from that of adenocarcinoma of the esophagus, but the symptoms, treatments, and prognoses are similar.

INCIDENCE AND EPIDEMIOLOGY

The American Cancer Society estimated that 12,300 new cases of esophageal cancer and 11,900 esophageal cancer deaths would occur in the United States in 1998. Esophageal cancer is rare among people less than 40 years of age, and the incidence increases with each subsequent decade. The incidence of SCC varies dramatically throughout the world: as low as 5 per 100,000 in the United States to over 700 per 100,000 in certain provinces in China. Men are more often affected than are women, and African-Americans have a fivefold increase in incidence. The cause of SCC is unknown, but environmental, dietary, and local esophageal factors have been implicated. Smoking and alcohol abuse are primary risk factors for SCC and for head and neck cancers in the United States. The combination of heavy smoking and alcohol ingestion may increase the risk of cancer 44-fold. Lye strictures, radiation injury, Plummer-Vinson syndrome, achalasia, tylosis, and celiac disease are also associated with an increased risk of SCC of the esopha-

gus. Adenocarcinoma of the esophagus is primarily a disease of white men; the white-to-black ratio is 4:1, and the male-to-female ratio is 7:1. The only known risk factor for adenocarcinoma is Barrett's esophagus, the replacement of the normal squamous mucosa lining the esophagus with intestinal epithelium. The only known cause of Barrett's esophagus is severe chronic gastroesophageal reflux disease. It is presumed that intestinal metaplasia progresses to low-grade dysplasia and variably to high-grade dysplasia and finally adenocarcinoma. Nearly 90% of adenocarcinomas develop in the distal esophagus, whereas 50% of SCCs occur in the middle third, and the other 50% are evenly distributed in the proximal and distal esophagus.

CLINICAL PRESENTATION

Early and curable esophageal carcinoma is frequently asymptomatic and detected serendipitously. The presence of symptoms heralds an advanced and most often incurable stage of disease. Under careful questioning, most patients will have had symptoms for a few months before they sought medical attention. Dysphagia is the most common symptom of esophageal carcinoma. It occurs when the esophageal lumen has been compromised by approximately 75% of its normal diameter. Difficulty swallowing solid foods precedes dysphagia to liquids. With complete obstruction, regurgitation, aspiration, and cough or pneumonia may occur. Pulmonary symptoms may also occur if a tracheoesophageal fistula is present. Patients uniformly have weight loss and anorexia. Chest pain, hiccups, or hoarseness indicate involvement of adjacent structures such as the mediastinum, diaphragm, and recurrent laryngeal nerve, respectively. If gastrointestinal bleeding occurs, it is often occult or associated with an iron deficiency anemia. Life-threatening gastrointestinal hemorrhage can occur if the tumor has invaded major vessels. Clubbing of the nails and paraneoplastic syndromes, such as hypercalcemia and Cushing's syndrome, are rarely seen.

DIAGNOSIS

Dysphagia should be evaluated by upper endoscopy or a double-contrast esophageal barium study. Esophageal carcinoma may appear as a plaque, an ulcer, a stricture, or a mass. The advantage of endoscopy includes the opportunity to obtain tissue of the cancer, either by biopsy or brush cytologic study. Computed tomographic scanning of the chest and abdomen is performed to detect invasion of local structures and metastases to the lung and liver. Endoscopic ultrasonography with its ability to image the esophageal wall as a five-layer structure that correlates with histologic layers, is more accurate than computed tomography for staging tumor depth, local invasion, and regional node involvement.

THERAPY

Stage is the most important prognostic factor for the survival of patients with esophageal cancer and influences the treatment options. Staging is based on the TNM classification system (Table 37–1). Only stage I (T1, N0, M0) and stage IIA (T2 or T3, N0, M0) lesions are potentially curable by surgery. In spite of significant reductions in the rate of operative mortality to 10% to 15% in experienced centers, the survival rate remains 25% at 1 year and 10% at 5 years after resection for surgical cure. Patients with locally advanced or regional nodal disease should be offered concurrent chemoradiotherapy, which has been shown to improve survival in comparison with radiotherapy alone. Patients with metastatic disease should be considered for palliative treatment of dysphagia. Local treatment with endoscopic methods (such as malignant stricture dilation), placement of an endoprosthesis (stent), and tumor ablation by laser or photodynamic therapy are often the methods of choice for rapid palliation. Palliative radiotherapy may provide significant partial, albeit short-term, relief of dysphagia.

Gastric Carcinoma

Gastric carcinoma is one of the leading causes of cancer-related deaths worldwide. For unknown reasons, the incidence of gastric cancer has declined dramatically in the United States since 1950. Unfortunately, gastric cancer is often advanced at the time of diagnosis; the 5-year survival rate is 5% to 15%.

INCIDENCE AND EPIDEMIOLOGY

More than 90% of gastric cancers are adenocarcinomas. The incidence of gastric cancer varies widely throughout the world. The incidence rate in America is 9 per 100,000, whereas it exceeds 100 per 100,000 in some areas in Japan. Migrant studies have shown a reduction in the incidence of the disease when populations move to an area of lower endemicity. The American Cancer Society estimated that there would be 22,600 new cases of gastric carcinoma and 13,700 cancer related deaths in Americans in 1998. Males in nonwhite ethnic groups, including African-Americans, Asians, Pacific Islanders, Native Americans, and Hispanic minorities, are affected twice as commonly as women and white men. The mean age at diagnosis is 63 years. Low socioeconomic status, improper food storage, and other dietary and local gastric factors are associated with the disease. Dietary factors include deficiencies in fats, protein, and vitamins A and C and excesses in salted meat/fish and nitrates. Atrophic gastritis, postgastrectomy states, achlorhydria, and pernicious anemia are associated with an increased incidence. The World Health Organization has classified *Helicobacter pylori* as a carcinogen and epidemiologically linked to gastric adenocarcinoma (Fig. 37–1). However, only a small proportion of patients infected with *H. pylori* develop gastric adenocarcinoma.

Gastric lymphomas account for fewer than 5% of primary gastric malignancies. The stomach is the most common site of extranodal non-Hodgkin's lymphoma, but Hodgkin's lymphoma of the stomach is rare. Gastric mucosa-associated lymphoid tissue (MALT) lymphomas are associated with *H. pylori* infection in 90% of cases and are reported to regress in 60% to 70% of cases after eradication of *H. pylori*.

CLINICAL PRESENTATION

The location, size, and growth pattern of gastric cancers may influence the presenting symptoms. Abdominal discomfort is the most frequent symptom; however, early satiety, nausea, and vomiting may occur, especially with

TABLE 37–1 TNM Classification of Esophageal Carcinoma

Primary Tumor (T)	
TX	Primary tumor cannot be assessed
T0	No evidence of primary tumor
T1S	Carcinoma in situ
T1	Tumor invades lamina propria or submucosa
T2	Tumor invades muscularis propria
T3	Tumor invades adventitia
T4	Tumor invades adjacent structures
Regional Nodes (N)	
NX	Regional lymph nodes cannot be assessed
N0	No regional lymph node metastasis
N1	Regional lymph node metastasis
Metastases (M)	
MX	Distant metastasis cannot be assessed
M0	No distant metastasis
M1	Distant metastases

Used with the permission of the American Joint Committee on Cancer (AJCC ®), Chicago, Illinois. The original source for this material is the AJCC Cancer Staging Manual, 5th ed. Philadelphia: Lippincott-Raven, 1997.

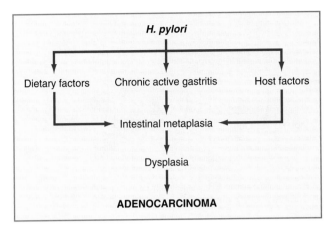

FIGURE 37–1   Model for the development of gastric adenocarcinoma.

gastric outlet obstruction. Gastrointestinal bleeding may manifest as iron deficiency anemia, occult bleeding, or frank upper gastrointestinal hemorrhage. Anorexia and weight loss often accompany other symptoms. The signs of metastatic disease, which may be found on physical examination and signify incurability, include a Virchow (left supraclavicular) node, a Blumer shelf (mass in the perirectal pouch, found on digital rectal examination), and a Krukenberg tumor (metastasis to the ovaries). A variety of paraneoplastic syndromes have been associated with gastric adenocarcinoma and warrant an investigation for a gastrointestinal malignancy. They include Trousseau's syndrome (thrombosis), acanthosis nigricans (pigmented dermal lesions), membranous nephropathy, microangiopathic hemolytic anemia, Leser-Trélat sign (seborrheic keratosis), and dermatomyositis.

DIAGNOSIS

The diagnostic tests for gastric carcinoma include double-contrast upper gastrointestinal radiography or endoscopy. Lesions detected on barium study require endoscopic biopsy and cytologic study for histologic evaluation. Gastric carcinomas may appear as ulcers, masses, enlarged gastric folds, or an infiltrative process with a nondistensible stomach wall (linitis plastica). The accuracy of endoscopic ultrasonography is 90% for determining the depth of invasion and 80% for predicting regional node involvement. Computed tomographic scanning of the chest and abdomen may detect metastases in the lung and liver but is otherwise poor for staging. Laparoscopy is increasingly being used for staging and determination of resectability with high accuracy.

THERAPY

The standard treatment of gastric cancer is complete surgical resection with removal of all gross and microscopic disease. The postoperative local-regional recurrence rate remains 80%. In the United States, up to two thirds of patients present with advanced disease, stages III to IV, with a survival rate of less than 5%. In these patients, palliative resection may be performed to prevent obstruction or treat bleeding. Chemotherapy, radiation, and endoscopy have proved neither curative nor of palliative benefit in gastric carcinoma.

Colorectal Polyps and Carcinoma

Carcinoma of the colon and rectum is the second most common cancer and the second most common cause of cancer deaths in American men and women. There are more than 130,000 new cases and 46,000 cancer-related deaths annually. The lifetime risk of developing invasive colorectal cancer is 6%. Since 1990, use of colorectal cancer screening with annual fecal occult blood testing and flexible sigmoidoscopy, as well as endoscopic polypectomy, has resulted in a decrease in colorectal cancer mortality through the detection of asymptomatic adenomas and early-stage cancers.

INCIDENCE AND EPIDEMIOLOGY

The majority of colorectal cancers are believed to arise from a benign neoplasm called an "adenoma" or "adenomatous" polyp (Table 37–2). Adenomas are seen in up to 40% of patients over the age of 60. Fortunately, only a minority of adenomas progress to colorectal cancer. It is unknown how long an adenoma takes to develop into an invasive cancer, but data from multiple observational studies suggest 10 years. Part of the molecular biology of colorectal carcinoma has been elucidated (Fig. 37–2). *Acquired* mutations in the oncogene *kras* (chromosome 12p) and in the tumor supressor genes APC (chromosome 5q), p53 (chromosome 17p), and DCC (chromosome 18q) have been identified in colorectal neoplasia. The frequency and number of mutations increase as adenomas progress in size and dysplasia to colorectal cancer. Dominantly *inherited* mutations in the "mismatch repair genes" that control DNA repair lead to hereditary nonpolyposis colorectal cancer (HNPCC), and those in the tumor supressor gene APC lead to familial adenomatous polyposis (FAP). In addition to somatic and germline genetic mutations, multiple epidemiologic studies have shown that dietary factors are associated with colorectal carcinogenesis. Populations

TABLE 37–2   Histologic Classification of Colon Polyps

Neoplastic	Non-neoplastic
Benign	Hyperplastic
Adenoma	Hamartoma
Tubular	Lymphoid aggregate
Tubulovillous	Inflammatory or pseudopolyps
Villous	
Malignant	
Carcinoma-in-situ	
Invasive adenocarcinoma	

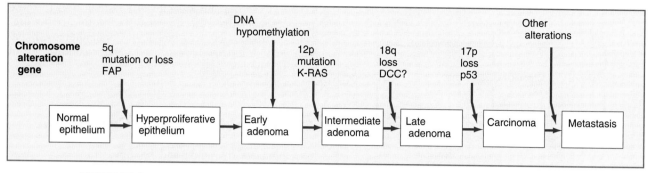

FIGURE 37–2   A genetic model for colorectal tumorigenesis. (From Fearon ER, Vogelstein B: A genetic model for colorectal tumorigenesis [review]. Cell 1990; 61:759–767. Copyright by Cell Press.)

that consume a diet low in fiber, fruits, and vegetables but high in fat, especially that from red meat, have a higher incidence of colorectal neoplasia.

The risk for adenomatous polyps and cancer is low in persons younger than 40 years and increases with age to a peak in the seventh and eighth decades. Colorectal cancer does not appear to have a gender or racial predilection, although African-Americans have a slightly higher incidence of stage IV disease. Only 25% of persons in whom colorectal cancer develops have a defined risk factor (Table 37–3).

CLINICAL PRESENTATION

The majority of colorectal neoplasms are asymptomatic until advanced. Gastrointestinal blood loss is the most common symptom and may include fecal occult blood, hematochezia, or unexplained iron deficiency anemia. Other symptoms include abdominal pain from obstruction or invasion, change in bowel habits, or unexplained anorexia or weight loss.

DIAGNOSIS

All patients with symptoms suggestive of colorectal neoplasia should undergo an evaluation of the colon by colonoscopy or by flexible sigmoidoscopy and air-contrast barium enema study. Populations with known risk factors for colorectal cancer should undergo periodic total colonic surveillance examinations based upon na-

TABLE 37–3   Risk Factors for Colorectal Cancer

Personal history of adenomatous polyps or colorectal cancer
Familial adenomatous polyposis (FAP)/Gardner's syndrome
Hereditary nonpolyposis colon cancer (HNPCC)
   Three relatives with colorectal cancer, one a first-degree relative of the other two
   Two generations affected
   One cancer detected at less than age 50 years
Ulcerative colitis or Crohn's colitis
First-degree relative with colon cancer or adenomatous polyps
Personal history of breast, ovarian, or uterine cancer

tional recommendations. Screening is recommended for asymptomatic, average-risk patients beginning at age 50 (Table 37–4). Approximately 50% of colorectal adenomas and cancers are located between the rectum and splenic flexure; however, in women and in elderly persons, a greater percentage are located in the proximal colon. Colorectal cancers may arise in sessile (flat) or pedunculated (on a stalk) polyps, or they may appear as a stricture, a fungating mass, or an ulcerated mass. Colonoscopy has greater accuracy than barium enema study in the detection of small polyps and early cancers, as well as the ability to remove neoplasms or biopsy lesions at the time of the examination. Lesions detected on barium enema study necessitate colonoscopic evaluation. Computed tomographic scanning of the abdomen and pelvis is used preoperatively to assess the extent of metastatic disease. Endoscopic ultrasonography is used for the preoperative staging of rectal cancer. Carcinoembryonic antigen (CEA) level is measured preoperatively for a baseline value and, if elevated, monitored to detect tumor recurrence postoperatively.

THERAPY

The rate of survival of patients with colorectal carcinoma is based on the stage of disease (Table 37–5). Unfortunately, 45% of patients first come to medical attention with stage III or IV disease. Surgery alone is curative for early-stage colorectal cancers. Surgery and adjuvant chemotherapy with 5-fluorouracil and leucovorin are recommended for stage III colon cancer. For patients with stage II and III rectal cancer, the combination of postoperative radiation and 5-fluorouracil has been found to significantly reduce the recurrence rate, cancer-related deaths, and overall mortality.

The Polyposis Syndromes

The rare, dominantly inherited disorders that result in multiple polyps throughout the gastrointestinal tract and impart an increased risk of gastrointestinal cancer include FAP and Peutz-Jeghers syndrome.

In FAP, hundreds to thousands of colonic adenomas

TABLE 37-4 **American Cancer Society Recommendations for Colorectal Cancer Screening**

Risk	Age to Begin	Diagnostic Option	Interval
Average	50 years	Fecal occult blood test	Annual
		Flexible sigmoidoscopy	Every 5 years
		Double-contrast barium enema*	Every 5–10 years
		Colonoscopy	Every 10 years

* Flexible sigmoidoscopy is recommended with double-contrast barium enema.
From Byers T, Levin B, Rothenberger D, et al: American Cancer Society guidelines for screening and surveillance for early detection of colorectal polyps and cancer: Update 1997. CA Cancer J Clin 1997; 47:154–160.

develop by the second decade of life. Colon cancer develops in all patients by age 40 unless prophylactic colectomy is performed. Duodenal adenomas are common and confer a significant risk of periampullary cancer. Gardner's syndrome is a phenotypic variant of FAP. Benign soft tissue tumors, osteomas, dental abnormalities, desmoid tumors, and congenital hypertrophy of the retinal pigmented epithelium may be found in addition to the colonic and duodenal adenomas.

Peutz-Jeghers syndrome manifests as gastrointestinal polyposis and mucocutaneous pigmentation. The causative gene mutation is currently being sought. Pigmented macules may be found on the buccal mucosa, lips, plantar surfaces of the feet, and dorsa of hands. Polyps may be located throughout the gastrointestinal tract. In contrast to the adenomatous polyps found in FAP, Peutz-Jeghers polyps are non-neoplastic hamartomas. Patients with Peutz-Jeghers syndrome have an increased risk of colonic and small bowel carcinoma. The commonest presenting features are bleeding and small bowel obstruction or intussusception secondary to the small bowel tumors.

TABLE 37-5 **Survival and Comparison of Dukes' and TNM Staging**

Dukes'	TNM Stage	5-Year Survival Rate
A	I	90%
B	II	75%
C	III	35%–60%
D	IV	<10%

Carcinoid Tumors

The overall incidence of carcinoid tumors in the United States is estimated at 1 to 2 cases per 100,000 people. The most common sites, in descending order of frequency, are the appendix, ileum, rectum, bronchi, stomach, and colon.

Carcinoid tumors arise from neuroendocrine cells and contain a variety of secretory granules containing various hormones and biogenic amines. Serotonin is synthesized from 5-hydroxytryptophan and metabolized in the liver to 5-hydroxyindoleacetic acid (5-HIAA), which is biologically inert and secreted in the urine. The release of serotonin and other vasoactive substances into the systemic circulation is thought to cause the carcinoid syndrome. Therefore, carcinoid metastases in the liver or other sites that drain into systemic veins may be associated with the carcinoid syndrome, as may primary carcinoids in the ovary or bronchus. The symptoms include episodic flushing, wheezing, diarrhea, right-sided valvular heart disease, and, potentially, vasomotor collapse.

Most carcinoids are indolent; however, the malignant potential is variable and appears to be related to the site and, often, the size of the primary tumor. Surgical resection is the only curative treatment for carcinoid tumors. Somatostatin analogues are highly effective in the management of the symptoms of carcinoid syndrome.

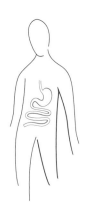

38

DISEASES OF THE PANCREAS

Darwin L. Conwell

Anatomy and Physiology

The pancreas is a retroperitoneal organ (Fig. 38–1), approximately 12 to 20 cm in length, that weighs between 70 and 120 g. The head of the pancreas is nestled in the C loop of the duodenum, and the tail extends obliquely posterior to the stomach toward the hilum of the spleen. The pancreas has a rich blood supply provided by branches of the celiac, superior mesenteric, and splenic arteries. Venous drainage is through the hepatic portal system. The pancreas has both sympathetic and parasympathetic efferent fibers supplied by the vagus and splenic nerves through the hepatic and celiac plexus.

PANCREATIC ACINUS

The functional unit of the pancreas is the *pancreatic acinus* (Fig. 38–2). It is composed of both acinar and ductal epithelial cells. The *acinar cells* have a rich and highly specialized intracellular matrix for the synthesis, storage, and secretion of large amounts of proteins, mainly in the form of precursor digestive enzymes. Enzymes secreted in an active form include lipase, amylase, and ribonuclease. The *ductal cells* primarily secrete water and electrolytes, which decrease the viscosity of the protein-rich acinar secretions and alkalinize gastric contents emptied into the duodenum. The concentrations of the two principal anions, namely, bicarbonate and chloride, vary reciprocally (Fig. 38–3). At maximal stimulation, bicarbonate-rich fluid neutralizes hydrochloric acid entering the second portion of the duodenum from the stomach and raises the intraduodenal pH to levels at which the pancreatic enzymes become catalytically active (pH ranges from >3.5 to 4). Inactive enzymes secreted into the duodenum are converted to an active form by enterokinase secreted from small bowel enterocytes. Enterokinase converts trypsinogen to tryp-sin. Trypsin then converts all the other proenzymes to their active form within the duodenum (Fig. 38–4).

PHASES OF PANCREATIC SECRETION

The three phases of pancreatic secretion are cephalic, gastric, and intestinal, and they account for 10%, 25%, and 50% to 75% of pancreatic secretion, respectively. The *cephalic phase* is stimulated by the thought, sight, taste, or smell of food through vagal cholinergic fibers. The *gastric phase* is in response to gastric distention, which is also mediated by vagal cholinergic reflexes. The *intestinal phase* provides the major component of pancreatic secretion and is primarily regulated by the release of the intestinal hormones secretin and cholecystokinin. These two hormones are found in the proximal duodenal enterocytes. *Secretin* is responsible for bicarbonate and water secretion from the pancreatic ductal cells. *Cholecystokinin* is responsible for protein enzyme secretion from the pancreatic acinar cells and also mediates secretin-stimulated electrolyte secretion from ductal epithelial cells. When maximally stimulated, the normal pancreas may secrete 7 L or less of fluid a day. A negative feedback loop exists whereby increased entero-duodenal protease activity (i.e., trypsin) suppresses circulating cholecystokinin levels and thus decreases pancreatic secretion. Supplemental pancreatic enzymes (proteases) are given to decrease cholecystokinin-mediated pancreatic secretion, an approach that alleviates pain in some patients with chronic pancreatitis.

STUDIES OF PANCREATIC STRUCTURE AND FUNCTION

Invasive and noninvasive techniques have been developed to study pancreatic physiology, parenchyma, and duct morphology. These methods are often needed in evaluating patients with pancreatic disease. Endoscopic retrograde cholangiopancreatography (ERCP) and endoscopic ultrasonography are invasive diagnostic and thera-

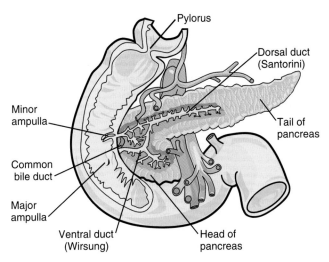

FIGURE 38-1 Normal anatomy of the pancreas.

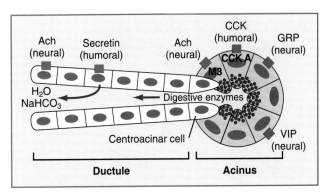

FIGURE 38-2 Functional unit of the exocrine pancreas. Acetylcholine (Ach), secretin, cholecystokinin (CCK), gastrin-releasing peptide (GRP), and vasoactive intestinal peptide (VIP) act as neural and humoral agents to activate the ductule or the acinus. Ach acts through an M3 receptor, and CCK acts through a CCK-A receptor. (Adapted from Pandol SJ, Raybould HE: The integrated response to a meal. *In* The Undergraduate Teaching Project in Gastroenterology and Liver Disease, Unit 24. Bethesda, MD: American Gastroenterological Association, 1995.)

peutic procedures that allow the study of pancreatic duct parenchyma and duct morphology. The major limitation of ERCP is the development of procedure-related acute pancreatitis in 5% to 7% of patients. Computed tomography (CT), transabdominal ultrasonography, and magnetic resonance imaging are noninvasive methods of studying the pancreas that do not carry the risk of pancreatitis. Magnetic resonance cholangiopancreatography is a noninvasive diagnostic imaging modality that provides visualization of the pancreatic and biliary systems with images similar to those seen by ERCP.

The current standard for studying pancreatic physiology and secretory reserve is the *secretin test*. This test involves placement of a drainage tube in the duodenum for aspiration of pancreatic fluid after secretin stimulation. This is the most sensitive test (>95%) for documenting pancreatic insufficiency. Peak bicarbonate levels of less than 80 mEq/L are diagnostic of chronic pancreatitis. This quantitative measure of pancreatic secretion and enzyme activity is primarily performed in patients

with chronic abdominal pain in whom the diagnosis of chronic pancreatitis is suspected and in whom results of imaging studies are negative or equivocal. The secretin test is available only at specialized research centers, it is labor intensive to perform, and it is uncomfortable for patients. Numerous less invasive tests have been developed, but they fall short of the accuracy of the secretin test, especially in the diagnosis of early chronic pancreatitis.

The *serum trypsinogen determination* has a high specificity of 98% but a variable sensitivity ranging from 20% to 80%. The *72-hour fecal fat determination* is the most definitive test to document steatorrhea (fecal fat >7 g/24 hours). However, pancreatic steatorrhea does not occur until more than 90% of pancreatic function is lost; therefore, this test is insensitive in the evaluation of early chronic pancreatitis.

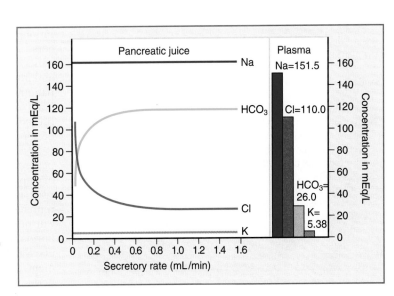

FIGURE 38-3 Relation between pancreatic juice ion concentrations and secretory flow rate. (Adapted from Bro-Rasmussen F, et al: The composition of pancreatic juice as compared to sweat, parotid saliva and tears. Acta Physiol Scand 1956; 37:97.)

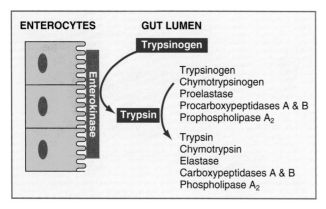

FIGURE 38–4 Mechanism of proenzyme activation in the intestinal lumen. (Adapted from Solomon TE: Exocrine pancreas: Pancreatitis. *In* The Undergraduate Teaching Project in Gastroenterology and Liver Disease, Unit 24. Bethesda, MD: American Gastroenterological Association, 1984.)

Acute Pancreatitis

Acute pancreatitis is an inflammatory disorder of the pancreas associated with edema, various amounts of autodigestion, necrosis, and hemorrhage. Clinically, acute pancreatitis is defined by a typical symptom complex of abdominal pain, nausea, and vomiting.

ETIOLOGY AND PATHOGENESIS

Gallstones (40%) and alcohol (35%) account for most cases of acute pancreatitis. Ten to 15% of cases are idiopathic, and miscellaneous causes account for 10% of cases (Table 38–1). The pathophysiology of acute pancreatitis in experimental models has been extensively studied. Disruption in the normal separation of lysosomal and pancreatic enzymes appears to result in the

TABLE 38–1   Conditions Associated with Acute Pancreatitis

Ethanol abuse*
Cholelithiasis
Abdominal trauma*
Abdominal surgery
Hypercalcemia
Hyperlipidemia
Drugs: anticonvulsant (valproic acid), antibiotics (sulfonamides, tetracycline), antimetabolite (6-mercaptopurine), diuretics (hydrochlorothiazide, furosemide)
Viral infections: mumps, coxsackie, hepatitis, others
Scorpion bite
Carcinoma of the pancreas
Pancreas divisum*
Peptic ulcer with posterior penetration
Hereditary (familial) pancreatitis*
Endoscopic retrograde cholangiopancreatography
Hypoperfusion (vasculitis)

* Associated with chronic pancreatitis.

formation of condensing vacuoles within the acinar cell. This exposure of pancreatic proenzymes to lysosomal enzymes activates trypsinogen and leads to premature activation of other pancreatic enzymes. The result is pancreatic autodigestion and the potential for profound systemic complications once activated enzymes are leaked into the blood stream.

CLINICAL MANIFESTATIONS

Classic symptoms of acute pancreatitis include acute abdominal pain, nausea, and vomiting. Physical examination may reveal reduced bowel sounds secondary to ileus, jaundice resulting from gallstones, abdominal tenderness, fever, or tachycardia. Acute injury to the pancreas results in leakage of pancreatic enzymes into the blood stream (Fig. 38–5). This condition is detected as an increase in serum amylase and/or lipase concentrations. Amylase and lipase levels greater than two to three times normal levels suggest acute pancreatitis. Laboratory features may include an elevated white blood cell count, hyperbilirubinemia, hypoglycemia, hypocalcemia, and mild elevations in serum alanine aminotransferase and alkaline phosphatase. Bilirubin and serum alanine aminotransferase levels twice normal strongly suggest gallstone disease. Other less common manifestations resulting from local peripancreatic inflammation include (1) left-sided pleural effusion, (2) discoloration of the flanks (Grey Turner's sign) or around the umbilicus (Cullen's sign), (3) ascites, (4) jaundice from impingement of the common bile duct, and (5) an epigastric mass from a pseudocyst. Systemic effects of pancreatic enzymes released into the blood stream include (1) respiratory distress syndrome, (2) renal failure, and (3) subcutaneous fat necrosis.

DIAGNOSIS

The diagnosis of acute pancreatitis is based on clinical findings of abdominal pain with associated nausea and vomiting and elevations of the serum amylase and lipase levels. The physician should consider other causes of hyperamylasemia such as small bowel obstruction, perforation, infarction of the bowel, perforated duodenal ulcers, salpingitis, choledocholithiasis, and ectopic pregnancy during an evaluation of patients with acute abdominal pain. The imaging modality of choice when a patient presents with acute pancreatitis is an ultrasound scan of the right upper quadrant. This study shows the presence or absence of gallstone disease and provides noninvasive imaging of the pancreatic head. A CT scan is recommended only for those patients with severe pancreatitis who are not improving after 48 to 72 hours of supportive therapy. The serum amylase level usually rises rapidly, as does the serum lipase level, and may remain elevated for 3 to 5 days. The serum lipase level can be elevated after the serum amylase has returned to normal. The degree of elevation of pancreatic enzymes does not correlate with severity of disease. Measurement of urinary clearance of amylase is of little diagnostic help, except in the diagnosis of macroamylasemia.

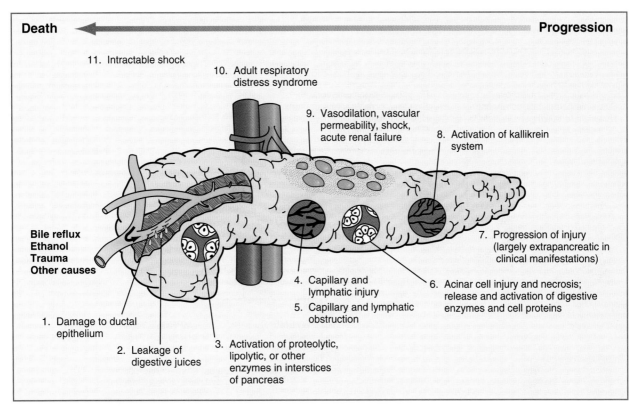

Death ← **Progression**

11. Intractable shock

10. Adult respiratory distress syndrome

9. Vasodilation, vascular permeability, shock, acute renal failure

8. Activation of kallikrein system

Bile reflux
Ethanol
Trauma
Other causes

7. Progression of injury (largely extrapancreatic in clinical manifestations)

4. Capillary and lymphatic injury

5. Capillary and lymphatic obstruction

6. Acinar cell injury and necrosis; release and activation of digestive enzymes and cell proteins

1. Damage to ductal epithelium

2. Leakage of digestive juices

3. Activation of proteolytic, lipolytic, or other enzymes in interstices of pancreas

FIGURE 38–5 The pathophysiology of acute pancreatitis is not fully understood, but as this schematic illustration implies, a cascade of events seems likely, beginning with the release of toxic substances into the parenchyma and ending with shock and death. Damage to the ductal epithelium or acinar cell injury may result from bile reflux, increased intraductal pressure, alcohol, or trauma. (Adapted from Grendell JH: The pancreas. *In* Smith LH Jr, Thier SO [eds]: Pathophysiology: The Biological Principles of Disease, 2nd ed. Philadelphia: WB Saunders, 1985, p 1228.)

TREATMENT AND PROGNOSIS

The treatment of acute pancreatitis is supportive, with intravenous fluids, intake of nothing by mouth, relief of pain with analgesics, nutritional support, and close clinical observation. In general, the mortality rate of acute pancreatitis is approximately 10%. An estimated 90% of patients recover within the first 2 weeks. Prognosis can be determined at the time of admission and 48 hours later using the Ranson criteria (Table 38–2). Patients with fewer than three criteria on admission have a mortality rate of less than 1%. Mortality increases to 40% when five or six signs are present, and it increases to 100% when seven or more signs are positive. After 48 hours of admission, the Ranson criteria are no longer valid, and the Apache II score is more reliable. An Apache II score of 8 or more is consistent with severe acute pancreatitis.

A dynamic CT scan is indicated for those patients who have severe pancreatitis (Ranson score, >3; Apache II score, >8) after 48 to 72 hours, to assess for pancreatic necrosis (Fig. 38–6). Uniform enhancement implies an intact microcirculation and suggests that the pancreatic injury is interstitial. Areas of nonenhancement indicate disruption of pancreatic microcirculation and strongly suggest pancreatic necrosis.

The distinction between interstitial and necrotic acute pancreatitis has important prognostic implications. The infection rate in interstitial pancreatitis is less than 1%, whereas the rate of infection in necrotizing pancreatitis

TABLE 38–2 Signs Used to Assess Severity of Acute Pancreatitis

At Time of Admission or Diagnosis
Age >55 yr
White blood cell count >16,000/mm³
Blood glucose >200 mg/dL
LDH >2× normal
ALT >6× normal
During Initial 48 hr
Decrease in hematocrit >10%
Serum calcium <8 mg/dL
Increase in blood urea nitrogen >5 mg/dL
Arterial Po₂ <60 mm Hg
Base deficit >4 mEq/L
Estimated fluid sequestration >600 mL

ALT = alanine aminotransferase; LDH = lactate dehydrogenase.
Modified from Ranson JH, Rifkind KM, Turner JW: Prognostic signs and nonoperative peritoneal lavage in acute pancreatitis. Surg Gynecol Obstet 1976; 43:209–219. By permission of Surgery, Gynecology and Obstetrics.

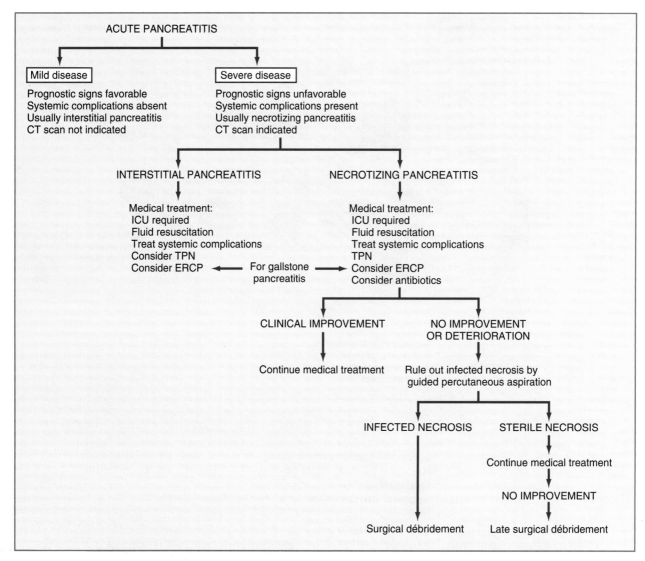

FIGURE 38–6 Therapeutic algorithm for evaluating acute pancreatitis. CT = computed tomography; ERCP = endoscopic retrograde colangiopancreatography; ICU = intensive care unit; TPN = total parenteral nutrition. (From Banks PA: Acute and chronic pancreatitis. *In* Feldman M, Scharschmidt BF, Sleisenger MH [eds]: Sleisenger and Fordtran's Gastrointestinal and Liver Disease: Pathophysiology/Diagnosis/Management, 6th ed. Philadelphia: WB Saunders, 1998, p 833.)

may be as much as 50%. Furthermore, infection with necrosis can have a mortality rate approaching 30%. Because of this significant infection rate and mortality, patients with areas of necrosis require aggressive management. Percutaneous aspiration and Gram's stain is recommended whenever necrosis is seen on a CT scan. A positive Gram stain (infected necrosis) requires surgical debridement. Patients with negative Gram's stains (sterile necrosis) can be followed with supportive therapy. The mortality rate of sterile necrosis can still be 10% or more.

COMPLICATIONS

Acute pancreatitis can have local and systemic complications. *Local complications* include the development of pancreatic pseudocyst, pancreatic abscess, and pancre-

atic ascites. Treatment of symptomatic pancreatic pseudocysts and abscesses requires radiographic, endoscopic, or surgical drainage. Asymptomatic pseudocysts should be followed. Pancreatic ascites is the result of duct disruption and is best treated with total parenteral nutrition, endoscopic stenting, and subcutaneous octreotide administration. Surgical intervention may be needed if this conservative approach is unsuccessful.

Systemic complications include renal failure, acute respiratory distress syndrome, gastrointestinal bleeding, and septic shock. Systemic complications are best managed in an intensive care unit with aggressive fluid administration and hemodynamic monitoring. Emergency ERCP for removal of impacted gallstones or establishment of biliary drainage is indicated for patients with evidence of biliary sepsis. This procedure should be followed by elective cholecystectomy.

Chronic Pancreatitis

Chronic pancreatitis represents a slowly progressive destruction of the pancreatic acinar cells with varying degrees of inflammation, fibrosis, and morphologic changes within the pancreatic ducts. Alcohol consumption, the most common cause, accounts for 70% of cases, and another 20% of cases are idiopathic. Other miscellaneous causes (10%) include trauma, pancreas divisum, cystic fibrosis, and metabolic disturbances such as hypercalcemia and hypertrygliceridemia. Chronic pancreatitis can also be inherited as an autosomal dominant disorder (i.e., hereditary pancreatitis).

ETIOLOGY AND PATHOGENESIS

The underlying physiology of chronic alcoholic pancreatitis involves basal hypersecretion of pancreatic proteins with a concomitant decrease of protease inhibitors. This process changes the biochemical composition of the pancreatic juice and predisposes patients to the formation of protein plugs and pancreatic stones. Blockages of small ducts result in premature activation of pancreatic enzymes, with the development of acute pancreatitis that eventually causes permanent structural damage to the gland. The discovery of the gene that causes hereditary pancreatitis shed further insight into the mechanisms of pancreatic injury. In *hereditary pancreatitis,* an Arg-His substitution at residue 117 of the cationic trypsinogen gene produces a mutant trypsin that cannot be shut down by trypsin inhibitor. This process results in unchecked activation of pancreatic enzymes within the acinar cell that leads to pancreatic injury.

CLINICAL MANIFESTATIONS

The most common signs and symptoms of chronic pancreatitis are abdominal pain, weight loss, diabetes, and steatorrhea. Other manifestations include obstructive jaundice secondary to compression of the distal common bile duct as it progresses through the scarred and fibrotic pancreatic head, chronic pseudocysts, pancreatic ascites, and gastrointestinal bleeding. Gastrointestinal bleeding is usually secondary to gastric varices as a result of splenic vein thrombosis. The etiologic mechanism for pain is controversial, but it may involve inflammation of the pancreas, increased intrapancreatic pressure, neural inflammation, or extrapancreatic causes such as stenosis of the common bile duct and duodenum. The weight loss seen in patients with chronic pancreatitis is usually the result of decreased food intake because of fear of precipitating abdominal pain. Later in the illness, as pancreatic insufficiency progresses, patients manifest malabsorption of ingested nutrients or diabetes with resultant weight loss. This condition usually occurs when more than 90% of the gland has been destroyed.

The diagnosis of chronic pancreatitis is strongly suggested by the patient's history and is confirmed through laboratory tests and imaging studies. The presence of diffuse calcifications throughout the pancreas seen on radiographs, ultrasonograms, or CT scans is diagnostic of chronic pancreatitis (Fig. 38–7). Plain film radiography of the abdomen should be the first diagnostic test performed when pancreatitis is suspected because it is both simple and inexpensive. Ultrasonography and CT scanning have a higher sensitivity, in the range of 70% and 90%, respectively. ERCP is the most sensitive and specific test for diagnosing chronic pancreatitis, but it also has a low but significant rate of procedure-related pancreatitis. ERCP should be reserved for patients in whom the diagnosis cannot be established clearly or for the evaluation of complications (stones, strictures) associated with chronic pancreatitis. Magnetic resonance cholangiopancreatography is a noninvasive diagnostic technique that does not require pancreatic duct cannulation and therefore carries no risk of precipitating acute pancreatitis.

The *pancreatic secretin test,* which directly measures pancreatic bicarbonate secretion, is the standard for diagnosing chronic pancreatitis. It is usually needed only in those patients with suspected chronic pancreatitis in whom results of imaging studies are negative or equivocal.

TREATMENT

The treatment of chronic pancreatitis usually involves control of pain, avoidance of alcohol, and pancreatic enzyme supplementation. Pancreatic enzymes decrease pancreatic secretion and ductal pressure and result in marked pain relief in some patients with chronic pancreatitis. Pancreatic enzymes are also effective in treating pancreatic steatorrhea. Celiac plexus blockade, octreotide, and pancreatic duct stenting are being evalu-

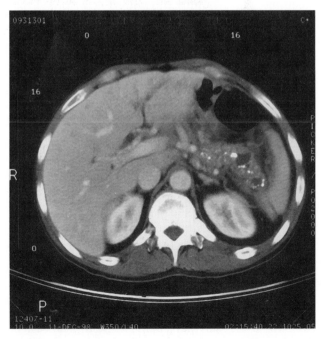

FIGURE 38–7 Computed tomography scan of a patient with calcifications and small pseudocysts in pancreas consistent with chronic pancreatitis.

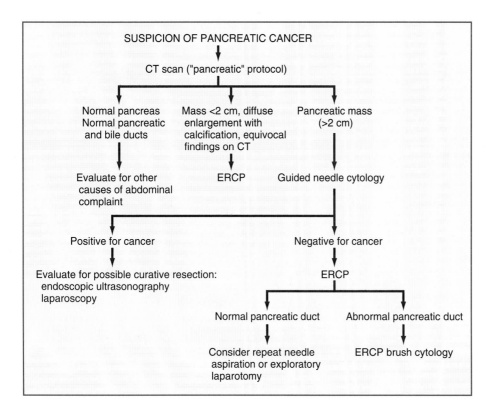

FIGURE 38–8 Diagnostic algorithm for evaluating a patient with suspected pancreatic carcinoma. CT = computed tomography; ERCP = endoscopic retrograde cholangiopancreatography. (From Cello JP: Pancreatic cancer. *In* Feldman M, Scharschmidt BF, Sleisenger MH [eds]: Sleisenger and Fordtran's Gastrointestinal and Liver Disease: Pathophysiology/Diagnosis/Management, 6th ed. Philadelphia: WB Saunders, 1998, p 865.)

ated in controlled studies for their efficacy in the treatment of chronic pancreatic pain. Surgical ductal drainage, usually with lateral pancreaticojejunostomy (Puestow's procedure), may effectively decrease pain in approximately 80% of patients. This procedure is safe and has an operative mortality rate of less than 5%; however, only 50% of patients are free of pain at 5-year follow-up.

COMPLICATIONS

The most common complications of chronic pancreatitis include the development of pancreatic pseudocysts, ascites, and splenic vein thrombosis. Treatment of pancreatic pseudocysts and pancreatic ascites is discussed earlier. Splenic vein thrombosis, a result of peripancreatic inflammation, occurs in 4% of patients and can result in gastrointestinal bleeding from gastric varices. The diagnosis is confirmed by mesenteric angiography, and splenectomy is curative.

Carcinoma of the Pancreas

Carcinoma of the pancreas accounts for approximately 5% of cancer deaths in the United States. Carcinoma of the pancreas is an almost uniformly fatal malignant disease. The 5-year survival is only 1%. More than 90% of these tumors are adenocarcinomas and arise from the ductal cells.

ETIOLOGY AND PATHOGENESIS

Risk factors for developing pancreatic carcinoma include cigarette smoking, a high-fat diet, chronic pancreatitis, hereditary pancreatitis, and industrial exposure to coal tar derivatives. Hereditary pancreatitis carries a fivefold increased risk for development of pancreatic cancer when compared with the general population.

CLINICAL MANIFESTATIONS

The clinical manifestations of pancreatic carcinoma may be nonspecific and are often insidious. The tumor has usually reached an advanced stage by the time of diagnosis. The most common presenting symptoms are epigastric pain and weight loss. The pain is usually constant, with radiation to the back. Because most cancers begin in the pancreatic head, patients may present with obstructive jaundice or a large, palpable gallbladder (Courvoisier's sign). Anorexia, nausea, and vomiting may also occur, along with emotional disturbances. Other, less common presenting symptoms include signs of migratory thrombophlebitis (Trousseau's sign), acute pancreatitis, diabetes, paraneoplastic syndromes (Cushing's syndrome), hypercalcemia, gastrointestinal bleeding, splenic vein thrombosis, and a palpable abdominal mass.

DIAGNOSIS

Pancreatic carcinoma should always be suspected in elderly patients with abdominal pain or new-onset diabetes, depression associated with weight loss, acute pancreatitis without other known risk factors, or obstructive jaundice. When an abdominal mass is identified by a CT scan or ultrasound, fine-needle aspiration biopsy is indicated (Fig. 38–8). Aspiration can be performed with ultrasound or CT guidance. Endoscopic ultrasonography is emerging as a useful diagnostic and therapeutic technique for determining operative resectability and for performing aspiration biopsy. The tumor marker CA 19-9 has a sensitivity of 80% to 90% and a specificity of 85% to 95% in diagnosing pancreatic cancer in patients presenting with signs and symptoms suggestive of pancreatic cancer.

TREATMENT

Surgery offers the only chance for cure. Only 10% of tumors are resectable at the time of diagnosis. The procedure of choice is Whipple's operation when the carcinoma is in the head of the pancreas. The rate of operative mortality is less than 5%. Palliative procedures such as gastrojejunostomy or endoscopic bile duct stenting are undertaken in patients with unresectable or metastatic lesions. Attempts at radiation and chemotherapy have met with little success and only modest improvements in patient survival.

REFERENCES

Conwell DL: Pancreatic diseases. *In* Stoller JK (ed): The Cleveland Clinic Intensive Review of Internal Medicine. Baltimore: Williams & Wilkins, 1998, pp 586–591.

Steer ML: Chronic pancreatitis. N Engl J Med 1995; 332:1482–1490.

Steinberg W: Acute pancreatitis. N Engl J Med 1994; 330:1198–1210.

Warshaw AL: Pancreatic carcinoma. N Engl J Med 1992; 326:455–465.

Whitcomb D: Hereditary pancreatitis is caused by a mutation in the cationic trypsinogen gene. Nat Genet 1996; 14:141–145.

SECTION VII

Diseases of the Liver and Biliary System

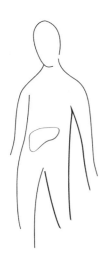

39

LABORATORY TESTS IN LIVER DISEASE

Michael B. Fallon • Brendan M. McGuire
Gary A. Abrams • Miguel R. Arguedas

The liver, the largest internal organ in the body, plays a central role in many essential physiologic processes, including glucose homeostasis, plasma protein synthesis, lipid and lipoprotein synthesis, bile acid synthesis and secretion, and vitamin storage (B_{12}, A, D, E, and K). In addition, it is vital in biotransformation, detoxification, and excretion of a vast array of endogenous and exogenous compounds. The clinical manifestations of liver disease are also varied and may be quite subtle. Clues to the existence, severity, and etiology of liver disease may be obtained from a careful history and physical examination as well as by routine laboratory screening tests. Clinical clues to the presence of liver disease are briefly mentioned here and are discussed more fully in other chapters. The focus in this chapter is on the use of laboratory tests in evaluating liver disease.

Clinical Approach to Liver Disease

Clinical clues to the presence of liver disease are outlined in Table 39–1. Other important historical information to be obtained includes a history of jaundice or liver disease in family members, recent travel, exposure to individuals or animals with liver or parasitic disease, blood transfusions, sexual promiscuity, use of intravenous drugs, and exposure to alcohol, toxins, or drugs.

Laboratory Tests of Liver Function and Disease

Understanding the utility of different types of laboratory tests of the liver is extremely important in characterizing the underlying liver disease. Unlike tests used to assess function of other organ systems (e.g., arterial blood gas, creatinine clearance), many so-called liver function tests do not directly measure hepatic function and may not accurately reflect etiology or severity of the liver disease process. Specific diagnostic tests such as serologic tests for viral, autoimmune, and inherited liver disease are covered in other chapters.

TESTS OF HEPATIC FUNCTION

The great variety of functions performed by the liver has made it difficult to devise a simple, inexpensive, reproducible, and noninvasive test that accurately reflects hepatic capacity for all functions. Instead, currently available tests of liver function are indirect, static measurements of serum levels of compounds that are synthesized, metabolized, and/or excreted by the liver. The liver has a large reserve capacity, and therefore results of "function" tests may remain relatively normal until liver dysfunction is severe.

The most widely available and useful liver function tests are outlined in Table 39–2. The serum albumin level and prothrombin time both reflect the hepatic capacity for protein synthesis. The prothrombin time, which responds rapidly to altered hepatic function because of the short serum half-lives of factors II and VII (hours), is useful as frequently as daily as a marker of hepatic function. However, coexistent vitamin K deficiency must be excluded and/or treated before using the prothrombin time as a measure of hepatic function. In contrast, the serum half-life of albumin is 14 to 20 days, and serum levels fall only with prolonged liver dysfunction. Malnutrition and renal or gastrointestinal losses merit consideration in the setting of significant hypoalbuminemia, especially if the prothrombin time is relatively well preserved.

TABLE 39–1   Clinical Manifestations of Liver Disease

Sign/Symptom	Pathogenesis	Liver Disease
Constitutional		
Fatigue, anorexia, malaise, weight loss	Liver dysfunction	Acute or chronic hepatitis Cirrhosis
Fever	Hepatic inflammation or infection	Liver abscess Alcoholic hepatitis Viral hepatitis
Fetor hepaticus	Sulfur compounds, produced by intestinal bacteria, not cleared by the liver	Acute or chronic liver failure
Cutaneous		
Spider telangiectasias, palmar erythema	Altered estrogen and androgen metabolism with altered vascular physiology	Cirrhosis
Jaundice	Diminished bilirubin excretion	Biliary obstruction Severe liver disease
Pruritus	Uncertain	Biliary obstruction
Xanthomas and xanthelasma	Increased serum cholesterol	Biliary obstruction/cholestasis
Endocrine		
Gynecomastia, testicular atrophy, diminished libido	Altered estrogen and androgen metabolism	Cirrhosis
Hypoglycemia	Decreased glycogen stores and gluconeogenesis	Acute liver failure Alcohol binge with fasting
Gastrointestinal		
Right upper quadrant abdominal pain	Liver swelling, infection	Acute hepatitis Hepatocellular carcinoma Liver congestion (heart failure) Acute cholecystitis Liver abscess
Abdominal swelling	Ascites	Cirrhosis, portal hypertension
Gastrointestinal bleeding	Esophageal varices	Portal hypertension
Hematologic		
Decreased red cells, white cells, and/or platelets	Hypersplenism	Cirrhosis, portal hypertension
Ecchymoses	Decreased synthesis of clotting factors	Liver failure
Neurologic		
Altered sleep pattern, subtle behavioral changes, somnolence, confusion, ataxia, asterixis, obtundation	Hepatic encephalopathy	Liver failure, portosystemic shunting of blood

SCREENING TESTS OF HEPATOBILIARY DISEASE

Screening tests of hepatobiliary disease (see Table 39–2) may be divided into two categories: (1) tests of biliary obstruction and/or cholestasis and (2) tests of hepatocellular damage, based on the mechanisms responsible for the abnormal test. However, none of the tests is specific for either category, and it is the overall pattern and the relative magnitude of abnormalities in these two categories of tests that often provide diagnostic clues to the type of liver disease present.

The *serum bilirubin* level reflects a balance between bilirubin production and its conjugation and excretion into bile by the liver. The differential diagnosis for hyperbilirubinemia (see Chapter 40) requires consideration of an extensive list of disorders in which bilirubin production (hematologic disorders), hepatic metabolism (congenital abnormalities of bilirubin, liver disease), or excretion (biliary obstruction) are altered. Hence, an elevated serum bilirubin determination is not specific for any etiology of liver disease. However, such an abnormality, especially in association with predominant elevations in other tests of biliary obstruction, should prompt an evaluation for potentially treatable biliary abnormalities. It is important to recognize that serum bilirubin levels may not return promptly to normal after relief of biliary obstruction or improvement in liver disease because some bilirubin binds covalently to albumin and is removed from the circulation only as albumin is catabolized.

Serum alkaline phosphatase activity reflects a group

TABLE 39–2   Clinical Tests of Hepatic Function

	Property Examined	Significance of Abnormal Results
Tests of Hepatic Function (Normal Values)		
Serum albumin (3.5–5.5 mg/dL)	Protein synthetic capacity (over days to weeks)	Decreased synthetic capacity Protein malnutrition Increased protein loss (nephrotic syndrome, protein-losing enteropathy) Increased extracellular fluid volume
Prothrombin time (10.5–13 sec)	Protein synthetic capacity (hours to days)	Decreased synthetic capacity (especially factors II and VII) Vitamin K deficiency Consumptive coagulopathy
Screening Tests of Hepatobiliary Disease		
Tests of Biliary Obstruction or Impaired Bile Flow		
Serum bilirubin (0.2–1.0 mg/dL) (3.4–17.1 mol/L)	Extraction of bilirubin from blood conjugation and excretion into bile	Hemolysis Diffuse liver disease Cholestasis Extrahepatic bile duct obstruction Congenital disorders of bilirubin metabolism
Serum alkaline phosphatase (also 5′-nucleotidase and γ-glutamyl transpeptidase) (56–176 U/L)	Increased enzyme synthesis and release	Bile duct obstruction Cholestasis Infiltrative liver disease (neoplasms, granulomas) Bone destruction/remodeling Pregnancy
Tests of Hepatocellular Damage		
Aspartate aminotransferase (AST, SGOT) (10–30 U/L)	Release of intracellular enzyme	Hepatocellular necrosis Cardiac or skeletal muscle necrosis
Alanine aminotransferase (ALT, SGPT) (5–30 U/L)	Release of intracellular enzyme	Same as AST; however, more specific for liver cell damage

of isoenzymes derived from liver, bone, intestine, and placenta. Serum levels are elevated in association with a variety of conditions, including cholestasis, partial or complete bile duct obstruction, bone regeneration, pregnancy, and neoplastic, infiltrative, and granulomatous liver diseases. An isolated elevated alkaline phosphatase level may be the only clue to partial obstruction of the common bile duct, to obstruction of ducts in a single lobe or segment of liver, or to neoplastic or granulomatous hepatic disease. In cholestasis, serum alkaline phosphatase levels rise as a result of retention of bile acids in the liver, which solubilize alkaline phosphatase off the hepatocyte plasma membrane as well as stimulate its synthesis. 5′-Nucleotidase and γ-glutamyl transpeptidase, other hepatocyte plasma membrane enzymes, are similarly released into the circulation during bile duct obstruction or cholestasis and are used to confirm that an elevated alkaline phosphatase level is caused by hepatobiliary disease.

Aspartate (AST, SGOT) and *alanine* (ALT, SGPT) *aminotransferases* are intracellular aminotransferring enzymes present in large quantities in hepatocytes. After injury or death of liver cells, they are released into the circulation. In general, the serum aminotransferases are sensitive (albeit nonspecific) tests of liver damage, and the height of the serum aminotransferase activity reflects the severity of hepatic necrosis, with important exceptions. For instance, both enzymes require pyridoxal 5′-phosphate as a cofactor, and the relatively low serum aminotransferase values seen in patients with severe alcoholic hepatitis (usually <300 U/L) may reflect deficiency of this cofactor. Although aminotransferase levels are increased in a wide array of liver diseases, high levels (>15 times the upper limit of normal) infrequently indicate acute bile duct obstruction or hepatic ischemia and generally indicate acute hepatocellular necrosis from viral or toxic causes. Patients who present with isolated asymptomatic elevations of aspartate aminotransferase and alanine aminotransferase may have fatty liver (caused by obesity or alcohol intake) and hepatocellular disease, such as hemochromatosis or chronic viral hepatitis. These patients should be screened for treatable diseases. Some patients may require liver biopsy.

Individual liver function tests frequently do not indicate the nature of the underlying liver disease. However, the overall *pattern* of liver test abnormalities and the relative magnitude of abnormalities in individual

TABLE 39–3 **Characteristic Patterns of Liver Function Tests**

Disorder	Bilirubin	Alkaline Phosphatase	Aspartate Aminotransferase	Alanine Aminotransferase	Prothrombin Time	Albumin
Gilbert's syndrome (abnormal bilirubin metabolism)	↑	NL	NL	NL	NL	NL
Bile duct obstruction (pancreatic cancer)	↑↑↑	↑↑↑	↑	↑	↑ – ↑↑	NL
Acute hepatocellular damage (toxic, viral hepatitis)	↑ – ↑↑↑	↑ – ↑↑	↑↑↑	↑↑↑	NL– ↑↑↑	NL– ↓↓
Cirrhosis	NL– ↑	NL– ↑	NL– ↑	NL– ↑	NL– ↑↑	NL– ↓↓

NL = normal; ↑ = increased; ↓ = decreased (arrows indicate extent of change: ↑ – ↑↑↑ = slight to large).

tests often provide significant insight into the nature of the liver disease. Table 39–3 outlines common patterns of liver test abnormalities.

Liver Biopsy

Biopsy and histologic examination of liver tissue are frequently valuable in the differential diagnosis and treatment of diffuse or localized parenchymal diseases (e.g., cirrhosis, hepatitis, hemochromatosis, tumors) or hepatomegaly. Liver biopsy is generally safe (serious complica-

tions <0.5%); however, it is contraindicated in uncooperative patients and those with significant coagulation abnormalities or thrombocytopenia.

REFERENCES

Friedman LS, Martin P, Munoz SJ: Liver function tests and the objective evaluation of the patient with liver diseases. *In* Zakim D, Boyer T (eds): Hepatology: A Textbook of Liver Disease, 3rd ed. Philadelphia: WB Saunders, 1996, pp 791–832.

Weisiger RA: Laboratory tests in liver disease. *In* Goldman L, Bennett JC (eds): Cecil Textbook of Medicine, 21st ed. Philadelphia: WB Saunders, 2000, pp 775–779.

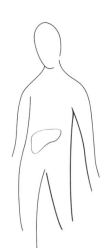

40

JAUNDICE

Michael B. Fallon • Brendan M. McGuire
Gary A. Abrams • Miguel R. Arguedas

The term *jaundice,* or *icterus,* describes the yellow pigmentation of skin, sclerae, and mucous membranes produced by increased serum bilirubin *(hyperbilirubinemia).* Jaundice is a common sign of a variety of liver and biliary diseases and serves as a starting point for evaluating many of these disorders. Serum bilirubin levels normally range from 0.5 to 1.0 mg/dL. Jaundice usually becomes clinically evident at levels higher than 2.5 mg/dL and is most readily detected in the sclerae.

Bilirubin Metabolism

About 4 mg/kg of bilirubin is produced each day, mainly (80% to 85%) derived from the catabolism of the hemoglobin heme group of senescent red blood cells. The heme ring is cleaved in the reticuloendothelial system to form biliverdin, which, in turn, is oxidized to bilirubin, a water-insoluble tetrapyrrole. A smaller proportion of bilirubin (15% to 20%) is derived from the destruction of maturing erythroid cells in the bone marrow *(ineffective erythropoiesis)* and from the heme groups of predominantly hepatic hemoproteins such as cytochrome P-450 and cytochrome *c* (Fig. 40–1).

This unconjugated bilirubin is released into the plasma and is transported to the liver while it is bound tightly but reversibly to albumin. Unconjugated bilirubin is apolar and insoluble in water and is virtually incapable of being excreted in the bile or urine. However, it readily dissolves in lipid-rich environments and traverses the blood-brain barrier and placenta. Three phases of hepatic bilirubin metabolism are recognized: (1) uptake, (2) conjugation, and (3) excretion into the bile, the last step being overall rate limiting. Uptake is reversible and follows dissociation of bilirubin from albumin.

Unconjugated bilirubin is rendered water soluble and is capable of being excreted in the aqueous bile by its conjugation with a sugar, glucuronic acid. Monoglucuronides and diglucuronides of bilirubin are formed in the hepatic endoplasmic reticulum catalyzed by the enzyme uridine diphosphate (UDP)–glucuronyl transferase. If the biliary excretion of conjugated bilirubin is impaired, then the pigment will regurgitate from hepatocytes into plasma. Conjugated bilirubin is both water soluble and less tightly bound to albumin than unconjugated pigment, so it is readily filtered by the glomerulus and appears in the urine when plasma levels are increased (see Fig. 40–1). In patients with sustained conjugated hyperbilirubinemia (e.g., obstructive jaundice), a proportion of the conjugated bilirubin becomes covalently bound to albumin and is therefore unavailable for renal or biliary excretion.

Conjugated bilirubin is excreted into bile by a multi-specific canalicular transporter identified as an isoform of the multidrug resistance protein (Mrp2). It is converted by bacterial action in the gut to colorless tetrapyrroles termed *urobilinogens.* Up to 20% of urobilinogen is reabsorbed and undergoes enterohepatic circulation, with a proportion excreted in the urine. Thus, both impaired hepatocellular excretion and marked overproduction of bilirubin may lead to increased appearance of urobilinogen in the urine.

Laboratory Tests for Bilirubin

The *van den Bergh reaction* is the most commonly used test for bilirubin in biologic fluids. When carried out in an aqueous medium, the test shows a colored reaction only with water-soluble bilirubin derivatives (called the *direct* van den Bergh fraction). The addition of methanol enables a colored reaction to take place with water-insoluble bilirubin (called the *indirect* van den Bergh fraction). Direct and indirect van den Bergh fractions provide clinically useful estimations of conjugated and unconjugated bilirubin, respectively. However, the correlation between actual levels of conjugated bilirubin and levels estimated by the direct-reacting fraction is poor. Normal plasma actually contains >95% unconjugated bilirubin.

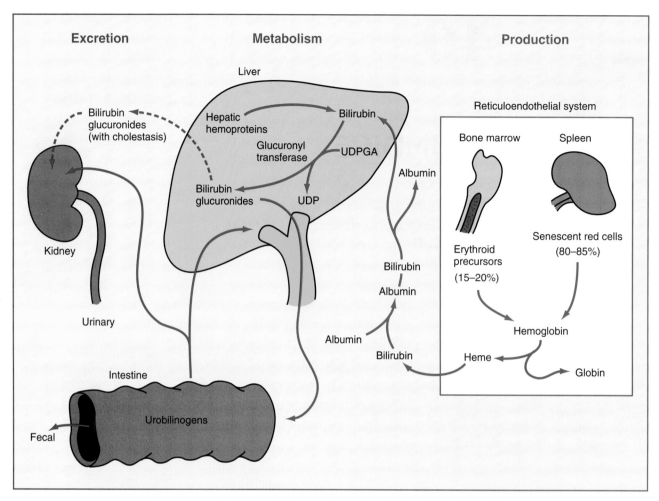

FIGURE 40–1   Bilirubin production, metabolism, and excretion. UDP = uridine diphosphate; UDPGA = uridine diphosphate glucuronic acid.

Clinical Classification

A logical first step in studying a jaundiced patient is to determine whether the patient has unconjugated or conjugated hyperbilirubinemia. This question is usually easily resolved by serum testing.

Classification of jaundice according to this distinction is shown in Table 40–1. Mechanisms contributing to predominantly unconjugated hyperbilirubinemia include (1) overproduction, (2) decreased hepatic uptake, and (3) decreased conjugation. Conjugated hyperbilirubinemia implies either (1) a defect in hepatocellular excretion of bilirubin or (2) mechanical obstruction to the major extrahepatic bile ducts. Occasionally, jaundice may result from a single abnormality in the pathway from bilirubin production to biliary excretion (hemolysis, inherited disorder of bilirubin metabolism), although more frequently, jaundice has multiple rather than isolated causes. For example, the jaundice occurring in patients with hepatocellular disease (i.e., hepatitis, cirrhosis) may result from a combination of diminished red cell survival and impairment of all three stages of hepatocellular bilirubin transport and metabolism.

UNCONJUGATED HYPERBILIRUBINEMIA

The causes of unconjugated hyperbilirubinemia are easily determined. These disorders are rarely associated with significant hepatic dysfunction. Several common causes of unconjugated hyperbilirubinemia are discussed here.

Overproduction

Hemolysis from a variety of causes may lead to bilirubin production sufficient to exceed the clearing capacity of the liver, with subsequent development of jaundice. This *hemolytic jaundice* is characteristically mild; serum bilirubin levels rarely exceed 5 mg/dL in the absence of coexistent hepatic disease. Ineffective erythropoiesis, which may be substantially increased in megaloblastic anemias, may also lead to mild jaundice.

Impaired Hepatic Uptake

Impaired uptake is rarely encountered as an isolated cause of clinical jaundice, but it may play a role in the mild jaundice that occurs after administration of certain

TABLE 40–1 Classification of Jaundice

Predominantly Unconjugated Hyperbilirubinemia
Overproduction
    Hemolysis (e.g., spherocytosis, autoimmune disorders)
    Ineffective erythropoiesis (e.g., megaloblastic anemias)
Decreased hepatic uptake
    Gilbert's syndrome
    Drugs (e.g., rifampin, radiographic contrast agents)
    Neonatal jaundice
Decreased conjugation
    Gilbert's syndrome
    Crigler-Najjar syndrome types I and II
    Neonatal jaundice
    Hepatocellular disease
    Drug inhibition (e.g., chloramphenicol)
Predominantly Conjugated Hyperbilirubinemia
Impaired hepatic excretion
    Familial disorders (Dubin-Johnson syndrome, Rotor syndrome, benign recurrent cholestasis, cholestasis of pregnancy)
    Hepatocellular disease
    Drug-induced cholestasis
    Primary biliary cirrhosis
    Sepsis
    Postoperative
Extrahepatic ("mechanical") biliary obstruction
    Gallstones
    Tumors of the head of the pancreas
    Tumors of bile ducts
    Tumors of the ampulla of Vater
    Biliary strictures (postcholecystectomy, primary sclerosing cholangitis)
    Congenital disorders (biliary atresia)

drugs, such as rifampin (competition for bilirubin uptake) and in Gilbert's syndrome (see later).

Impaired Conjugation

A genetically determined decrease or absence of UDP-glucuronyl transferase is encountered in the Crigler-Najjar syndrome, whereas mild, acquired defects in the enzyme may be produced by drugs (e.g., chloramphenicol).

Neonatal Jaundice

All steps of hepatic bilirubin metabolism are incompletely developed in the neonate, whereas production is also increased. The major defect is in conjugation, however, leading to the common finding of mild to moderate unconjugated hyperbilirubinemia between the second and fifth days of life. When significant increased production of bilirubin occurs in the neonatal period (hemolytic disease secondary to blood group incompatibility), the infant may have severe unconjugated hyperbilirubinemia, which is associated with a risk of neurologic damage *(kernicterus)*.

Gilbert's Syndrome

This common disorder affects up to 7% of the population, with a marked male predominance. It commonly manifests during the teens or 20s as mild unconjugated hyperbilirubinemia, exacerbated by fasting, and noted clinically as an incidental laboratory finding. The genetic defect involves a mutation in the promoter region of the UDP-glucuronyl transferase gene, and its clinical expression results from increased production and/or diminished hepatic uptake of bilirubin. Nonspecific gastrointestinal symptoms and fatigue are commonly associated, but the condition is entirely benign. The diagnosis is strongly suggested by unconjugated hyperbilirubinemia with normal hepatic enzymes and the absence of overt hemolysis. Liver biopsy is generally not indicated to confirm the diagnosis.

CONJUGATED HYPERBILIRUBINEMIA

Conjugated hyperbilirubinemia indicates either impaired hepatic excretion or altered biliary drainage of bilirubin. This finding frequently occurs in the setting of impaired formation or excretion of all components of bile, a situation termed *cholestasis*. However, it may also result from hepatocellular injury independent of cholestasis. Frequently, the clinical challenge in patients with *cholestatic jaundice* is in distinguishing whether hyperbilirubinemia results from an intrahepatic defect or from extrahepatic biliary obstruction.

Typically in cholestatic jaundice, the alkaline phosphatase level is increased to three to four times normal along with conjugated hyperbilirubinemia (see Chapter 39). When prolonged, cholestasis may lead to hypercholesterolemia, malabsorption of fat and fat-soluble vitamins, and retention of bile salts, which may cause pruritus. Biochemical evidence of liver cell damage (elevated transaminases, prolonged prothrombin time uncorrected by administration of vitamin K) may be minimal or marked, depending on the cause of the cholestasis. In some forms of cholestasis, bilirubin metabolism and excretion are well preserved, and these patients may have all the features of cholestasis without jaundice.

Impaired Hepatic Excretion

This pathogenetic category of jaundice, also called *intrahepatic cholestasis,* is applied to all disorders in the transport of conjugated bilirubin from the hepatocyte to the radiologically visible intrahepatic bile ducts. Thus, it includes a wide range of conditions from drug-induced cholestasis (impaired canalicular transport) to primary biliary cirrhosis (destruction of the small intrahepatic bile ductules). The following are some important causes of intrahepatic cholestasis.

Drug-Induced Cholestasis. Typical cholestatic jaundice may be produced by a wide array of drugs, including phenothiazines, oral contraceptives, and methyltestosterone. Eosinophilia may accompany drug-induced jaundice.

Sepsis. Systemic sepsis, mainly from gram-negative organisms, may produce a predominantly conjugated hyperbilirubinemia, usually accompanied by mildly elevated serum alkaline phosphatase levels.

Postoperative Jaundice. This increasingly recognized syndrome has an incidence of 15% after heart surgery and 1% after elective abdominal surgery. Occurring 1 to 10 days postoperatively and multifactorial in origin, the elevated bilirubin is predominantly of the conjugated variety, with increased alkaline phosphatase and minimally abnormal transaminase levels.

Hepatocellular Disease. Hepatocellular disease (i.e., hepatitis and cirrhosis) from a variety of causes (see Chapters 41 and 43) may result in typical cholestatic jaundice. Evidence of hepatocellular damage and dysfunction is usually prominent and includes elevated transaminases, prolonged prothrombin time, hypoalbuminemia, and clinical features of hepatic dysfunction. In hepatocellular disease, all three steps of hepatic bilirubin metabolism are impaired. Excretion, the rate-limiting step, is usually the most profoundly disturbed, leading to a predominantly conjugated hyperbilirubinemia. Jaundice may be profound in acute hepatitis (see Chapter 41) without adverse prognostic implications. In contrast, in chronic liver disease, persistent jaundice usually implies decompensation of hepatic function and a poor prognosis.

Extrahepatic Biliary Obstruction

Complete or partial obstruction of the extrahepatic bile ducts may result from a variety of causes, including impaction of gallstones, carcinoma of the head of the pancreas, tumors of the bile ducts, bile duct strictures, and chronic pancreatitis with bile duct compression. In complete obstruction, conjugated hyperbilirubinemia is prominent and usually plateaus at 30 to 40 mg/dL in the absence of renal failure, hepatocellular damage, or infection within the bile ducts, all of which may develop during the course of mechanical obstruction and may cause a further rise in bilirubin. Stools may become clay colored as a result of the failure of bile to enter the intestine. In partial obstruction, jaundice may be mild or even absent, to become prominent when infection of the ducts (cholangitis) complicates the obstruction.

Approach to Diagnosis

The differential diagnosis of hepatic causes of jaundice applies to those patients with predominant conjugated hyperbilirubinemia. A history of darkened urine invariably implies conjugated hyperbilirubinemia and should prompt evaluation. A careful history and physical examination and judicious use of laboratory studies are of paramount importance in obtaining clues to the nature of jaundice and specifically in determining whether hepatocellular injury, impaired hepatic excretion, or biliary obstruction is involved. A history of pale stools and pruritus suggests cholestasis rather than hepatocellular injury. An inquiry about the use of drugs or alcohol, risk factors for viral hepatitis, and preexisting liver disease may also provide information regarding potential causes of cholestasis and hepatocellular injury. Recurrent abdominal pain and nausea (gallstones) and epigastric pain radiating to the back with weight loss and gallbladder distention (carcinoma of the pancreatic head) suggest biliary obstruction. Serum transaminases are usually elevated less than 5-fold to 10-fold, and the alkaline phosphatase levels are usually greater than two to three times normal in patients with biliary obstruction. Conversely, serum transaminases are often elevated more than 10-fold to 15-fold, and the alkaline phosphatase levels are less than 2 to 3 times normal in hepatocellular disease. Further serologic testing for hepatitis (see Chapter 41) and autoantibody testing (antimitochondrial antibody for primary biliary cirrhosis) may also be helpful.

Once initial evaluation has established the presence of cholestatic jaundice, more sophisticated diagnostic procedures are frequently used to distinguish intrahepatic cholestasis from biliary obstruction and to provide potential treatment in cases of biliary obstruction. A diagnostic approach is outlined in Figure 40–2. If extrahepatic obstruction is suspected, noninvasive means should be used to determine whether bile ducts are dilated. In jaundiced patients, dilation of the ducts is usual when a mechanical obstruction is present but is absent in cases of intrahepatic cholestasis. Either ultrasonography or computed tomography may be used to assess bile ducts, and ultrasonography is preferred be-

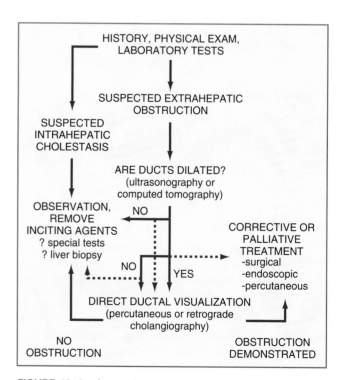

FIGURE 40–2 Approach to the patient with cholestatic jaundice. The algorithm demonstrates the systematic consideration of the available diagnostic options.

cause of its lower cost and the absence of radiation. Additional definitive clues, such as the presence of stones in the common duct or gallbladder, may be found as well. If dilated ducts are found on noninvasive imaging, direct cholangiography will provide the most reliable approach to nonoperative management and potential treatment of cholestatic jaundice. This may be accomplished by either percutaneous puncture of the intrahepatic biliary tree (percutaneous transhepatic cholangiography) or by endoscopic retrograde cholangiography.

If intrahepatic cholestasis is suspected clinically and extrahepatic obstruction is excluded by noninvasive means and/or direct cholangiography, then liver biopsy will sometimes be useful in determining the cause of cholestasis. Regardless, when a potential inciting agent is found, an ideal approach is to discontinue the agent and observe for resolution of jaundice.

REFERENCE

Scharschmidt BF: Bilirubin metabolism, hyperbilirubinemia and the approach to the jaundiced patient. *In* Goldman L, Bennett JC (eds): Cecil Textbook of Medicine, 21st ed. Philadelphia: WB Saunders, 2000, pp 770–775.

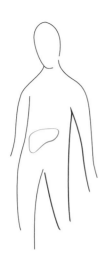

41

ACUTE AND CHRONIC HEPATITIS

Michael B. Fallon • Brendan M. McGuire
Gary A. Abrams • Miguel R. Arguedas

The term *hepatitis* is applied to a broad category of clinicopathologic conditions that result from the damage produced by a viral, toxic, pharmacologic, or immune-mediated attack on the liver. The common pathologic features of hepatitis are hepatocellular necrosis, which may be focal or extensive, and inflammatory cell infiltration of the liver, which may predominate in the portal areas or may extend into the parenchyma. Physical examination may show an enlarged tender liver and icteric mucous membranes. Laboratory evidence of hepatocellular damage is invariably found in the form of elevated transaminase levels. Independent of the cause of hepatitis, the clinical course may range from subclinical or mild to severe hepatocellular dysfunction with evidence of impairment of coagulation, marked jaundice, and disturbance of neurologic function.

Acute hepatitis implies a condition lasting less than 6 months, culminating either in complete resolution of the liver damage with return to normal liver function and structure or a rapid progression of the acute injury toward extensive necrosis and a fatal outcome.

Chronic hepatitis is defined as a sustained inflammatory process in the liver lasting longer than 6 months and is often impossible to differentiate from acute hepatitis on histologic criteria alone. Inflammatory cells extending beyond the limits of the portal tracts surrounding isolated nests of hepatocytes (*piecemeal necrosis*) and portal and/or central areas of the hepatic lobules connected by inflammation, necrosis, and collapse of architecture (*bridging necrosis*) are seen in severe forms of chronic hepatitis. However, these features may also be noted in uncomplicated acute hepatitis that ultimately resolves completely. A purely histologic diagnosis of chronic hepatitis usually requires evidence of progression toward cirrhosis, such as significant fibrous deposition and disruption of the hepatic lobular architecture.

Acute Hepatitis

Agents commonly causing acute hepatic injury are listed in Table 41–1. The mechanisms whereby these agents produce hepatic damage include direct toxin-induced necrosis (e.g., acetaminophen, *Amanita phalloides* toxin) and host immune-mediated damage. Massive hepatic necrosis is the dominant process in cases of *Amanita* poisoning, and the clinical course is more aptly described as fulminant hepatic failure (see Chapter 42) than as acute hepatitis. Such a course is less common but well recognized with all the causative agents listed in Table 41–1.

ACUTE VIRAL HEPATITIS

Etiology

Viral hepatitis is caused by at least seven viruses. Hepatitis viruses A (HAV), B (HBV), C (HCV), D (HDV), E (HEV), and G (HGV) (Table 41–2) have been characterized at the molecular level. Hepatitis F virus is another potential infectious agent that has been experimentally transmitted from human stool to primates and is currently being characterized. Cytomegalovirus and Epstein-Barr virus occasionally cause hepatitis. HDV, an incomplete RNA virus, causes hepatitis only in patients with either acute (HDV *coinfection*) or chronic hepatitis B (HDV *superinfection*). HCV accounts for most cases of hepatitis previously designated "non-A, non-B." HBV has been extensively characterized. The complete HBV (Dane particle) consists of several antigenically distinct components (Fig. 41–1), including a surface coat (hepatitis B surface antigen [HBsAg]) and a core of circular DNA, DNA polymerase, hepatitis B core antigen (HBcAg), and hepatitis B e antigen (HBeAg). HBsAg

TABLE 41-1   Causes of Acute Hepatitis

Viral Hepatitis
Hepatitis A virus
Hepatitis B virus
Hepatitis C virus
Hepatitis D virus ("delta agent")
Hepatitis E virus
Epstein-Barr virus
Cytomegalovirus

Alcohol

Toxins
Amanita phalloides mushroom poisoning
Carbon tetrachloride

Drugs
Acetaminophen
Isoniazid
Halothane
Chlorpromazine
Erythromycin

Other
Wilson's disease
Herbs

may exist in serum either as part of the Dane particle or as free particles and rods. HBsAg, HBcAg, and HBeAg elicit distinct antibody responses from the host that are used to diagnose and characterize the state of virus replication in the liver.

Transmission

HAV is excreted in the feces during the incubation period (Fig. 41–2) and is transmitted by the fecal-oral

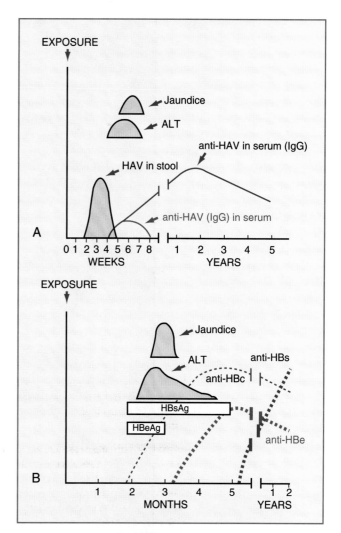

FIGURE 41–2 Sequence of clinical and laboratory findings in *(A)* a patient with acute hepatitis A virus (HAV) and *(B)* a patient with hepatitis B. ALT = alanine transaminase; HBc = hepatitis B core; HBe = hepatitis B e; HBeAg = hepatitis B e antigen; HBs = hepatitis B surface; HBsAg = hepatitis B surface antigen.

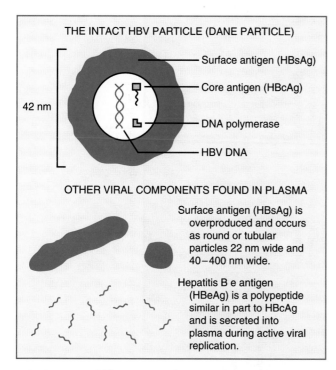

FIGURE 41–1 Different types of hepatitis B virus (HBV) particles in plasma.

route. It is thus implicated in most instances of water-borne and food-transmitted infection and in epidemics of viral hepatitis.

HBV is present in virtually all body fluids and excreta of carriers and is transmitted mainly by parenteral routes. Thus, transmission occurs most commonly by blood and blood products, contaminated needles, and sexual contact. High-risk transmission groups include the following: *sexual partners* of acutely as well as chronically infected persons, with male homosexuals being at particularly high risk; *health professionals*, particularly surgeons, dentists, and workers in clinical laboratories and dialysis units; *intravenous drug abusers;* and infants of infected mothers (*"vertical transmission"*). Patients with increased exposure to blood or blood products and/or with impaired immunity (e.g., patients undergoing dialysis, patients with leukemia or Down's syndrome) are also highly susceptible to HBV infection.

HCV, similar to HBV, is largely parenterally transmit-

TABLE 41-2 Characteristics of Common Causative Agents of Acute Viral Hepatitis

	Hepatitis A	Hepatitis B	Hepatitis C	Hepatitis D	Hepatitis E	Hepatitis G
Causative agent	27-nm RDA virus	42-nm DNA virus; core and surface components	Flavivirus-like RNA agent	36-nm hybrid particle with HBsAg coat	27–34 nm nonenveloped RNA virus	Single-strand RNA virus
Transmission	Fecal-oral; waterborne or foodborne	Parenteral inoculation or equivalent; direct contact	Similar to HBV	Similar to HBV	Similar to HAV	Parenteral
Incubation period	2–6 wk	4 wk–6 mo	5–10 wk	Similar to HBV	2–9 wk	2–4 wk
Period of infectivity	2–3 wk in late incubation and early clinical phase	During HBsAg positivity (occasionally only with anti-HBc positivity)	During anti-HCV positivity	During HDV RNA or anti-HDV positivity	Similar to HCV	Unknown
Massive hepatic necrosis	Rare	Uncommon	Uncommon	Yes	Yes	Unclear
Carrier state	No	Yes	Yes	Yes	No	Unknown
Chronic hepatitis	No	Yes	Yes	Yes	No	Possible: viremia persistent but hepatitis uncertain
Prophylaxis	Hygiene, immune serum globulin, vaccine	Hygiene, hepatitis B immune globulin, vaccine	Hygiene	Hygiene, HBV vaccine	Hygiene, sanitation	Hygiene

HAV = hepatitis A virus; HBc = hepatitis B core; HBsAg = hepatitis B surface antigen; HBV = hepatitis B virus; HCV = hepatitis C virus; HDV = hepatitis D virus.

TABLE 41–3   Serologic Markers of Viral Hepatitis

Agent	Marker	Definition	Significance
Hepatitis A virus (HAV)	Anti-HAV	Antibody to HAV	
	IgM type		Current or recent infection or convalescence
	IgG type		Current or previous infection; conferring immunity
Hepatitis B virus (HBV)	HBsAg	HBV surface antigen	Positive in most cases of acute or chronic infection
	HBeAg	e antigen; a component of the HBV core	Transiently positive in acute hepatitis B
			May persist in chronic infection
			Reflection of presence of viral replication, whole Dane particles in serum, and high infectivity
	Anti-HBe	Antibody to e antigen	Transiently positive in convalescence
			Possibly persistently present in chronic cases
			Usually a reflection of low infectivity
	Anti-HBc (IgM or IgG)	Antibody to HBV core antigen	Positive in all acute and chronic cases
			Reliable marker of infection, past or current
			IgM anti-HBc a reflection of active viral replication
			Not protective
	Anti-HBs	Antibody to HBV surface antigen	Positive in late convalescence in most acute cases
			Conferring immunity
Hepatitis C virus (HCV)	Anti-HCV	Antibodies to a group of recombinant HCV peptides (C22-3, C200)	Positive on average 15 wk after exposure; not protective
			Persistent in chronic infection
Hepatitis D virus (HDV)	Anti-HDV (IgM or IgG)	Antibody to HDV antigen	Acute or chronic infection; not protective

ted. HCV is the main cause of post-transfusion hepatitis, it is a common cause of hepatitis in intravenous drug users, and it accounts for at least 50% of cases of sporadic, community-acquired hepatitis. In these cases, the mode of virus transmission is unclear. HEV is the cause of an epidemic, waterborne hepatitis that has been associated with outbreaks, mainly in Asia and Africa.

Clinical and Laboratory Manifestations

Acute viral hepatitis typically begins with a prodromal phase lasting several days and characterized by constitutional and gastrointestinal symptoms including malaise, fatigue, anorexia, nausea, vomiting, myalgia, and headache. A mild fever may be present. Symptoms suggestive of "flu" may be prominent; arthritis and urticaria, attributed to immune complex deposition, may be present, particularly in hepatitis B. Smokers often describe an aversion to cigarettes. Jaundice soon appears with bilirubinuria and acholic (pale) stools, often accompanied by an improvement in the patient's sense of well-being. Jaundice may be absent (*anicteric hepatitis*), and in such cases medical attention is often not sought. The liver is usually tender and enlarged; splenomegaly is found in about one fifth of patients.

Transaminases (alanine transaminase and aspartate transaminase) are released from the acutely damaged hepatocytes, and serum transaminase levels rise, often to levels >20-fold normal. An elevated serum bilirubin (>2.5 to 3.0 mg/dL) results in jaundice and defines *icteric hepatitis*. Values higher than 20 mg/dL are uncommon and approximately correlate with the severity of disease. Elevations in serum alkaline phosphatase are usually limited to three times normal levels, except in cases of cholestatic hepatitis. A complete blood cell count most commonly shows mild leukopenia with atypical lymphocytes. The icteric phase of acute viral hepatitis may last days to weeks, followed by gradual resolution of symptoms and laboratory values.

Serodiagnosis

The ability to detect the presence of viral components in hepatitis B and C and antibodies to components of hepatitis A, B, C, and D has fostered progress in the epidemiology of viral hepatitis. These viral markers can be diagnostic of the cause of acute viral hepatitis (Table 41–3). An etiologic diagnosis is of great importance in planning preventive and public health measures pertinent to the close contacts of infected patients and in evaluating prognosis. The time course of appearance of these markers in acute hepatitis A and B is shown in Figure 41–2. Epstein-Barr virus and cytomegalovirus hepatitis may also be diagnosed by the appearance of specific antibodies of the IgM class. In acute hepatitis B, HBsAg and HBeAg are present in serum. Both are usually cleared within 3 months, but HBsAg may persist in some patients with uncomplicated cases for 6 months to 1 year. Clearance of HBsAg is followed after a variable "window" period by emergence of anti-HBs, which confers long-term immunity. Anti-HBc and anti-HBe appear in the acute phase of the illness, but neither provides immunity. Uncommonly, during the serologic window period, anti-HBc may be the only evidence of hepatitis B infection, and IgM anti-HBc, a marker of active viral replication, suggests recent infection. HDV infection superimposed on HBV infection may be detected by specific antibody to this agent. Acute hepatitis C can be detected using a sensitive polymerase chain reaction assay for HCV RNA. Serum antibodies to

HCV develop within 15 weeks of exposure or within 6 to 7 weeks after biochemical abnormalities are discovered.

Complications

Cholestatic Hepatitis. In some patients, most commonly during HAV infection, a self-limited period of cholestatic jaundice may supervene that is characterized by marked conjugated hyperbilirubinemia, elevation of alkaline phosphatase, and pruritus. Investigation may be required to differentiate this condition from mechanical obstruction of the biliary tree (see Chapter 45).

Fulminant Hepatitis. Massive hepatic necrosis occurs in <1% of patients with acute viral hepatitis and leads to a devastating and often fatal condition called *fulminant hepatic failure*. This is discussed in detail in Chapter 42.

Chronic Hepatitis. Hepatitis A does not progress to chronic liver disease, although occasionally it has a relapsing course. Persistence of transaminase elevation beyond 6 months in patients with hepatitis B and C suggests evolution to chronic hepatitis, although slowly resolving acute hepatitis may occasionally lead to abnormal liver function tests for up to 12 months, with eventual complete resolution. Chronic hepatitis is considered in detail later in this chapter. HBV infection without evidence of any liver damage may persist, resulting in asymptomatic or "healthy" hepatitis B carriers. In Asia and Africa, many such carriers appear to have acquired the virus from infected mothers during infancy.

Rare Complications. Acute viral hepatitis may be followed by *aplastic anemia*, which affects mostly male patients and results in a mortality of greater than 80%. Pancreatitis, myocarditis, and neurologic complications including Guillain-Barré syndrome, aseptic meningitis, and encephalitis have also been reported. Cryoglobulinemia, glomerulonephritis, and polyarteritis nodosa are associated with hepatitis B.

Management

No specific treatment exists for acute viral hepatitis. Management is largely supportive and includes rest, maintenance of hydration, and adequate dietary intake. Most patients show a preference for a low-fat, high-carbohydrate diet. Vitamin supplementation is of no proven value, although vitamin K may be indicated if prolonged cholestasis occurs. Activity is restricted to limit fatigue. Alcohol should be avoided until liver enzymes return to normal. Measures to combat nausea can include small doses of metoclopramide and hydroxyzine. Hospitalization is indicated in patients with severe nausea and vomiting or in those with evidence of deteriorating liver function, such as hepatic encephalopathy or prolongation of the prothrombin time. In general, hepatitis A may be regarded as noninfectious after 2 to 3 weeks, whereas hepatitis B is potentially infectious to sexual contacts throughout its course, although the risk

is low once HBsAg has cleared. Although hepatitis C may also be transmitted to sexual contacts, the risk of this is considered less than for hepatitis B.

Prevention

Both feces and blood from patients with hepatitis A contain virus during the prodromal and early icteric phases of the disease. Raw shellfish concentrate the virus from sewage pollution and may serve as vectors of the disease. General hygienic measures should include handwashing by contacts and careful handling, disposal, and sterilization of excreta and contaminated clothing and utensils. Close contacts of patients with hepatitis A should receive immune serum globulin (ISG) as soon as possible but no later than 6 weeks after exposure. Travelers to endemic areas where sanitation facilities are poor may be protected by prior administration of ISG or by using hepatitis A vaccines. The use of such vaccines in other high-risk groups is currently under study.

Hepatitis B is rarely transmitted by body fluids other than blood, but nonetheless one should avoid contact with the excreta of patients. Far more important is the meticulous disposal of contaminated needles and other blood-contaminated utensils.

Efforts at preventing hepatitis B have involved the use of ISG enriched in anti-HBs (hepatitis B immune globulin [HBIG]) and the recombinant hepatitis B vaccine. Postexposure prophylaxis with HBIG after blood or mucosal exposure (e.g., needlestick, eye splash, sexual contacts of acute hepatitis B patients, neonates born to mothers with acute or chronic infection) should be given within 7 days and subsequently with hepatitis B vaccine. Preventive vaccination is currently recommended for high-risk groups and individuals (health care professionals, patients undergoing dialysis, patients with hemophilia, residents and staff of custodial care institutions, sexually active homosexual men) and is advocated universally for children.

No accepted prevention strategies are available for HCV. Because ISG does not contain HCV-neutralizing antibodies, it is of no use for postexposure prophylaxis. However, evidence indicates that early treatment of acute hepatitis C with agents such as interferon-α may significantly reduce the development of chronic infection. The advent of widespread blood product screening for anti-HCV has significantly reduced the incidence of post-transfusion hepatitis.

ALCOHOLIC FATTY LIVER AND HEPATITIS

Alcohol abuse is the most common cause of liver disease in the Western world. Three major pathologic lesions resulting from alcohol abuse are (1) fatty liver, (2) alcoholic hepatitis, and (3) cirrhosis. The first two lesions are potentially reversible and may sometimes be confused clinically with viral hepatitis or gallbladder and biliary tract disease. Alcoholic cirrhosis is discussed in Chapter 43.

Mechanism of Injury

Alcohol appears to produce liver damage by several mechanisms that are still incompletely understood. Fatty liver may be related to increased nicotinamide-adenine dinucleotide phosphate generated during alcohol metabolism, which promotes fatty acid synthesis and triglyceride formation. Because alcohol also impairs the release of triglycerides in the form of lipoproteins, fat accumulates in hepatocytes. Acetaldehyde, produced from oxidation of alcohol, may be directly hepatotoxic and is implicated in the production of the more severe hepatic lesions seen in alcoholic patients. Immune-mediated hepatic damage may also play a role in producing the lesion of alcoholic hepatitis.

Hepatic toxic effects from alcohol vary considerably among individuals. Nevertheless, consumption by men of 40 to 60 g of ethanol per day (one beer or one mixed drink = 10 g of ethanol) for 10 to 15 years carries a substantial risk of the development of alcoholic liver disease, whereas women appear to have a lower threshold of injury. Malnutrition may potentiate the toxic effects of alcohol on the liver, and genetic factors may contribute to individual susceptibility.

Clinical and Pathologic Features

Alcoholic fatty liver may present as an incidentally discovered tender hepatomegaly. Some patients consult a physician because of pain in their right upper quadrant. Jaundice is rare. Transaminase levels are mildly elevated (less than five times normal). Liver biopsy shows diffuse or centrilobular fat occupying most of the hepatocyte.

Alcoholic hepatitis, a severe and prognostically ominous lesion, is characterized by the following histologic triad: (1) Mallory bodies (intracellular eosinophilic aggregates of cytokeratins), usually seen near or around the cell nuclei of hepatocytes; (2) infiltration by polymorphonuclear leukocytes; and (3) a network of intralobular connective tissue surrounding hepatocytes and central veins (*spider fibrosis*). Patients with this histologic lesion may be asymptomatic or extremely ill with hepatic failure. Anorexia, nausea, vomiting, weight loss, and abdominal pain are common presenting symptoms. Hepatomegaly is present in 80% of patients with alcoholic hepatitis, and splenomegaly is often present. Fever is common, but bacterial infection should always be excluded, because patients with alcoholic liver disease are prone to develop pneumonia as well as infection of the urinary tract and peritoneal cavity. Jaundice is commonly present and may be pronounced, with cholestatic features that require differentiation from biliary tract disease (see Chapter 40). Cutaneous signs of chronic liver disease may be found, including spider angiomas, palmar erythema, and gynecomastia. Parotid enlargement, testicular atrophy, and loss of body hair may be prominent (see Chapter 43). Ascites and encephalopathy may be present and indicate severe disease. The white blood cell count may be strikingly elevated, whereas transaminase levels are modestly increased (range, 200 to 400 U/L), an important differentiating feature from

other forms of acute hepatitis. The ratio of aspartate transaminase to alanine transaminase frequently exceeds 2, in contrast to viral hepatitis, in which the transaminase levels are usually increased in parallel. Prolonged prothrombin time, hypoalbuminemia, and hyperglobulinemia may be found.

Diagnosis

A history of excessive prolonged alcohol intake is often difficult to obtain from patients with alcoholic liver disease. However, historical, clinical, and biochemical features of alcoholic hepatitis are often sufficient to establish the diagnosis. Many patients suspected or found to imbibe alcohol excessively may have causes other than alcohol for their liver disease (e.g., chronic viral hepatitis). Thus, when other causes of liver disease are suspected and the patient's alcohol intake is uncertain, a liver biopsy may be extremely helpful in establishing the diagnosis.

Complications and Prognosis

Alcoholic fatty liver completely resolves with cessation of alcohol intake. Alcoholic hepatitis can also resolve, but more commonly it progresses either to cirrhosis, which may already be present at the time of initial presentation, or to hepatic failure and death. The development of encephalopathy, ascites, deteriorating renal function (*hepatorenal syndrome*), and gastrointestinal bleeding from varices often complicates alcoholic hepatitis.

Treatment

Treatment of acute alcoholic hepatitis is supportive. A high-calorie diet with vitamin (particularly thiamine) supplementation is instituted and may require administration by nasogastric tube in severely anorectic patients. Protein should be included, but it may need to be restricted in patients with encephalopathy (see Chapter 43). Treatment with corticosteroids may be of benefit in selected patients with severe disease.

DRUG-INDUCED AND TOXIN-INDUCED HEPATITIS

A broad spectrum of hepatic disease may result from a variety of therapeutic drugs or toxins (Table 41–4). The pathophysiologic mechanisms whereby these hepatic lesions are produced are complex. At one end of the spectrum is a predictable, dose-dependent, direct toxic effect on hepatocytes that leads to frank centrilobular hepatocellular necrosis typical of acetaminophen and carbon tetrachloride toxicity. Other reactions are generally not predictable and usually occur for unknown reasons in susceptible persons (*idiosyncratic drug reaction*). In some instances, genetically determined differences in pathways of hepatic drug metabolism may result in metabolites with greater toxic potential. Examples include viral hepatitis–like reactions (halothane, isoniazid), cho-

TABLE 41-4   Classification of Drug-Induced Liver Disease

Category	Examples
Predictable hepatotoxins with zonal necrosis	Acetaminophen Carbon tetrachloride
Nonspecific hepatitis	Aspirin Oxacillin Herbs (chaparral, germander)
Viral hepatitis–like reactions	Halothane Isoniazid Phenytoin
Cholestasis	Estrogens
Noninflammatory	17α-Substituted steroids
Inflammatory	Chlorpromazine Antithyroid agents
Fatty liver	
Large droplet	Ethanol Corticosteroids
Small droplet	Amiodarone Allopurinol
Chronic hepatitis	Methyldopa Nitrofurantoin
Tumors	Estrogens Vinyl chloride
Vascular lesions	6-Thioguanine Anabolic steroids Herbs (senna, comfrey)
Fibrosis	Methotrexate
Granulomas	Allopurinol Sulfonamides

lestatic hepatitis (chlorpromazine), granulomatous hepatitis (allopurinol), chronic hepatitis (methyldopa), and pure cholestasis without inflammatory cell infiltration or hepatocellular necrosis (estrogens, androgens). Immune-mediated hepatic damage may contribute in some cases, possibly when the drugs or their metabolites act as a hapten on the surface of hepatocytes. A few important examples of drug-induced hepatitis are discussed here.

Acetaminophen

Acetaminophen is metabolized by the hepatic cytochrome P-450 system to a potentially toxic metabolite that is subsequently rendered harmless through conjugation with glutathione. When massive doses are taken (>10 to 15 g), the formation of excess toxic metabolites depletes the available glutathione and produces necrosis. Acetaminophen overdose, commonly taken in a suicide attempt, leads to nausea and vomiting within a few hours. These symptoms subside and are followed in 24 to 48 hours by clinical and laboratory evidence of hepatocellular necrosis (raised transaminase levels) and hepatic dysfunction (prolonged prothrombin time, hepatic encephalopathy). Similar findings may occur with therapeutic doses of acetaminophen in patients with chronic alcoholism. Extensive liver necrosis may lead to fulminant hepatic failure and death. Severe liver damage may

be predicted on the basis of acetaminophen blood levels from 4 to 12 hours after ingestion. Treatment with N-acetylcysteine given orally (140-mg/kg bolus followed by 70 mg/kg × 17 doses), thought to promote hepatic glutathione synthesis, may be life-saving.

Isoniazid

Isoniazid, as single-drug prophylaxis against tuberculosis, commonly produces subclinical hepatic injury (20% incidence), as evidenced by raised serum transaminase levels. This effect appears to be transient and self-limiting in most patients. However, a 1% incidence exists of clinical hepatitis, which progresses to fatal hepatic necrosis in 10% of affected patients. Individual and age-related differences in hepatic acetylation of potentially toxic isoniazid metabolites may be important in this injury. Thus, the incidence of severe hepatic damage increases with age, such that significant elevation of transaminase levels in persons who are more than 35 years of age is an indication for discontinuing the drug.

Halothane

Historically, this anesthetic agent caused an uncommon acute viral hepatitis–like reaction several days after exposure in susceptible persons. Hepatic injury was caused in part by an allergic response to hepatic neoantigens produced by halothane metabolism, and the severity of this reaction increased with repeated exposure. Newer, commonly used halogenated anesthetic agents (isoflurane, enflurane) are hepatotoxic in a much smaller number of patients.

Chlorpromazine

Chlorpromazine produces a cholestatic reaction, often weeks to months after administration of the drug is begun. Fever, anorexia, and a rash may accompany jaundice and pruritus. Eosinophilia is common. Erythromycin may produce a similar picture, but pain in the right upper quadrant that mimics acute cholecystitis is often prominent.

Herbs

Herbal supplements are taken throughout the world, and approximately 5 billion dollars per year are spent in the United States alone on herbal agents. Incorrectly considered to be safe because they are "natural," many herbs are hepatotoxic. *Senecio, Heliotropium, Crotalaria,* and comfrey contain pyrrolizidine alkaloids that cause hepatic veno-occlusive disease. Hepatotoxicity ranging from mild hepatitis to massive necrosis and fulminant hepatic failure has been associated with the use of chaparral, germander, pennyroyal oil, mistletoe, and skullcap. Milk thistle, often taken by patients with chronic hepatitis and cirrhosis, has not been associated with hepatotoxicity, but its benefit is undefined because of the lack of controlled studies.

Chronic Hepatitis

Chronic hepatitis is defined as a hepatic inflammatory process that fails to resolve after 6 months.

ETIOLOGY

Acute viral hepatitis can ultimately lead to chronic hepatitis, with the notable exceptions of HAV and HEV (Table 41–5). Several drugs may produce chronic hepatitis, the best recognized being methyldopa. In contrast to acute hepatitis, an etiologic agent is sometimes difficult to identify in cases of chronic hepatitis. The pathogenesis of these idiopathic forms may represent quiescent autoimmune disease, undetected past drug-induced injury, antibody-negative viral infections, or misdiagnosed cholestatic liver injury (e.g., primary biliary cirrhosis, primary sclerosing cholangitis).

CLASSIFICATION

The initial classification of chronic hepatitis was developed in the mid-1970s. Chronic persistent hepatitis (inflammatory activity confined to portal areas) and chronic lobular hepatitis (inflammatory activity and necrosis scattered throughout the lobule) were thought to have a generally good prognosis. Chronic active hepatitis (inflammatory activity in portal areas that spill out into the lobule [periportal hepatitis, piecemeal necrosis] in association with necrosis and fibrosis) was thought to have a significant risk for progression to cirrhosis and liver failure.

Although histologic criteria remain generally useful, we recognize that many causes of chronic hepatitis and their natural histories are independent of histologic features, and the realization that the development of progressive disease may occur regardless of histologic stage has prompted a reclassification of chronic hepatitis. This classification is based on the *etiologic agent* responsible for disease, the *grade* of injury (determined by the numbers and location of inflammatory cells), and the *stage* of disease (determined by the degree, location,

and distortion of normal architecture by fibrosis). It allows integration of knowledge of the natural history of specific causes with histologic features of present and past hepatic damage to assess the severity and prognosis of the process. Thus, in general, both serologic studies and liver biopsy are used in the diagnosis of and in planning treatment for chronic hepatitis.

CHRONIC VIRAL HEPATITIS

Chronic hepatitis B follows acute HBV in about 5% of adults in the United States. Patients who are HBsAg and HBeAg positive are considered to be in a high replicative phase in comparison with those who are HBsAg and HBeAb positive (low replicative phase). Therapy is administered to patients with a high replication phase of HBV. Chronic hepatitis C is estimated to affect 2% of the United States population, and about 45% of these patients develop chronic hepatitis. Approximately 30% of these patients may develop cirrhosis. Subjects with either HBV or HCV infection are at a greater risk of developing hepatocellular carcinoma. Treatment of chronic HBV infection with interferon-α and of chronic HCV infection with a combination of interferon-α and ribavirin has decreased inflammatory activity and has suppressed viral activity in 30% to 40% of patients.

AUTOIMMUNE HEPATITIS

Autoimmune liver disease has several forms; however, the typical disease is characterized by significant hepatic inflammation with plasma cells and fibrosis in a young woman. The presence of hypergammaglobulinemia, as well as antinuclear or anti–smooth muscle antibodies, represents the classic variant. Extrahepatic manifestations including amenorrhea, rashes, acne, vasculitis, thyroiditis, and Sjögren's syndrome are common. Evidence of hepatic failure and the presence of chronic disease on biopsy at the time of diagnosis are frequent. Treatment with corticosteroids, often with azathioprine for steroid sparing, is efficacious and in many cases prolongs survival.

GENETIC AND METABOLIC HEPATITIS

Wilson's disease and α_1-antitrypsin deficiency generally present before the age of 35 years, and a family history of liver disease may be present. Diagnostic evaluation for Wilson's disease includes low serum ceruloplasmin and high urinary copper and hepatic copper levels. Therapy is with D-penicillamine (copper chelation), and patients are treated indefinitely. A low serum α_1-antitrypsin level and diastase-positive staining of hepatocellular inclusions on liver biopsy suggest α_1-antitrypsin deficiency. A homozygous phenotype (PiZZ) supports the diagnosis, and no specific medical therapy exists.

Nonalcoholic steatohepatitis has become increasingly recognized and most commonly occurs in persons who are overweight and who have diabetes and hyperlipidemia, although it can occur in persons of normal weight.

TABLE 41–5   Causes of Chronic Hepatitis

Viral
Hepatitis B
Hepatitis B with superimposed hepatitis D
Hepatitis C

Drugs and Toxins
Methyldopa
Nitrofurantoin
Amiodarone
Isoniazid

Autoimmune

Genetic and Metabolic Disorders
Wilson's disease
α_1-Antitrypsin deficiency
Nonalcoholic steatohepatitis

Histologic criteria include macrovesicular fatty infiltration (mainly triglyceride), inflammation including polymorphonuclear leukocytes, and hepatocyte injury (ballooning degeneration or necrotic hepatocytes) with or without fibrosis. The pathogenesis is still under investigation, but the disorder is thought to result from mitochondrial fatty oxidation impairment. Clinical trials are investigating the efficacy of weight reduction, vitamin E (as an antioxidant), and antihyperlipidemic agents.

REFERENCES

Bass NM: Toxic and drug-induced liver disease. *In* Goldman L, Bennett JC (eds): Cecil Textbook of Medicine, 21st ed. Philadelphia: WB Saunders, 2000, pp 779–783.

Boyer JL, Reuben A: Chronic hepatitis. *In* Schiff L, Schiff E (eds): Diseases of the Liver, 7th ed. Philadelphia: JB Lippincott, 1993, pp 586–637.

Dasmet VJ, Gerber M, Hoofnagle JH, et al: Classification of chronic hepatitis: Diagnosis, grading and staging. Hepatology 1994; 19:1513.

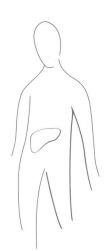

42

FULMINANT HEPATIC FAILURE

Michael B. Fallon • Brendan M. McGuire
Gary A. Abrams • Miguel R. Arguedas

Fulminant hepatic failure (FHF) is defined as the onset of encephalopathy occurring within 8 weeks of the onset of acute liver disease in a patient with acute liver disease. "Late-onset hepatic failure" is recognized as the development of encephalopathy in patients between 8 and 24 weeks after the onset of jaundice. The pathogenesis of FHF involves severe widespread hepatic necrosis, commonly resulting from acute viral infection with hepatitis A, B, C, or D viruses. It may also result from exposure to hepatotoxins such as acetaminophen, isoniazid, halothane, valproic acid, mushroom toxins (e.g., those of *Amanita phalloides*), or carbon tetrachloride. Reye's syndrome, a disease predominantly of children, and acute fatty liver of pregnancy, both of which are characterized by microvesicular fatty infiltration and little hepatocellular necrosis, often resemble FHF. In a number of patients with FHF, no cause is found, although a viral infection is usually presumed to be responsible.

Diagnosis

The diagnosis of FHF rests on the combination of hepatic encephalopathy and liver failure. This is evident with elevated serum bilirubin and transaminase levels and prolongation of the prothrombin time.

Treatment

Treatment of FHF remains supportive, because the underlying etiology of liver failure is rarely treatable. However, most processes that result in widespread liver cell necrosis and FHF are transient events, and liver cell regeneration with recovery of liver function often occurs if patients do not die from the complications of liver failure in the interim. Meticulous supportive treatment in an intensive care unit setting has been shown to improve survival. Patients with FHF should be cared for in centers with experience with this disease and with a liver transplantation program. Numerous complications (Table 42–1) result from FHF, and careful identification and treatment of each are essential.

Hepatic encephalopathy is often the first and most dramatic sign of liver failure. The pathogenesis of hepatic encephalopathy, discussed in Chapter 43, remains unclear. Hepatic encephalopathy that accompanies FHF differs from that associated with chronic liver disease in two important aspects: (1) It often responds to therapy only when liver function improves, and (2) it is frequently associated with two other potentially treatable causes of coma: hypoglycemia and cerebral edema. Therapy for hepatic encephalopathy in FHF differs slightly from the principles outlined in Chapter 43. Lactulose may be given orally, per nasogastric tube, or rectally, but the oral route should not be used if the patient is at risk for aspiration. Lactulose should be discontinued if no improvement is noted after several doses are administered. Intubation is often necessary to protect the airway from aspiration and to allow ventilation in patients with advanced encephalopathy.

Cerebral edema, the pathogenesis of which is unknown, is a common complication and the leading cause of death in FHF. Clinically, it is difficult to differentiate from hepatic encephalopathy, and computed tomography of the head is often unreliable. Therefore, most liver centers use intracranial monitoring to detect and monitor intracranial pressures. The goal is to maintain an intracranial pressure of less than 20 mm Hg. Management includes control of agitation, head elevation of 20 to 30 degrees, hyperventilation, administration of mannitol, treatment of barbiturate-induced coma, and urgent liver transplantation.

Hypoglycemia is a common complication of liver failure resulting from impaired hepatic gluconeogenesis and

TABLE 42-1   Management of Selected Problems in Fulminant Hepatic Failure

Complications	Pathogenesis	Management
Hepatic encephalopathy	Liver failure	Search for treatable causes, i.e., hypoglycemia, drugs used for sedation, sepsis, gastrointestinal bleeding, electrolyte imbalance, decreased Po_2, increased Pco_2; lactulose
Cerebral edema	Unknown	Elevate head of bed 20–30 degrees; hyperventilate (Pco_2 25–30 mm Hg); mannitol, 0.5–1 g/kg IV bolus over 5 min; pentobarbital infusion; urgent liver transplantation
Coagulopathy and gastrointestinal hemorrhage	Decreased synthesis of clotting factors Gastric erosions	Vitamin K; fresh-frozen plasma if actively bleeding and for prevention of bleeding; IV H_2-antagonist prophylaxis
Hypoglycemia	↓ Gluconeogenesis Insulin degradation	IV 10% dextrose, monitor every 2 hours; 30%–50% dextrose may be needed
Agitation	May be due to: Encephalopathy ↑ Intracranial pressure Hypoxemia	Search for treatable causes (i.e., ↓ Po_2, skin ulcers, lacerations, or abscesses); soft restraints; if severely agitated and a concern of injury, consider sedation along with mechanical ventilation to protect airway

insulin degradation. All patients should receive 10% glucose intravenous infusions with frequent monitoring of blood glucose levels. Other metabolic abnormalities commonly occur, including *hyponatremia, hypokalemia, respiratory alkalosis,* and *metabolic acidosis.* Thus, frequent monitoring of blood electrolytes and pH is indicated.

Gastrointestinal hemorrhage occurs frequently and is commonly caused by gastric erosions and impaired synthesis of clotting factors. All patients should receive vitamin K and prophylactic intravenous H_2-receptor antagonists to maintain gastric pH above 5. Fresh-frozen plasma should be used if clinically significant bleeding occurs or if major procedures, including intracranial pressure monitoring and central line placement, are performed.

Hepatic Transplantation

Hepatic transplantation (see Chapter 43) has been performed with considerable success in patients with FHF and is the treatment of choice for patients who appear unlikely to recover spontaneously. Because of the urgent need for transplantation, potential candidates should be transferred to transplant centers before significant complications develop (e.g., coma, cerebral edema, hemorrhage, or infection).

Transplantation is usually indicated in patients with severe encephalopathy or coagulopathy or in those whose clinical course is protracted and subacute. The cause is also important in determining prognosis. Patients with FHF resulting from viral hepatitis A, B, and D or acetaminophen overdose are more likely to recover spontaneously, whereas those with FHF secondary to drugs or of indeterminate cause or who have Wilson's disease rarely survive without transplantation.

Many other forms of therapy for FHF have been tried, including corticosteroid administration, exchange transfusion, plasmapheresis, hemodialysis, charcoal hemoperfusion, and extracorporeal perfusion through a human cadaver or pig liver. None has been shown to offer any advantage over conventional supportive therapy or liver transplantation.

Prognosis

Short-term prognosis without liver transplantation is very poor, the average reported survival rate being about 20%. Long-term prognosis for those who survive is excellent. Follow-up studies have shown normal liver function and histology in virtually all surviving patients, regardless of the cause of the fulminant failure. One-year survival is in the range of 80% to 90% after liver transplantation for FHF.

REFERENCES

Diehl AM: Acute and chronic liver failure and hepatic encephalopathy. *In* Goldman L, Bennett JC (eds): Cecil Textbook of Medicine, 21st ed. Philadelphia: WB Saunders, 2000, pp 813–816.

Hoofnagle JH, Carithers RL Jr, Shapiro C, et al: Fulminant hepatic failure: Summary of a workshop. Hepatology 1995; 21:240–252.

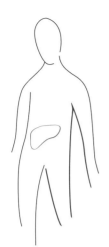

43

CIRRHOSIS OF THE LIVER AND ITS COMPLICATIONS

Michael B. Fallon • Brendan M. McGuire
Gary A. Abrams • Miguel R. Arguedas

Cirrhosis is the irreversible end result of the fibrous scarring and hepatocellular regeneration that constitute the major responses of the liver to a variety of long-standing inflammatory, toxic, metabolic, and congestive insults. In cirrhosis, the normal hepatic lobular architecture is replaced by interconnecting bands of fibrous tissue surrounding nodules derived from foci of regenerating hepatocytes.

Regenerative nodules may be small (<3 mm, *micronodular cirrhosis*), a typical feature of alcoholic cirrhosis, or large (>3 mm, *macronodular cirrhosis*). The latter, also termed *postnecrotic cirrhosis,* is more commonly seen as a sequel to chronic active hepatitis. The pathologic features of cirrhosis determine its natural history and clinical manifestations. Thus, fibrous scarring and disruption of the hepatic architecture distort the vascular bed and lead to portal hypertension and intrahepatic shunting. Normal hepatocyte function is disturbed by the resulting inadequacy of blood flow and ongoing direct toxic, inflammatory, and/or metabolic damage to hepatocytes.

Clinical and Laboratory Features

Clinical features of cirrhosis (often called "stigmata of chronic liver disease") are attributable to hepatocellular dysfunction and portal hypertension (Table 43–1). *Hepatocellular dysfunction* leads to impaired protein synthesis (hypoalbuminemia and prolongation of prothrombin time), hyperbilirubinemia, which may result in jaundice, low blood urea nitrogen levels, and elevated ammonia levels. *Hypersplenism,* resulting from splenomegaly, results in thrombocytopenia and leukopenia, but it is usually of little clinical significance and does not warrant splenectomy.

Specific Causes

Most of the conditions that may lead to cirrhosis (Table 43–2) are rarely encountered. Alcohol consumption and hepatitis C virus infection are by far the most common causes of cirrhosis in the Western world, whereas hepatitis B is a major cause in developing countries. Cryptogenic cirrhosis remains a diagnosis of exclusion.

ALCOHOL

Alcoholic cirrhosis may coexist with alcoholic hepatitis (see Chapter 41). Features of hepatocellular dysfunction are thus often marked and may improve with abstinence. Micronodular cirrhosis is the rule but is not specific for alcoholic cirrhosis. Data suggest that hepatitis C virus infection in patients with alcoholism may cause a more severe and rapidly progressive liver disease. Evidence of malnutrition and vitamin deficiency is frequently found, particularly in patients with severe alcoholism. Anemia of mixed origin is common, often with macrocytic indices.

PRIMARY BILIARY CIRRHOSIS

Primary biliary cirrhosis is seen more commonly in women, with a male-to-female ratio of 1:9. It typically presents in patients between the ages of 30 and 65 years and results from progressive, immune-mediated destruction of the interlobular bile ducts. Cholestatic features predominate, with high serum levels of alkaline phosphatase and γ-glutamyltransferase. Fatigue and pruritus are major early symptoms, followed later in the course of the disease by xanthomas, hyperpigmentation, steatorrhea, and bone pain resulting from osteoporosis or osteomalacia. Commonly associated conditions in-

TABLE 43-1 **Causes of Cirrhosis**

> Alcohol
> Nonalcoholic steatohepatitis
> Hepatitis viruses (B and C)
> Drugs and toxins
> Autoimmune chronic active hepatitis
> Biliary cirrhosis
>   Primary biliary cirrhosis
>   Secondary biliary cirrhosis
>   Bile duct strictures
>   Sclerosing cholangitis
>   Biliary atresia
>   Tumors of the bile ducts
>   Cystic fibrosis
> Chronic hepatic congestion
>   Budd-Chiari syndrome
>   Chronic right heart failure
>   Constrictive pericarditis
> Genetically determined metabolic diseases
>   Hemochromatosis
>   Wilson's disease
> α_1-Antitrypsin deficiency
>   Galactosemia
> Cryptogenic

clude Sjögren's syndrome, scleroderma, and the CREST syndrome (*c*alcinosis, *R*aynaud's syndrome, *e*sophageal dysfunction, *s*clerodactyly, *t*elangiectasia). Antimitochondrial antibodies are present in high titer, and serum IgM levels are elevated. Serum cholesterol levels are elevated in >50% of patients with primary biliary cirrhosis, mainly because of elevations of high-density lipoproteins. Liver biopsy may show characteristic destructive lesions of the bile ducts and is of value in confirming the diagnosis. Jaundice is a prominent feature late in the course of the disease. Treatment with ursodeoxycholic acid (replaces endogenous toxic bile acids) improves pruritus, slows the progression of disease, and thus delays the need for liver transplantation and prolongs life.

CHRONIC ACTIVE HEPATITIS

See Chapter 41.

HEMOCHROMATOSIS

See Chapter 61.

WILSON'S DISEASE

See Chapter 61.

....

Major Complications

The major sequelae of cirrhosis are as follows:

1. Portal hypertension and hepatocellular dysfunction, which may result in
   a. Variceal hemorrhage.
   b. Ascites, which can be further complicated by spontaneous bacterial peritonitis.
   c. Hepatic encephalopathy.
   d. Hepatorenal syndrome.
   e. Hepatopulmonary syndrome.
2. Hepatocellular carcinoma.

The pathophysiologic interrelationships among these complications are shown diagrammatically in Figure 43–1.

PORTAL HYPERTENSION

The distortion of hepatic architecture in cirrhosis leads to a marked increase in resistance to portal venous flow, which, in turn, leads to an increase in portal venous pressure. In alcoholic liver disease, increased resistance to sinusoidal blood flow may also result from hepatocyte swelling (*hydropic degeneration*).

Although cirrhosis is the most important cause of portal hypertension, any process leading to increased resistance to portal blood flow into (presinusoidal) or through the liver (sinusoidal) or to hepatic venous outflow from the liver (postsinusoidal) results in portal hypertension (Table 43–3). Hydrostatic pressure within any vascular system is proportional to both resistance and blood flow. In cirrhosis, increases in splanchnic blood flow may also result from increased cardiac output, which further aggravates portal hypertension.

Portal hypertension leads to the formation of venous collateral vessels between the portal and systemic circulations. Collateral vessels may form at several sites, the most important clinically being those connecting the portal vein to the azygos vein that form dilated, tortuous veins (varices) in the submucosa of the gastric fundus and esophagus. The normal portal pressure gradient (hepatic vein–portal vein) is 4 to 6 mm Hg. When the gradient is more than 12 mm Hg, esophageal varices may rupture.

TABLE 43-2 **Clinical and Laboratory Features of Cirrhosis**

Clinical	Laboratory
Hepatocellular Dysfunction	
Jaundice	Hyperbilirubinemia
Spider angiomas	Edema
Palmar erythema	Low serum blood urea nitrogen
Gynecomastia	Prolonged prothrombin time
Loss of body hair	Hyperammonemia
Testicular atrophy	Thrombocytopenia
Dupuytren's contracture	Leukopenia
Muscle wasting	—
Hypoalbuminemia	Low serum albumin
Bruising	—
Signs of hepatic encephalopathy	—
Fetor hepaticus	
Portal Hypertension	
Splenomegaly	—
Ascites	—
Caput medusae	—
Variceal bleeding	—

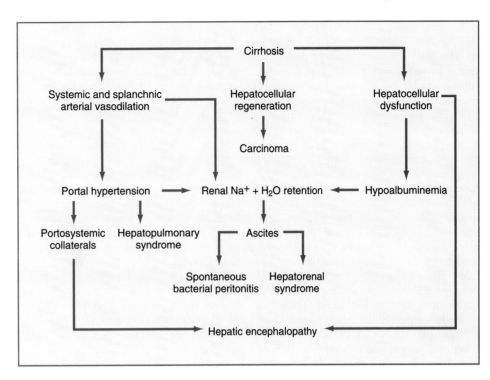

FIGURE 43–1 Interrelationships among the complications of cirrhosis.

VARICEAL HEMORRHAGE

Hemorrhage occurs most frequently from varices in the esophagus and is a common and serious complication of portal hypertension that has a mortality rate of 30% to 60%. Large varices bleed most commonly, and bleeding occurs when high tension in the walls of these vessels leads to rupture. Bleeding may present as hematemesis, hematochezia, melena, or any combination of these entities (see Chapter 32). Bleeding may lead to shock, it may stop spontaneously, or it may recur. Impaired hepatic synthesis of coagulation factors (hepatocellular dysfunction) and thrombocytopenia (hypersplenism) may further complicate the management of variceal bleeding. The management of esophageal varices includes early

medical intervention to prevent bleeding as well as the treatment of acute variceal hemorrhage (Fig. 43–2). Nonselective β blockers (propranolol and nadolol) and mononitrates (isosorbide mononitrate) are effective in

TABLE 43–3 Causes of Portal Hypertension

Increased resistance to flow
  Presinusoidal
    Portal or splenic vein occlusion (thrombosis, tumor)
    Schistosomiasis
    Congenital hepatic fibrosis
    Sarcoidosis
  Sinusoidal
    Cirrhosis (all causes)
    Alcoholic hepatitis
  Postsinusoidal
    Veno-occlusive disease
    Budd-Chiari syndrome
    Constrictive pericarditis
Increased portal blood flow
  Splenomegaly not due to liver disease
  Arterioportal fistula

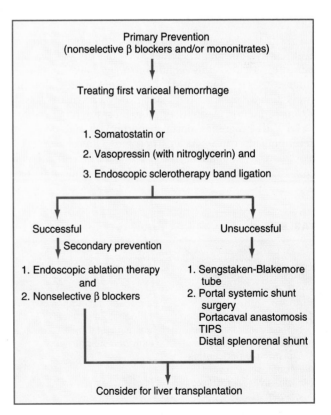

FIGURE 43–2 Primary prevention of variceal bleeding. TIPS = transjugular intrahepatic portosystemic shunt.

preventing variceal hemorrhage by reducing portal blood flow and pressure. Screening for varices is appropriate in patients with cirrhosis who have clinical features of portal hypertension, particularly those patients who have telangiectasias on physical examination and thrombocytopenia. Somatostatin (or its synthetic analogue, octreotide) and vasopressin are given intravenously to reduce splanchnic blood flow and are used in the acute setting of esophageal hemorrhage until endoscopic or surgical therapy is performed. Intravenous nitroglycerin should be given with vasopressin to minimize systemic vasoconstrictive toxicity. Endoscopic therapy includes injection with sclerosing solutions and/or band ligation. A meta-analysis has shown that band ligation may be more effective to prevent recurrent bleeding, and it is associated with fewer adverse effects. Repeated courses can lead to variceal obliteration. Balloon tamponade (Sengstaken-Blakemore tube, Linton tube, or Minnesota tube) is an effective temporary measure for patients in whom endoscopic therapy has failed. These patients may need to undergo portal decompression either by a variety of surgical procedures or by transjugular intrahepatic portosystemic shunt placement. The patient's candidacy for liver transplantation affects the surgeon's choice of portal decompressive procedure.

HEPATIC DYSFUNCTION

Cirrhosis results in impaired synthesis of proteins by hepatocytes and leads to hypoalbuminemia and deficient production of coagulation factors and diminished capacity for hepatic detoxification (see Chapters 39 and 42).

ASCITES

Ascites is the accumulation of excess fluid in the peritoneal cavity. Although cirrhosis is the most common cause of ascites, this condition may have numerous other causes (Table 43–4). The serum-ascites albumin gradient has replaced the exudative-transudative classification of ascites. A high serum-ascites albumin gradient ($\geq$1.1 g/dL) signifies portal hypertension but does not determine its cause. Ascites becomes clinically detectable when accumulations reach >500 mL. Shifting dullness to percussion is the most sensitive clinical sign of

ascites, but ultrasonography more readily detects small fluid volumes.

Several theories explain the formation of ascites in cirrhosis. Initially, systemic arterial vasodilatation (*peripheral arterial vasodilation theory*) results in excess renal reabsorption of sodium and water and leads to hypervolemia and overflow of fluid into the peritoneum (*overflow theory*), thus causing ascites. Ascites causes an "ineffective" intravascular volume (*underflow theory*) that results in enhanced production of renin, aldosterone, and antidiuretic hormone and thereby further increases sodium and water retention and perpetuates ascites formation.

Treatment of ascites consists initially of sodium restriction, preferably less than 2 g/day. Restricted fluid intake may be necessary if hyponatremia (<120 mEq/L) is present. The administration of spironolactone, an aldosterone antagonist, supplemented with a loop diuretic (e.g., furosemide) is often effective. Diuresis should be monitored closely, because aggressive diuretic therapy may result in hypokalemia and a depleted plasma volume, leading to hepatic encephalopathy and impaired renal function. *Refractory ascites* occurs in about 10% of patients with cirrhosis and is defined as persistent tense ascites despite maximal diuretic therapy (spironolactone, 400 mg/day, and furosemide, 160 mg/day) or if azotemia develops (creatinine >2 mg/dL) while the patient is receiving submaximal doses. Treatment in these patients includes repeated large-volume paracentesis (many physicians simultaneously give intravenous albumin, at 6 to 8 g/L of ascitic fluid removed, but whether this is of any benefit is unclear and may not be necessary if $\leq$5 L is removed), surgically implanted peritoneovenous shunts (LeVeen or Denver), transjugular intrahepatic portosystemic shunt, portacaval anastomoses, or liver transplantation.

Two important complications occur in patients with cirrhotic ascites: spontaneous bacterial peritonitis and the hepatorenal syndrome. These complications are discussed in the next two sections.

SPONTANEOUS BACTERIAL PERITONITIS

Infection of ascitic fluid, usually with Enterobacteriaceae or *Pneumococcus,* may occur in patients with cirrhosis. Fever, abdominal pain, and tenderness may be present, or the infection may be clinically silent. Hepatic encephalopathy may be precipitated. The diagnosis is strongly suspected if the ascitic fluid polymorphonuclear leukocyte count is more than 250/μL, and the diagnosis may be confirmed by culture. Treatment with a third-generation cephalosporin for 5 to 7 days is usual. Prophylactic therapy is indicated in patients with a prior episode of spontaneous bacterial peritonitis, in patients with cirrhosis and ascites who are hospitalized with upper gastrointestinal bleeding, and in other selected patients (i.e., patients with an ascitic fluid total protein concentration <1 g/dL and candidates for liver transplantation). Prophylaxis with norfloxacin (400 mg/day), ciprofloxacin (750 mg once weekly), or trimethoprim-sulfamethoxazole (160 mg/800 mg Monday through Friday) has been shown to be effective.

TABLE 43–4 **Causes of Ascites**

Serum-Ascites Albumin Gradient	
High: >1.1 g/dL	**Low: <1.1 g/dL**
Cirrhosis	Peritoneal carcinomatosis
Chronic hepatic congestion	Peritoneal tuberculosis
Right-sided heart failure	Pancreatic and biliary disease
Budd-Chiari syndrome	Nephrotic syndrome
Constrictive pericarditis	—
Nephrotic syndrome	—
Massive liver metastases	—
Myxedema	—
Mixed ascites	—

HEPATORENAL SYNDROME

Serious liver disease from any cause may be complicated by a form of functional renal failure termed the *hepatorenal syndrome*. It almost invariably occurs in the presence of significant hepatic synthetic dysfunction and severe ascites. This syndrome occurs in approximately 4% of patients with decompensated cirrhosis, and some prospective series have determined that the probability of developing it in patients admitted to the hospital for the treatment of ascites may be as high as 32% at 2 years. Typically, the kidneys are histologically normal, with the capacity of regaining normal function in the event of recovery of liver function. Severe cortical vasoconstriction has been demonstrated angiographically, and it reverses when these kidneys have been transplanted in patients who do not have cirrhosis. The renal dysfunction is characterized by a declining glomerular filtration rate, oliguria, low urine sodium (<10 mEq/L), normal urinary sediment, and azotemia, often with a disproportionately high ratio of blood urea nitrogen to creatinine. The decline in renal function often follows one of three events in a patient with cirrhosis and ascites: sepsis, a vigorous attempt to reduce ascites with diuretics, or large-volume paracentesis.

The hepatorenal syndrome is usually progressive and fatal, with a mortality of 95%. It should be diagnosed only after plasma volume depletion (a common cause of reversible, prerenal azotemia in patients with cirrhosis, particularly with diuretic use) and other forms of acute renal injury have been excluded.

Patients should be given volume expanders to treat possible prerenal azotemia. Successful reversal of hepatorenal syndrome has been documented using low-dose vasopressin, octreotide, or norepinephrine, which raise systemic vascular resistance and thereby increase renal blood flow. Liver transplantation has become an accepted treatment for the hepatorenal syndrome.

HEPATIC ENCEPHALOPATHY

Hepatic encephalopathy (also called *hepatic coma* or *portosystemic encephalopathy*) is a complex neuropsychiatric syndrome that may complicate advanced liver disease and/or extensive portosystemic collateral formation (*shunting*). Two major forms of hepatic encephalopathy are recognized: acute and chronic.

Acute hepatic encephalopathy usually occurs in the setting of fulminant hepatic failure. Cerebral edema plays a more important role in this setting: coma is common and mortality is extremely high (see Chapter 42). *Chronic hepatic encephalopathy* usually occurs with chronic liver disease, commonly manifests as subtle disturbances of neurologic function, and is often reversible.

The pathogenesis of hepatic encephalopathy is thought to involve the inadequate hepatic removal of predominantly nitrogenous compounds or other toxins ingested or formed in the gastrointestinal tract. Inadequate hepatic removal results from impaired hepatocyte function, as well as the extensive shunting of splanchnic blood directly into the systemic circulation by portosystemic collateral vessels. Nitrogenous and other absorbed compounds are thought to gain access to the central nervous system and to lead to disturbances in neuronal function. Ammonia, derived from both amino acid deamination and bacterial hydrolysis of nitrogenous compounds in the gut, has been strongly implicated in the pathogenesis of hepatic encephalopathy, but its blood levels correlate poorly with the presence or degree of encephalopathy. Investigators have suggested that ammonia generated in the stomach (especially in the presence of hypochloridia) by *Helicobacter pylori* may contribute to the development of encephalopathy. Other proposed neurotoxins include γ-aminobutyric acid, mercaptans, short-chain fatty acids, and benzodiazepine-like compounds. Mercaptans are also thought to produce the characteristic breath odor (*fetor hepaticus*) of patients with chronic liver failure. Another hypothesis suggests that an imbalance between plasma branched-chain and aromatic amino acids, a common consequence of severe liver disease, leads to decreased synthesis of normal neurotransmitters and to increased formation of "false neurotransmitters" from aromatic amino acids in the central nervous system. In addition, altered cerebral metabolism (disturbed Na^+,K^+-ATPase activity), zinc deficiency causing decreased activity of urea-cycle enzymes, and deposition of manganese in the basal ganglia have been implicated as possible mechanisms.

The clinical features of hepatic encephalopathy include disturbances of higher neurologic function (intellectual and personality disorders, dementia, inability to copy simple diagrams [*constructional apraxia*], disturbance of consciousness), disturbances of neuromuscular function (asterixis, hyperreflexia, myoclonus), and rarely, a Parkinson-like syndrome and progressive paraplegia. As with other metabolic encephalopathies, which may show many of the signs of hepatic encephalopathy, asymmetric neurologic findings are unusual but can occur, and brain stem reflexes (pupillary light, oculovestibular, and oculocephalic responses) are preserved until extremely late in the course of the disease. Hepatic encephalopathy is usually divided into stages according to its severity (Table 43–5). Subtle disorders of psychomotor function may exist in as many as 50% to 70% of patients with cirrhosis in whom a conventional neurologic examination is normal. Such subclinical encephalopathy (termed *stage 0* encephalopathy) is important in that it may impair work performance. One of the earliest manifestations is the alteration of the patient's normal sleep-wake cycle. The differential diagnosis of hepatic encephalopathy includes hypoglycemia, subdural hematoma, meningitis, and sedative drug overdose, all of which are common in patients with liver disease, particularly patients with alcoholism.

Treatment

Treatment of hepatic encephalopathy is based on four simple principles.

Identify and Treat Precipitating Factors
Table 43–6 lists several important factors that may precipitate or severely aggravate hepatic encephalopathy in patients with severe liver disease. Gastrointestinal bleed-

TABLE 43-5 Stages of Hepatic Encephalopathy

Stage*	Clinical Manifestations
I	Apathy
	Restlessness
	Reversal of sleep rhythm
	Slowed intellect
	Impaired computational ability
	Impaired handwriting
II	Lethargy
	Drowsiness
	Disorientation
	Asterixis
III	Stupor (arousable)
	Hyperactive reflexes, extensor plantar responses
IV	Coma (response to painful stimuli only)

*Stage 0 encephalopathy is used to describe subclinical impairment of intellectual function.

ing and increased protein intake may provide increased substrate for the bacterial or metabolic formation of nitrogenous compounds that induce encephalopathy. Patients prone to develop hepatic encephalopathy have increased sensitivity to drugs that depress the central nervous system, and the use of these drugs should be avoided in these patients.

Reduce and Eliminate Substrate for the Generation of Nitrogenous Compounds

Restrict Dietary Protein. Patients in coma should receive no protein, whereas those with mild encephalopathy may benefit from restriction of protein intake to 40 to 60 g/day. Vegetable protein diets also appear to be less encephalopathogenic. Treatment with formulas rich in branched-chain amino acids have shown no benefit in improving encephalopathy or mortality. Their primary role appears to be in the treatment of severely malnourished patients in whom aggressive protein supplementation is desired but who are intolerant to standard protein preparations.

Cleanse Bowels. This recommendation is important mainly in patients with encephalopathy precipitated by

TABLE 43-6 Hepatic Encephalopathy: Precipitating Factors

Gastrointestinal bleeding
Increased dietary protein
Constipation
Infection
CNS-depressant drugs (benzodiazepines, opiates, tricyclic antidepressants)
Deterioration in hepatic function
Hypokalemia: Most often induced by diuretics
Azotemia: Most often induced by diuretics
Alkalosis: Most often induced by diuretics
Hypovolemia: Most often induced by diuretics

CNS = central nervous system.

acute gastrointestinal bleeding or constipation and is achieved by administration of enemas.

Reduce Colonic Bacteria

Neomycin administered orally reduces the number of bacteria that are responsible for production of ammonia and other nitrogenous compounds, but its use may be associated with the development of nephrotoxicity and ototoxicity. Other antibiotics effective in the treatment of hepatic encephalopathy include metronidazole and rifaximin (a nonabsorbable rifamycin derivative).

Prevent Ammonia Diffusion from the Bowel

This is achieved by administration of lactulose, lactitol, and lactose (in lactase-deficient patients). These are nonabsorbable disaccharides that, when fermented to organic acids by colonic bacteria, lead to a lower stool pH. This lowered pH traps ammonia in the colon as nondiffusible NH_4^+ ions, but other mechanisms such as inhibition of bacterial ammonia production, and the promotion of the growth of non–urease-producing lactobacilli may also be important.

HEPATOPULMONARY SYNDROME

Hepatopulmonary syndrome is an increasingly recognized clinical entity (in 10% to 15% of patients with cirrhosis), characterized by abnormalities of arterial oxygenation in patients with chronic liver disease and/or portal hypertension. The pathophysiology of this syndrome involves intrapulmonary vascular dilatation in the absence of architectural damage. These vascular abnormalities consist of precapillary dilatation, direct arteriovenous communications, and dilated pleural vessels. Intrapulmonary vascular dilatation is detected by contrast echocardiography, which shows delayed visualization of microbubbles in the left heart chambers. The vascular dilatation leads to impaired oxygen transfer from alveoli to the central stream of red blood cells within capillaries, with a resulting "functional" intrapulmonary right-to-left shunt that improves with 100% oxygen. Clinical features range from subclinical abnormalities in gas exchange to profound hypoxemia causing dyspnea at rest. Patients often require supplemental oxygen and have significant limitations in their performance of usual daily activities. No proven medical therapy exists. As in hepatorenal syndrome, hepatopulmonary syndrome is a functional disorder that reverses in most patients after liver transplantation.

HEPATOCELLULAR CARCINOMA

Hepatocellular carcinoma and its relation to cirrhosis are discussed in Chapter 44.

Hepatic Transplantation

Liver transplantation is a highly successful procedure in patients with progressive, advanced, and otherwise untreatable liver disease. Advances in surgical techniques and supportive care, the use of cyclosporine and tacrolimus for immunosuppression, and careful selection of patients have all contributed to the encouraging results of liver transplantation. From 70% to 80% of patients undergoing liver transplantation survive at least 3 years, usually with good quality of life. The most common indication for liver transplantation in the United States is chronic liver disease resulting from hepatitis C virus infection. Other liver diseases for which transplantation is commonly performed include cirrhosis from alcoholic liver disease, autoimmune hepatitis, primary biliary cirrhosis, and primary sclerosing cholangitis. Patients with hepatitis B undergo liver transplantation if they do not have hepatitis e antigen and/or hepatitis B virus DNA in their serum. Hepatitis B immunoglobulin is given after liver transplantation to help prevent recurrence. Trials evaluating the efficacy of nucleoside analogues in lowering replication of hepatitis B virus and in facilitating liver transplantation are under way. Excellent results have also been obtained in selected patients with fulminant hepatic failure (see Chapter 42). Liver transplantation for malignant hepatobiliary disease has been less successful because of recurrent disease in the transplanted liver.

The timing of liver transplantation presents a particular challenge. Liver-assist devices for temporary support are currently being evaluated. The survival of ambulatory patients undergoing liver transplantation electively is greater than that of those who are critically ill at the time of the operation. Thus, liver transplantation is usually considered when the patient has refractory ascites and/or spontaneous bacterial peritonitis, recurrent variceal hemorrhage, intractable pruritus, or an unacceptable quality of life.

REFERENCES

Friedman S: Alcoholic liver disease, cirrhosis, and its major sequelae. In Goldman L, Bennett JC (eds): Cecil Textbook of Medicine, 21st ed. Philadelphia: WB Saunders, 2000, pp 804–812.

LaBrecque D: Portal hypertension. Clin Liver Dis 1997; 1:1–278.

Laffi G, La Villa G, Gentilini P: Pathogenesis and management of the hepatorenal syndrome. Semin Liver Dis 1994; 14:71–80.

Neuberger J, Lucey MR (eds): Liver Transplantation: Practice and Management. London: BMJ, 1994, pp 34–100.

Riordan SM, Williams R: Treatment of hepatic encephalopathy. N Engl J Med 1997; 337:473–479.

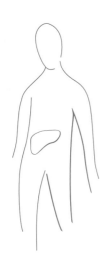

44

NEOPLASTIC, INFILTRATIVE, AND VASCULAR DISEASES OF THE LIVER

Michael B. Fallon • Brendan M. McGuire
Gary A. Abrams • Miguel R. Arguedas

Hepatic Neoplasms

Hepatic neoplasms can be divided into three groups: (1) benign neoplasms, (2) hepatocellular carcinoma, and (3) tumor metastases to the liver. In this chapter we provide a brief review of all three categories of hepatic neoplasms, describe liver abscesses and granulomatous liver disease, describe diagnostic approaches, and conclude with a brief discussion of the diagnostic approach to these lesions.

BENIGN NEOPLASMS

The category of benign neoplastic lesions includes hemangioma, hepatocellular adenoma, nodular regenerative hyperplasia, focal nodular hyperplasia, and rare mesenchymal tumors (e.g., fibromas, lipomas, leiomyomas).

Hemangiomas are the most common mesenchymal hepatic neoplasms, with a prevalence in the general population of 2% to 5%. They are usually located in the right lobe of the liver and are most often asymptomatic and, thus, incidentally discovered. Large lesions may cause right upper quadrant abdominal pain owing to intratumoral thrombosis, and acute spontaneous hemoperitoneum has been described in a few patients with large lesions located near the surface of the liver. Diagnosis is readily made when a hyperechoic lesion on ultrasound evaluation corresponds to a peripheral enhancing lesion that eventually completely fills during dynamic computed tomography, when magnetic resonance imaging reveals a high-intensity signal on T2-weighted images (most sensitive test), or when a technetium-99m

red blood cell scan (most specific test) shows retention of the isotope in the tumor. Treatment is usually not necessary unless lesions are very large (>4 cm) or symptomatic.

Adenomas almost exclusively occur in women of childbearing age, are associated with estrogen and oral contraceptive use, and may enlarge during pregnancy. In men, the development of adenomas has been closely associated with the use of anabolic steroids. They are usually incidentally identified, but patients may have signs or symptoms of an abdominal mass that can spontaneously hemorrhage during menstruation, pregnancy, or post partum, causing shock and requiring surgical resection. Adenomas consist of normal hepatocytes without portal tracts and Kupffer cells. The diagnosis is suggested by the appearance of a cold spot on technetium-99m sulfur colloid scans (resulting from absence of Kupffer cells) and of vascular lesions on angiography. The appearance on computed tomography and magnetic resonance imaging may be of variable density or intensity. Management of asymptomatic adenomas is controversial; however, because of potential rupture and potential malignant transformation, elective segmental liver resection may be performed. A trial period of observation may be warranted if oral contraceptives can be discontinued and regression of tumor is noted.

HEPATOCELLULAR CARCINOMA

Hepatocellular carcinoma (HCC) is rare in the United States, with a yearly incidence of approximately 3 per 100,000 population. It accounts for less than 2.5% of all malignancies. In other areas of the world, including sub-Saharan Africa, China, Japan, and Southeast Asia, it is one of the most frequent malignancies and is an important cause of mortality, particularly in middle-aged men. HCC often arises in a cirrhotic liver and is closely associated with chronic hepatitis B or C. Hepatitis B virus DNA has been shown to integrate in the host cell genome, where it may disrupt tumor suppressor genes and/or activate oncogenes. The advent and widespread use of vaccination to prevent infection with hepatitis B virus has begun to reduce the incidence of this disease. The exact role of hepatitis C in the pathogenesis of HCC is unknown. The risk of HCC is low in primary biliary cirrhosis and Wilson's disease, intermediate in cirrhosis caused by alcohol abuse, and high in hemochromatosis. Other risk factors for development of HCC, as well as its clinical manifestations, are listed in Table 44–1. Currently used imaging techniques for the detection of HCC and the most common appearance of the tumor are listed in Table 44–2. A tissue specimen may be necessary to confirm the diagnosis of HCC in some cases but may not be needed if characteristic features of HCC are present on imaging procedures and are accompanied by a rise in serum α-fetoprotein levels. Diagnosis of small, surgically resectable lesions in high-risk areas is possible with intensive screening programs

TABLE 44–1 Hepatocellular Carcinoma

Incidence

From 1–7 per 100,000 to >100 per 100,000 in high-risk areas

Sex

4:1 to 8:1 male preponderance

Associations

Chronic hepatitis B infection
Chronic hepatitis C infection
Hemochromatosis (with cirrhosis)
Cirrhosis (alcoholic, cryptogenic)
Aflatoxin ingestion
Thorotrast
α_1-Antitrypsin deficiency
Androgen administration

Common Clinical Presentations

Abdominal pain
Abdominal mass
Weight loss
Deterioration of liver function

Unusual Manifestations

Bloody ascites
Tumor emboli (lung)
Jaundice
Hepatic or portal vein obstruction
Metabolic effects
  Erythrocytosis
  Hypercalcemia
  Hypercholesterolemia
  Hypoglycemia
  Gynecomastia
  Feminization
  Acquired porphyria

Clinical/Laboratory Findings

Hepatic bruit or friction rub
Serum α-fetoprotein level >400 ng/mL

TABLE 44–2 Ultrasonographic, Radiographic, and MRI Characteristics of HCC

Ultrasonography

Mass lesion with varying echogenicities but usually hypoechoic

Dynamic Computed Tomography

Arterial phase: tumor enhances quickly
Venous phase: quick de-enhancement of the tumor relative to the parenchyma

MRI

T1-weighted images: hypointense
T2-weighted images: hyperintense
After gadolinium administration, the tumor increases in intensity

HCC = hepatocellular carcinoma; MRI = magnetic resonance imaging.

that employ ultrasound examinations and serum α-fetoprotein levels, although the long-term outcome and cost-effectiveness of this strategy remain unclear. Most patients present with widespread, often multifocal disease, and the median survival from the time of diagnosis is less than 6 months. Systemic and intra-arterial chemotherapy, arterial embolization, intratumor ethanol injection, radiation therapy, and hepatic transplantation have yielded disappointing results.

Other primary hepatocellular malignancies include cholangiocarcinoma, angiosarcoma (related to exposure to vinyl chloride, arsenic, or Thorotrast), hepatoblastoma (the most common hepatic tumor in children), and cystadenocarcinoma.

TUMOR METASTASES TO THE LIVER

Metastatic tumors constitute the majority of hepatic masses in the United States and, in decreasing order, most commonly originate from the lung, colon, pancreas, breast, stomach, unknown primary, ovary, prostate, and gallbladder.

Liver Abscess

Pyogenic and amebic liver abscesses are important mass lesions of the liver. Unlike hepatic neoplasms, abscesses often manifest as a relatively acute febrile illness associated with pain in the right upper quadrant of the abdomen. Lesions can be localized by radionuclide scan, ultrasonography, or computed tomography. The clinical presentation, diagnosis, and treatment of these lesions are discussed in Chapter 102.

Granulomatous Liver Disease

Hepatic granulomas are common, being found in 2% to 10% of all liver biopsy specimens, often in association with an elevated serum alkaline phosphatase level. However, they are rarely a specific finding and have been reported in association with a variety of infections, systemic illnesses, hepatobiliary disorders, drugs, and toxins, some of which are listed in Table 44–3. Although granulomas are a nonspecific finding, occasionally specific features are seen, such as acid-fast bacilli in tuber-

TABLE 44–3 Diseases Associated with Hepatic Granulomas

Infections
Bacterial, Spirochetal
Tuberculosis and atypical *Mycobacterium* infections
Tularemia
Brucellosis
Leprosy
Syphilis
Whipple's disease
Listeriosis
Viral
Infectious mononucleosis
Cytomegalovirus infections
Rickettsial
Q fever
Fungal
Coccidioidomycosis
Histoplasmosis
Cryptococcal infections
Actinomycosis
Aspergillosis
Nocardiosis
Parasitic
Schistosomiasis
Clonorchiasis
Toxocariasis
Ascariasis
Toxoplasmosis
Amebiasis
Hepatobiliary Disorders
Primary biliary cirrhosis
Granulomatous hepatitis
Jejunoileal bypass
Systemic Disorders
Sarcoidosis
Wegener's granulomatosis
Inflammatory bowel disease
Hodgkin's disease
Lymphoma
Drugs/Toxins
Beryllium
Parenteral foreign material (e.g., starch, talc, silicone)
Phenylbutazone
α-Methyldopa
Procainamide
Allopurinol
Phenytoin
Nitrofurantoin
Hydralazine

culosis, ova in schistosomiasis, larvae in toxocariasis, and birefringent granules in starch, talc, or silicone granulomas. The differential diagnosis of hepatic granulomas is one of the most extensive in medicine, and the work-up requires meticulous attention to details of the history, physical examination, and laboratory tests. Indeed, in 10% to 20% of patients, no cause for granulomas is found despite extensive investigation. A subset of these patients have a syndrome consisting of fever, hepatomegaly, and hepatic granulomas that responds to corticosteroids, described as hepatic granulomatous disease or "granulomatous hepatitis." These patients may possibly have a variant of sarcoidosis.

Liver biopsy (and culture, particularly for acid-fast bacteria) is of considerable value in the diagnosis of sarcoidosis, miliary tuberculosis, and histoplasmosis, because virtually all patients with these disorders have hepatic granulomas. Characteristic granulomas are seen in many patients with primary biliary cirrhosis, and granulomas may be the first clue to Hodgkin's disease.

Diagnostic Approach to Hepatic Lesions

The patient's clinical presentation and the presence of specific risk factors and coexisting illnesses help dictate the diagnostic approach of a liver mass. In general, ultrasonography is the first test ordered because it is inexpensive, noninvasive, and useful for differentiating cystic from solid tumors. Once a solid tumor is identified, radionuclide scanning may be reasonable, although lesions less than 3 cm are often too small to be detected. A solid lesion that exhibits uptake in a subject with cirrhosis most likely represents a regenerative nodule. If a lesion does not exhibit uptake, further evaluation using rapid-sequence computed tomography, magnetic resonance imaging, red blood cell scan, or angiography will be necessary to diagnose hemangiomas, adenomas, and/ or HCC. Often these tests are nondiagnostic, and a tissue specimen, obtained by percutaneous liver biopsy, computed tomography, ultrasound-guided fine-needle aspiration, or laparoscopy, is needed to confirm a diagnosis.

Vascular Disease of the Liver

Portal vein thrombosis, hepatic vein thrombosis (Budd-Chiari syndrome), and veno-occlusive disease are uncommon disorders of the hepatic vasculature. Affected patients usually present with portal hypertension with or without associated liver dysfunction.

Portal vein thrombosis may develop after abdominal trauma, umbilical vein infection and neonatal sepsis, and inflammatory diseases (e.g., pancreatitis) or in association with cirrhosis or hypercoagulable states. In most cases, however, particularly in children, the cause is unknown. The disease produces the manifestations of portal hypertension (see Chapter 43); however, liver histology is usually normal. The diagnosis is established by angiography, but Doppler ultrasonography may reveal an echogenic thrombus, collateral circulation near the porta hepatis, and splenomegaly. In long-standing portal vein thrombosis tortuous venous channels develop within the organized clot, leading to "cavernous transformation." Thrombolysis may be attempted in acute portal vein thrombosis. Although controversial, long-term anticoagulation may be used in chronic thrombosis secondary to hypercoagulable states. Variceal hemorrhage is managed with endoscopic obliteration. Prophylaxis with β blockers is not recommended because portal inflow decreases, potentially propagating the thrombus. If endoscopic treatment fails, surgical management with portosystemic shunting may be attempted, but it is often difficult because of the absence of suitable patent vessels.

The Budd-Chiari syndrome is associated with hematologic disease (e.g., polycythemia vera, paroxysmal nocturnal hemoglobinuria, myeloproliferative disorders), tumors, pregnancy, use of oral contraceptives, other hypercoagulable states, abdominal trauma, and congenital webs of the vena cava. Illness may manifest acutely as right upper quadrant abdominal pain, hepatomegaly, and ascites, whereas the chronic form manifests as portal hypertension. Doppler ultrasonography may show decreased or absent hepatic vein blood flow and is established angiographically by the inability to catheterize and visualize the hepatic veins. On venography, there is a characteristic "spider web" pattern of collateral vessels and the inferior vena cava may appear compressed, owing to hepatomegaly or an enlarged caudate lobe. On liver biopsy, centrilobular necrosis is seen. Although elevation of serum bilirubin and transaminase levels may be mild, liver function is often poor, and mortality rates of 40% to 90% are reported. Thrombolysis followed by anticoagulation may be useful in selected patients (i.e., in patients presenting early after developing symptoms); however, transjugular intrahepatic portacaval and side-to-side portacaval shunts, performed to relieve hepatic congestion, may improve survival, and liver transplantation may be curative.

REFERENCES

Fallon M: Hepatic tumors. *In* Goldman L, Bennett JC (eds): Cecil Textbook of Medicine, 21st ed. Philadelphia: WB Saunders, 2000, pp 819–821.

Kew MC: Hepatic tumors and cysts. *In* Feldman M, Scharschmidt BF, Sleisenger MH (eds): Gastrointestinal and Liver Disease: Pathophysiology/Diagnosis/Management, 6th ed. Philadelphia: WB Saunders, 1998, pp 1364–1387.

Khakoo SI, Grellier LFL, Soni PN, et al: Etiology, screening and treatment of hepatocellular carcinoma. Med Clin North Am 1996; 80:1121–1145.

Schafer DF, Sorrell MF: Vascular Diseases of the Liver. *In* Feldman M, Scharschmidt BF, Sleisenger MH (eds): Gastrointestinal and Liver Disease: Pathophysiology/Diagnosis/Management, 6th ed. Philadelphia: WB Saunders, 1998, pp 1188–1198.

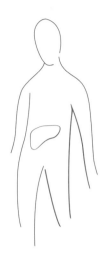

45

DISORDERS OF THE GALLBLADDER AND BILIARY TRACT

Michael B. Fallon • *Brendan M. McGuire*
Gary A. Abrams • *Miguel R. Arguedas*

The liver produces 500 to 1500 mL of bile per day. The major physiologic role of the biliary tract and gallbladder is to concentrate this material and to conduct it in well-timed aliquots to the intestine. In the intestine, bile acids participate in normal fat digestion, whereas cholesterol and a variety of other endogenous and exogenous compounds carried in bile are excreted in the feces. In this chapter we briefly outline the normal physiology of the biliary system and then focus on the pathophysiology and clinical consequences of gallstones, the most important biliary tract disorder. A brief discussion of neoplasms and other causes of bile duct obstruction is also provided. The reader is referred to Chapter 40 for a detailed discussion of the diagnostic approach to jaundice and biliary obstruction and to Chapter 33 for a review of the various imaging techniques used to study the biliary tract.

Normal Biliary Physiology

Bile, a complex fluid secreted by hepatocytes, passes through the hepatic bile ducts into the common hepatic duct. Tonic contraction of the sphincter of Oddi during fasting diverts about half of the bile through the cystic duct into the gallbladder, where it is stored and concentrated. Cholecystokinin, released after food is ingested, causes the gallbladder to contract and the sphincter of Oddi to relax, allowing delivery of a timed bolus of bile, rich in bile acids, into the intestine. Bile acids, detergent molecules possessing both fat-soluble and water-soluble moieties, convey phospholipids and cholesterol from the liver to the intestine, where cholesterol undergoes fecal excretion. In the intestinal lumen, bile acids solubilize dietary fat and promote its digestion and absorption. Bile acids are, for the most part, efficiently

reabsorbed by the small intestinal mucosa, particularly in the terminal ileum, and are recycled to the liver for re-excretion, a process termed *enterohepatic circulation* (Fig. 45–1).

Pathophysiology of Gallstone Formation (Cholelithiasis)

Gallstones, the most common cause of biliary tract disease in the United States, occur in 20% to 35% of persons by age 75 years and are of two types: (1) cholesterol stones, which account for 75% of gallstones, and (2) pigment stones, which account for the remaining 25%, and are composed of calcium bilirubinate and other calcium salts. Cholesterol, which is insoluble in water, normally is carried in bile solubilized by bile acids and phospholipids. However, in most individuals, many of whom do not develop gallstones, bile contains more cholesterol than can be maintained in stable solution (Fig. 45–2); that is, it is supersaturated with cholesterol. In the supersaturated bile of some individuals, microscopic cholesterol crystals form. The interplay of nucleation (mucus, stasis) and "antinucleating" (apolipoprotein A-I) factors may determine whether cholesterol gallstones form in supersaturated bile. Gradual deposition of additional layers of cholesterol leads to the appearance of macroscopic cholesterol gallstones.

The gallbladder is key to gallstone formation; it constitutes an area of bile stasis in which slow crystal growth can occur, and it also may provide mucus or other material to act as a nidus to initiate cholesterol crystal formation. Many of the recognized predisposing factors for cholelithiasis can be understood in terms of the pathophysiologic scheme just outlined: (1) biliary cholesterol saturation is increased by estrogens, multi-

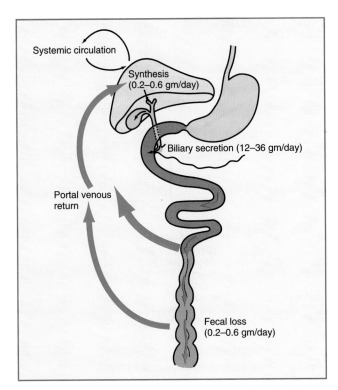

FIGURE 45–1 The enterohepatic circulation of bile salts. The liver secretes 12 to 36 g of bile salts per day in bile. Ninety-five percent of these bile salts are reabsorbed, with specific bile salt transporters in the terminal ileum accounting for much of the uptake. Bile salts recycle to the liver through portal blood, where they are efficiently extracted by hepatocytes and resecreted into bile. The liver also synthesizes sufficient bile salts to equal daily fecal losses (0.2 to 0.6 g/day). Because of efficient uptake of bile salts by both intestine and liver, delivery of 12 to 36 g of bile salts to the intestine daily is achieved by recycling a small pool (3 g) of bile salts 4 to 12 times per day. (Modified from Carey MC: The enterohepatic circulation. *In* Arias IM, Popper H, Schacter D, et al [eds]: The Liver: Biology and Pathobiology. New York, Raven Press, 1982.)

parity, oral contraceptives, obesity, rapid weight loss, and terminal ileal disease (which decreases the bile acid pool); and (2) bile stasis is increased by bile duct strictures, parenteral hyperalimentation, fasting, and choledochal cysts. Pregnancy also promotes lithogenesis because of gallbladder hypomotility.

The pathophysiology of pigment stones is less well understood; however, increased production of bilirubin conjugates (hemolytic states), increased biliary Ca^{2+} and CO_3^{2-}, cirrhosis, and bacterial deconjugation of bilirubin to a less soluble form are all associated with pigment stone formation.

Clinical Manifestations of Gallstones

Most individuals with gallstones are asymptomatic. Duct obstruction is the underlying cause of all manifestations of gallstone disease. Obstruction of the cystic duct distends the gallbladder and produces biliary pain, while

superimposed inflammation or infection leads to acute cholecystitis. Obstruction of the common duct may produce pain, jaundice, infection (cholangitis), pancreatitis, and/or hepatic damage and secondary biliary cirrhosis. The natural history of gallstone disease is outlined in Figure 45–3.

ASYMPTOMATIC GALLSTONES

Sixty to 80% of patients with gallstones in the United States are asymptomatic. Over a 20-year period it appears that only about 18% of these individuals develop biliary pain and only 3% require cholecystectomy. Asymptomatic patients should be followed expectantly, with prophylactic cholecystectomy considered in three high-risk groups: (1) diabetics, who have a greater mortality (10% to 15%) from acute cholecystitis; (2) persons with a calcified (porcelain) gallbladder, which may be associated with carcinoma of the gallbladder; and (3) persons with sickle cell anemia, in whom hepatic crises may be difficult to differentiate from acute cholecystitis. Dissolution of cholesterol gallstones by orally administered chenodeoxycholic acid or ursodeoxycholic acid is successful in some selected patients; however, a policy of expectant management followed by cholecystectomy if symptomatic disease develops is probably more cost effective. Alternative methods to eliminate gallstones include (1) dissolving cholesterol stones by instilling methyl-tert-butyl ether or ethyl propionate into the gallbladder and (2) fragmenting stones by extracorporeal shock wave lithotripsy.

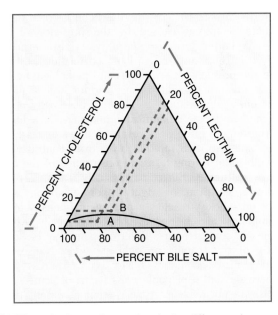

FIGURE 45–2 Phase diagram for plotting different mixtures of bile salt, lecithin, and cholesterol. The curved line represents the boundary of the micellar zone for aqueous solutions containing 4% to 10% solids. Any mixture, such as A, falling within this area contains cholesterol in solution. Any mixture, such as B, falling outside this area has excess cholesterol as a precipitate or supersaturated solution. The points A and B actually depict the average composition of gallbladder bile obtained from normal persons and patients with cholesterol gallstones, respectively.

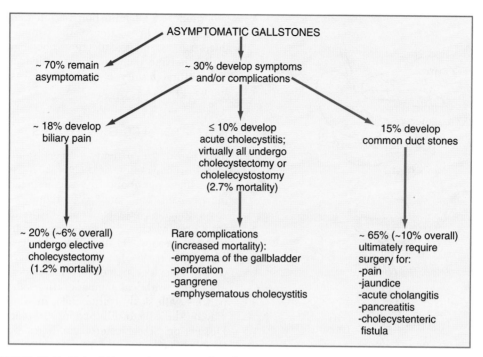

FIGURE 45-3 Natural history of asymptomatic gallstones. The clinical syndromes associated with gallstones are shown here, and the numbers represent the approximate percentage of adults who develop one or more of these symptoms or complications over a 15- to 20-year period. Over this period, approximately 30% of individuals with gallstones undergo surgery. (The risk of developing complications of gallstones varies considerably among series. The figures shown here represent those derived from more recent studies.)

CHRONIC CHOLECYSTITIS AND BILIARY PAIN

The term *chronic cholecystitis* has been used to denote nonacute symptoms caused by the presence of gallstones. A better term is *biliary pain* (also misnamed biliary colic), because only a loose correlation exists between the presence of symptoms and pathologic findings such as inflammation in the gallbladder wall. Gallbladders from symptomatic patients may be grossly normal with mild histologic inflammation and may show fibrosis and thickening, often as a result of previous attacks of acute cholecystitis. Symptoms arise from contraction of the gallbladder during transient obstruction of the cystic duct by gallstones. Biliary pain usually is a steady ache in the epigastrium or right upper quadrant, which comes on quickly, reaches a plateau of intensity over a few minutes, and begins to subside gradually over 30 minutes to several hours. Referred pain may be felt at the tip of the scapula or right shoulder. Nausea and vomiting may accompany biliary pain, whereas fever, leukocytosis, and a palpable mass (signs of acute cholecystitis) are not evident. Attacks occur at variable intervals (days to years). Other symptoms such as dyspepsia, fatty food intolerance, bloating and flatulence, heartburn, and belching may occur in patients with gallstones; however, they are nonspecific and frequently occur in individuals with normal gallbladders.

Gallstones can be best demonstrated by ultrasonography (sensitivity and specificity > 95%). Oral cholecystography (sensitivity 90%, specificity 75%) is reserved for ensuring cystic duct patency in patients whom dissolution therapy or extracorporeal shock wave lithotripsy is planned.

Laparoscopic cholecystectomy is the treatment of choice for recurrent biliary pain and may be accompanied by preoperative endoscopic or radiologic (transoperative) examination of the common bile duct for concomitant choledocholithiasis. Open cholecystectomy, which carries a mortality rate of less than 0.5%, may be necessary because of difficulties encountered during a laparoscopic procedure and in certain patients such as those with prior abdominal surgery who may have adhesions and those who may be obese. Surgery relieves symptoms of biliary pain in virtually all patients and prevents development of future complications, such as acute cholecystitis, choledocholithiasis, and cholangitis. Alternative approaches to eliminating gallstones, including dissolution and fragmentation, are less commonly used because of their lower efficacy, cost, and higher gallstone recurrence rate. Several reports and trials have suggested that the use of nonsteroidal anti-inflammatory agents during biliary pain may provide adequate pain relief and decrease the rate of progression to acute cholecystitis.

ACUTE CHOLECYSTITIS

Acute cholecystitis refers to acute right subcostal pain and tenderness resulting from obstruction of the cystic duct and subsequent distention, inflammation, and secondary infection of the gallbladder. Acalculous cholecystitis, accounting for 5% of cases, is associated with the triad of "prolonged fasting, immobility, and hemodynamic instability," such as occurs in critically ill patients (especially patients with burns, trauma, and sepsis) and with parenteral hyperalimentation. Acute cholecystitis usually begins with epigastric or right upper quadrant pain that gradually increases in severity and usually localizes to the area of the gallbladder. Unlike biliary pain, the pain of acute cholecystitis does not subside spontaneously. Low-grade fever, anorexia, nausea, vomiting, and right subcostal tenderness are commonly present, as is Murphy's sign (increased subhepatic tenderness and inspiratory arrest during a deep breath). In approximately one third of patients, a tender, enlarged gallbladder may be felt. Mild jaundice occurs in about 20% of patients as a result of concomitant common duct stones or bile duct edema. Complications of acute cholecystitis include emphysematous cholecystitis (especially in diabetics with bacterial gas present in the gallbladder lumen and wall), empyema of the gallbladder, gangrene, and perforation. Profound jaundice may result from Mirizzi's syndrome, in which extrinsic common bile duct compression occurs from an impacted stone in the gallbladder neck. Approximately 10% of patients present with or develop one of these complications and require emergency surgery. The onset of severe fever, shaking chills, increased leukocytosis, increased abdominal pain or tenderness, or persistent severe symptoms, alone or in combination, indicates progression of disease and suggests development of one of these complications.

Radionuclide scanning after intravenous administration of ^{99m}Tc-DISIDA or HIDA is the most accurate test with which to confirm the clinical impression of acute cholecystitis (cystic duct obstruction). If the gallbladder fills with the isotope, acute cholecystitis is unlikely, whereas if the bile duct is visualized but the gallbladder is not, the clinical diagnosis is strongly supported. An ultrasonographic examination that shows the presence of gallstones (or sludge in acalculous cholecystitis), along with localized tenderness over the gallbladder (ultrasonographic Murphy's sign), pericholecystic fluid, and gallbladder wall thickening, provides strong supportive evidence for acute cholecystitis. Oral cholecystograms are of no value in this clinical setting, because they are unreliable in the acutely ill patient.

Patients with acute cholecystitis may improve over 1 to 7 days with conventional expectant management, which includes nasogastric suction for patients with profound vomiting and/or abdominal distention, intravenous fluids, antibiotics, and analgesics. Because of the high risk of recurrent acute cholecystitis, most patients need to undergo cholecystectomy, often performed within the first 24 to 48 hours or, less often, 4 to 8 weeks after an acute episode, as either conventional or laparoscopic cholecystectomy (Fig. 45–4).

Emergency surgery is performed on patients with advanced disease and complications, usually associated with infection and sepsis. Cholecystostomy (either operative or percutaneous), rather than cholecystectomy, may be a useful technique in patients in whom there is a high operative risk. Patients who are good operative

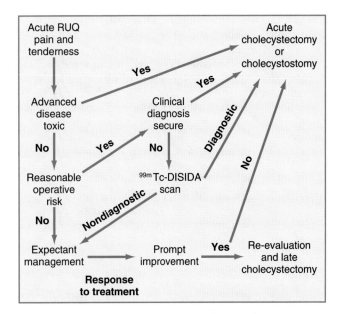

FIGURE 45–4 Scheme for managing patients with right upper quadrant pain and tenderness who are thought to have acute cholecystitis. This scheme is based on a policy of early operation (conventional or laparoscopic) for appropriate patients and use of cholecystostomy (operative or percutaneous) for patients who are poor operative risks.

risks and in whom the diagnosis is certain are scheduled for prompt cholecystectomy within 24 to 48 hours. Antibiotics are used in patients with suppurative complications. Expectant management is reserved for those with uncomplicated disease who are not good operative candidates or those in whom the diagnosis is not clear.

The mortality of acute cholecystitis of 5% to 10% is almost entirely confined to patients older than age 60 with serious associated diseases and to those with suppurative complications. Complications of acute cholecystitis include infectious complications and cholecystoenteric fistula resulting in gallstone ileus.

CHOLEDOCHOLITHIASIS AND ACUTE CHOLANGITIS

In the United States, most gallstones in the common duct come from the gallbladder; this occurs in up to 15% of persons with cholelithiasis. Less commonly, stones may form de novo in the biliary tree. Ductal stones may be asymptomatic (30% to 40%) or may produce biliary colic, jaundice, cholangitis, pancreatitis, or a combination of these. Secondary hepatic effects include secondary biliary cirrhosis and pyogenic hepatic abscesses.

Intermittent cholangitis, consisting of biliary pain, jaundice, and fever plus chills (Charcot's triad), is a common manifestation of choledocholithiasis. Biliary infection may be mild, or it may be severe, with suppurative cholangitis, sepsis, and shock. Suppurative cholangitis has a mortality of 50%, reflecting the age of the patients generally affected, the speed with which sepsis develops, and the frequent failure to identify the biliary tree as the source of sepsis. Diagnosis is based on a compatible clinical picture and radiologic or endoscopic evidence of ductal stones. Treatment includes hospitalization, treatment of infection, and prompt removal of stones. The latter may be accomplished surgically in patients with an intact gallbladder by cholecystectomy and choledochotomy. Alternatively, endoscopic sphincterotomy and stone extraction may be combined with laparoscopic cholecystectomy. In individuals with a previous cholecystectomy or those who are poor surgical candidates, endoscopic stone extraction and sphincterotomy, which opens the sphincter of Oddi and allows passage of gallstones up to 1 cm, is the preferred approach. In some patients, long-term ursodeoxycholic acid has been administered to prevent the recurrence of stones.

OTHER DISORDERS OF THE BILIARY TREE

A number of other processes, all of which may present as biliary obstruction, jaundice, or infection, may involve the biliary tree. The approach to evaluating these entities is outlined in Chapter 33.

Benign biliary strictures usually result from surgical injury and may cause symptoms days to years later. Early diagnosis is important, because strictures that partially obstruct and are clinically asymptomatic may cause secondary biliary cirrhosis. Biliary stricture should be suspected in anyone with a history of surgery of the right upper quadrant and persistently elevated serum alkaline phosphatase and γ-glutamyltransferase levels. A similar type of benign stricture is seen in alcoholics in whom the intrapancreatic portion of the common bile duct is compressed by pancreatic fibrosis. Endoscopic balloon catheter dilatation and/or stenting is useful in many of these patients, and surgical repair or bypass may also be considered.

Sclerosing cholangitis is an idiopathic condition of nonmalignant, nonbacterial chronic inflammatory narrowing of the intrahepatic and extrahepatic bile ducts. It most commonly occurs in males, often in association with ulcerative colitis. Patients frequently present with pruritus and jaundice, although asymptomatic elevations in the serum alkaline phosphatase and γ-glutamyltransferase levels may also be seen. Endoscopic retrograde cholangiopancreatography shows characteristic changes ("beading") of the bile ducts. Therapy includes prophylactic antibiotics for bacterial cholangitis, medical treatment of cholestasis (ursodeoxycholic acid, treatment of pruritus, fat-soluble vitamin repletion), attempts at improving biliary drainage (if a "dominant stricture" is present), and liver transplantation.

Structural abnormalities such as choledochal cysts, Caroli's disease (saccular intrahepatic bile duct dilation), and duodenal diverticuli may also cause bile duct obstruction, often with secondary choledocholithiasis resulting from bile stasis. Hemobilia with intermittent bile duct obstruction by blood clots may be caused by hepatic injury, neoplasms, or hepatic artery aneurysms.

Biliary neoplasms are rare but include carcinoma of the gallbladder, cholangiocarcinoma, and carcinoma of the ampulla of Vater. The last two neoplasms usually present as unremitting painless jaundice, although necrosis and sloughing of tumor may cause intermittent obstruction and the appearance of occult fecal blood. Carcinoma of the gallbladder often presents as advanced disseminated disease with weight loss, jaundice, pruritus, and large right upper quadrant mass. Symptoms also may resemble those of acute or chronic cholecystitis, particularly when the tumor is small. The incidence of cholangiocarcinoma is increased in patients with primary sclerosing cholangitis. Resection offers the only chance for cure, but it is difficult in most of these tumors and, thus, prognosis is poor. For patients with unresectable tumor, the goal is palliation; and for those with severe symptoms caused by obstruction, percutaneous or endoscopic stenting of the biliary tree may be helpful.

Motility disorders of the biliary tree were not well recognized in the past. With the use of newer endoscopic techniques for measuring biliary pressures and motility, it has become apparent that a small group of patients with biliary-type pain have symptoms resulting from "sphincter of Oddi dysfunction"; and in a selected group of patients, endoscopic or surgical sphincterotomy is of value.

REFERENCES

Evangelos A, Akriviadis A, Hatzigavriel M, et al: Treatment of biliary colic with diclofenac: A randomized, double blind, placebo-controlled trial. Gastroenterology 1997; 113:225–231.

Phillips JO, Wiesner RH, LaRusso NF: Sclerosing cholangitis. In Kirsner JB (ed): The Growth of Gastroenterologic Knowledge During the Twentieth Century. Baltimore: Williams & Wilkins, 1994.

Feldman M, Scharschmidt BF, Sleisenger MH (eds): Sleisenger and Fordtran's Gastrointestinal and Liver Disease: Pathophysiology/Diagnosis/Management, 6th ed. Philadelphia: WB Saunders, 1998.

Vlahcevic ZR, Heuman DM: Diseases of the gallbladder and bile ducts. In Goldman L, Bennett JC (eds): Cecil Textbook of Medicine, 21st ed. Philadelphia: WB Saunders, 2000, pp 821–833.

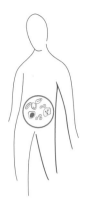

SECTION VIII

Hematologic Disease

46

HEMATOPOIESIS AND HEMATOPOIETIC FAILURE

Eunice S. Wang • Nancy Berliner

Hematopoiesis is the process that determines the formation and development of the wide variety of cellular elements of the blood. The constituents of peripheral blood arise by a complex and carefully regulated process of ontogeny. The pluripotent hematopoietic stem cell both maintains itself by self-renewal and undergoes multilineage differentiation to generate the appropriate numbers and types of cells within the circulating blood compartment (Table 46–1). The hematopoietic system is unique in that it is constantly undergoing this full cycle of maturation by which a primitive cell develops into a variety of highly specialized end-stage cells, all of which have different lifespans and are present in different quantities. The bone marrow must have the capacity to produce cells to compensate for the normal rapid turnover of hematopoietic cells that results from senescence, utilization, and migration into tissue spaces. Furthermore, it must have a reserve capacity to produce increased cells in response to unusual demands that arise from bleeding, infection, or other stresses. Understanding of the repeated cycle of cellular ontogeny and self-renewal that meets these challenges provides important insights into normal and pathologic mechanisms in hematology.

Hematopoietic Tissues

Hematopoiesis commences in the embryonic yolk sac, in which early erythroblasts in blood islands form the first hemoglobinized cells. After 6 weeks of gestation, the fetal liver begins producing primitive lymphocytoid cells, megakaryocytes, and erythroblasts, and the spleen becomes a secondary site of erythropoiesis. Hematopoiesis then shifts to its definitive long-term site in the *bone marrow*, the principal site for lifelong hematopoiesis in the normal host. Early in life, all fetal bones contain this regenerative bone marrow, but the marrow becomes progressively replaced by fat with age. In adults, active marrow resides only in the axial skeleton (sternum, vertebrae, pelvis, ribs) and in the proximal ends of the femur and humerus. Consequently, bone marrow samples, needed for many hematologic diagnoses, are usually obtained from the iliac crest or sternum. Under pathologic conditions that stress the capacity of the marrow space, as seen in diseases associated with marrow fibrosis (myeloproliferative diseases) or in severe inherited hemolytic anemia (thalassemia major), extramedullary hematopoiesis may be reestablished in sites of fetal hematopoiesis, especially the spleen.

Stem Cell Theory of Hematopoiesis

All mature hematopoietic cells are hypothesized to derive from a small population of *pluripotent stem cells*. Composing less than 1% of all cells in the bone marrow, these cells bear no distinctive morphologic markings and are best defined by their unique functional properties. Stem cells have two distinctive characteristics. First, they are highly resilient and productive, capable of continuously replenishing huge numbers of granulocytes, lymphocytes, and erythrocytes throughout life. The demand for a continuous fluctuating supply of blood cells requires a hematopoietic system capable of producing large numbers of selected cells in a short time. For example, overwhelming infection by invading microorganisms triggers the release of neutrophils, whereas hypoxia or acute blood loss leads to increased red blood cell production. Second, stem cells represent a self-renewing cell population that is able to maintain its numbers while also providing a continued supply of progenitor cells of multiple different lineages.

In spite of their vast proliferative potential, under normal conditions, most stem cells are paradoxically quiescent, and few cells undergo expansion or differentiation at any one time. However, their ability to prolifer-

TABLE 46-1 Normal Values for Peripheral Blood Cells

Cell Type/Size	Mean	Range
Hemoglobin	Women: 14.0 g/dL	Women: 12–16 g/dL
	Men: 15.5 g/dL	Men: 13.5–17.5 g/dL
Hematocrit	Women: 41%	Women: 36–46%
	Men: 47%	Men: 41–53%
Reticulocyte count	1%	0.5–1.5%
	60,000/μL	35,000–85,000/μL
Mean corpuscular volume		80–100
Platelet count	250,000/μL	150,000–400,000/μL
Total white count	7400/μL	4500–11,000/μL
Neutrophils	4400/μL (60%)	1800–7700/μL
Lymphocytes	2500/μL (35%)	1000–4800/μL
Monocytes	300/μL (<5%)	

ate is striking. Studies with lethally irradiated mice have demonstrated the ability of a few transplanted cells (termed *colony-forming unit–spleen* [CFU-S] cells) to regenerate multilineage hematopoiesis.

The signals regulating the differentiation of pluripotent stem cells into committed progenitors are unknown. Data suggest that the first step toward lineage commitment is a *stochastic* (chance) event; subsequent stages of maturation are hypothesized to occur under the influence of growth factors, or cytokines (Table 46–2). Cytokines act on different cells through specific cytokine receptors. Activation of these receptors induces signal transduction pathways that lead to gene transcription and eventual cell proliferation and differentiation. These growth factors have also been shown to act as survival factors for the developing hematopoietic cells by preventing *apoptosis* (programmed cell death). This process occurs in the cellular milieu of the bone marrow, and it is well recognized that hematopoiesis also depends in part on the nonhematopoietic cells (fibroblasts, endothelial cells, osteoblasts, and fat cells) that make up the bone marrow microenvironment. Stem cell biology is also regulated by hematopoietic cytokines produced locally and by cell surface ligand interactions between stem cells and the surrounding parenchyma.

Hematopoietic Differentiation Pathway

Hematopoiesis proceeds along a tightly regulated hierarchy. As more primitive cells mature under the influence

TABLE 46-2 Cytokines and Their Activities

Abbreviation	Name	Effects on Hematopoiesis
EPO	Erythropoietin	Stimulation of proliferation and maturation of erythroid progenitors; produced by the kidney in response to anemia/hypoxia; important clinically for treatment of anemia associated with low EPO levels (renal failure, some anemia of chronic disease)
G-CSF	Granulocyte colony-stimulating factor	Stimulation of proliferation and maturation of granulocytes; more broad-based effect, because also increases release of "stem cells" in peripheral blood; clinically important for treatment of neutropenia and mobilization of stem cells for transplant
GM-CSF	Granulocyte-monocyte colony-stimulating factor	Proliferation of granulocyte and monocyte precursors; role unclear in steady-state hematopoiesis, because knockout has no hematopoietic phenotype
TPO	Thrombopoietin	Proliferation of megakaryocytes; results in disappointing clinical studies
M-CSF	Monocyte colony-stimulating factor	Proliferation of monocytes
IL-2	Interleukin-2	Proliferation of T cells
IL-3	Interleukin-3 (multi-CSF)	Proliferation of granulocytes, monocytes; broad-based effects, appearing to increase the proliferation of "stem cells"; not in use clinically
IL-4	Interleukin-4	Proliferation of B cells
IL-5	Interleukin-5	Proliferation of T cells, B cells; proliferation and differentiation of eosinophils
IL-11	Interleukin-11	Proliferation of megakaryocytes; undergoing clinical testing
LIF	Leukemia inhibitory factor	Proliferation of stem cells and megakaryocytes
SCF	Stem cell factor (kit ligand)	Proliferation of progenitor cells; broad-based effects on multiple lineages

of specific cytokines, they undergo several cell divisions and become *progenitor cells* committed to one lineage. They also lose their self-renewal capacity. Morphologically, these cells are transformed from nonspecific blast-like cells into cells that can be identified by their color, shape, and granular and nuclear content. Functionally, they acquire distinguishing cell surface receptors and responses to specific signals. Maturing *granulocytes* and *erythroid cells* undergo several more cell divisions in the bone marrow, whereas *lymphocytes* travel to the thymus and lymph nodes for further development. *Megakaryocytes* cease cellular division but continue with nuclear replication. Eventually, these cells are released from the marrow as fully functional *erythrocytes, mast cells, granulocytes, monocytes, eosinophils, macrophages,* and *platelets.*

PLURIPOTENT STEM CELL

The pluripotent stem cell is morphologically indistinguishable and is best identified by its expression of the cell differentiation antigen, CD34, and by its ability to form pluripotent colonies in vitro. Under the influence of interleukin-1 (IL-1), IL-3, IL-6, and a specific stem cell factor (*c-kit* ligand or steel factor), this cell matures into either a myeloid-lineage stem cell (CFU–granulocyte/erythrocyte/macrophage/megakaryocyte [CFU-GEMM]) or a lymphoid-lineage stem cell. In the presence of granulocyte-macrophage colony-stimulating factor (GM-CSF) and IL-3, the myeloid stem cell will further differentiate into daughter cells of its named lineages (Fig. 46–1).

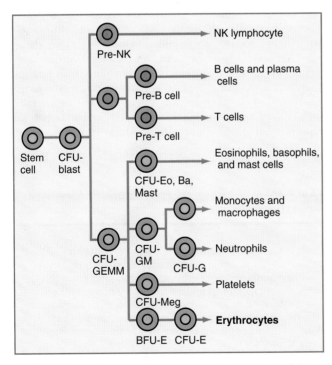

FIGURE 46–1   Schema of the development of the cells of the bone marrow. Ba = basophil; BFU = blast-forming unit; CFU = colony-forming unit; E = erythroid; Eo = eosinophil; G = granulocyte; GEMM = granulocyte/erythrocyte/macrophage/megakaryocyte; GM = granulocyte-macrophage; Meg = megakaryocyte; NK = natural killer.

The lymphopoietic stem cell, on the other hand, will become either a pre–B cell or a prothymocyte (pre–T cell) and will leave the marrow for further maturation.

ERYTHROID LINEAGE

Primitive erythroid precursors arising from the myeloid stem cell are called *burst forming unit–erythroid* (BFU-E) cells. These cells then differentiate into CFU-E (colony-forming unit–erythroid) cells, which are the committed progenitor cells of erythrocytes. CFU-E cells express receptors for erythropoietin (EPO), an 18-kd molecule produced by renal interstitial cells in response to low oxygenation states or anemia. EPO upregulates proliferation of CFU-E cells and promotes their maturation into proerythroblasts and reticulocytes, which begin to synthesize hemoglobin.

GRANULOCYTE AND MONOCYTE LINEAGES

Human GM-CSF acts early in the hematopoietic pathway to regulate maturation of the CFU-GEMM stem cell. Differentiation of this myeloid precursor into specific committed progenitors occurs under the direction of granulocyte-CSF (G-CSF) and monocyte-CSF (CSF). Granulocyte-CFU (CFU-G) cells undergo sequential transformation into easily recognizable myeloblasts, myelocytes, and eventually early polymorphonuclear neutrophils with their characteristic polysegmented nuclei. Monocyte-CFU (CFU-M) cells, on the other hand, retain a single nucleus as they mature from monoblasts to promonocytes to monocytes and sometimes macrophages.

OTHER LINEAGES

Eosinophils and basophils develop from CFU-GEMM cells under the influence of IL-5 and IL-3/IL-4, respectively. The acquisition of their specific granular contents helps in distinguishing their precursors from those of early monocytes.

Thrombopoietin has been identified as a cytokine that influences the development of the megakaryocytic lineage. CFU-GEMM cells become CFU-Meg (megakaryocyte) cells, so named because this cell line ceases cell division early but not nuclear replication. Over the course of several cell cycles, the maturing megakaryocyte eventually acquires severalfold the nuclear content of other cells in preparation for its eventual dissolution into platelets with a fraction of the cytoplasm of other hematopoietic cells.

GROWTH FACTORS IN CLINICAL USE

The discovery of the factors influencing normal hematopoiesis has led to important applications to the treatment of patients with defects in hematopoietic cell production. The discovery that committed hematopoietic cells of each lineage can be stimulated to proliferate and differentiate in the presence of specific cytokines has been of great clinical utility. Advances in DNA technology have led to the synthesis and purification of recombinant proteins with similar biologic activity in vivo. The administration of these products to patients has allowed the successful manipulation of the numbers of mature cells in the peripheral blood. For example, exogenous EPO is now considered a mainstay in the management of anemia caused by renal failure. The use of recombinant G-CSF in neutropenic patients after chemotherapy or radiation therapy has been shown to reduce hospital stays and to shorten the period of high infection risk. Technologies using high-dose regimens to ablate bone marrow and using stem cell transplants (discussed in Chapter 47) rely on the ability of cytokines to enhance stem cell proliferation greatly. Recombinant thrombopoietin is undergoing trials as an agent for the treatment of thrombocytopenia.

Disorders of Hematopoiesis

PATHOPHYSIOLOGY

Diseases of the hematopoietic stem cell disrupt the normal regulated pattern of stem cell development and can result in underproduction of mature progeny (*aplastic anemia*), overproduction of mature progeny (*myeloproliferative disease*), or failed differentiation with production of too many immature forms (*myelodysplasia* and *acute leukemia*). Myeloproliferative, myelodysplastic, and leukemic disorders are discussed in Chapter 47.

HEMATOPOIETIC FAILURE: APLASTIC ANEMIA

Hematopoietic stem cell failure leads to *aplastic anemia,* characterized by pancytopenia (decreased production of all blood cell lineages) with a markedly hypocellular bone marrow. This disease was first described by Paul Erhlich in 1888, who noted that autopsy bone marrow specimens from a young woman who died of severe anemia and neutropenia were extremely hypoplastic. More recent studies demonstrated that patients with severe aplastic anemia possess less than 1% of normal pluripotent stem cell numbers even though these patients have functional marrow stromal cells and normal or even elevated levels of stimulatory cytokines.

Clinical Presentation and Diagnosis

Clinical onset of aplastic anemia can be insidious. Patients often complain of symptoms related to their cytopenias: weakness, fatigue, dyspnea, or palpitations resulting from anemia; gingival bleeding, epistaxis, petechiae, or purpura caused by low platelet counts; or recurrent bacterial infections caused by low or nonfunctioning neutrophils. Physical examination is often normal. The degree of pancytopenia on peripheral blood counts helps to define the severity of the disease (Table 46–3). In general, patients have a low reticulocyte count (from low red blood cell production) with macrocytic anemia.

TABLE 46–3 Diagnosis of Severe Aplastic Anemia

Peripheral blood: At least two of the following:
  Neutrophil count <500/μL (0.5 × 109/L)
  Platelet count <20,000/μL (20 × 109/L)
  Anemia with corrected reticulocyte counts <1%
Bone marrow: Cellularity <25%; often <5–10%

Confirmation of the diagnosis requires bone marrow biopsy and evaluation to confirm hypocellularity and to rule out other marrow infiltrative processes. The bone marrow in severe aplastic anemia reveals <5% cellularity with increased fat accumulation and few, if any, hematopoietic cells. Although present in markedly decreased numbers, the progenitor and precursor cells that are found in the aplastic marrow are morphologically and genetically normal, an important fact in distinguishing this disease from hematologic disorders such as myelodysplasia or leukemia (see Chapter 47).

Etiology and Pathophysiology

Aplastic anemia is an uncommon disease. The incidence ranges from 1 to 5 cases per million in the general population, predominantly in the young (20 to 25 years old) and the elderly (60 to 65 years old). Most cases of aplastic anemia are idiopathic. Some of the known and suspected causes of the disease are listed in Table 46–4.

Prior bone marrow toxicity resulting from drugs, chemicals, or radiation predisposes to aplastic anemia. These agents directly injure proliferating and differentiating hematopoietic stem cells by inducing DNA damage. Agents such as benzene and cyclic hydrocarbons (found in petroleum products, rubber glue, insecticides, chemical dyes) cause aplastic anemia by this mechanism. Therapies such as cytotoxic chemotherapy (especially with alkylating agents) or radiation therapy target all rapidly cycling cells and often induce reversible bone marrow aplasia.

TABLE 46–4 Causes of Acquired Aplastic Anemia

Drugs:
  Dose-related: chemotherapeutic agents, antibiotics (chloramphenicol, trimethoprim-sulfamethoxazole)
  Idiosyncratic (many unproven): chloramphenicol, quinacrine, nonsteroidal anti-inflammatory drugs, anticonvulsants, gold, sulfonamides, cimetidine, penicillamine
Toxins: benzene and other hydrocarbons, insecticides
Viral infection: hepatitis, Epstein-Barr virus, human immunodeficiency virus
Immune disease: graft-versus-host disease in immunodeficiency, hypogammaglobulinemia
Paroxysmal nocturnal hemoglobinuria
Radiation
Pregnancy

Aplastic anemia also occurs in diseases of immune dysregulation and after viral infections and drug use, findings suggesting a second, immune-mediated mechanism for the disease. One hypothesis is that antigens presented to the immune system by viruses or drugs trigger cytotoxic T-cell responses that then persist to destroy normal stem cells. Patients may develop aplastic anemia as an idiosyncratic drug reaction and may unknowingly possess a certain genetic predisposition to sensitivity to drugs such as chloramphenicol, nonsteroidal anti-inflammatory drugs, sulfonamides, anticonvulsants, quinacrine, penicillamine, or gold salts. The presumed immune mechanism for drug-induced aplasia and the observation that aplastic anemia can occur in autoimmune disease have provided the impetus for immunosuppressive approaches to the treatment of aplastic anemia.

Treatment

Median survival of untreated patients with aplastic anemia is poor, ranging from 2 to 6 months. Supportive care with broad-spectrum antibiotics as well as antifungal and antiviral agents may be warranted in extremely neutropenic patients. Red blood cell and platelet transfusions are helpful in profoundly symptomatic patients (with care given to patients eligible for transplantation). Because endogenous cytokine production is usually high in patients with aplastic anemia, use of growth factors such as G-CSF and EPO is generally ineffective.

All young patients with severe aplastic anemia and an human leukocyte antigen (HLA)–compatible bone marrow donor should be considered for allogeneic bone marrow transplantation. This procedure (see Chapter 47) aims to restore normal stem cell function and offers the only chance of definitive cure of the disease. Although long-term survival is excellent (75% to 90%), morbidity from the transplant itself is a continuing problem. Evidence for the immune-mediated causes of aplastic anemia is seen in the high rate of responses of patients to immunosuppressive therapy. Treatment with antithymocyte globulin, antilymphocyte globulin, and cyclosporine (a specific T-cell inhibitor) allows for restoration of marrow function and prolonged survival in 60% to 80% of those patients who are not eligible for bone marrow transplantation. Success with high-dose cyclophosphamide suggests that durable remissions may be achievable without transplantation. Side effects of antithymocyte globulin include serum sickness (to horse or rabbit antigens in the antisera) but are generally self-limited. Unfortunately, relapses occur in up to half these patients, and late emergence of myelodysplasia may occur after immunosuppressive therapy for aplastic anemia. The relation of such clonal disorders to the pathogenesis of the original aplastic anemia remains controversial.

REFERENCES

Marsh JC, Gordon-Smith EC: Treatment options in severe aplastic anaemia. Lancet 1998; 351:1830–1831.

Moore M: Clinical implications of positive and negative hematopoietic stem cell regulators. Blood 1991; 78:1–19.

Quesenberry PJ: Hematopoietic stem cells, progenitor cells, and cytokines. *In* Beutler E (ed): Williams' Hematology, 5th ed. New York: McGraw-Hill, 1995.

Rafii S, Mohle R, Shapiro F, et al: Regulation of hematopoiesis by microvascular endothelium. Leuk Lymphoma 1997; 27:375–386.

Whetton AD, Spooncer E: Role of cytokines and extracellular matrix in the regulation of haematopoietic stem cells. Curr Opin Cell Biol 1998; 10:721–726.

Young NS: Aplastic anaemia. Lancet 1995; 346:228–232.

Young NS, Jaroslaw M: The pathophysiology of acquired aplastic anemia. N Engl J Med 1997; 336:1365–1372.

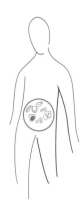

CLONAL DISORDERS OF THE HEMATOPOIETIC STEM CELL

Eunice S. Wang • Nancy Berliner

Malignant transformation involves combined defects in cellular maturation and differentiation. The multistep theory of oncogenesis suggests that these defects are often separable and may contribute to a stepwise progression from a normal to a fully transformed cell. The continuous cycling of hematopoietic cells provides a milieu for the development of clonal genetic abnormalities that support this model. Clonal defects of the hematopoietic stem cell give rise to an array of preleukemic and leukemic disorders. Primary defects of maturation give rise to the *myelodysplastic* disorders, whereas loss of normal control of proliferation results in *myeloproliferative* disease. All these disorders are preleukemic, with a variable but definite rate of transformation to acute leukemia.

Myelodysplastic Disorders

The myelodysplastic syndromes (MDS) are characterized by ineffective and disordered hematopoiesis. Patients have pancytopenia, despite the presence of normal or increased numbers of hematopoietic cells in the bone marrow. Disordered maturation is accompanied by increased intramedullary *apoptosis* (programmed cell death), which contributes to the decreased release of mature cells into the periphery.

Primary MDS is predominantly a disease of elderly persons and occurs in approximately 1 in 500 patients between the ages of 60 and 75 years. Most cases are idiopathic, although the incidence is increased in persons with prior exposure to radiation, chemotherapy, and organic chemicals (benzene). MDS may also occur in patients of any age after chemotherapy (alkylating agents, anthracyclines), ionizing radiation, and bone marrow transplantation. As therapies for primary cancers

prolong survival, the incidence of secondary myelodysplasia is likely to rise.

DIAGNOSIS

Most patients with MDS are referred for evaluation of an incidental finding of peripheral cytopenias. Symptomatic patients usually present with findings related to the secondary effects of cytopenias: bleeding, bruising, infection, fatigue, weakness, and dyspnea related to thrombocytopenia, leukopenia, and anemia. Physical examination is usually unremarkable, although 25% or more of patients may have splenomegaly.

In addition to cytopenias, the peripheral blood smear may show characteristic morphologic abnormalities. Erythroid cells are usually macrocytic, often with basophilic stippling. Neutrophils are often hypogranular and hypolobulated, with a characteristic bilobed nuclear morphology termed *pseudo–Pelger-Huët abnormality*. Pelger-Huët anomaly should be suspected when automated differential cell counts report an unusually large numbers of bands.

The bone marrow in MDS is usually normocellular or hypercellular, although 10% of patients may have a hypocellular marrow. Dysplastic changes usually occur in all three cell lines. Erythroid cells appear megaloblastic, with multinucleated cells or asynchronous nuclear-cytoplasmic development. The myeloid series shows poor maturation with a "left shift" to earlier myeloid forms. Elevated numbers of myeloblasts are common, and these cells increase with progression toward acute leukemia. Extremely small "micromegakaryocytes" and agranular megakaryocytes may also be present. Electron microscopy of the marrow shows cellular changes (prominent nuclear chromatin, cytoplasmic vacuoles, and blebs) characteristic of increased apoptosis.

Other causes of marrow dysplasia such as vitamin B_{12}

TABLE 47–1 French-American-British (FAB) Classification of Myelodysplastic Disorders

Subtype	Blood	Marrow	Leukemic Evolution (%)	Median Survival (mo)
Refractory anemia (RA)	Blasts <1%	Blasts <5%	16	50
Refractory anemia with ringed sideroblasts (RARS)	Blasts <1%	Blasts <5%	15	65
Refractory anemia with excess blasts (RAEB)	Blasts <1%	Blasts 5–20%	48	15
Refractory anemia with excess blasts in transformation (RAEB-T)	Blasts <1%	Blasts 20–30%	62	9
Chronic myelomonocytic leukemia (CMML)	Monocytes >1 × 10⁹/L	Any number of blasts	29	23

or folate deficiency, alcohol use, chemotherapy, and human immunodeficiency virus infection should be considered. In a patient with suspected MDS who has a hypocellular bone marrow, the syndrome must be distinguished from aplastic anemia. Cytogenetic analysis of the bone marrow confirms clonal chromosomal abnormalities in one third to one half of all patients. The identification of some gene deletions and translocations identical to those found in acute myeloid leukemias points to similar mechanisms of clonal myeloid stem cell injury (see Table 47–5).

CLASSIFICATION AND PROGNOSIS

The disease course of MDS varies widely. Some patients may live normal lifespans, but most die prematurely of cytopenia-related complications. Fifteen to 20 percent die of acute leukemia. As in acute leukemia (see later discussion), the natural history of the disease has been correlated with certain cytogenetic abnormalities. For example, patients with an isolated deletion of the long arm of chromosome 5 have a well-characterized clinical course. Persons with 5q− syndrome are predominantly female patients who present with refractory macrocytic anemia. Survival is prolonged by red blood cell transfusions alone, and the risk of eventual leukemic transformation is low. In contrast, other cytogenetic abnormalities similar to those in poor-prognosis leukemia, such as monosomy 7 or trisomy 8, correlate with poor prognosis (see Table 47–5).

Traditionally, MDS has been classified according to the French-American-British (FAB) system into five subtypes based on marrow cellular morphology and percentage of blasts. These subtypes are (1) refractory anemia (RA), (2) refractory anemia with ringed sideroblasts (RARS), (3) refractory anemia with excess blasts (RAEB), (4) refractory anemia with excess blasts in transformation (RAEB-T), and (5) chronic myelomonocytic leukemia (CMML). Although this classification does correlate with overall survival (Table 47–1), the International MDS Risk Analysis Workshop developed the International Prognostic Scoring System (IPSS) in 1998 in an attempt to define prognostic categories of MDS better. The IPSS divides MDS patients into prognostic categories based on cytogenetic abnormalities. These categories were combined with other variables such as cytopenias, advanced age, and percentage of bone marrow blasts, to predict clinical prognosis (Table 47–2).

Median length of survival in MDS is usually less than 2 years. Unfortunately, options for therapy of this disorder are limited. As in other hematologic stem cell disorders, the only curative therapy is allogeneic stem cell transplantation (see later). All patients less than 40 years of age and who have human leukocyte antigen (HLA)–matched sibling donors should be offered this procedure, and such patients are also candidates for consideration of mismatched or unrelated donor transplants. Long-term survival rates in young patients who receive matched sibling donor transplants are 45% to 75%.

TABLE 47–2 International Prognostic Scoring System (IPSS) Classification of Myelodysplastic Disorders

Score	Blasts	Karyotype	Cytopenias*	Overall Score	Median Survival (yr)
0	<5%	Normal, Y-,5q-,20q-	0–1 cytopenias	0	5.7
0.5	5–10%	All other abnormalities	2–3 cytopenias	0.5–1.0	3.5
1.0	—	Abnormal 7, >3 abnormalities		1.5–2.0	1.2
1.5	11–20%			≥2.5	0.4
2.0	21–30%				

*Cytopenias defined as follows: hemoglobin <10; neutrophils <1500; platelets <100,000.

Therapeutic regimens for most patients ineligible for stem cell transplantation are varied. Elderly patients may not tolerate or desire aggressive intervention without hope of cure. Patients with MDS who are considered to be at low risk for disease transformation are best managed supportively with red blood cell and platelet transfusions. Administration of recombinant growth factors (granulocyte colony-stimulating factor, granulocyte-monocyte colony-stimulating factor, erythropoietin [EPO]) has been successful in treating MDS-related anemia and neutropenia in some patients.

Patients with cytogenetic abnormalities that predispose them to leukemia or high levels of circulating blasts are treated as if they had acute myeloid leukemia. Standard chemotherapeutic regimens, however, result in low remission rates, short disease-free intervals, and a high relapse rate in 12 to 18 months. Overall, treatment is not associated with significant prolongation of survival, even in patients who achieve remission. Secondary MDS is especially difficult to treat and often progresses to refractory myeloid leukemia. Use of differentiating agents, use of low-dose chemotherapy, and immunomodulatory regimens are still considered experimental.

Myeloproliferative Disorders

The myeloproliferative diseases (MPDs) are clonal stem cell disorders characterized by leukocytosis, thrombocytosis, erythrocytosis, splenomegaly, and bone marrow hypercellularity. They are divided into polycythemia vera (PV), essential thrombocytosis (ET), agnogenic myeloid metaplasia or myelofibrosis, and chronic myelogenous leukemia (CML), based on the predominant hyperproliferative cell type. All can be associated with clonal evolution to acute leukemia, although with the exception of CML, acute leukemia is an infrequent and late complication. The hallmark of MPD is the failure of the stem cell to respond to normal feedback mechanisms regulating hematopoietic cell mass. Stem cells from patients with MPD demonstrate colony growth in vitro when these cells are grown in the presence of serum without the addition of exogenous cytokines. This technique has become a standard means of establishing a diagnosis of MPD.

POLYCYTHEMIA VERA

Normal early erythroid progenitor cells are stimulated to differentiate from pluripotent stem cell precursors by EPO, a growth factor produced by kidneys in response to hypoxia. The body's ability to increase red blood cell production in hypoxemia, anemia, hemolysis, and acute blood loss ensures continual oxygen delivery to tissues. When sufficient numbers of red blood cells are produced, a negative feedback mechanism suppresses further EPO production, and erythropoiesis is reduced. *Polycythemia* is defined as an increased red blood cell mass in the peripheral blood. This may be primary,

resulting from a stem cell defect, or secondary, from increased levels of erythropoiesis in response to physiologic stimuli.

PV is a primary clonal stem cell disorder of unknown origin that is characterized by predominant erythrocytosis associated with other hematopoietic abnormalities. Half of all patients have concurrent leukocytosis and/or thrombocytosis. Diagnosis of PV was formerly one "of exclusion"; diagnostic criteria were based on exclusion of hypoxemia and other secondary causes of polycythemia, with some weight given to detection of splenomegaly and documentation of elevated levels of other cell lineages. The identification of the key role of EPO in red blood cell proliferation and the ability to measure serum levels of EPO changed these diagnostic criteria. A suspected diagnosis of PV can be confirmed by documentation of low EPO levels and by the ability of in vitro erythroid colonies to proliferate independent of EPO.

PV occurs in 1 to 3 in 100,000 people, with a median age at onset of 65 years. Early recognition and treatment of PV are important because untreated patients with PV are at high risk of significant morbidity and mortality from thromboembolic disease. Twenty percent of patients present with symptoms of arterial and venous thrombosis. Typically, patients complain of headache, visual problems, mental clouding, and pruritus after bathing. Occlusive vascular events such as stroke, transient ischemic attacks, myocardial ischemia, and digital pain, paresthesias, or gangrene are common. In addition, pulmonary, deep venous, hepatic, and portal venous thromboses may occur. Paradoxically, patients are also predisposed to hemorrhagic events, which are presumed to be caused by abnormal platelet function, and such patients may present with gastrointestinal bleeding. Physical examination often shows retinal vein occlusion, ruddy cyanosis, and splenomegaly. Peripheral blood often appears microcytic, with or without iron deficiency. Bone marrow examination shows a hypercellular marrow. Cytogenetic features at the time of diagnosis are usually normal; the development of clonal cytogenetic abnormalities heralds transformation in the later stages of disease.

Without treatment, half of all patients with PV die of thrombotic complications within 18 months of diagnosis. With therapy, PV is a chronic, progressive disease. The risk of transformation to myelofibrosis and myeloid leukemia is 5% to 20% over 20 years. Patients with advanced age, prior history of thrombosis, and high hematocrit values are at high risk of subsequent vascular events. Therefore, intermittent phlebotomy is the mainstay of treatment. Low-dose chemotherapeutic agents are frequently added to treat leukocytosis and thrombocytosis. Older therapies included use of alkylating agents and radioactive phosphorus (^{32}P). Current therapies depend more heavily on hydroxyurea and interferon. Goals of therapy are hematocrit values less than 45% in men and less than 42% in women. Nonsteroidal anti-inflammatory drugs and aspirin should be used judiciously because of the risk of gastrointestinal hemorrhage. With effective therapy, the rate of long-term survival of these patients is high.

ESSENTIAL THROMBOCYTOSIS

ET is a pluripotent stem cell disorder resulting in elevated levels of platelets and white blood cells. Platelet function and length of survival remain normal. As with PV, the origin is unknown. Because elevated platelet counts can be related to underlying bacterial infections, sepsis, iron deficiency, autoimmune diseases, and other malignant diseases, these other causes of disease should be excluded before a diagnosis of ET is considered. In general, diagnosis requires a platelet count exceeding 600,000 $\mu g/L$, with normal red blood cell mass, normal iron studies, and bone marrow examination excluding the presence of myelodysplasia, myelofibrosis, or the Philadelphia chromosome diagnostic of CML. Unlike in other MPDs, bone marrow cells from patients with ET frequently do not show factor-independent colony growth.

ET is an uncommon disorder with an increasing number of cases found in asymptomatic patients on routine laboratory testing. Although the median age at presentation is 60 to 65 years, 10% to 25% of patient are less than 40 years old. Up to two thirds of patients are symptomatic. Vasomotor symptoms include headache, dizziness, visual changes, and *erythromelalgia* (burning pain and erythema of feet and hands). Serious arterial thrombotic complications such as transient ischemic attacks, strokes, seizures, angina, and myocardial infarcts may occur. Patients may rarely have purpuric skin lesions or hematomas. The risk of gastrointestinal bleeding is less than 5%.

In general, patients with this disorder have long-term survival rates similar to those of age-matched control subjects. The risk of leukemic transformation is extremely low (3% to 4%) in comparison with other MPDs. However, morbidity from recurrent hemorrhagic and thrombotic complications is high. Treatment is determined by clinical symptoms and signs. Low-dose enteric aspirin is effective in relieving neurologic symptoms and has a minimal risk of causing bleeding. Patients with advanced age, prior history of thrombosis, and long disease duration are predisposed to future vascular events and are treated with platelet-lowering agents. Hydroxyurea, a nonspecific myelosuppressive agent, is most commonly used to lower platelet and leukocyte counts, but it has unknown long-term leukemogenic and teratogenic effects. For this reason, young and/or pregnant patients are often not treated until they become symptomatic. Other drugs include anagrelide, an oral antiplatelet agent that directly inhibits megakaryocyte maturation, and interferon.

A significant fraction of patients with ET consists of young women of childbearing age. Management of pregnancy in such patients is a unique problem. Patients with ET have a high incidence of fetal wastage. Although large studies are not available, studies in small numbers of patients and anecdotal reports suggest that interferon and aspirin can improve the chances for the successful outcome of pregnancy.

MYELOFIBROSIS (AGNOGENIC MYELOID METAPLASIA)

Myelofibrosis is a clonal stem cell disorder characterized by abnormal excess marrow fibrosis leading to marrow failure. An abnormal myeloid precursor is believed to give rise to dysplastic megakaryocytes that produce increased levels of fibroblast growth factors. These cytokines act on normal fibroblasts and other stromal cells, a process that stimulates excessive proliferation and collagen deposition. Over time, increasing fibrosis of the bone marrow leads to premature release of multipotent hematopoietic precursors into the periphery. These cells then migrate and reestablish themselves in other sites, thereby shifting hematopoiesis out of the bone marrow and into other tissues, especially the spleen and liver. This process is termed *extramedullary hematopoiesis.*

Myelofibrosis (agnogenic myeloid metaplasia) is a rare chronic disease of elderly persons with an annual incidence of 0.5 cases per 100,000. Early in the disease, patients may be asymptomatic. Later, patients complain of progressive fatigue and dyspnea related to anemia or early satiety and left upper quadrant fullness or pain associated with splenomegaly and splenic infarction. More than half these patients develop massive hepatosplenomegaly. In more advanced disease, patients may have constitutional symptoms such as fever, weight loss, and night sweats. As bone marrow failure evolves, complications of neutropenia and thrombocytopenia develop. Bleeding from occult disseminated intravascular coagulation is a risk. Extramedullary hematopoiesis in the peritoneal and pleural cavities as well as in the central nervous system (CNS) and spinal cord may also cause symptoms.

Diagnosis of agnogenic myeloid metaplasia is made by demonstration of bone marrow fibrosis with normal red blood cell mass, lack of Philadelphia chromosome (diagnostic of CML), splenomegaly, anemia, and evidence of extramedullary hematopoiesis. Variable degrees of cytopenias are present. Teardrop-shaped erythrocytes and nonleukemic immature myeloid, erythroid, and leukocyte cells are commonly seen in the peripheral blood.

Median length of survival is poor, ranging from 2 to 5 years. Adverse prognostic factors include age greater than 60 years, higher percentage of circulating blasts, leukocytosis, anemia, thrombocytopenia, hepatomegaly, cytogenetic abnormalities, and presence of systemic symptoms. Leukemic transformation occurs in 8% to 10% of patients. Other causes of death include heart failure, infection, intracranial hemorrhage, and pulmonary embolism.

No curative therapy for myelofibrosis exists. Young patients with disease may be considered for experimental allogeneic stem cell transplantation. Palliative transfusion therapy and administration of androgens and/or corticosteroids are given to maintain red blood cell levels. Hydroxyurea may be used to decrease thrombocytosis and leukocytosis. Splenectomy is offered to patients with symptomatic splenomegaly, refractory thrombocytopenia, hypermetabolic symptoms, and portal hypertension, and results are generally good. Nonsurgical patients may benefit from palliative splenic irradiation. However, no treatment prolongs survival or significantly retards disease progression.

Chronic Myelogenous Leukemia

CML is an MPD characterized by a predominantly increased granulocytic cell line, associated with concurrent erythroid and platelet hyperplasia. It is unique among the MPDs in its characteristic natural history, including an inevitable transformation to acute leukemia.

EPIDEMIOLOGY AND NATURAL HISTORY

CML accounts for 15% of all leukemias and occurs in 1 in 100,000 people. The median age of onset is 53 years, but patients of any age may be affected. Up to 40% of patients are initially asymptomatic. Others present with fatigue, lethargy, shortness of breath, weight loss, easy bruising, and early satiety. Physical examination usually shows splenomegaly. Laboratory values are significant for a markedly elevated white blood cell count with mature and immature myeloid cells, low alkaline phosphatase levels, high uric acid and lactate dehydrogenase levels, and thrombocytosis.

The natural history of CML is characterized by a chronic phase that evolves into an acute blast crisis. Patients are typically diagnosed during the chronic phase, an indolent stage lasting 3 to 5 years. Peripheral white blood counts are elevated, but few blasts are seen. With control of peripheral blood cell counts, patients are essentially asymptomatic during this period. Eventually, the disease enters an accelerated phase characterized by fever, weight loss, worsening splenomegaly, and bone pain related to rapid marrow cell turnover. The last phase of CML, termed *blast crisis*, marks an evolution to acute leukemia, in which marrow is replaced by blasts, with accompanying loss of normal mature cellular elements in the marrow and periphery. Death occurs in a few weeks to months. Two thirds of patients develop myeloid leukemia, whereas the rest develop lymphoid leukemia, a finding confirming that the initial neoplastic cell is an early stem cell capable of multilineage differentiation.

GENETICS

CML was the first hematologic malignant disease shown to be associated with a specific chromosomal abnormality. More than 95% of patients with CML have a clonal expansion of a stem cell that has acquired the Philadelphia chromosome, a balanced translocation between chromosomes 9 and 22 t(9;22). This translocation joins the *abl* (abelson leukemia virus) gene on chromosome 9 to the *bcr* (breakpoint cluster region) gene on chromosome 22, and the result is the production of a fusion protein termed bcr-abl. A subset of patients with CML lack a detectable Philadelphia chromosome but have the fusion product for the *bcr-abl* translocation detectable by reverse transcriptase–polymerase chain reaction (RT-PCR), indicating a subchromosomal translocation that results in the same pathologic gene product. The bcr-abl product is a constitutively active cytoplasmic tyrosine kinase that has been found to induce leukemia in hematopoietic cells. The bcr-abl fusion protein activates signal transduction mechanisms to permit cell growth independent of cytokine regulation and the influence of the bone marrow stroma. CML cells are resistant to chemotherapy and are protected from normal programmed cell death (*apoptosis*).

TREATMENT

Advances in treatment of CML have prolonged survival. Identification of the Philadelphia chromosome has allowed for easier diagnosis and monitoring of disease. Exquisitely sensitive PCR procedures allow for detection of up to a single bcr-abl–positive cell in 10^5 to 10^6 peripheral cells. Responses to treatment regimes in CML are now described, to distinguish among hematologic (return of peripheral blood cell counts), cytogenetic (loss of the Ph chromosome), and molecular (loss of the *bcr-abl* gene) remissions.

Oral chemotherapeutic agents such as hydroxyurea and busulfan are effective in reducing myeloid cell numbers in patients during the chronic phase of CML. Although this decreases disease complications, it does not alter long-term prognosis. Use of interferon-α achieves similar rates of hematologic remissions but also induces cytogenetic responses in a small percentage of cases. The combination of chemotherapy with interferon has been shown to increase the rate of cytogenetic responses further. Major cytogenetic responses to interferon-containing regimens are associated with prolonged survival. Patients treated with interferon-α still possess cells with the *bcr-abl* translocation by PCR chain reaction and are therefore still at risk of disease relapse; however, many patients remain in hematologic and cytogenetic remission for many years despite detectable molecular disease. The mechanism by which the disease is controlled with these regimens despite detectable bcr-abl–positive cells remains unknown.

Eradication of all cells that contain detectable levels of the *bcr-abl* translocation occurs only after allogeneic stem cell transplantation. Allogeneic transplantation is a procedure whereby abnormally functioning hematopoietic bone marrow is eradicated and is replaced with normal bone marrow or stem cells from an HLA-compatible source, from either a related or an unrelated donor. High-dose chemotherapy with or without radiation is administered to destroy the patient's bone marrow, followed by the infusion of new stem cells that engraft and restore normal hematopoiesis. Treatment-related morbidity is significant, with a procedure-related mortality of 10% to 30%; however, improvements in supportive care and immunomodulatory therapy designed to suppress graft-versus-host disease are continuing to improve outcome. In general, younger patients (<50 years old) are considered best candidates for this intensive therapy, although this, too, is changing in the setting of newer supportive modalities. Patients who have undergone stem cell transplantation have a 10-year median survival rate of 70%. For reasons that are not clear, the outcome of transplantation is improved in patients who undergo the procedure within a year of diagnosis.

In the setting of CML, increasing evidence indicates that the excellent response of patients with CML to stem cell transplantation is partly related to the active suppression of the disease by the newly transplanted graft, referred to as the *graft-versus-leukemia effect* (GVL). After allogeneic bone marrow transplantation for CML, RT-PCR reveals that most patients continue to have detectable *bcr-abl* transcripts, especially within the first 6 months after the transplantation procedure. However, detection of *bcr-abl* in this setting is not predictive of imminent hematologic or cytogenetic relapse. Eventually, many patients become *bcr-abl* negative, although low levels of *bcr-abl* transcripts have been shown to persist in some patients in long-term remission. That this is related to GVL is supported by several observations. Patients with *graft-versus-host disease* (an autoimmune phenomenon in which intact lymphocytes in the transplanted marrow attack the host tissues) have a decreased rate of relapsed CML. Studies have also resulted in the compelling observation that infusion of donor lymphocytes can restore remission in patients with evidence of relapse after allogeneic transplantation for CML. Conversely, procedures that minimize the reactivity between donor and host increase disease relapse. For example, the rate of relapse in patients who receive syngeneic (identical twin) transplants and in patients who receive T-cell–depleted marrow in an attempt to reduce graft-versus-host disease is increased. Because this reduces the allogeneic reactivity of the donated stem cells, these patients have a relapse rate of up to 60%, heralded by increasing levels of PCR positivity before hematologic and cytogenetic relapse.

Median length of survival in CML has risen dramatically, from a few month to years in the first half of the twentieth century, to 6 years for interferon-treated patients, to more than 10 years in patients who undergo allogeneic transplantation.

Acute Leukemias

The *acute leukemias* are clonal hematopoietic malignant diseases that arise from the malignant transformation of an early hematopoietic stem cell. Leukemias occur in 8 to 10 in 100,000 people (in comparison with 42 in 100,000 for prostate cancer and 62 in 100,000 for breast cancer). Acute leukemias are classified by cell lineage into *acute myelogenous leukemia* (AML) or *acute lymphoblastic leukemia* (ALL) based on morphology, cytogenetics, cell surface and cytoplasmic markers, and molecular studies. Ninety percent of adult leukemia is AML (10% ALL), whereas 90% of childhood leukemia is ALL (with 10% AML). The distinction between AML and ALL is crucial diagnostically, therapeutically, and

prognostically. Morphologic subgroups of both ALL and AML have been defined by the FAB group (Table 47–3).

The pathogenesis of acute leukemia is unknown. Unregulated proliferation of immature cells incapable of further differentiation *(blasts)* results in marrow replacement and hematopoietic failure. Many patients with acute leukemia have detectable characteristic clonal chromosomal abnormalities, but the role of these aberrations in malignant transformation is unknown. Known risk factors for leukemia are high-dose radiation exposure, occupational exposure to benzene, and prior chemotherapy (especially with alkylating agents such as chlorambucil, melphalan, and nitrogen mustard). An increased incidence of leukemia is also found in patients with chromosomal instability disorders such as Bloom's syndrome, Fanconi's anemia, Down's syndrome, and ataxia telangiectasia.

Patients present clinically with evidence of bone marrow failure (similar to other hematopoietic disorders). Complications of disease include anemia, infection, and bleeding from peripheral cytopenias. In addition, proliferating blasts infiltrating the bone marrow may cause bone pain. Blasts also invade other organs and lead to peripheral, mediastinal, and abdominal lymphadenopathy, hepatosplenomegaly, skin infiltration, and meningeal involvement.

Therapy of acute leukemias is divided into several stages. *Induction therapy* is directed at reducing numbers of leukemic blasts to an undetectable level and restoring normal hematopoiesis *(complete remission)*. At complete remission, however, significant subclinical disease persists, requiring further therapy. Subsequent *consolidation therapy* involves continuing chemotherapy with the same agents to induce elimination of further leukemic cells. With development of a wider range of effective agents, *intensification therapy* has been introduced, involving the use of high-dose therapy with different "noncross-reactive" drugs, to eliminate cells with potential primary resistance to the induction regimen.

TABLE 47–3 French-American-British (FAB) Classification of Acute Leukemia

Acute Myelocytic Leukemia

M_1—Acute myelocytic leukemia without differentiation
M_2—Acute myelocytic leukemia with differentiation (predominantly myeloblasts and promyelocytes)
M_3—Acute promyelocytic leukemia
M_4—Acute myelomonocytic leukemia
M_5—Acute monocytic leukemia
M_6—Erythroleukemia
M_7—Megakaryotic leukemia

Acute Lymphocytic Leukemia

L_1—Predominantly "small" cells (twice the size of normal lymphocyte), homogeneous population; childhood variant
L_2—Larger than L_1, more heterogenous population; adult variant
L_3—"Burkitt-like" large cells, vacuolated abundant cytoplasm

Maintenance therapy employs low-dose intermittent chemotherapy given over a prolonged period to prevent subsequent disease relapse.

Adverse prognostic factors for AML and ALL are similar despite widely different treatment approaches. In general, age exceeding 35 years, secondary leukemia or prolonged preleukemic states, high initial leukocyte count, unfavorable cytogenetic abnormalities, and prolonged time to achieve response to initial treatment are associated with unfavorable outcomes.

ACUTE LYMPHOBLASTIC LEUKEMIA

Classification

The FAB classification system divides ALL into three subtypes (L1, L2, and L3) based on the morphology of cells. L1 cells are small, uniform lymphoblasts with indistinct nucleoli and make up 25% to 30% of cases. L2 cells are larger, more pleomorphic, and occur more commonly in adults (65%), whereas the L3 subtype with large basophilic cells and vacuoles is the most infrequent type, occurring in 2% to 3% of patients. Identification of specific cell surface antigens found on cells during normal maturation allows further classification of disease into B-cell or T-cell lineage, with some prognostic significance (Table 47–4).

Treatment

Progress in the understanding and treatment of this disease in the 1990s has led to cure rates of up to 80% in children and 40% of adults. Poorer outcomes in adults may reflect the higher incidence of cytogenetic abnormalities associated with poor prognosis. For example, the Philadelphia chromosome, t(9,22), also found in patients with CML, is seen much more commonly in adult patients and is associated with poor prognosis.

Treatment of ALL is lengthy. Induction chemotherapy typically involves a combination of vincristine and prednisone with L-asparaginase. Adult patients benefit from the addition of an anthracycline. Complete remission rates are 97% to 99% in children and 75% to 90% in adults. On the return of normal hematopoiesis, patients then undergo consolidation and intensification therapy with multiple drugs to eradicate disease. For unknown reasons, ALL tends to relapse several months to years after initial remission, but the frequency of relapse may be reduced by maintenance chemotherapy given for 2 to 3 years. Such prolonged treatment may eliminate slow-growing leukemic clones, may prevent further transformation, and/or may destroy occult disease in other sites. The CNS and testes provide common "sanctuaries" for residual leukemia cells that can lead to disease relapse. Therefore, intrathecal methotrexate or brain irradiation is given in most patients with ALL as an adjunct of treatment.

Most relapses of disease occur within 2 years of initial treatment, with leukemic cells in the bone marrow, CNS, or testes. Although relapsed ALL responds to local irradiation and further chemotherapy, the duration of second remissions is usually less than 6 months, with an overall 3-year survival rate of less than 10% with chemotherapy alone. All patients whose disease has relapsed and for whom appropriate donors are found should be considered for allogeneic stem cell transplantation.

ACUTE MYELOGENOUS LEUKEMIA

Classification

The FAB classification of AML divides the disease into eight subtypes (M0 to M7) based on morphologic criteria and stage of cellular differentiation (myeloblastic, monocytic, erythroleukemic, megakaryoblastic). In contrast to ALL, some of these FAB subsets correlate with specific clinical syndromes that help to determine treatment approaches as well as prognosis. For example, patients with M3 (acute promyelocytic leukemia) often present with spontaneous bleeding from disseminated intravascular coagulation. Patients with M4 or M5 dis-

TABLE 47–4   Laboratory Aids to Distinguish Between Acute Myeloblastic Leukemia (AML) and Acute Lymphoblastic Leukemia (ALL)

	AML	ALL
Morphology of leukemic blasts	Granules in cytoplasm; Auer rods* may be present	Agranular, basophilic cytoplasm
	Multiple nucleoli	Regular, folded nucleus with one prominent nucleolus
	FAB (see Table 47–3) subclassification M_1–M_7	FAB subclassification, L_1–L_3
Histochemistry	Myeloperoxidase-positive	Myeloperoxidase-negative; PAS-positive
Cytoplasmic markers	—	Terminal deoxynucleotidyl transferase (Tdt)–positive
Surface markers (% of cases)	—	B-cell markers (5%)
		T-cell markers (15–20%): CD 2, 3, or 5
		CALLA (50–65%): CD 10
Cytogenetic and oncogenetic abnormalities	M_3: t(15,17) Abnormal retinoic acid receptor gene	L3: t(8,14) abnormal c-*myc*
	M_5: t(9,11)	Some ALL: Ph[1] *bcr-abl* fusion gene

*Auer rods are a linear coalescence of cytoplasmic granules that stain pink with Wright's stain.
CALLA = common acute lymphoblastic leukemia antigen; FAB = French-American-British classification system; PAS = periodic acid–Schiff.

ease (monocytic leukemias) have high levels of circulating white blood cells and may have swollen gums as a result of infiltration with blasts. Patients with megakaryoblastic leukemia (M7) have significant marrow fibrosis and usually present with organomegaly and pancytopenia similar to those seen in patients with myelofibrosis and myeloid metaplasia.

Laboratory evaluation shows blast cells in the bone marrow and peripheral blood. White blood cell counts range from neutropenic levels ($1.0 \times 10^9/L$) to extreme leukocytosis ($200 \times 10^9/L$). Severe thrombocytopenia and normocytic anemia are also common. Bone marrow biopsy shows 30% to 100% blast cells with depressed production of normal mature cells. AML can be distinguished from ALL by cell morphology and by the presence of *Auer rods,* formed by the aggregation of myeloid granules. Further immunophenotyping using cell surface antigens and histochemistry confirms cells as being of either myeloid or lymphoid origin. Cytogenetic abnormalities such as t(15,17) found in promyelocytic leukemia and the t(8,21) found in M2 disease are helpful diagnostically and influence therapy.

Leukemic Emergencies

Patients newly diagnosed with AML may present with acute emergencies requiring immediate stabilization. *Leukostasis* caused by high levels of circulating blasts (>80,000 to 100,000) leads to diffuse pulmonary infiltrates and acute respiratory distress. Blast cells may injure surrounding vasculature and may lead to life-threatening CNS bleeding. In addition, high cell numbers result in the release of cellular breakdown products, hypokalemia, acidosis, and hyperuricemia that may cause renal failure. Treatment of these complications should be instituted as soon as possible with leukopheresis, hydroxyurea, and induction chemotherapy to reduce circulating cell numbers, along with hydration and urine alkalinization to reduce urine crystallization. Red blood cell transfusions are contraindicated in patients with high numbers of circulating blast cells because of the risk of further increases in blood viscosity. CNS complications such as intracranial bleeding, cranial nerve invasion, and leukemic meningitis are treated with emergency irradiation of the CNS. Patients with AML, especially with acute promyelocytic leukemia (M3), may present with disseminated intravascular coagulation resulting from procoagulant factors released from malignant cells. Low-dose heparin and supportive platelet transfusions may help to treat this complication.

Treatment

Treatment of AML differs from that of ALL in many ways. Therapy involves induction chemotherapy with consolidation and intensification over 4 to 6 months. Unlike in ALL, maintenance chemotherapy has no established role in prolonging remissions in AML. Routine CNS prophylaxis is also not necessary in AML. Various chemotherapeutic regimens employing an anthracycline (daunorubicin or idarubicin) and cytosine arabinoside have led to complete remissions in 60% to 80% in adults. Patients in whom this induction therapy fails have a poor prognosis, but they are usually treated with non–cross-reactive drugs such as epidophyllotoxins or high-dose cytosine arabinoside.

Long-term cure rates (defined as length of survival >5 years after remission) range from 15% to 30% with chemotherapy alone, although some subtypes of leukemia have a much higher rate of cure with chemotherapy alone (Table 47–5). Notably, t(8,21)- and inv(16)-associated AML is unusually responsive to consolidation therapy with high-dose cytosine arabinoside and can be cured in 50% to 70% of patients with chemotherapy alone. Acute promyelocytic leukemia is discussed in the next paragraph. Patients with these favorable subtypes of AML are not considered candidates for transplantation procedures unless they have a disease relapse after chemotherapy. By contrast, use of chemotherapy alone in primary resistant disease or to induce a second remission after disease relapse in poor-prognosis leukemia is rarely successful, and such patients should be offered transplantation procedures during first remission if age and donor availability permit. Elderly patients with major comorbidities and/or secondary leukemia after prior diseases may not tolerate aggressive chemotherapeutic regimens to induce remission, and it may be appropriate to use supportive therapy, given the low response rates and high mortality.

Treatment of Acute Promyelocytic Leukemia (M3). Treatment of acute promyelocytic leukemia differs from that of other acute leukemias because of the unique biology of this disease. Acute promyelocytic leukemia cells (APL cells) are promyelocytic cells containing large granules and the characteristic Auer rods of AML. Complications include life-threatening coagulopathy induced by release of granule contents. APL cells possess a unique chromosomal translocation, t(15,17), which results in a unique fusion protein (PML/RARα). This protein, a combination of a nuclear transactivating protein, PML, with a retinoic acid receptor on chromo-

TABLE 47–5 Prognostically Significant Cytogenetic Abnormalities in Acute Myelogenous Leukemia

Abnormality	Frequency	Complete Remission/ Continuous Complete Remission
Good Prognosis		
inv(16)	5%	>90% (50–80%)
t(8,21)	5%	>90% (50–80%)
t(15,17)	5–10%	70–95% (60–85%)
Intermediate Prognosis		
Normal	30–50%	50–80% (15–25%)
Poor Prognosis		
5-,5q-,7-,7q-	15%	30–50% (<5%)
8+	10–15%	40–65% (<5%)

some 17, results in arrested promyelocytic differentiation and enhanced proliferation. Treatment of acute promyelocytic leukemia with all-*trans*-retinoic acid (ATRA) has been shown to overcome this effect, by allowing differentiation of immature blast cells into mature neutrophils and by inducing clinical remission of disease in up to 90% of patients. However, ATRA-related toxicity (high levels of circulating leukocytes with leukostasis and pulmonary infiltrates) and high relapse rates after ATRA therapy alone have led to the combination of ATRA with intense chemotherapy. This regimen has led to long-term remission rates in two thirds of treated patients. Promising data suggest that the use of arsenic can also induce remission in patients with relapsed acute promyelocytic leukemia by inducing further leukemic cell death.

STEM CELL TRANSPLANTATION

Allogeneic transplantation offers the only hope for long-term cure in many patients with de novo AML and relapsed ALL. Overall cure rates with chemotherapy alone in patients with AML are 15% to 30%. For patients less than 60 years old, allogeneic bone marrow transplantation offers an overall long-term cure rate of 40% to 60%, with a procedure-related mortality rate of 20% to 25%. Results are better when patients undergo bone marrow transplantation after initial induction chemotherapy (in the first remission), rather than after disease relapse (the second remission). However, chemotherapeutic regimens are also more effective in the first remission than after transplantation, and cure from transplantation performed during second remissions are still 25%. Decisions about the best time to perform bone marrow transplantation in patients are probably best guided by cytogenetic data that predict those patients at high risk of disease relapse (see Table 47–5). Eligible patients with poorer prognoses are recommended for earlier transplantation, whereas those with favorable disease features may benefit from further chemotherapy before transplantation or may undergo bone marrow transplantation only after relapse has occurred.

In ALL, as in AML, the worse the prognosis, the earlier transplantation should be offered. Studies have shown that patients with Philadelphia chromosome positivity, high white blood cell counts, or prolonged time to first remission have benefited from bone marrow transplantation in first remission. Early transplantation has achieved 5-year survival rates of 40% to 44%, in comparison with 20% with other therapies. Patients with ALL who have a disease relapse after second remission have few options other than bone marrow transplantation or experimental treatments.

Patients with AML who are ineligible for allogeneic transplants because of advanced age or lack of compatible HLA donors may be offered autologous bone marrow or stem cell transplantation. Marrow or peripheral stem cells are harvested from patients and are purged in vitro to remove neoplastic cells before their reinfusion into patients after myeloablative high-dose chemotherapy and radiation. Up to 10% patients die as a result of lack of marrow engraftment and other complications. However, an overall long-term survival rate between 20% and 40% offers a slightly better chance of cure than with chemotherapy alone.

REFERENCES

Appelbaum FR: Allogeneic hematopoietic stem cell transplantation for acute leukemia. Semin Oncol 1997; 24:114–123

Bishop JF: The treatment of adult acute myeloid leukemia. Semin Oncol 1997; 24:57–69

Cassileth PA, Harrington DP, Appelbaum FR, et al: Chemotherapy compared with autologous or allogeneic bone marrow transplantation in the management of acute myeloid leukemia in first remission. N Engl J Med 1998; 339:1649–1656

Fenaux P, Chomienne C, Degos L: Acute promyelocytic leukemia: Biology and treatment. Semin Oncol 1997;24:92–102.

Ganser A, Hoelzer D: Clinical use of hematopoietic growth factors in the myelodysplastic syndromes. Semin Hematol 1996; 33:186–195

Gorin NC: Autologous stem cell transplantation in acute myelocytic leukemia. Blood 1998; 92:1073–1085

Greenberg P, Cox C, LeBeau MM, et al: International scoring system for evaluating prognosis in myelodysplastic syndromes. Blood 1997; 89:2079–2088

Guilhot F, Chastang C, Michallet M, et al: Interferon alfa-2b combined with cytarabine versus interferon alone in chronic myelogenous leukemia. N Engl J Med 1997; 337:223–229

Heaney ML, Golde DW. Myelodysplasia. N Engl J Med 1999; 340: 1649–1660.

Kolb HJ, Mitlermüller J, Clemm C, et al: Donor leukocyte transfusions for treatment of recurrent chronic myelogenous leukemia in marrow transplant patients. Blood 1990; 76:2462–2465

Levitt L, Lin R: Biology and treatment of adult acute lymphoblastic leukemia. West J Med 1996; 164:143–155.

Liesner RJ, Goldstone AH: The acute leukemias. BMJ 1997; 314:733–736

Mathias C, Wakoff A, Porter D: Chronic myelogenous leukemia: Extending the prospects for cure. Hosp Pract 1998; 33:137–151

Messinezy M, Pearson TC: Polycythemia, primary (essential) thrombocytopenia and myelofibrosis. BMJ 1997; 314:587–590

Pui AH, Evans WE: Acute lymphoblastic leukemia. N Engl J Med 1998; 339:605–615

Sawyers CL: Chronic myeloid leukemia. N Engl J Med 1999; 340: 1330–1340

Soignet SL, Maslak P, Wang ZG, et al: Complete remission after treatment of acute promyelocytic leukemia with arsenic trioxide. N Engl J Med 1998; 339:1341–1348

Tefferi A: Pathogenetic mechanisms in chronic myeloproliferative disorders: Polycythemia vera, essential thrombocytopenia, agnogenic myeloid metaplasia, and chronic myelogenous leukemia. Semin Hematol 1999; 36(Suppl 2):3–8

Tefferi A, Litzow MR, Noel P, et al: Chronic granulocytic leukemia: recent information on pathogenesis, diagnosis, and disease monitoring. Mayo Clin Proc 1997; 72:445–452

Tefferi A, Silverstein MN, Noel P: Agnogenic myeloid metaplasia. Semin Oncol 1995; 22:327–333

Warrell RP Jr, Frankel SR, Miller WH Jr, et al: Differentiation therapy of acute promyelocytic leukemia with tretinoin (all-*trans*-retinoic acid). N Engl J Med 1991; 324:1385–1393.

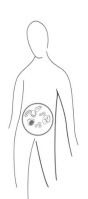

48

DISORDERS OF RED BLOOD CELLS

Nancy Berliner

Normal Red Blood Cell Structure and Function

The red blood cell delivers oxygen to all the tissues in the body and carries carbon dioxide back to the lungs for excretion. The erythrocyte is uniquely adapted to this function. It has a biconcave disc shape that maximizes the membrane surface area for gas exchange, and it has a cytoskeleton and membrane structure that allow it to deform sufficiently to pass through the microvasculature. Passage through capillaries that have a diameter that may be one fourth the resting diameter of the erythrocyte is made possible by interactions between proteins in the membrane (band 3, glycophorin) and underlying cytoplasmic proteins that make up the erythrocyte cytoskeleton (spectrin, ankyrin, protein 4.1).

The mature red blood cell (RBC) contains no nucleus and depends throughout its lifespan on proteins synthesized before extrusion of the nucleus and release into the peripheral circulation. Ninety-eight percent of the cytoplasmic protein of the mature erythrocyte is hemoglobin (Hb). The remainder is composed mainly of enzymatic proteins, such as those required for anaerobic metabolism and the hexose monophosphate shunt.

As discussed later, defects in any of the intrinsic structural features of the erythrocyte can result in hemolytic anemia. Abnormalities of the membrane or cytoskeletal proteins alter erythrocyte shape and flexibility, inborn defects in the enzymatic pathways for glucose metabolism decrease the resistance to oxidant stress, and inherited abnormalities of Hb structure and synthesis lead to polymerization of abnormal Hb (sickle cell disease [SCD]) or to precipitation of unbalanced Hb chains (thalassemia). All these changes decrease RBC survival.

Oxygen is transported by Hb, a tetramer composed of two α chains and two β-like (β, γ, or δ) chains. In fetal life, the main Hb is fetal Hb (HbF) ($\alpha_2\gamma_2$); the switch from fetal HbF to adult HbA ($\alpha_2\beta_2$) occurs in the perinatal period. By 4 to 6 months of age, the level of HbF falls to about 1% of total Hb. HbA$_2$ ($\alpha_2\gamma_2$) is a minor adult Hb, comprising around 1% of adult Hb.

Clinical Approach to Anemia

Anemia, the reduction in RBC mass, is an important sign of disease. It may reflect decreased production of erythrocytes, either because of primary hematologic disease or in response to systemic illness. Alternatively, it may reflect increased cellular turnover from hemolysis. This condition, in turn, may occur as a result of intrinsic abnormalities of the RBC, because of primary immune RBC destruction, or as a part of a systemic vascular process. The analysis of anemia is therefore a critical component of the evaluation of any patient, and it may provide important insight into systemic illness.

CLINICAL PRESENTATION

The symptoms of anemia usually reflect the rapidity with which the reduction in erythrocyte mass has occurred. Patients with acute hemorrhage or massive hemolysis may present with symptoms of hypovolemic shock. However, most patients develop anemia more slowly, and they may have few symptoms. Usual complaints are fatigue, decreased exercise tolerance, dyspnea, and palpitations. In patients with coronary artery disease, anemia may precipitate increasing symptoms of chest pain. On physical examination, the major sign of anemia is pallor. Patients may be tachycardic and often have audible flow murmurs. Patients with hemolysis often present with jaundice and splenomegaly.

LABORATORY EVALUATION

The key components of the laboratory evaluation of anemia are the reticulocyte count, the peripheral blood smear, erythrocyte indices, and the bone marrow aspirate.

The *reticulocyte count* allows the critical distinction between anemia arising from a primary failure of RBC production and that resulting from increased RBC destruction. Erythrocytes newly released from the bone marrow still contain small amounts of RNA; these cells are termed *reticulocytes,* and they can be detected by staining the peripheral blood smear with methylene blue or other supravital stains. In response to the stress of anemia, erythropoietin (EPO) production increases and promotes the production and release of increased numbers of reticulocytes. The number of reticulocytes in the peripheral blood therefore reflects the response of the bone marrow to anemia. The reticulocyte count can be expressed either as a percentage of the total RBC number or as an absolute number. In patients without anemia, a normal reticulocyte count is 1%, with an absolute count of 50,000/μL. When anemia is caused by decreased RBC survival, appropriate marrow response results in a reticulocyte count over 2%, with an absolute reticulocyte count of over 100,000/μL. When the reticulocyte count is not elevated, that should prompt a search for a cause of a failure of RBC production. Reticulocyte counts that are expressed as a percentage of total RBCs must be corrected for anemia, because decreasing the number of circulating cells will increase the reticulocyte percentage without any increase in release from the marrow. The corrected reticulocyte count is calculated by multiplying the reticulocyte count by the ratio of the patient's hematocrit (Hct) to a normal Hct. The advantage of the absolute reticulocyte count is that this correction is not necessary. This test is becoming increasingly available and will probably eventually supersede the standard reticulocyte count.

Evaluation of the *peripheral blood smear* may provide important clues to the origin of anemia. RBC morphology is especially critical in the evaluation of anemia associated with reticulocytosis, in which examination of the smear is essential to distinguishing between immune hemolysis (which results in spherocytes) and microangiopathic hemolysis (which causes *schistocytes,* or erythrocyte fragmentation). Characteristic changes associated with other causes of anemia include sickle and target cells characteristic of hemoglobinopathies, teardrop cells and nucleated RBCs associated with myelofibrosis and marrow infiltration, intracorpuscular parasites in malaria and babesiosis, and pencil-shaped deformities associated with severe iron deficiency. In addition, examination of myeloid cells and platelets may also be helpful. Hypersegmented neutrophils and large platelets support the diagnosis of megaloblastic anemia, and presence of immature blast forms may be diagnostic of leukemia.

The *mean corpuscular volume* (MCV) is an extremely helpful tool in the diagnosis of hypoproliferative anemias. In patients with anemia and a low reticulocyte count, the size of the RBCs is used to characterize the anemia as microcytic (MCV < 80), normocytic (MCV = 80 to 100), or macrocytic (MCV > 100). The differential diagnosis of hypoproliferative anemia based on this division is described later.

In patients with anemia and an elevated reticulocyte count, the vigorous production of new erythroid cells suggests that bone marrow function is normal and is increased in response to the stress of the anemia. Bone marrow examination in this situation is rarely indicated, because the marrow simply shows erythroid hyperplasia, usually without revealing any primary marrow disorder. Evaluation should be focused on determining the cause of RBC consumption, either by bleeding or by hemolysis. In contrast, bone marrow examination is often required for the evaluation of hypoproliferative anemia. In patients in whom common abnormalities such as iron deficiency have been ruled out, bone marrow aspiration and biopsy are indicated to search for abnormalities such as marrow infiltration, marrow involvement with granulomatous disease, marrow aplasia, or myelodysplasia.

Evaluation of Hypoproliferative Anemia

EVALUATION OF MICROCYTIC ANEMIA

The differential diagnosis of microcytic anemia is outlined in Table 48–1. Microcytosis and hypochromia are the hallmarks of anemias caused by defects in Hb synthesis. This disorder can reflect either failure of heme synthesis or abnormalities in globin production. The leading cause of microcytic anemia is iron deficiency, in which lack of heme synthesis results from the absence of iron to incorporate into the porphyrin ring. Iron deficiency is discussed in detail in the next section. Lead poisoning blocks incorporation of iron into heme. Sid-

TABLE 48–1 Differential Diagnosis of Anemia with Low Reticulocyte Count

Microcytic Anemia (MCV <80)
Iron deficiency
Thalassemia minor
Sideroblastic anemia
Lead poisoning

Macrocytic Anemia (MCV >100)
Megaloblastic anemias
    Folate deficiency
    Vitamin B$_{12}$ deficiency
    Drug-induced megaloblastic anemia
Nonmegaloblastic macrocytosis
    Liver disease
    Hypothyroidism

Normocytic Anemia (MCV 80–100)
Early iron deficiency
Aplastic anemia
Myelophthysic disorders
Endocrinopathies
Anemia of chronic disease
Uremia
Mixed nutritional deficiency

MCV = mean corpuscular volume.

eroblastic anemias arise from failure to synthesize the porphyrin ring, usually because of inhibition of the heme synthetic pathway enzymes. Congenital sideroblastic anemia may respond to pyridoxine, a cofactor for several of the heme synthetic pathway enzymes. A more common cause of acquired sideroblastic anemia is alcohol abuse; ethanol inhibits nearly every enzyme in the heme synthetic pathway. Failure of globin synthesis occurs in thalassemic syndromes, as described in detail later. All these disorders lead to decreased mean corpuscular Hb concentration (low MCHC), with consequent hypochromia and decrease in RBC size (low MCV).

Iron Deficiency Anemia

Iron deficiency is the leading cause of anemia worldwide. Although classic iron deficiency anemia presents as microcytic anemia, early iron deficiency is associated with normocytic anemia. Consequently, iron deficiency should be considered in all anemic patients, and iron indices should be a part of the evaluation of any patient with hypoproductive anemia, regardless of the MCV.

Iron is acquired in the diet from either heme (found in meat) or nonheme (derived from vegetables such as spinach) sources. Iron from heme is better absorbed than nonheme iron. Iron absorption is increased in iron deficiency and in patients with ineffective erythropoiesis. Iron is absorbed from the proximal small intestine bound to transferrin, which mediates its uptake into RBC precursors through the transferrin receptor. The iron is released and incorporated into heme. Iron outside of Hb-producing cells is stored in ferritin. Men and women have 50 and 40 mg/kg of total iron, respectively. From 60% to 75% of total iron is found in Hb. A small amount (2 mg/kg) is found in heme and nonheme enzymes, and 5 mg/kg may be found in myoglobin. The remainder is stored in ferritin, which resides primarily in liver, bone marrow, spleen, and muscle. The capacity for excreting iron is limited, and exposure to increased iron, as a result of transfusion, hemochromatosis, or ineffective erythropoiesis, leads to increased iron deposition in these tissues and secondary deposition in endocrine organs and results in liver dysfunction, diabetes, and other endocrine abnormalities.

The most frequent cause of iron deficiency is occult blood loss. All men and postmenopausal women who are found to have iron deficiency should have evaluation for a source of gastrointestinal blood loss, regardless of the detection of occult blood at the time of evaluation. In premenopausal women, iron deficiency is most frequently secondary to loss of iron with menstruation (about 15 mg/month) and during pregnancy (about 900 mg/pregnancy). Dietary deficiency of iron is most commonly seen in young children whose growth outstrips their intake of iron and in babies who drink mostly milk at the expense of intake of iron-containing foods.

Laboratory Evaluation. As stated earlier, early iron deficiency does not present with the hallmark microcytosis and hypochromia that characterize classic iron deficiency. Evaluation of the blood smear may therefore be unrevealing, although severe iron deficiency may result in bizarre RBC forms, including pencil-shaped elongated cells. It is frequently associated with reactive thrombocytosis.

The mainstay of the diagnosis of iron deficiency is the peripheral blood iron indices. These include iron and total iron binding capacity (TIBC) and ferritin. The transferrin saturation is the ratio of serum iron to transferrin concentration (TIBC) and is normally at least 20%. Iron deficiency results in a decrease in serum iron and an increase in TIBC, leading to a decrease in this ratio to less than 10%. Chronic inflammatory conditions (infection, inflammation, malignancy) often decrease both iron and TIBC, but the transferrin saturation usually remains higher than 20%.

The ferritin level reflects total-body iron stores. Ferritin is synthesized by the liver in proportion to total-body iron, and a level of less than 12 ng/mL strongly supports a diagnosis of iron deficiency. Unfortunately, ferritin is an acute phase reactant, and levels rise in the setting of fever, inflammatory disease, infection, or other stresses. However, in the presence of iron deficiency, ferritin levels in response to stress should not rise higher than 50 to 100 ng/mL; therefore, ferritin levels greater than 100 usually rule out iron deficiency.

If the indirect measurement of iron indices does not definitively confirm or refute a diagnosis of iron deficiency, then bone marrow examination will provide direct assessment of marrow iron stores. The presence of iron in the bone marrow excludes iron deficiency, because marrow iron stores are depleted before any fall in RBC production caused by iron deficiency; conversely, complete absence of bone marrow iron confirms iron deficiency.

Treatment. Treatment of iron deficiency is with oral iron supplementation, with administration of ferrous sulfate or ferrous gluconate three times daily. Patients may complain of diarrhea or constipation, and they should be treated symptomatically. Reduction of the dose and gradual reinstitution of full doses may allow oral therapy to be continued. Iron should be administered for several months after resolution of anemia, to allow reconstitution of iron stores.

In patients with malabsorption, complete inability to tolerate oral iron, or iron demands that outstrip the replacement with oral supplements, parenteral iron may be administered. The parenteral administration of iron has been associated with anaphylaxis, and some cases have been fatal. However, administration of an initial dose under careful supervision allows the safe administration of iron to most patients in whom it is necessary. As previously stated, all male patients and all postmenopausal women with iron deficiency require evaluation for a source of gastrointestinal bleeding.

Thalassemia

The thalassemic syndromes are a heterogeneous group of disorders associated with decreased or absent synthesis of either α or β globin chains. Severe thalassemic syndromes are associated with severe hemolytic anemia and are diagnosed in early childhood. However, mild forms of thalassemia minor frequently cause mild microcytic anemia with little or no evidence of hemolysis. These syndromes are often confused with iron deficiency because of the decreased MCV.

β-Thalassemia. More than 100 mutations have been described that lead to β-thalassemia, in which mutations decrease or eliminate expression from the β globin locus. The decreased expression of β globin can be caused by structural mutations in the coding region of the gene, resulting in nonsense mutations, truncated mRNA, and no expression of intact globin from the affected allele (β^0 thalassemia). However, many mutations that result in decreased transcription, translation, or altered splicing of the β globin mRNA may result in reduction, but not elimination, of globin chain expression from the affected allele (β^+ thalassemia).

Defective globin chain synthesis in β-thalassemia causes both decreased normal Hb production and the production of a relative excess of α chains. The decrease in normal Hb synthesis results in hypochromic anemia, and the excess α chains form insoluble α chain tetramers and cause hemolysis. In mild thalassemic syndromes, the excess α chains are insufficient to cause significant hemolysis, and the primary presenting finding is microcytic anemia. In severe forms of thalassemia, hemolysis occurs both in the periphery and in the marrow, with intense secondary expansion of the marrow production of RBCs. The expansion of the marrow space causes severe skeletal abnormalities, and the ineffective erythropoiesis also provides a powerful stimulus to iron absorption.

The clinical spectrum of β-thalassemia reflects the heterogeneity of the molecular lesions causing the disease (Table 48–2). β-Thalassemia major results from homozygous β^0-thalassemia, leading to severe hemolytic anemia; such patients are diagnosed in infancy and depend on transfusions from birth. Patients with β-thalassemia intermedia also have two β-thalassemia alleles, but at least one of them is a mild β^+ mutation. These patients have severe chronic hemolytic anemia, but they do not require transfusions. Because of ineffective erythropoiesis, these patients chronically hyperabsorb iron, and they may develop iron overload in the absence of transfusions. β-Thalassemia minor usually results from heterozygous β-thalassemia, although it may reflect the inheritance of two mild thalassemic mutations. These are the patients in whom iron deficiency is often misdiagnosed. Iron studies show normal to increased iron values with a normal iron saturation. Diagnosis can be confirmed by documenting a compensatory increase in HbA_2 and HbF.

α-Thalassemia. α-Thalassemia is nearly always caused by mutations that delete one or more of the α chain loci on chromosome 16. Four α chain loci have been identified, with two nearly identical copies of the α globin gene on each chromosome. The spectrum of α-thalassemia therefore reflects whether the patient lacks one, two, three, or all four α globin genes (see Table 48–2). In general, the clinical manifestations of α-thalassemia are milder than those of β-thalassemia, for two reasons. First, the presence of four α chain genes allows for adequate α chain synthesis unless three or four loci are deleted. Second, β chain tetramers are much more soluble than their α chain counterparts, and they do not cause hemolysis. Patients with loss of a single α chain gene are silent carriers, and they have normal Hct and MCV values. Patients with deletion of two α chains, either on the same chromosome ($--/\alpha\alpha$, α-thal 1) or on different chromosomes ($\alpha-/\alpha-$, α-thal 2), are microcytic and mildly anemic. Patients who inherit one α-thal 1 allele and one α-thal 2 allele ($--/\alpha-$) have HbH disease. HbH is the product of excess β chain production, β_4; it causes mild hemolytic anemia and minimal or no intramedullary erythrocyte destruction. Inheritance of the homozygous α-thal 2 allele results in no functional α chain loci and is incompatible with life. The fetus is unable to make any functional Hb beyond embryonic development, because HbF also requires α chains. Free γ chains form tetramers, termed HbBarts. HbBarts has an extremely high oxygen affinity, and failure to release oxygen in peripheral tissues results in

TABLE 48–2   Thalassemic Syndromes

Disorder	Genotypic Abnormality	Clinical Phenotype
β-Thalassemia		
Thalassemia major (Cooley's anemia)	Homozygous β^0 thalassemia	Severe hemolysis, ineffective erythropoiesis, transfusion dependency, iron overload
Thalassemia intermedia	Compound heterozygous β^0 and β^+ thalassemia	Moderate hemolysis, severe anemia, but not transfusion dependent; main life-threatening complication is iron overload
Thalassemia minor	Heterozygous β^0 or β^+ thalassemia	Microcytosis, mild anemia
α-Thalassemia		
Silent carrier	$\alpha-/\alpha\alpha$	Normal complete blood count
α-Thalassemia trait	$\alpha\alpha/-$ (α-thalassemia 1) OR $\alpha-/\alpha-$ (α-thalassemia 2)	Mild microcytic anemia
Hemoglobin H	$\alpha-/--$	Microcytic anemia and mild hemolysis; not transfusion dependent
Hydrops fetalis	$--/--$	Severe anemia, intrauterine anasarca from congestive heart failure; death in utero or at birth

severe congestive heart failure and anasarca, a clinical picture termed *hydrops fetalis*. Affected fetuses are still-born or die soon after birth.

EVALUATION OF MACROCYTIC ANEMIA

Two categories of hypoproductive macrocytic anemias are recognized. *Megaloblastic anemia* arises from a failure of DNA synthesis and results in asynchronous maturation of the nucleus and cytoplasm of all rapidly dividing cells. *Nonmegaloblastic macrocytic anemias* usually reflect membrane abnormalities resulting from abnormalities in cholesterol metabolism, seen most commonly with advanced liver disease or severe hypothyroidism.

Megaloblastic Anemia

Megaloblastic anemia usually results from a block to synthesis of critical nucleotide precursors of DNA that leads to a cell cycle arrest in S phase. Cytoplasmic maturation occurs, but maturation of the nucleus is arrested. Cells take on a bizarre appearance, with large, immature nuclei surrounded by mature-appearing cytoplasm. Megaloblastic anemia is not an isolated anemia, because these changes affect all rapidly dividing cells. Patients with megaloblastic syndromes usually have pancytopenia and gastrointestinal symptoms such as diarrhea and/or malabsorption. In women, megaloblastic changes of the cervical mucosa occur and may cause alarmingly abnormal Papanicolaou smears. The most common causes of megaloblastic anemia are deficiencies of vitamin B_{12} or folate, medications that inhibit DNA synthesis or that block folate metabolism, and myelodysplasia.

Vitamin B_{12} (Cobalamin) Deficiency. Cobalamin (Cbl) is absorbed from animal protein in the diet. The process of Cbl absorption and metabolism is complex, because Cbl is always bound to other proteins. In the stomach, protein-bound vitamin is released by digestion with pepsin and immediately becomes bound to transcobalamin I. Transcobalamins I and III, termed *R binders* because of their rapid electrophoretic mobility, are found in all secretions, in plasma, and within the secondary granules of neutrophils. Although they are presumed to be involved with storage of Cbl, their function is unknown, and isolated congenital deficiency of R binders is clinically silent. Within the proximal duodenum, pancreatic proteases digest Cbl away from the R-binder proteins, and Cbl becomes bound to intrinsic factor (IF). IF is secreted by the parietal cells of the stomach and mediates absorption of Cbl through IF-specific receptors in the distal ileum. Within the ileal mucosal cell, the IF-Cbl complex is again digested, and Cbl is released into the plasma bound to transcobalamin II, the carrier protein that mediates cellular uptake of Cbl by transcobalamin II–specific receptors.

Within the cell, Cbl is a cofactor for two intracellular enzymes. It is the coenzyme for methylmalonyl coenzyme A (CoA) mutase, a mitochondrial enzyme that functions in the citric acid cycle to convert methylmalonyl CoA to succinyl CoA. Deficiency of this pathway interferes with the metabolism of odd-chain fatty acids. Cbl is also a coenzyme for the cytoplasmic enzyme homocysteine-methionine methyltransferase. The methyltransferase enzyme is necessary for the transfer of methyl groups from *N*-methyltetrahydrofolate to homocysteine to form methionine. Demethylated tetrahydrofolate is necessary as a carbon donor in the conversion of deoxyuridine to deoxythymidine; absence of Cbl results in a "trapping" of tetrahydrofolate in its methylated form and blocks the synthesis of thymidine triphosphate for incorporation into DNA. The megaloblastic changes induced by Cbl deficiency are mediated through this functional folate deficiency; this finding explains the similarity between the hematologic lesion induced by Cbl deficiency and that found in folate deficiency.

Causes. The causes of Cbl deficiency are outlined in Table 48–3. The most common cause of Cbl deficiency is pernicious anemia. Pernicious anemia is an autoimmune disease associated with gastric parietal cell atrophy, defective gastric acid secretion, and absence of IF. Antiparietal cell and anti-IF antibodies are frequently found in patients with PA, and it is also associated with other autoimmune diseases, such as Graves' disease, Addison's disease, and hypoparathyroidism. Many other lesions in the gastrointestinal tract can interfere with the absorption of Cbl (see Table 48–3). Gastrectomy interferes with absorption by loss of parietal cell function and IF secretion. Pancreatic insufficiency interferes with the digestion of the R-binder–Cbl complex and hinders binding to IF and ileal absorption. Resection of the terminal ileum prevents vitamin B_{12} absorption, as do diseases that affect ileal mucosal function such as Crohn's disease, sprue, intestinal tuberculosis, and lymphoma. Because the stores of Cbl are large, and daily loss of Cbl is low, the body stores of Cbl are adequate for 3 to 4 years if intake stops abruptly. Consequently, signs of Cbl deficiency do not develop until defective absorption has occurred over several years. Because of the ample body stores of Cbl, nutritional Cbl deficiency is also rare, and it is only seen in persons who have been on strict vegan diets, excluding all animal products, for many years. Infants born to vegan mothers and who are breast-fed are also at risk of developing Cbl deficiency.

Folate Deficiency. Folate is widely present in food, in leafy vegetables, fruits, and animal protein. However, because prolonged cooking destroys it, raw fruits and vegetables are the most reliable source of folate. Folate

TABLE 48–3   **Causes of Cobalamin Deficiency**

Malabsorption of vitamin B_{12}
Pernicious anemia
Partial or total gastrectomy
Pancreatic insufficiency
Bacterial overgrowth
Diseases of the terminal ileum
Tapeworm infection
Congenital intrinsic factor or transcobalamin II deficiency
Nutritional (vegans)

is absorbed in the proximal small intestine, and it is present in much lower supply than Cbl. Consequently, nutritional folate deficiency is extremely common in malnourished persons who eat few fresh fruits and vegetables. Folate deficiency can also be caused by increased demand, as occurs with pregnancy, hemolysis, and exfoliative dermatitis. Malabsorption of folate and increased losses, which occur with dialysis, can also lead to folate deficiency. Causes of folate deficiency are outlined in Table 48–4.

Other Causes. Drugs and toxins are the most common other causes of megaloblastic anemia. Some drugs, such as methotrexate and sulfa drugs, act as direct folate antagonists and mimic folate deficiency. Purine and pyrimidine analogue chemotherapeutic agents (e.g., azathioprine, 5-fluorouracil) are direct DNA synthesis inhibitors. Antiviral agents cause megaloblastic changes by unclear mechanisms. Alcohol interferes with folate metabolism and increases the impact of frequent concomitant folate deficiency.

Myelodysplasia commonly presents as macrocytic anemia, with megaloblastic changes in the erythroid series. Unlike other megaloblastic anemias, the megaloblastic changes tend to be restricted to the erythroid lineage. Megakaryocytes in myelodysplasia are dysplastic, but large platelets are unusual. Similarly, myeloid cells tend to show a left shift, but not the classic hypersegmented morphology seen in megaloblastic anemia (see later).

Clinical Manifestations. The development of megaloblastic anemia is usually gradual and allows adequate time for concomitant plasma expansion to prevent hypovolemia. Consequently, patients are frequently severely anemic at the time of presentation. They may have yellowish skin, resulting from a combination of pallor and jaundice. Some patients have glossitis and cheilosis. With severe anemia, patients usually have an MCV greater than 110, although concomitant iron deficiency may decrease the macrocytosis. Patients frequently have mild to severe pancytopenia.

Peripheral smear shows large, oval cells (macro-ovalocytes), hypersegmented neutrophils, and large platelets. Hypersegmented polymorphonuclear cells are a unique diagnostic feature of megaloblastic anemia. As previously noted, hypersegmented neutrophils are not a typical feature of myelodysplasia, and the presence of these cells helps to distinguish these entities. The bone marrow is hypercellular, with abnormally large precursors. Also evident is marked ineffective hematopoiesis, with elevated bilirubin and lactate dehydrogenase levels as a result of intramedullary destruction of erythrocytes.

Cbl deficiency is associated with neurologic abnormalities that are not seen with other causes of megaloblastic anemia. The neurologic signs may range widely, from subtle loss of vibratory sensation and position sense to frank dementia and neuropsychiatric disease. The neurologic changes may present without anemia, and they may progress if a patient with Cbl deficiency is treated with folate, which corrects the hematologic manifestations of megaloblastic anemia but does not treat the neurologic abnormalities. The neurologic manifestations of Cbl deficiency are thought to be attributable to changes related to absence of function of the mitochondrial enzyme methylmalonyl CoA mutase. One proposed explanation is that failure to metabolize odd-chain fatty acids results in their improper incorporation into myelin and causes neurologic dysfunction. This may explain why these findings are seen uniquely in Cbl deficiency and not in other megaloblastic anemias restricted to the folate pathway.

Diagnosis of megaloblastic anemia may be made by measuring levels of Cbl and folate in the peripheral blood. Because megaloblastic changes in the gut mucosa can cause concomitant folate or Cbl deficiency in the setting of a deficiency of the other, great care should be taken to be certain that both levels are measured.

In the setting of Cbl deficiency, the Schilling test may help to establish the origin of the deficiency. Radioactive Cbl is given orally with a large parenteral dose of unlabeled Cbl. The absorption of orally administered Cbl is then measured by determining the excretion of radioactivity into the urine. Cbl bound to IF and labeled with a different isotope can be given simultaneously. Selective absorption of IF-bound Cbl supports a diagnosis of pernicious anemia. If neither isotope is absorbed, the test may be repeated after a course of antibiotics (to treat potential bacterial overgrowth) or after administration of pancreatic enzymes (to rule out pancreatic insufficiency). The use of the Schilling test has decreased with the availability of assays of antiparietal cell antibodies and anti-IF antibodies, particularly because the necessity of an adequate urine collection makes it frequently unreliable.

Treatment. Patients with megaloblastic anemia frequently present with extremely low Hct values. Consequently, if the diagnosis is suspected, treatment should be initiated as soon as the folate and Cbl levels have been drawn. Patients with Cbl deficiency should initially receive daily parenteral therapy, with 100 μg IV for 7 days. Alternatively, therapy can be given subcutaneously, 1 mg/day. Long-term therapy should be with 1 mg IM monthly. Rare patients with nutritional Cbl deficiency can receive oral replacement therapy. Oral therapy with crystalline vitamin B_{12} may overcome blocks to normal Cbl absorption, and oral therapy may be an option in

TABLE 48–4   **Causes of Folate Deficiency**

Dietary insufficiency
Increased folate requirements
   Pregnancy
   Lactation
   Hemolysis
   Exfoliative dermatitis
   Malignancy
Malabsorption
   Sprue
   Crohn's disease
   Short bowel syndrome
Antifolate medications
   Methotrexate
   Sulfa drugs

patients who refuse parenteral supplementation. Therapy with Cbl should be accompanied by folate therapy because patients often have concomitant secondary folate deficiency.

Patients with folate deficiency can receive replacement therapy with 1 to 5 mg/day of oral folate. As noted previously, it is critical to be certain that patients do not have Cbl deficiency, because replacement of folate corrects the hematologic parameters in patients with Cbl deficiency, but it does not improve the neurologic sequelae.

After treatment for megaloblastic anemia, patients usually have a rapid response. Reticulocytosis is seen as early as 2 days after therapy, and it peaks within 7 to 10 days. Despite rapid resolution of neutropenia, hypersegmentation of neutrophils may persist for several days. During this period, rapid cellular proliferation and turnover may precipitate hypokalemia, hyperuricemia, or hypophosphatemia. Patients should also be followed for development of iron deficiency in the face of increased demand with the rapid cellular proliferation in response to replacement therapy. Anemia and other cytopenias should respond completely within 1 to 2 months, but the neurologic manifestations of Cbl deficiency may be irreversible.

EVALUATION OF NORMOCYTIC ANEMIA

Differential Diagnosis

The differential diagnosis of normocytic hypoproductive anemia is long. Most nutritional anemias that classically cause microcytosis or macrocytosis begin as normocytic anemia. Combined nutritional deficiencies may also cause normalization of the MCV. The measurement of EPO levels may be helpful in the diagnosis of normocytic anemia. In addition to helping in the diagnosis of anemia resulting from unsuspected occult renal failure, many of the anemias associated with chronic inflammation and endocrinopathies may present with a depressed EPO level. An elevated EPO level suggests inadequate marrow response to anemia and increases the likelihood of a diagnosis of myelophthisis or primary bone marrow failure. In patients in whom the diagnosis is not clear on routine iron studies and EPO determination, a bone marrow examination is indicated to rule out these primary marrow disorders.

Anemia of Chronic Disease

The anemia of chronic disease occurs in patients with chronic inflammatory, infectious, malignant, and autoimmune diseases. It is caused by absolute or relative EPO deficiency and is often associated with relative EPO resistance and poor iron incorporation into developing erythrocytes. Patients have low serum iron levels, a finding that explains why the anemia of chronic disease is often included in the differential diagnosis of iron deficiency anemia even though it is not microcytic. In contrast to the iron indices in iron deficiency, patients usually also have depressed TIBC, with a transferrin saturation of greater than 10%. Ferritin levels are usually elevated, both as an acute phase reactant and as a reflection of decreased iron incorporation.

The anemia of chronic disease will resolve if the underlying chronic condition is treated. In the absence of primary treatment, anemia often responds to therapy with EPO. EPO levels may be helpful in defining those patients who are likely to respond. Interpretation of EPO levels is difficult in patients with mild anemia, because EPO levels do not usually rise to more than the normal range until the Hct is depressed to less than 30%. At Hct levels of less than 30%, the EPO level is often in the normal range. However, such levels are inappropriate in the setting of a depressed Hct. In general, therapy with EPO may be successful in patients with levels lower than 150 U, although therapy is most successful if the level is less than 50 U. Responses to EPO are most dramatic in patients with certain malignant diseases, especially multiple myeloma, in rheumatoid arthritis, and in the anemia of human immunodeficiency virus infection.

Treatment of the anemia of chronic renal failure depends on EPO replacement. Treatment of other causes of normocytic anemia is dictated by the primary cause of the disorder. The evaluation and treatment of primary marrow failure syndromes and hematologic malignancy are discussed in Chapters 46 and 47, respectively.

EVALUATION OF ANEMIA WITH RETICULOCYTOSIS

An elevated reticulocyte count in the setting of anemia signals a compensatory response of a normal marrow to premature loss of erythrocytes. *Hemolysis* is the premature destruction of RBCs in the reticuloendothelial system *(extrinsic hemolysis)* or in blood vessels *(intrinsic hemolysis)*. The only other condition that causes anemia with reticulocytosis is acute bleeding. The differential diagnosis of hemolytic anemia is outlined in Table 48–5.

Although examination of the peripheral blood smear is frequently helpful in characterizing any anemia, it is absolutely critical in the evaluation of patients with hemolytic anemia. As noted earlier, the morphology of the erythrocytes is helpful in distinguishing immune hemolysis from microangiopathic hemolytic anemia. In addition, other abnormalities of RBC morphology are characteristic for specific diseases such as SCD (sickled cells), enzyme defects ("bite" cells), or erythrocyte membrane abnormalities (spherocytes, elliptocytes).

IMMUNE HEMOLYTIC ANEMIA

Immune-mediated hemolysis results from coating of the erythrocyte membrane with antibodies and/or complement. It may be mediated by IgG antibodies ("warm" antibody) or by IgM antibodies ("cold" antibody). The designation "warm" and "cold" denotes the temperature at which maximal antibody binding takes place, and the clinical syndromes caused by the two types of antibodies are distinct.

The diagnosis of hemolytic anemia is based on the direct and indirect antiglobulin (Coombs) test. To per-

TABLE 48–5 **Differential Diagnosis of Hemolytic Anemia**

Immune Hemolytic Anemia
Immunoglobulin G (warm antibody)–mediated hemolysis
Immunoglobulin M (cold antibody)–mediated hemolysis
Other Causes of Hemolysis from Causes Extrinsic to the Erythrocyte
Microangiopathic hemolysis
Disseminated intravascular coagulation
Thrombotic thrombocytopenic purpura
Preeclampsia, eclampsia, HELLP
Drugs (mitomycin, cyclosporine)
Valvular hemolysis
Splenomegaly
Infection
Hemolytic Anemia Caused by Disorders of the Erythrocyte Membrane
Inherited membrane abnormalities
Hereditary spherocytosis
Hereditary elliptocytosis
Hereditary pyropoikilocytosis
Acquired membrane abnormalities
Paroxysmal nocturnal hemoglobinuria
Spur cell anemia
Hemolysis Caused by Erythrocyte Enzymopathies
Glucose-6-phosphate dehydrogenase deficiency
Other enzyme deficiencies
Hemoglobinopathies
Sickle cell disease
Other sickle syndromes
Thalassemia

HELLP = hemolysis, elevated liver enzymes, and low platelet count.

form a direct Coombs test, patient erythrocytes are mixed with rabbit antisera directed against either human IgG or human complement. The cells are then monitored for agglutination, the presence of which confirms the presence of antibody and/or complement on the patient's RBCs. The indirect Coombs test is performed by mixing patient serum with ABO compatible erythrocytes and then mixing with rabbit antisera against IgG; this is a test for antibody in the patient's serum.

Immunoglobulin G–Mediated (Warm) Immune Hemolysis

Classic autoimmune hemolytic anemia is caused by IgG antibody directed against erythrocyte antigens. Warmtype hemolysis may be primary (idiopathic) or associated with autoimmune disease, lymphoproliferative disorders, or drugs. Patients present with acute anemia, jaundice, and an elevated reticulocyte count. Some patients present with splenomegaly. Laboratory analysis confirms the presence of IgG on the erythrocyte membrane, as demonstrated by a positive Coombs test; some cases are also associated with complement. Occasional patients do not have reticulocytosis; in such patients, the antibody destroys reticulocytes as well as mature erythrocytes.

The mainstay of therapy of autoimmune hemolytic anemia is corticosteroid administration. Patients are usually treated with 1 to 2 mg/kg of prednisone, and doses in responding patients are tapered slowly over several months. Patients who fail to respond to prednisone can be treated with other immunosuppressive agents, such as cyclophosphamide, azathioprine, or chlorambucil. Occasional patients respond to intravenous immunoglobulin. Splenectomy may be effective in some patients who are refractory or resistant to steroids; however, some evidence indicates that patients who do not respond and who have ongoing hemolysis after splenectomy are at high risk of secondary thromboembolic events.

Drug-induced hemolysis is mediated by warm antibodies. Drugs may induce autoimmune hemolytic anemia by several mechanisms (Table 48–6). Penicillin produces hemolysis by binding to erythrocytes and acting as a hapten; the antibody is directed against the drug, and hemolysis occurs only in the presence of the drug. Type

TABLE 48–6 **Drug-Induced Autoimmune Hemolytic Anemia**

Type	Mechanism	Drugs Implicated	Direct Coombs	Indirect Coombs
1	Hapten-mediated	Penicillin Cephalothin (and others)	IgG+ Complement +/−	+ Only in the presence of drug
2	Immune complex–mediated	Quinine Quinidine Phenacetin Rifampin Isoniazid Tetracycline Chlorpromazine (and others)	IgG− Complement +	+ Only in the presence of drug
3	"True" anti-RBC antibody	Methyldopa Levodopa Procainamide Ibuprofen Interferon-α (and others)	IgG+ Complement −	+

2 hemolysis is caused by formation of an antibody-drug complex that binds to the erythrocyte membrane and activates complement. Drugs associated with this type of hemolysis include quinidine, quinine, and rifampin. Still other drugs, including methyldopa and procainamide, cause hemolysis by inducing the production of "true" antierythrocyte antibodies directed against Rh and other RBC antigens. Antibody may persist in the absence of the drug, but not all patients with a positive Coombs test have evidence of hemolysis.

Immunoglobulin M–Mediated (Cold) Hemolytic Anemia

Cold-type immune hemolysis is usually postinfectious. The most common associated illnesses are *Mycoplasma pneumoniae* and Epstein-Barr virus. IgM antibodies are produced that are directed against the RBC antigen I (*Mycoplasma*) or i (Epstein-Barr virus). The antibodies bind at lower temperatures, usually in the distal circulation, and bind complement. During the return to the central circulation, the IgM falls off the RBC and leaves complement bound. The Coombs test is negative for IgG or IgM, but it is positive for complement. Hemolysis is self-limited, rarely severe, and resolves with supportive therapy. In cases of severe hemolysis requiring transfusion, blood should be administered through a blood warmer to minimize further hemolysis.

Cold agglutinin disease is a chronic IgM antibody-mediated hemolysis usually seen in association with lymphoproliferative disease. This is usually associated with chronic low-grade hemolysis, although it may occasionally be severe. Patients respond poorly to steroids and splenectomy. Acute severe IgM-mediated hemolysis may respond to plasmapheresis. Supportive therapy includes avoidance of exposure to the cold.

OTHER CAUSES OF HEMOLYSIS FROM CAUSES EXTRINSIC TO THE ERYTHROCYTE

Microangiopathic Hemolysis

Microangiopathic hemolytic anemia is caused by traumatic destruction of RBCs as they pass through small vessels. The leading causes of this disorder (see Table 48–5) include disseminated intravascular coagulation and thrombotic thrombocytopenic purpura/hemolytic uremic syndrome. Other causes include pregnancy-related syndromes including preeclampsia, eclampsia, and the HELLP (hemolysis, elevated liver enzymes, and low platelets) syndrome, drugs, and metastatic cancers. A similar hemolytic picture can be seen in traumatic hemolysis on a damaged cardiac valve.

Diagnosis of microangiopathic hemolytic anemia is made by the finding of schistocytes (fragmented erythrocytes) on the peripheral blood smear. The presence of a normal prothrombin time and of a normal partial thromboplastin time supports a diagnosis of thrombotic thrombocytopenic purpura/hemolytic uremic syndrome over that of disseminated intravascular coagulation. Treatment is described in Chapter 52.

Infection

Hemolysis can be caused by direct infection of RBCs by parasites, as seen in malaria, babesiosis, and bartonellosis. Severe, overwhelming hemolysis can be seen in clostridial sepsis, in which direct damage to the membrane by bacterial toxins occurs.

HEMOLYTIC ANEMIAS CAUSED BY DISORDERS OF THE ERYTHROCYTE MEMBRANE

Inherited Membrane Abnormalities

Hereditary Spherocytosis. Hereditary spherocytosis is caused by heterogeneous congenital abnormalities in proteins of the erythrocyte cytoskeleton. Most have dominantly inherited mutations in spectrin or ankyrin. Hereditary spherocytosis is characterized by hemolytic anemia, splenomegaly, and prominent spherocytes in the peripheral blood. Spherocytes are formed in the spleen, which removes portions of the abnormal membrane. The loss of membrane decreases the membrane-to-cytoplasm ratio, and the erythrocyte loses its biconcave morphology and assumes a spherocytic shape. Spherocytes are less flexible and may be destroyed in the microvasculature. The laboratory characteristic of hereditary spherocytosis is the finding of increased osmotic fragility, caused by the loss of distensibility associated with decrease in surface membrane. Hereditary spherocytosis is usually a mild disorder, with well-compensated hemolysis. Patients typically have exacerbations during infections or when given marrow-suppressing medication. Patients with significant hemolysis should receive folate supplementation. Many patients require cholecystectomy for pigment stones. Severe, symptomatic anemia is treated with splenectomy.

Hereditary Elliptocytosis. Hereditary elliptocytosis is typically caused by dominantly inherited mutations affecting the interaction between membrane proteins with underlying cytoplasmic proteins. The most common abnormalities affect the interaction with spectrin and protein 4.1. This process causes the RBCs to assume an elliptic shape. As in hereditary spherocytosis, patients usually have mild hemolysis and splenomegaly.

Hereditary Pyropoikilocytosis. Hereditary pyropoikilocytosis is a rare recessive disorder that is frequently caused by inheritance of two different membrane disorders (e.g., one allele for hereditary spherocytosis and one for hereditary elliptocytosis). Patients have much more severe hemolysis, with microspherocytes and elliptocytes on smear. As in hereditary spherocytosis, treatment of symptomatic anemia in hereditary elliptocytosis and hereditary pyropoikilocytosis is splenectomy.

Acquired Membrane Abnormalities

Paroxysmal Nocturnal Hemoglobinuria. Paroxysmal nocturnal hemoglobinuria (PNH) is an acquired clonal disease that is associated with an abnormality of complement regulation. All hematopoietic cells in these patients have a defect in the ability to synthesize the membrane glycoprotein anchor (glycan-phosphoinositol anchor) that stabilizes decay-accelerating factor and membrane inhibitor of reactive lysis on the membrane. These proteins protect cells from surface complement activation. Absence of the glycan-phosphoinositol anchor from erythrocytes renders them susceptible to complement-mediated lysis. Traditional tests for PNH were functional assays based on the increased susceptibility of erythrocytes to lysis by acidic serum (Ham's test) or hypotonic medium (sucrose lysis test). Now that the underlying molecular abnormality in PNH has been defined, diagnosis can be made by flow cytometric documentation of the absence of decay-accelerating factor or membrane inhibitor of reactive lysis on the surface of RBCs or leukocytes.

PNH is manifested by episodic acute intravascular hemolysis, with release of free Hb that results in the hemoglobinuria for which the disease is named. The disease is considered to be part of the spectrum of myeloproliferative diseases: it is a clonal stem cell disorder associated with thrombotic risk and with a risk of developing leukemia and/or myelofibrosis. Patients are susceptible to thrombotic complications typical of those seen in myeloproliferative disorders, including Budd-Chiari syndrome, portal vein thrombosis, and cerebrovascular thrombosis. PNH also has an association with aplastic anemia: patients may develop aplasia, and patients with aplastic anemia who respond to immunosuppressive therapy frequently recover with PNH-like clones. Treatment is largely supportive. However, young patients should be considered for allogeneic stem cell transplantation.

Spur Cell Anemia. Spur cells (*acanthocytes*) are cells with abnormal membrane morphology that are found in patients with advanced liver disease, severe malnutrition, malabsorption, and asplenia. The membrane acquires protrusions as a result of the presence of abnormal lipids. The changes may be associated with mild hemolysis, although in patients with advanced liver disease, distinguishing hemolysis from hypersplenism may be difficult. Similar changes may be seen in patients with abetalipoproteinemia.

HEMOLYTIC ANEMIAS CAUSED BY DISORDERS OF ERYTHROCYTE ENZYMES

Glucose-6-Phosphate Dehydrogenase Deficiency

Glucose-6-phosphate dehydrogenase (G6PD) is a critical enzyme in the hexose monophosphate shunt pathway, which is required to maintain intracellular stores of reduced glutathione to protect erythrocytes from membrane oxidation and Hb oxidation. The gene for G6PD resides on the X chromosome, and nearly all patients with the disorder are male. However, an occasional heterozygous female patient with skewed lyonization appears deficient. Most G6PD genes are found in Africa

and the Mediterranean, and they are thought to have been selected for because they confer resistance to malaria. The African form of G6PD deficiency is relatively mild, whereas that in the Mediterranean is more severe.

Absence of G6PD renders erythrocytes sensitive to oxidative stress. In the setting of infection, acidosis, or oxidant drugs, Hb may precipitate within the cells and may cause hemolysis. Many drugs are associated with hemolysis in the setting of G6PD deficiency, including sulfonamides, antimalarials, dapsone, aspirin, and phenacetin. Diagnosis should be suspected in men of African-American or Mediterranean extraction in the setting of acute infection or recent exposure to oxidant drugs. Cells with precipitated Hb contain *Heinz's bodies* that can be visualized with crystal violet staining of the peripheral blood smear. These inclusions are removed in the spleen and result in the finding of "bite cells" in the blood smear. Diagnosis can be confirmed with measurement of G6PD levels in the peripheral blood. However, reticulocytes and young RBCs in patients with G6PD deficiency have a higher enzyme level; consequently, if the diagnosis is suspected, patients with a normal G6PD level should be retested at a time removed from the acute episode. The mainstay of preventing hemolysis in these patients is avoidance of oxidative stress, especially related to drugs implicated in causing hemolysis. Splenectomy is recommended only for patients with severe episodic or chronic hemolysis.

Other Enzyme Deficiencies

Deficiencies have been reported involving nearly all the enzymes of the glycolytic pathway as rare causes of hemolytic anemia. The most common of these is *pyruvate kinase deficiency*. These enzymes are encoded by autosomal genes, and the pattern of inheritance is therefore autosomal recessive.

HEMOGLOBINOPATHIES

Hemoglobinopathies are mutations that result in the synthesis of abnormal Hb. The most common of these are the sickle syndromes, which, like thalassemia and G6PD deficiency, arose in areas of the world in which malaria is endemic.

Sickle Cell Disease

SCD is the most common of the sickle syndromes and arises from a point mutation that results in a glutamic acid to valine substitution in the sixth amino acid of the β globin gene. It has arisen as an independent mutation in diverse populations in Africa, India, the Mediterranean, and the Middle East. The substitution of a hydrophobic for a hydrophilic residue renders the deoxygenated sickle Hb less soluble, as well as susceptible to polymerization and precipitation. The rate of precipitation of sickle Hb is exquisitely sensitive to the intracorpuscular concentration of deoxygenated Hb. Sickling is therefore increased in settings in which that concentration is increased either by changes in cellular hydration (dehydration) or by changes in the oxygen dissociation curve (hypoxia, acidosis, high altitude).

Acute Manifestations. Most of the acute complications of SCD are related to vaso-occlusion (Table 48–7). Painful crises, caused by ischemic pain in organs with occlusions of the microvasculature, can occur anywhere, with pain most common in the extremities, chest, abdomen, and back. Painful crises are commonly precipitated by infections, dehydration, rapid changes in temperature, and pregnancy. However, patients often have no obvious precipitating cause for an acute painful crisis. Vaso-occlusion in the pulmonary circulation can be a particularly ominous complication of SCD and can result in *acute chest syndrome*. The acute chest syndrome is characterized by chest pain, hypoxemia, and chest infiltrates. The roles of infection, infarction, and in situ thrombosis in the acute chest syndrome are indistinguishable, but all patients should receive antibiotics for presumed pneumonia. Because hypoxemia predisposes to further sickling and increasing respiratory compromise, the acute chest syndrome is life-threatening and is an indication for emergency exchange transfusion.

Neurologic events are a major cause of morbidity in patients with SCD. Acute large-vessel occlusions occur in children, with a recurrence rate of 70% if these patients are untreated; such strokes are an indication for long-term exchange transfusion, which has been shown to decrease the rate of repeated occlusions. For reasons that are poorly understood, such large-vessel occlusions rarely occur in adults. Adults may suffer hemorrhagic strokes as a result of aneurysmal dilatation of proliferative vessels that form in response to repeated microocclusions in the cerebral vessels.

TABLE 48–7 Clinical Manifestations of Sickle Cell Disease

Acute Manifestations
Vaso-occlusive crisis
Painful crisis
Acute chest syndrome
Priapism
Cerebrovascular events
Thrombotic stroke
Hemorrhagic stroke
Aplastic crisis
Splenic sequestration
Osteomyelitis
Chronic Manifestations
Chronic renal disease
Isosthenuria
Chronic renal failure
Chronic pulmonary disease
Sickle hepatopathy
Proliferative retinopathy
Avascular necrosis
Skin ulcers

Any toxic or infectious insult that transiently suppresses bone marrow activity may cause an *aplastic crisis*. The shortened survival of the RBC in SCD renders these patients highly dependent on vigorous ongoing marrow activity, and short intervals of decreased reticulocyte formation can cause profound decreases in Hb and Hct. Most dramatic are infections associated with parvovirus B19, which directly infects erythroid precursors. Supportive care is usually all that is required. However, some patients may go on to develop bone marrow necrosis, with a leukoerythroblastic picture; this situation may be complicated further by bone marrow embolization to the lungs.

Certain vascular beds are especially prone to complications of SCD. The renal medulla is highly susceptible to damage by vaso-occlusion because high tonicity and low oxygen tension both markedly increase the concentration of deoxygenated HbS. All patients with SCD develop defects in urinary concentration ability, and by adulthood, these patients are uniformly isosthenuric. Acute episodes of hematuria secondary to papillary necrosis are common.

Recurrent sickling uniformly occurs in the spleen. By adulthood, all patients have become functionally asplenic from repeated infarctions of the microvasculature. This is one of the contributing factors to the increased susceptibility of patients with SCD to infections with encapsulated organisms. Acute infection remains a significant cause of death in patients with SCD. For unclear reasons, patients with SCD are particularly prone to osteomyelitis, with an unusually high incidence of *Salmonella* as the responsible organism.

Chronic Manifestations. SCD used to be a disease of childhood. As more patients survive to adulthood, it has become clear that repeated episodes of vaso-occlusion damage nearly every end organ (see Table 48–7). Renal failure and pulmonary failure are leading causes of death in adult patients with SCD. Other long-term complications include chronic skin ulcers, retinopathy, and liver dysfunction. In addition, most patients require cholecystectomy for pigment stones.

Treatment. Treatment of SCD remains largely supportive. Painful crises are treated with fluid, oxygen supplementation, and analgesics. Patients with any indication of infection should receive antibiotics. Patients with symptomatic anemia should receive transfusion therapy. Exchange transfusion is indicated for patients with chest syndrome, stroke, bone marrow necrosis, and priapism. More controversial indications for exchange transfusion include intractable pain and slow response to other supportive measures. The goal of exchange transfusion is to achieve a level of 30% to 40% HbS. As previously noted, patients who have sustained a thrombotic large-vessel stroke should undergo exchange transfusions on a long-term basis.

Studies have shown that treatment with hydroxyurea, an agent that increases the concentration of HbF in patients with SCD, reduces the incidence of vaso-occlusive crises. The efficacy of hydroxyurea has been shown in a randomized study. The effect is attributed to the formation of Hb tetramers containing one B^S chain and one γ chain ($\alpha_2\beta^S\gamma$), which will not undergo polymerization. Studies have suggested that response is also related to decreases in leukocyte count and to changes in endothelial adherence properties.

Other Sickle Syndromes

Hemoglobin C. HbC is caused by another substitution, glutamic acid to lysine, in the sixth position of the β globin chain. Homozygous HbC causes mild sickle symptoms and is usually nearly clinically silent. Patients with HbSC are more symptomatic, although the clinical manifestations are milder than those of patients with HbSS. Patients have a higher Hct, and the higher viscosity increases the degree of retinopathy. They do not have splenic infarctions, and unlike patients with HbSS, they usually have splenomegaly. Consequently, they occasionally have episodes of acute splenomegaly associated with profound decreases in Hb and Hct (splenic sequestration crisis); although such crises can also occur in children with HbSS, functional asplenia prevents this complication in adults with homozygous HbS.

Hemoglobin E. HbE occurs primarily in Southeast Asia and results from a mutation in amino acid 26 of β globin. This mutation does not significantly affect the function of the Hb. However, the mutation activates a cryptic splice site in the globin mRNA, and the resultant phenotype resembles thalassemia. Patients have mild anemia with microcytosis.

Sickle-β-Thalassemia. Patients who are double heterozygotes for HbS and β-thalassemia have a spectrum of disease dependent on the level of β globin that they produce. Sickle β^+-thalassemia is a milder disease than HbSS, probably because of the decreased intracorpuscular concentration of HbS. Patients with sickle β^0-thalassemia have essentially the same phenotype as patients with homozygous HbS.

REFERENCES

Berliner N, Duffy TP, Abelson H: Approach to the adult and child with anemia. *In* Benz EJ, Cohen HJ, Furie B, et al (eds): Hematology: Basic Principles and Practice. New York: Churchill Livingstone, 1994, pp 468–483.

Rose M, Berliner N: Red blood cells. *In* Fred J. Schiffman (ed): Hematologic Pathophysiology. Philadelphia: Lippincott-Raven, 1998, pp 49–96.

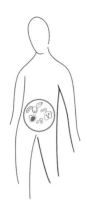

49

CLINICAL DISORDERS OF NEUTROPHILS

Nancy Berliner

Leukocytes provide the main defense against bacterial infection. Monocytes and granulocytes are phagocytic cells that can kill ingested bacteria through the generation of reactive intermediates. Monocytes also release inflammatory mediators that increase the activity of lymphocytes. Lymphocyte function is discussed in Chapter 50.

Normal Granulocyte Development, Structure, and Function

NEUTROPHILS

Neutrophils (polymorphonuclear leukocytes) are the predominant white blood cell in the peripheral blood. They are morphologically recognizable by their characteristic segmented nucleus. They also contain various cytoplasmic granules that both give them a characteristic appearance and are also functionally important.

Neutrophil killing of bacteria requires chemotaxis, phagocytosis, and intracellular killing. *Chemotaxis* is the ordered movement of the cell toward an attracting stimulus, such as bacterial formyl peptides, or complement fragments (C3b, C5a). Neutrophils adhere to endothelial cells by interaction of neutrophil surface glycoproteins (CD11b/CD18) with endothelial adhesion molecules (intracellular adhesion molecule-1 [ICAM-1], endothelial leukocyte adhesion molecule-1 [ELAM-1]), termed *margination*. In response to a chemotactic stimulus, these adherent neutrophils move toward the target along the endothelial surface. The importance of neutrophil adhesion as the first step in bacterial killing is underscored by the syndrome of leukocyte adhesion deficiency. This rare disease is caused by the absence of surface expression of the CD11b/CD18 complex on neutrophils. Neutrophils fail to adhere to endothelium, are unable to undergo chemotaxis, and do not phagocytose or kill bac-

teria. Patients have severe, life-threatening bacterial infections, despite high levels of circulating neutrophils.

Phagocytosis requires recognition of target bacteria or debris by the neutrophil. Targets are *opsonized* by the surface binding of immunoglobulin or complement factor C3b. The neutrophil has surface receptors for C3b and the Fc portion of IgG, which allows recognition and binding to the opsonized target. The target then becomes engulfed in a phagocytic vacuole, which fuses with neutrophil granules.

Intracellular killing occurs by both oxygen-dependent and oxygen-independent mechanisms. Contents of the primary granule, including cathepsin G, defensins, and lysozyme, act to break down the bacterial cell wall and kill the target organism. The major mechanism of bacterial killing, however, is through the *respiratory burst*. Stimulation of the neutrophil activates a membrane-bound oxidase complex, which generates superoxide through transfer of an electron from reduced nicotinamide-adenine dinucleotide (NADPH); interaction of superoxide with water generates hydroxyl ions. In addition, myeloperoxidase catalyzes the formation of hypochlorite ion from hydrogen peroxide and chloride. The NADPH oxidase is a multisubunit enzyme. Absence or decreased activity of any one subunit impairs bacterial killing and results in chronic granulomatous disease, another serious illness in which patients are predisposed to life-threatening bacterial infections.

The granules that give neutrophils their characteristic appearance have important functions in the process of neutrophil activation and killing. *Primary granules* arise early in myeloid differentiation and are found in both neutrophils and monocytes. They contain a large number of proteins, including myeloperoxidase, acid hydrolases, and neutral proteases. These granules fuse with the phagocytic vacuole and aid in digestion of ingested bacteria. *Secondary granules* arise later in the differentiation pathway and give the neutrophil its characteristic granular appearance. These granules contain lactoferrin, transcobalamin, and the matrix-modifying enzymes collagenase and gelatinase. On neutrophil stimulation, these granules are released into the extracellular space. Lactoferrin and transcobalamin act as antibacterial proteins by sequestering iron and vitamin B_{12} away from bacteria, and collagenase and gelatinase break down connective tissue at the site of inflammation. Abnormalities in neutrophil granules have been described in rare clinical syndromes. Absence of myeloperoxidase produces surprisingly mild symptoms and may be associated with defects in control of fungal infection. Secondary granule deficiency is extremely rare and is associated with a slight increase in the risk of bacterial infections.

EOSINOPHILS and BASOPHILS

Eosinophils and *basophils* arise from myeloid precursors in the bone marrow. They transit rapidly from the marrow to the blood into the peripheral tissues, where they play a role in allergic and inflammatory reactions. Like neutrophils, they have characteristic secondary granules that give them their characteristic appearance and that are also functionally important. Both cell types are present in small numbers under normal conditions. Elevated levels of basophils may be seen in myeloproliferative syndromes.

Although eosinophils are capable of phagocytosis, most of the activity of these cells is mediated through the release of their granules. Their numbers are elevated in parasitic and helminthic infections, in which these cells are thought to play a role in the allergic response to those organisms. Numbers of these cells are also elevated in allergic reactions and in collagen vascular diseases, again linking their function to immunomodulation. *Hypereosinophilic syndromes,* in which extremely high levels of eosinophils can be seen, are rare, and they can be associated with damage to the lung, peripheral nervous system, and endocardial tissues.

MONOCYTES

Monocytes arise from a common myeloid precursor with granulocytes, under the influence of granulocyte-macrophage colony-stimulating factor (GM-CSF) and macrophage-CSF (M-CSF). Most circulating monocytes are marginated along the walls of vessels, from which they migrate into tissues, where they develop into macrophages. The monocyte-macrophage lineage has many diverse functions. These phagocytic cells undergo chemotaxis, phagocytosis, and intracellular killing in much the same manner as neutrophils. They are especially important in the killing of mycobacteria, fungi, and protozoal species.

In addition to their role in killing of infectious organisms, monocytes have an important interaction with the immune system. They are antigen-presenting cells for T lymphocytes, they are capable of cellular cytotoxicity, and they secrete certain cytokines. Monocytes that migrate into tissues give rise to macrophages that process antigens and "present" them to T lymphocytes. These cells include the Langerhans cells of the skin, interdigitating cells of the thymus, and dendritic cells in lymph nodes. Antigen-presenting cells are nonphagocytic cells, and the process by which they internalize antigen is not fully understood. Protein antigens are partially digested and are expressed on the cell surface in association with human leukocyte (HLA) or Ia antigens. This feature permits interaction with and activation of helper T cells. Other macrophages, such as Kupffer's cells of the liver and alveolar macrophages of the lung, play an important role in removing particulate and cellular debris and senescent erythrocytes from the circulation.

Monocytes have a role in tumor cell cytotoxicity. They are capable of both antibody-dependent and antibody-independent cytotoxicity against tumor cells. The cytotoxicity is increased by tumor necrosis factor, interleukin-1, and interferon, all of which are also secreted by monocytes. Monocytes secrete a large number of proteins. These include immunomodulatory proteins (tumor necrosis factor, interleukin-1, interferon), cytokines (G-CSF, GM-CSF), coagulation proteins, cell adhesion proteins, and proteases.

Determinants of Peripheral Neutrophil Number

Most granulocyte precursors are in the bone marrow, where maturation occurs over 6 to 10 days. Marrow precursors represent 20%, and the storage pool represents 75%, of the granulocyte mass. Therefore, peripheral neutrophils comprise only 5% of the total granulocyte mass. Furthermore, neutrophils circulate in transit between the marrow and peripheral tissues. Of circulating neutrophils, more than half are adherent to the vascular endothelium. This characteristic is termed margination. The half-life of a neutrophil in the circulation is short, usually only 6 to 12 hours; the neutrophil may then migrate into tissues, where it may survive another 1 to 4 days. Therefore, the peripheral neutrophil count represents a sampling of less than 5% of the total granulocyte pool and is taken during a period of less than 5% of the total neutrophil lifespan. The peripheral white cell count is therefore a poor reflection of granulocyte kinetics. Abnormalities in neutrophil number can occur rapidly and may reflect either a change in marrow granulocyte production or a shift among various cellular compartments. An elevated peripheral white cell count may result from increased marrow production, or it may reflect mobilization of neutrophils from the marginated pool or release from the marrow storage pool. Similarly, a low granulocyte count may reflect decreased marrow production, increased margination and/or sequestration in the spleen, or increased destruction of peripheral cells.

The *total peripheral white cell count* represents the sum of lymphocyte and granulocytes. The significance of an elevated or depressed leukocyte count therefore depends on the nature of the cellular elements that are increased or decreased. *Leukocytosis* is a nonspecific term that may denote an increase in either lymphocytes (*lymphocytosis*) or neutrophils (*granulocytosis*). In rare cases, increases may reflect excessive numbers of monocytes or eosinophils. Leukocytosis related to an elevation in the neutrophil count is referred to as neutrophil leukocytosis, or *neutrophilia*. Extreme elevation of the white blood cell count to more than 50,000/μL with the premature release of early myeloid precursors is termed a *leukemoid reaction;* this may be associated with chronic inflammatory reactions and chronic infections, but it requires consideration of a diagnosis of myeloproliferative disease, especially chronic myelogenous leukemia. Evaluation of the peripheral blood smear may reveal characteristic changes that provide clues to the underlying disorder. A *leukoerythroblastic* smear shows the presence of immature granulocytes, teardrop-shaped erythrocytes, nucleated erythrocytes, and increased platelets. Such changes are reflective of marrow infiltration (*myelophthysis*) by fibrous tissue, granulomas, or neoplasm. As with leukocytosis, *leukopenia* may reflect either lymphopenia or *neutropenia*. Neutropenia is defined as an absolute neutrophil count of less than 1500/μL.

Evaluation of Leukocytosis (Neutrophilia)

Leukocytosis is usually secondary to other processes, and it rarely indicates a primary hematologic disorder (Table 49–1). Patients with persistent elevation of the neutrophil count, especially in association with elevation of the hematocrit and/or platelet count, should be evaluated to rule out a primary myeloproliferative disorder. A leukocyte alkaline phosphatase determination is helpful in ruling out chronic myelogenous leukemia.

Once primary hematologic disorders are eliminated, patients should be evaluated for acute and chronic infectious or inflammatory processes. Neutrophilia related to acute infection, stress, or acute steroid administration

TABLE 49–1 **Differential Diagnosis of Neutrophilia**

Primary Hematologic Disease
Congenital disorders
Myeloproliferative disorders
Secondary to Other Disease Processes
Infection
Acute
Chronic
Acute stress
Drugs
Steroids
Lithium
Cytokine stimulation (e.g., G-CSF)
Chronic inflammation
Myelophthysis
Marrow hyperstimulation
Chronic hemolysis, immune thrombocytopenia
Recovery from marrow suppression
After splenectomy

G-CSF = granulocyte colony-stimulating factor.

TABLE 49–2 **Differential Diagnosis of Leukopenia**

Decreased Production of Neutrophils
Congenital/constitutional conditions
Benign cyclic neutropenia
Postinfectious conditions
Nutritional deficiency (vitamin B$_{12}$, folate)
Drug-induced conditions
Primary marrow failure
Aplastic anemia
Myelodysplasia
Acute leukemia
Increased Peripheral Destruction
Overwhelming infection
Immune destruction
Drug-related
Associated with collagen vascular disease
Isoimmune (in newborn)
Hypersplenism/Sequestration

(as in asthma) primarily reflects demargination and is usually transient. Persistent neutrophilia usually reflects chronic bone marrow stimulation. Nevertheless, bone marrow aspirate and biopsy are rarely indicated. The exception is in those patients who demonstrate leukoerythroblastic changes, who should be evaluated with bone marrow examination, including culture, to rule out chronic tuberculosis or fungal infection, marrow infiltration with tumor, or marrow fibrosis. Cytogenetic studies should also be performed to help eliminate a diagnosis of myeloproliferative disorder.

Evaluation of Leukopenia (Neutropenia)

Neutropenia can reflect decreased production, increased sequestration, or peripheral destruction of neutrophils (Table 49–2). Patients should first be evaluated for splenomegaly to rule out the possibility of sequestration. In patients who are completely asymptomatic and in whom previous studies are unavailable, the possibility of congenital or cyclic neutropenia should be entertained and can be evaluated by serial peripheral counts. The normal neutrophil count varies among ethnic groups, and the normal neutrophil count in African-Americans is lower than that in whites.

If a diagnosis of benign or cyclic neutropenia is not clear, then the evaluation of the patient with neutropenia should include stopping all potentially offending drugs and performing serologic studies to rule out collagen vascular disease. Unlike in patients with leukocytosis, bone marrow examination is indicated early in the evaluation and is frequently diagnostic. Neutropenia much more often reflects primary hematologic disease, and bone marrow examination enables one to diagnose marrow failure syndromes, leukemia, and myelodysplasia. In the absence of bone marrow failure, other causes of neutropenia also may give a characteristic bone marrow picture. Drug-induced neutropenia produces a characteristic "maturation arrest" of the myeloid series. Rather than an actual inhibition of neutrophil maturation, this feature reflects the immune destruction of myeloid precursors that leaves only the earliest cells behind. All patients should have cytogenetic studies performed to aid in the diagnosis of myelodysplasia.

The therapeutic approach to patients with neutropenia depends on the degree of depression of the neutrophil count. Neutrophil counts between 1000 and $1500/\mu L$ are not associated with any significant impairment in the host response to bacterial infection and require no intervention beyond what is demanded for diagnosis and indicated therapy of the underlying cause. Patients with neutrophil counts between 500 and 1000/μL should be alerted to their slightly increased risk of infection, although serious problems are rarely encountered in patients with neutrophil counts higher than $500/\mu L$. Patients with neutrophil counts lower than 500/μL are at significant risk of infection. Such patients must be instructed to notify the physician at the first signs of infection and/or fever, and they must be managed aggressively with intravenous antibiotics regardless of the documentation of a source or infecting organism. Patients with a markedly depressed neutrophil count may exhibit few signs of infection, because much of the inflammatory response at the site of infection is generated by the neutrophils themselves. In patients with severe immune-mediated neutropenia, steroids and intravenous immunoglobulin may be helpful in elevating the neutrophil count and in improving infectious complications. G-CSF may help to increase the peripheral white count and may help to resolve infections in neutropenia induced by drugs, including chemotherapy. It has also been efficacious in some patients with immune neutropenia, as well as in patients with myelodysplasia.

REFERENCES

Coates T, Baehner R: Leukocytosis and leukopenia. *In* Benz EJ, Cohen HJ, Furie B, et al (eds): Hematology: Basic Principles and Practice. New York: Churchill Livingstone, 1994, pp 769–784.

Curnutte JT: Disorders of phagocyte function. *In* Benz EJ, Cohen HJ, Furie B, et al (eds): Hematology: Basic Principles and Practice. New York: Churchill Livingstone, 1994, pp 792–818.

Newburger PE, Parmley RT: Neutrophil structure and function. *In* Benz EJ, Cohen HJ, Furie B, et al (eds): Hematology: Basic Principles and Practice. New York: Churchill Livingstone, 1994, p 738.

50

DISORDERS OF LYMPHOCYTES

Jill Lacy

The central cell of the immune system is the lymphocyte. Lymphocytes mediate the adaptive immune response, providing specificity to the immune system by responding to specific pathogens and conferring long-lasting immunity to reinfection. Lymphocytes are derived from pluripotent hematopoietic stem cells that reside in the bone marrow and give rise to all of the cellular elements of the blood. There are two major functional classes of lymphocytes: B lymphocytes, or B cells, and T lymphocytes, or T cells, which are distinguished by their site of development, antigenic receptors, and function. The major disorders of lymphocytes include (1) neoplastic transformation of specific subsets of lymphocytes resulting in an array of lymphomas or leukemias, (2) congenital and acquired defects in lymphocyte development or function with resultant immunodeficiency syndromes, and (3) physiologic responses to infection or antigenic stimulation that may lead to lymphadenopathy, lymphocytosis, or lymphocytopenia.

Cells of the Immune System: Lymphocyte Development, Function, and Localization

B CELLS

B cells are characterized by the presence of cell surface immunoglobulin (or antibody). Their major function is to mount a humoral immune response to antigens by producing antigen-specific antibody. B cells develop in the bone marrow in a series of highly coordinated steps that involve sequential rearrangement of the heavy and light chain immunoglobulin genes and expression of B cell–specific cell surface proteins (Fig. 50–1). Rearrangement of the immunoglobulin genes results in the generation of a huge repertoire of B cells that are each characterized by an immunoglobulin molecule with unique antigenic specificity. Mature B cells migrate

from the bone marrow to lymphoid tissue throughout the body and are readily identified by the presence of cell surface immunoglobulin and antigens that are B cell specific, including CD19, CD20, and CD21. In response to antigen binding to cell surface immunoglobulin, mature B cells are activated to proliferate and undergo differentiation into end-stage plasma cells, which lose most of their B cell surface markers and produce large quantities of soluble antibodies. Neoplastic disorders of B cells arise from B cells at different stages of development, and thus B-cell lymphomas can be highly varied in their morphology and cell surface expression of B-cell antigens, or immunophenotype.

T CELLS

T cells perform an array of functions in the immune response, including those that are classically regarded as cellular immune responses. T-cell precursors migrate from the bone marrow to the thymus, where they differentiate into mature T-cell subsets. In the thymus, T-cell precursors undergo a coordinated process of differentiation that involves rearrangement and expression of the T-cell receptor (TCR) genes and acquisition of cell surface proteins that are unique to T cells, including CD3, CD4, and CD8. As T cells mature in the thymus, they ultimately lose either the CD4 or CD8 protein, and thus mature T cells are composed of two major groups: CD4$^+$ and CD8$^+$ cells. These two groups mediate distinct immune functions. CD8$^+$ cells are cytotoxic T cells that kill target cells or suppress immune functions and are designated cytotoxic or suppressor T cells. CD4$^+$ cells activate other immune response cells such as B cells and macrophages and thus are considered helper T cells. Like B cells, T cells express unique TCR molecules that recognize specific peptide antigens. In contrast to B cells, T cells only respond to peptides that are processed intracellularly and bound to (or presented by) specialized cell surface antigen–presenting proteins, designated major histocompatibility complex (MHC)

435

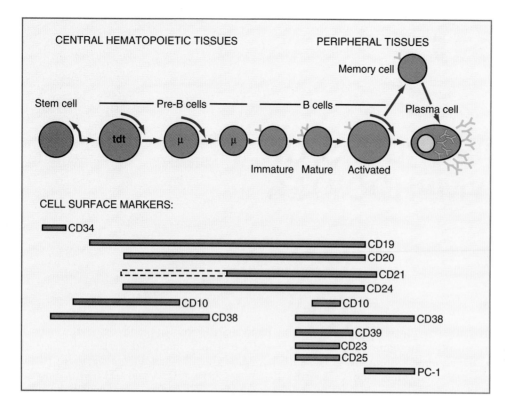

CELL SURFACE MARKERS:

FIGURE 50–1 The maturation of B lymphocytes. *Top,* The changes in immunoglobulin production and maturation are shown. *Bottom,* The appearance and disappearance of surface markers are shown. (Adapted from Handin RI, Lux SE, Stossel TP [eds]: Blood Principles and Practice of Hematology. Philadelphia: JB Lippincott, 1995.)

molecules. Binding of the TCR by a specific peptide/MHC complex triggers T-cell activation of helper or cytotoxic effector functions in $CD4^+$ and $CD8^+$ cells, respectively.

THE LYMPHOID SYSTEM

Lymphocytes localize to the peripheral lymphoid tissue, which is the site of antigen/lymphocyte interaction and lymphocyte activation. The peripheral lymphoid tissue is composed of lymph nodes, the spleen, and mucosal lymphoid tissue. Lymphocytes circulate continuously through these tissues through the vascular and lymphatic systems.

The lymph nodes are highly organized lymphoid tissues that are sites of convergence of the lymphatic drainage system that carries antigens from draining lymph to the nodes where they are trapped. A lymph node consists of an outer cortex and an inner medulla (Fig. 50–2). The cortex is organized into lymphoid follicles composed predominantly of B cells; some of the follicles contain central areas or germinal centers, where activated B cells are undergoing proliferation after encountering a specific antigen, surrounded by a mantle zone. The T cells are distributed more diffusely in paracortical areas surrounding the follicles. The spleen traps antigens from blood rather than the lymphatic system and is the site of disposal of senescent red cells. The lymphocytes in the spleen reside in the areas described as the white pulp, which surround the arterioles entering the organ. As in lymph nodes, the B and T cells are segregated into a periarteriolar lymphoid sheath that is composed of T cells and flanking follicles composed

of B cells. The mucosa-associated lymphoid tissues (MALTs) collect antigen from epithelial surfaces and include the gut-associated lymphoid tissue or GALT (tonsils, adenoids, appendix, Peyer's patches of the small intestine) as well as more diffusely organized aggregates of lymphocytes at other mucosal sites.

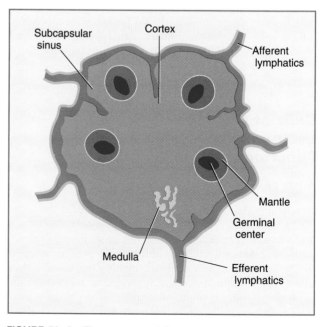

FIGURE 50–2 The structure of the normal lymph node. The cortical area contains the follicles, which consist of a germinal center and a mantle zone. The medulla contains a complex of channels that lead to the efferent lymphatics.

Lymphocytes circulate in the peripheral blood and comprise 20% to 40% of peripheral blood leukocytes in adults (the proportion is higher in newborns and children). Eighty percent to 90% of peripheral blood lymphocytes are T cells, and the remainder are largely B cells. The majority of peripheral blood lymphocytes are mature, resting lymphocytes that morphologically are small with scant cytoplasm and inconspicuous nucleoli. A small percentage of peripheral blood lymphoid cells represent a third category of lymphoid cells that are referred to as natural killer (NK) cells. These cells do not bear the characteristic cell surface molecules of B or T cells, and their immunoglobulin or TCR genes have not undergone rearrangement. Morphologically, these cells are large, with abundant cytoplasm containing azurophilic granules, and thus they are often called large granular lymphocytes. Functionally, they are part of the innate immune system, responding nonspecifically to a wide range of pathogens without requiring prior antigenic exposure.

Neoplasia of Lymphoid Origin

Malignant transformation of lymphocytes can lead to a diverse array of neoplasia of lymphoid origin, including tumors that arise from T cells or B cells and tumors that represent different stages of lymphocyte development. Lymphoid malignancies usually involve lymphoid tissues, but they can arise in or spread to any site. The major clinical groupings of lymphoid malignancies include non-Hodgkin's lymphomas (NHLs), Hodgkin's disease, lymphoid leukemias, and plasma cell dyscrasias.

The most common clinical presentation of a lymphoid malignancy in adults is painless enlargement of lymph nodes, or lymphadenopathy. There are many causes of lymphadenopathy, in addition to lymphoid malignancies (Table 50–1). Thus, it is important to take a thorough history and perform a careful physical examination before performing a lymph node biopsy. The investigation of lymphadenopathy can be organized according to the location of the enlarged nodes (localized or generalized) and the presence of clinical symptoms. Cervical lymphadenopathy is most often caused by infections of the upper respiratory tract, including infectious mononucleosis syndromes and other viral syndromes as well as bacterial pharyngitis. Unilateral axillary, inguinal, or femoral adenopathy may be caused by skin infections involving the extremity, including cat-scratch fever. Generalized lymphadenopathy may be caused by systemic infections, such as human immunodeficiency virus (HIV) or cytomegalovirus infection, drug reactions, autoimmune diseases, one of the systemic lymphadenopathy syndromes, or lymphoma. If the cause of persistent lymphadenopathy is not apparent after a careful evaluation, an excisional lymph node biopsy should be undertaken. An enlarged supraclavicular lymph node is highly suggestive of malignancy and should always be sampled.

The accurate diagnosis of lymphoma requires excisional biopsy of a lymph node or generous biopsy of

TABLE 50–1 Common Causes of Lymphadenopathy

Infectious Diseases

Viral: infectious mononucleosis syndromes (cytomegalovirus, Epstein-Barr virus), acquired immunodeficiency syndrome, rubella, herpes simplex, infectious hepatitis
Bacterial: localized infection with regional adenopathy (streptococci, staphylococci), cat-scratch disease, brucellosis, tularemia, listeriosis, bubonic plague *(Yersinia pestis),* chancroid *(Haemophilus ducreyi)*
Fungal: coccidioidomycosis, histoplasmosis
Chlamydial: lymphogranuloma venereum, trachoma
Mycobacterial: scrofula, tuberculosis, leprosy
Protozoan: toxoplasmosis, trypanosomiasis
Spirochetal: Lyme disease, syphilis, leptospirosis

Immunologic Diseases

Rheumatoid arthritis
Systemic lupus erythematosus
Dermatomyositis
Serum sickness
Drug reactions—phenytoin, hydralazine, allopurinol

Malignant Diseases

Lymphomas
Metastatic solid tumors to lymph nodes: melanoma, lung, breast, head and neck, gastrointestinal tract, Kaposi's sarcoma, unknown primary tumor, renal, prostate

Atypical Lymphoid Proliferations

Giant follicular lymph node hyperplasia
Angioimmunoblastic lymphadenopathy
Castleman's disease

Miscellaneous Diseases and Diseases of Unknown Cause

Sinus histiocytosis
Dermatopathic lymphadenitis
Sarcoidosis
Amyloidosis
Mucocutaneous lymph node syndrome
Lymphomatoid granulomatosis
Multifocal Langerhans cell (eosinophilic) granulomatosis
Lipid storage diseases: Gaucher's and Niemann-Pick diseases

involved lymph tissue. Fine-needle aspiration or needle biopsy is rarely sufficient for the diagnosis of malignant lymphoma. Analysis of the pathologic specimen should include routine histologic examination and immunophenotyping. Immunophenotyping involves the characterization of the immunologic cell surface antigens that are expressed on the malignant lymphocyte by means of a panel of monoclonal antibodies. Immunophenotyping permits a determination of cell of origin (B cell, T cell, NK cell, or nonlymphoid cell), and the pattern of cell surface antigens. In the case of B-cell NHLs, immunophenotyping can also reveal whether the process is monoclonal in origin (i.e., neoplastic) by determining whether the surface immunoglobulin is restricted to either kappa or lambda light chains. Immunophenotyping has become an essential aspect of the diagnosis and classification of lymphomas and can be accomplished by flow cytometric analysis or by immunohistochemical studies on tissue specimens. In some cases, cytogenetic analysis or molecular studies for immunoglobulin or TCR gene rearrangement may be required to determine the pathologic subtype of lymphoma or to establish a monoclonal (i.e., malignant) process. If a lymph node biopsy is nondiagnostic, and unexplained lymph node enlargement persists, the biopsy should be repeated.

NON-HODGKIN'S LYMPHOMAS

The NHLs comprise a heterogeneous group of lymphoid malignancies that differ with respect to their histologic appearance, cell of origin and immunophenotype, molecular biology, clinical features, prognosis, and outcome with therapy. In view of the heterogeneity of NHLs, classification schemes have been devised to identify specific pathologic subtypes that correlate with distinct clinical entities. The most widely used classifications are the Working Formulation (WF), which was introduced in 1982, and the Revised European American Lymphoma (REAL) classification, introduced in 1994 (Table 50–2). The WF classifies NHLs on the basis of the architecture of the node (the presence of follicles vs. diffuse infiltrate) and the morphology of the malignant lymphocyte (small cell vs. large cell, with cleaved or noncleaved nucleus) and organizes the pathologic subtypes into low, intermediate, or high grade based on their natural history and clinical behavior. In general, the low-grade histologies are associated with an indolent course and relatively long survival but are incurable, whereas the intermediate- and high-grade histologies are biologically aggressive (i.e., short natural history if left untreated) but are potentially curable with current treatment modalities. With the widespread use of immunophenotyping and molecular characterization of lymphomas, it is apparent that the WF does not adequately define specific pathologic and clinical entities. The more recent REAL classification incorporates not only histologic features but also immunophenotype, cytogenetics, and epidemiologic/etiologic factors. Thus, the REAL classification identifies several NHL subtypes that are not easily classified within the WF (see Table 50–2). These subtypes include the mantle cell lymphomas; the MALT lymphomas and monocytoid B-cell lymphomas, which are both derived from cells in the marginal zone of lymph nodes; and the various T-cell lymphomas, including human T-cell lymphotrophic virus I (HTLV-I)–associated leukemia/lymphoma, cutaneous T-cell lymphoma (mycosis fungoides/Sézary's syndrome), and the biologically aggressive peripheral T-cell lymphomas. The most common NHLs encountered in the United States include the low-grade follicular lymphomas of the WF (follicular small cleaved and follicular mixed lymphomas), small lymphocytic lymphoma/leukemia (also known as chronic lymphocytic leukemia [CLL]), mantle cell lymphomas of the REAL classification, and diffuse large cell lymphomas, including immunoblastic sarcoma.

The cause of most NHLs is not known. In the majority of patients with NHL, no apparent genetic predisposition or epidemiologic/environmental factor can be identified. Many of the NHL subtypes carry pathognomonic chromosomal translocations that often involve an

TABLE 50–2 Classification of Non-Hodgkin's Lymphomas

Working Formulation

Low Grade
A. *Small lymphocytic, diffuse; consistent with chronic lymphocytic leukemia*
B. *Follicular, small cleaved cell*
C. *Follicular, mixed small cleaved cell and large cell*

Intermediate Grade
D. Follicular, large cell
E. Diffuse, small cleaved cell
F. Diffuse, mixed small cleaved cell and large cell
G. *Diffuse, large cell*

High Grade
H. *Diffuse large cell, immunoblastic*
I. Lymphoblastic
J. Small non–cleaved cell
    Burkitt's
    Non-Burkitt's

REAL Classification: The More Common Entities

B-Cell Neoplasms
Precursor B-lymphoblastic leukemia/lymphoma (B-cell acute lymphocytic leukemia/lymphoblastic lymphoma)
Mature (Peripheral B-Cell Neoplasms)
    Chronic lymphocytic leukemia/small lymphocytic lymphoma
    Plasma cell myeloma/plasmacytoma
    *Extranodal marginal zone B-cell lymphoma of mucosa-associated lymphoid tissues (MALT) type
    *Mantle cell lymphoma
    Follicular lymphoma
    Diffuse large B-cell lymphoma
    Burkitt's lymphoma
T- and NK-Cell Neoplasms
Precursor T-lymphoblastic lymphoma/leukemia (T-cell acute lymphocytic leukemia/lymphoblastic lymphoma)
Mature (peripheral) T-cell neoplasms
    *Adult T-cell lymphoma/leukemia
    *Mycosis fungoides/Sézary syndrome
    *Peripheral T-cell lymphoma
    *Anaplastic large cell lymphomas

Note: The most common entities in the Working Formulation that are encountered in the United States are in italics. The entities in the REAL classification marked with an asterisk cannot be readily identified in the Working Formulation.

immunoglobulin locus (or *TCR* locus in the case of T cell–derived NHLs) and an oncogene or growth regulatory gene. The cause of these aberrant chromosomal rearrangements is unknown. Patients with congenital immunodeficiency syndromes or autoimmune disorders are at increased risk of developing NHL. Viral cofactors have been identified for some of the less common NHL variants. Epstein-Barr virus (EBV) is causally linked to several biologically aggressive NHLs, including acquired immunodeficiency syndrome (AIDS)–related diffuse aggressive lymphomas, the lymphoproliferative disorders that arise in immunosuppressed patients after organ transplantation, and the form of Burkitt's lymphoma that is endemic in Africa. HTLV-I is associated with an aggressive form of T-cell leukemia/lymphoma that is endemic in areas of Japan and the Caribbean basin. The herpesvirus of Kaposi's sarcoma has been implicated in a variant of diffuse aggressive NHL that arises in serosal cavities and is encountered almost exclusively in HIV-infected patients. *Helicobacter pylori* infection is causally linked to gastric MALT lymphomas, and eradication of infection with antibiotics is often associated with regression of the lymphoma.

Clinical Presentation, Evaluation, and Staging

As described in the preceding section, the majority of patients with NHL present with painless lymphadenopathy involving one or more of the peripheral nodal sites. Additionally, NHL can involve extranodal sites, and thus patients can present with a variety of symptoms reflective of the site of involvement. The most common sites of extranodal disease are the gastrointestinal tract, bone marrow, liver, and Waldeyer's ring, although virtually any site potentially can be involved with NHL. In general, the aggressive subtypes of NHL (diffuse large cell, lymphoblastic, Burkitt's) are more likely than the indolent lymphomas to involve extranodal sites. Central nervous system involvement, including leptomeningeal spread, rarely occurs in the indolent subtypes but does occur in the aggressive variants. The most aggressive NHLs (Burkitt's and lymphoblastic) have a particular propensity to spread to the leptomeninges. Constitutional symptoms such as fevers, weight loss, or night sweats occur in about 20% of patients with NHL at the time of presentation, and these symptoms are more common in patients with aggressive subtypes of NHL.

The diagnosis of NHL requires an adequate biopsy of the involved nodal tissue or extranodal site. In patients with bone marrow and peripheral blood involvement, such as small lymphocytic lymphoma/CLL, it is often possible to make the diagnosis from immunophenotyping of peripheral blood lymphocytes by flow cytometry. Once the diagnosis of a lymphoma has been made, patients should undergo a complete staging evaluation (Table 50–3). Staging determines the extent of involvement, provides prognostic information, and may influence the choice of therapy. The modified Ann Arbor staging classification is used to stage patients with both NHL and Hodgkin's disease (Table 50–4). Standard staging evaluation includes a careful history to elicit symptoms referable to the lymphoma including the presence of constitutional symptoms (fevers, night sweats, or weight loss, designated "B" symptoms); a complete physical examination with documentation of the size and distribution of enlarged lymph nodes; blood work, including lactate dehydrogenase (LDH) evaluation; computed tomography (CT) of chest, abdomen, and pelvis; and bone marrow aspirate and biopsy. A gallium scan be helpful in assessing response to therapy in those lymphomas that are gallium avid (usually the aggressive subtypes) and is often included in the staging evaluation of the aggressive NHLs. Lumbar puncture for cytologic analysis should be performed only in those patients at risk for leptomeningeal disease, which includes all patients with Burkitt's and lymphoblastic lym-

TABLE 50–3   Staging Evaluation for Lymphomas

Required Evaluation Procedures

Biopsy of lesion with review by an experienced hematopathologist
History with attention to the presence or absence of "B" symptoms
Physical examination with attention to node-bearing areas (including Waldeyer's ring) and size of liver and spleen
Standard blood work, including
    Complete blood cell count
    Lactate dehydrogenase and β_2-microglobulin
    Evaluation of renal function
    Liver function tests
    Calcium, uric acid
Radiologic studies, including
    Chest radiograph (posteroanterior and lateral)
    Chest-abdominal pelvic CT
    Gallium scan (in Hodgkin's and intermediate- and high-grade lymphomas)
Bilateral bone marrow aspirates and biopsies

Procedures Required Under Certain Circumstances

Abdominal ultrasonogram or gastrointestinal contrast studies to supplement CT scans or investigate sites of unexplained symptoms
Bone scan if bone symptoms
Plain bone radiographs of symptomatic or abnormal areas on bone scan
Brain or spinal CT or MRI if neurologic signs and symptoms
Serum and urine protein electrophoresis

CT = computed tomography; MRI = magnetic resonance imaging.

TABLE 50–4   Staging System for Lymphomas

Stage	Description
Stage I	Involvement of a single lymph node region or structure (I), or a single extralymphatic site (IE)
Stage II	Involvement of two or more lymph node regions on the same side of the diaphragm (II), or localized involvement of a contiguous extralymphatic site and lymph node region (IIE)
Stage III	Involvement of lymph node regions on both sides of the diaphragm (III), which may be accompanied by localized involvement of one extralymphatic site (IIIE) or spleen (IIIS) or both (IIISE)
III₁	With or without involvement of splenic, hilar, celiac, or portal nodes
III₂	With involvement of para-aortic, iliac, and mesenteric nodes
Stage IV	Diffuse or disseminated involvement of one or more extralymphatic organs with or without associated lymph node involvement
	Identification of the presence or absence of symptoms should be noted with each stage designation. A = asymptomatic; B = fever, sweats, weight loss > 10% of body weight

phoma, and those patients with diffuse large cell lymphoma with involvement of bone marrow, testes, or structures directly abutting the central nervous system (e.g., paranasal sinus, calvarium). A variety of ancillary tests may be performed in specific situations. For example, a test for HTLV-I or HIV should be performed if adult T-cell leukemia/lymphoma or AIDS-related lymphoma is suspected, respectively. A gastrointestinal series or endoscopic evaluation may be warranted in any patients with gastrointestinal symptoms or in patients at risk for gastrointestinal tract involvement (lymphomas involving the Waldeyer's ring). Serum protein electrophoresis and determination of β_2-microglobulin and quantitative immunoglobulins should be performed in patients suspected of having plasma cell dyscrasias. A laparotomy for the sole purpose of staging patients with NHL is never performed, because it rarely influences therapeutic decision making.

A variety of prognostic variables have been identified for NHL. In general, the predictors for poor survival in most subtypes of NHL include advanced stage at presentation (stage III or IV), involvement of multiple extranodal sites of disease, elevated LDH levels, the presence of "B" symptoms, and poor performance status.

Natural History, Prognosis, and Treatment

Low-Grade NHLs. The common low-grade or indolent histologies include the follicular lymphomas (small cleaved cell and mixed cell types) and small lymphocytic lymphoma (the latter is identical to CLL and is discussed later), which account for about 30% and 5% of all NHLs, respectively. The low-grade follicular lymphomas are mature clonal B-cell neoplasms with an immunophenotype that is positive for surface immunoglobulin (kappa or lambda chain restricted) and the mature B-cell markers (CD19, CD20, CD21) and negative for CD5. Follicular lymphomas are characterized cytogenetically by the t(14;18) translocation that juxtaposes the immunoglobulin heavy chain with the antiapoptotic gene *BCL2; BCL2* is uniformly expressed in follicular lymphomas. Although the follicular lymphomas are low grade, indolent neoplasms with a long natural history (median survival approaches 10 years), the majority of patients (80%–90%) present with an advanced stage (stage III or IV), often with bone marrow involvement, and cannot be cured with standard treatment modalities. Most patients with follicular NHL eventually experience transformation of their disease to a more aggressive lymphoma, characterized pathologically by a diffuse large cell infiltrate and clinically by rapidly expanding nodes or other tumor masses, rising LDH levels, and the onset of disease-related symptoms.

The management of the follicular lymphomas is determined by the stage. For those few patients who are considered to have early-stage (I or II) disease after clinical staging, the appropriate treatment is radiation therapy. With the use of subtotal or total lymphoid irradiation, more than half of patients with early-stage disease will achieve a durable remission and appear to be cured. For patients with advanced-stage disease, the management is more controversial. Although advanced-

stage indolent NHL is responsive to a variety of treatment modalities, the incurability and the long natural history has led to the practice of deferring treatment until the patient develops symptoms. This strategy is referred to as the "watch and wait" approach. Indications for treatment include cosmetic or mechanical problems caused by enlarging lymph nodes, constitutional symptoms, and evidence of marrow compromise. The appropriate treatment of advanced-stage disease, when necessary, is systemic chemotherapy. The follicular lymphomas are responsive to a variety of single and multidrug programs. Single alkylating agents (cyclophosphamide or chlorambucil), multidrug regimens containing an alkylating agent (e.g., CVP: cyclophosphamide, vincristine, prednisone), or single-agent fludarabine all are effective initial regimens for this disease. The majority of patients respond to chemotherapy, and at least one third achieve a clinical complete remission that may last 1 to 3 years. Treatment should be discontinued when the maximum response has been achieved to minimize cumulative toxicity. Once a patient relapses, subsequent remissions may be achieved but are usually less durable than the first remission. Therapeutic options for patients who relapse include re-treatment with chemotherapy, often with a different drug or combination than that used initially. Alternatively, patients in relapse can be treated with rituximab, a humanized monoclonal antibody to the CD20 antigen. Rituximab is a highly effective nontoxic agent for use in patients with relapsed follicular lymphoma, inducing responses that are often durable in the majority of patients; its role as first-line treatment of follicular NHL remains to be defined. For patients who have clinical or pathologic evidence of transformation to a higher grade of lymphoma, treatment that is appropriate for a diffuse aggressive histology should be offered (see later discussion). The role of high-dose chemotherapy with autologous or allogeneic stem cell transplant for follicular NHLs remains unclear and should be considered experimental.

In addition to the follicular NHLs, the MALT lymphomas and closely related marginal zone lymphomas are also considered low-grade, indolent subtypes. Given the excellent prognosis, localized nature, and long natural history of the MALT lymphomas, they are generally managed conservatively with local treatment modalities (irradiation or surgery) and avoidance of systemic chemotherapy. Importantly, the gastric MALT lymphomas are highly associated with *H. pylori* infection, and remissions can often be achieved with eradication of this infection. Thus, antibiotic therapy is the first-line treatment for early gastric MALT lymphoma.

Intermediate-Grade NHLs. The common intermediate-grade NHLs in the United States include the diffuse large cell histologies and immunoblastic sarcoma, accounting for about one third of all NHLs. Although immunoblastic sarcoma was originally classified as a high-grade NHL in the WF, it behaves similarly to the diffuse large cell histologies and is managed in an identical manner. These entities are often referred to simply as diffuse aggressive NHLs, which also includes the anaplastic large cell NHL of the REAL classification. The majority of the diffuse aggressive large cell lymphomas are B cell in origin; the T-cell diffuse aggressive lesions, or peripheral T-cell lymphomas, are managed similarly but may have a worse prognosis compared with their B-cell counterparts.

The diffuse aggressive NHLs are biologically aggressive entities; if left untreated, the median survival is less than 1 to 2 years. Compared with the follicular NHLs, a higher percentage of patients with diffuse aggressive histologies will present with early-stage disease (30% to 50%) or with an extranodal site of involvement (50%). The outcome and likelihood of cure of patients with diffuse aggressive histologies is directly related to the total number of adverse prognostic features that are present at presentation: age older than 60, advanced stage (III or IV), elevated LDH levels, poor performance status, and the presence of two or more extranodal sites of disease. The likelihood of cure and long-term disease-free survival ranges from more than 75% in patients with one or fewer adverse factors to less than 30% in patients with four or more adverse factors.

In contrast to patients with low-grade follicular NHLs, all patients with diffuse aggressive histologies should be offered immediate therapy, because these are potentially curable lymphomas. The standard initial therapy for all patients with diffuse aggressive NHL is a multidrug chemotherapy regimen that includes an anthracycline. The most widely used regimen is designated CHOP (cyclophosphamide, doxorubicin, vincristine, prednisone). This regimen appears to be equivalent to more complex and intensive regimens such as M-BACOD, Pro-MACE, and MACOP-B, and thus CHOP remains the standard. Patients with early-stage disease (I or II) do benefit from local radiation therapy after a minimum of three cycles of CHOP. Patients with advanced-stage disease require six cycles of CHOP; the role of local radiation to sites of bulky disease in the setting of advanced-stage disease is not established. Complete remissions can be achieved with the CHOP or similar regimens, and 30% to 40% of patients are cured. Patients who experience relapse after achieving a remission often can be cured with high-dose chemotherapy with autologous peripheral stem cell support, or "transplant," particularly if their relapsed disease remains responsive to standard doses of chemotherapy. The morbidity and mortality of this procedure have diminished substantially since 1990 with the use of colony-stimulating factor support, and it can be safely performed in patients without serious comorbid conditions. High-dose chemotherapy with autologous stem cell transplant is superior to standard doses of a salvage regimen and is considered standard therapy for patients with relapsed chemosensitive diffuse aggressive NHL.

Mantle cell lymphoma has been recognized with increasing frequency since immunophenotyping has become standard practice for classifying NHLs, and it is included in the REAL classification. Mantle cell NHL was not recognized in the WF and was often designated as a diffuse small cleaved cell or diffuse mixed cell lymphoma in the WF classification. It accounts for 5% to 8% of all NHLs. Mantle cell lymphomas are mature B-cell neoplasms that appear to arise in the mantle zone of the lymphoid follicle and display a highly characteristic immunophenotype. Mantle cells express the CD5 antigen, as well as the mature B-cell markers (CD19, CD20, CD21) but typically are negative for CD23 expression. Because mantle cell lymphomas can be easily confused pathologically and clinically with CLL, which is the only other B-cell NHL that is CD5⁺, the absence of CD23 is important for distinguishing mantle cell lymphoma from CLL, which is typically CD23⁺. Mantle cell lymphomas are also characterized by a pathognomonic t(11;14) chromosomal translocation that juxtaposes the immunoglobulin heavy chain with the *BCL1* or *PRAD1* gene that encodes the growth-promoting protein cyclin D1. Mantle cell lymphomas are in many ways similar to indolent lymphomas in that patients usually present with advanced-stage disease with frequent bone marrow involvement. These lymphomas have a peculiar propensity to involve Waldeyer's ring and the gastrointestinal tract. As with the low-grade follicular lymphomas, mantle cell lymphomas are treatable but not curable. However, in contrast to the indolent lymphomas, these are biologically aggressive neoplasms with a median survival of just 2 to 3 years. These patients are generally treated with systemic chemotherapy at diagnosis because of the more aggressive nature of mantle cell lymphomas compared with follicular lymphomas, but durable remissions are difficult to achieve. The optimal therapy for this challenging subtype remains to be established, and these patients should be considered for experimental therapies, including immunotherapy or transplantation.

High-Grade NHL. The two high-grade subtypes, Burkitt's or small non–cleaved cell and lymphoblastic lymphoma, are quite rare in the adult population. Nonetheless, these subtypes are important because they are potentially curable with appropriate therapy and often require urgent, inpatient treatment at the time of diagnosis because of their highly aggressive nature, rapid growth, and tumor lysis on initiation of therapy. Lymphoblastic lymphoma is an aggressive lymphoma that is closely related to T-cell acute lymphocytic leukemia and readily distinguished from most NHLs by its T-cell immunophenotype and the presence of terminal deoxynucleotide transferase (TdT). It usually afflicts young adult males and involves the mediastinum and bone marrow, with a propensity to relapse in the leptomeninges. Burkitt's, or small non–cleaved cell lymphoma, is a rare B-cell lymphoma in adults that is highly aggressive with a propensity to involve the bone marrow and central nervous system. Burkitt's lymphoma is characterized cytogenetically by the pathognomonic t(8;14) translocation that juxtaposes the *Ig* locus with the *myc* oncogene. In central Africa, where Burkitt's lymphoma is endemic in children, it is usually associated with EBV, but in the United States it is uncommon for sporadic Burkitt's lymphoma to be Epstein-Barr virus (EBV) positive. Burkitt's lymphoma and lymphoblastic lymphomas both require treatment with intensive multiagent chemotherapy, including intrathecal chemotherapy to prevent leptomeningeal relapse. These lymphomas undergo rapid tumor lysis on initiation of chemotherapy, and it is imperative that all patients receive prophylaxis against tumor lysis syndrome before and during their first course of chemotherapy. Prophylaxis includes hydration, alkalinization of the urine, and allopurinol.

HODGKIN'S DISEASE

Hodgkin's disease (HD) is the most common lymphoma in young adults. It has a bimodal distribution in the United States and industrialized countries, with the larger peak occurring between ages 15 and 35 and a second smaller peak occurring in patients older than 50. The etiology of Hodgkin's disease remains enigmatic. Although EBV is frequently present in the malignant cell of Hodgkin's disease, a direct causal link between EBV and Hodgkin's disease has not been established. HD does not appear with increased frequency in patients with congenital immunodeficiency syndromes or in immunosuppressed organ transplant recipients, but there does appear to be an increased risk of HD in HIV-infected patients.

The diagnosis of HD is made by identifying the Reed-Sternberg (RS) cell in involved lymphoid tissue. The classic RS cell is large and binucleate, with each nucleus containing a prominent nucleolus, suggesting the appearance of "owl's eyes." Although the cellular origin of the RS cell was debated for many decades, molecular studies have confirmed that RS cells are B cell in nature with clonal rearrangement of germline Ig locus, despite the absence of cytoplasmic or cell surface immunoglobulin. In contrast to NHL and other malignancies, the bulk of the infiltrate in lymph nodes involved with HD is usually composed of benign reactive inflammatory cells, and often the diagnostic RS cells can be difficult to find. Immunophenotyping of classic RS cells reveals that they are CD30 (Ki-1) and CD15 positive and negative for CD20, CD45, and cytoplasmic or surface immunoglobulin; EBV is identified in the RS cells in about half of the cases of HD.

There are four pathologic variants of HD. Nodular sclerosing (NS) is by far the most common (80% of HD cases) and is characterized by the presence of fibrous bands separating the node into nodules and the "lacunar" type of RS cells. It is the predominant type encountered in adolescents and young adults and typically involves the mediastinum and other supradiaphragmatic nodal sites. In the mixed cellularity (MC) type, which accounts for about 15% of HD cases, band-forming sclerosis is absent and RS cells are easily identified in a diffuse infiltrate that is more heterogeneous than that seen in the NS variant. The MC variant may be encountered in any age group, and advanced-stage disease with subdiaphragmatic involvement is more common with MC variant HD than with NS variant HD. The lymphocyte-depleted type is rare, accounting for less than 1% of the HD cases, and is characterized by sheets of RS cells with a paucity of inflammatory cells. This variant is most common in the elderly, in HIV-infected patients, and in persons in nonindustrialized countries. The lymphocyte-predominant (LP) type has emerged as a distinct entity that may be more closely related to indolent NHL than HD, although it is managed as a true HD. The LP type is characterized by a nodular growth pattern with variants of RS cells that have polylobated nuclei and are referred to as "popcorn" cells; classic RS cells are usually absent. The immunophenotype of the atypical cells is distinct from classic RS cells, with expression of B-cell antigens (CD19, CD20) and CD45 but absence of the classic RS markers CD15 and CD30. The LP type of HD accounts for about 5% of cases, has a strong male preponderance, and tends to involve peripheral nodes with sparing of the mediastinum. The prognosis is excellent, although late relapses are more common than in the other types of HD.

HD arises in lymph nodes, most commonly in the mediastinum or neck, and spreads to adjacent contiguous or noncontiguous nodal sites, including retroperitoneal nodes and the spleen. As the disease progresses, it spreads hematogenously to involve extranodal sites, including bone marrow, liver, and lung. In contrast to NHL, it is exceedingly rare for HD to arise in extranodal sites, although HD can involve extranodal sites by contiguous spread from an adjacent lymph node (e.g., involvement of vertebrae from adjacent retroperitoneal lymph nodes or involvement of pulmonary parenchyma from adjacent hilar nodes).

HD usually presents as painless enlargement of lymph nodes, most often in the neck. Mediastinal adenopathy may be found incidentally in an asymptomatic patient on routine chest radiography. Massive mediastinal or hilar adenopathy, with or without adjacent pulmonary involvement, may cause respiratory symptoms such as cough, shortness of breath, wheezing, or stridor. Approximately one third of patients with HD have constitutional symptoms of fever, night sweats, or weight loss—"B" symptoms—which can be the presenting complaint. In addition to the "B" symptoms, generalized pruritus is also associated with HD and correlates with the NS type. Occasionally, patients give a history of troubling pruritus for months to years before the diagnosis of HD. Although HD is associated with functional T-lymphocyte defects, manifested as cutaneous anergy to intradermal skin tests, patients rarely present with opportunistic infections. If left untreated, the natural history of HD is one of inexorable, albeit often slow, progression to involve multiple nodal sites, followed by hematogenous spread to bone marrow, liver, and other viscera. As the disease advances, patients experience "B" symptoms, malaise, cachexia, and infectious complications, and patients with progressive HD ultimately die of complications of bone marrow failure or infection.

Accurate staging of patients with newly diagnosed HD is important for treatment planning, prognosis, and assessing response to therapy. A modification of the Ann Arbor classification is used (see Table 50–4), and the suffix "A" or "B" is appended to denote the absence or presence, respectively, of fever, night sweats, or weight loss. The staging work-up of a patient with newly diagnosed HD is similar to that for patients with NHL (see Table 50–3). Patients should undergo a thorough history and physical examination; complete blood work, including an erythrocyte sedimentation rate; chest radiography; CT of the chest, abdomen, and pelvis; bone marrow aspirate and biopsy; and gallium scan. A lymphangiogram can be useful in assessing subdiaphragmatic adenopathy if the expertise is available to perform and interpret this test. Additional tests, such as bone films, bone scan, and spinal magnetic resonance imaging should be obtained only if symptoms suggest involvement of these structures. The information derived from this noninvasive work-up defines the clinical stage of a patient with HD. The role of the staging laparotomy to more accurately determine involvement below the diaphragm waned substantially during the 1990s, as therapy for early-stage disease has evolved. This procedure entails a laparotomy with splenectomy, liver biopsy, and a sampling of retroperitoneal nodes; the information derived from this procedure defines the pathologic stage of the disease. A staging laparotomy should no longer be considered routine. However, if a patient with clinical stage I or II supradiaphragmatic disease will be treated with radiation therapy as the sole modality, a staging laparotomy is an option to rule out occult involvement of the spleen and retroperitoneal nodes. Occult HD can be found below the diaphragm in as many as 30% of patients with clinical stage I or II disease, mandating treatment with chemotherapy. Patients who do undergo staging laparotomy with splenectomy are at risk for overwhelming bacterial infection with encapsulated organisms and should receive pneumococcal and *Haemophilus influenzae* vaccine before surgery.

A variety of prognostic factors that influence risk of relapse or survival have been identified in HD. The most important adverse prognostic factors are mixed cellularity or lymphocyte-depleted histologies, male sex, large number of involved nodal sites, advanced stage (age >40), the presence of "B" symptoms, high erythrocyte sedimentation rate, and bulky disease (widening of the mediastinum by more than one third or the presence of a nodal mass measuring more than 10 cm in any dimension). The presence of any of these factors in patients with early-stage disease places them at increased risk of occult abdominal involvement or relapse after primary radiation therapy and thus influences the decision to include chemotherapy in the initial treatment.

The treatment of HD has evolved considerably since 1980. HD is highly curable; the cure rate exceeds 80% with the use of current treatment modalities. Because most patients with HD are young adults and will experience long-term disease-free survival, the emphasis has shifted toward using therapies that minimize treatment-related morbidity and mortality without sacrificing curative potential. Radiation therapy in moderate doses (>3.5 Gy) to involved sites of disease plus contiguous nodal regions is curative for the majority of patients with low-risk, early-stage disease (nonbulky stages I and IIA without adverse risk factors) and remains a viable treatment option for these patients. However, the long-term follow-up of patients treated with standard doses of radiation therapy has revealed a substantially increased risk of developing a variety of solid tumors within or at the margin of the radiation field more than a decade later. Chest irradiation for HD is associated with a particularly high risk of breast cancer in women and of lung cancer in both men and women. Additional long-term sequelae of standard radiation therapy for

HD include thyroid dysfunction (usually hypothyroidism) and accelerated coronary artery disease. Thus, enthusiasm for primary radiation therapy in standard doses for low-risk, early-stage Hodgkin's disease is diminishing in patients who will require chest irradiation, which represents the overwhelming majority of early-stage patients.

In response to the recognition of the long-term carcinogenic effects of standard dose radiation, the approach to the treatment of patients with low-risk, early-stage HD is evolving. Increasingly, the trend has been to combine chemotherapy (e.g., the ABVD regimen, described later) with a low dose of radiation therapy (<3.0 Gy), which has not been associated with an increased risk of secondary solid tumors. The optimal duration of chemotherapy in combination with low-dose irradiation for early-stage HD remains unsettled. Alternatively, patients with early-stage HD can be treated with a full course of chemotherapy alone (described later).

Patients with advanced-stage HD (III or IV) or with early-stage disease with adverse risk factors (e.g., bulky disease, "B" symptoms, mixed cellularity type) are not candidates for radiation therapy as the sole treatment modality, because of the high rate of relapse. These patients should be treated with chemotherapy. The multiagent chemotherapy program designated MOPP (nitrogen mustard, vincristine [Oncovin], procarbazine, and prednisone) was demonstrated to be highly curative in patients with advanced-stage disease in the 1970s. MOPP remains a highly effective regimen, but it is rarely used in current practice because of the long-term toxic effects associated with MOPP. These include sterility in nearly all males and infertility in a significant percentage of women who receive MOPP and a high risk of developing acute myeloid leukemia. The ABVD—doxorubicin (Adriamycin), bleomycin, vinblastine, dacarbazine—regimen is now the most widely used program in the United States. ABVD is as effective as MOPP but does not cause sterility or infertility or treatment-induced leukemias. ABVD has been associated with pulmonary fibrosis in a small percentage of patients (<5%) because of the inclusion of bleomycin in this regimen; the risk of pulmonary fibrosis is highest in patients who have underlying lung disease or who receive chest irradiation as a part of the treatment program. Patients who have an underlying cardiomyopathy are not candidates for ABVD, because of the potential risk of further cardiac injury from doxorubicin, and MOPP may be the preferred regimen in these patients. Radiation therapy in combination with chemotherapy is not generally used in the treatment of advanced-stage Hodgkin's disease. However, in patients with bulky mediastinal disease, consolidative radiation to the mediastinum after completion of chemotherapy has been shown to decrease the rate of relapse. Thus, combined modality therapy (chemotherapy plus radiation therapy) is considered standard for patients with bulky mediastinal disease.

Evaluating the patient's response to therapy in HD involves repetition of the staging evaluation (physical examination, CT, gallium scan, and bone marrow biopsy if positive at diagnosis) during and at the completion of treatment. Patients may be cured despite the presence of a residual radiographic abnormality on chest radiography or CT (e.g., enlarged nodes or residual mediastinal mass). Patients with residual radiographic abnormalities after an initial response to therapy should not be subjected to salvage therapy without additional corroborating evidence of persistent HD, such as biopsy confirmation or radiographic progression over time. A persistently positive gallium scan in patients with residual radiographic abnormalities is associated with a high rate of subsequent relapse, and those patients should be followed closely or considered for immediate repeat biopsy and/or salvage therapy. The majority of patients destined to relapse will do so within 2 years; relapses after 5 years are exceedingly rare.

Patients who relapse or fail to respond after initial therapy should be offered salvage therapy, because the majority of these patients can now be cured if treated appropriately. Approximately 20% of patients with early-stage HD who receive standard-dose radiation therapy (without chemotherapy) will relapse. These patients can be salvaged with standard chemotherapy (e.g., ABVD). Patients who relapse after standard chemotherapy should be treated with high-dose chemotherapy with autologous peripheral stem cell support. More than 50% of patients with HD who do not respond to standard chemotherapy can be cured with high-dose chemotherapy with autologous peripheral stem cell support.

LYMPHOID LEUKEMIAS

Acute Lymphocytic Leukemias

The acute lymphocytic leukemias that arise from precursor B or T cells are described in detail in Chapter 47.

Chronic Lymphocytic Leukemia

B-cell CLL is a malignant disorder of lymphocytes characterized by expansion and accumulation of small lymphocytes of B-cell origin. CLL is essentially identical to B-cell small lymphocytic lymphoma in the REAL and WF classifications. CLL is the most common form of leukemia in the United States and affects twice as many men as women. Although it can occur at any stage of life, the incidence increases with age, and more than 90% of cases are diagnosed in adults older than 50. The etiology of CLL is unknown. There does not appear to be a genetic basis for the disease, and environmental factors, such as radiation and exposure to carcinogens, have not been implicated.

The common form of CLL is a clonal proliferation of mature B cells expressing characteristic mature B-cell markers and low levels of surface IgM that is light chain restricted, reflecting the clonal origin of this malignancy. In addition, CLL B cells express the CD5 molecule, which marks a minor subset of normal B cells, and CD23 (the Fc receptor for IgE). Thus, the diagnostic immunophenotype of CLL is that of a mature B-cell population that is clonal (by light chain restriction or immunoglobulin gene rearrangement studies), expresses the characteristic mature B-cell markers (CD19, CD20,

CD21), and is positive for both CD5 and CD23. Although a pathognomonic chromosomal abnormality has not been identified in CLL, 30% to 50% of patients have cytogenetic abnormalities. The most frequent abnormalities involve chromosome 12 (often trisomy 12), 13, or 14, and the presence of cytogenetic abnormalities is associated with a poorer prognosis. Smears of the bone marrow or peripheral blood reveal a predominance of small lymphocytes with inconspicuous nucleoli, and involved lymph nodes reveal a diffuse infiltrate of these cells ablating normal architecture.

CLL cells accumulate in bone marrow, peripheral blood, lymph nodes, and spleen, resulting in lymphocytosis, decreased bone marrow function, lymphadenopathy, and splenomegaly. CLL is also frequently associated with immune dysregulation, manifested as hypogammaglobulinemia with an increased risk of bacterial infections and autoimmune phenomena such as Coombs-positive hemolytic anemia or immune thrombocytopenia. The diagnosis is often made incidentally on a routine blood cell count that shows a leukocytosis with a predominance of small lymphocytes; flow cytometric analysis of peripheral blood or a bone marrow aspirate will reveal the characteristic clonal B-cell population that is CD5 and CD23 positive. Some patients present with lymphadenopathy, symptoms related to cytopenias, or, occasionally, recurrent infections. As the disease progresses, patients develop generalized lymphadenopathy, hepatosplenomegaly, and bone marrow failure. Death often results from infectious complications or bone marrow failure in patients who have become refractory to treatment. In about 5% of cases, CLL transforms to a highly malignant diffuse large cell lymphoma, which is usually rapidly fatal; this transformation is commonly referred to as Richter's syndrome.

CLL is a low-grade leukemia/lymphoma that typically is characterized by a long natural history with slow progression over years or even decades; the median survival is in excess of 6 years. The extent of disease, or stage, at presentation is the best predictor of survival. Table 50–5 shows the widely used Rai and Binet staging systems for CLL; the majority of patients present with stage 0, I, or II disease. Given that standard therapy is not curative, and because CLL may have a long asymptomatic phase lasting years, specific treatment can be withheld until the patient develops symptoms (e.g., bulky lymphadenopathy, constitutional symptoms such as fevers, or cytopenias caused by either bone marrow infiltration or autoimmune phenomenon). When treatment is required, initial therapy is either with an alkylating agent such as chlorambucil in combination with prednisone or with the nucleoside analogue fludarabine. The majority of patients respond to either of these interventions with significant reductions in tumor burden. Fludarabine therapy is associated with a higher rate of complete remissions compared with therapy with chlorambucil and thus is emerging as the preferred initial treatment. Patients who develop autoimmune phenomena require treatment with corticosteroids, and intravenous gammaglobulin may be used to reduce the frequency of infections in patients who have developed hypogammaglobulinemia.

TABLE 50-5 Staging System for Chronic Lymphocytic Leukemia

Stage	Lymphocytosis	Lymphadenopathy	Hepatomegaly or Splenomegaly	Hemoglobin (g/dL)	Platelets (×10³/μL)
RAI System					
0	+	−	−	≥11	≥100
I	+	+	−	≥11	≥100
II	+	±	+	≥11	≥100
III	+	±	±	<11	≥100
IV	+	±	±	Any	<100
BINET System					
A	+	± (<3 lymphatic groups* positive)	±	≥10	≥10
B	+	± (≥3 lymphatic groups* positive)	±	≥10	≥10
C	+	±	±	<10	<10

* Cervical, axillary, inguinal nodes, liver and spleen are each considered one group whether unilateral or bilateral.

Hairy Cell Leukemia

Hairy cell leukemia is a biologically indolent neoplastic lymphoid disorder characterized by an accumulation of neoplastic B cells in the bone marrow, peripheral blood, and spleen that morphologically have a characteristic appearance described as "hairy cells." Hairy cells are lymphoid cells with fine cytoplasmic projections that are readily identified by the presence of tartrate-resistant acid phosphatase (TRAP), B-cell immunophenotype, and rearranged heavy and light chain immunoglobulin genes. The diagnosis is made by identifying typical hairy cells in the peripheral blood or on bone marrow biopsy. The bone marrow is often inaspirable, because of the extensive reticulin fibrosis typically present in the marrow.

This disease superficially may resemble CLL, but it has unique clinical features and requires different therapy. Hairy cell leukemia may by diagnosed in an asymptomatic patient on routine blood cell count; symptomatic patients usually present with symptoms referable to splenomegaly, infection caused by impaired host defenses, or associated autoimmune syndromes such as vasculitis or arthritis. Osteolytic bone lesions can occur and may cause pain. "B" symptoms are rare. On examination, splenomegaly is present in more than 80% of patients; hepatomegaly is less common, and lymphadenopathy is distinctly unusual. Pancytopenia is typically present at diagnosis. The course of hairy cell leukemia is generally indolent, with slowly progressive pancytopenia and splenomegaly. However, there is a considerable variability in severity and rate of disease progression. Before effective therapy, bacterial and fungal infections occurred frequently and were the major cause of death.

Asymptomatic patients without significant cytopenias or other complications of the disease require no immediate therapy and can be monitored closely for progression or infectious complications. Patients who present with moderate cytopenias, history of infections, rapidly progressive disease, symptomatic splenomegaly, bone involvement, or autoimmune syndromes should undergo therapy. First-line therapy is the purine nucleoside analogue 2-chlorodeoxyadenosine (2-CDA). In 90% of patients, one course of treatment given as a continuous infusion over 7 days results in a complete response that

is usually durable. 2-CDA is considered the treatment of choice and has largely supplanted older therapies such as interferon-α, pentostatin, and splenectomy.

PLASMA CELL DISORDERS

The plasma cell disorders or "dyscrasias" comprise a group of B-cell neoplasms that are related to each other by virtue of their production and secretion of monoclonal immunoglobulin (or part of an immunoglobulin molecule), or M protein. The tumor cell of these disorders exhibits features of a differentiated plasma cell that is adapted to synthesize and secrete immunoglobulin at a high rate. The laboratory hallmark of plasma cell dyscrasias is the presence of a homogeneous immunoglobulin molecule (or part of an immunoglobulin molecule) that can be detected in the serum or urine by protein electrophoresis. Clinically, these disorders are often characterized by the systemic effects of the M protein, as well as by the direct effects of bone and bone marrow infiltration. The classification of plasma cell dyscrasias is determined in part by the immunoglobulin class (IgG, IgA, IgD, IgE, or IgM) or component of immunoglobulin (heavy chain or light chain) that is produced (Table 50–6). The most common plasma cell neoplasms are multiple myeloma and the closely related plasmacytoma, which is a solitary myeloma of bone and extramedullary soft tissue; other less common plasma cell neoplasms include Waldenström's macroglobulinemia, heavy chain disease, and primary amyloidosis.

M proteins can be found in benign and malignant conditions other than the plasma cell dyscrasias (see Table 50–6). Approximately 10% of patients with CLL have detectable monoclonal IgG or IgM in their serum. M proteins can be detected in a variety of autoreactive or infectious disorders. In addition, an M protein on serum protein electrophoresis can be found in individuals with no apparent associated disease and in the absence of any other laboratory or clinical evidence of a plasma cell dyscrasia. This finding is designated "monoclonal gammopathy of unknown significance" (MGUS) and increases in frequency with age older than 60 years. Although MGUS is often considered a premalignant

TABLE 50–6 **Classification of Disorders Associated with Monoclonal Immunoglobulin (M Protein) Secretion**

Disorder	M Protein	Antibody Activity of M Protein
Plasma Cell Neoplasms		
Multiple myeloma	IgG > IgA > IgD; ±free light chain or light chain alone ($\kappa > \lambda$)	
"Solitary" myeloma of bone	IgG > IgA > IgD; ±free light chain or light chain alone ($\kappa > \lambda$)	
Extramedullary plasmacytoma	IgG > IgA > IgD; ±free light chain or light chain alone ($\kappa > \lambda$)	
Waldenström's macroglobulinemia	IgM ± free light chain ($\kappa > \lambda$)	
Heavy-chain disease	γ, α, or μ heavy chain or fragment	
Primary amyloidosis	Free light chain ($\lambda > \kappa$)	
Monoclonal gammopathy of unknown significance	IgG > IgM > IgA, usually without urinary light chain secretion	
Other B-Cell Neoplasms		
Chronic lymphocytic leukemia	M protein occasionally secreted; IgM > IgG	
B-cell non-Hodgkin's lymphomas; Hodgkin's disease	M protein occasionally secreted; IgM > IgG	
Nonlymphoid Neoplasms		
Chronic myelogenous leukemia	No consistent patterns	
Carcinomas (e.g., colon, breast, prostate)	No consistent patterns	
Autoimmune or Autoreactive Disorders		
Cold agglutinin disease	IgMκ most common	Anti-I antigen
Mixed cryoglobulinemia	IgM or IgA	Anti-IgG
Sjögren's syndrome	IgM	
Miscellaneous Inflammatory, Storage, or Infectious Disorders		
Lichen myxedematosus	IgGλ	
Gaucher's disease	IgG	
Cirrhosis, sarcoid, parasitic diseases, renal acidosis	No consistent pattern	

Modified from Salmon SE: Plasma cell disorders. *In* Wyngaarden JB, Smith LH Jr (eds): Cecil Textbook of Medicine, 18th ed. 1988, p 1026.

condition, only about 10% of these patients subsequently develop a frank plasma cell neoplasm.

Multiple Myeloma

Multiple myeloma is a malignant plasma cell disorder characterized by neoplastic infiltration of the bone marrow and bone and the presence of monoclonal immunoglobulin or light chains in the serum or urine. The diagnosis of multiple myeloma is made by identifying an increase in the number of plasma cells in the bone marrow (>30%) and a serum M protein other than IgM exceeding 3.5 g/dL for IgG or 2 g/dL for IgA or a urine M protein exceeding 1 g/24 hours. In patients with lower levels of M protein and bone marrow plasmacytosis, the major differential diagnosis is usually between MGUS and myeloma; in some cases, the distinction can only be made by serial follow-up of the patient with evidence of rising M-protein levels or the development of associated clinical manifestations of myeloma. About 20% of patients with multiple myeloma do not have detectable serum M protein but have free light chains in the urine (Bence Jones protein) that can be detected in a 24-hour urine collection by urine protein electro-

phoresis ("light chain disease"). In rare cases, patients with "nonsecretory" myeloma have neither detectable serum nor urine M protein, but in these patients a monoclonal population of plasma cells can be detected by immunohistochemical identification of cytoplasmic light-chain restricted immunoglobulin.

The clinical manifestations of multiple myeloma relate to the direct effects of bone marrow and bone infiltration by malignant plasma cells, the systemic effects of the M protein, or the effects of the concomitant deficiency in humoral immunity that occurs in this disease. The most common symptom in multiple myeloma is bone pain. Bone radiographs typically show pure osteolytic "punched out" lesions, often in association with generalized osteopenia and pathologic fractures. Bony lesions can present as expansile masses associated with spinal cord compression. Hypercalcemia caused by extensive bony involvement is common in myeloma and may dominate the clinical picture. Anemia occurs in the majority of patients as a result of marrow infiltration and suppression of hematopoiesis; granulocytopenia and thrombocytopenia are less common. Patients with myeloma are susceptible to bacterial infections because of impaired production and increased catabolism of normal immunoglobulins. Respiratory tract infections from *Streptococcus pneumoniae*, *Staphylococcus aureus*, *H. influenza*, and *Klebsiella pneumoniae* and gram-negative urinary tract infections are common. Renal insufficiency occurs in about 25% of patients with myeloma. The cause of renal failure in these patients is often multifactorial; hypercalcemia, hyperuricemia, infection, and amyloid deposition can contribute. However, direct tubular damage from light chain excretion is invariably present. M proteins can also cause a host of diverse effects because of their physicochemical properties. These include cryoglobulinemia, hyperviscosity, amyloidosis, and clotting abnormalities resulting from interaction of the M protein with platelets or clotting factors.

The three-tier staging system for myeloma is a functional system that correlates with survival (Table 50–7). In contrast to the anatomic staging systems used for lymphomas and solid tumors, myeloma staging is based on clinical (bone radiographs) and laboratory tests (hemoglobin, serum calcium, serum or urine M protein levels, and serum creatinine) that correlate with tumor burden. Adverse prognostic factors include advanced stage, impaired renal function, elevated LDH levels, and elevated β_2-microglobulin levels. The last is the single most powerful predictor of survival.

The vast majority of patients with myeloma present with symptomatic, advanced-stage disease and require therapy. However, about 10% of patients have stage I disease and an indolent course. These patients do not require immediate therapy, but they should be monitored for disease progression by serial quantification of the M protein. For patients with solitary bone or extramedullary plasmacytomas, local radiation therapy can induce long-term remissions and is the treatment of choice. Patients with symptomatic, advanced-stage (II or III) myeloma require systemic chemotherapy as well as meticulous attention to supportive care. Although myeloma is not a curable malignancy, systemic chemotherapy can prolong survival and dramatically improve quality of life. The standard treatment has consisted of pulses of an alkylating agent (most commonly melphalan) with prednisone or, alternatively, the three-drug VAD—vincristine, doxorubicin (Adriamycin), and dexamethasone—regimen, which is less toxic to bone marrow stem cells. The majority of patients respond to initial therapy with a reduction in bone pain, hypercalcemia, and anemia, in association with a decline in the M protein level. In recent years, the use of high-dose chemotherapy with alkylating agents followed by autologous peripheral stem cell infusion has been shown to improve survival and quality of life compared with standard doses of chemotherapy. Although this approach is not curative, it does represent an important treatment option for some patients. Allogenic bone marrow transplant may represent the only potentially curative treatment for myeloma, but the associated excessive morbidity and mortality in elderly or heavily pretreated patients have limited its use in this disease. Patients who experience relapse and are refractory to alkylating drugs can be treated with high doses of corticosteroids or experimental therapies.

Supportive care directed toward anticipated complications of myeloma is an important aspect of the management of this disease. Bone resorption can be reduced with regular injections of the diphosphonate pamidronate, reducing pain and pathologic fractures. Bony lesions, particularly those involving weight-bearing bones, may require palliative radiation for pain control and prevention of pathologic fractures. Vertebral bony lesions may lead to spinal cord compression, with increasing back pain and neurologic symptoms. Any symptoms suggestive of cord compression require prompt evaluation with spinal magnetic resonance imaging and, if necessary, local radiation to involved areas. Avoidance of nephrotoxins, including intravenous dyes, is important to prevent renal failure. Acute renal failure caused by light chain deposition may improve with plasmapheresis to acutely reduce protein load. All patients should receive pneumococcal and *H. influenzae* vaccine, and intravenous gamma globulin may be useful in preventing recurrent infections in patients with profound hypogammaglobulinemia. Use of erythropoietin may alleviate anemia and decrease the need for blood transfusions.

Waldenström's Macroglobulinemia

Waldenström's macroglobulinemia is a malignancy of plasmacytoid lymphocytes that secrete large quantities of IgM. It is a chronic disorder affecting elderly patients (median age is 64) that shares features of the low-grade lymphomas and myeloma. In contrast to myeloma, Waldenström's macroglobulinemia is associated with lymphadenopathy and hepatosplenomegaly, and although bone marrow involvement is invariably present, lytic lesions and hypercalcemia are distinctly rare. The major clinical manifestation of Waldenström's macroglobulinemia is usually the hyperviscosity syndrome caused by the physical properties of IgM. In contrast to IgG, IgM remains largely confined to the intravascular space, and

TABLE 50–7   Myeloma Staging System

Stage	Criteria
I	All of the following:
	1) Hemoglobin >10 g/dL
	2) Serum calcium <12 mg/dL
	3) Normal bone radiograph or solitary lesion
	4) Low M-component production
	a) IgG level <5 g/dL
	b) IgA level <3 g/dL
	c) Urine light chain <4 g/24 h
II	Fitting neither I nor III
III	One or more of the following:
	1) Hemoglobin <8.5 g/dL
	2) Serum calcium >12 mg/dL
	3) Advanced lytic bone lesions
	4) High M-component production
	a) IgG level >7 g/dL
	b) IgA level >5 g/dL
	c) Urine light chains >12 g/24 h

Subclassification
  A Serum creatinine <2 mg/dL
  B Serum creatinine >2 mg/dL

as IgM levels rise, plasma viscosity increases. Epistaxis, retinal hemorrhages, dizziness, confusion, and congestive heart failure are common symptoms of the hyperviscosity syndrome. Approximately 10% of IgM proteins have properties of cryoglobulins, and these patients present with symptoms of cryoglobulinemia or cold agglutinin syndrome manifested as acrocyanosis, Raynaud's phenomenon and vascular symptoms, or hemolytic anemia precipitated by exposure to cold. Some patients with Waldenström's macroglobulinemia may develop a peripheral neuropathy that may antedate the appearance of the neoplastic process.

The approach to and treatment of Waldenström's macroglobulinemia is similar to that of other low-grade B-cell lymphomas. The use of nucleoside analogs (2CDA and fludarabine) or an alkylating agent, alone or in combination with prednisone, is effective in decreasing adenopathy and splenomegaly and controlling the M spike but is not curative. Plasmapheresis is highly effective in acutely decreasing serum IgM levels and is often needed initially to treat hyperviscosity. Although complete remissions are rare, patients who respond to therapy have median survivals of 4 years, and some patients survive more than a decade.

Rare Plasma Cell Disorders

Heavy chain disease is a rare lymphoplasmacytoid neoplasm characterized by production of a defective heavy chain of the gamma, alpha, or mu type. The clinical manifestations vary with the type of heavy chain secreted. Gamma heavy chain disease is associated with lymphadenopathy, Waldeyer's ring involvement with palatal edema, and constitutional symptoms. Alpha chain disease, also known as Mediterranean lymphoma, is characterized by lymphoid infiltration of the small intestine with associated diarrhea and malabsorption. Mu chain disease is associated with CLL. Primary amyloidosis is a systemic illness characterized by deposition of immunoglobulin light chain in organs and tissue, resulting in an array of symptoms caused by organ dysfunction. Congestive heart failure, bleeding diathesis, nephrotic syndrome, and peripheral neuropathy are common complications. Primary amyloidosis responds poorly to the treatments used for myeloma, and treatment is largely supportive.

CONGENITAL AND ACQUIRED DISORDERS OF LYMPHOCYTE FUNCTION

There are a number of congenital disorders that affect lymphocyte maturation or function, resulting in immunodeficiency disorders. Acquired disorders of lymphocyte function are far more common than congenital disorders. HIV infection is the most important infectious cause of acquired immunodeficiency and is discussed in Chapter 108. Patients who have undergone an allogeneic organ transplant require potent immunosuppressive drugs (cyclosporine, tacrolimus, azathioprine, corticosteroids, methotrexate) to prevent graft-versus-host disease

in the case of bone marrow recipients or allograft rejection in the case of solid organ transplantation. These medications can cause profound defects in T-cell function with an associated acquired immunodeficiency state. Transplant recipients are susceptible to a host of viral and protozoal infections, including an EBV-associated lymphoproliferative syndrome that can behave as an aggressive lymphoma.

INFECTIOUS DISORDERS

Lymphocytes play an essential role in the adaptive response to infection. This response can be manifested clinically with an increase in lymphocytes in the peripheral blood (reactive lymphocytosis) and lymph node enlargement. Reactive lymphocytosis is always polyclonal and usually predominantly T cell and is usually easily distinguishable from the common monoclonal B-cell neoplastic processes. Some infections are typically associated with a prominent lymphocytosis (e.g., EBV-associated infectious mononucleosis, cytomegalovirus, toxoplasmosis in immunocompetent hosts, viral hepatitis). Enlargement of lymph nodes, either local/regional or generalized lymphadenopathy, is a common manifestation of some infections (see Table 50–1). Lymph node enlargement may be striking and associated with tenderness. In most cases, the adenopathy is reactive and the organism cannot be readily cultured from the node; in other cases (e.g., tuberculosis, fungal disease), the organism can be identified by culture or appropriate staining in lymph node tissue. Biopsy of the node generally will confirm the non-neoplastic nature of the process, showing a normal architecture and cellular pattern and absence of a monoclonal population of lymphoid cells.

REFERENCES

Canellos GP, Anderson JR, Propert KJ, et al: Chemotherapy of advanced Hodgkin's disease with MOPP, ABVD, or MOPP alternating with ABVD. N Engl J Med 1992; 327:1478–1484.

DeVita, VT Jr, Mauch P, Harris NL: Hodgkin's disease. In DeVita VT Jr, Hellman S, Rosenberg SA (eds): Cancer—Principles and Practice of Oncology. Philadelphia: Lippincott-Raven, 1997, pp 2242–2283.

Fisher RI, Gaynor ER, Dahlberg S, et al: Comparison of a standard regimen (CHOP) with three intensive chemotherapy regimens for advanced non-Hodgkin's lymphoma. N Engl J Med 1993; 328:1002–1006.

Gaidano G, Dalla-Favara R: Molecular biology of lymphomas. In DeVita VT Jr, Hellman S, Rosenberg SA (eds): Cancer—Principles and Practice of Oncology. Philadelphia: Lippincott-Raven, 1997, pp 2131–2145.

Harris N, Jaffe E, Stein H, et al: A revised European-American classification of lymphoid neoplasms: A proposal from the International Lymphoma Study Group. Blood 1994; 84:1361–1392.

Philip T, Guglielmi C, Hagenbeek A, et al: Autologous bone marrow transplantation as compared with salvage chemotherapy in relapses of chemotherapy-sensitive non-Hodgkin's lymphoma. N Engl J Med 1995; 33:1540–1545.

Salmon SE, Cassady JR: Plasma cell dyscrasias. In DeVita VT Jr, Hellman S, Rosenberg SA (eds): Cancer—Principles and Practice of Oncology. Philadelphia: Lippincott-Raven, 1997, pp 2344–2387.

Shipp MA, Mauch PM, Harris NL: Non-Hodgkin's Lymphomas. In DeVita VT Jr, Hellman S, Rosenberg SA (eds): Cancer—Principles and Practice of Oncology. Philadelphia: Lippincott-Raven, 1997, pp 2165–2220.

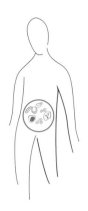

51

NORMAL HEMOSTASIS

Henry M. Rinder

Normal hemostasis involves the physiologic balance of procoagulant and anticoagulant factors that maintains liquid blood flow and the structural integrity of the vasculature. Vascular damage results in initiation of clotting with the goal of producing a *localized* platelet/fibrin plug to prevent blood loss; this is followed by processes that lead to clot containment, wound healing, clot dissolution, and tissue regeneration and remodeling. In healthy persons, all these reactions occur continuously and in a balanced fashion such that bleeding is contained, but blood vessels remain patent and deliver adequate organ blood flow. When one or several of these processes are disrupted because of inherited defects or acquired abnormalities, disordered hemostasis may result either in bleeding or thromboembolic complications.

Blood flow in the arterial and venous systems is disparate and imposes different needs on the coagulation system. In the pressurized arteries, relatively minor vascular damage can rapidly result in massive blood loss; thus, the coagulant response in arteries must be capable of arresting bleeding rapidly. Platelets are critical to this response; they initially contain blood loss and then provide an active surface that both localizes and accelerates the fibrin formation that ultimately produces hemostasis. By contrast, in the venous circulation, the lesser flow rates produce slower bleeding, a feature that makes platelets less critical; the pivotal reaction controlling the balance of venous hemostasis is the rate of thrombin generation. These differences are also underscored by the anticoagulant agents used in these settings, that is, antiplatelet agents such as aspirin to prevent coronary artery thrombus and antithrombin-based interventions, such as heparins and warfarin, for prophylaxis against deep vein thrombosis.

This chapter briefly details the physiology of vascular hemostasis, including the normal balance of procoagulant and anticoagulant functions of the blood vessel wall, platelet physiology and receptor-ligand interactions critical for hemostasis, and the highly complex, interwoven processes that comprise the coagulation cascade.

Vascular Wall Physiology

Vascular endothelial cells (ECs) function as a barrier to contain and prevent blood from contacting the highly thrombogenic subendothelial contents. In addition, normal intact ECs possess strong anticoagulant functions and secrete prostacyclin, nitric oxide, ADPase, and plasminogen activator (Table 51–1). Prostacyclin and nitric oxide have dual mechanisms to prevent thrombosis; both affect smooth muscle cells to induce vasodilation and thereby increase blood flow and minimize platelet contact with the vessel wall. At the same time, prostacyclin and nitric oxide are secreted into the blood stream, where they promote cyclic AMP generation within platelets and thereby inhibit platelet activation and aggregation.

However, when ECs are damaged or activated, the balance of coagulant properties quickly shifts to favor a procoagulant status. This function is mediated by both the ECs themselves and by the subendothelial matrix, which is exposed by vascular injury. Activated ECs express on their surface adhesive ligands that include the selectins (both E-selectin and P-selectin), β_1-integrin and β_2-integrin, platelet-EC adhesion molecule-1, and von Willebrand factor (vWF; see Table 50–1). On the EC surface, these proteins localize and promote platelet adhesion and also mediate migration of leukocytes into the tissues. Exposed subendothelial matrix binds vWF (Fig. 51–1) and contains other procoagulant adhesive moieties, including thrombospondin, fibronectin, and collagen. These function both as ligands to capture platelets and as activators of adherent platelets; collagen in particular is a strong platelet agonist causing platelets to undergo dense granule release and to express conformationally active ligands such as glycoprotein IIb/IIIa (GPIIb/IIIa; see later). Another critical procoagulant mediator exposed by EC damage is tissue factor (TF), which is constitutively expressed by subendothelial smooth muscle cells and fibroblasts. As outlined later

TABLE 51–1 Endothelial Cell Coagulant Properties

Procoagulant	Anticoagulant
Collagen	Vasodilation
Factor VIII	ADPase
Fibronectin	Heparan sulfates
Integrins	Nitric oxide
Platelet-endothelial cell adhesion molecule-1	Prostacyclin
Selectins (E- and P-)	Thrombomodulin
von Willebrand factor	Tissue factor pathway inhibitor
Vasoconstriction	Tissue plasminogen activator

(Fig. 51–2), TF is the major initiator of the soluble coagulation system that results in the formation of a definitive fibrin clot.

These procoagulant properties of the EC and subendothelial matrix ensure plugging of the endothelial injury and cessation of bleeding. At the same time, the normal ECs that surround the site of injury exert anticoagulant properties (see Table 51–1) that prevent propagation of clot beyond the injury, thereby avoiding thrombosis of the entire vessel. These anticoagulant functions may be constitutive, as noted earlier with prostacyclin and nitric oxide, or they may be initiated by vessel damage and the clotting cascade itself. Thrombin generated at the site of endothelial damage or clotting diffuses and binds to normal ECs, where it is bound to surface thrombomodulin. Once bound to thrombomodulin, thrombin acts as an initiator of the natural anticoagulant system, rather than as a primary soluble procoagulant factor. The thrombin-thrombomodulin complex converts protein C to its activated form (APC) which, in conjunction with its coenzyme, protein S, inactivates factors Va and VIIIa to downregulate further thrombin formation (Fig. 51–3). In addition, EC constitutive secretion of tissue-type plasminogen activator (t-PA), the primary initiator of fibrinolysis, converts plasminogen to the active enzyme, plasmin, which degrades formed fibrin clots. The finding that t-PA must be bound directly to clot to express full activity helps to limit the fibrinolytic response to areas of clot formation. ECs also secrete ADPase that degrades platelet-released ADP and results in inhibition of additional platelet activation and recruitment, thus limiting clot propagation. Furthermore, ECs release TF pathway inhibitor (TFPI), which is a potent inhibitor of the extrinsic procoagulant pathway and, to a lesser extent, factor Xa. TFPI complexes with Xa and TF to inhibit their activity and to downregulate thrombin generation. The balance of procoagulant and anticoagulant vascular function localizes and regulates activation of platelets and soluble coagulation factors.

Platelet Physiology

The platelet functions as the cellular-based platform for hemostasis. Platelet membrane receptors mediate primary hemostasis and allow platelets to bind directly to endothelium and subendothelium at sites of damage. Platelet adhesion causes transmembrane signaling through surface receptors to induce platelet activation and to further procoagulant function through translocation of receptors to the membrane surface, receptor conformational change, release of granule contents, and exposure of membrane phospholipid. The procoagulant surface of

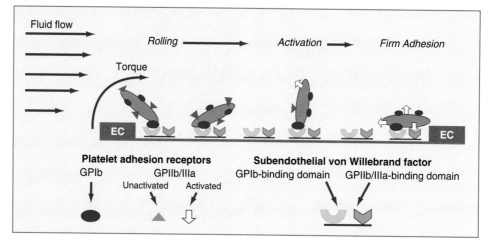

FIGURE 51–1 The adhesive interactions producing stable platelet attachment to subendothelial von Willebrand factor (vWF). The initial attachment between glycoprotein Ib (GPIb) and its binding domain on vWF is rapid but has a short half-life, and the result is a rolling movement from torque generated by flowing blood. The vWF-GPIb interaction produces transmembrane signaling that activates the platelet and transforms GPIIb/IIIa into a conformation capable of binding to the arginine-glycine-aspartate (RGD) domain on vWF. This secondary adhesion is nearly irreversible and anchors the platelet to the exposed subendothelium. EC = endothelial cell.

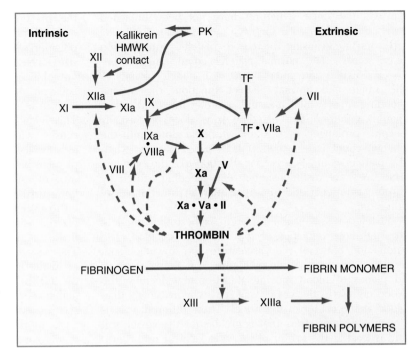

FIGURE 51–2 The coagulation cascade. The extrinsic and intrinsic pathways converge to a common procoagulant pathway that results in thrombin generation and fibrin clot formation. The ability of thrombin to amplify its own formation by positive feedback on factor activation is demonstrated by the *dotted lines.* HMWK = high-molecular-weight kininogen; PK = prekallikrein; TF = tissue factor.

the platelet then serves as a platform for assembly of the coagulation cascade and formation of thrombin, which (1) feeds back on platelets and the clotting cascade to amplify the procoagulant response and (2) produces fibrin to provide secondary, long-lasting hemostasis. Finally, the platelet assists in clot consolidation and protection from fibrinolysis, respectively, by contributing factor XIII and platelet factor 4 to the clot milieu (Table 51–2).

Platelets in the circulation are anucleate cells be-

tween 2 and 4 μm in diameter with a volume between 6 and 11 fL. Platelets are derived from the megakaryocyte cytoplasm after a maturation time of about 4 days. When platelets are released into the circulation, they survive for 7 to 10 days; platelets are removed from the circulation by a combination of senescence and the normal maintenance of vascular structural integrity. For the latter, approximately 7100 platelets/μL are required per

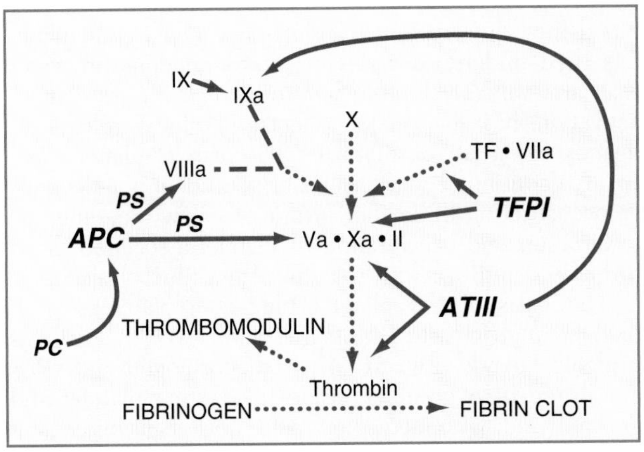

FIGURE 51–3 Endogenous anticoagulant pathways. Activation of the clotting cascade is downregulated by antithrombin III (ATIII) inhibition of Xa and thrombin and by tissue factor pathway inhibitor (TFPI) blockade of Xa and TF-VIIa. The complex of thrombin and thrombomodulin activates protein C (APC), which combines with protein S (PS) to cleave and inactivate Va and VIIIa. Fibrin clot combined with tissue plasminogen activator induces plasmin formation; plasmin then degrades formed fibrin clot into soluble fibrin peptides.

TABLE 51–2 Procoagulant Properties of Platelets

Receptor-Ligand Interactions Promoting Adhesion
GPIb/IX : vWF
GPIIb/IIIa : fibrinogen and GPIIb/IIIa : vWF
GPIa/IIa : collagen
P-selectin : P-selectin glycoprotein ligand-1
Receptor-Ligand Interactions Mediating Activation
GPV : thrombin
GPVI : collagen
Secreted α-Granule Proteins
Ligands (fibrinogen, fibronectin, thrombospondin, vitronectin, vWF)
Enzymes (α₂-antiplasmin, factors V, VIII, and XI)
Antiheparin (platelet factor 4)
Secreted Dense Granule Agonists
ADP, serotonin
Secreted Cytosolic Factor XIII Membrane Components
Thromboxane A₂ formation, phosphatidylserine expression

GPIb/IX complex = CD42; GPIIb/IIIa ($\alpha_2\beta_3$) complex = CD41; GPIa/IIa = complex of glycoprotein 1a and CO29; P-selectin = CD62P; P-selectin glycoprotein ligand-1 = CD162; vWF = von Willebrand factor.

day when vascular structures have not been breached (as would happen with surgery) and when no additional stressors are causing increased platelet consumption (e.g., sepsis). The normal platelet count range is between 150,000 and 450,000/μL; with platelet counts in this range and normal platelet function, the normal bleeding time (which measures platelet function) is less than 8 minutes. The bleeding time does not usually become prolonged by thrombocytopenia alone until the platelet count is less than 100,000/μL. However, when the platelet count is less than 100,000/μL, the bleeding time does not distinguish between bleeding caused by thrombocytopenia and abnormal platelet function/vessel adhesion.

Platelet–vessel wall interaction is best illustrated at the high-flow velocities of the arterial circulation. The interaction between the vasculature and flowing blood, as shown on the left side of Figure 51–1, creates parallel planes of blood moving at different velocities; the blood closest to the vessel wall moves more slowly than blood at the center of the vessel. These different velocities create shear stress that is greatest at the vessel wall and is least at the center of the vessel. Shear rate therefore changes inversely with the vessel diameter, with levels estimated to vary between 500 sec^{-1} in larger arteries to 5000 sec^{-1} in the smallest arterioles. Shear rates at the surface of atherosclerotic plaques with modest (50%) stenosis reach 3000 to 10,000 sec^{-1}, with even greater shear in clinically significant stenoses. The high-velocity arterial blood flow opposes tendencies to clot by (1) limiting the time available for procoagulant reactions to occur and (2) disrupting cells and proteins that are not tightly adherent to the vessel wall. However, once the vessel wall is damaged and bleeding occurs, platelets can rapidly and decisively respond to the loss of endothelial integrity, while they simultaneously resist the tendency to be swept downstream.

One of the forces enhancing platelet readiness for wall adhesion in the arterial circulation is *radial dispersion*, the tendency of larger cells (erythrocytes and leukocytes) to stream in the center of the vessel where shear is lowest; this process effectively pushes the smaller platelets toward the vessel wall and optimally positions them to respond to hemostatic challenges. This size-dependent flow may also explain the seemingly paradoxical ability of red blood cell transfusions to slow or stop bleeding simply by correcting severe anemia. This effect also underscores the importance of platelets in arterial hemostasis; reductions in platelet number or function may be associated with catastrophic arterial hemorrhage. By contrast, the lesser shear forces experienced in the venous circulation permit more random cell movement and greater time for coagulation reactions to occur and make the minimum requirements for platelet number and function correspondingly less stringent.

In the setting of high-velocity blood flow at an arterial bleeding site, platelets must activate and adhere to the injured vessel nearly instantaneously. Two molecules present in the subendothelium are critical for this process: vWF and collagen. Control of bleeding in vessels under the highest shear stresses absolutely depends on the presence and function of vWF. vWF is a large molecule synthesized in ECs and megakaryocytes that polymerizes in the blood to form a range of multimer sizes. The largest multimeric forms of vWF, which are immobilized by adherence to exposed subendothelial collagen, bind to the GPIb receptor on the platelet surface in response to high shear stress (see Fig. 51–1). This is an extremely rapid but low-affinity binding that causes platelets to become slowed, but it leaves them only weakly adherent to the subendothelium. With platelets no longer streaming by, but instead, tumbling over the subendothelium, the high shear stress in tandem with transmembrane signaling produced by the GPIb-vWF interaction results in loss of the normal platelet discoid shape (shape change) and conformational change in another platelet receptor, GPIIb/IIIa. The activated GPIIb/IIIa now binds either to fibrinogen or to the larger vWF multimers at a site removed from the GPIb binding site. This secondary adhesion is a higher-affinity interaction than the GPIb-vWF bond and secures the platelet firmly to the subendothelium.

At more moderate shear rates, vWF-GPIb adhesion is supplemented by platelet binding to subendothelial collagen, an adhesive moiety that is capable of arresting the platelet by binding to GPIa/IIa (see Table 51–2). Thus, subendothelial vWF and collagen act cooperatively to initiate platelet adhesion, with the former predominating at higher shear. Collagen is unique in that it can anchor platelets at one locus by binding to platelet GPIa/IIa and can activate platelets at a second locus by binding to platelet GPVI. The congenital absence of any of the critical platelet adhesion receptors—GPIIb/IIIa, GPIb, GPVI, or GPIa/IIa—results in a significant hemostatic defect, correctable only by platelet transfusion. Similarly, decreases in vWF, especially the larger multimeric forms, can predispose to bleeding. Once a layer of platelets is adherent to the site of bleeding, vWF bound to GPIb on the uppermost adherent platelets serves to recruit additional platelets from the flowing blood into the growing platelet plug. The bound platelets then undergo a series of interdependent processes that are collectively referred to as *activation*. Platelet activation has five major effects: (1) local release of ligands essential to stabilizing the platelet-platelet matrix, (2) continued recruitment of additional platelets, (3) vasoconstriction of smaller arteries to slow bleeding, (4) localization and acceleration of platelet-associated fibrin formation, and (5) clot protection from fibrinolysis.

The basis of the platelet plug is a platelet-ligand-platelet matrix with fibrinogen and vWF serving as bridging ligands (Fig. 51–4). Both fibrinogen and vWF are stored in α granules inside the resting platelet and are released with activation, and both can bind to a GPIIb/IIIa receptor on each of two platelets, thereby linking them. As mentioned earlier, platelet GPIIb/IIIa undergoes a calcium-dependent conformational change that allows it to bind to a locus containing the amino acid sequence arginine-glycine-aspartate (RGD) on either fibrinogen or vWF. Each fibrinogen molecule has two RGD sites on its polar ends, and the larger vWF multimers have several RGD sites, all capable of binding to conformationally altered GPIIb/IIIa and creating

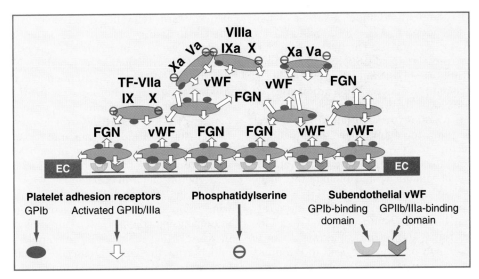

FIGURE 51–4 Assembly of coagulation factors on the platelet plug promotes thrombin generation. Platelets are adherent to subendothelial von Willebrand factor (vWF) and to one another, through both vWF and fibrinogen (FGN). Assembly of the intrinsic (VIIIa-IXa-X) and extrinsic tenase complexes (TF-VIIa-IX-X), and the prothrombinase (Xa-Va) complex occurs on platelet membranes by binding to specific platelet receptors for factors Va, IXa, and Xa. The function of these coagulation complexes also depends on the phospholipid-rich milieu provided by activated platelet surface expression of phosphatidylserine. EC = endothelial cell; GP = glycoprotein.

the platelet-ligand-platelet matrix. GPIIb/IIIa is the most abundant glycoprotein on the platelet surface, with approximately 50,000 copies on the *resting* platelet, and additional GPIIb/IIIa receptors within the cytosol that are mobilized to the surface after activation.

Platelets are also recruited and then are cemented into the platelet plug by local agonists (collagen, epinephrine, and thrombin) and by platelet release of agonists into the local microenvironment. Both collagen (as noted previously) and thrombin interact with their specific platelet receptors to activate platelets strongly; although epinephrine alone is not a powerful platelet agonist, stimulation of the α-adrenergic receptor on platelets primes them for synergistic activation to even relatively weak agonists such as ADP. Activating compounds released directly from the platelet include thromboxane A_2, which is formed in the platelet cytosol after cyclooxygenase cleavage of arachadonic acid and then released into the clot milieu. Thromboxane A_2 is both a platelet agonist and a vasoconstrictor, and it is rapidly degraded to its inert by-product, thromboxane B_2. Cyclooxygenase activity is *irreversibly* inhibited by aspirin, thereby blocking thromboxane A_2 formation for the lifetime of that platelet; this is in contrast to other nonsteroidal anti-inflammatory drugs (e.g., indomethacin), which *reversibly* inhibit cyclooxygenase activity. Other platelet agonists are liberated into the extracellular fluid by fusion of the dense granules and α granules with the platelet canalicular membrane, and the result is extrusion of granule contents. The dense granules contain serotonin that, like thromboxane A_2, is both a platelet agonist and a vasoconstrictor. Another dense granule constituent, ADP, acts purely as a platelet agonist without vasoactive properties (see Table 51–2). The importance of thromboxane A_2-induced and serotonin-induced

vasoconstriction is not entirely clear. However, vasoconstriction, by decreasing the vessel diameter, may increase shear stress and may thereby facilitate recruitment of platelets to the injured site. The importance of dense granule release to the maintenance of hemostasis is underscored by the severe bleeding seen in congenital dense granule deficiencies (e.g., Hermansky-Pudlak syndrome and storage pool disease). Platelet activation therefore serves to amplify platelet adhesion and, as detailed later, to optimize the platelet surface for fibrin-generating procoagulant activity by interaction with the coagulation cascade.

Coagulation Cascade

The *coagulation cascade* is characterized by continuous factor activation and coordinated assembly of enzyme complexes, held in check by circulating inhibitors. These enzyme complexes consist of serine proteases, cofactors, and zymogen substrates assembled on a membrane (phospholipid) surface. Under normal circumstances, formation of these complexes is relatively slow, and inactivation of the complexes by circulating inhibitors balances their procoagulant activity and prevents clot formation. However, once a procoagulant stimulus occurs that allows a burst of activated factor formation, formation of these enzyme complexes is rapidly amplified and leads to intense thrombin formation.

The liver is the major site of synthesis of most of the coagulation factors. In severe liver disease, all coagulation factor levels are diminished, except for factor VIII, a finding suggesting that factor VIII is produced not only by the liver but also by ECs and cells of the reticuloendothelial system. In addition, a subset of factors is vitamin K dependent, that is, prothrombin (factor II) and factors VII, IX, and X. The naturally occurring anticoagulants, proteins C and S, also have vitamin K–dependent synthesis. Post-translational modification (through a vitamin K–dependent carboxylase) of the N-terminal domain of these proteins adds 10 to 12 γ-carboxyglutamate residues; these residues are critical for calcium binding and for determining the functional 3-dimensional structure of the proteins and their proper binding orientation to membrane surfaces. Warfarin blocks liver uptake of vitamin K and inhibits the function of this carboxylase.

From the perspective of laboratory testing, the coagulation cascade can be divided into what are traditionally termed the extrinsic and intrinsic pathways, which converge on the common pathway and lead to thrombin and fibrin generation (see Fig. 51–2). The physiologic extrinsic pathway initiator, TF, is constitutively expressed on subendothelial fibroblasts and smooth muscle cells that are only exposed to blood by EC damage. TF is also expressed on peripheral blood monocytes and vascular ECs after exposure to activating or inflammatory stimuli such as endotoxin. In the laboratory, the extrinsic pathway is assayed by measuring the interaction of circulating factor VIIa with exogenously added TF/thromboplastin and is measured as the prothrombin time (PT). The PT is highly sensitive to deficiencies of factors involved in both the extrinsic (factor VII) and common pathways (factors V and X and prothrombin), and all these deficiencies are associated with significant bleeding complications. Because three of these factors are vitamin K dependent, including the factor with the shortest half-life, factor VII, the PT is the most sensitive assay of the therapeutic efficacy of warfarin. The PT is completely unaffected by deficiencies of factors XII, XI, IX, or VIII. The degree of prolongation of the PT by warfarin partly depends on the strength of the thromboplastin used in the assay, which varies by manufacturer and in its particular activity with each coagulation instrument. Therefore, the international normalized ratio (INR) was devised to standardize the variations in the PT induced by warfarin among laboratories, to allow for global application of anticoagulant recommendations. The INR is based on the international sensitivity index (ISI) of each thromboplastin and is calculated for each patient as follows: (patient PT/mean control PT)^{ISI}. Therapeutic INRs with warfarin vary according to the specific disease indication and are covered in Chapter 52. In contrast to warfarin, the PT is relatively insensitive to unfractionated heparin at therapeutic levels.

The intrinsic, or contact activation, pathway is measured as the partial thromboplastin time (PTT) in the laboratory; testing is initiated by plasma stimulation with a negatively charged compound such as kaolin. The PTT assay is sensitive to deficiencies of intrinsic pathway factors (prekallikrein [PK], high-molecular-weight kininogen [HMWK], and factors XII, XI, IX, and VIII) and to common pathway deficiencies (factors V and X and prothrombin). However, deficiencies of PK, HMWK, and factor XII do not result in clinical bleeding, so it is unlikely that these particular initiators of the intrinsic

pathway are relevant to physiologic hemostasis, even though they are detected by laboratory testing. By contrast, deficiencies of factor XI, and especially factors IX and VIII, cause significant bleeding. The PTT is sensitive to the presence of unfractionated heparin and is used as a rapid monitoring assay for therapeutic heparin levels. Unlike in warfarin therapy, the range for therapeutic PTT levels with heparin is much wider and not as well standardized. Therapeutic unfractionated heparin levels (measured by assays of anti-Xa activity) correspond to a PTT of more than 1.5 to 2.5 times the initial PTT (before heparin is begun).

Although the traditional schema of independent intrinsic and extrinsic pathways of coagulation reflects a reasonable paradigm for the purposes of in vitro testing, in vivo clotting follows a more complex path. Physiologic initiation of the clotting cascade is caused by tissue injury and low levels of circulating activated factors, and coagulation events are also bidirectionally linked to inflammation; activated monocytes express functional TF, and factor Xa induces inflammatory responses. The coagulation cascade in vivo is propagated by enzyme complexes that function effectively only on phospholipid membrane surfaces. The appropriate phospholipid surface appears to be predominantly supplied by the platelet. Low levels of circulating activated factor VII (VIIa) are generated by thrombin (see Fig. 51–2) and by the factor Xa–phospholipid complex and, to a lesser extent, by factor VIIa–TF itself. TF expressed after EC injury binds to circulating factor VIIa, and the factor VIIa–TF complex subsequently binds to its zymogen substrates, factors IX and X, on the activated platelet membrane to form the *extrinsic* tenase complex (see Fig. 51–4).

In addition to providing an essential negative phospholipid surface for tenase and the prothrombinase reactions (described later), activated platelets provide specific receptors for factors Xa, IXa, and Va. Factor V is also secreted from the α granule of the activated platelet, although evidence indicates that most secreted factor V is derived from the plasma pool. Membrane association of these coagulation factors in their ideal spatial orientation with negatively charged, platelet-expressed phosphatidylserine (see Fig. 51–4) accelerates procoagulant enzymatic reactions and simultaneously protects the activated factors from circulating inhibitors; this process culminates in accelerated thrombin generation. TF–factor VIIa converts factor X to Xa and factor IX to IXa, both of which are bound to platelet receptors. The platelet factor Xa receptor is closely associated with platelet-bound factor Va; together with free calcium and platelet membrane phosphatidylserine, these factors bind prothrombin (factor II) to form the prothrombinase complex, thereby generating thrombin, albeit in relatively small amounts. This initially formed thrombin feeds back to activate factor VIII to VIIIa (which binds to membrane-bound factor IXa), factor V to Va (which binds to its platelet receptor), and factor XI to XIa.

Up to this point in the cascade, the rate of factor Xa and thrombin generation formed is relatively slow. However, once these initial amounts of thrombin generate appreciable quantities of factor XIa and cofactors Va and VIIIa on the platelet surface, activation of the more kinetically favorable intrinsic pathway occurs and eventually becomes dominant, especially after circulating TFPI closes down the extrinsic pathway. Because of thrombin feedback activation, the intrinsic pathway massively amplifies the clotting cascade, thus increasing the rate of factor Xa and thrombin generation exponentially. The *intrinsic* tenase complex is formed initially by TF-induced factors IXa and X; subsequent *extrinsic* tenase formation is mediated by sustained factor XIa–based activation of factor IX. Factor IXa binds to its cofactor, VIIIa, and its zymogen substrate X to further amplify production of factor Xa on the membrane surface (see Fig. 51–2). The burst of factor Xa formation that follows amplifies the formation of the prothrombinase complex and results in much higher rates of thrombin generation. As noted earlier, what role factor XII, HMWK, and prekallikrein have in the in vivo generation of clot remains uncertain.

With rapid thrombin generation, fibrinogen is cleaved to fibrin monomers that rapidly combine to form a fibrin matrix integrated with the platelet plug. Factor XIIIa, a transamidase produced by the action of thrombin on either plasma or platelet-released XIII, converts the soluble fibrin clot into an insoluble fibrin polymer and also binds α_2-antiplasmin to the fibrin to protect the clot from plasmin-mediated dissolution (Fig. 51–5). Finally, the platelet plug undergoes clot retraction, which additionally protects the platelet-fibrin matrices from lysis by plasmin. These antilytic mechanisms, largely linked to platelet activation, may explain the relative resistance of platelet-rich clots to thrombolysis.

At the same time the tenase and prothrombinase complexes are forming on the platelet and EC membranes, the natural inhibitors of coagulation are activated to downregulate clotting. In the intact circulation and at the perimeter of a newly formed clot, certain endogenous mechanisms, including an intact EC barrier, limit clotting to the area of injury and maintain the surrounding flowing blood in a liquid form. In the arterial circulation, vessel occlusion by the growing clot is counteracted by the high-velocity blood flow that dilutes and disperses coagulation factors. Antiplatelet factors are also part of the anticoagulant activity intrinsic to the healthy EC lining and limit extension of the platelet plug past the area of damage. These include the following: (1) net negative surface charge, which repels similarly charged platelets; (2) constitutive release of nitric oxide and prostacyclin that inhibits platelet aggregation; and (3) constitutive surface expression of an ADPase that inactivates platelet-released ADP and thus limits recruitment of additional platelets (see Table 51–1).

Once the platelet plug and associated fibrin deposition have halted the bleeding and have covered any exposed endothelium, reining in the coagulation cascade becomes critical. Clot limitation occurs by several mechanisms (see Fig. 51–3): (1) tenase and TF–factor VIIa neutralization by TFPI; (2) thrombin, factor IXa, Xa, and XIa neutralization by antithrombin III (ATIII); (3) elimination of thrombin-activated cofactors Va and VIIIa by APC and its cofactor protein S; and (4) dissolution of the formed fibrin clot by t-PA and urokinase (see Fig. 51–5). ATIII and TFPI are circulating, constitutive protease inhibitors. ATIII inhibits the activity of thrombin and factors Xa, IXa, and XIa by complexing with these proteins; both the antithrombin and anti-Xa activity of ATIII are amplified about 2000-fold by unfractionated heparin. ECs synthesize an endogenous glycosaminoglycan, heparan sulfate, which associates with the extracellular matrix; heparan sulfate then complexes with blood ATIII to amplify neutralization of locally developed thrombin. Because heparan sulfates are bound to the extracellular matrix associated with neighboring intact endothelium, ATIII-heparan interactions help to prevent the clot from extending away from the damaged area. ECs constitutively release TFPI that also inhibits circulating factor Xa activity but mainly acts to downregulate TF-induced tenase function. This is accomplished through binding of the TFPI–factor Xa complex to the

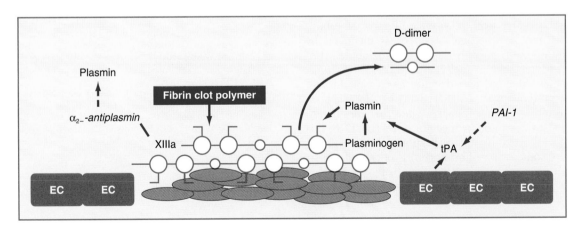

FIGURE 51–5 Balanced fibrinolysis limiting the platelet-fibrin clot. The platelet plug and fibrin matrices are strengthened by incorporation of factor XIIIa into the fibrin clot. Factor XIIIa also binds α_2-antiplasmin to the clot to protect it from plasmin-mediated fibrinolysis. At the same time, nearby intact endothelial cells (EC) secrete tissue-type plasminogen activator (t-PA). t-PA that evades plasminogen activator inhibitor-1 (PAI-1) converts clot-bound plasminogen to plasmin and leads to fibrin clot degradation and release of soluble fibrin peptides and D-dimer. Thus, detection of circulating D-dimer indicates active fibrinolysis.

TF–factor VIIa complex and inactivation of TF–factor VIIa activity through this quaternary complex formation, thereby shutting down the extrinsic tenase pathway.

Thrombomodulin is another EC surface-associated protein. Thrombin that escapes antithrombin neutralization binds to thrombomodulin on the membranes of nearby intact ECs, and this enzyme complex activates protein C (see Fig. 51–3). APC cleaves non–platelet-associated factors Va and VIIIa and thereby inactivates the respective prothrombinase and intrinsic tenase complexes and downregulates thrombin formation. The vitamin K–dependent factor, protein S, serves as a cofactor for APC and increases its biologic activity for cleavage of factors Va and VIIIa by 20-fold and 5-fold, respectively. Protein S functions only when it is circulating in the free state and not when it is complexed with the C4b-binding protein; in acute illness, the C4b-binding protein may be increased as an acute phase reactant. Increased binding of protein S may therefore occur in acute illnesses; this process may decrease free protein S levels and may lead to a relative decrease in natural anticoagulant activity and a procoagulant state.

Endothelial-Associated Fibrinolysis

Intravascular fibrinolytic activity results from a balance between plasminogen activators, such as t-PA and urokinase-PA (u-PA), and inhibitors, such as plasminogen activator inhibitor-1 (PAI-1) and α_2-antiplasmin (see Fig. 51–5). Regulation of fibrinolysis occurs at the endothelial surface. Vascular ECs synthesize and secrete t-PA and PAI-1. Plasminogen activation to plasmin is boosted by cell surface–associated t-PA, especially in the presence of fibrin clot, and to a lesser extent by the relatively small circulating amounts of u-PA. Plasmin facilitates degradation of fibrin and matrix components in the pericellular environs. PAI-1 is present in relatively large concentrations in the circulation compared with t-PA, and it effectively blocks any circulating t-PA function that could otherwise lead to systemic fibrinolysis. Inhibition of plasmin, a procoagulant effect, is mediated by α_2-antiplasmin and possibly by α_2-macroglobulin. Besides ECs, other cells, namely macrophages, are critical to fibrinolysis. Macrophages degrade fibrin clot through lysosomal proteolysis by a mechanism that does not involve plasmin. The macrophage binds to fibrin(ogen) through its surface integrin receptor, CD11b/CD18; this binding is followed by internalization of the complex into the lysosome, where fibrin(ogen) is degraded.

Tissue repair and regeneration eventually require dissolution of the fibrin-based clot. t-PA and urokinase act on the circulating zymogen plasminogen to generate the active fibrinolytic enzyme, plasmin. In addition, the intrinsic pathway activators, kallikrein, factor XIIa, and factor XIa, help to convert plasminogen to plasmin. Plasminogen binding to cell surface receptors promotes its own activation by placing it in proximity to t-PA and fibrin clot, as well as by protecting plasmin from inactivation by circulating (but not clot-bound) α_2-antiplasmin (see Fig. 51–5). Plasmin dissolves the fibrin matrix and produces soluble fibrin peptides and D-dimer, and plasmin also activates metalloproteinases that degrade damaged tissue. Fibroblasts and leukocytes migrate into the wound, the latter mediated by E-selectin and P-selectin binding, and these cells act in concert with growth factors secreted by leukocytes and activated platelets (e.g., transforming growth factor-β) to promote vascular repair and tissue regeneration.

All these procoagulant and anticoagulant processes operate together continuously to maintain balanced hemostasis; these pathways maintain vascular integrity and continuous blood flow through the circulation. By amplifying these processes in a way that consistently restricts the hemostatic response to the site of injury, systemic complications are minimized. Furthermore, redundancy in the coagulant pathways of the vascular tissues, platelets, and the coagulation cascade has allowed for survival even in patients with severe inherited or acquired disorders of hemostasis.

REFERENCES

Banner EW: The factor VIIa/tissue factor complex. Thromb Haemost 1997; 78:512–515.

Cines DB, Pollak ES, Buck CA, et al: Endothelial cells in physiology and in the pathophysiology of vascular disorders. Blood 1998; 91:3527–3561.

Collen D, Lijnen HR: Basic and clinical aspects of fibrinolysis and thrombolysis. Blood 1991; 78:3114.

Esmon CT, Johnson AE, Esmon NL, et al: Initiation of the protein C pathway. N Y Acad Sci 1991; 614:30.

Ikeda Y, Handa M, Kawano K: The role of von Willebrand factor and fibrinogen in platelet aggregation under varying shear stress. J Clin Invest 1991; 87:1234.

Loscalzo J. The macrophage and fibrinolysis. Semin Thromb Hemost 1996; 22:503–506.

Mann KG, Bovill EG, Krishnaswamy S: Surface-dependent reactions in the propagation phase of blood coagulation. In Ruggeri ZM, Fulcher CA, Ware J (eds): Progress in Vascular Biology, Hemostasis, and Thrombosis. New York: New York Academy of Sciences, 1991, p 63.

Ofosu FA, Longbin L, Freedman J: Control mechanisms in thrombin generation. Semin Thromb Haemost 1996; 22:303–308.

Rapaport SI: Regulation of the tissue factor pathway. In Ruggeri ZM, Fulcher CA, Ware J (eds): Progress in Vascular Biology, Hemostasis, and Thrombosis. New York: New York Academy of Sciences, 1991, p 51.

Ruggeri ZM: Mechanisms initiating platelet thrombus formation. Thromb Haemost 1997; 78:611–616.

Ruggeri ZM: Von Willebrand factor. J Clin Invest 1997; 99:559–564.

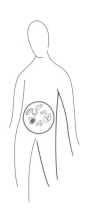

52

DISORDERS OF HEMOSTASIS: BLEEDING

Henry M. Rinder

Clinical Evaluation of Bleeding

The evaluation of bleeding requires a careful history, physical examination, and laboratory evaluation. The patient's history should include a description of bleeding (epistaxis, menorrhagia, hematoma formation), the circumstances under which bleeding occurred (association with trauma, surgery, or dental procedures), and whether any blood products (and what kind of products) were required to staunch bleeding. The clinician should determine whether the temporal addition of medications, such as aspirin, was associated with the bleeding, and whether the patient had any concomitant medical illnesses such as infection or liver disease. Finally, determining whether the patient has any family history of bleeding is critical; the physician may need to query several generations and second-degree relations, such as maternal uncles when hemophilia is suspected in a boy.

The physical examination may yield some clues to the origin of bleeding and may help to distinguish between small vessel bleeding, such as petechial (pinpoint) hemorrhage, and larger vessel bleeding, which usually produces hematomas and purpura (large bruises). Small vessel bleeding in the skin, mucous membranes, or gastrointestinal (GI) tract tends to occur more often in patients with thrombocytopenia, qualitative platelet defects, vascular abnormalities, and von Willebrand's disease (vWD). In women, menorrhagia may be the only symptom. Large vessel bleeding in solid organs, joints, or muscles is more commonly associated with factor deficiencies, such as hemophilia A or B. Screening laboratory assays are often useful in the initial assessment of the bleeding patient (Table 52–1). Such assays should include the following: (1) *blood cell counts* (especially the platelet count) and examination of the peripheral blood smear; (2) the *prothrombin time* (PT), which is highly sensitive to the extrinsic pathway and defects in vitamin K–dependent coagulation factors; and (3) the *partial thromboplastin time* (PTT), which detects deficiencies in factors VIII, IX, and XI, as well as the initiators of the intrinsic pathway, prekallikrein, high-molecular-weight kininogen, and factor XII. Abnormalities of the common pathway result in elevations of both the PT and the PTT. Another readily available test for the bleeding patient is the *thrombin time;* this test directly measures the conversion of fibrinogen to fibrin by exogenous thrombin and assays both the fibrinogen level and its functional capability. The *bleeding time* is prolonged by thrombocytopenia (platelet count <100,000/μL) and by qualitative platelet defects. If the PT or the PTT is prolonged, patient plasma should be combined with normal plasma *(mixing study),* and the clotting time study should be repeated. The mixing study enables one to distinguish between factor deficiency (the PT or the PTT corrects into the normal range) and a circulating inhibitor (the clotting time remains prolonged).

A rapid approach to identifying possible causes of bleeding (Fig. 52–1) should consider the following major disease categories: (1) thrombocytopenia or abnormal platelet function; (2) low levels of multiple coagulation factors resulting from vitamin K deficiency or liver disease; (3) single factor deficiency, either inherited or acquired; (4) consumptive coagulopathies such as disseminated intravascular coagulation (DIC); and (5) circulating inhibitors to coagulation factors, such as antibody to factor VIII. In addition, disorders intrinsic to the blood vessels themselves may cause a bleeding diathesis.

Vascular Causes of Bleeding

Vascular purpura (bruising) is defined as bleeding caused by intrinsic structural abnormalities of blood vessels or by inflammatory infiltration of blood vessels (*vas-*

TABLE 52-1   Screening Hemostasis Assays

Laboratory Test	Aspect of Hemostasis Tested	Causes of Abnormalities
Blood counts/peripheral blood smear	Platelet count and morphology	Thrombocytopenia; thrombocytosis; gray platelet and giant platelet syndromes
Prothrombin time	Extrinsic/common pathways	Vitamin K deficiency/warfarin; liver disease, DIC, factor deficiency (VII, V, X), factor inhibitor
Partial thromboplastin time	Intrinsic/common pathways	Heparin; DIC; lupus anticoagulant*; vWD; factor deficiency (XI, IX, VIII, V, X, XII, HMWK, PK), factor inhibitor
Thrombin time	Fibrinogen	Heparin; DIC; hypofibrinogenemia; dysfibrinogenemia
Bleeding time	Platelet function	Aspirin; thrombocytopenia; vWD; storage pool disease
Mixing study	Presence of an inhibitor	Abnormal clotting time corrects with a deficiency, does not correct with an inhibitor

* Lupus anticoagulant is not associated with bleeding.
DIC = disseminated intravascular coagulation; HMWK = high-molecular-weight kininogen; PK = prekallikrein; vWD = von Willebrand's disease.

culitis). Although vascular purpura usually causes bleeding in the setting of normal platelet counts and normal coagulation studies, vasculitis and vessel damage may be severe enough to cause secondary consumption of platelets and coagulation factors. Abnormalities of the subcutaneous tissue that overlies blood vessels is often seen in older patients and is termed *senile purpura;* similar skin changes leading to fragile blood vessels are also common effects of steroid therapy. In this setting, collagen breakdown and thinning of subcutaneous tissue lead to bruising as a result of atrophy. Another acquired cause of vascular purpura is scurvy or vitamin C deficiency.

Scurvy is characterized by bleeding around individual hair fibers *(perifollicular hemorrhage)* and corkscrew-shaped hairs. Bruising occurs in a classic "saddle" pattern, distributed over the upper thighs. The bleeding gums seen with scurvy are caused by gingivitis and not by the subcutaneous tissue defect; thus, edentulous patients with scurvy do not have bleeding gums, and scurvy should not be excluded on this basis.

Congenital defects of the vessel wall may cause bruising. These rare syndromes include *pseudoxanthoma elasticum,* a defect of the elastic fibers of the vasculature that is associated with severe GI and genitourinary

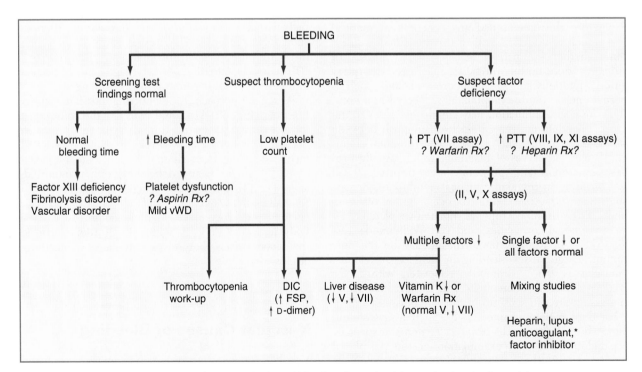

FIGURE 52-1   Algorithm for the evaluation of bleeding. Screening laboratories for platelet and factor deficiencies are used to narrow the work-up for bleeding, followed by specific factor and other coagulation studies (e.g., mixing studies, D-dimer) to confirm the diagnosis.

bleeding, and *Ehlers-Danlos syndrome,* characterized by abnormal collagen molecules in both blood vessels and subcutaneous tissue. Both these syndromes present with bruising in the skin, but only patients with pseudoxanthoma elasticum develop significant GI bleeding. Another inherited vessel wall defect associated with GI bleeding is *hereditary hemorrhagic telangiectasia (Osler-Weber-Rendu syndrome);* this disorder is characterized by degeneration of the blood vessel wall that results in angiomatous lesions resembling blood blisters on mucous membranes, including the lips and GI tract. The frequency of bleeding caused by breakdown of these lesions increases with age, and GI lesions commonly cause significant, chronic bleeding, often resulting in iron deficiency.

The sudden onset of *palpable purpura* (localized, raised hemorrhages in the skin) in association with rash and fever may be caused by vasculitis (either aseptic or septic). *Septic vasculitis* may be caused by meningococcemia and other bacterial infections and is often accompanied by thrombocytopenia and prolongation of clotting times. One cause of aseptic vasculitis in young children and adolescents is *Henoch-Schönlein purpura,* a vasculitis of the skin, GI tract, and kidneys, which is usually accompanied by abdominal pain (caused by bleeding into the bowel wall). This syndrome may occur after a viral prodrome and appears to be caused by an IgA hypersensitivity reaction, as evidenced by serum IgA immune complexes and renal histopathologic features resembling IgA nephropathy. *Drug hypersensitivity* (e.g., to allopurinol) can present with extensive cutaneous purpura as well.

The therapy of bleeding from vascular disorders is straightforward. Senile purpura and steroid-induced purpura usually do not require treatment. Scurvy is corrected by oral ascorbic acid. In the case of congenital disorders, including Ehlers-Danlos syndrome, hereditary hemorrhagic telangiectasia, and pseudoxanthoma elasticum, patients should avoid medications that may aggravate their bleeding tendencies, such as aspirin, and they should receive supportive therapy, such as iron supplementation. Systemic administration of estrogen in hereditary hemorrhagic telangiectasia may help to decrease epistaxis by inducing squamous metaplasia of the nasal mucosa and thereby protecting lesions from trauma. Treatment of septic vasculitis obviously focuses primarily on appropriate antibiotic therapy; in the case of aseptic vasculitis, steroids and/or immunosuppressive agents are most effective. When vasculitis is severe enough to cause consumption of platelets and coagulation factors (see later discussion of DIC), transfusions of platelets, cryoprecipitate, or fresh-frozen plasma may be indicated.

Bleeding Caused by Platelet Disorders: Thrombocytopenia

Thrombocytopenia (platelet count $<150,000/\mu L$) is one of the most common problems in hospitalized patients. The initial diagnostic approach to thrombocytopenia involves classifying whether the low platelet count is caused by (1) decreased platelet production, (2) increased platelet sequestration, or (3) increased peripheral platelet destruction (Fig. 52–2).

THROMBOCYTOPENIA CAUSED BY DECREASED MARROW PRODUCTION

Decreased production of platelets in the bone marrow is characterized by decreased or absent megakaryocytes on the bone marrow aspirate and biopsy. Suppression of normal megakaryocytopoiesis occurs in the following situations: (1) marrow damage and destruction of stem cells, as seen with cytotoxic chemotherapy; (2) destruction of the normal marrow microenvironment and replacement of normal stem cells by invasive malignant disease, aplasia, infection (e.g., miliary tuberculosis), or myelofibrosis; (3) specific intrinsic defects of the megakaryocytic stem cells; and (4) metabolic abnormalities affecting megakaryocyte maturation.

Thrombocytopenia may result from cytotoxic or immunosuppressive chemotherapy for malignant or autoimmune disease. Thrombocytopenia is usually reversible, and platelet production rebounds as megakaryocytic stem cells recover and regenerate. However, repeated and/or intensive chemotherapy (e.g., stem cell transplantation) may permanently damage the megakaryocytic stem cells and supporting stromal environment and may cause chronic thrombocytopenia. This condition is usually accompanied by leukopenia and anemia suggestive of refractory anemia *(myelodysplasia).* Commonly used drugs such as thiazide diuretics, alcohol, and estrogens (Table 52–2) may also damage bone marrow megakaryocytes. Nutritional disorders, especially alcoholism and abnormal folate or B_{12} metabolism, are also commonly associated with thrombocytopenia; platelet counts respond to abstinence from alcohol and to appropriate multivitamin replacement therapy.

Platelet production is suppressed by intrinsic malignant diseases of the bone marrow such as leukemia and multiple myeloma and by malignant diseases that secondarily invade the bone marrow (non-Hodgkin's lymphoma, small cell lung cancer, breast and prostate cancer, and many others). The bone marrow aspirate under these circumstances shows decreased megakaryocytes and, occasionally, malignant cells; bone marrow biopsy has a much higher yield for diagnosing malignant involvement of the marrow. Flow cytometric evaluation for clonal B cells in the marrow aspirate is highly sensitive for detecting lymphoproliferative disease in the marrow.

Myelofibrosis, an increase in the reticulin fibers (and sometimes collagen) of the marrow, may lead to thrombocytopenia or pancytopenia. Myelofibrosis occurs most commonly in myeloproliferative disorders, in mastocytosis, and in mycobacterial and other infections involving the marrow. It may also occur occasionally in patients with myelodysplasia or acute leukemia (especially megakaryocytic FAB M7) and, rarely, on a congenital basis *(osteogenesis imperfecta).* Thrombocytopenia is also seen in patients with severe aplastic anemia, and the bone marrow shows decreased or absent megakaryocytes, with other cell lineages similarly affected.

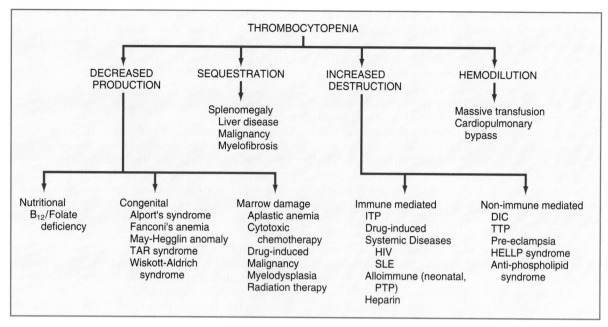

FIGURE 52–2 Differential diagnosis of thrombocytopenia. Disorders resulting in a decrease in circulating platelet number can be divided into four main pathophysiologic mechanisms, namely, hypoproduction, sequestration, peripheral destruction, and hemodilution. The history, physical examination, and bone marrow evaluation usually narrow the range of possible causes.

Thrombocytopenia in children can also result from congenital defects of megakaryocyte production as seen with the *thrombocytopenia–absent radii syndrome* and *Fanconi's anemia (congenital aplastic anemia with renal hypoplasia and skin hyperpigmentation)*. Disorders that are intrinsic to the bone marrow include the *May-Hegglin anomaly,* characterized by giant platelets and Döhle's bodies (basophilic inclusions in leukocytes and platelets) on the peripheral blood smear. *Wiskott-Aldrich syndrome* is an X-linked disorder presenting with eczema, immunodeficiency, and thrombocytopenia with small platelets. The few other congenital platelet hypoproduction syndromes are not well characterized but appear to be autosomal dominant (thrombocytopenia and decreased or absent megakaryocytes noted in family members); when accompanied by nerve deafness and nephritis, congenital hypoproductive thrombocytopenia is part of *Alport's syndrome.*

Platelet transfusions are used to support patients with hypoproductive thrombocytopenia of any origin but especially those receiving induction or maintenance chemotherapy for malignant diseases. The *prophylactic* use of platelet transfusions for thrombocytopenia in patients receiving chemotherapy is much more common than transfusion for actual bleeding. Although the platelet count trigger for such prophylactic transfusions was set in the past at 20,000/μL, data from some studies have confirmed that a threshold of 10,000/μL is both safe and appropriate in patients with relatively uncomplicated clinical pictures (no fever, sepsis, or GI bleeding). If complicating circumstances are present or if patients are about to undergo a procedure, then prophylactic platelet transfusions should be given when counts are lower than 20,000/μL. Using a threshold of 10,000/μL has been shown to be safe and efficacious with respect to the frequency of bleeding complications. This approach also significantly decreases the frequency of platelet transfusion. This reduction in platelet transfusions may decrease alloimmunization in chronically transfused patients, although this effect of lowering the prophylactic transfusion threshold has not yet been studied.

In thrombocytopenic patients without any cause for increased peripheral platelet destruction, each unit of random donor platelet concentrates raises the platelet count by about 10,000/μL. Thus, 6 U of platelets trans-

TABLE 52–2 Drugs Commonly Causing Thrombocytopenia

Immune-Mediated Peripheral Platelet Destruction
Anticonvulsants
Antihypertensives
Gold salts
Heparin
Procainamide
Psychotropics
Quinidine and quinine
Sulfonamides
Decreased Platelet Production by Suppressing Megakaryopoiesis
Anticonvulsants
Estrogens
Ethanol
Thiazide diuretics
Chemotherapeutic agents

fused into a patient with a platelet count of 10,000/μL would be expected to raise the count to near 70,000/μL. However, concomitant fever, sepsis, alloimmunization, use of amphotericin B, graft-versus-host disease, or DIC in thrombocytopenic patients will increase platelet consumption and blunt the platelet rise. With the exception of alloimmunization, the foregoing conditions generally decrease overall transfused platelet survival but not what is termed *immediate platelet recovery*. Thus, the platelet count rises significantly by 1 hour after transfusion and then declines at a steeper rate than in patients swith asymptomatic thrombocytopenia. In contrast, in an allo-immunized patient, the platelet rise at 1 hour after transfusion may be minimal or absent. Because alloimmunized patients often require single-donor apheresis platelets, with or without donor screening by platelet crossmatching, or human leukocyte antigen matching, obtaining a 1-hour posttransfusion platelet count may be an important test to maximize the response to transfused platelets. In patients with these conditions, efforts should be made to transfuse type-specific platelets, if available, to minimize any clearance caused by ABO determinants carried on platelet glycoproteins and glycolipids.

THROMBOCYTOPENIA CAUSED BY SEQUESTRATION

Up to 30% of circulating platelets are normally contained within the spleen at any given time. Conditions that lead to splenomegaly cause increased trapping of platelets; this *platelet sequestration* causes thrombocytopenia, often dropping the platelet count into the range of 50,000 to 100,000/μL, but rarely lower. Thrombocytopenia from sequestration is common in advanced liver disease, myeloproliferative disorders accompanied by splenomegaly (chronic myelogenous leukemia, agnogenic myeloid metaplasia with myelofibrosis), and malignant disease involving the spleen. Splenectomy may be indicated in patients with malignant disease. In contrast, splenectomy is rarely used to treat thrombocytopenia resulting from portal hypertension; variceal bleeding in these patients is not caused by thrombocytopenia. The decision to perform splenectomy for thrombocytopenia in patients with myeloproliferative syndromes must be individualized to each case and weighed against its complications, both surgical and those related to the specific disease process.

THROMBOCYTOPENIA CAUSED BY PERIPHERAL PLATELET DESTRUCTION

Increased peripheral platelet destruction (caused by immune or nonimmune mechanisms) commonly leads to thrombocytopenia. Autoimmune thrombocytopenia may present as a primary immune disorder directed only at platelets or as a secondary complication of another autoimmune disease, such as systemic lupus erythematosus. The pathophysiology of immune platelet destruction involves increased levels of polyclonal antiplatelet antibodies in the circulation and coating the platelet. These antibodies are usually directed against platelet mem-

brane glycoprotein receptors, most often glycoprotein IIb/IIIa (gpIIb/IIIa) or Ib (gpIb). Coating of the platelet with these antibodies leads to opsonization of the platelets by Fc receptors on cells of the reticuloendothelial system (RES). Antibody-coated platelets are cleared by the spleen and, to a lesser extent, by the liver. These disorders generally involve a dramatic increase in marrow platelet production reflected by increased numbers of marrow megakaryocytes. The younger platelets produced have relatively high granule contents providing increased hemostatic function. Bone marrow examination for the presence of increased or normal megakaryocyte numbers is the traditional means of distinguishing platelet destruction from decreased production. However, data suggest that increased percentages of *reticulated platelets* in the circulation are associated with destructive, especially immune-mediated, thrombocytopenia and may be sufficient for diagnosing platelet destruction. Thrombocytopenia resulting from immune clearance may be severe, and platelet survival is reduced from the normal 7 to 10 days often to less than 1 day. Despite severe thrombocytopenia, even in the range of 1000 to 2000/μL, serious bleeding or hemorrhagic death is rare, partly because the function of young platelets is increased and partly because the number of circulating platelets required to maintain vascular integrity is relatively low, only 7100/μL/day.

IMMUNE THROMBOCYTOPENIC PURPURA

In children, *acute immune thrombocytopenic purpura* (ITP) is often preceded by a viral infection, such as varicella. Patients with ITP present with petechial hemorrhage, mucosal bleeding, and thrombocytopenia with counts often lower than 20,000/μL. The peripheral blood smear shows large platelets and no other abnormal cells (such as blasts, which would accompany childhood leukemia); the bone marrow demonstrates increased, or occasionally normal, numbers of megakaryocytes. The diagnosis of ITP is partly made by exclusion: fever, organomegaly, pancytopenia, lymphadenopathy, or abnormal peripheral blood cells should prompt an evaluation for malignant disease, such as leukemia, neuroblastoma, or Wilms' tumor, or other nonmalignant bone marrow disorders. Laboratory tests may complement the clinical evaluation, but they are not required to make the diagnosis of ITP. These include the demonstration of an increased percentage of reticulated platelets in the peripheral blood or the detection of platelet autoantibodies in serum or on the platelet (*platelet-associated immunoglobulin*). However, assays of platelet-associated antibodies are not specific for ITP, because immunoglobulins that bind nonspecifically to platelets are often increased in patients with thrombocytopenia secondary to other causes. Techniques that measure specific platelet glycoprotein reactivity of antibodies hold greater promise for diagnostic use. An increase in mean platelet volume is also a relatively insensitive and nonspecific indicator of destructive thrombocytopenia, in part because of the wide range of normal values.

Acute ITP in children can resolve without therapy, but most clinicians prefer to treat children with steroids or intravenous immunoglobulin (IVIG). IVIG therapy for ITP is thought to work by multiple mechanisms: (1) high IgG concentrations block Fc receptors on phagocytes of the RES and on cellular effectors of antibody-dependent cytotoxicity; (2) infusion of IgG increases the fractional rate of IgG catabolism and thereby increases the destruction of antiplatelet IgG in direct proportion to its concentration; and (3) IVIG may increase clearance of antiplatelet Ig through anti-idiotypic effects. More than 80% of children with acute ITP have a rapid remission, and ITP does not recur. A subset of 10% to 20% go on to develop recurrent thrombocytopenia (i.e., chronic ITP); however, more than 70% of such children respond completely to splenectomy. For those with chronic courses after splenectomy, episodic IVIG, RhoGAM (see later discussion), and, in severe cases, immunosuppressive therapy are used. Hemorrhagic deaths are rare in childhood ITP (<2%), but some mortality (2% to 5%) is associated with chronic, refractory ITP.

As with children, the diagnosis of ITP in adults is made largely by exclusion, but unlike in children, acute ITP in adults rarely remits spontaneously and is much more likely to become a chronic disorder, evolving to chronic ITP in more than 50% of patients. Petechial hemorrhage and mucosal bleeding are accompanied by platelet counts commonly lower than 20,000/μL and often as low as 1000 to 2000/μL. Hemorrhagic deaths occur in fewer than 10% of adults with ITP. In adults, ITP may be associated with other diseases, such as human immunodeficiency virus (HIV) infection. ITP is often the presenting manifestation of HIV infection, whereas thrombocytopenia in more advanced stages of HIV infection is more often caused by bone marrow failure resulting from megakaryocyte infection with HIV, mycobacterial infection of the bone marrow, and nutritional deficiencies of end-stage HIV disease. ITP also occurs in patients with autoimmune disorders such as systemic lupus erythematosus, inflammatory bowel disease, and hepatitis. As in de novo ITP, thrombocytopenia in these autoimmune disorders is caused by increased peripheral platelet destruction, with normal or increased megakaryocytes on bone marrow examination, and increased platelet-associated immunoglobulin. Antibody may be directed against platelet gpIIb/IIIa or gpIb, or clearance by nonspecific immune complex deposition on the platelet membrane may occur. Therapy of both ITP and the underlying autoimmune disorder is usually complementary.

Immune platelet destruction can also be associated with drugs (see Table 52–2). Some drugs (especially quinidine or quinine-based formulations) bind to platelets and create a *hapten*, a neoantigen of the platelet and drug together. Antibody is directed against this neoantigen and causes rapid clearance of platelets by the RES. Development of thrombocytopenia is temporally related to exposure to the drug and is usually rapid; discontinuation of the drug causes an equally rapid rise in the platelet count. Other medications that cause immune thrombocytopenia include sulfa compounds, gold salts, and psychotropic drugs. Discontinuing the medication is always necessary but may need to be accompanied by steroid or IVIG therapy.

The first-line treatment of acute ITP in adults is steroids, usually prednisone, 1 to 2 mg/kg/day. Platelet transfusions are not generally used in ITP because transfused platelet survival is brief and bleeding complications are uncommon; however, in patients with significant bleeding or the need for surgery, platelet transfusions have been safely used and may transiently increase the platelet count, although usually for less than 24 hours. In patients with acute ITP with severe thrombocytopenia (<5000/μL) or with life-threatening bleeding, high-dose methylprednisolone (1 g/day for 3 days) may be used alone or in combination with IVIG (2 g/kg in divided doses over 2 to 5 days). In recurrent ITP, chronic steroid treatment is often necessary but is usually accompanied by significant side effects. Evidence indicates that patients, both children and adults, with chronic ITP who initially responded to IVIG therapy respond well to subsequent splenectomy, whereas those who did not respond to IVIG are less likely to have a disease remission after splenectomy. More than 50% of patients with chronic ITP have some degree of disease remission after splenectomy, although about one third of patients who undergo splenectomy will continue to have chronic ITP. If ITP does recur after splenectomy, one must rule out the presence of an accessory spleen, usually by liver and spleen scanning, because Howell-Jolly bodies may still be present. Recurrent disease may often be episodic, especially after viral infections, and these patients can be treated with IVIG, or RhoGAM in patients who are Rh-positive. *RhoGAM* is antibody to the blood group Rh D antigen, which induces mild hemolysis, presumably causing Fc receptor blockade of the RES in the same manner as IVIG and thereby decreased platelet uptake by the spleen and liver. RhoGAM is generally ineffective in patients who have undergone splenectomy. In patients who fail to respond to splenectomy, steroid dosage may be spared by the addition of danazol, colchicine, and immunosuppressive therapy (most often cyclophosphamide). About 5% of adults with ITP die of chronic, refractory disease.

ALLOIMMUNE THROMBOCYTOPENIA

Neonatal alloimmune thrombocytopenia occurs when the mother is homozygous for an uncommon platelet alloantigen, most often Pl^{A2} on gpIIIa, and the fetus expresses the Pl^{A1} haplotype inherited from the father (Table 52–3). The pathogenesis of alloimmune thrombocytopenia is analogous to the mechanism by which Rh sensitization induces hemolytic disease of the newborn. The mother is exposed to the Pl^{A1} antigen during a first pregnancy, and in second and subsequent pregnancies, she produces high-titer IgG antibody against Pl^{A1}. These antibodies cross the placenta, react with Pl^{A1}-positive fetal platelets, and cause peripheral platelet destruction by the RES. Neonatal alloimmune thrombocytopenia may be severe, but this does not necessarily predict whether bleeding will occur in utero, at delivery, or in the first days of life. Maternal platelets (lacking Pl^{A1}) and IVIG are used to treat bleeding and to restore the platelet count.

Alloimmune thrombocytopenia can also occur in

TABLE 52–3   Human Platelet Alloantigens

Glycoprotein	Alleles (Alloantigens)	Phenotype Frequency	Amino Acid and Location
GPIIIa	Pl^{A1}/Pl^{A2}	0.98/0.25	Leucine/proline; 33
GPIIIa	Pen^a/Pen^b	0.99/0.01	Arginine/glutamine; 143
GPIIb	Bak^a/Bak^b	0.91/0.70	Isoleucine/serine; 843
GPIb	Ko^b/Ko^a	0.99/0.14	Threonine/methionine; 145
GPIa	Br^b/Br^a	NA/0.21	Glutamic acid/lysine; 505

NA = data not available.

adults after transfusion (*posttransfusion purpura*). As in neonates, this condition is based on exposure to a common platelet alloantigen such as Pl^{A1} that is not present on the patient's native platelets. This disorder most commonly occurs after red blood cell or platelet transfusions in a woman who is homozygous for Pl^{A2} and who is alloimmunized to Pl^{A1} as a result of previous pregnancy or more rarely in any patient alloimmunized because of prior transfusion. More than 90% of blood donors express Pl^{A1}, and Pl^{A1} is shed by platelets. Consequently, even red blood cell products with little platelet contamination contain Pl^{A1}. The anamnestic response to the blood product causes destruction of residual donor platelets and, even more interestingly, destruction of native platelets *that do not express the Pl^{A1} alloantigen*. The pathophysiology of this aspect of posttransfusion purpura is unclear, although evidence suggests that native platelets may be destroyed either nonspecifically by the RES or by adsorption of Pl^{A1} onto host platelets. As with neonates, these patients are treated with IVIG, and any further transfusions must be derived from homozygous Pl^{A2} donors. Although Pl^{A2} is the most common cause of alloimmune thrombocytopenia, other platelet alloantigens have been found to cause this clinical syndrome (see Table 52–3).

Thrombocytopenia in neonates can also be caused by maternal ITP. Antiplatelet antibodies are commonly IgG antibodies that may cross the placenta and induce thrombocytopenia in the fetus. However, significant neonatal thrombocytopenia is rare with maternal ITP and occurs in fewer than 10% of those at risk, although some evidence indicates that the incidence of neonatal thrombocytopenia is increased when the mother has ITP and maternal platelet counts lower than 75,000/μL. Sometimes, the mother needs to be treated for ITP with the goal of decreasing placental transfer of the maternal autoantibody, although in most instances of maternal ITP, fetal thrombocytopenia is uncommon or mild, and safe vaginal delivery may be accomplished.

HEPARIN-INDUCED THROMBOCYTOPENIA

Although also immune in nature, heparin-induced thrombocytopenia (HIT) must be distinguished from other drug-induced forms of ITP because of its potentially catastrophic *thrombotic* complications and its unique pathophysiology. Nearly 25% of patients who are exposed to unfractionated heparin will develop antibodies (detected by enzyme-linked immunosorbent assay) that recognize the complex of heparin and platelet factor 4 (PF4), the latter released from the α granule after platelet activation. When such patients receive heparin again, about 20% of these patients develop HIT, most with platelet counts between 50,000 and 100,000/μL. The mechanism of thrombocytopenia appears to be platelet Fc receptor binding of this antibody-heparin-PF4 complex. Fc binding then causes signal transduction in the platelet and induces activation, granule release, platelet destruction, and resultant thrombocytopenia. Although this procoagulant response can be reproduced in vitro in most patients with HIT, fewer than 10% to 20% of HIT patients will actually develop thrombotic complications, but these complications may be severe. Although thrombosis is more frequent in patients with concomitant cardiovascular disease who are receiving full-dose heparin, any heparin dose (even heparin flushes) can result in thrombosis in these patients. HIT has been reported in association with Swan-Ganz catheters embedded with heparin as the only source of ongoing heparin exposure. Arterial and venous thromboemboli can occur while the patient is receiving heparin and even after heparin is discontinued, an effect perhaps mediated by the continued circulation of procoagulant platelet microparticles. Discontinuation of heparin is critical; moreover, although the antibody may have been induced by treatment with *unfractionated* heparin, more than 80% of these antibodies cross-react with low-molecular-weight heparins, and approximately 15% of them react with heparinoid. Thus, the preferred therapies for short-term anticogulation in patients with HIT are the hirudin-like compounds (e.g., lepirudin) and argatroban. These direct thrombin inhibitors do not cross-react with the heparin-PF4 antibodies in HIT; warfarin is the usual choice for long-term anticogulation. Warfarin, given on a short-term basis in HIT, especially without additional anticoagulant coverage, may result in catastrophic limb thrombosis in these patients, perhaps because of a mechanism mediated by protein C deficiency, similar to the warfarin skin necrosis syndrome (see Chapter 53).

DISSEMINATED INTRAVASCULAR COAGULATION

One of the most common and potentially life-threatening causes of nonimmune peripheral platelet destruction is DIC; DIC is associated with sepsis, malignancy, advanced liver disease, and other disorders that trigger endotoxin release or cause severe tissue damage (Table 52–4). In DIC caused by bacterial sepsis, the extrinsic pathway is activated by circulating endotoxin that induces expression of tissue factor on circulating monocytes and endothelial cells, a process leading to overwhelming thrombin and fibrin generation. Deposition of fibrin occurs throughout the vasculature, with relatively inadequate concurrent fibrinolysis, and leads to a thrombotic or microangiopathic vasculopathy and subsequent organ damage. Thrombin activation of platelets and circulating factors eventually overwhelms the bone marrow and liver synthetic capability, respectively, and results in thrombocytopenia and prolongation of the PT and PTT. Thus, although the primary lesion of DIC is clot generation, the clinical end point is usually *consumptive coagulopathy*. The thrombocytopenia and low factor levels resulting from the consumptive coagulopathy cause mucosal bleeding, especially in the GI tract, and characteristic oozing from intravenous puncture sites.

In the consumptive coagulopathy of DIC, fibrinogen levels are usually low, but they may be normal or slightly high; the acute phase reaction to sepsis or the underlying disorder may actually increase fibrinogen secretion and may lead to normal levels in the midst of DIC. Therefore, DIC should not be ruled out because fibrinogen is in the normal range. Fibrinolysis in DIC is triggered by fibrin clot and tissue-type plasminogen activator; laboratory testing usually shows increased levels of fibrin split products to more than 40 μg/mL (cleavage of fibrin monomers) and D-dimer to more than 0.5 μg/mL (cleavage of fibrin-fibrin bonds). Although fibrin split products are usually elevated in DIC, this finding is nonspecific; in contrast, an elevated D-dimer is more specific for DIC and is often used to confirm the elevated fibrin split product screening assay.

TABLE 52–4 Causes of Disseminated Intravascular Coagulation

Sepsis or Endotoxin
Gram-negative bacteremia

Tissue Damage
Trauma
Closed head injury
Burns
Hypoperfusion or hypotension

Malignant Disease
Adenocarcinoma
Acute promyelocytic leukemia

Primary Vascular Disorders
Vasculitis
Giant hemangioma (Kasabach-Merritt)
Aortic aneurysm
Cardiac mural thrombus

Exogenous Causes
Snake venom
Activated factor infusions (prothrombin complex concentrate)

Chronic DIC may be triggered by consumption of platelets and factors into large clots found in aneurysms, hemangiomas, and mural thrombi. A unique cause of chronic DIC is malignant disease, often adenocarcinoma or acute promyelocytic leukemia; malignant cells in these disorders secrete substances that either activate factor X or simulate factor Xa activity. Xa activation leads to formation of the prothrombinase complex, production of thrombin, and platelet activation and clearance; chronic DIC in this circumstance usually causes enough factor consumption that both the PT and the PTT are slightly prolonged. Clinically, such patients present with *migratory thrombophlebitis (Trousseau's syndrome)* or *nonbacterial thrombotic (marantic) endocarditis.*

Therapy of DIC should be aimed at the following: (1) the underlying disorder, such as antibiotics for sepsis or chemotherapy for malignant disease; (2) supportive hemostatic therapy including platelets, cryoprecipitate (for fibrinogen), and fresh-frozen plasma; and (3) disrupting activation of coagulation factors and platelets. For the last approach, anticoagulation is generally not indicated unless the balance of procoagulant versus anticoagulant activity actively favors clotting, such as arterial thromboemboli with mural thrombus or migratory thrombophlebitis with Trousseau's syndrome. These thrombotic complications of chronic DIC are often resistant to warfarin therapy; resolution of DIC generally requires more intensive anti-Xa therapy (unfractionated or low-molecular-weight heparin), as well as successful treatment of the underlying malignant disease or consumptive disorder. Besides anti-Xa agents, experimental therapies for controlling the coagulation disorder have included infusions of antithrombin III, activated protein C, and tissue factor pathway inhibitor. Although the extensive studies of antithrombin III have not shown a significant benefit for decreasing mortality associated with DIC, studies of activated protein C and tissue factor pathway inhibitor are ongoing and show promise.

THROMBOTIC THROMBOCYTOPENIC PURPURA

Another nonimmune cause of thrombocytopenia resulting from platelet activation and clearance is *thrombotic thrombocytopenic purpura* (TTP). In patients with congenital relapsing TTP, the normal von Willibrand factor (vWF)–cleaving protease is absent. Patients with acquired TTP without a family history usually have an antibody, often IgG, which blocks the normal function of this vWF-cleaving protease. Deficient protease function leads to decreased clearance and higher circulating levels of the larger, high-molecular-weight vWF multimers; these, in turn, cause increased platelet adhesion and clearance *without* activating the coagulation cascade. Therefore, the PT and the PTT are normal. TTP after chemotherapy (mitomycin C) and in association with HIV infection seems to have a similar pathogenesis. Thrombocytopenia (often severe) is accompanied by microangiopathy with schistocytes on the peripheral smear and increased serum lactate dehydogenase resulting from red blood cell lysis. Microvascular occlusions in multiple organs cause many of the symptoms, especially in the kidney and brain. The classic pentad of signs (fever, thrombocytopenia, microangiopathic hemolysis, neurologic symptoms, and renal insufficiency) is present in fewer than 25% of patients with TTP.

Treatment of TTP is based on removal of the antibody and replenishment of cleaving protease activity. These goals are generally accomplished by plasma exchange whereby patient plasma is removed and replaced with fresh-frozen plasma, often "cryo-poor" (to reduce vWF multimer levels in transfused plasma). Steroids and antiplatelet drugs (aspirin, dipyridamole) are often administered simultaneously, but the relative benefit of both agents remains controversial. Platelet transfusions are absolutely contraindicated in TTP.

Most authorities consider the *hemolytic uremic syndrome* (HUS) to be part of the TTP spectrum of disease; however, the hemolytic anemia and renal failure of HUS are not usually accompanied by neurologic impairment, and HUS generally does not have the same degree of thrombocytopenia or schistocytosis as TTP. Moreover, this is *not* associated with defective vWF-cleaving protease activity. Unlike TTP, HUS is primarily seen in children, and less commonly adults, with hemorrhagic colitis caused by Shiga-like toxin-producing bacteria, especially the *Escherichia coli* 0157.H7 serotype. The similar pathophysiology of microvascular platelet thrombi suggests that HUS is part of the TTP continuum, and indeed, patients with HUS respond to plasmapheresis with plasma exchange, as well as to maintenance dialysis until renal function recovers.

THROMBOCYTOPENIA WITH PREGNANCY-INDUCED HYPERTENSION

Mild thrombocytopenia in pregnant women is most often related to hemodilution and the normal physiology of pregnancy that commonly brings platelet counts into the range of 100,000 to 150,000/μL; these counts are not associated with maternal or fetal complications. In contrast, autoimmune causes of platelet destruction (as noted earlier) and pregnancy-induced hypertension can result in platelet counts lower than 100,000/μL with complications. The spectrum of *pregnancy-induced hypertension* includes hypertension progressing to proteinuria and renal dysfunction (*preeclampsia*) or to cerebral edema and seizures (*eclampsia*). Thrombocytopenia may appear as a late finding accompanying pregnancy-induced hypertension, most often at the time of delivery or late in the third trimester. The related *HELLP syndrome* in pregnancy is characterized by *h*emolysis, *el*evated *l*iver enzymes, and *l*ow *p*latelet counts. The thrombocytopenia associated with pregnancy-induced hypertension and HELLP is probably caused by abnormal vascular prostaglandin metabolism that leads to platelet consumption, vasculopathy, and microvascular occlusions. These disorders are usually reversed by delivery of the fetus and placenta. Occasionally, IVIG or plasmapheresis has been required to treat the disorder successfully. When thrombocytopenia does not resolve

after delivery, other processes, such as TTP, must be considered in the differential diagnosis.

ANTIPHOSPHOLIPID SYNDROME

Distinct from ITP associated with systemic lupus erythematosus, the antiphospholipid syndrome is not associated with bleeding. The *antiphospholipid syndrome* is characterized by destructive thrombocytopenia, recurrent thrombosis, or fetal loss and is diagnosed by the demonstration of a lupus anticoagulant and/or anticardiolipin antibody. The antiphospholipid syndrome can be a primary disorder, without diagnostic criteria for systemic lupus erythematosus, or it can occur secondary to true systemic lupus erythematosus. Thrombocytopenia in the antiphospholipid syndrome is caused by increased peripheral platelet destruction, not as a result of platelet-specific antibodies, but rather because of vascular angiopathy and increased platelet consumption in the microvasculature. Long-term, intensive anticoagulation with warfarin or low-molecular-weight heparin, sometimes with the addition of aspirin or other antiplatelet drugs, may prevent thrombotic complications and may restore platelet counts to normal (see Chapter 53).

DILUTIONAL THROMBOCYTOPENIA

In addition to sequestration and hypoproductive and destructive causes of thrombocytopenia, thrombocytopenia can also result from *hemodilution*. This circumstance usually follows massive red blood cell and plasma transfusions, especially for trauma, or cardiopulmonary bypass, in which significant hemodilution occurs by addition of the extracorporeal circuit to the normal circulatory system. Moreover, in addition to the hemodilution of bypass, platelets exposed to the cardiopulmonary bypass circuit become temporarily dysfunctional because of activation and loss of membrane receptors; this defect may be mild and transient, but occasionally it is severe and leads to bleeding, especially after long bypass procedures. After the conclusion of bypass or once the acute trauma is resolved, the platelet count rebounds within 48 to 72 hours; however, platelet transfusions may be needed to treat significant bleeding in these patients while the platelet count recovers.

Bleeding Caused by Platelet Disorders: Qualitative Platelet Defects

ASPIRIN AND ACQUIRED CAUSES OF PLATELET DYSFUNCTION

The ability of platelets to adhere to damaged vasculature and to recruit additional platelets into the clot is critical for primary hemostasis, especially when patients are challenged by surgery. One critical question for preoperative screening is whether patients are taking medi-

TABLE 52-5 Disorders Causing Abnormal Platelet Aggregation

	Response to Agonist				
	Epinephrine	**ADP**	**Collagen**	**Arachadonic acid**	**Ristocetin**
Aspirin/NSAIDs	#	#	NL, ↓*	↓	NL
Glanzmann's disease	Absent	Absent	Absent	Absent	#
Bernard-Soulier syndrome	NL	NL	NL	NL	Absent
Storage pool disease	↓	#	↓	NL, ↓	#
Hermansky-Pudlak syndrome	↓	#	↓	NL	#
Gray platelet syndrome	↓	↓	↓	NL	NL
vWD	NL	NL	NL	NL	↓, NL†

* Aspirin results in decreased aggregation with low-dose collagen, but aggregation is normal with high-dose collagen.

† In vWD type 2B, patients have increased aggregation with low-dose ristocetin, and decreased or normal aggregation with standard doses of ristocetin.

↓ = decreased; # = primary wave aggregation only; NL = normal; NSAIDs = nonsteroidal anti-inflammatory drugs; vWD = von Willebrand's disease.

cations that interfere with platelet function, such as aspirin. *Aspirin* irreversibly acetylates cyclooxygenase and thereby blocks normal arachidonic acid metabolism. All exposed platelets are irreversibly affected and do not respond to arachidonic acid even after aspirin is discontinued. The characteristic aspirin-induced platelet aggregation pattern is shown in Table 52–5. In contrast, *other nonsteroidal anti-inflammatory drugs* (e.g., indomethacin) *reversibly* inhibit cyclooxygenase, and platelet function is restored within 24 to 48 hours after discontinuation of the drug. Bleeding associated with aspirin or nonsteroidal drugs is usually mild, and aspirin may not need to be discontinued, especially because aspirin-induced platelet dysfunction is desirable in patients at risk of stroke or myocardial infarction. However, when bleeding caused by aspirin requires treatment, transfusion of platelets is appropriate. In most cases, a single platelet transfusion of 4 to 6 random donor units restores primary hemostasis. Platelet dysfunction and bleeding caused by other drugs (Table 52–6) are similarly treated by discontinuation of the drug and platelet transfusion when needed.

TABLE 52-6 Drugs Affecting Platelet Function

Strong Inhibitors
Abciximab (and other anti-gpIIb/IIIa or anti-RGD compounds)
Aspirin (often contained in over-the-counter medications)
Clopidogrel/ticlopidine (ADP receptor blockers)
Nonsteroidal anti-inflammatory drugs

Moderate Inhibitors
Antibiotics (penicillins, cephalosporins, nitrofurantoin)
Dextran
Fibrinolytics
Heparin
Hetastarch

Weak Inhibitors
Alcohol
Nitroglycerin
Nitroprusside

Uremic platelet dysfunction is caused by proteins that accumulate in renal failure and poison platelet adhesive function. Control of renal failure with dialysis and maintenance of the hematocrit are usually adequate to preserve platelet function. However, uremic bleeding is a common inpatient problem, especially in the setting of acute renal failure. Short-term treatment of uremic platelet dysfunction includes desmopressin (DDAVP), which has been shown to shorten the bleeding time significantly, and cryoprecipitate. Conjugated estrogens are of some benefit for long-term treatment. Platelet transfusions may be useful in patients with life-threatening bleeding and renal failure, but the effect of this treatment is short-lived because the transfused platelets rapidly acquire the uremic defect.

CONGENITAL PLATELET DYSFUNCTION

Inherited qualitative platelet defects include abnormalities of platelet receptors and granules. Two rare but well-characterized platelet receptor disorders are *Bernard-Soulier syndrome* and *Glanzmann's thrombasthenia*. Bernard-Soulier syndrome is caused by decreased surface expression of platelet GPIb (the primary vWF receptor) and more rarely by diminished GPIb function. The syndrome is characterized by mild thrombocytopenia, increased bleeding time, large platelets, and a mild to moderate bleeding disorder. The diagnosis is usually made in children, but occasionally the condition may not be manifest until adulthood. Laboratory testing for Bernard-Soulier syndrome shows an absent platelet aggregation response to ristocetin (see Table 52–5) despite adequate vWF levels and vWF function, such as normal ristocetin cofactor (Rcof) activity. Glanzmann's thrombasthenia is characterized by an increased bleeding time and abnormally low levels of platelet GPIIb/IIIa expression (the receptor for both vWF and fibrinogen) or, more rarely, normal expression but absent GPIIb/IIIa function. Patients commonly present with bleeding in childhood. Platelet aggregation testing in Glanzmann's thrombasthenia shows absent or diminished response to all agonists except ristocetin (see Table 52–5). Platelet transfusions correct the bleeding in both Bernard-Soulier syndrome and Glanzmann's thrombasthenia. However, because of the high risk of alloimmunization with frequent platelet transfusions, this therapy should be used sparingly.

Inherited platelet granule disorders are defined by the type of granule that is absent or defective. *Storage pool disease* is characterized by a relative decrease or absence of dense granules and correspondingly moderate to severe mucosal bleeding. Because of the defect in dense granules, release of granule constituents that recruit and activate platelets is impaired. Thus, storage pool disease is characterized by a diminished or absent secondary wave aggregation to most agonists (see Table 52–5). *Hermansky-Pudlak syndrome* is a similar dense granule deficiency associated with oculocutaneous albinism and mild thrombocytopenia. Patients have significant bleeding, which may occur spontaneously but more often in association with surgical procedures. *Chédiak-Higashi disease* is a general granule disorder characterized by mild bleeding, partial albinism, and recurrent pyogenic infections. *Gray platelet syndrome* is characterized by colorless or gray platelets that lack normal staining on the peripheral smear; electron microscopy confirms the loss of α granules and/or their contents. Patients with gray platelet syndrome have a mild bleeding history, and aggregation testing exhibits diminished responses to epinephrine, ADP, and collagen. All the platelet granule disorders are successfully treated by avoidance of aspirin and other antiplatelet drugs, by hormonal control of menses in women, and, when bleeding occurs, by platelet transfusions.

VON WILLEBRAND'S DISEASE

Disorders of plasma proteins, which are the functional ligands for platelet adhesion to the vasculature, cause bleeding that clinically resembles the bleeding associated with platelet or vascular disorders (epistaxis, GI bleeding). vWF is synthesized in endothelial cells and megakaryocytes and functions in plasma to mediate platelet rolling along damaged vessels and subsequent platelet adhesion to the damaged site (see Fig. 51–1). vWf is a large molecule that polymerizes to form multimeric proteins of varying size; the largest multimers contain the greatest number of adhesive sites and thus confer greater hemostatic ability than smaller vWF molecules. In patients with abnormal or low vWF levels, platelet adhesion to damaged vessels is delayed, and the results are mucosal bleeding and a prolonged bleeding time. vWF also serves as the carrier protein for factor VIII; deficiency of vWF or abnormal vWF-VIII binding leads to rapid clearance of factor VIII, decreased factor VIII levels, and a prolonged PTT. Many mutations in the vWF gene have been described; these have been phenotypically grouped into three major subtypes of vWD (Table 52–7).

Most patients have *type 1 vWD*, a mild to moderate *quantitative* decrease in all vWF multimers. This condition is commonly caused by a heterozygous mutation and shows a dominant pattern of inheritance. Type 1 vWD is characterized by equivalent decreases in factor VIII, vWF antigen, and Rcof activity; Rcof measures the ability of patient plasma (which contains vWF) to agglutinate normal platelets in the presence of ristocetin. Patients with type 1 vWD usually have mild to moderate bleeding, often only in relation to surgery or dental procedures. Historically, patients with type 1 vWD were treated with cryoprecipitate, which is rich in vWF. However, because cryoprecipitate cannot be virally inactivated, alternatives are now used. DDAVP stimulates endothelial cells to release stored vWF and leads to an increase in plasma vWF antigen, Rcof, and factor VIII levels. DDAVP, at 0.3 μg/kg given subcutaneously, is commonly used in type 1 vWD with excellent results. However, tachyphylaxis to DDAVP may occur, because endothelial cells require time to synthesize new vWF after repeated DDAVP dosing. Thus, VWF concentrates must sometimes be used in patients with more severe type 1 vWD or in those who are undergoing a more prolonged hemostatic challenge. Virally inactivated, *intermediate-purity* factor VIII products (not recombinant or monoclonal antibody-purified) contain large amounts of vWF (e.g., Humate-P) and are the preferred therapy after DDAVP. Bleeding in type 1 vWD during pregnancy is exceedingly rare. Because vWF rises markedly in pregnancy, vWF antigen and Rcof levels usually normalize during the second or third trimester and eliminate the bleeding risk for that time. Most pregnant

TABLE 52–7   Classification of von Willebrand's Disease (vWD)

	Type 1	Type 2A	Type 2B	Type 2M	Type 2N	Type 3	Pseudo-vWD	BSS
Inheritance	AD	AD/AR	AD/AR	AD	AR	AR/AD	AD	AR
Platelet count	NL	NL	NL, ↓	NL	NL	NL	↓, NL	↓, NL
Bleeding time	NL, ↑	↑	↑	↑	NL, ↑	↑↑	↑	↑
PTT	NL, ↑	↑, NL	↑, NL	↑	↑↑	↑↑	↑, NL	NL
VIII	NL, ↓	NL, ↓	↓, NL	NL, ↓	↓↓	↓↓	↓, NL	NL
vWF:Ag	NL, ↓	NL, ↓	↓, NL	NL	NL	Absent	↓, NL	NL
vWF: Rcof	NL, ↓	↓↓	↓, NL	↓↓	NL	Absent	↓, NL	NL
Multimers	NL, ↓	↓ H/I	↓↓ H	NL	NL	Absent	↓↓ H	NL
RIPA	N1, ↓	↓↓	↑*	↓	NL	↓↓	↑*	↓↓

↑ = increased; ↓ = decreased; ↑* = increased agglutination to low-dose ristocetin; AD = autosomal dominant; AR = autosomal recessive; BSS = Bernard-Soulier syndrome; H = high-molecular-weight multimers; I = intermediate-molecular-weight multimers; NL = normal; PTT = partial thromboplastin time; RIPA = ristocetin-induced platelet agglutination; vWF:Ag = von Willebrand factor antigen level; vWF:Rcof = von Willebrand factor: ristocetin cofactor activity.

women with type 1 vWD have no bleeding complications with delivery and do not require therapy during pregnancy or in the early postpartum period.

Type 2 vWD is characterized by heterozygous mutations of variable penetrance that produce a *qualitative* defect in the vWF molecule; the most common type 2 disorders are characterized by a relative lack of the larger vWF multimers (see Table 52–7). High- and intermediate-molecular-weight vWF multimers by electrophoresis are absent in *type 2A disease*, and platelet-associated function is moderately decreased; patients with type 2A vWD show disproportionately low ristocetin cofactor activity compared with vWF antigen. Patients with type 2A vWD respond to vWF concentrate and less commonly to DDAVP. The abnormal vWF molecule in *type 2B vWD* has increased affinity for platelets, a situation that causes loss of high-molecular-weight multimers from the circulation and often produces thrombocytopenia. Platelet aggregometry in type 2B vWD (see Table 52–7) shows an abnormal increase in low-dose ristocetin-induced platelet agglutination; in the laboratory, the addition of patient vWF to normal platelets similarly increases ristocetin-induced platelet agglutination and confirms the abnormal vWF. DDAVP would induce release of the abnormal vWF in patients with type 2B vWD and therefore is contraindicated in this disorder; vWF concentrate should be used instead.

Type 2M vWD demonstrates decreased platelet-dependent function with laboratory findings similar to those in type 2A, but high-molecular-weight multimers are present by electrophoresis. Some patients with type 2M vWD respond to DDAVP, but most require vWF concentrate. In *type 2N vWD*, the abnormal vWF molecule has decreased binding affinity for factor VIII, a characteristic that decreases VIII survival and produces a phenotype similar to that of hemophilia A. The low factor VIII levels do not respond to high-purity factor VIII infusions, unlike in true hemophilia A, but they improve with vWF concentrate. Rcof and vWF antigen levels are normal in type 2N vWD because the mutation in the factor VIII binding site does not affect vWF function or survival.

The rare patient with *type 3 vWD* has a complete deficiency of vWF as a result of inheritance of two abnormal vWF alleles; these compound heterozygotes have absent or extremely low levels of both Rcof and vWF antigen and factor VIII levels of 3% to 10%. Patients with type 3 vWD usually have severe bleeding that may mimic hemophilia. Type 3 vWD does not respond to DDAVP and requires vWF concentrates for bleeding.

vWD occasionally presents as an acquired defect, usually as a severe, type 2A–like defect with absent larger vWF multimers. *Acquired vWD* is caused by abnormal clearance of the larger vWF multimers and is commonly associated with monoclonal gammopathies, lymphoproliferative disorders, or myeloma, as well as with other malignant and myeloproliferative diseases characterized by thrombocytosis. Acquired vWD has been successfully treated with IVIG and therapy of the underlying disease.

Fibrinogen Disorders

Fibrinogen functions as a bridging ligand for the platelet receptor gpIIb/IIIa in the platelet-platelet matrix at sites of vascular damage. Fibrinogen also functions in the final steps of the coagulation cascade to form fibrin clot. Low fibrinogen levels are most commonly seen with consumptive disorders such as *DIC*, although rare congenital hypofibrinogenemias and afibrinogenemias are recognized. *Dysfibrinogenemia* is defined as an abnormal fibrinogen protein. Patients with dysfibrinogenemia usually bleed because of decreased adhesive function, but some patients have a hypercoagulable state. Dysfibrinogenemia is occasionally inherited, but it is more often acquired with liver disease. Both the PT and the PTT are prolonged by abnormalities of fibrinogen quantity or function because it is in the common pathway of coagulation (Table 52–8). A prolonged thrombin time is more specific for a low fibrinogen level or abnormal molecule, although inhibitors such as heparin and fibrin

TABLE 52-8   Screening Laboratory Results in Coagulation Factor Deficiencies

Deficient Factor	Frequency	PT	PTT	TT
I (fibrinogen)	Rare	↑	↑	↑
II (prothrombin)	Very rare	↑	↑	↑
V	1:1,000,000	↑	↑	NL
VII	1:500,000	↑	NL	NL
VIII	1:5000 (male)	NL	↑	NL
IX	1:30,000 (male)	NL	↑	NL
X	1:500,000	↑	↑	NL
XI	Rare*	NL	↑	NL
XII† or HMWK† or PK†	Rare	NL	↑	NL
XIII	Rare	NL	NL	NL

* Except in those of Ashkenazi Jewish descent (approximately 4% are heterozygous for factor XI deficiency).
† Not associated with clinical bleeding.

↑ = increased over normal range; HMWK = high-molecular-weight kininogen; NL = normal; PK = prekallikrein; PT = prothrombin time; PTT = partial thromboplastin time; TT = thrombin time.

split products also prolong the thrombin time. The *reptilase time,* which is insensitive to heparin, can be used to eliminate the possibility of an increased thrombin time resulting from heparin contamination of the sample. Both hypofibrinogenemia and dysfibrinogenemia are treated with cryoprecipitate, the blood product most enriched for fibrinogen.

Bleeding Caused by Coagulation Factor Disorders

HEMOPHILIA AND OTHER INHERITED FACTOR DEFICIENCIES

With normal platelet function, primary hemostasis initiates plugging of vascular lesions and maintains mucosal integrity. However, if abnormalities of coagulation factors are present, then the initial platelet plug is not solidified by normal secondary hemostasis, and the effects are clot breakdown and bleeding. This bleeding differs from platelet-type bleeding; coagulation deficiencies lead to bleeding in deep tissues and joints, and milder deficiencies may present as bleeding in a delayed fashion after surgery. Most patients with significant factor deficiencies present with abnormal results of screening laboratory tests (see Table 52–8), although patients with mild deficiencies can still present with bleeding and normal coagulation screens.

The X-linked deficiencies of factor VIII *(hemophilia A)* and factor IX *(hemophilia B)* are the most common factor deficiencies, after vWD. Hemophilia A is about six times more frequent than hemophilia B. Approximately 50% or more of cases of severe hemophilia A arise as a result of an inversion of a major portion of the gene that results in complete loss of activity. Other mutations tend to result in milder disease. Most patients with hemophilia B have mutations that result in a functionally abnormal factor IX with absent activity. The combined results of antigenic and functional assays can resolve whether deficiency is due to loss of the protein or loss of its normal function. Both hemophilia A and hemophilia B are categorized by their factor levels: severe deficiency is characterized by absent (<1%) factor VIII or IX, whereas patients with moderate and mild hemophilia have factor levels of 1% to 5% and more than 5%, respectively. Severe hemophilia A and hemophilia B present in childhood with bleeding into muscles, joints, and soft tissue. Because they are X-linked

disorders, they are seen primarily in males; the mother of an affected male is a carrier, and 50% of maternal uncles have the disease. About 25% to 30% of cases of hemophilia, however, result from new mutations and hence have no relevant family history. In exceedingly rare instances, a female carrier with extremely skewed X-inactivation may have a mild bleeding disorder. Bleeding in severe hemophilia is often spontaneous, as well as common after any type of surgery or even mild trauma.

Bleeding in hemophilia frequently occurs in joints and the retroperitoneum; hematuria and mucosal and intracranial bleeding also occur. Patients with moderate hemophilia have less spontaneous bleeding, but they are still at significant risk of hemorrhagic complications of surgery or trauma. Patients with mild hemophilia may be undetected into adulthood and may present only with bleeding after major surgery. The complications of hemophilia stem from chronic bleeding into joints and muscles that leads to severe deformities, arthritis, muscle atrophy, and contractures; these complications require intensive physical therapy and orthopedic care, often culminating in joint replacement. In addition, patients with hemophilia who received pooled factor concentrates before the era of viral inactivation have complications related to transfusion-transmitted infections, especially HIV and hepatitis B and C. Current therapy uses factor concentrates that are virally inactivated or recombinant. Rapid factor replacement is the key to effective therapy. Patients with severe hemophilia often infuse low doses of prophylactic factor on a regular basis (25 to 40 U/kg 3 times per week) and boost their dose or the frequency of infusion when they sense internal bleeding, sustain trauma, or undergo dental procedures (Table 52–9).

Patients with mild hemophilia A may not need factor infusions for minor surgery; indeed, such patients are often managed with ϵ-aminocaproic acid (EACA), 4 g q4–6h, with or without infusions of DDAVP of 0.3 μg/kg. However, most patients with hemophilia require factor infusions, if not prophylactically, then at times of surgery or trauma. Factor VIII products are infused every 8 to 12 hours, and 1 U/kg of factor VIII concentrate raises plasma factor VIII activity by 2%; thus, 50 U/kg of factor VIII theoretically will yield 100% factor VIII activity in a patient with severe hemophilia. Factor IX has a longer half-life and is infused every 18 to 24 hours; factor IX requires 2 U/kg for a 2% increase in factor IX activity: that is, 100 U/kg for 100% activity. Major surgery in patients with hemophilia requires intensive factor therapy to achieve normal factor levels

TABLE 52–9   Factor Replacement Guidelines in Hemophilia A and B

| Injury | Factor VIII (U/kg) | | Factor IX (U/kg) | |
	Initial dosing	Maintenance	Initial dosing	Maintenance
Dental prophylaxis	20	10–20 q12h	10–20	20 q12h
Hemarthrosis	10–20	10–20 q12h	30–60	20 q24h
Muscle hematoma	20–30	20 q12h	30–50	30 q24h
Trauma or surgery	50	20–30 q8h	60–100	40–80 q24h

(>80%) in both the intraoperative period and the early postoperative period to prevent wound hematoma formation. The dosing of factors (see Table 52–9) is adjusted downward from this intensity, depending on the severity of the insult, the patient's response to previous factor infusions, and whether inhibitors to factor have developed.

INHERITED FACTOR DEFICIENCIES OTHER THAN HEMOPHILIA

Inherited bleeding disorders caused by deficiencies of coagulation factors V, VII, X, and XI (see Table 52–8) are much rarer than hemophilia. Patients with *factor V deficiency* usually lack both plasma factor V and platelet factor V and have joint and muscle bleeding like patients with hemophilia. Some plasma V–deficient persons are asymptomatic until they are challenged with the stress of surgery or trauma, and these patients are thought to have normal platelet factor V levels. Patients with factor V deficiency can be treated either with fresh-frozen plasma or with platelets; platelets are especially useful in patients who have developed inhibitors to factor V after receiving long-term plasma therapy. Rarely, patients inherit factor deficiencies in tandem, such as combined factor V and factor VIII deficiencies.

Patients with *factor XI deficiency* have a milder bleeding disorder than do patients with hemophilia (even with factor XI levels <5%) and are treated with plasma infusions, whereas *factor X deficiency* is usually more severe and is also treated with plasma. *Factor XI deficiency* is an autosomal recessive disorder seen with increased frequency among Ashkenazi Jews. *Acquired factor X deficiency* can occur in association with amyloidosis, a condition in which the abnormal circulating light chains adsorb to and clear factor X and produce low levels and occasional bleeding. The rare *factor VII– deficient patient* with levels of less than 10% can be treated with prothrombin complex concentrate (Proplex T has the highest factor VII levels) or with recombinant factor VIIa. The development of purified or recombinant factors was important because replacement of factor levels with fresh-frozen plasma is difficult at best. Factor concentrations in fresh-frozen plasma are similar to in vivo concentrations; thus, a patient may require 4 U of fresh-frozen plasma to increase factor levels from 0% to 30%. This high fluid load is problematic in patients with heart disease, liver failure, or renal insufficiency.

ACQUIRED COAGULATION FACTOR DISORDERS

Factor Inhibitors

Over time, about 25% of patients with hemophilia A develop autoantibodies to transfused factor VIII. An inhibitor acts functionally in vivo such that previously therapeutic infusions of factor concentrate result in lower factor levels and do not arrest bleeding. Inhibitors are measured in the United States as Bethesda units (BU); 1 BU is designated to be an inhibitor unit that neutralizes 50% of the factor activity in vitro under standard conditions. Inhibitor titers of less than 10 BU in hemophilia A can be overcome by infusion of high doses of concentrate. However, titers may be initially high or may increase over time with therapy to levels exceeding 10 BU. High-level inhibitors neutralize the activity of infused factor concentrates, even at extremely high doses. Bleeding in the presence of high inhibitor titers in hemophilia A requires treatment with *porcine* factor VIII, factor VIII inhibitor bypass activity (FEIBA), or recombinant factor VIIa (now approved in the United States). Unfortunately, many inhibitors recognize and block porcine factor VIII, either immediately or after prolonged exposure. In addition, like IVIG, porcine factor VIII is rationed and is difficult to acquire. Thus, FEIBA (an activated prothrombin complex concentrate) and recombinant factor VIIa are the treatments of choice for acute bleeding with significant factor VIII inhibitors. Long-term suppression of an inhibitor is accomplished by a combination of IVIG, immunosuppressive therapy, plasmapheresis, and induction of immune tolerance using high-dose concentrate infusions. Patients with hemophilia B have a lower incidence of inhibitors (2% to 6%), but otherwise they are treated in a similar fashion with high-dose prothrombin complex concentrate, FEIBA, or factor VIIa to bypass the inhibitor and with similar strategies for long-term suppression of the antibody.

Acquired inhibitors to factor VIII (and more rarely to other coagulation factors) occasionally occur in persons who do not have hemophilia. These patients do not have a bleeding history until the development of the inhibitor. They usually present suddenly with hemophilia-like bleeding into joints and muscles. Acquired inhibitors are usually seen in older persons, and factor VIII inhibitor titers can be extremely high. Acquired factor inhibitors are commonly associated with malignant diseases, especially lymphoproliferative disorders. Patients with acquired inhibitors to factor VIII are similarly treated with factor VIIa, FEIBA, or porcine factor VIII. Intensive immunosuppressive therapy (cyclophosphamide and prednisone) is the mainstay of successful treatment and should be started as soon as possible to eradicate the inhibitor.

Vitamin K Deficiency

Inpatients and severely ill outpatients may have bleeding resulting from acquired coagulation factor deficiencies. Foremost among the causes of low factor levels is vitamin K deficiency. Vitamin K deficiency may be caused by any of the following: (1) biliary tract disease interfering with enterohepatic circulation and leading to decreased absorption of vitamin K; (2) drugs, especially antibiotics that sterilize the gut and reduce bacterial sources of vitamin K or other drugs (cholestyramine) that directly block vitamin K absorption; this category includes cephalosporins, which interfere with intrahepatic metabolism of this fat-soluble vitamin; and (3) poor nutritional status induced by malabsorptive disease (sprue), chronic disease, or poor oral intake in acutely ill patients. As noted previously, factors II, VII, IX, and X are vitamin K–dependent procoagulant factors, as are proteins C and S. Warfarin blocks vitamin K–dependent γ-carboxylation of these factors and causes an acute decrease in functional factor VII levels because factor VII has the shortest half-life (6 hours) of all vitamin K–dependent factors. Parenteral replacement of vitamin K (10 mg/day for 3 days) restores coagulation factor synthesis in the presence of a normal liver.

Bleeding in Patients with Liver Disease

Patients with mild to moderate liver disease have prolongation of the PT and usually normal PTT values. Severe liver disease prolongs both the PT and the PTT. Unlike patients with vitamin K deficiency or those receiving warfarin, patients with liver disease have low levels of nearly all factors, not just the vitamin K–dependent factors; the exception is factor VIII. Although liver transplantation increases factor VIII levels in patients with hemophilia, factor VIII levels usually *rise* with liver disease, a finding suggesting the presence of sources of factor VIII production outside the liver. If factor VIII levels are decreased in patients with liver disease, one should consider whether DIC is superimposed. Therefore, when one evaluates a prolonged PT for its cause, measurement of factor VII and a non–vitamin K–dependent factor such as factor V is most useful. In vitamin K deficiency, factor VII is low and factor V is normal; in contrast, levels of both factor VII and factor V should be low in patients with generalized liver disease. The PT is a sensitive measure of liver function and becomes elevated in patients with even mild liver disorders; this elevation precedes a significant decrease in the albumin or prealbumin levels and is usually coincident with transaminase changes. In patients with mild to moderate liver disease, the PT is prolonged, but the PTT usually remains in the normal range; when severe liver disease is present, the PT becomes even more prolonged, and the PTT becomes abnormal as well. Causes of bleeding in liver disease other than decreased factor synthesis include (1) decreased clearance of fibrin split products and/or associated DIC, (2) inhibition of platelet function, and (3) increased tissue plasminogen activator levels. Replacement of coagulation factors with fresh-frozen plasma is the treatment of choice. Although factor VII can be replaced with prothrombin complex concentrates rather than with fresh-frozen plasma, the activated factors in the concentrate are contraindicated in liver disease because they may actually precipitate DIC.

Bleeding in Patients with a Normal Laboratory Screen

Occasionally, patients with bleeding disorders present without any abnormalities in screening laboratory assays (PT, PTT, platelet count). As noted previously, these disorders include the vascular purpuras, but patients with other bleeding variants present in this fashion (see Fig. 52–1). Patients with bleeding caused by mild vWD may have a normal PTT, but additional studies usually show mild decreases in factor VIII, vWF antigen, or vWF Rcof; multimeric analysis may also be abnormal in patients with mild type 2A vWD. Similarly, mild factor deficiencies (factor II, V, VII, VIII, IX, or XI) may not prolong the PT or PTT, but specific factor assays demonstrate levels lower than the normal range. Mild bleeding, often with a delayed onset after surgery or trauma, may occur in patients with clot instability resulting from factor XIII deficiency or dysfibrinogenemia; in neonates, factor XIII deficiency may present with late umbilical stump bleeding. Factor XIII deficiency results in increased clot solubility in urea; if the clot dissolves in 8 mol/L urea, enzyme-linked immunosorbent assay for the factor XIII level should be performed. Factor XIII deficiency is treated with fresh-frozen plasma. Low fibrinogen levels or abnormal fibrinogen function will prolong both the thrombin time and the reptilase time. The thrombin time is also prolonged by heparin, but the reptilase time is insensitive to heparin and therefore can enable one to rule out the presence of contaminating heparin or to test fibrinogen levels and function in the presence of heparin. Finally, bleeding in patients with normal platelet counts and clotting times should be evaluated by testing of platelet qualitative function; inherited deficiencies of platelet receptors or granules and acquired platelet abnormalities with drugs or uremia can be diagnosed by demonstration of abnormal platelet aggregation results.

REFERENCES

Bolan CD, Alving BM: Pharmacologic agents in the management of bleeding disorders. Transfusion 1990; 30:541.

Burrows RF, Kelton JG: Fetal thrombocytopenia and its relation to maternal thrombocytopenia. N Engl J Med 1993; 329:1463–1466.

Dunlop LC, Andrews RK, Lopez JA, et al: Congenital disorders of platelet function. *In* Loscalzo J, Shafer A (eds): Thrombosis and Hemorrhage. Baltimore: Williams & Wilkins, 1998, pp 685–689.

Furie BC, Furie B: Vitamin K: Metabolism and disorders. *In* Hoffman R, Benz EJ Jr, Shattil SJ, et al (eds): Hematology: Basic Principles and Practice. New York: Churchill Livingstone, 1995, pp 1737–1741.

Furlan M, Robles R, Galbusera M, et al: von Willebrand factor–cleaving protease in thrombotic thrombocytopenic purpura and the hemolytic uremic syndrome. N Engl J Med 1998; 339:1578–1584.

Galanakis DK: Inherited dysfibrinogenemia: Emerging abnormal structure associations with pathologic and nonpathologic dysfunctions. Semin Thromb Hemost 1993; 19:386–395.

George JN, Shattil SJ: The clinical importance of acquired abnormalities of platelet function. N Engl J Med 1991; 324:27.

George JN, Woolf SH, Raskob GE, et al: Idiopathic thrombocytopenic purpura: A practice guideline developed by explicit methods for the American Society of Hematology. Blood 1996; 88:3–40.

Kasper CK, Boylen AL, Ewing NP: Hematologic management of hemophilia A for surgery. JAMA 1985; 253:1279.

Law C, Marcaccio M, Tam P, et al: High-dose intravenous immune globulin and the response to splenectomy in patients with idiopathic thrombocytopenic purpura. N Engl J Med 1997; 336:1494–1498.

Levi M, ten Cate H: Disseminated intravascular coagulation. N Engl J Med 1999; 341:586–592.

Nichols WC, Coone KA, Ginsburg, et al: von Willebrand disease. *In* Loscalzo J, Shafer A (eds): Thrombosis and Hemorrhage. Baltimore: Williams & Wilkins, 1998, pp 729–756.

Rinder MR, Richards RE, Rinder HM: Acquired von Willebrand's disease: A concise review. Am J Hematol 1997; 54:139–145.

Rock GA, Shumack KH, Buskard NA: Comparison of plasma exchange with plasma infusion in the treatment of thrombotic thrombocytopenic purpura. N Engl J Med 1991; 325:393.

Scaradavou A, Bussel JB: Clinical experience with anti-D in the treatment of idiopathic thrombocytopenic purpura. Semin Hematol 1998; 35(Suppl 1):52–57.

Slichter SJ: Optimizing platelet transfusions in chronically thrombocytopenic patients. Semin Hematol 1998; 35:269–278.

Sullivan CA, Martin JN Jr: Management of the obstetric patient with thrombocytopenia. Clin Obstet Gynecol 1995; 38:521–534.

Tsai HM, Lian ECY: Antibodies to von Willebrand factor–cleaving protease in acute thrombotic thrombocytopenic purpura. N Engl J Med 1998; 339:1585–1594.

Warkentin TE, Hayward CP, Boshkov LK, et al: Sera from patients with heparin-induced thrombocytopenia generate platelet-derived microparticles with procoagulant activity: An explanation for the thrombotic complications of heparin-induced thrombocytopenia. Blood 1994; 84:3691–3699.

Zalusky R, Furie B: Hematologic complications of liver disease and alcoholism. *In* Hoffman R, Benz EJ Jr, Shattil SJ, et al (eds): Hematology: Basic Principles and Practice. New York: Churchill Livingstone, 1995, pp 2096–2103.

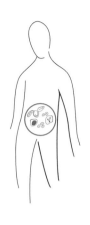

53

DISORDERS OF HEMOSTASIS: THROMBOSIS

Henry M. Rinder

Clinical Evaluation of Thrombosis

The approach to patients with thromboembolism is defined by clinical history, physical findings, and laboratory studies. Events that trigger deep venous thrombosis (DVT) include immobilization, orthopedic and other surgical procedures, use of oral contraceptives, and pregnancy. Venous thrombosis that is recurrent (thrombophilia), presents at an early age, occurs in unusual sites (e.g., cerebral vessels), or is accompanied by a family history of thromboembolism may indicate an inherited disorder. In contrast, acquired venous thrombotic risk may be associated with systemic disorders such as hemolysis (paroxysmal nocturnal hemoglobinuria, autoimmune hemolytic anemia), collagen vascular disorders, or various malignant diseases. Arterial thrombotic disease is more commonly superimposed on ruptured atherosclerotic plaque (e.g., coronary artery disease) and atheroembolic disorders (e.g., ischemic stroke). The clinical approach to thrombotic disease should consider the location of the disease (arterial versus venous and the specific vascular bed) and whether abnormalities of the vascular endothelium, platelets, or soluble coagulation factors predispose to thromboembolism.

Vascular Causes of Thrombosis

Virchow's triad defines the phenotypic mechanisms underlying thrombosis: diminished blood flow, damage to the vascular wall, and an imbalance favoring procoagulant over anticoagulant forces. The first two aspects are clearly localized to specific vascular beds; although the last element of the triad may be systemic, data now show at least partial vascular bed–specific regulation of the hemostatic balance. For example, congenital deficiencies of antithrombin III (ATIII), protein C, or protein S predispose to DVT of the lower, but not upper, extremities. In contrast, the inherited hypercoagulable disorders associated with factor V Leiden and the prothrombin 20210A mutation predispose not only to lower extremity DVT but also to venous thrombosis of the brain. Such differences in hypercoagulability appear to be regulated by the interaction of these systemic factors with dynamic signal transduction and the microenvironment of distinct vascular tissues. This hemostatic regulation in vascular tissues is mediated by multiple factors that include the following: (1) microenvironmental signals, such as shear stress, which affect endothelial cell (EC) expression of thrombomodulin, tissue factor, and nitric oxide synthase; (2) EC subtype–specific signaling; for example, shear stress upregulates aortic but not pulmonary artery nitric oxide synthase; and (3) differences in EC transcriptional regulation of proteins such as von Willebrand factor (vWF).

Atherothrombosis

This section briefly discusses those factors that predispose to thrombosis in the setting of atherosclerotic plaque (atherothrombosis); the pathophysiology of atherogenesis is discussed in another chapter. In addition to EC-intrinsic regulation of hemostasis, the interaction of ECs with the fibrinolytic system is important in the development of atherothrombotic disease. Deficiency in EC release of tissue-type plasminogen activator (t-PA) may predispose patients to arterial thrombosis, especially in the coronary arteries. For example, cardiac allografts that were depleted of t-PA had a higher incidence of coronary artery occlusion and lesser graft survival than allografts with normal t-PA levels. Aprotinin, which decreases blood loss during cardiopulmonary bypass through its antifibrinolytic effects, is associated with increased risk of vein graft occlusion and myocardial infarction after cardiopulmonary bypass. Although cardiovascular risk factors may affect plasminogen activator inhibitor (PAI-1) synthesis, whether increased PAI-1 levels convey an increased risk of atherosclerotic disease or coronary events, with the exception of late restenosis after angioplasty, is controversial.

HYPERHOMOCYSTEINEMIA

One disorder linked to atherothrombosis and venous thrombosis is hyperhomocysteinemia. Investigators recognized early that extremely high plasma homocysteine (HCY) levels, as are found in rare congenital syndromes characterized by homocystinuria and severe hyperhomocysteinemia syndromes, (e.g., cystathionine β-synthase deficiency), are associated with thromboembolism and severe premature atherosclerosis. HCY may damage ECs or may downregulate the normal anticoagulant function of ECs. However, studies support that even mild elevation in HCY (present in about 5% of the general population) leads to increased coronary, peripheral, and cerebral arterial disease. HCY in plasma can be measured after patients have fasted or after they have received a methionine load. Evidence indicates that both measures are important in that they are affected by different abnormalities of HCY metabolism, involving either the remethylation cycle or the transsulfuration pathway, respectively. Mildly elevated HCY levels are often associated with a thermolabile form of the N^5,N^{10}-methylene tetrahydrofolate reductase (MTHFR) enzyme. This protein results from a point polymorphism (C677T) in the coding region of the MTHF binding site. This mutation occurs in up to 30% to 40% of the general population and is correlated with modest elevations in HCY. Patients homozygous for the polymorphism have even higher HCY levels. Furthermore, HCY levels are more likely to be elevated when such persons are relatively folate deficient. In fact, deficiency of any of the vitamin cofactors of HCY metabolism (folate, vitamin B_6, and vitamin B_{12}) may lead to mild hyperhomocysteinemia. Reduction in HCY levels by supplementation with vitamin B_6, vitamin B_{12}, and folate is probably the most effective therapy for reducing both the HCY level and the concomitant atherothrombotic risk, regardless of the cause of hyperhomocysteinemia.

ROLE OF PLATELETS

Although these EC-associated abnormalities clearly influence hemostasis, platelet activation and adhesion are critical to the development of atherothrombosis, especially in patients with myocardial infarction, unstable angina, and ischemic stroke. In addition, both acute and chronic antiplatelet therapies are the primary modalities for maintaining patency after coronary revascularization. Antiplatelet therapy can be targeted against specific platelet functions, including cyclooxygenase-mediated

thromboxane A_2 formation, interaction of adenosine diphosphate (ADP) with its platelet receptor, and glycoprotein IIb/IIIa (GPIIb/IIIa)–fibrinogen binding for aggregation (Table 53–1). Aspirin has long been a mainstay in treatment of myocardial infarction, angina, and stroke because of its irreversible inhibition of platelet cyclooxygenase, a process leading to blockade of thromboxane A_2 release. Some drugs used to treat stroke and coronary disease specifically block the platelet ADP receptor from interaction with ADP in the clot milieu and thereby blunt platelet recruitment by preventing locally released ADP from activating additional platelets. Two thienopyrimidine derivatives, ticlopidine and clopidogrel, are used to antagonize ADP-induced platelet effects through their metabolites, which block ADP from binding to the platelet ADP receptor. Both drugs are highly inhibitory to platelet function and produce bleeding times that are more prolonged than with aspirin. Both drugs are effective in combination with aspirin for preventing ischemic stroke and for blocking stent thrombosis after revascularization, although the hematologic side effects of ticlopidine are a concern.

One of the first GPIIb/IIIa inhibitors was the modified monoclonal antibody abciximab, which prevents GPIIb/IIIa from binding to fibrinogen and blocks platelet aggregation. Abciximab successfully prevented restenosis after angioplasty, stent placement, or pharmacologic thrombolysis, and it has been used to block infarct extension and to resolve unstable angina. Other GPIIb/IIIa blockers (both parenteral and oral) that interfere with the GPIIb/IIIa arginine-glycine-aspartate (RGD) binding sites have been approved or are in clinical trials of patients with acute coronary events. The successful use of such blockers in patients at risk of coronary arterial events further reinforces the importance of platelet receptor–ligand interactions in thrombus formation. Currently, these GPIIb/IIIa inhibitors are indicated for acute intravenous use in patients with unstable angina and myocardial infarction and for maintenance of coronary patency after revascularization. However, if

TABLE 53–1   Antiplatelet Therapies

Inhibitors of Cyclooxygenase
Aspirin
Nonaspirin nonsteroidal anti-inflammatory drugs

ADP-Receptor Antagonists
Clopidogrel
Ticlopidine

Phosphodiesterase Inhibitors
Dipyridamole
Prostacyclin

GPIIb/IIIa and RGD Blockers
Abciximab
Integrilin
Lamifiban
Tirofiban
Xemilofiban

RGD = arginine-glycine-aspartate amino acid sequence.

oral anti-GPIIb/IIIa formulations show efficacy for preventing angina and infarction, long-term treatment may be part of future strategies for preventing acute coronary syndromes.

Not only is GPIIb/IIIa clearly critical for platelet-dependent atherothrombosis, it also now appears that a specific platelet GPIIb/IIIa allotype, PLA^2 (discussed in Chapter 52) is an emerging risk factor for coronary thrombosis. Studies have shown that the PLA^2 allotype of the GPIIIa molecule is associated with an increased incidence of coronary events, both myocardial infarction and unstable angina. Although these findings are controversial, the predominance of studies has found that the PLA^2 allotype is a coronary risk factor. Evidence also suggests that PLA^2 and other platelet receptor allotypes associated with thrombosis may promote increased platelet responsiveness to agonists and shear. Therefore, future studies probably will be aimed at determining not only the relative thrombotic potential of different platelet receptor allotypes but also their functional correlates, to examine possible inhibitors for these epitopes.

Inherited Risk Factors for Venous Thrombosis

The balance between thrombin formation and anticoagulant pathways has been extensively studied in patients with inherited deficiencies of naturally occurring anticoagulants (Table 53–2). These patients are predisposed to venous thrombosis and pulmonary embolism (PE).

FACTOR V LEIDEN

The most common inherited disorder leading to DVT is the factor V Leiden mutation. About 5% of the general population is heterozygous for factor V Leiden. The factor V mutation occurs at a site where activated protein C (APC) cleaves and inactivates normal factor Va (Arg506); abolition of this cleavage site results in APC resistance. Failure to inactivate the mutant factor Va allows the prothrombinase complex to be relatively uninhibited and leads to increased thrombin generation and a thrombophilic phenotype. Inheritance of heterozy-

gous factor V Leiden conveys an approximately fivefold increased risk of DVT or PE. Nearly one fourth of patients presenting with an initial occurrence of DVT or PE will have heterozygous factor V Leiden, and this percentage increases to nearly 60% in those with recurrent DVT or a strong family history of DVT. APC resistance can be demonstrated by specialized clotting tests showing that the addition of APC does not adequately prolong the partial thromboplastin time (PTT). Genotyping can then determine whether the factor V Leiden allele is present and whether it is heterozygous or homozygous.

Factor V Leiden is a weak hypercoagulable risk factor. At 50 years of age, only 25% of persons with heterozygous factor V Leiden have had DVT or PE, compared with much higher percentages in persons with other inherited thrombophilias. In addition, DVT or PE in persons with factor V Leiden is typically associated with concomitant "acquired" risk factors, such as immobilization, pregnancy, or oral contraceptive use. Occasional reports exist of patients with homozygous factor V Leiden who are asymptomatic into old age, although homozygous factor V Leiden is generally associated with a 90-fold increased risk of DVT compared with persons who have wild-type factor V. In addition, a few patients have demonstrated APC resistance *without* the factor V Leiden mutation. Factor V Cambridge, although much rarer than V Leiden, has a similar mutation at an APC cleavage site (Arg306) and is associated with APC resistance and thrombosis. Acquired APC resistance may be caused by the presence of a lupus anticoagulant yielding spuriously low APC results.

PROTHROMBIN G20210A

Another mutation associated with inherited thrombophilia is the prothrombin G20210A mutation, which occurs in the 3′ untranslated region of the prothrombin gene; this mutation leads to higher prothrombin levels than normal and about a twofold increased risk of DVT or PE. The heterozygous mutation is present in about 3% of European-derived populations. The mutation does not appear to convey any functional difference in the prothrombin molecule, and the elevated prothrombin levels are not sufficiently different from levels in healthy persons to warrant measurement. Thus, how this prothrombin mutation affects thrombus development is unknown. The diagnosis of the G20210A genotype is made by examining DNA for this specific mutation.

INHERITED DEFICIENCY OF NATURAL ANTICOAGULANT PROTEINS

Deficiencies in the naturally occurring anticoagulants (ATIII, protein C, and protein S) are less common than factor V Leiden or prothrombin G20210A, but they are more likely to produce symptomatic venous thrombosis at an earlier age. Only about half the thromboses that occur with these deficiencies are associated with acquired risk factors such as pregnancy, surgery, or immobilization. Deficiencies of ATIII, protein C, or protein S are detected by functional and/or antigenic assays, be-

---

TABLE 53–2   Inherited Causes of Thrombophilia

Activated protein C resistance/factor V Leiden (20–60%)*
Homocyst(e)inemia (10–15%)
Prothrombin 20210A (5–15%)
Antithrombin III deficiency (1–4%)
Protein C deficiency (2–6%)
Protein S deficiency (2–5%)
Tissue plasminogen activator deficiency (rare)
Plasminogen activator inhibitor excess (rare)
Dysfibrinogenemia (rare)
Decreased plasminogen (very rare)

* Prevalence in patients presenting with deep venous thrombosis or pulmonary embolism.

cause some mutations cause decreased antigenic factors and some produce dysfunctional proteins. Many mutations have been associated with these deficiencies, but none are predominant. Deficiencies of ATIII, protein C, and protein S in the aggregate account for fewer than 5% to 10% of all patients presenting with DVT and/or PE.

ATIII is a naturally occurring anticoagulant that complexes with endogenous heparan sulfates to inhibit both formed thrombin and factor Xa. Heterozygous ATIII deficiency leads to ATIII levels of less than 50% and is associated with thrombosis that occurs exclusively in the venous circulation. However, reports have noted a homozygous mutation in the heparin-binding site of ATIII that results in arterial thrombosis. Thrombosis occurs by the age of 25 years in 50% of heterozygous patients. ATIII has a low molecular weight and may be lost through the kidney in the proteinuria of nephrotic syndrome, a process leading to symptomatic acquired ATIII deficiency. Acquired ATIII deficiency (as well as protein C deficiency) may also be associated with severe hepatic veno-occlusive disease after stem cell transplantation; investigators have hypothesized that ATIII and protein C are consumed in the damaged hepatic microvasculature. ATIII replacement with or without heparin appears to be useful in resolving platelet consumption and the fluid disorders of veno-occlusive disease after stem cell transplantation. Successful treatment of symptomatic patients with heterozygous ATIII deficiency has included short-term replacement of ATIII with plasma or concentrate, usually coupled with heparin. Long-term therapy for such patients has consisted primarily of warfarin.

The complex of thrombin and thrombomodulin on the EC surface activates protein C; APC coupled with its cofactor, protein S, cleaves and inactivates factors Va and VIIIa. These actions downregulate the prothrombinase and tenase complexes, respectively, to slow the rate of thrombin generation. Like ATIII deficiency, heterozygous protein C and protein S deficiencies present with venous, and occasionally arterial, thrombosis at a young age (median occurrence, 20 to 40 years). Homozygous protein C deficiency does occur and presents in the neonate as *purpura fulminans* with widespread venous thrombosis and skin necrosis. A similar clinical presentation has been reported in adults after institution of warfarin therapy *without* simultaneous heparinization, so-called *warfarin-induced skin necrosis*. About one-third of such patients are found to be deficient in protein C on a hereditary basis, whereas the rest appear to have an acquired protein C deficiency. Warfarin inhibits production of vitamin K–dependent protein C synthesis, and because of the factor's short half-life, protein C levels rapidly fall before a decline in the levels of the procoagulant factors II, IX, and X. This imbalance shortly after starting warfarin may favor a procoagulant state and occasionally results in widespread microvascular thrombosis. Although protein C deficiency, either inherited or acquired, is relatively infrequent, most clinicians prefer that a patient with venous thrombosis be fully anticoagulated with heparin (either unfractionated [UFH] or of low molecular weight [LMWH]) before concurrent warfarin therapy is begun. Inherited defi-

ciency of protein S has similarly been implicated in warfarin-induced skin necrosis. Protein S deficiency can also be acquired in acute illness. Protein S circulates in a free form and is bound to C4b-binding protein; only free protein S is active as a cofactor for protein C. C4b-binding protein is an acute phase reactant, and increased C4b-binding protein levels with severe illness therefore decrease free protein S levels. Short-term therapy for homozygous or doubly heterozygous protein C or S deficiency, especially in the setting of neonatal *purpura fulminans*, has included plasma or protein C concentrate with full-dose heparin anticoagulation. As with ATIII deficiency, long-term treatment with warfarin has been successful in patients with protein C or S deficiency.

Acquired Risk Factors for Venous Thrombosis

SURGERY

Many medical and surgical illnesses convey an increased thrombotic risk; these "acquired" risk factors are acknowledged, even though the pathophysiologic features favoring thrombosis are unclear in most instances (Table 53–3). Several of these risk factors, including surgery (especially orthopedic) and trauma, are associated with immobilization with stasis of lower extremity blood flow. When evidence of thrombosis is actively sought, both surgery and trauma can be shown to be associated with extremely high (>50%) incidences of DVT. Besides immobilization, other pathophysiologic factors may contribute to the risk of DVT with surgery and trauma, including fat embolism and tissue damage, the latter especially after closed head injuries that result in massive tissue factor release. In some institutions, prophylactic inferior vena cava filters placed in patients who have undergone

TABLE 53–3 Acquired Causes of Thrombosis

Medical and Surgical Illnesses
Antiphospholipid antibody/lupus anticoagulant
Artificial heart valves
Atrial fibrillation
Hemolytic anemia (sickle cell, thrombotic thrombocytopenic purpura)
Hyperlipidemia
Immobilization
Malignancy
Myeloproliferative disorders/thrombocytosis
Nephrotic syndrome
Orthopedic procedures
Pregnancy
Trauma/fat embolism

Medications
Heparin-induced thrombocytopenia
Oral contraceptives
Prothrombin complex concentrates

trauma have been shown to protect against PE, especially in high-risk patients in whom anticoagulation is contraindicated because of the increased risk of bleeding. Stasis of blood flow in the left atrial appendage with atrial fibrillation is another source of systemic thromboembolism (usually stroke) in untreated patients.

PREGNANCY AND ORAL CONTRACEPTIVE USE

Both pregnancy and oral contraceptive use convey an increased risk of DVT and PE. Cigarette use or concomitant heterozygosity for factor V Leiden further increases the risk of DVT and PE in women who take oral contraceptives.

PROTHROMBOTIC STATES

As noted earlier, thrombosis in nephrotic syndrome appears to be associated with loss of ATIII through the kidneys. Other prothrombotic states appear to mediated through blood cell destruction, perhaps by increasing exposure to procoagulant membrane phospholipids; these states include artificial heart valves, sickle cell disease, and other hemolytic anemias. Platelet activation and clearance appear to be the primary prothrombotic manifestations of heparin-induced thrombocytopenia and thrombotic thrombocytopenic purpura (see Chapter 52), and abnormal platelet physiology is probably present in myeloproliferative disorders associated with thrombosis. Although chronic disseminated intravascular coagulation is present in some malignant diseases (Trousseau's syndrome), malignant diseases in general appear to be associated with an increased risk of DVT and PE that is not related to disseminated intravascular coagulation.

ANTIPHOSPHOLIPID ANTIBODY SYNDROME

Another acquired prothrombotic disorder is the antiphospholipid antibody (APA) syndrome. APA syndrome may present as a primary disorder, or it may be secondarily associated with other autoimmune diseases such as systemic lupus erythematosus. All the manifestations of APA syndrome are related to hypercoagulability, including recurrent venous or arterial thrombosis, thrombocytopenia caused by platelet clearance, and recurrent fetal loss resulting from placental vascular insufficiency. The serologic markers of APA syndrome include *anticardiolipin antibodies* and/or the *lupus anticoagulant*. Anticardiolipin antibodies are usually detected by enzyme-linked immunosorbent assay, whereas lupus anticoagulants are defined by prolongation of a phospholipid-dependent clotting test (prothrombin time, PTT, or Russell's viper venom clotting time), which is then corrected by addition of excess phospholipid. Thus, the lupus anticoagulant is actually a misnomer, because its presence predisposes to clotting rather than to bleeding. Another misleading aspect of this nomenclature is that phospholipid-reactive antibodies are actually directed against phospholipid-binding proteins in plasma, β_2-GPI, and prothrombin. Furthermore, the risk of thrombosis appears to be strongest when antibodies (especially IgG but also IgM or IgA) are directed specifically against β_2-GPI.

Hypercoagulability and Platelet Disorders

Essential thrombocythemia, chronic myelogenous leukemia, and polycythemia vera are clonal myeloproliferative disorders that are wholly (essential thrombocythemia) or partially (chronic myelogenous leukemia, polycythemia vera) characterized by an elevated platelet count, so-called *primary* thrombocytosis. Platelet aggregometry in these disorders often shows abnormal responses, especially to weak agonists such as epinephrine and ADP; however, the abnormal aggregation does not correspond well to bleeding risk or thrombosis risk. Patients with myeloproliferative disorders are at risk for thrombosis. Patients with polycythemia vera in particular have a high incidence of thrombosis in the mesenteric, portal, and hepatic venous circulation. Thrombotic complications, both arterial and venous, occur in essential thrombocythemia, even in young patients. However, no clear risk factors predict which patients with myeloproliferative disorders will develop thrombosis. High platelet counts, especially more than $1,000,000/\mu L$, are thought to increase the risk of thrombosis, and evidence indicates that increased platelet turnover in thrombocytosis is associated with thromboembolic complications. The latter has been demonstrated by radioactive platelet survival studies and an increase in the percentage of reticulated platelets associated with thrombosis. Antiplatelet agents may cause bleeding in patients with myeloproliferative disorders; thus, aspirin is indicated only in patients with *symptomatic* thrombosis, such as those with erythromelalgia. Successful treatment with aspirin of symptomatic patients increases platelet survival by decreasing platelet clearance. Other therapies to prevent thrombotic complications of thrombocytosis include lowering the platelet count with hydroxyurea or anagrelide. Patients with reactive (secondary) thrombocytosis resulting from iron deficiency anemia, chronic infection, rheumatoid arthritis, or the postsplenectomy state do not generally have significantly increased thrombotic risk.

Laboratory Evaluation of Thrombosis

Recurrent venous thromboembolism is a strong indication for laboratory testing for causes of thrombophilia, especially in patients less than 50 years old, in patients with unexplained DVT, and in those with a family history of venous thrombosis. In such patients, one must define any risk factors that may predispose to recurrence and to define any inherited disorders that may necessitate family counseling or avoidance of additional environmental risks. The current assays in the work-up of venous thrombophilia include the following: (1) APC

TABLE 53-4 **Laboratory Evaluation of Venous Thrombosis**

Activated protein C resistance
Factor V Leiden
Lupus anticoagulant
Homocyst(e)ine level: fasting or following methionine load
Prothrombin 20210A mutation
Antithrombin III level
Protein C level
Protein S level (total and free)

resistance using a dilute factor V method; (2) genotyping for prothrombin 20210A; (3) lupus anticoagulant assay and anticardiolipin antibodies; (4) ATIII level; and (5) protein C and protein S (total and free) levels (Table 53–4). Genotyping for the factor V Leiden mutation should be done when APC resistance is present to define whether factor V Leiden is truly present, and if so, to determine whether the patient is heterozygous or homozygous. Testing for antibodies specifically to β_2-GPI can be used to confirm the APA syndrome after positive screening for a lupus anticoagulant or anticardiolipin antibody; whether anti–β_2-GPI testing should be performed when APA screening tests are negative is not clear.

The utility of laboratory testing in the setting of atherothrombosis and arterial thromboembolism is unclear. Identification of elevated HCY levels is probably important because specific therapy (folate, vitamin B_6, and vitamin B_{12} supplementation) is indicated. Platelet-specific risk factors for both arterial and venous thrombosis have not been defined adequately for available sophisticated laboratory tests to give meaningful or prognostic data. Therefore, platelet aggregation studies and examination of platelet receptor allotypes are not indicated. In the setting of a myeloproliferative disorder, the platelet count is the only available useful test. In patients with recurrent thromboses or a strong family history, assays for rarer entities can be justified, including testing for low t-PA levels, high PAI-1 levels, dysfibrinogenemia (prolonged thrombin or reptilase time), and low plasminogen levels, all of which should be done in consultation with specialists in hemostasis.

Therapy for Venous Thromboembolism

Prophylaxis for DVT should be administered in patients undergoing surgical procedures that carry an increased risk of venous thrombosis, especially orthopedic procedures or major operations requiring significant postoperative immobilization. Prophylactic therapies include lower extremity intermittent compression and pharmacologic treatment with low doses of UFH or LMWHs. Once thromboembolism is diagnosed, immediate therapy is required. Thrombolytic therapy is indicated for

patients with extensive proximal venous clots or PE. Inferior vena cava filters are used in patients with contraindications to anticoagulation, usually because of active bleeding or the potential for bleeding. In most other patients with venous thrombosis, anticoagulation is accomplished on a short-term basis with heparin compounds and on a long-term basis with warfarin.

UFH is still the therapy of choice for inpatients requiring acute anticoagulation because of its low cost, ease of monitoring, and short half-life. Heparin is begun as a bolus intravenous infusion of 80 U/kg, followed by a continuous infusion of 18 U/kg/hr; heparin doses in excess of 30,000 U/day have been shown to be most efficacious at preventing recurrent thrombosis. Heparin is monitored by the PTT. A therapeutic PTT for heparin is more than 1.5 and less than 2.5 times the patient's initial PTT value. This PTT range should correspond to therapeutic anti-Xa levels of 0.4 to 0.7 U/mL. Adjustment of the heparin infusion should be based on the patient's weight and the PTT (Table 53–5); discontinuation of the heparin infusion, even for a brief period, may allow the PTT to normalize because of heparin's short half-life (about 4 hours). UFH should be continued for ≥4 days, longer in patients with extensive clots, and UFH can be discontinued when patients are fully anticoagulated with warfarin (international normalized ratio [INR] ≥2.0 for 2 consecutive days). Some patients may receive large doses of heparin (usually >40,000 U/day), and yet, the PTT does not become therapeutic. This *heparin resistance* is caused by a dissociation of the PTT and the true heparin level (measured as anti-Xa activity); monitoring of anti-Xa levels is indicated in heparin resistance. Heparin resistance is only rarely caused by ATIII deficiency; more often, heparin resistance occurs in patients with inflammatory diseases and is caused by increased plasma levels of factor VIII and other heparin-binding proteins.

LMWHs are rapidly gaining in use in the United States. The advantages of LMWH over UFH include the following: (1) reduced binding to macrophages and EC, a process that increases the plasma half-life of LMWH; (2) less nonspecific binding to plasma proteins that leads to a more predictable dose-response and allows for intermittent fixed dosing; (3) reduced binding to platelets and platelet factor 4, with a resulting lower

TABLE 53-5 **Unfractionated Heparin Dose Adjustment Based on Partial Thromboplastin Time (PTT) and Weight***

PTT Value (Times Baseline)	Heparin Adjustment
1.2–1.5	40 U/kg bolus, ↑ infusion by 4 U/kg/hr
>1.5–2.4	No change
>2.4–3.0	↓ infusion by 2 U/kg/hr
>3.0	Hold infusion for 1 hr, ↓ infusion by 3 U/kg/hr

* After initial therapy with 80 U/kg bolus and 18 U/kg/hr infusion.
↑ = Increase; ↓ = decrease.

incidence of heparin-induced thrombocytopenia; and (4) reduced bone loss. Although the incidence of heparin-induced thrombocytopenia is lower with initial use of LMWH when compared with UFH, once heparin-induced thrombocytopenia is established, antibody cross-reactivity with all the LMWH preparations is more than 75% (see Chapter 52). All the LMWH preparations (dalteparin, enoxaparin, nadroparin, and tinzaparin) have been shown to be as safe and effective as UFH in prophylaxis for DVT, treatment of uncomplicated DVT, and treatment of symptomatic PE, when these drugs are given in a subcutaneous, weight-adjusted dose. In particular, outpatient therapy with LMWH for uncomplicated DVT provides a significant cost saving (when compared with hospitalization for intravenous UFH) without compromising patient outcome. Because of its predictable dose-response curve, LMWH therapy in most studies has not required monitoring. LMWH therapy does not prolong the PTT and is monitored, if necessary, by anti-Xa levels. Peak anti-Xa levels generally occur between 3 and 5 hours after subcutaneous LMWH injection and vary according to the dosage given. For example, 4000 U of enoxaparin subcutaneously results in a mean peak concentration of 0.4 U/mL of anti-Xa activity 4 hours after injection, and significant anti-Xa activity persists in plasma for 12 hours after subcutaneous injection. As with UFH, switching from LMWH to warfarin for long-term management can be accomplished after therapeutic INR values are present for 2 to 3 days.

Warfarin is the treatment of choice for long-term anticoagulation and for preventing early recurrence of thrombus. Warfarin should be begun in the first 24 hours after presentation with venous thromboembolism and concurrent with heparin treatment. The prothrombin time is prolonged within hours by warfarin because of a rapid decrease in factor VII levels; however, therapeutic warfarin anticoagulation does not occur until other vitamin K–dependent factors (II, IX, and X) also decrease. Therapeutic warfarin anticoagulation usually requires at least 4 to 5 days of adequate warfarin dosing starting at 7.5 to 10 mg daily for 2 to 3 days; UFH or LMWH can be discontinued after at least 4 days of therapy and only when the INR is between 2.0 to 3.0 for at least 2 consecutive days. The intensity of warfarin dosing, evaluated by the INR, depends on the condition predisposing to thromboembolism. Treatment of uncomplicated DVT in a patient without known risk factors does not require an INR exceeding 3.0; in contrast, prophylaxis for recurrent thrombosis in patients with APA syndrome requires INR values between 3.0 and 4.0 (Table 53–6).

The duration of warfarin treatment also varies depending on the circumstances of the venous thromboembolism, the estimated clinical risk of bleeding, and the potential for recurrence. In general, the longer the anticoagulation with warfarin, the less is the chance of recurrence; short-term warfarin (6 weeks) is not as effective at preventing recurrence as longer courses (6 months). Patients with definite, transient risk factors such as orthopedic surgery have low recurrence rates even with short-term therapy; in contrast, patients with

TABLE 53–6 Therapeutic International Normalized Ratio (INR) Ranges for Warfarin According to Patient Subgroup

Subgroup	INR Range
Venous thrombosis	
Treatment	2.0–3.0
Prophylaxis	1.5–2.5
Artificial heart valves	
Tissue	2.0–2.5
Mechanical	3.0–4.0
Atrial fibrillation	
Prophylaxis	1.5–2.5
Lupus anticoagulant	
Treatment/prophylaxis	3.0–4.0

idiopathic thromboembolism have significant recurrence rates even after 3 to 6 months of warfarin. Evidence indicates that inherited hypercoagulable disorders, such as factor V Leiden, lead to a lifelong increased risk of DVT or PE. However, no studies are available that address whether the bleeding risks incurred by long-term warfarin use are favorably balanced by the threat of recurrent thrombosis. The presence of inherited thrombophilia such as factor V Leiden may warrant continuing warfarin for a longer period, depending on the patient's other medical illnesses and whether certain circumstances may have predisposed the patient to venous thrombosis. Patients who develop recurrent venous thrombosis after discontinuation of warfarin should receive long-term anticoagulation, regardless of whether they have a defined cause of thrombophilia. Table 53–7 suggests guidelines for the duration of warfarin therapy in specific patient subgroups. Warfarin is a teratogen; effective contraception should be used concurrently in women of childbearing age.

Supratherapeutic INR levels commonly occur with

TABLE 53–7 Guidelines for Duration of Anticoagulation in Venous Thromboembolism

Condition	Duration of Therapy
Distal or superficial vein thrombus	3 mo
First proximal DVT/PE	
No risk factors	Long-term*
Correctable risk factor (e.g., surgery, trauma)	3–6 mo
Malignancy	Long-term
Antiphospholipid antibody	Long-term
Inherited risk factor†	6 mo
Recurrent DVT/PE	Lifelong

* Long-term therapy must be adjusted individually according to other diseases, risks of bleeding, presence of transient risk factors, and ease of compliance.

† Inherited risk factors include factor V Leiden; prothrombin 20210A; deficiencies of antithrombin III, protein C, or protein S; and hyperhomocysteinemia.

DVT/PE = deep venous thrombosis; pulmonary embolism.

TABLE 53-8 Drugs that Affect Warfarin Levels

Drugs that Increase Warfarin Levels: Prolonged INR
↓ Warfarin clearance
  Disulfiram
  Metronidazole
  Trimethoprim-sulfamethoxazole
↓ Warfarin-protein binding
  Phenylbutazone
↑ Vitamin K turnover
  Clofibrate

Drugs that Decrease Warfarin Levels: Subtherapeutic INR
↑ Hepatic metabolism of warfarin
  Barbiturates
  Rifampin
↓ Warfarin absorption
  Cholestyramine

INR = international normalized ratio. ↑ = Increased; ↓ = decreased.

warfarin therapy, with or without bleeding. In patients with moderately elevated INR values (<1.0 elevation over therapeutic levels) with little or no bleeding, discontinuation of warfarin for 2 to 3 days and reinstitution of the drug at a lower maintenance dose may be sufficient. Patients with higher INR values without serious bleeding should have warfarin withheld and should receive low doses (1 mg/day) of vitamin K to reach therapeutic INR levels. When serious active bleeding occurs with high INR values, especially if surgery is required to correct the bleeding, a combination of vitamin K and plasma will rapidly correct the INR. The INR can become elevated as a result of concurrent use of drugs that increase free warfarin levels (Table 53–8). Whenever bleeding occurs as a complication of anticoagulation, serious consideration must be given to future bleeding risks and to whether the patient requires filter placement instead of anticoagulation.

Venous Thromboembolism During Pregnancy

The risk of DVT and PE during pregnancy and in the postpartum period is about fivefold higher than for nonpregnant women. Pregnancy is a hypercoagulable state associated with significant venous stasis, as well as alterations in procoagulant proteins (fibrinogen, vWF). DVT can occur at any time during pregnancy or the puerperium. Heparins, both UFH and LMWH, are the safest therapy for venous thrombosis during pregnancy; neither crosses the placenta, unlike warfarin, which causes a characteristic fetal embryopathy. Warfarin also causes fetal hemorrhage and placental abruption and should be avoided during pregnancy. DVT or PE during pregnancy should be treated with intravenous UFH for 5 to 10 days, followed by an adjusted-dose regimen of subcutaneous UFH, starting with 20,000 U q12h and adjusted to achieve a PTT higher than 1.5 times baseline at 6

hours after injection. An attractive alternative to UFH during pregnancy is LMWH that can be given subcutaneously once or twice daily and does not require monitoring. Suprarenal inferior vena cava filters have also been used successfully during pregnancy without significant morbidity.

Heparin should be discontinued at the time of labor and delivery, although the risk of hemorrhage is not high during delivery, especially if anti-Xa levels are less than 0.7 U/mL. One concern with residual anticoagulation at delivery is the risk of spinal hematoma with epidural anesthesia; this has been reported with both UFH and LMWH. The anti-Xa level that is safe for an epidural procedure is not known. Protamine sulfate can be used to neutralize UFH if the PTT is prolonged during labor and delivery; unfortunately, LMWH is not reversed by protamine.

Anticoagulation during the postpartum period can be carried out with heparin or warfarin; neither drug is contraindicated during breast-feeding. Women who become pregnant and who are at risk of developing a thromboembolism should receive more intensive heparin therapy, followed by warfarin in the postpartum period; this category includes women with a history of previous DVT or PE or women with APA syndrome without previous thrombus. Women receiving long-term warfarin therapy (e.g., for valvular heart disease) who wish to become pregnant will need to be switched to a fully anticoagulating dose of UFH or LMWH; warfarin treatment can be restarted post partum.

Perioperative Anticoagulation

A common clinical problem is the management of anticoagulation in patients who require surgery. The principles of care in this situation reflect the need for adequate hemostasis during and immediately after surgical procedures and the critical importance of restarting anticoagulation as soon as possible postoperatively, especially because surgery itself represents a relative hypercoagulable state. In patients with thromboembolism who are anticoagulated on a short-term basis (<1 month), elective surgical procedures should be postponed; if such patients must undergo surgery, discontinuation of anticoagulation and placement of an inferior vena cava filter may be the best option. In most patients receiving long-term anticoagulation for venous thromboembolism, preoperative heparin is not generally used; warfarin should be discontinued for at least 4 days preoperatively, to allow the INR to decrease gradually to less than 1.5, a level that is safe for surgery. Postoperatively, intravenous heparin can be safely used for anticoagulation until therapeutic INR levels are reached after restarting warfarin. These guidelines obviously should be tailored to individual patient care. Patients with arterial thromboembolic disease may need heparin therapy right up until the time of the surgical procedure and shortly thereafter. On the other hand, heparin therapy immediately after a major surgical procedure may be contraindicated because of the high risk of hemorrhage; anticoagulation may need to be delayed in this instance for 12 to 24 hours postoperatively.

Future Anticoagulant Strategies

The critical roles of platelet adhesion and thrombin generation, especially in arterial thrombogenesis, provide a rationale for future antithrombotic strategies. LMWH is actively being investigated for its efficacy in unstable angina and other acute coronary artery disease syndromes. More recent insights into the regulation of coagulation and fibrinolysis may provide new targets for antithrombotic strategy, including thrombin-regulated and thrombomodulin-mediated inhibition of fibrinolysis. Newer antithrombotic therapies are becoming available. The direct thrombin inhibitors, hirudin and argatroban, are already in clinical use for heparin-induced thrombocytopenia (see Chapter 52). Like LMWH, direct thrombin inhibitors lack the limitations of heparin. Moreover, these agents inhibit fibrin-bound, as well as plasma, thrombin and produce a predictable anticoagulant response. Especially in acute coronary artery disease syndromes, studies are now focusing on the optimal *combinations* of antiplatelet and antithrombin therapies to (1) prevent recurrent thrombosis and (2) maintain graft or stent patency; such studies include the use of multiple antiplatelet agents (aspirin, clopidogrel, and abciximab) and antithrombin agents (bivalirudin, LMWH, UFH). The future of thromboembolism therapy may lie in optimizing "combination chemotherapies" for distinct arterial and venous thrombosis syndromes.

REFERENCES

Bertina RM: The prothrombin 20210 G to A variation and thrombosis. Curr Opin Hematol 1998; 5:339–342.
Dahlback B: Inherited thrombophilia: Resistance to activated protein C as a pathogenic factor of venous thromboembolism. Blood 1995; 85:607.
de Moerloose P, Bounameaux HR, Mannucci PM: Screening test for thrombophilic patients: Which tests, for which patient, by whom, when, and why? Semin Thromb Hemost 1998; 24:321–327.
De Stefano V, Leone G, Mastrangelo S, et al: Clinical manifestations and management of inherited thrombophilia: Retrospective analysis and follow-up after diagnosis of 238 patients with congenital deficiency of antithrombin III, protein C, protein S. Thromb Haemost 1994; 72:352–358.
Ginsberg JS: Management of venous thromboembolism. N Engl J Med 1996; 335:1816–1828.
Harker LA: Platelets in thrombotic disorders: Quantitative and qualitative platelet disorders predisposing to arterial thrombosis. Semin Hematol 1998; 35:241–252.
Kearon C, Hirsh J: Current concepts: Management of anticoagulation before and after elective surgery. N Engl J Med 1997; 336:1506–1511.
Pengo V, Biasiolo A, Brocco T, et al: Autoantibodies to phospholipid-binding plasma proteins in patients with thrombosis and phospholipid-reactive antibodies. Thromb Haemost 1996; 75:721–724.
Price DT, Ridker PM: Factor V Leiden mutation and the risks for thromboembolic disease: A clinical perspective. Ann Intern Med 1997; 127:895–903.
Ravandi-Kashani F, Schafer AI: Microvascular disturbances, thrombosis, and bleeding in thrombocythemia: Current concepts and perspectives. Semin Thromb Hemost 1997; 23:479–488.
Silverstein RL, Nachman RL: Cancer and clotting: Trousseau's warning. N Engl J Med 1992; 327:1163.
Thomas DP, Roberts HR: Hypercoagulability in venous and arterial thrombosis. Ann Intern Med 1997; 126:638–644.
Toglia MR, Weg JG: Venous thromboembolism during pregnancy. N Engl J Med 1996; 335:108–114.
Weinmann EE, Salzman EW: Deep vein thrombosis. N Engl J Med 1994; 331:1630–1641.
Welch GN, Loscalzo J: Homocysteine and atherothrombosis. N Engl J Med 1998; 338:1042–1050.

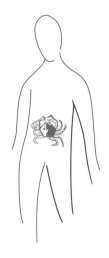

Oncologic Disease

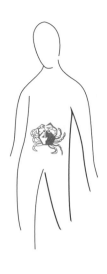

54

CANCER ETIOLOGY: ONCOGENES AND ENVIRONMENTAL/TOXIC FACTORS

Christopher E. Desch

Cancer is a general term for many different diseases. All cancers have an unrestrained growth pattern and a propensity to detach and metastasize. Since the mid-1970s, tremendous amounts of basic knowledge about the cell cycle, molecular genetics, angiogenesis, and cell adhesion have led to a greater understanding of the pathophysiology of cancer. This understanding has initiated a wave of research designed to correct the cellular and molecular events that produce cancer. This chapter highlights significant cellular and genetic events that cause cancer and relates these findings to a clinical context.

Cancer Phenotype

A malignant tumor is observably different from normal cells in the body. Table 54–1 shows some of the ways that cancer is different from normal cells and organs. Cancer cells can live independently in a test tube or culture dish (in vitro). Most cancers do not need growth factors and hormones that normal tissues would require to grow outside the body. Further, cultured cancer cells tend to grow in vitro in a disorganized fashion, frequently growing over the top of one another unlike normal cells which exhibit contact inhibition. Some malignant cells do not undergo normal programmed cell death, or apoptosis. Consequently, they become immortal and are resistant to chemotherapy and ionizing radiation. Malignant tumors also have the ability to create their own blood supply, a process called *angiogenesis*.

Cancer Genetics

Most of the events that lead to the cancer phenotype are under genetic control. Specific mutations or major gene deletions result in uncontrolled cellular proliferation. Several classes or families of these mutations and deletions are recognized. Table 54–2 shows the clinical consequences of several specific mutations.

ONCOGENES

Proto-oncogenes are evolutionarily conserved genes that play an important role in normal cellular proliferation. When proto-oncogenes mutate, they can become oncogenes that produce protein products or turn on a nearby gene, and the results are profound changes in cellular growth. For example, chronic myelogenous leukemia occurs when the proto-oncogene *abl* from chromosome 9 translocates to the *bcr* gene on chromosome 22. The new protein formed by the union of the *bcr* and *abl* oncogenes, called *bcr-abl*, plays a role in coupling cell surface receptors to the signal transduction pathway, with resulting unchecked growth-promoting signals to the nucleus. The precise cause of the translocation that results in the malignant process in chronic myelogenous leukemia is not known.

TUMOR SUPPRESSOR GENES

Tumor suppressor genes are recessive genes that keep cellular growth in check. When tumor suppressor genes

485

TABLE 54–1 Cancer Phenotype

Loss of differentiation
Uncontrolled growth
Loss of contact inhibition in vitro
Invasive capacity
Reduced apoptosis
Induction of angiogenesis

undergo mutation or deletion, the rate of neoplastic transformation is much higher. *TP53* is one of the best-known tumor suppressor genes. This gene deletion can be inherited, and progeny have a much higher rate of a variety of cancers including breast and brain tumors, leukemia, and sarcoma, a pattern termed the *Li-Fraumeni syndrome*. If *TP53* is deleted in a specific organ or cell through an acquired insult, tumors then may occur in that organ, such as in breast, bladder, and colon. In vitro experiments show that when *TP53* is added to a clone of cancer cells, malignant growth ceases, and the cells revert to a normal pattern.

RESISTANCE TO APOPTOSIS

Apoptosis, or programmed cell death, appears to result in a delicate interplay between the oncogene *bcl-2* and another oncogene, *bax*. Interference with apoptosis by various mutations can cause malignant transformation of cells. When cells are severely disturbed after the administration of chemotherapy or radiation, the expression of the *bax* gene is increased. This change results in a sequence of events ending in cell death. *Bcl-2*, however, is an inhibitor of *bax* or the effect of *bax* on the nucleus. In chronic lymphocytic leukemia, the overexpression of *bcl-2* and therefore the resistance to apoptosis appear to be responsible for the signs, symptoms, and relatively refractory nature of this B-cell malignant disease.

INTERRUPTION OF THE CELL CYCLE

Mature cells spend the majority of their time in the resting phase (G_0) of the cell cycle. Certain transcription factors, such as the product of the *c-myc* proto-onco-

gene, are sufficient to drive the cell from the resting phase into the replication phase (S_1). When the expression of the *myc* oncogene becomes aberrant or the gene itself undergoes mutation, uncontrolled growth occurs. Burkitt's lymphoma, a high-grade tumor of children and adults, is characterized by the accumulation of abnormal *myc* forms and rapid tumor growth.

Cancer is rarely the result of a single mutation or loss of a suppressor allele. Certain solid tumors such as colon cancer result from a cascade of events that occur over many years. The molecular events occurring between the development of an adenomatous polyp and its later transformation to colon adenocarcinoma have been defined. In the early development of colonic neoplasms, tumor suppressor genes such as *TP53* and *FAP* are lost. Later, other mutations in other oncogenes such as *DCC* occur. These events develop within a growing polyp. Removing polyps before the occurrence of neoplastic transformation should reduce or eliminate the later development of colon cancer.

Etiology

Despite growing understanding of cancer genetics, the mechanisms by which mutations, loss of suppressors, and gene alterations occur is not known. Some persons probably have a predisposition to DNA breaks and the inability to repair errors. Further, epidemiologic studies have uncovered relationships among specific factors in the diet, environment, and certain infections that are associated with the later development of cancer. The specific gene locations at which various agents such as tobacco, benzene, or ionizing radiation cause sufficient damage to result in the development of cancer are not known. The following section outlines important carcinogens and their influence on the development of cancer (Table 54–3).

TOBACCO

Long-term use of tobacco, whether smoked, dipped, or sniffed, leads to the development of cancers in areas

TABLE 54–2 Cancers Associated with Selected Genetic Mutations

Type of Cancer	Specific Mutation	Cellular Event and Consequence
Chronic myelogenous leukemia	Translocation of *abl* gene to *bcr* gene forming the "Philadelphia chromosome" (oncogene)	Production of p210 protein Rapid expansion of bone marrow, predominantly myeloid cells
Chronic lymphocytic leukemia	Mutation of *bcl-2* gene (oncogene)	Reduction in apoptosis Increased cell survival; increased resistance to radiation, chemotherapy
Breast, ovarian	Mutation in *BRCA1* gene (oncogene)	Unknown event Increased cell growth
Many, including sarcoma, and breast, brain, and adrenal cancers	Loss or mutation of *TP53* gene (tumor suppressor gene)	Loss of a growth suppressor Unchecked growth
Burkitt's lymphoma, neuroblastoma	Mutation of *c-myc* (transcription factor)	Movement of cells from G_0 to S in cell cycle Rapid growth

TABLE 54-3   Etiologic Factors Promoting Neoplasia

Agent	Specific Cancer	Specific Genetic Effect	Strength of Association
Tobacco	Lung, esophagus, head and neck, renal cell, bladder, pancreatic cancer	Possible effect near *TP53* site	High
Asbestos	Mesothelioma, lung cancer	Unknown	High
Ionizing radiation	Leukemia, thyroid cancer, sarcoma	Increased mutation rate	High
Solar radiation	Melanoma, squamous cell skin cancers	DNA breaks	Moderate
Human papillomavirus 16 and 18	Cervical cancer	Unknown	Moderate
Diet	Breast, prostate, colon cancer	Unknown	Low
Estrogen	Breast, endometrial, vaginal cancer in female children of mothers taking compound during pregnancy	Many effects on intracellular and paracrine growth factors	Low

exposed to carcinogens in tobacco. Consequently, to-bacco users have much higher rates of cancers of the head and neck, lung, bladder, cervix, esophagus, and pancreas. The highest rates occur for lung cancer, the organ that receives the greatest concentration of the offending agents. A tobacco by-product, benzopyrene di-olepoxide, causes changes at a specific gene locus near the *TP53* oncogene and links epidemiologic observations relating smoking to cancer to a specific molecular event.

Genetics factors also contribute to the addiction to tobacco. Population genetic studies using monozygotic (identical) and dizygotic (fraternal) twins, both concordant and discordant for a history of smoking, show that many persons smoke because they have an inherited tendency to nicotine addiction. The exact gene, or group of genes, that confers addictive behavior is not known.

OTHER HABITS AND ENVIRONMENTAL EXPOSURES

Various other habits and environmental exposures may increase the risk of cancer. Consumption of alcoholic beverages potentiates the effect of smoking on the upper airways and gastrointestinal tract. However, whether prolonged alcohol consumption increases cancer risk because of a component of the beverage, an effect on the metabolism of a carcinogenic compound, or a deficiency that results from an abnormal diet is not yet clear. Certain occupational exposures increase cancer risk. Benzene exposure increases the risk of leukemia. Asbestos fibers increase the rate of mesothelioma and lung cancers, particularly in cigarette smokers. Radon, acquired from high levels in the home, can also increase the risk of lung cancer. Exposure to ionizing radiation, either accidental or therapeutic, also increases the risk of cancer. For example, patients who undergo therapeutic radiation, particularly in conjunction with alkylating agents for Hodgkin's disease, have almost a 5% chance of acquiring acute leukemia within 10 years of initial treatment.

MEDICATIONS

Various medications can increase the risk of cancer. For instance, synthetic estrogens such as diethylstilbestrol,

given to mothers during pregnancy, may result in the development of vaginal cancer in their offspring. Conjugated estrogens taken for less than 5 years to 10 years appear to increase the risk of breast cancer. Endometrial cancer is almost five times more common in postmenopausal women who take estrogens than in those who do not. Progestins, on the other hand, appear to protect the uterus from the malignant transformation of estrogen. Immunosuppressive agents also increase cancer risk. For example, pharmacologic immunosuppression in organ transplant recipients results in a much higher rate of cervical, lymphoid, and skin cancers. Kaposi's sarcoma, usually a rare disease in elderly men of Mediterranean descent, is much more common in transplant recipients as well as those with the human immunodeficiency virus.

INFECTIOUS AGENTS

Various infectious agents predispose to the development of cancer although the pathophysiology of malignant transformation is undetermined. *Helicobacter pylori* and gastric cancer, the Epstein-Barr virus and Burkitt's lymphoma, hepatitis B virus and hepatocellular carcinoma, and the human papillomaviruses 16 and 18 and cervical cancer are examples of cancers related to specific infections.

DIET

Last, important links may exist between diet and cancer, but the specific agents and molecular mechanisms have not been elucidated. Circumstantial evidence suggests that dietary fat plays a role in the development of colon, prostate, and breast cancers. However, nagging questions remain, such as which specific component of fat is the culprit, or, conversely, whether total caloric intake is more of an issue than a specific food component. Just as fat may play a role in causing cancer, various micronutrients are under study as chemopreventive agents (see Chapter 55).

Eventually, the implications of genetic and environmental causes of cancer will facilitate interventions that capitalize on the ability to manipulate DNA. It is already possible to prevent cancer by avoiding carcinogens and to detect it through genetic studies. Investigators may soon be able to repair genetic mistakes before or after cancer develops.

REFERENCES

Brown MA: Tumor suppressor genes and human cancer. Adv Hum Genet 1997; 36:45–135.

Fitzgerald MG, MacDonald DJ, Krainer M, et al: Germline *BRCA1* mutations in Jewish and non-Jewish women with early-onset breast cancer. N Engl J Med 1996; 334:143–149.

Shattuck-Eidens D, McClure M, Simared J, et al: A collaborative survey of 80 mutations in the *BRCA1* breast and ovarian cancer susceptibility gene. JAMA 1995; 272:535–541.

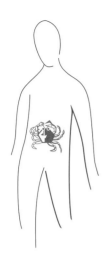

55

CANCER EPIDEMIOLOGY AND CANCER PREVENTION

Jennifer J. Griggs

Cancer Epidemiology

Cancer incidence rates (the number of new cases each year) are expressed as the number of new cases per 100,000 people. Because the incidence of most cancers increases with age, rates are age adjusted to account for the age distribution of the population under study. The risk of developing a particular type of cancer is described as a *lifetime risk* or as an *age group–specific risk*. For example, the risk of developing breast cancer between the ages of 40 and 59 years is 4%, or 1 in 25, and the lifetime risk is 12.5%, or 1 in 8 (Table 55–1). *Disease-specific mortality rates* are also expressed as rates per 100,000 or as risk percent.

Survival rates are usually expressed as relative survival rates, for example, as the percentage of people with the disease who are alive 5 years (for example) after the cancer is diagnosed. Survival rates are often broken down by the stage of disease. People who have limited-stage disease (confined to the organ of origin) have better 5-year survival rates than those with regional disease (involving regional lymph nodes), and people with regional disease have better survival rates than do patients with metastatic disease.

Except for lung cancer in African-American women, the mortality rates for all cancers are consistently higher among African-Americans than among any other ethnic or racial group in the United States. African-American men are 50% more likely to develop prostate cancer than men of any other group, and colon cancer is more common among African-American men and women. The differences in mortality are not accounted for by differences in the stage of presentation of the disease; even within the same stage, the mortality differences persist. Socioeconomic factors are probably the greatest determinant of the difference in outcome.

The *prevalence* of a disease is the number of people (e.g., per 100,000) living with the disease. Cancers associated with a longer life expectancy have a higher prevalence than those associated with shorter life expectancy.

Cancer Prevention

The three levels of disease prevention are primary, secondary, and tertiary. *Primary* prevention keeps the disease from occurring by reducing risk factor exposure. *Secondary* prevention detects the disease before it is symptomatic and when intervention can prevent illness. *Tertiary* prevention reduces the complications of a disease once the disease is clinically evident.

PRIMARY PREVENTION

Primary prevention of cancer is achieved by either avoidance of a causative agent or by use of an agent that prevents development of the malignant process. Primary prevention includes lifestyle risk reduction measures (avoidance of tobacco exposure, ingestion of a low-fat, high-fiber diet, use of sunscreen) and chemopreventive agents. Chemopreventive agents are drugs or micronutrients (minerals and vitamins) used to prevent the development of cancer. Many agents are being considered through epidemiologic studies and randomized controlled trials for prevention of breast, ovarian, lung, prostate, and colon cancers (Table 55–2). Chemopreventive agents have side effects and are generally considered for people at high risk of developing the disease.

SECONDARY PREVENTION

Secondary prevention of cancer is achieved with screening tests to detect disease in asymptomatic patients with

TABLE 55–1   Probability of Developing Cancer by Age Group and Sex, 1993–1995

		Lifetime	Ages 40–59 yr	Ages 60–79 yr
All Sites	Male	45% (1 in 2)	8% (1 in 12)	35% (1 in 3)
	Female	38% (1 in 3)	9% (1 in 11)	22% (1 in 5)
Lung cancer	Male	8% (1 in 12)	1.3% (1 in 75)	6.6% (1 in 15)
	Female	5% (1 in 18)	.97% (1 in 103)	3.9% (1 in 25)
Colorectal cancer	Male	5.7% (1 in 18)	.9 (1 in 115)	4% (1 in 25)
	Female	5.6% (1 in 18)	.7 (1 in 150)	3% (1 in 32)
Breast cancer	Female	12.5% (1 in 8)	4% (1 in 25)	6.9% (1 in 15)
Prostate cancer	Male	17% (1 in 6)	1.8% (1 in 55)	15% (1 in 7)

early-stage disease. Examples include mammography to detect breast cancer, Papanicolaou (Pap) smears to detect cervical cancer, and sigmoidoscopy to detect colon cancer. Screening tests do not prevent disease and are not diagnostic on their own. Instead, they identify patients who need additional diagnostic tests and may need treatment for the disease. For most types of cancers, no effective screening tests exist. Diseases for which screening tests are available and recommended are listed in Table 55–3.

For screening to be recommended for a disease, these criteria must be met: (1) the disease must be associated with substantial morbidity and mortality in the studied population; screening for rare diseases does not improve the health of the population; (2) the disease must have a long asymptomatic (preclinical) phase during which time intervention is likely to be beneficial; (3) an effective intervention must be available, and early treatment must be more effective than later treatment; and (4) the test should be highly sensitive and specific, inexpensive, and safe.

The *sensitivity* of a screening test is the likelihood of a positive test result in a person with the disease. A 100% sensitive test is never negative in a person who has the disease, that is, it has a 0% false-negative rate. The *specificity* of a test is the likelihood of a negative test result in a person who does not have the disease. A 100% specific test is never positive in a person without the disease and has a 0% false-positive rate. The *positive predictive value* of a test is the likelihood that a person with a positive test result has the disease, and

the *negative predictive value* of a test is the likelihood that a person with a negative test result does not have the disease. Both depend on the sensitivity and specificity of the test and the prevalence of the disease in the population screened:

$$PPV = \frac{\text{prevalence} \times \text{sensitivity}}{(\text{prevalence} \times \text{sensitivity}) + (1 - \text{specificity}) \times (1 - \text{prevalence})}$$

Because screening is used in large numbers of asymptomatic people, the prevalence of the disease is usually low. The positive predictive value of screening tests is often low, and many people with positive test results but without disease must undergo further testing to determine whether the disease is truly present. The costs and risks of additional testing need to be included in cost-effectiveness evaluations of screening tests.

Randomized trials are theoretically the best way to demonstrate the effectiveness of cancer screening, but these trials require large numbers of people, take years to complete, and are vulnerable to errors, such as unplanned screening among subjects randomized to the nonscreening arm of the study or noncompliance with screening among study subjects randomized to the screening arm of the trial. Case-control and cohort studies are alternative study designs, but a suitable control group is essential.

TABLE 55–2   Cancer Chemopreventive Agents

Malignant Disease	Chemopreventive Agent
Breast cancer	Tamoxifen*
Ovarian cancer	Oral contraceptives*
Colon cancer	Folic acid
	Nonsteroidal anti-inflammatory agents*
Melanoma	Topical sunscreens
Prostate cancer	Lycopene

*In high-risk patients.

TABLE 55–3   Cancer with Demonstrated Benefit Screening Tests

Cancer	Recommendations for People at Average Risk
Breast cancer	Annual mammogram in women ≥50 yr; possible benefit in women ages 40–49 yr Annual health care with breast examination Monthly self-breast examination
Cervical cancer	Annual Pap test for women ages 18 and over
Colon cancer	Annual fecal occult blood testing (three specimens); flexible sigmoidoscopy and barium enema every 5 years *or* colonoscopy every 10 years

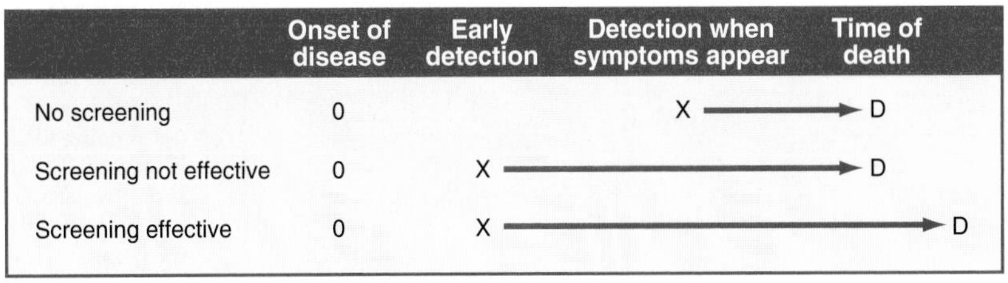

	Onset of disease	Early detection	Detection when symptoms appear	Time of death
No screening	0		X ⟶	D
Screening not effective	0	X ⟶		D
Screening effective	0	X ⟶⟶⟶		D

FIGURE 55–1 Effect of lead time bias. Both effective and ineffective screening tests can increase survival time from diagnosis to death without increasing life expectancy. An effective screening test improves life expectancy.

Three types of bias may occur in studies of effectiveness of screening tests: lead time bias, length time bias, and compliance bias. *Lead time* is the time between detection of disease by screening and the actual appearance of symptomatic disease. For rapidly progressive diseases with a short asymptomatic period, such as pancreatic cancer, treatment of disease detected by screening does not alter outcome much more than treatment when symptoms appear. Diagnosing the disease earlier with screening may make it appear that the patient lived longer, but the survival of the patient from the onset of disease is not altered (Fig. 55–1). To avoid lead time bias, analyses of screening tests must demonstrate improvements in age-specific mortality among the screened population.

Length time bias occurs when subsets of the cancer under study have different growth rates. Screening is more likely to detect the tumors that grow more slowly because of the greater prevalence of asymptomatic people with slow-growing tumors than fast-growing tumors. People with fast-growing tumors present for medical attention before screening can be performed and have shorter life expectancy because of the nature of their tumor. Thus, patients with cancer that is detected with screening appear to have longer survival as a result of screening when the longer course of their disease results from the behavior of the tumor itself (Fig. 55–2). Length time bias can be avoided by randomized controlled trials because a mixture of people with slow-growing and fast-growing tumors is included in the trials.

Compliance bias is seen in nonrandomized studies of screening tests in which volunteers present for testing. Such studies may suggest that screening tests lead to better health. However, because people who request screening studies tend to be healthier and have longer life expectancy, such a conclusion is flawed. Randomized, controlled studies of screening interventions are needed to circumvent compliance bias.

Screening tests have risks as well as benefits. False-negative results miss the diagnosis, and the patient does not benefit from having had the screening test. False-positive results are expensive, inconvenient, and may have health risks. False-positive test results can cause the patient to be labeled with a disease that is not truly present. Moreover, true-positive test results for a disease that cannot be treated satisfactorily cause anxiety without health benefit.

GENETIC SCREENING

DNA testing is available for several types of cancer. In general, this testing is reserved for people with a strong family history of the disease (Table 55–4). If a mutation is found in an affected family member, other family members can be tested to assess their risk of developing the disease. Most genes associated with a predisposition to cancer are large, and mutations can occur anywhere within the gene. Screening is therefore impractical unless an affected family member is available for testing.

Patients having genetic testing must receive counseling before and after the test so they know the test limitations, the prevention options available if the test result is positive, and the risks of having a positive test result. Discrimination by employers, by friends, and by family, psychosocial issues, and side effects of the prevention measures should all be discussed fully with patients before DNA testing. Patients who have a negative test result must understand that their risk of cancer is not zero but approaches that of the general population.

TABLE 55–4 Hereditary Cancer Syndromes for Which Genetic Testing is Available

Cancer and Involved Gene(s)	Prevention Measures
Breast: *BRCA1, BRCA2*	Prophylactic mastectomy Tamoxifen Lifestyle risk reduction
Ovarian: *BRCA1*	Prophylactic oophorectomy Oral contraceptives

Colon cancer syndromes
  Familial adenomatous polyposis coli: *APC* gene
  Hereditary nonpolyposis colon cancer: *SDH2, MLH1, PMS1, PMS2*
	Prophylactic colectomy
	Nonsteroidal anti-inflammatory drugs
	Lifestyle risk reduction

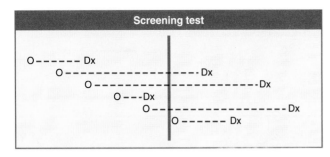

FIGURE 55-2 Length time bias. Screening is more likely to detect tumors with longer time from onset of disease (O) to diagnosis (Dx) than it is to detect fast-growing tumors. Concluding that the screening test has led to improved survival would be erroneous because improved survival is actually the result of tumor biology.

REFERENCES

Aaltonen LA, Salovaara R, Kristo P, et al: Incidence of hereditary nonpolyposis colorectal cancer and the feasibility of molecular screening for the disease. N Engl J Med 1998; 338: 1481–1487.

Elmore JG, Barton MB, Moceri VM, et al: Ten-year risk of false positive screening mammograms and clinical breast examinations. N Engl J Med 1998; 338: 1089–1096.

Giovannucci E, Stampfer MJ, Colditz GA, et al: Multivitamin use, folate, and colon cancer in women in the Nurses' Health Study. Ann Intern Med 1998; 129: 517–524.

Hartmann LC, Schaid DJ, Woods JE, et al: Efficacy of bilateral prophylactic mastectomy in women with a family history of breast cancer. N Engl J Med 1999; 340: 77–84.

Narod SA, Risch H, Moslehi R, et al: Oral contraceptives and the risk of hereditary ovarian cancer: Hereditary Ovarian Cancer Clinical Study Group. N Engl J Med 1998; 339: 424–428.

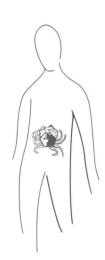

56

SOLID TUMORS

Jennifer J. Griggs • Christopher E. Desch

Lung Cancer

Lung cancer is a devastating malignant disease of adults. Although the rate of increase of new lung cancers has leveled, the mortality rate for lung cancer is the highest of all the cancers.

EPIDEMIOLOGY

Lung cancer is the most common malignant disease in the United States. More than 170,000 new cases of lung cancer and almost 160,000 deaths occur each year. Although cases of lung cancer have decreased in men since 1980, by 1988 lung cancer had become the most common cause of cancer death in women.

Tobacco smoke accounts for more than 90% of all lung cancers. One metabolite of cigarette smoke, benzopyrene diolepoxide, binds to areas near the *TP53* suppressor gene. This finding provides a link between the genetics of lung cancer and the epidemiologic association between smoking and cancer. Second-hand smoking is also associated with a higher risk of lung cancer. A nonsmoking spouse has a relative risk of lung cancer of 1.5 to 2.0 compared with nonexposed control subjects.

In addition to cigarette smoke, household exposure to radon seeping through the ground into enclosed spaces and asbestos exposure increase cancer risk. Cigarette smoking enhances the risk of cancer from both these toxic exposures.

PATHOLOGY

The two major types of lung cancer are *non–small cell lung cancer* (NSCLC) and *small cell lung cancer* (Table 56–1). NSCLC includes several histologic subtypes, including squamous cell, adenocarcinoma, and large cell.

Squamous cell carcinoma usually presents as a centrally located endobronchial lesion and is the subtype most commonly associated with paraneoplastic hypercalcemia. *Adenocarcinomas* are the most common lung cancers and are the type seen most often in nonsmokers. Adenocarcinomas present more often with a peripheral lung nodule. *Bronchioalveolar lung cancer* is a histologic variant of adenocarcinoma characterized by multiple nodules and interstitial infiltration. Sputum production with this subtype can be prolific. *Large cell tumors* are the least common; some have histologic features of neuroendocrine tumors. Although differences are noted in the clinical presentation of various subtypes, the natural history and response to treatment are similar.

Small cell lung cancer is highly linked to cigarette exposure. The cell of origin is derived from the neuroendocrine family. This finding probably explains its proclivity to cause paraneoplastic syndromes such as syndrome of inappropriate antidiuretic hormone and Cushing's syndrome. Small cell lung cancer often presents with a large, central tumor with mediastinal involvement.

GENETICS

Many genetic abnormalities are associated with lung cancer. Mutations in the *ras* gene are common in adenocarcinomas and predict a poorer prognosis. The oncogene *myc* is commonly amplified in small cell lung cancer and is also associated with resistance to therapy. Abnormalities in the tumor suppressor genes on chromosome 3 as well as *TP53* are common.

CLINICAL PRESENTATION

All types of lung cancer commonly present with a cough, hemoptysis, chest pain, and weight loss in a chronic smoker. Approximately 60% of patients with small cell lung cancer present with metastatic disease. Common metastatic sites include the brain, liver, skeleton, and bone marrow. Small cell lung cancer may also present with the superior vena cava syndrome as well as with paraneoplastic syndromes. NSCLC presents with metastatic disease less than one third of the time, most often in the bone and adrenal glands. NSCLC is associated with paraneoplastic syndromes such as pulmonary

493

TABLE 56-1   Lung Cancer

Tumor	Staging Tests	Standard Treatment	Outcome
Non–small cell lung cancer	Computed tomography of chest through adrenal glands, bronchoscopy, mediastinoscopy if enlarged lymph nodes	Early stage: surgery only Later stage (unresectable): combined chemotherapy/radiation or chemotherapy alone	Early stage: stage II patients have a 40%–50% survival with surgery Late stage: stage IV patients have 1-yr survival rates near 20% with chemotherapy
Small cell lung cancer	Computed tomography scans of chest, abdomen, and head; bone marrow biopsy if no other indication of extensive disease	Limited: cisplatin-based chemotherapy followed by chest radiation and (consider) prophylactic cranial radiation Extensive: chemotherapy for palliation	Limited: 20%–30% 5-yr survival Extensive: median survival 10 mo with treatment

hypertrophic osteoarthropathy, disseminated intravascular coagulation, and hypercalcemia.

STAGING

Staging of lung cancer requires a computed tomography (CT) scan to determine the extent of disease in the mediastinum as well as to uncover any occult signs of metastatic disease. CT scan of the chest should extend through the liver and adrenal glands, common sites of metastases. Bronchoscopy or fine-needle aspiration is frequently used to make the histologic diagnosis. Patients with NSCLC who have enlarged mediastinal lymph nodes should undergo mediastinoscopy to determine resectability (mediastinal nodes are rarely resectable). If the adrenal gland is enlarged, it should be examined by biopsy to determine whether the enlargement results from metastases. In patients with resectable disease, surgical treatment may offer a chance for cure.

Staging for lung cancer is shown in Table 56–2. For NSCLC, tumor size, proximity to central structures, and the location of lymph nodes are the most important features. Staging for small cell lung cancer is slightly different. Because surgical resection is rarely performed, the focus of the staging evaluation is to uncover signs of metastatic disease that would preclude aggressive local therapy to the chest and prophylactic radiation to the brain. Therefore, a patient with small cell lung cancer should undergo additional tests such as a bone scan, bone marrow biopsy, and CT scan of the head before treatment is initiated.

TREATMENT

Non–Small Cell Lung Cancer

Because complete removal of the tumor provides the best chance for long-term survival, the focus of primary

TABLE 56-2   Staging for Lung Cancer

Stage	Type
Non–Small Cell Lung Cancer	
I	No lymph node involvement; tumor may be any size but not closer than 2 cm from carina
II	Tumor may be any size, not closer than 2 cm from carina Peribronchial and/or hilar nodes involved
IIIA	Any size tumor and may invade chest wall, but not heart, great vessels, trachea, and esophagus; may be close to carina but not invading it; involves ipsilateral mediastinal nodes and/or subcarinal nodes
IIIB	Any size tumor and may invade any structure; nodes extend to contralateral mediastinum or supraclavicular or scalene area
IV	Presence of metastases
Small Cell	
Limited	Tumor confined to one lung; nodes may involve contralateral lung but all cancer must be encompassed in one radiation portal
Extensive	Metastatic disease or disease not encompassed in one radiation field

treatment for NSCLC should begin with an assessment of resectability. Resectability depends on the anatomic location of the tumor as well as on the patient's medical condition and pulmonary reserve. In general terms, the risk of pneumonectomy is small if the patient has a forced expiratory volume in 1 second greater than 2 L, carbon dioxide diffusing capacity of more than 60%, a maximum voluntary ventilation of more than 50% of predicted values, or the ability to walk up three flights of stairs. Lesser resections (i.e., lobectomy) may require less stringent criteria. Occasionally, patients with severe obstructive disease cannot undergo a curative procedure because they lack pulmonary reserve.

Patients with stage I and II tumors (localized lesions or involvement of hilar lymph nodes only) should undergo surgical treatment. Peripheral tumors are removed by lobectomy; more central tumors, if resectable, require pneumonectomy. Postoperative chemotherapy or radiation does not benefit this population. Stage III tumors may be operable in some situations. In patients with significant mediastinal lymph node involvement detected during tumor resection or at the time of mediastinoscopy, the chance of long-term survival is less than 20% even with surgical treatment.

Almost 80% of lung cancers are unresectable. If the tumor cannot be resected and has not spread to distant organs (stages IIIA and IIIB), chemotherapy is given, followed by radiation. This treatment leads to better median survival and 5-year disease-free survival rates than radiation alone, but combined therapy for unresectable disease should be reserved for patients with good functional status. Aggressive treatment is much less effective in patients who have lost more than 5% of their body weight or who are active less than 50% of the day. The median survival for patients with locally advanced, unresectable lung cancer is approximately 10 months.

Patients with metastatic disease may benefit from chemotherapy. The most active agents are cisplatin, paclitaxel, gemcitabine, vinorelbine, and cyclophosphamide. Chemotherapy improves survival and quality of life compared with supportive measures and can relieve pain and cough, and it also leads to a reduction in tumor volume in 50% or fewer of patients.

Small Cell Lung Cancer

The cornerstone of treatment of small cell lung cancer is combination chemotherapy. Active agents for this cancer include cyclophosphamide, doxorubicin, vincristine, cisplatin, and etoposide. Patients with limited-stage small cell lung cancer (defined as limited to the thorax and encompassed in a single radiation therapy portal) should undergo four to six cycles of chemotherapy as long as they are responding to treatment. Approximately 50% of patients have a complete response; another 20% to 30% may have a partial response. Concomitant or sequential radiation therapy provides longer survival than either modality alone in patients with limited-stage disease. Because almost 40% of patients with small cell lung cancer have brain involvement, prophylactic cranial radiation should be considered for those patients who have a complete response in the lung to primary che-

moradiotherapy. Oral etoposide may palliate extremely elderly or infirm patients with small cell lung cancer. Approximately 20% to 30% of patients with small cell lung cancer are alive and free of disease 3 years after diagnosis. These patients are, however, still at risk for late relapses and other tobacco-related cancers.

Both NSCLC and small call lung cancer have high relapse rates. The use of second-line chemotherapy for these patients is controversial. Although these cancers are likely to respond to subsequent agents, the use of these drugs outside a clinical trial should be restricted to palliation. No evidence indicates a survival benefit with the use of second-line or third-line treatments.

Gastrointestinal Cancers

Cancers of the gastrointestinal tract are among the most common tumors. Advances in the treatment of colorectal cancer have improved survival and quality of life for patients with these diseases. Cancers of the esophagus, pancreas, liver, and stomach are less common. Table 56–3 outlines the common signs and symptoms, treatments, and prognosis of gastrointestinal tumors.

ESOPHAGEAL CANCER

Epidemiology and Natural History

The two types of esophageal cancer are squamous cell and adenocarcinoma. *Squamous cell cancers* are most common in the cervical and thoracic esophagus, and *adenocarcinomas* commonly occur in the lower esophagus down to the gastroesophageal junction. Squamous cell cancers are more common in African-Americans and are associated with predisposing factors including smoking, caustic injury, achalasia, and alcohol intake. Squamous cell cancers are associated with other tobacco-related cancers in the upper airways and digestive tract. Adenocarcinomas, conversely, are most common in the lower esophagus. The rate of adenocarcinoma is increasing; this increase is related to Barrett's esophagus, adenomatous metaplasia of the distal esophagus often caused by gastroesophageal reflux disease. Almost 25% of patients with severe Barrett's esophagus eventually have esophageal adenocarcinoma. The most useful intervention for patients with Barrett's esophagus is frequent endoscopic screening and biopsy; pharmacologic treatment of acid reflux disease does not prevent neoplastic transformation.

Symptoms

The most common symptom of esophageal cancer is dysphagia. As the lumen of the esophagus narrows, the patient loses normal swallowing capacity and has a sensation that solid food becomes "stuck." Eventually, the patient may become unable to swallow liquids. Patients commonly become afraid to eat because of frequent regurgitation at mealtime. Significant weight loss is therefore common.

TABLE 56–3   Gastrointestinal Cancers

Tumor Site	Common Findings	Standard Treatments	Expected Outcome
Esophageal	Dysphagia, chest pain, weight loss	Early stage-surgery alone; later stages combinations of chemotherapy and radiation therapy +/− surgery	Early stage ≈30% 5-yr survival Later stage <13% 5-yr survival
Gastric	Pain, supraclavicular adenopathy, vomiting, melena	Early stage: surgery alone; later stage chemotherapy +/− radiation	Early >90% 5-yr survival
Hepatocellular	Elevated α-fetoprotein; pain or liver function test changes	Resection for early lesions	Node-positive 20%–50% 5-yr survival for tumors <2 cm Always fatal in later-stage disease
Pancreas	Weight loss, boring midline pain through back, jaundice	Early stage: Whipple's procedure ± radiation therapy; late stage: chemotherapy plus radiation or chemotherapy alone	Resectable: median survival 6–12 mo Unresectable: median survival 4–6 mo
Colon/rectal	Abdominal pain, occult or overt bleeding in stool, change in bowel habits	Early stage: resection alone If nodal involvement, add chemotherapy Patients with rectal cancers should receive chemotherapy and radiation therapy before/after surgery	Early stage >70% at 5 yr Nodal involvement: 40%–60% at 5 yr Metastatic: median <1 yr
Anal	Constipation, bleeding, rectal pain/urgency	Early stage: chemotherapy plus radiation therapy; later stage: abdominoperineal resection	Localized: 70% at 5 yr

Diagnosis

An upper gastrointestinal radiographic series or endoscopy demonstrates an esophageal lesion, which then undergoes biopsy. The most effective staging tool is endoscopic ultrasonography, an accurate tool in assessing local lymph node metastases. CT scanning is also required to ensure that the tumor has not already metastasized to the chest or liver, the two most common sites of spread.

Treatment

The most common treatment of esophageal cancer is surgical. Resection of the involved esophagus includes a wide margin on either side. The stomach is then pulled up to join the remainder of the esophagus. Alternatively, part of the intestine may be transposed to the chest to create another digestive pathway. Approximately 10% to 30% of patients with stage II disease who are treated by surgical resection alone are alive and free of cancer at 5 years. If surgical treatment is not possible, either because the cancer is technically unresectable or the patient is medically unfit for surgery, the standard of care is to provide chemotherapy and radiation. This approach leads to a median survival of 12.5 months compared with 9 months with radiation alone. Whether chemotherapy and radiation provide an outcome as good as with surgical resection alone is not clear.

For patients with unresectable esophageal cancer, radiation alone or the combination of chemotherapy and radiation may provide useful palliation. For patients with severe dysphagia that cannot be treated adequately with radiation or surgery, endoscopic placement of a metal or plastic stent results in reasonable palliation.

GASTRIC CANCER

Epidemiology and Natural History

Gastric cancer rates are highest in poor countries that use smoked meats and meats high in nitrates. Other predisposing conditions include pernicious anemia, achlorhydria, gastric ulcers, and prior gastric surgery. Except for cancers of the gastroesophageal junction, gastric cancer rates have decreased in the United States. A recognized risk factor for gastric cancer is infection with *Helicobacter pylori*. Whether early treatment of *H. pylori* infection changes the rate of cancer in infected populations is not clear, however.

Diagnosis

Patients with gastric cancer commonly present with abdominal pain, early satiety, anemia, hematemesis, weakness, and weight loss. Frequently, the cancer has already involved local lymph nodes by the time the diagnosis is made. Physical examination may show a gastric mass, an umbilical node (Sister Mary Joseph's node), or a left supraclavicular node (Virchow's node). Pathologic analysis shows an adenocarcinoma that can be localized or spread throughout the gastric lining *(linitis plastica)*. Required staging includes a CT scan, upper gastrointestinal endoscopic examination, and endoscopic ultrasonography.

Treatment

Gastric cancer is most often treated surgically. When the tumor and all relevant lymph nodes have been removed, patients have a 40% or lower chance of 5-year survival. If gastric cancer recurs, the most common sites are local extension or hematogenous spread through the portal vein to the liver. No clear role exists for postoperative therapy with chemotherapy or radiation. Patients with metastatic gastric cancer may opt for chemotherapy to palliate symptoms. Chemotherapy usually provides a response rate of 20% to 40%, but it has no discernible impact on the expected survival of 5 to 7 months.

COLORECTAL CANCER

Epidemiology and Natural History

Approximately 1 in 20 people will be diagnosed with colon cancer. This tumor has a strong familial tendency; several genes discovered to play a role in the development of adenomas and cancers include *DCC, MCC,* and *APC.* Among the predisposing factors are familial cancer syndromes, ulcerative colitis, and familial polyposis. A clear relationship exists between adenomatous polyps and the later development of colon cancer. Because the removal of polyps is probably the most important way to prevent the development of invasive colon cancer, the most reliable way to reduce colon and rectal cancer mortality is to perform periodic sigmoidoscopy and regular fecal occult blood testing. For patients with a strong family history (familial adenomatous polyposis, Gardner's syndrome, hereditary nonpolyposis colon cancer) or who have other diseases associated with colorectal cancer such as ulcerative colitis, total colon imaging should begin before 40 years of age. Research efforts are under way in the primary prevention of colorectal cancers using interventions such as diet, daily aspirin, and other chemopreventive agents to reduce cancer incidence. Enthusiasm for promoting a high-fiber diet to reduce the risk of colon cancer has waned.

Symptoms

Colon and rectal cancers commonly present with rectal bleeding. Patients with right-sided colon lesions often complain of a change in stool color or pain and transient bloating. Left-sided lesions may become friable and may result in red blood along the length of a stool. Occasionally, colon and rectal cancers are asymptomatic until they totally obstruct the bowel or perforate the peritoneal cavity. The most common recurrence pattern for rectal cancer is local pelvic extension; colon cancer tends to recur with metastases to the lung or liver.

Diagnosis

The work-up for colon cancer requires measurement of serum carcinoembryonic antigen, palpation of the liver at operation or an abdominal CT scan, and imaging of the colon to ensure that all polyps and cancers are removed near the time of the primary operation. Table 56–4 describes staging for colon and rectal cancer.

Treatment

Treatments for colon cancer and rectal cancer differ. Even in patients with metastatic disease, the most appropriate treatment for colon cancer is surgical. Surgical resection treats or prevents obstruction and pain. If cancer has spread to the lymph nodes, adjuvant chemotherapy with 5-fluorouracil (5-FU) and levamisole or leucovorin is indicated and reduces the chance of tumor recurrence by approximately 40%. For patients with rectal cancer, any lesion that invades the muscle or lymph nodes should be treated with chemotherapy and radiation before or after surgery to reduce the chance of local and distant recurrence of the disease. 5-FU has been used more than any other drug for treatment of colon cancer. Irinotecan, a camptothecin, has shown impressive activity in the setting of metastatic disease that has failed to respond to 5-FU.

ANAL CARCINOMA

Anal cancers are increasing in frequency. Persons infected with the human papillomavirus as well as human immunodeficiency virus (HIV) are more likely to develop anal cancer. Patients with anal cancer usually present with rectal bleeding or complaints of rectal fullness.

Combined chemotherapy with 5-FU and mitomycin and radiation therapy comprise the standard approach to a patient with localized anal cancer. Results with combined therapy are superior to those with local resection, with the additional benefit of sparing the anal sphincter. Abdominoperineal resection is reserved for patients in whom local therapy fails.

PANCREATIC CANCER

Epidemiology and Natural History

Pancreatic cancer is often associated with cigarette smoking and excessive intake of alcohol. Epithelial pan-

TABLE 56–4 Staging for Colon and Rectal Cancer

Stage	Tumor Size	Nodal Status	Metastases
0	In situ	No	No
1	Invades mucosa only	No	No
2	May invade muscularis or through serosa	No	No
3	Any size tumor or any level of invasion	Yes	No
4	Any size or depth	Positive nodes present or absent	Yes

creatic cancer is an adenocarcinoma with an extremely high mortality rate because it usually presents when the tumor is beyond the capability of surgical resection. The less common type of pancreatic cancer originates in endocrine cells. These tumors are characterized by symptoms related to secretion of peptides such as gastrin, vasointestinal polypeptide, and insulin.

Symptoms

The most common presentation of pancreatic cancer is abdominal pain accompanied by rapid weight loss. Characteristically, the pain is located in the periumbilical region and pierces or stabs through to the back. The pain is often explained by the frequent invasion of the celiac plexus deep in the retroperitoneum. Other symptoms of pancreatic cancer are the recent onset of diabetes, intestinal angina reflecting encasement of the superior mesenteric artery, a palpable gallbladder (Courvoisier's sign), and jaundice from blockage of the distal common bile duct. Migrating thrombophlebitis (Trousseau's sign) is a common paraneoplastic complication of pancreatic adenocarcinoma. The tumor marker CA 19-9 is elevated in ≤75% of all cases.

Treatment

The only curative treatment for pancreatic cancer is pancreaticoduodenectomy (Whipple's procedure), an extensive operation requiring numerous anastamoses and splenectomy that carries a high mortality rate in centers with less experience with the procedure. The 5-year survival for patients with localized pancreatic cancer is 25% to 50%. Patients with unresectable disease may benefit from local radiation therapy with concurrent 5-FU; more than 30% of patients treated this way may have some improvement in their symptoms. When patients have progressive disease, the use of palliative chemotherapy with weekly gemcitabine has been shown to improve quality of life and survival to a small degree (5.7 months with gemcitabine, 4.4 months without).

HEPATOCELLULAR CARCINOMA

Although it is uncommon in the United States, hepatocellular carcinoma (HCC) is one of the most common cancers throughout the world; more than 1 million cases are diagnosed per year. The common causes of HCC are viral hepatitis (both B and C) and cirrhosis secondary to alcoholism. Although this approach is unproved, considerable interest exists in screening patients who are at extremely high risk of HCC for α-fetoprotein (AFP) levels. Even in early-stage HCC, AFP levels are commonly elevated.

Treatment of early-stage HCC is surgical. Cure rates are more than 75% for patients with tumors less than 2 cm. Patients with severe cirrhosis and who have small liver cancers may benefit from liver transplantation. Patients with cancers that are more extensive rarely benefit from chemotherapy or radiation.

Breast Cancer

EPIDEMIOLOGY

Breast cancer is the most common cancer in women and the second leading cause of cancer death (after lung cancer) among women in the United States. Each year, approximately 175,000 newly diagnosed cases of invasive breast cancer are reported, and more than 43,000 women die of the disease. Breast cancer in men is rare.

Risk factors for breast cancer include older age, positive family history, early menarche, late menopause, first term pregnancy after age 25 years, nulliparity, and perhaps use of exogenous estrogen. Exposure to ionizing radiation, as is used in the treatment of Hodgkin's disease, also increases the risk. Although epidemiologic studies suggest that a diet high in fat increases the risk, no causal role has been established. Only 5% to 10% of cases of breast cancer are associated with the breast cancer susceptibility genes, *BRCA1* and *BRCA2*.

PATHOLOGY

Most breast cancers are infiltrating ductal adenocarcinomas. A smaller proportion consists of infiltrating lobular adenocarcinomas. The latter are more likely to be bilateral. Tubular and mucinous carcinomas are associated with a better prognosis. Ductal carcinoma in situ (DCIS, or intraductal carcinoma) is increasing in frequency, most likely because of increased mammographic screening.

CLINICAL PRESENTATION

Breast cancer is diagnosed when a patient or her physician notices a palpable mass or when routine mammography demonstrates a lesion. Fewer than 10% of women present with metastatic disease. Recurrent breast cancer presents most commonly with metastases in the bone, liver, lung, and central nervous system, but breast cancer can recur in any organ of the body. Women with a history of breast cancer are also at increased risk of breast cancer in the contralateral breast. Inflammatory breast cancer presents with breast induration and erythema, often without a palpable mass.

STAGING

Breast cancer staging requires removal of the primary tumor and ipsilateral axillary lymph node dissection. Women with tumors more than 2 cm and those with positive axillary lymph nodes should have additional staging tests, including a chest radiograph, bone scan, and CT of the abdomen if liver function tests are abnormal. Patients with small tumors and negative lymph nodes do not need to have these additional tests unless they have symptoms suggestive of metastatic involvement, such as skeletal pain.

TREATMENT

For women with small breast tumors, breast-conserving surgery with lumpectomy followed by radiation therapy

TABLE 56-5   Recommendations for Treatment of Metastatic Breast Cancer

Hormonal Therapy*	Chemotherapy
Estrogen receptor–positive disease Lymph node, skin, bone metastases >2 yr from completion of adjuvant therapy	Estrogen receptor–negative disease Lung, liver involvement <2 yr from completion of adjuvant therapy Progression after use of first- and second-line chemotherapy

* Ovarian ablation in premenopausal women; tamoxifen or aromatase inhibitors (anastrazole or letrozole) in postmenopausal women.

is standard therapy. Women with larger tumors or two or more tumors in separate quadrants of the breast should undergo mastectomy. Some women also prefer mastectomy, with or without breast reconstruction. Chemotherapy given before surgical treatment (*neoadjuvant* or *primary chemotherapy*) may allow breast conservation in women with large tumors who would otherwise not be able to have lumpectomy. Preoperative hormone therapy can be considered in frail patients with estrogen receptor–positive tumors, but it should not replace surgical treatment. Adjuvant therapy with the hormonal agent tamoxifen and with chemotherapy improves relapse-free and overall survival rates in premenopausal and postmenopausal women with high risk of recurrent, systemic breast cancer.

Metastatic disease is treated with either hormone therapy or chemotherapy (Table 56–5). Life expectancy is longer in women with lymph node or bone metastases than in those with liver, lung, or central nervous system metastases. Bisphosphonates, such as pamidronate, decrease the pain associated with bone metastases and the risk of fracture in women with skeletal metastases.

DCIS is treated with either lumpectomy followed by radiation therapy or mastectomy. Women with multifocal or palpable DCIS should have axillary lymph node dissection because a small but measurable proportion will have positive lymph nodes that indicate foci of invasive cancer. Women with DCIS who have invasive cancer in the lymph nodes are treated with systemic therapy as if they had an infiltrating primary tumor.

Prophylactic bilateral mastectomy is offered to women with the *BRCA1* or *BRCA2* breast cancer susceptibility genes. An alternative approach is close clinical surveillance including monthly self-breast examination, frequent examination by a physician, and regular mammography. Tamoxifen may decrease the risk of breast cancer in these women and in other women at high risk of the disease.

Genitourinary Cancers (Table 56–6)

PROSTATE CANCER

Epidemiology and Natural History

Prostate cancer is the most common cancer in men; in the United States, nearly 180,000 new cases are diagnosed and 37,000 deaths occur per year. Other than increasing age, no clear risk factors or habits are related to prostate cancer. The incidence of prostate cancer is highest in countries with a high consumption of dietary fat. The exact component of the diet that causes prostate cancer has yet to be determined. Some investigators have suggested that α-linoleic acid may increase the risk, whereas vitamins such as α-tocopherol, genistein (isoflavanoid), and retinoids may offer some protection. Other risk factors, such as high mean testosterone level, black race, and a positive family history, also increase the risk of developing this tumor.

Symptoms

Prostate cancer presents with a prostate mass on digital rectal examination, with voiding difficulties, or with elevation of the prostate specific antigen (PSA) test. Some patients present with bone pain from metastatic disease.

Diagnosis

If a screening PSA is elevated, or if the digital rectal examination is abnormal, a transrectal ultrasound study is commonly performed. Although a specific lesion may be visible on an ultrasound scan, more commonly the physician performs six biopsies along a grid, three from each lobe of the prostate gland. The Gleason system, a 1 to 10 scale, is used for histologic grading. High Gleason's scores correlate with a worse prognosis. Patients with involvement of a large portion of the prostate gland or who have extremely high PSA levels should undergo a bone scan to look for the presence of metastatic disease.

Treatment

The treatment of organ-confined prostate cancer in men less than 75 years of age remains a major uncertainty in urologic oncology. Although several published studies have estimated outcomes using models of disease progression and treatment effect, only a few trials have compared surgery with radiation therapy. Furthermore, older patients with early-stage prostate cancer are more likely to die of other medical causes than of their tumor. Therefore, the contributions of treatment to outcome remain subject for debate.

Men less than 65 years of age who have organ-confined tumors and Gleason's score of 7 or higher should undergo definitive treatment with radiation or surgical resection. Elderly patients with low Gleason's scores and low PSA levels probably do not benefit from surgery or radiation until disease progression is clearly identified. Those patients can be monitored regularly with a PSA test and digital rectal examination. Patients who present with locally advanced disease, involvement of the seminal vesicles, or bone metastases are not cured with surgical resection or radiation therapy. These patients should be given hormonal treatment.

Bilateral orchiectomy (surgical castration) or administration of a gonadotropin-releasing hormone (GnRH) analogue such as leuprolide acetate (medical castration), given every 1 to 3 months, usually suppresses growth of the neoplastic prostate gland. Testosterone levels fall, and men may have adverse effects such as hot flashes, impotence, and loss of muscle tone. The duration of hormonal control varies. Some patients may have adequate suppression of their cancer for years. In other patients, the tumor may undergo further genetic changes that allow it to escape hormonal control and grow to produce new symptoms.

Long-term control of metastatic prostate cancer can be achieved in many patients with GnRH compounds. When the disease progresses, some patients may benefit from chemotherapy such as prednisone and mitoxantrone, an anthracycline. Bone pain from metastatic prostate cancer frequently requires radiation therapy to the affected area. Compounds such as radioactive strontium-83 or samarium-153, given intravenously, may markedly reduce bone pain.

TESTICULAR CANCER

Epidemiology and Natural History

This tumor is most common in men from the ages of 15 to 30 years. The only known predisposing factor is cryptorchidism; 5% to 20% of males with cryptorchidism develop testicular cancer. These cancers derive from the malignant transformation of premeiotic germ cells. Occasionally, germ cell tumors present in the retroperitoneum or mediastinum and reflect the track these cells take during embryologic development.

The tumor derived from premeiotic germ cells is termed *seminoma*. Other tumors derived from testicular supporting structures, including embryonal cell cancer, choriocarcinoma, and mature teratoma, are termed *nonseminomatous germ cell tumors* (NSGCTs). Only NSGCTs make AFP. Both seminomas (rarely) and choriocarcinomas (commonly) secrete measurable amounts of human choriogonadotropin (hCG). The short arm of chromosome 12 is duplicated in more than 80% of all germ cell tumors.

Symptoms

The most common complaint of patients presenting with testicular cancer is painless swelling of the testicle. Occasionally, hormone-secreting tumors produce gynecomastia, and tumors metastatic to the lungs at diagnosis can produce respiratory symptoms.

Diagnosis

Treatment of suspected germ cell tumors requires inguinal orchiectomy. Transscrotal biopsy of testicular tumors is associated with iatrogenic spread to the groin and should be avoided. Routine staging includes CT scans of the chest, abdomen, and pelvis to assess the common metastatic sites, as well as serum testing for hCG, AFP, and lactate dehydrogenase. Serum levels of hCG, AFP, and lactate dehydrogenase are reliable tumor markers; elevation of these markers or failure of marker levels to fall after primary treatment is an important indicator of an incomplete resection or relapse. Several different staging systems exist for testicular cancer. In general, prognosis of NSGCT depends on tumor size, magnitude of tumor marker elevation, and presence of mediastinal or visceral metastases.

Treatment

In general, patients with stage I and II testicular cancer benefit from radical orchiectomy. Controversy exists over who should undergo retroperitoneal lymph node dissection. This treatment is indicated in patients with nodes less than 3 cm and is curative in many patients. Patients who do not undergo lymph node dissection require close monitoring of serum markers and CT scans. Patients with seminomas, even those with spread to the retroperitoneal nodes, can be cured with radiation therapy. Patients with large retroperitoneal lymph nodes or metastatic disease from NSGCT clearly benefit from chemotherapy. The standard approach is intravenous administration of cisplatin, etoposide, and bleomycin.

BLADDER CANCER

Epidemiology and Natural History

Approximately 50,000 cases of new bladder cancer occur per year in the United States. The disease is much less common in women than in men. About one fifth of affected patients will die of their disease. The most important risk factor is cigarette smoking, which accounts for at least two thirds of all cases. Other risk factors include exposure to polycyclic hydrocarbons in the dye, rubber, and paint industries, as well as long-term exposure to cyclophosphamide and phenacetin and chronic infection with *Schistosoma haematobium*.

Transitional cell carcinoma is the most common type of bladder cancer. These tumors can occur outside the bladder as well, at any point from the renal pelvis through the bladder covered by urothelial lining. Squamous cell cancers and adenocarcinomas of the bladder and renal pelvis account for only 10% of all tumors in this region.

Symptoms

The most common presentation is gross or microscopic hematuria. Approximately 30% of bladder cancers present with symptoms of bladder irritation or spasms.

TABLE 56–6 Genitourinary Cancers

Tumor Site	Common Findings	Standard Treatments	Expected Outcomes
Testicle	Testicular swelling, pain, back pain or cough if metastatic	Inguinal (not scrotal) orchiectomy for either type	Early-stage seminoma >90% 5-yr survival
		Node-positive seminoma: radiation therapy	Stage III NSGCT ≈75% 5-yr survival
		Node-positive NSGCT: RPLND or chemotherapy	Poor risk tumors <50%
Prostate	Elevated prostate-specific antigen, decreased urinary stream; bone pain with metastatic presentation	Early-stage: prostatectomy, radiation therapy, or watchful waiting, depending on age, likelihood of spread, and tumor grade	Early-stage ≈80%–90% 5-yr survival with surgery and radiation
		Patients with later-stage tumors may receive hormones, radiation therapy or both	Stage C and D2 have worse prognosis, but time to relapse is variable
Bladder	Hematuria, cystitis	Superficial cancers: cytoscopic resection; biopsy as well as intravesical chemotherapy	10%–30% of superficial tumors progress to invasive cancer
		Muscle invasion: radical cystectomy or bladder sparing chemotherapy/radiation	Muscle invasive disease: 20%–50% 5-yr survival; <20% node-positive patients live 5 yr
Renal cell	Triad of hematuria, abdominal pain, and flank mass occurs <10%	Early-stage: radical nephrectomy	Organ confined ≈80% 5-yr survival
		Advanced or metastatic disease: moderate-to-high dose interleukin-2 interferon	Metastatic disease: median survival = 1 yr; 5-yr survival 0%–10%

NSGCT = nonseminomatous germ cell tumor; RPLND = retroperitoneal lymph node dissection.

When this cancer extends beyond the confines of the bladder, the symptoms relate to compression of local structures and may include leg swelling, pelvic pain, or compression of the nerves in the pelvic plexus.

Diagnosis

Bladder cancers are divided into superficial, invasive, and metastatic tumors. The evaluation of bladder cancer requires direct imaging and biopsy to determine the level of tumor invasion. Depth of invasion correlates with prognosis and determines the type of treatment required. Therefore, cystoscopy is the most important diagnostic tool. In patients at high occupational risk of developing the disease, urine cytologic examination may be helpful in the absence of symptoms that require cystoscopy. Furthermore, an intravenous pyelogram may be needed if cystoscopy does not localize a tumor in the ureters or renal pelvis.

The most important determinant of prognosis and treatment is whether the tumor has invaded the muscular wall of the bladder. Because the relationship between the depth of invasion detected by cystoscopy and that detected by cystectomy is only 50%, other tools such as CT scan, magnetic resonance imaging, and bone scan are important to help to define the presence of invasion, nodal involvement, or metastases. Tumor grade

is important because low-grade tumors rarely invade muscle, whereas high-grade tumors do so frequently.

Treatment

Superficial tumors are treated by transurethral resection of the bladder. Cystoscopy is performed every three months to assess response and perform resections when required. For frequent relapses, or when superficial cancer involves most of the surface of the bladder, intravesicle therapy is recommended. Here, bacille Calmette-Guérin, or another chemotherapeutic agent such as thiotepa, is instilled in the bladder through a Foley catheter, is allowed to remain for a short time, and is expelled. This process is repeated every week for 6 weeks and is followed by cystoscopy to assess response.

Tumors that invade the muscle require more invasive treatment. If the tumor has invaded muscle but is not through the bladder wall, the standard approach is cystectomy. The bladder, prostate, seminal vesicles, and proximal urethra are removed in men, and hysterectomy, bilateral salpingo-oophorectomy, and partial removal of the anterior vaginal wall are performed in women, and an ileal conduit is formed to store and expel urine. Not all patients with tumors that invade the bladder wall require removal of the bladder. Bladder preservation may be considered for patients with localized tumors away from the trigone or tumors that have been resected through the cystoscope, although studies have not proven that the outcomes of chemoradiation are equivalent to those with surgical treatment alone. Patients with tumors invading through the wall of the bladder should be treated by a combination of radiation and chemotherapy instead of cystectomy. Highly selected series of patients treated with combined chemotherapy and radiation show a 5-year survival rate of almost 50%. Patients with metastatic disease frequently respond to combination chemotherapy containing cisplatin, but the tumor invariably relapses.

RENAL CELL CARCINOMA

Epidemiology and Natural History

Renal cell adenocarcinoma, one of the least common tumors of the genitourinary system, accounts for about 3% of all cancers. Some relationship exists between kidney cancer and exposure to cadmium, perhaps in cigarette smoke. Renal cell carcinoma occurs commonly in the Von Hippel–Lindau syndrome, in which synchronous, bilateral renal carcinomas occasionally occur. Abnormalities of the long arm of chromosome 3 are seen in more than 90% of cases.

The natural history of kidney cancers is erratic. Some tumors progress relentlessly and are refractory to all interventions, whereas some patients can have spontaneous regressions of metastases.

Symptoms

The "classic" presentation, consisting of hematuria, flank pain, and an abdominal mass, is seen in only 10% of patients. More often, hematuria alone or persistent back pain prompts the patient to seek attention. Occasionally, bilateral lower extremity edema occurs when the tumor has completely occluded the inferior vena cava. Renal cell adenocarcinoma is also associated with some unusual paraneoplastic syndromes including fever, polycythemia (from erythropoietin production), and hypercalcemia from ectopic hormone production.

Diagnosis

The most common tool to diagnose renal cell adenocarcinoma is CT scanning of the abdomen. A large, dense, contrast-enhancing mass occupies a substantial amount of one kidney and is frequently accompanied by nodal or venous involvement. Magnetic resonance imaging is recommended to assess inferior vena cava involvement. Because resection is the only curative treatment, CT scanning of the lungs should be performed to rule out metastatic disease.

Treatment

Resection is the most common treatment for cancer limited to the kidney. Surgical treatment may be possible even if parts of the renal vein and vena cava are involved.

Renal cell adenocarcinoma is notably resistant to chemotherapy and radiation. However, data show that renal tumors may respond to biologic response modifiers such as interleukin-2 and interferon-α in approximately 10% to 15% of cases. Occasionally, these agents induce complete responses. Similar dramatic events have occurred spontaneously.

OVARIAN CANCER

Epidemiology

Ovarian cancer occurs in 1 in 70 women in the United States. More than 25,000 cases are diagnosed each year, and 14,000 women die each year of the disease, a statistic that makes this disease the fifth most common cause of cancer death in women. As with most cancers, the incidence of ovarian cancer increases with age. Other risk factors include a personal history of breast cancer (twice the risk), nulliparity, and a family history of ovarian cancer. Familial ovarian cancers account for 5% to 10% of the cases of ovarian carcinoma. Exposure to talc may increase the risk of ovarian cancer. Use of oral contraceptives decreases the risk of ovarian cancer, as do more than one pregnancy and breast-feeding.

Pathology

Most malignant ovarian tumors arise from celomic epithelium. The tumor can arise in any part of the peritoneal cavity; thus, prophylactic oophorectomy does not prevent the disease. Epithelial ovarian tumors are classified histologically as benign, malignant, or borderline. The most common histologic types of ovarian cancer are serous, mucinous, and endometroid. Stromal tumors, most often granulosa cell tumors, and germ cell tumors account for fewer than 15% of ovarian tumors. Cancers from other sites such as breast and gastrointestinal tract can metastasize to the ovaries.

Clinical Presentation

Symptoms of early ovarian cancer include vague pelvic or abdominal pain, early satiety, and indigestion, but the symptoms are so nonspecific that most cases are not diagnosed until the disease is advanced. No effective screening tests exist for ovarian cancer, although transvaginal ultrasound may be helpful in women with an affected first-degree relative. Advanced ovarian cancer causes abdominal swelling and pain, intestinal obstruction, and vaginal bleeding. Patients with malignant pleural effusions have stage IV disease.

Staging and Treatment

Ovarian cancer is surgically staged with a total abdominal hysterectomy and bilateral salpingo-oophorectomy, omentectomy, lymph node sampling, and peritoneal biopsies. Stage I disease involves only the ovaries; stage II disease involves extension to the uterus or fallopian tubes; peritoneal or inguinal lymph node involvement is stage III disease. Many patients have clearly visible peritoneal tumor implants, but in those who do not, representative biopsy specimens from all areas of the peritoneum should be removed for microscopic examination. Disease outside the pelvis, except for implants on the surface of the liver, is stage IV disease.

The mainstay of treatment for ovarian cancer is surgery; women whose total residual disease after surgery is less than 2 cm in diameter have an improved prognosis compared with women who have greater amounts of residual disease.

Combination chemotherapy with paclitaxel and cisplatin or carboplatin is given postoperatively to women with locally advanced but nonmetastatic ovarian cancer. If first-line therapy fails, additional chemotherapy can be given; responses occur in 60% of women. Women with metastatic disease at presentation should also have "debulking" surgery; chemotherapy can palliate symptoms of pleural effusions.

ENDOMETRIAL CANCER

Epidemiology

Endometrial cancer is the fourth most common malignant disease among women in the United States; more than 37,000 cases are diagnosed each year. The tumor usually presents with early-stage disease and is usually curable with 5-year survival rates more than 80%. Risk factors for endometrial cancer include increasing age, late menopause, nulliparity, obesity, and previous pelvic radiation. Women who are treated with estrogen without concomitant progesterone and those who do not ovulate are also at increased risk of the disease. Most endometrial cancers are adenocarcinomas.

Clinical Presentation

Most women with endometrial carcinoma have abnormal uterine bleeding. Even minimal postmenopausal bleeding should prompt an evaluation for endometrial cancer. Advanced disease can cause urinary symptoms or back or pelvic pain.

Staging and Treatment

Staging is achieved by surgical exploration. Most endometrial cancers are stage I, with invasion into less than half the uterine wall. More advanced tumors involve the cervix, vagina, pelvic or periaortic lymph nodes, bladder, and rectal mucosa. Metastases outside the pelvis (stage IV disease) are unusual.

Treatment of endometrial cancer is with abdominal hysterectomy, bilateral salpingo-oophorectomy, and peritoneal washings for histologic examination. Lymph node sampling is done in patients with high-grade tumors. Radiation therapy is given to women with histologically high-grade tumors and those with deep myometrial in-

volvement. Women with advanced disease are treated with megestrol acetate and chemotherapy.

CERVICAL CANCER

Because of widespread screening for cervical cancer with the Papanicolaou (Pap) smear, the incidence of invasive cervical cancer and mortality from cervical cancer have continued to decline in the United States. Cervical cancer and its precursor, cervical intraepithelial neoplasia, are more common in women with HIV infection and infection with human papillomavirus subtypes 16, 18, 31, 33, and 35. Most women with cervical intraepithelial neoplasia or cervical cancer are asymptomatic and are found to have the disease by Pap smear. Vaginal bleeding, postcoital bleeding, vaginal discharge, and pelvic pain may occur in women with invasive disease. Advanced disease presents with signs and symptoms of local pelvic involvement, including leg edema or back and leg pain. Metastatic disease is rare.

Biopsy of the cervix confirms the diagnosis of cervical cancer in a woman with an abnormal Pap smear. Some women may need cone biopsy if the colposcopy-directed biopsy is inconclusive, does not confirm invasive disease, or shows cervical dysplasia or if the sample is inadequate. The use of other staging tests depends on the extent of local involvement, as determined by pelvic and rectal examination.

Treatment of cervical cancer depends on the stage of the disease. Cone biopsy may be sufficient in women with minimal microscopic invasion into the cervix. Women with more advanced disease undergo radical hysterectomy with lymph node dissection. Combination chemotherapy with 5-FU and cisplatin and radiation therapy are recommended for women with locally advanced disease.

Melanoma

EPIDEMIOLOGY

The incidence of melanoma is increasing at a rate of 4% per year in the United States. Each year, more than 44,000 new cases are diagnosed, and there are more than 7000 deaths. Incidence rates increase with age and are 10-fold higher in white persons than in African-Americans. Melanoma is related to ultraviolet B radiation exposure, particularly to sunburn in childhood. A history of dysplastic nevi and a family history of melanoma also increase the risk.

PATHOLOGY

Most melanomas are superficial spreading melanomas. The antigenic markers S-100 and HMB-45 can be used to confirm the diagnosis of undifferentiated melanomas, although S-100 is nonspecific and HMB-45 is not 100% sensitive. Ulceration indicates a worse prognosis.

CLINICAL PRESENTATION

Patients with melanoma most often present with a change in a pigmented skin lesion. Although 90% of melanomas arise in the skin, melanomas can arise from any area where melanocytes reside, including the choroid of the eye, the meninges, and along the mucosa of the alimentary and respiratory tracts. Approximately 5% of melanomas arise from unknown primary sites. Melanomas can also present with metastatic disease in lymph nodes, lung, bone, liver, and brain.

STAGING

Melanoma is staged according to the thickness of the primary tumor, as measured both in millimeters of the tumor and in the depth of invasion into the skin. The tumor thickness is the single most important prognostic factor. Dissection of any palpable lymph node is required for full staging of the disease. In-transit lymph node metastases are those between the primary lesion and the first major regional lymph node basin.

TREATMENT

Surgical excision with wide margins is required for cure of primary cutaneous lesions. The location and thickness of the lesion determine the optimal surgical margin. Locally recurrent lesions are surgically resected if possible; radiation therapy is given if surgical resection is not possible. Intralesional injection of bacille Calmette-Guérin can lead to tumor regression in 40% of lesions. In patients with regional lymph node involvement, adjuvant immunotherapy with 12 months of interferon-α improves relapse-free and overall survival rates. Many patients have severe side effects, such as myalgias and fever, and need to discontinue treatment early. Metastatic melanoma may be treated with immunotherapy, combination chemotherapy, or surgical resection of isolated metastases. Radiation therapy is used to treat metastases to the brain, spinal cord, and bone.

REFERENCES

Early Breast Cancer Trialists' Collaborative Group: Tamoxifen for early breast cancer: An overview of the randomised trials. Lancet 1998; 351:1451–1467.

Eisenberger MA, Blumenstein BA, Crawford ED, et al: Bilateral orchiectomy with or without flutamide for metastatic prostate cancer. N Engl J Med 1998; 339:1036–1042.

Goldberg RM, Fleming TR, Tangen CM, et al: Surgery for recurrent colon cancer: Strategies for identifying resectable recurrence and success rates after resection. Eastern Cooperative Oncology Group, the North Central Cancer Treatment Group, and the Southwest Oncology Group. Ann Intern Med 1998; 129:27–35.

Pritchard RS, Anthony SP: Chemotherapy plus radiotherapy compared with radiotherapy alone in the treatment of locally advanced, unresectable, non–small-cell lung cancer: A meta-analysis. Ann Intern Med 1996; 125:723–729.

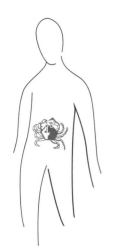

57

COMPLICATIONS OF CANCER

Jennifer J. Griggs

Cancer cells can metastasize to any organ, including the central nervous system. Direct compression by tumor and systemic effects of the cancer often require treatment in addition to standard chemotherapy and radiation.

Spinal Cord Compression

EPIDEMIOLOGY

After brain metastases, spinal cord compression is the most common neurologic complication of cancer. Approximately 20,000 cases of spinal cord compression occur each year. Most patients who develop spinal cord compression already have a known diagnosis of a malignant disease. Lung and breast cancers cause approximately 20% of cases. Lymphoma, sarcoma, multiple myeloma, and prostate and renal cell cancers each account for 6% to 7% of the cases of spinal cord compression. In only 10% of patients is spinal cord compression the first manifestation of cancer. Although the risk of spinal cord compression in a patient with cancer is only 1%, the effects are devastating but usually preventable.

PATHOGENESIS

Most compressive tumors occur at the anterior aspect of the spinal cord. Tumor cells disseminate through the blood stream to the bone marrow, where they multiply within the vertebral body and eventually extend posteriorly. Tumors cause necrosis and demyelination of predominantly the lateral and posterior white matter columns. This observation suggests that obstruction of venous outflow is the cause of the congestion, edema, and hemorrhage within the spinal cord.

CLINICAL PRESENTATION

Approximately 70% of cases of spinal cord compression are thoracic, 20% are lumbosacral, and only 10% occur in the cervical region. In 50% of patients, only one vertebral body is involved; in 25% of people, contiguous vertebral bodies are involved, and in the remaining cases, multiple noncontiguous vertebral bodies are involved. Most patients present with back pain that is constant, dull, aching, and progressive. The pain is often exacerbated by sneezing, coughing, or neck flexion. In contrast to the pain associated with disc herniation, the pain is usually worse when the patient is in the supine position. Radicular pain may be constant or intermittent and usually localizes to the level of the compression. Bilateral bandlike pain is more common with thoracic disease, whereas unilateral radicular pain is more common with lumbosacral and thoracic lesions.

Neurologic signs develop insidiously: weakness occurs in about 80% of patients, particularly difficulty with proximal leg function leading to difficulty in climbing stairs; paresthesias; ataxia, the result of proprioceptive impairment; and autonomic dysfunction, including loss of bowel and bladder function. Weakness, sensory loss, ataxia, and autonomic dysfunction can all progress rapidly and may lead to paraplegia if treatment is not instituted rapidly.

DIAGNOSIS

Physical examination can usually suggest the diagnosis and identify the level of spinal cord involvement. Radiologic tests should focus on the suspected area of involvement. The rapidity and severity of symptoms and signs determine how quickly diagnostic tests should be performed.

Plain radiographs are abnormal in 70% of patients with spinal cord compression. Among patients with pain, more than 80% will have abnormal radiographs. Typical radiographic findings include destruction of the pedicle and vertebral body collapse. Magnetic resonance imaging and computed tomography (CT) provide more information than do plain radiographs, and CT scans are superior in evaluating vertebral stability and bone destruction in patients undergoing surgical decompression.

TABLE 57-1   Management of Hypercalcemia

Outpatient Management of Hypercalcemia

Preferably given with cytotoxic therapy, e.g., chemotherapy, radiation therapy

Clear instructions about oral intake of fluids

Avoidance of diuretics

Pamidronate once a week

Gallium nitrate subcutaneously each day possibly helpful after acute normalization

Inpatient Management of Hypercalcemia

Immediate intravenous fluids

Antiresorptive therapy once good urine output
  Pamidronate × 2 q48–72h
  Gallium nitrate × 1 (5-day infusion)

Crossover to other therapy if no response

Calcitonin for coma or cardiac irritability

Mithramycin only for nonresponders

Consideration of dialysis in patients with renal insufficiency

---

TREATMENT

Loss of ambulation or sphincter function before treatment predicts a poor response to treatment. Goals of treatment are to prevent loss of neurologic function, to palliate pain, to prevent local recurrence, and to preserve spinal stability.

Few randomized trials on the optimal management of spinal cord compression have been done. Corticosteroids should be given immediately. An intravenous bolus of dexamethasone, 10 mg, with subsequent doses of 4 to 24 mg q6h, is recommended for most patients. Most studies favoring surgery over radiation therapy are nonrandomized and may reflect selection bias. Surgical treatment is clearly needed in patients with spinal instability, in those who need a histologic diagnosis, or those who again develop epidural compression after or during radiation therapy. Radiation therapy is effective in treating radiosensitive tumors, such as cancers of the breast and prostate, lymphoma, myeloma, seminoma, and small cell lung cancer. Radiation is usually preferable in patients with few or no deficits and a gradual onset of symptoms, with a radiosensitive tumor, or with a contraindication to surgery (e.g., bleeding diathesis, severe bone disease, and severe heart or lung disease).

Superior Vena Cava Syndrome

Superior vena cava (SVC) syndrome results from obstruction of blood flow by compression or invasion of the SVC by tumor thrombi. The SVC is a thin-walled, low-pressure vessel surrounded by rigid structures that make it vulnerable to metastatic disease in adjacent lymph nodes. The SVC collateral vessels, including the azygos vein and the internal mammary, paraspinous, lateral thoracic, and esophageal veins, lessen the obstruction of flow. The azygos vein is the most important of these collateral vessels; SVC obstruction below the level of the azygos vein is not well tolerated.

Cancer causes 80% of cases of SVC syndrome. Lung cancer is responsible for 80% of the cases, and lymphoma, breast cancer, and germ cell tumors account for most of the others. Nonmalignant causes include mediastinal fibrosis (e.g., histoplasmosis) and thrombosis of central venous catheters and pacemakers.

CLINICAL FINDINGS

Symptoms begin insidiously and are often worse on bending, stooping, or lying down. Symptoms include dyspnea, occurring in 60% to 70% of patients, and facial fullness, which occurs in 50%. Cough, arm swelling, chest pain, and dysphagia may occur. Physical findings include venous distention of the neck and chest wall (60%), facial edema (50%), plethora and cyanosis (each in 20% of patients), and arm edema (10%).

DIAGNOSIS AND TREATMENT

Chest radiography shows mediastinal widening in two thirds of these patients and a pleural effusion in one fourth. A right hilar mass is be seen in up to 15% of patients. CT can demonstrate the size, shape, and location of a mass, the extent of obstruction, and options for biopsy. Venography is no longer routinely obtained, but it may show patency of an SVC initially thought to be completely obstructed.

Treatment of the SVC syndrome requires a histologic diagnosis of the tumor before radiation or chemotherapy. Biopsy of a palpable supraclavicular or cervical node, thoracentesis, sputum cytology, and percutaneous needle biopsy of the obstructing tumor are options for diagnosis.

The goals of treatment are to alleviate the obstruction and to attempt a cure. SVC occlusion does not change the prognosis of the underlying tumor. Small cell lung cancer, lymphoma, and germ cell tumors are best treated with chemotherapy alone or chemotherapy combined with radiation therapy. Radiation therapy alone is preferred for tumors of all other histologic types.

Hypercalcemia

Hypercalcemia occurs with all types of cancer but most commonly in multiple myeloma and breast cancer. In patients with extensive osteolytic bone disease, hypercalcemia is caused by the secretion of parathyroid hormone–related polypeptide by the tumor, along with other cytokines such as transforming growth factor-α, interleukin-6, and tumor necrosis factor.

CLINICAL PRESENTATION

The symptoms of hypercalcemia depend less on the absolute serum calcium level than on the time course

TABLE 57-2 Paraneoplastic Syndromes

Syndrome	Associated Tumors	Mechanism
Ectopic ACTH production	Small cell lung cancer, pancreatic cancer, pheochromocytoma	Tumor secretion of ACTH precursor
SIADH	Lung cancer, head and neck tumors, brain tumors	Ectopic production of antidiuretic hormone
Cerebellar degeneration and peripheral neuropathy	Lung, ovarian, breast cancers, lymphoma (especially Hodgkin's disease)	Autoantibodies, including antibodies to Purkinje cells ("anti-YO" antibodies) and antineuronal ("anti-Hu") antibodies
Opsoclonus-myoclonus	Lung cancer Neuroblastoma (in children)	No consistent findings; some patients have anti-HU antibodies
Lambert-Eaton syndrome (myasthenic)	Small cell lung cancer	Antibody production against calcium channels in presynaptic nerve terminal
Erythrocytosis	Renal cell carcinoma, hepatoma	Tumor production of erythropoietin
Thrombophlebitis	Pancreatic cancer, adenocarcinomas	Uncertain

ACTH = Adrenocorticotropic hormone; SIADH = syndrome of inappropriate antidiuretic hormone.

over which the hypercalcemia develops. Common symptoms are constipation, polydipsia, polyuria, fatigue, nausea, vomiting, and bradycardia. Most patients with hypercalcemia have volume depletion. Patients are often confused and may be obtunded. Muscle stretch reflexes are often hyperactive.

TREATMENT

Treatment of hypercalcemia uses two strategies: increasing urinary calcium excretion and decreasing bone resorption (Table 57–1). Drugs such as thiazide diuretics, those that decrease renal blood flow (H_2-blockers and nonsteroidal anti-inflammatory drugs), calcium-containing drugs, and vitamins A and D should be stopped immediately.

Fluid replacement at a rate of 300 to 400 mL per hour for 3 to 4 hours should be given with frequent monitoring of electrolytes. Such rapid fluid replacement should be seen as rehydration rather than as primary therapy. Drugs that decrease bone resorption should be given as soon as the patient is rehydrated. Bisphosphonates are the most commonly used antiresorptive drugs; pamidronate, at a dose of 60 to 90 mg, is administered over 2 to 4 hours. The major side effects of pamidronate are fever and myalgias.

Gallium nitrate is a more potent inhibitor of bone resorption and induces normocalcemia in 70% to 90% of patients. Calcitonin, at a dose of 6 to 8 U/kg IM q6h for 48 hours, is a weak hypocalcemic agent but has a rapid onset of action. Calcitonin can be used concurrently with pamidronate and gallium. Corticosteroids can be used to treat hypercalcemia caused by hematologic malignancies; patients with breast cancer occasionally respond to steroids.

Patients can be treated as outpatients if the serum calcium concentration is less than 12 mg/dL, if they have no significant nausea and only mild constipation, if they are able to take fluids orally, if mentation is intact, if creatinine levels are normal, if they have a stable cardiac rhythm, and if a companion is available to observe them. Immediate inpatient management is indicated in all other situations.

Unless the underlying malignant disease is treated, hypercalcemia will persist or recur. Appropriate management of hypercalcemia therefore requires an attempt to control the cancer itself.

Paraneoplastic Syndromes

Tumors have disease manifestations through immunologic and metabolic factors that are not the direct result of invasion by neoplastic cells. These paraneoplastic syndromes may appear before the diagnosis of cancer is made. Because detection and treatment of the underlying malignant disease may improve the syndrome and occasionally may facilitate cure of the cancer, recognition of paraneoplastic syndromes is important. Table 57–2 lists the endocrinologic, neurologic, and hematologic paraneoplastic syndromes. Gastrointestinal and cutaneous syndromes also exist.

REFERENCES

Bundred NJ, Ratcliffe WA, Walker RA, et al: Parathyroid hormone–related protein in malignancy-associated hypercalcemia. BMJ 1991; 303:1506.
Hahn SM: Oncologic emergencies. In Bennett JC, Plum F (eds): Cecil Textbook of Medicine, 20th ed. Philadelphia: WB Saunders, 1996, pp 1049–1054.
Portenoy RK, Lipton RB, Foley KM: Back pain in the cancer patient: An algorithm for evaluation and management. Neurology 1987; 37: 134.

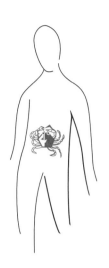

58

PRINCIPLES OF CANCER TREATMENT

Christopher E. Desch

Modern cancer treatment requires a coordinated effort among medical, surgical, and radiologic specialties, as well as nursing and allied health care in symptom management and rehabilitation. In the past, the sequence of care was linear: treatment modalities were chosen sequentially. Today, treatment is increasingly integrated, and new findings of tumor cell biology are exploited by combining treatment modalities in a coordinated regimen.

Radiology

Radiologic techniques of ultrasonography and computed tomographic scanning may guide fine-needle aspiration or core-needle biopsy to facilitate diagnosis and staging before surgery, thereby enabling precise preoperative planning. Similarly, using computed tomography, positive emission tomographic scans, magnetic resonance imaging, and sophisticated vascular imaging, radiologists now have a much greater capability to detect metastases as well as define more clearly the limits of resectability. Interventional radiologists can embolize cancers of the liver, bone, and kidney and permit safer resection or better palliation.

Surgery

Surgical procedures include making the diagnosis by biopsy, beginning definitive treatment by removing the cancer, staging the cancer by assessing regional nodes and metastases, reconstructing the limb or organ sacrificed in the surgery, providing permanent or temporary intravenous access for chemotherapy or feeding, and palliating the symptoms of cancer when resection or intestinal bypass is required.

The goal of cancer surgery is the total removal of the tumor, including adjacent tissue that may be involved. At surgery, the tumor is isolated and almost never opened during the procedure. The surgeon dissects an adequate margin of normal tissue around the tumor and removes regional lymph nodes. In some cases, the surgeon leaves an outline of the tumor bed with radiopaque clips, which helps the radiation therapist define the fields for subsequent treatment.

Tumor staging, required before a management plan is developed, most often follows the TNM method developed by the International Union Against Cancer and the American Joint Committee on Cancer. This system requires three measurements: (1) the size and local invasion of the primary tumor (T score); (2) the number, location, or fixation of lymph nodes (the N score); and (3) the presence or absence of metastases (M score). For instance, a 2.5-cm breast cancer and two involved axillary lymph nodes without evidence of metastatic disease would be staged as a T2,N1,M0 cancer. All the TNM scores can be grouped into prognostic categories. In this example, the breast cancer is stage II.

Radiation Therapy

The goals of radiation therapy are to provide definitive treatment in which radiation is the sole curative local modality, to allow organ preservation after organ-sparing surgical resection, to decrease the likelihood of both local and regional recurrence after attempted surgical extirpation, and to provide palliation of symptoms from unresectable primary or metastatic tumor.

Radiation therapy exploits the effect of ionizing radiation on cellular division. The goal is to deliver the highest dose to the tumor without permanently damaging the normal tissues that surround it. Specific cellular features of most cancers, such as a reduced ability to repair sublethal damage and a faster mitotic rate, make tumor cells more susceptible to radiation than are normal tissues. Several factors affect the sensitivity of a tumor and of normal tissues to radiation. This sensitivity is modified by the amount of oxygen in the irradiated tissue, the dose per unit time of radiation, the proportion of the cells in a susceptible phase of the cell cycle during exposure to the beam, and the tumor size and type.

The radiation therapist controls three variables: the radiation dose, the number of fractions, and the volume of tissue under treatment. The dose of radiation is measured in radiation-absorbed doses (rads); the common nomenclature is a unit called a Gray (Gy), which represents 100 rads. Daily fraction schedules are the standard approach that minimizes normal tissue damage and yet "hits" the tumor cell frequently enough to minimize neoplastic cell repair. For instance, a common approach to lung cancer administers 1.8 Gy of photons each day for 35 fractions (Monday through Friday for 7 weeks) to the tumor, a margin of normal tissue, and mediastinal nodes, providing a total of 63 Gy.

Ionizing radiation is delivered in a variety of ways. The most common is external beam therapy. A linear accelerator creates and delivers electrons and photons of different amounts of energy. The higher the energy, the deeper the particle can penetrate the body. The source of the radiation is external to the body, and the rays must transverse normal tissue as they enter and exit the target. Electrons (beta rays) penetrate only a few centimeters and are used to treat superficial lesions, whereas high-energy photons (gamma rays) deliver radiation deeper into the body. Brachytherapy is the direct application of a radiation source to the tumor. For instance, cesium 137, directly inserted around the cervix, delivers a very high dose of radiation to a locally advanced cervical cancer. In this example, there is less local toxicity because the photons do not need to cross normal tissues before hitting the cancer. Iridium seeds can be placed into catheters embedded in the prostate gland to safely deliver many times the dose obtainable by external beam therapy. Radiation can be injected intravenously through the use of elements that collect in certain organs. For instance, radioactive strontium 89 replaces calcium in bone and is used in the treatment of diffuse bone metastases from prostate cancer.

The complications of radiotherapy are divided into acute and late (Table 58–1). The acute effects occur mainly in rapidly proliferating tissues such as skin and gastrointestinal mucosa. The severity depends on frac-

tion size and overall treatment time. For example, breast radiotherapy commonly provokes redness and swelling of the skin over the radiated site. This complication lasts for several weeks and is a result of the sensitivity of the skin as well as of the angles used to encompass the breast and tumor bed. Late effects, including necrosis, fibrosis, and damage to specific organs such as the retina and the spinal cord are the dose-limiting factors in radiation therapy and do not appear to depend on the rapidity of cellular proliferation. These effects are not as well understood, but radiation-induced apoptosis probably plays a role. Late effects are dependent on total dose and fraction size and less dependent on overall treatment time. A specific late effect of radiotherapy is the development of secondary malignancies, which have been documented after radiation therapy for Hodgkin's disease and breast cancer.

Chemotherapy

Chemotherapy can cure some cancers and can palliate others. An intimate knowledge of the pharmacology and side effects of each agent, as well as their interactions with one another, is essential for their use. Wise use of chemotherapeutic agents also requires familiarity with the guidelines for withholding further treatment if the patient's quality of life will not benefit or if preexisting renal, hepatic, or cardiac dysfunction exists.

More than 60 drugs are used to treat or support the care of cancer patients. New drugs capitalize on recently understood biologic mechanisms or provide a toxicity profile superior to those of the first and second generations of chemotherapy medications. Combining drugs with different mechanisms of action and different patterns of resistance is generally more beneficial than single-agent therapy, but if a drug is not active by itself, it should not be used in a combination. In general, chemotherapy drugs should be given at the highest tolerated dose.

The mechanism of action of chemotherapy varies by the type of agent used. In general, treatment is designed to interrupt the growth and division of cancer cells. Chemotherapy is an attempt to exploit differences between the growth rate and susceptibility of cancer cells and those of normal tissue. Furthermore, new con-

TABLE 58-1 **Acute and Late Complications of Radiation Therapy**

Organ	Acute	Late	Dose (Gy) Associated with Adverse Effects
Bone marrow	Aplasia	Leukemia, myelodysplasia	25
Spinal cord	None	Myelopathy from vascular damage	45
Heart	None	Pericarditis, cardiomyopathy, coronary disease	45
Rectum	Diarrhea, tenesmus	Stricture, obstruction	60
Eye	None	Cataracts, retinopathy	55
Lung	Pneumonitis	Chronic pneumonitis and fibrosis	35

TABLE 58-2   Commonly Used Chemotherapy Agents

Drug	Cancers Treated	Common Side Effects
Cyclophosphamide	Breast, ovarian, lymphoma, leukemia, lung	N, V, alopecia, hematuria, BMS
Doxorubicin	Breast, lung, lymphoma	N, V, alopecia, cardiomyopathy, stomatitis, BMS
Paclitaxel	Breast, lung, Kaposi's sarcoma, ovarian	Alopecia, anaphylaxis, peripheral neuropathy, cardiotoxicity, myalgias, BMS
Cisplatin	Lung, bladder, ovarian, cervical, head and neck	Nephrotoxicity, neuropathy, N, V, BMS
Gemcitabine	Pancreatic, lung	N, V, BMS
Vincristine	Lymphoma, lung, leukemia,	Peripheral neuropathy
Fluorouracil	Gastrointestinal malignancies, head and neck	BMS, stomatitis, skin disorders, enteritis
Irinotecan	Colon	BMS, diarrhea
Carmustine	Brain	BMS, N, V, pulmonary disorders, skin disorders
Methotrexate	Leukemia, head and neck, lymphoma	BMS, N, V, pulmonary disorders, stomatitis, enteritis, renal disorders
Vinorelbine	Lung, breast	BMS, ileus, neuropathy
Etoposide	Lung, testicular, lymphoma	BMS, N, V

BMS = bone marrow suppression; N = nausea; V = vomiting.

cepts of chemotherapy have identified the ability of certain agents such as paclitaxel to initiate the apoptosis pathway and facilitate the genetic programs coding for death of the cell. Table 58–2 lists 10 common chemotherapy agents, their side effects, and their most common applications.

The role of chemotherapy varies according to the disease under treatment. For example, chemotherapy by itself is curative in the majority of patients with advanced testicular cancer and in young children with acute lymphoblastic leukemia. Multiagent chemotherapy cures more than 80% of these cancers. In these cases, the cellular sensitivity to chemotherapy is extraordinarily high. In other circumstances, chemotherapy is employed to delay or prevent recurrent cancer after a mastectomy or breast-conserving surgery in women at high risk of relapse. Adjuvant therapy of breast cancer reduces the recurrence rate of node-positive breast cancer by about 33%. Finally, chemotherapy can relieve symptoms. For unresectable lung cancer, only 5% to 10% of patients with this disease have long-term disease-free survival. However, chemotherapy, used in conjunction with radiation therapy, can alleviate symptoms such as dyspnea and pain in more than half the patients and prolong survival by a few months. The use of chemotherapy

improves quality of life for most patients under these circumstances.

The chief obstacle to chemotherapy is drug resistance. Many cancers are able to exclude the intracellular distribution of certain drugs by producing a specific protein that pumps the agent from the cell. To overcome drug resistance, higher doses are employed to eradicate greater fractions of the tumor. The results of efforts to provide higher chemotherapy doses, then rescuing the hematopoietic system with bone marrow transplantation, has become well established in lymphoma and leukemia but to a far lesser extent in breast cancer, lung cancer, and other solid tumors. The future of chemotherapy requires the design of new agents that have greater cellular specificity and target cellular messages that encourage proliferation.

Hormonal Therapy

Cancers originating from tissue under the influence of hormones, such as breast, prostate, and endometrium, often respond to agents that block the hormone receptor or antagonize the effect of the hormonal agonist (Table 58–3).

TABLE 58-3   Hormonal Therapy

Agent	Common Use	Side Effects
Tamoxifen	Metastatic breast cancer	Endometrial cancer, hot flashes, deep venous thrombosis
LHRH agonist	Prostate cancer	Hot flashes, muscle weakness
Progesterone	Endometrial cancer	Headaches, weight gain, vaginal bleeding

LHRH = luteinizing hormone–releasing hormone.

Both the luteinizing hormone–releasing hormone (LHRH) agonists leuprolide and goserelin induce signals that modulate androgen production and result in levels of testosterone seen in castrated men. Most prostate cancers respond to these medications with a reduction in bone pain and prostate-specific antigen levels, but these drugs also have adverse effects, such as hot flashes, muscle weakness, and loss of libido. Newer agents such as bicalutamide and flutamide are nonsteroidal antiandrogens that inhibit adrenal synthesis of testosterone. The combination of an LHRH agonist and an agent to reduce adrenal synthesis, termed *total androgen blockade,* has not appreciably improved survival of patients with metastatic prostate cancer.

In the majority of breast cancers, an estrogen receptor is present on the surface of the tumor cell. Women with estrogen receptor–positive metastatic breast cancer respond over 50% of the time to the use of tamoxifen or the aromatase inhibitors, anastrozole and letrozole, agents synthesized to alter hormone receptors. Furthermore, tamoxifen has been shown to reduce the chance of breast cancer recurrence in the adjuvant treatment of estrogen receptor–positive localized breast cancers. Tamoxifen has both estrogen agonist and antagonist properties, which explains its tendency to reduce bone loss and cardiac events in postmenopausal women and to increase the rates of endometrial cancer and thromboembolic events.

Supportive Care

Supportive care interventions can improve the safety and comfort of cancer treatments. These agents reduce bone marrow suppression, suppress nausea and vomiting, and spare normal cells the destructive consequences of chemotherapy and radiation. Erythropoietin, granulocyte or granulocyte-macrophage colony-stimulating factor, and megakaryocyte colony-stimulating factor represent three cytokines designed to stimulate erythroid, myeloid, and platelet proliferation, respectively. Treatment of cancer- or chemotherapy-related anemia can ameliorate the fatigue common in these patients. Cytokines that stimulate neutrophil and macrophage production reduce the duration of neutropenia and shorten hospitalizations of patients treated with myelosuppressive regimens. Platelet growth factor can shorten the time to platelet recovery during bone marrow transplantation. Although these agents do not clearly reduce mortality, they are thought to be cost effective (by decreasing hospital days) under a variety of circumstances.

Chemoprotective agents are drugs that decrease the side effects associated with cancer therapy by protecting normal tissues. Dexrazoxane is one such agent; this drug binds intracellular iron and prevents free radical formation. It reduces the incidence of cardiac failure in patients who receive high doses of anthracyclines. Amifostine, a thiophosphate compound that acts as a free radical scavenger, reduces the toxicity of radiation therapy and the renal damage produced by cisplatin.

Biologic Therapy

Interferons, interleukin-2 (IL-2), and monoclonal antibodies are examples of biologic therapies. Interferons have immunomodulatory, antiviral, and antiangiogenic effects. First used in the treatment of the rare hematologic malignancy hairy cell leukemia, interferons are now used more often in the treatment of chronic myelogenous leukemia (CML). Interferon reduces cellular proliferation and controls the leukocytosis in CML in approximately 70% patients. Up to 40% of patients have a bone marrow response and lose some or all of the metaphases containing the Philadelphia chromosome. About 25% of these responses are long-lasting. Interferon may also lengthen disease-free survival among patients with multiple myeloma and chronic lymphocytic leukemia.

IL-2 is used in patients with metastatic renal cell carcinoma. This immunomodulator binds to a receptor on T cells and activates cells that kill the tumor. Malignant melanoma and renal cell carcinoma are the two tumors that have shown an objective response to this agent, but IL-2 rarely results in a complete remission. Side effects of this agent include edema, hypotension, anorexia, emotional depression, and renal dysfunction; severe side effects occur much more frequently at the highest doses.

Monoclonal antibodies are used in the treatment of some patients with low-grade lymphoma and breast cancer. In patients with CD20$^+$-positive lymphoma, an antibody to the CD20 antigen results in a high proportion of tumor responses in patients whose disease has not responded to chemotherapy. The epidermal growth factor receptor, also termed HER2-neu, is present on approximately 25% of all breast cancer cells. Antibody (anti–Her2-neu) to this cellular protein results in a 20% rate of tumor shrinkage in women with metastatic disease.

Bone Marrow Transplantation

One of the major obstacles to delivering higher doses of chemotherapy is the toxicity of these agents to normal cells. Bone marrow cells, at least partly because of the high cellular turnover of bone marrow, are particularly vulnerable. Normal cells can be harvested from the patient (autologous cells) or from a human leukocyte antigen–matched related or unrelated donor (allogeneic cells) and reinfused after the completion of ablative doses of chemotherapy or radiation therapy. Bone marrow transplantation improves survival of patients with chronic myelogenous leukemia, relapsed Hodgkin's and non-Hodgkin's lymphoma, and acute leukemia. The complications of bone marrow transplantation are primarily those of chemotherapy toxicity to the lungs, liver, and bone marrow. Treatment-related mortality is usually the result of bacterial and viral infection. Patients undergoing allogeneic and unrelated bone marrow transplantation can develop graft-versus-host disease, an immunologic reaction of the donated marrow cells on the recipients' skin, liver, and gastrointestinal system.

REFERENCES

Beck WT, Dalton WS: Mechanism of drug resistance. *In* DeVita VT, Hellman S, Rosenberg SA (eds): Cancer: Principles and Practice of Oncology, 5th ed. Philadelphia: Lippincott-Raven, 1997, pp 498–512.

Purdy JA, Glasgow GP, Lightfoot DA: Principles of radiologic physics, dosimetry and treatment planning. *In* Perez CA, Brady LW (eds): Principles and Practice of Radiation Oncology, 2nd ed. Philadelphia: JB Lippincott, 1992, pp 183–207.

Salmon SE, Bertino JR: Principles of cancer therapy. *In* Bennett JC, Plum F (eds): Cecil Textbook of Medicine. Philadelphia: WB Saunders, 1996, pp 1036–1049.

SECTION X

Metabolic Disease

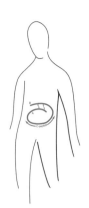

59

EATING DISORDERS

Peter N. Herbert

Obesity

A United States government task force has set a body mass index (BMI) equal to or greater than 27.3 for women and 27.8 for men as defining the term *overweight*. These values correspond to a 20% excess over ideal body weight.

Clinicians most frequently use body weight or, preferably, the BMI (weight [kg]/height [m²]) to judge whether a patient is "overweight." Very muscular persons may be moderately overweight and not obese. Others with small frames and low muscle mass may be obese without fulfilling criteria for being overweight. Nevertheless, most seriously overweight patients are also obese. An obesity classification scheme based on BMI is presented in Table 59–1. Up to 50 million Americans are overweight and 12 million are severely obese. Between 1980 and 1990, the prevalence of overweight in the United States increased by 8% and mean body weight by almost 4 kg. Minority populations are disproportionately affected. Almost 50% of African-American women are overweight.

Obesity is, to a great extent, genetically determined and is strongly influenced by the availability of palatable food and a sedentary lifestyle. A child of two obese parents has about an 80% chance of becoming obese, whereas the risk is only 15% for the offspring of two parents of normal weight. Moreover, a correlation between parents' and children's BMIs is found across a broad spectrum of values, which suggests both polygenic inheritance of obesity and several contributing metabolic mechanisms. The precise causative mechanisms remain unknown.

PATHOGENESIS

How does obesity occur? Fat accounts for 26% to 42% of the weight of middle-aged men and women (Table 59–2). At some time in life, the obese individual consumed more calories than he or she expended *and* appetite was not subsequently reduced to compensate for the increase in stored energy. The usual tight regulation of the size of the adipose organ indicates that neural or humoral signals from the adipose organ are transmitted to the brain, which in turn regulates food seeking and consumption (Fig. 59–1). Failure of fat cells to send adequate signals or failure of the brain to respond to appropriate signals causes obesity (Table 59–3).

Mechanisms controlling fat cell size and numbers are being discovered. Several facts are clear. The enzyme lipoprotein lipase, produced by the adipocyte and residing on its capillary endothelium, permits fat cells to take up fatty acids from circulating chylomicrons (dietary fat) and very-low-density lipoproteins. Fat cells with enhanced lipoprotein lipase activity may have a competitive advantage in assimilating lipoprotein triglycerides. The enzyme is very active in mesenteric fat and may contribute to abdominal obesity in men. It is less active in gluteal fat. Adipocytes can also take up fatty acids bound to albumin.

Breakdown and release of adipocyte triglycerides are regulated by a second enzyme, hormone-sensitive lipase, which responds to signals (i.e., circulating or neuronally derived catecholamines, prostaglandins, glucagon, gonadotropins) by increasing intracellular cyclic adenosine monophosphate and is inhibited by insulin (see Fig. 59–1). The adipocytes of obese persons may resist lipolytic stimuli from nerves or circulating catecholamines. Gluteal fat in both men and women, for example, has a lower lipolytic response to β_1-adrenergic stimulation than does abdominal fat. Abdominal fat in men appears to have more α_2-adrenergic receptor function (antilipolytic) than does abdominal fat in women, which thus leads to the "beer belly" in men more often than in women.

Well-fed fat cells can grow to a maximum of 1 μg. Storage of more fat requires an increase in adipocyte number by differentiation of preadipocytes (see Fig. 59–1). The signal for this hyperplasia is unknown and is a critical link if excess caloric consumption can drive an increase in adipocyte number. The converse, that increased adipocyte number drives increased food intake, is also possible. When fat depot mass results from increased cell numbers, as in gluteal and femoral obesity,

TABLE 59-1   Obesity Classification Based on Body Mass Index (BMI)

Classification	BMI (kg/m²)
Underweight	<20
Normal	20–25
Overweight	25–30
Obese	30–40
Severely obese	>40

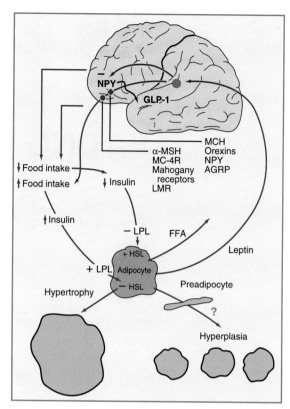

FIGURE 59-1   Pathogenesis of obesity. Increased food intake stimulates insulin secretion. Insulin, in turn, stimulates lipoprotein lipase (+LPL), permitting uptake of circulating triglyceride by the adipocyte, and insulin simultaneously inhibits hormone-sensitive lipase (−HSL) and the release of adipocyte free fatty acids (FFA). The overfed adipocyte may hypertrophy, or a stimulus, currently unknown, may trigger differentiation of preadipocytes. The well-fed adipocyte secretes leptin, which circulates and binds to receptors in the hypothalamus, causing glucagon-like peptide-1 (GLP-1) release and inhibiting neuropeptide-Y (NPY), a powerful stimulator of appetite and feeding. Reduced food intake, in contrast, lowers insulin, leading to LPL suppression (−LPL), activation of HSL (+HSL), and FFA release.

fat depots are very resistant to depletion, as evident in the condition called steatopygia, and in the so-called cellulite discussed often in periodicals. Fat depots with hyperplastic cells, in contrast, such as those in the abdominal wall and viscera, are much more metabolically active. These are more readily depleted by hypocaloric diets and contribute to the metabolic abnormalities of abdominal obesity. Finally, moderate obesity (BMI < 40) appears more associated with increased fat cell size, and severe obesity (BMI > 40) with high adipocyte number.

Single-gene effects do not account for most cases of human obesity, but biologically important genes, their products, and their regulators are rapidly being identified. Leptin, a hormone produced primarily by fat cells, circulates to the brain, binds to receptors, and causes release of glucagon-like peptide-1 and other neurotransmitters. These directly or indirectly suppress appetite. Leptin synthesis is induced by hyperglycemia, hyperlipidemia, and a replete fat cell mass; and leptin suppresses insulin production. Mice and humans with congenital leptin deficiency develop hyperphagia and severe obesity. Similarly, mice and humans with homozygous mutations in the leptin receptor gene also develop severe obesity and, in addition, hypogonadotropic hypogonadism. Among most obese persons, however, leptin levels are high rather than low. Thus, common forms of human obesity actually appear to be leptin-resistant. Leptin's primary role in the body economy may be, when levels are low, to signal starvation and induce feeding.

Central mechanisms controlling feeding are localized primarily to the hypothalamus. Output from the ventromedial hypothalamus inhibits feeding, whereas that from the lateral hypothalamus promotes feeding. A number of novel neuropeptides and receptors were identified in the hypothalamus in the 1990s. Activity levels and quantitative interactions among these may eventually explain much of the pathogenesis of obesity. Neuropeptide Y, produced in the arcuate nucleus, is a powerful central nervous system stimulant of appetite. Orexins in the lateral hypothalamus, like neuropeptide Y, also increase with starvation and cause hyperphagia and obesity after intracerebroventricular administration. Agouti-related peptide, also in the arcuate nucleus, is highly expressed when leptin levels are low. Agouti-related peptide inter-

TABLE 59-2   Variation of Fat and Lean Body Mass (LBM) with Age

Age	Men		Women	
	LBM (% Body Weight)	Fat (% Body Weight)	LBM (% Body Weight)	Fat (% Body Weight)
25	81	19	68	32
45	74	26	58	42
65	65	35	51	49

TABLE 59–3 Possible Causes of Obesity

Neurologic
Reduced sympathetic activity
Increased parasympathetic activity
Leptin receptor deficiency
Increased neuropeptide Y secretion/neuronal activity
Melanocortin receptor deficiency
Increased agouti-related peptide activity
Melanocortin deficiency
Increased activity of melanin-concentrating hormone neurons
Increased activity of orexin neurons
Decreased activity of the "mahogany" receptor

Adipocyte
Increased stimulus/response to preadipocyte differentiation
Increased lipoprotein lipase activity
Diminished hormone-sensitive lipase
Reduced leptin secretion
β_3-Adrenergic receptor hypofunction

Other
Insulin resistance/hyperinsulinemia

acts with the melanocortin-4 receptor and antagonizes the effect of α-melanocyte–stimulating hormone; α-melanocyte–stimulating hormone, unopposed, reduces appetite and increases metabolic rate. The "mahogany" receptor may interact in some way with the melanocortin-4 receptor and seems to have capacity to suppress diet-induced obesity. Finally, melanocortin-concentrating hormone, which does not interact with the melanocortin-4 receptor, is confined to neurons in the lateral hypothalamus, is highly expressed in leptin deficiency and starvation, and may project to higher centers, thereby integrating effects of other neurotransmitters. There are now many potential targets for pharmacologic control of feeding, and these should lead to novel drugs for controlling appetite and obesity.

Whatever the cause of obesity, the condition itself is nearly intractable once it occurs. Increased fat cell size and numbers are maintained, and fat cells, when deprived of calories, seem to communicate their underfed status to the brain, thus stimulating appetite. Moreover, caloric restriction to achieve weight loss is associated with reductions in energy expenditure in the obese to levels far below those in naturally lean individuals.

ANATOMY

Regional depots of body fat, as noted earlier, differ markedly in their metabolic features and in their relation to the adverse health consequences of obesity. The form of obesity that characteristically occurs in men, android or abdominal obesity, is closely associated with metabolic complications such as hypertension, insulin resistance, hyperuricemia, and dyslipoproteinemia (syndrome X). Mutation of the β_3-adrenoreceptor gene, which is expressed predominantly in visceral fat depots, has been linked to increased waist-to-hip circumference, glucose intolerance, and high blood pressure. The

mechanism involved may be enhanced sensitivity of visceral fat to catecholamine-mediated lipolysis. Increased free fatty acid release may drive very-low-density lipoprotein production by the liver and, by increasing skeletal muscle triglyceride, may promote insulin resistance.

It appears that the typical female or gynecoid obesity, with fat deposited in the hips and gluteal and femoral regions, has much less metabolic significance. The waist-to-hip circumference ratio has been used to distinguish these forms of obesity. A ratio above 1.0 in men and above 0.6 in women suggests the undesirable android obesity pattern. Thus, it is healthier to be shaped like a pear than like an apple.

MEDICAL CONSEQUENCES

Clinically Severe Obesity

Subjects weighing 45 kg (100 lb), or approximately 60%, more than desirable are designated as being severely obese. This corresponds to a weight of 240 lb (109 kg) in a woman 63 inches (157 cm) tall and to a weight of 260 lb (118 kg) in a man 68 inches (173 cm) tall. Cardiorespiratory problems present the greatest risk (Table 59–4). Chronic hypoventilation is common and leads to hypercapnia, pulmonary hypertension, and right-sided heart failure. Left ventricular dysfunction also occurs and may be related to both hypertension and hypervolemia. Severe episodic hypoxia can cause arrhythmias, and sudden death is 10 times more common among the severely obese as among people of normal weight. Most devastating, however, are the psychosocial consequences of the disorder. Self-esteem and body image are impaired, immobility greatly limits work and recreational activities, and humiliation is a daily experience when body size is too large for conventional scales, furniture, vehicles, and clothes.

Moderate Obesity

There is wide variation in body habitus between BMIs of 19 and 27, and within this broad range there is little association between BMI and health. Above a BMI of 27, however, important relations exist. Mild degrees of overweight in younger subjects are associated with increased total and cardiovascular mortality rates, and the effect is evident at lower BMIs in men than in women (Table 59–5). It should be remembered, however, that most deaths occur at more advanced ages. A BMI of 27 to 28 in men and women aged 60 years is associated

TABLE 59–4 Medical Complications of Severe Obesity

Sudden death
Obstructive sleep apnea
Pickwickian syndrome: daytime hypoventilation, somnolence, polycythemia, and cor pulmonale
Congestive heart failure
Nephrotic syndrome/renal vein thrombosis
Immobility limiting daily activities

TABLE 59-5 BMI Associated with a 50% Increase in Total and Cardiovascular Mortality, Over a 12-Year Period, in Men and Women

Age (Years)	Total Population		BMI with 50% Increased Mortality	
	Absolute Mortality Rate	Population Mean BMI	Total Mortality	CV Mortality
Men				
30–44	3%	25.6	27.2	26.3
55–64	17%	25.6	29.1	27.5
65–74	40%	25.1	42.1	33.2
Women				
30–44	2%	23.8	32.1	26.5
55–64	10%	25.2	32.0	30.3
65–74	27%	25.0	40.8	38.7

BMI = Body mass index (kg/m²); CV = cardiovascular.
Data for subjects who never smoked; derived from Stevens J, Cai J, Pamuk ER, et al: The effect of age on the association between body-mass index and mortality. N Engl J Med 1998; 338:1–7. A BMI of 21.0 was used as the reference point of comparison.

with more than a 20% increase in 12-year mortality, and 50% to 60% of this mortality is from cardiovascular disease.

Some disorders are clearly related to obesity. Hypertension is more frequent in obese people than in those of normal weight. This may result from sympathetic hyperactivity or to hyperinsulinemia, but neither mechanism is clearly established. Type II diabetes mellitus can be unmasked and aggravated by excess weight, and this may be the most important medical complication of moderate obesity. The cause appears to be insulin resistance, but many obese individuals never develop hyperglycemia. Obesity is often associated with high triglyceride levels and low levels of high-density lipoproteins, particularly when mild glucose intolerance is also present. Finally, obesity clearly increases the risk of cholelithiasis, endometrial carcinoma, and pseudotumor cerebri.

TREATMENT

Moderate Obesity

Americans spend $30 to $50 billion annually on weight-loss programs and diet products, and at any time, 15% to 35% of Americans are dieting. Low-calorie diets remain the most widely advocated treatment for obesity. The recommendation to count calories and eat less of everything has intuitive appeal but little success. Behavior modification techniques, focusing on stimulus control, the obese eating style, group and spouse support, reinforcement procedures, and exercise are probably more effective. These yield losses of about 6 kg after a year of follow-up. Nevertheless, at least 90% of graduates of such programs return to their initial weight within 5 years. More popular but even less successful are innumerable eating plans based on marked diet imbalance (e.g., rice diet, ice cream diet, Fit-for-Life diet). These are only transiently helpful because a diet very low in either fat or carbohydrate rapidly becomes monotonous and unpalatable. Diets very low in carbohydrate are also ketogenic and inhibit appetite. Most dramatic in effect, but potentially hazardous, are the very-low-calorie diets that approximate a supplemented fast, rely on withdrawal of most conventional foods, and involve purchase and consumption of an expensive diet supplement. No diet calling for 800 or fewer calories should be undertaken without medical supervision. More than 50 deaths, some from documented ventricular tachycardia and fibrillation, occurred with the early "liquid protein," very-low-calorie diets. No program consisting of caloric restriction alone has been generally successful beyond 12 to 18 months, despite the enormous commercial success of diet books and systems.

Anorectic drugs are potentially addicting, often unsafe, and only marginally effective. The medical profession and the public have been considerably chastened by the recognition that the fenfluramine/phentermine combination marketed in the 1990s caused valvular heart disease. Patients with any history of drug abuse should avoid all amphetamines. Anorectic agents may be useful in the short term when incorporated in a program that includes diet counseling, behavior modification, and close medical supervision.

As the pathophysiology of obesity is better elucidated, more specific and effective measures should emerge.

Clinically Severe Obesity

Severe caloric restriction to 200 to 800 kcal/day, with or without anorectic drugs, should be tried first. A 90% failure rate is the rule. Subjects more than 100 lb (45 kg) overweight in whom medical treatment has failed may be candidates for surgery to reduce stomach size. Vertical-banded gastroplasty consists of constructing a small pouch, with restricted outlet, high along the lesser curvature of the stomach. Gastric bypass procedures involve creation of a similar small pouch but with drainage into a loop of jejunum rather than into the the lower stomach. Patients in general lose 40% to 50% of excess weight within a year of gastric surgery, but some consume calorically dense liquids and regain weight. The long-term safety and efficacy of this surgery are not certain. The once common intestinal bypass surgery for morbid obesity has been abandoned because of unacceptable long-term complications.

Anorexia Nervosa and Bulimia Nervosa

These two psychiatric disorders are characterized by a distorted perception of body image and abnormal eating patterns. Neither has a distinctive pathognomonic feature; the two disorders share some common features, and they may overlap (Table 59–6). Bulimia nervosa is not associated with cachexia, whereas this is the most prominent aspect of anorexia nervosa. The primary treatment of both disorders is psychiatric, although they may manifest important medical complications.

ANOREXIA NERVOSA

Prevalence

The overall prevalence of anorexia nervosa is estimated to be 0.3% to 0.6% in the general population. In amenorrhea clinics, between 5% and 15% of patients may be affected, and in a Minnesota study the prevalence in the general population was 0.25% to 0.50%. The disorder affects girls at least 10 times as often as boys; the onset occurs typically during adolescence, but it may occur as late as the menopause. Many affected boys are homosexual or bisexual. There is little relation to socioeconomic factors.

Pathogenesis and Clinical Features

In the United States, concern over body image is often voiced by 8- to 10-year-old children and sometimes younger. Some persons can recall life situations or events that triggered their preoccupation with thinness. The usual pubertal weight increase may be critical in most affected girls. The restriction of food intake is initially voluntary, and a compulsion to lose weight may

TABLE 59–6 Diagnostic Criteria for Anorexia Nervosa and Bulimia Nervosa

Anorexia Nervosa
A. Refusal to maintain body weight at or above a minimally normal weight for age and height (e.g., weight loss leading to maintenance of body weight less than 85% of that expected or failure to make expected weight gain during period of growth, leading to body weight less than 85% of that expected).
B. Intense fear of gaining weight or becoming fat, even though underweight.
C. Disturbance in the way in which own body weight or shape is experienced, undue influence of body weight or shape on self-evaluation, or denial of the seriousness of the current low body weight.
D. In postmenarchal females, amenorrhea, i.e., the absence of at least three consecutive menstrual cycles (a woman is considered to have amenorrhea if her periods occur only following hormone administration, e.g., estrogen).
Bulimia Nervosa
A. Recurrent episodes of binge eating; an episode of binge eating is characterized by both of the following:
1. Eating, in a discrete period of time (e.g., within any 2-hour period), an amount of food that is definitely larger than most people would eat during a similar period of time and under similar circumstances.
2. A sense of lack of control over eating during the episode (e.g., a feeling that one cannot stop eating or control what or how much one is eating).
B. Recurrent inappropriate compensatory behavior in order to prevent weight gain, such as self-induced vomiting; misuse of laxatives, diuretics, enemas, or other medications; fasting; or excessive exercise.
C. The binge eating and the inappropriate compensatory behaviors both occur, on average, at least twice a week for 3 months.
D. Self-evaluation is unduly influenced by body shape and weight.
E. The disturbance does not occur exclusively during episodes of anorexia nervosa.

From American Psychiatric Association: *Diagnostic and Statistical Manual of Mental Disorders*, 4th ed. Washington, DC: American Psychiatric Association, pp 549–550. Copyright 1994 by the American Psychiatric Association. Reprinted by permission.

lead to self-induced vomiting, abuse of purgatives and diuretics, and exhausting exercise. Patients view their own body dimensions as excessive, but their view of other people is not abnormal. Treated anorectic patients have high cerebrospinal fluid levels of serotonin, which experimentally reduces feeding, but it is unclear whether this is a cause or an effect of anorexia nervosa.

In typical cases, the diagnosis of anorexia nervosa presents little difficulty. In atypical cases—occurring for example, in men and older women—careful evaluation for malignancy, acquired immunodeficiency syndrome, malabsorption, and hyperthyroidism may be necessary. Weight loss in anorexia nervosa usually begins within a few years of menarche, although onset may occur even later than 40 years. Amenorrhea is the rule and is secondary to weight loss and low gonadotropin levels. The latter may in turn be secondary to low leptin levels. Men complain of poor libido and impotence. Stunted growth and fractures of vertebrae and long bones may occur when the disease begins in early adolescence.

Physical examination shows little subcutaneous fat, with gaunt facies, atrophic breasts and buttocks, and often extensive growth of fine lanugo-like hair on neck and extremities. Extremities may be cold, cyanotic, and mildly edematous. Skin is often yellow from hypercarotenemia. Bradycardia and hypothermia may occur, presumably because of low triiodothyronine (T_3) levels. Hypovolemia from starvation and mild diabetes insipidus may cause hypotension.

Laboratory findings are not diagnostic but usually include low levels of gonadotropins and gonadal hormones, hypercortisolism, and low T_3 and increased reverse T_3, as in *sick euthyroidism*. On occasion there are pancytopenia, rarely with an increased number of severe infections; hypoglycemia, occasionally with coma; and, uncommonly, hypoalbuminemia and hypercholesterolemia. Hypokalemia is rare in patients who are not purging. Abdominal radiographs may show gastric distention and megaduodenum, and echocardiography may show mitral valve motion abnormalities and reduced left ventricular mass.

Treatment and Prognosis

All anorectic patients should be evaluated by a psychiatrist or psychologist experienced in treating anorexia nervosa. Patients weighing at least 65% of ideal body weight may be successfully managed as outpatients. Those under 65% of ideal body weight are candidates for inpatient psychiatric and nutritional care. If the patient is unable or unwilling to consume 500 kcal more than needed for daily energy requirements, use of peripheral parenteral nutritional supplementation (see Chapter 60) or tube feeding should be considered.

Hypothalamic and endocrine problems generally resolve when 85% of normal body weight is restored. Amenorrhea may persist for several more months, but menses usually return without specific intervention.

The mortality rate among patients with anorexia nervosa is about 6% per decade. At least 50% to 60% regain normal weight and eating habits and have return

of menses. In 20%, the condition remains chronic despite therapy. Prognosis is poorer in those with bulimic features or long duration of illness.

BULIMIA NERVOSA

Prevalence

The lifetime prevalence of bulimia, in a large Canadian study, was 1.1% among women and 0.1% among men. Less comprehensive studies have suggested that up to 20% of college students report bulimic symptoms. Within families of patients with bulimia, serious depression and substance abuse, particularly alcoholism, occur six times more frequently than expected by chance. The increase in weight and adiposity at puberty is probably the stimulus for bulimia, just as for anorexia nervosa. The hallmark of bulimia is not induced vomiting but binge eating; bulimia is synonymous with paroxysmal hyperphagia. Binges leave the patient embarrassed, guilty, and focused again on maintaining weight below an arbitrary level. This end is achieved by prolonged fasting, self-induced vomiting, use of nonprescription anorectic drugs, and use of emetics, diuretics and laxatives. In marked contrast to patients with anorexia nervosa, bulimic patients generally feel out of control and often welcome help.

Because bulimic patients may be normal or overweight, physical findings may be subtle or absent. Calluses or scratches on the dorsum of the hand may result from abrasion by teeth during induced gagging. Puffy cheeks from parotid or other salivary gland enlargement are present in up to 50% of patients, and serum salivary amylase levels may be elevated. Erosions occur on the lingual, palatal, and posterior occlusal surfaces of the teeth from acid-induced enamel dissolution and decalcification.

Frequent binge eating and vomiting may cause gastric or esophageal perforation or bleeding, pneumomediastinum, or subcutaneous emphysema. Heavy use of ipecac to induce vomiting may cause myopathic weakness and electrocardiographic abnormalities from emetine toxicity. Loss of gastric fluids can result in metabolic alkalosis with elevated carbon dioxide levels and hypochloremia. Diuretic abuse can produce both hypokalemia and hyponatremia. Menstrual irregularities are common, but amenorrhea is rare.

Treatment and Prognosis

Bulimic patients, in general, do not need hospitalization, but outpatient psychiatric treatment is beneficial. Cognitive behavioral therapy, in which the way the patient thinks is examined, followed by deliberate modification of the thought process, is probably superior to therapy directed at managing anxiety or to treatment with antidepressant drugs. Prescription of desipramine, followed if necessary by fluoxetine, may also work as well as does cognitive behavioral therapy. At least a third of patients experience relapse within a 2-year follow-up period, most within the first 6 months, and require additional treatment. Successfully treated bulimic patients still remain at high risk for alcohol and other drug dependences.

REFERENCES

Brownell KD, Fairburn CG (eds): Eating Disorders and Obesity. A Comprehensive Handbook. New York: Guilford Press, 1995.

Flier, JS, Maratos-Flier E: Obesity and the hypothalamus: Novel peptides for new pathways. Cell 1998; 92:437–440.

Herzog DB, Copeland PM: Eating disorders. N Engl J Med 1985; 313:295–303.

National Task Force on the Prevention and Treatment of Obesity: Long-term pharmacotherapy in the management of obesity. JAMA 1996; 276:1907–1915.

Pi-Sunyer FX: Obesity. *In* Goldman L, Bennett JC (eds): Cecil Textbook of Medicine, 21st ed. Philadelphia: WB Saunders, 2000, pp 1155–1162.

Rosenbaum M, Leibel RL, Hirsch J: Obesity. N Engl J Med 1997; 337:396–407.

Stevens J, Cai J, Pamuk ER, et al: The effect of age on the association between body-mass index and mortality. N Engl J Med 1998; 338: 1–7.

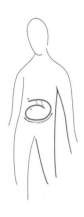

60

PRINCIPLES OF NUTRITIONAL SUPPORT IN ADULT PATIENTS

Peter N. Herbert

Nutritional Assessment

Every hospitalized patient deserves objective consideration of nutritional status. Severely malnourished patients have poorer outcomes, regardless of the disease entity or reason for hospitalization. Types of patients benefiting from nutritional support have been identified (Table 60–1). In general, patients who have recently lost 10% of their body weight or more and those 30% or more below ideal body weight are considered candidates for nutritional support. Patients who will be without adequate nutrition for 7 days or more should be supported from the time of admission. Finally, patients with a variety of specific disease entities (see Table 60–1) have quicker recoveries and shorter hospital stays if nutritional needs are met.

A number of aspects of nutritional assessment and support are controversial. Laboratory markers of malnutrition are capricious. Hypoalbuminemia may result from protein-calorie malnutrition but is equally likely to result from fluid shifts in recumbent and overhydrated patients; from losses in the urine, gastrointestinal tract, or third space; and from cytokine effects that reduce hepatic albumin production. Lymphopenia similarly has causes other than malnutrition, particularly the corticotropin (ACTH) and corticosteroid response to acute biologic stress. Parenteral nutrition was previously provided to a wide variety of surgical patients in the belief it supported rapid recovery and wound healing. It is now clear that surgical patients with severe malnutrition benefit from total parenteral nutrition (TPN), whereas in those with borderline or mild degrees of malnutrition, survival is not improved by TPN, and they suffer more infectious complications than do patients not given TPN.

Route of Nutritional Support

Support should be administered by the enteral route unless contraindications (Fig. 60–1) are present. Most critically ill patients tolerate enteral feeding. Use of the gut avoids gut starvation, gut atrophy, and undesirable increases in mucosal permeability to bacteria. Absorption through the small intestine presents most nutrients to the enterohepatic circulation, reduces tides of glycemia and lipemia, permits first-pass hepatic extraction of nutrients, and stimulates physiologic endocrine responses to feeding. Conversely, central parenteral nutrition, through subclavian or internal jugular veins, is plagued by mechanical complications of catheter insertion in 4% to 6% of cases. These complications include pneumothorax, hemothorax, and injury to vessels, brachial plexus, and thoracic duct. Infectious complications occur in about 5% of patients receiving parenteral nutrition and include tunnel and line sepsis, metastatic abscess, and right-sided endocarditis. Severe hyperglycemia and fluid, acid-base, and electrolyte disturbances, as well as nutritional deficiencies, are more common with parenteral nutrition unless great attention is paid to detail.

Peripheral parenteral nutrition (PPN) through a vein in the arm or hand may be used to provide partial or total nutrition for up to 2 weeks. Thereafter, venous access becomes difficult. PPN solutions cannot contain more than 10% dextrose, and 5% is typically used (Table 60–2). Solutions of high osmolality cause painful thrombophlebitis. Therefore, relatively high volumes of PPN are necessary to deliver a modest number of calories, and patients must be able to tolerate these volumes.

TABLE 60-1 Indications for Enteral Nutritional Support (ENS) and Parenteral Nutritional Support (PNS) in Adults

Strongly Supported by Outcome Studies	Moderately Supported by Research Studies	Recommended by Expert Panels
Acute respiratory failure with mechanical ventilatory support (ENS or PNS)	Acute or chronic alcoholic liver disease (ENS or PNS) Acute renal failure (ENS or PNS) Support of patients with acquired immunodeficiency syndrome (ENS or PNS)	Severely malnourished cancer patients suffering time-limited radiation or chemotherapy enteritis (ENS or PNS)
Acute exacerbation of Crohn's disease (ENS)	Severe but stable chronic obstructive pulmonary disease and cystic fibrosis (ENS)	Chronic renal failure (ENS or PNS) Prolonged (>7 days) acute pancreatitis (ENS)
Short bowel syndrome (PNS or ENS)	Chronic Crohn's disease (ENS)	Intensive care/critically ill patients (>7 days) (ENS or PNS)
Severely malnourished patients preoperatively (PNS or ENS)	Acute ulcerative colitis (ENS or PNS)	Neurologic impairment of oral intake (ENS)
	Blunt trauma/head trauma (ENS)	Anorexia nervosa with 30% recent weight loss or ≤65% of ideal body weight (ENS or PNS)
	Enterocutaneous fistulas (PNS)	Any patient with predicted severe inadequate nutrition >7 days (ENS or PNS)

Clinicians frequently have limited options in selecting the route of administration. Nasogastric feeding tubes are never practical for more than 4 to 6 weeks even when small-diameter (6- to 12-French) silicone or polyurethane tubes are employed. Thereafter, insertion of percutaneous endoscopic gastrostomy (PEG) or jejunostomy (PEJ) tubes is necessary. Patients with severe inflammatory bowel disease or those with bowels shortened from superior mesenteric artery infarction or other causes often require parenteral nutrition.

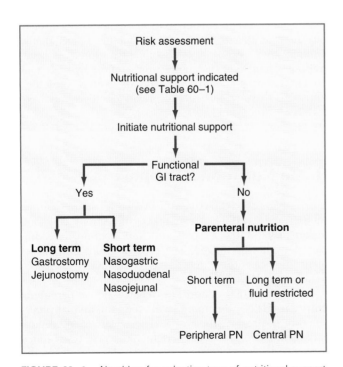

FIGURE 60-1 Algorithm for selecting type of nutritional support. GI = Gastrointestinal; PN = parenteral nutrition.

Water

Adults daily require about 30 mL of water per kilogram of body weight, or approximately 1 mL/kcal of energy. Elderly patients and other persons incapable of expressing their thirst require careful attention to serum osmolality. This should be routinely calculated and adjusted, if indicated, by increasing or decreasing total fluid volume (see Chapter 26). Patients with ascites, edema, heart failure, or intrinsic kidney disease may have low urine output and require less water. Those with fistulas, gastrointestinal drainage, or impaired renal water conservation may require large volumes of water and electrolytes.

Calories and Protein

Protein and carbohydrates provide about 4 kcal of energy per gram, and fat provides 9 kcal/g. In a typical American diet, about 16% of calories are protein, 37% fat, and 47% carbohydrate. Nonstressed patients should be provided total energy at 30 kcal/kg ideal body weight, and protein should constitute at least 4 kcal/kg or 1 g/kg/day. Stressed patients, such as those with major trauma, burns, inflammatory bowel disease, or infections, may require increasing protein up to 1.5 g/kg/day to avoid catabolism of muscle protein.

Peripheral and central parenteral nutrition solutions (see Table 60-2) are formulated with amino acids rather than proteins. Two liters of a 5% amino acid solution is equivalent to about 80 g of protein. Disease-specific amino acid mixtures are commercially available for parenteral nutrition, but their superiority over balanced mixtures of essential and nonessential amino acids

TABLE 60–2　Typical Nutrient Contents of Peripheral Parenteral Nutrition (PPN) or Central (CPN) Solutions

Nutrient	CPN and PPN	CPN	PPN
Nonprotein calories		1 kcal/mL	0.5 kcal/mL
Dextrose		20% (680 kcal/L)	5.0% (170 kcal/L)
Fat		3% (272 kcal/L)	3.8% (340 kcal/L)
Electrolytes (per liter)			
Cations			
Sodium	45.0 mEq		
Potassium	31.0 mEq		
Calcium	4.5 mEq		
Magnesium	5.0 mEq		
Anions			
Chloride	35.0 mEq		
Phosphate	12.5 mmol		
Acetate	29.5 mEq		
Trace elements (per day)			
Zinc	2.5 mg		
Copper	1.0 mg		
Manganese	0.25 mg		
Chromium	0.01 mg		
Multivitamins (per day)	One vial		
(A, D, E, B$_1$, B$_2$, niacin, B$_6$, C, K, biotin, pantothenic acid)			

is uncertain. Preparations for patients with renal disease contain only essential amino acids to limit the nitrogen load, whereas those for patients with liver failure are enriched in branched-chain amino acids (valine, leucine, and isoleucine). Chronic liver disease is associated with low plasma levels of these amino acids.

Most of the calories in parenteral nutrition formulations are derived from dextrose and fat (see Table 60–2). Dextrose concentrations as high as 25% to 30% can be infused through centrally placed catheters, whereas 10% is the practical maximum through peripheral catheters. Lipid emulsions, unless contraindicated by pancreatitis or severe hypertriglyceridemia, can be used to advantage to provide 20% to 40% of total calories. Lipid emulsions are isotonic rather than hypertonic and provide essential fatty acids. In certain patients, lipid also limits the risk of severe hyperglycemia, hepatic steatosis, and hypercapnia from excessive dextrose administration.

Most commercially available enteral feeding formulas also contain about 1 kcal/mL energy, but products as calorically dense as 1.5 kcal/mL are available. Calories are generally supplied by soy protein, cornstarch or syrup, and vegetable oil. Because much of their carbohydrate is complex, these formulas have relatively low osmolality (300 to 500 mOsm), and moderate volumes do not cause diarrhea. Most of the formulas are also lactose- and gluten-free and have little residue.

Vitamins and Minerals

Commercial enteral solutions contain sufficient vitamins, electrolytes, and trace minerals to guarantee adequate

nutrition when provided in 2- to 3-L volumes each day. The majority contain less than 2 g of sodium and are acceptable when salt intake must be limited.

Parenteral solutions routinely have water-soluble and miscible vitamins as well as standard additions of trace minerals. Notable exceptions are vitamin B$_{12}$, which should be administered intramuscularly every month during long-term parenteral nutrition, and selenium and molybdenum, which may become deficient after several months.

Hospitals often recommend a standard electrolyte mix such as that in Table 60–2, but physicians should monitor these carefully and stipulate different concentrations when indicated. Potassium uptake by cells may be large during the first 10 days of central parenteral nutrition, thereby necessitating relatively high initial potassium infusion rates.

Home Nutritional Support

More than 300,000 Americans receive home enteral tube feeding (HETF). The major indications cited are malignancy (~40% of patients) and neurologically impaired swallowing (30%). The ease of endoscopic placement of gastrostomy tubes has dramatically increased demand for HETF.

At least 50,000 Americans receive home parenteral nutrition (HPN); this number exceeds the annual prevalence in the rest of the world. The usual accepted indications are Crohn's disease, ischemic bowel disease, fistulas, and gastrointestinal motility disorders. In the United States, about 40% of patients receiving HPN have cancer, and 5% have acquired immunodeficiency syndrome. The annual cost of HPN is approximately $55,000, whereas the cost for HETF approximates $10,000.

Home nutritional support in Crohn's disease has been provided for up to 20 years and generally leads to long-term survival. HETF or HPN is also justified in a few other conditions. The use of home nutritional support to prolong life by weeks or months in the terminally ill and very elderly, however, is widely debated. Cost aside, physicians must ask whether nutritional support in such patients actually prolongs life or merely prolongs the dying process.

REFERENCES

Howard L, Malone M: Clinical outcome of geriatric patients in the United States receiving home parenteral and enteral nutrition. Am J Clin Nutr 1997; 66:1364–1370.

Joillet P, Pichard C, Biolo G, et al: Enteral nutrition in intensive care patients: A practical approach. Working Group on Nutrition and Metabolism, ESICM. European Society of Intensive Care Medicine. Intensive Care Med 1998; 24:848–859.

Klein S, Kinney J, Jeejeebhoy K, et al: Nutritional support in clinical practice: Review of published data and recommendations for future research directions. JPEN J Parenter Enteral Nutr 1997; 21:133–156.

The Veterans Affairs Total Parenteral Nutrition Cooperative Study Group: Perioperative total parenteral nutrition in surgical patients. N Engl J Med 1991; 325:525–532.

61

DISORDERS OF LIPID METABOLISM

Peter N. Herbert

Plasma Lipoprotein Physiology

The major properties of the plasma lipoproteins are summarized in Table 61–1. Normal men and women consume 80 to 120 g of fat (triglyceride [TG]) daily. Dietary fat is hydrolyzed by pancreatic lipase, absorbed by the intestinal mucosal cells, and secreted into the mesenteric lymphatics as chylomicrons (Fig. 61–1). One hundred grams of dietary fat mixed in an adult plasma volume of 25 dL can theoretically increase plasma TG by 4000 mg/dL! The liver also transforms plasma free fatty acids, which are unneeded when there is a surfeit of calories from the diet, into TG and daily secretes an additional 10 to 30 g of very-low-density lipoprotein (VLDL) TG into the plasma. This process can further increase TG by 1000 mg/dL. Both chylomicrons and VLDL acquire apolipoprotein C-II (apo C-II) from plasma high-density lipoproteins (HDL). Apo C-II is a critical cofactor for lipoprotein lipase, which is located on the capillary endothelium of muscle and adipose tissue. After hydrolysis of chylomicron and VLDL TG, excess phospholipid, cholesterol, and apoproteins transfer to HDL and increase HDL mass. The remnants remaining after hydrolysis of chylomicron TG are cleared very rapidly by the liver and do not normally accumulate in plasma. This process is mediated by apolipoprotein E (apo E) on the chylomicron surface, which binds to hepatic heparan sulfate proteoglycans and accounts for the rapid clearance of chylomicron remnants from the blood stream. Apo E on the chylomicron surface is then specifically bound to the low-density lipoprotein (LDL) receptor–related protein (LRP) in the hepatocyte cell membrane and internalized (see Fig. 61–1).

Some VLDL remnants (30% to 50%) are also cleared directly by the liver, and the remainder are converted to intermediate-density lipoprotein (IDL). IDL are normally short-lived and, by the action of lipases, are converted to the final VLDL catabolic product, LDL (see Fig. 61–1). In contrast to VLDL, which survive about 20 minutes in plasma, LDL circulate for 2 to 4 days. Although LDL normally account for 70% of the total plasma cholesterol, they are basically metabolic garbage. Most LDL clearance from plasma takes place when apo B on the LDL surface binds to the B,E receptor (LDL receptor) on membranes of many tissues, particularly the liver. About 75% of LDL are cleared by the LDL receptor pathway, and approximately two thirds are removed by the liver.

Lipoprotein(a) (Lp[a]) lipoproteins are secreted by the liver, constitute 10% or less of the total plasma lipoprotein mass, possess regions homologous to plasminogen, and are associated with vascular disease risk. Genetic heterogeneity produces 100-fold concentration differences among individuals, and levels are little affected by diet, habits, and most lipid-lowering drugs.

HDL are secreted into plasma by both intestine and liver. HDL accept cholesterol and phospholipid transported out of cells by an ATP-binding cassette (ABC) transporter. This process is critical to the production of HDL. Cholesterol is initially absorbed onto the HDL surface, where it is substrate for the plasma enzyme lecithin-cholesterol acyltransferase (LCAT). LCAT transfers a fatty acid from phosphatidyl choline to the 3-hydroxyl group of cholesterol. This produces cholesteryl esters that move from the hydrophilic HDL surface into the hydrophobic HDL core. The HDL surface is then free to accept more cholesterol from cells or other lipoproteins. The cholesteryl esters in the HDL core can be removed and transferred by a plasma protein and are the major source of cholesteryl esters contained in chylomicrons, VLDL, and LDL.

At least 10 well-characterized apolipoproteins are located on lipoprotein surfaces. These stabilize the lipoprotein micelle, are recognized by cell membrane receptors, and serve as enzyme cofactors. Their major lipoprotein associations are listed in Table 61–1. The usefulness of quantifying these apolipoproteins in clinical practice is uncertain.

TABLE 61–1   Properties of Lipoproteins

Liproprotein Class	Origin	Major Apoprotein Groups	Major Core Lipid
Chylomicrons	Intestine	B-48, C, E	Dietary triglycerides
VLDL	Liver	B-100, C, E	Hepatic triglycerides
LDL	VLDL catabolism	B-100	Cholesteryl esters
Lp(a)	Liver	B-100, (a)	Cholesteryl esters
HDL	Liver, intestine	A, C	Cholesteryl esters

HDL = High-density lipoprotein; LDL = low-density lipoprotein; Lp(a) = lipoprotein(a); VLDL = very-low-density lipoprotein.

Evaluation of Serum Lipoprotein Concentrations

Cholesterol levels should be measured in children who have a parent with hyperlipidemia or coronary heart disease that developed before age 55. Routine screening of other children is not recommended. Every adult should have total serum cholesterol and HDL-cholesterol levels determined during his or her 20s. A total cholesterol value of less than 200 mg/dL at any time of day does not necessitate retesting for 5 years. A level higher than 200 mg/dL should lead to measurement of total cholesterol, TG, and HDL-cholesterol after a 14-hour fast. Similar testing is indicated in adults who have first-degree relatives with vascular disease or lipid disorders. An HDL-cholesterol level lower than 35 mg/dL in men and lower than 45 mg/dL in women signifies clearly increased risk. If TG levels are over 500 mg/dL, specific treatment of hypertriglyceridemia should be undertaken. The highest total cholesterols commonly encountered (600 to 2000 mg/dL) are usually due to increases in chylomicrons and VLDL. Elevated cholesterol levels therefore cannot be interpreted without knowledge of TG levels.

If TG levels are lower than 400 mg/dL, the LDL-cholesterol (LDL-C) is calculated as follows:

$$LDL\text{-}C = Total\ C - (HDL\text{-}C + VLDL\text{-}C)$$
$$= Total\ C - (HDL\text{-}C + TG/5)$$

where C = cholesterol.

A therapeutic strategy based on LDL is indicated in Table 61–2.

Elevated HDL levels are thought to confer protection against coronary heart disease (CHD) and do not

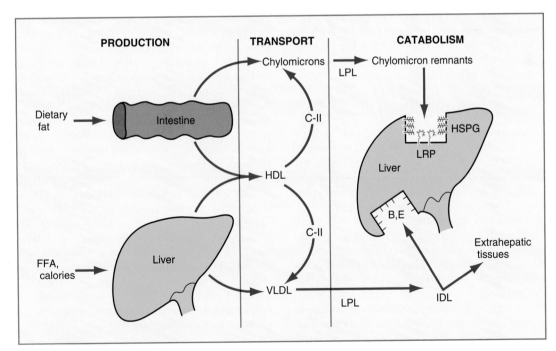

FIGURE 61–1   Normal metabolism of plasma lipoproteins. See text for details. B,E = Membrane receptor for lipoproteins containing apo B and apo E (synonymous with the LDL receptor); C-II = apolipoprotein C-II; FFA = free fatty acids; HDL = high-density lipoproteins; HSPG = heparan sulfate proteoglycan; IDL = intermediate-density lipoproteins; LDL = low-density lipoproteins; LPL = lipoprotein lipase; LRP = LDL-receptor–related protein; VLDL = very low density lipoproteins.

TABLE 61-2 **Approach to Elevated LDL-Cholesterol (LDL-C) Levels in Adults Without Coronary Heart Disease (CHD)***

LDL-C Level	Approach
<130 mg/dL	Desirable; repeat in 5 yr
130–159 mg/dL	Diet
160–189 mg/dL	Diet; consider drugs if two CHD risk factors present
190–220 mg/dL	Intensive diet in men <35 years and premenopausal women; diet and drugs in all others

*Recommendations of the Adult Treatment Panel, National Cholesterol Education Program. CHD risk factors include male aged ≥45 yr, female aged ≥55 yr, or menopause without estrogen replacement, family history of CHD before age 55 yr, smoking, hypertension, diabetes mellitus, and HDL-cholesterol <35 mg/dL. Subtract a risk factor if HDL-cholesterol ≥60 mg/dL.

require treatment. Low HDL levels justify aggressive modification of other factors, including even mild LDL elevations (>130 mg/dL).

Elevated Chylomicrons, VLDL, and IDL

DISORDERS MANIFEST IN CHILDHOOD

The occurrence of eruptive xanthomas, lipemia retinalis, hepatosplenomegaly, and abdominal pain in an infant or a small child suggests a primary defect in clearance of chylomicrons and VLDL. This may be due to a deficiency of lipoprotein lipase (assayed in plasma after heparin injection) or of apo C-II, the cofactor for lipoprotein lipase. These abnormalities have a prevalence less than one or two in 1 million.

DISORDERS MANIFEST IN ADULTHOOD

Both chylomicrons and VLDL are catabolized by lipoprotein lipase, and the enzyme is saturable. The enzyme prefers chylomicrons, so VLDL usually accumulate first until TG levels exceed 500 mg/dL. At higher levels, both VLDL and chylomicrons contribute to the hypertriglyceridemia. Testing to resolve the independent contribution of these two lipoproteins is rarely indicated, and tests for lipoprotein lipase and apo C-II should be reserved for cases arising in childhood. Most hypertriglyceridemia in adults appears to be due to VLDL overproduction, although defective catabolism is responsible in a subset of patients.

Moderate to severe hypertriglyceridemia is relatively common in men and women older than 30 years. The disorder is usually genetic and is commonly associated with hypertension, hyperuricemia, and abnormal glucose tolerance (syndrome X). Hypertriglyceridemia may be aggravated by obesity, even moderate alcohol consumption, exogenous estrogens, and drugs such as diuretics and β-adrenoreceptor blockers. Common secondary causes of hypertriglyceridemia are renal disease with proteinuria, both hyperthyroidism and hypothyroidism, exogenous and endogenous glucocorticoids, and type II diabetes mellitus. A very severe form of hypertriglyceridemia (TG levels, 2000 to 6000 mg/dL) can occur in patients with chronic insulin deficiency and very mild acidosis. This abnormality is completely corrected by insulin administration. The hypertriglyceridemia occurring in acute diabetic ketoacidosis is usually milder (TG levels, 250 to 800 mg/dL) and also responds to insulin.

The importance of hypertriglyceridemia in vascular disease risk is controversial. A National Institutes of Health consensus conference concluded that TG levels less than 250 mg/dL were normal, those 250 to 500 mg/dL were borderline, and only higher values were abnormal. Nevertheless, TG levels in the upper normal range (120 to 250 mg/dL) are very prevalent in CHD populations, and within this range the inverse relationship between TG and HDL-cholesterol is strongest. The association of hypertriglyceridemia and diabetes mellitus, obesity, and hypertension has further confounded efforts to define its independent role in vascular disease.

DYSBETALIPOPROTEINEMIA

This disease is characterized by the accumulation of chylomicron remnants and IDL in plasma. It is caused by homozygosity for a variant of apo E (E$_2$), which does not bind normally to the B,E receptor and probably also does not bind to the LRP (see Fig. 61–1). This leads to defective hepatic clearance of chylomicron remnants and ineffective catabolism of IDL to LDL. Less commonly, heterozygosity for a variant apo E results in an autosomal dominant form of dysbetalipoproteinemia.

Apo E$_2$ differs from normal apo E$_3$ and apo E$_4$ because of a point mutation that causes a substitution of cysteine for arginine. Homozygosity for apo E$_2$ occurs in 1% to 2% of the population, but fewer than 1 in 1000 of the total population develops hyperlipidemia. Dysbetalipoproteinemia occurs only if the E$_2$ homozygote also has an additional disorder such as hypothyroidism or familial hypertriglyceridemia. This abnormality is suspected in persons who have elevated levels of both cholesterol and TG. Diagnosis requires demonstration of the apo E$_2$ homozygosity (a test for which is not generally available) or unusual cholesterol enrichment of the VLDL. If the ratio of cholesterol to TG in VLDL, isolated by ultracentrifugation, is higher than 0.40, dysbetalipoproteinemia is likely to be present. This form of hyperlipoproteinemia causes palmar and tuberoeruptive xanthomas as well as coronary and peripheral vascular disease. The condition is worth identifying because it is exquisitely sensitive to weight reduction, cholesterol-lowering diets, and drugs such as gemfibrozil, fenofibrate, and hydroxymethylglutaryl–coenzyme A (HMG-CoA) reductase inhibitors.

FAMILIAL COMBINED HYPERLIPOPROTEINEMIA

Familial combined hyperlipoproteinemia has been used to describe families with a mixture of lipoprotein abnormalities that appear to segregate as an autosomal dominant trait. Affected members may have high VLDL levels, high LDL levels, or elevations of both VLDL and LDL. The basic abnormality is probably VLDL overproduction. Patients who do not effectively catabolize VLDL manifest only hypertriglyceridemia. Those who are very efficient in VLDL catabolism manifest only increased cholesterol and LDL levels. Others exhibit combined elevations of TG (VLDL) and cholesterol (LDL). Family screening is required for a confident diagnosis, but the label is often loosely used to describe the combination of both VLDL and LDL elevations. The abnormality occurs frequently in patients with CHD, and affected patients often require diet and several lipid-lowering drugs to achieve normal lipid concentrations. This is one of the most difficult treatment problems.

Treatment of Hypertriglyceridemia

GENERAL PRINCIPLES

The treatment of the hyperlipoproteinemias requires a systematic approach (Table 61–3). In general, the abnormality should be documented twice before treatment is undertaken. About half of affected persons are sensitive to diet (>10% reduction in lipids), and the extent of sensitivity should be defined by administering a fish-vegetarian diet for 2 to 3 weeks (Table 61–4). Patients are retested once or preferably twice while on this diet, and the results provide a point of reference for all future diet and drug interventions. If diet reduces cholesterol and LDL to target values (see Table 61–2) or TG values to less than 120 mg/dL, it may be liberalized to give greater menu variety. Skinned, defatted fowl may substitute for some fish entrees, and lean red meat may be consumed once or twice each week. If target values are not achieved, drug treatment is considered (Table

TABLE 61–3 **Treatment of Hyperlipoproteinemia**

1. Document abnormality twice after a 14-hr fast while on typical American diet. Provisionally classify as cholesterol or TG problem. Test total cholesterol, TG, HDL-C.
2. Evaluate potential for control with diet modification fish-vegetarian diet for 3 wk; retest after 2 and 3 wk.
3. Return to conventional lipid-lowering diet (30% fat with equal proportions of polyunsaturated, monounsaturated, and saturated fats) for 4 wk; retest.
4. If target values are not achieved, add lipid-lowering medicine or food supplements. Retest 4 wk after each change in regimen.

Maintenance

5. Patient keeps lipid record on flow sheet and has rapid access to test results.
6. Minimum follow-up test frequency is every 4 mo.

HDL-C = High-density lipoprotein cholesterol; TG = triglyceride.

TABLE 61–4 **Fish-Vegetarian Diet**

Permissible Foods/Beverages

Seafood (including fish, clams, oysters, lobster, shrimp, and scallops)
Bread
Pasta (with vegetable oil, tomato sauce, or clam sauce if desired)
Potato (with margarine)
Rice
Vegetables (all)
Fruits (except avocado) and fruit juices
Vegetable oils, margarine, and mayonnaise
Peanut butter
Nuts (except for coconut and macadamia)
Cereal (except granola-type "natural" cereals)
Low-fat crackers (matzo, Ry Krisp, Stoned Wheat Thins)
Angel food cake (plain)
Skim (not 1%) milk
Coffee, tea, soda
Alcohol
Nondairy creamers (Coffee-Rich, Poly-Rich, Poly-Perx)

Foods to Be Omitted

Meat (including fowl)
Baked goods (including desserts and "chips")
Dairy products (including eggs, butter, and cheese)

Restaurants

None

Fast Foods

None

61–5). Compliance is best when patients chart their lipid levels, have ready access to test results, and undergo follow-up testing every 3 to 4 months. Assessment of drug effects takes no more than 1 to 2 months, and in general the efficacy of individual agents should be established before combinations are prescribed.

TABLE 61–5 **Drugs for Hyperlipoproteinemia**

Problems	Mechanism
Cholesterol Problems	
Resins (cholestyramine, colestipol)	Deplete bile acids, upregulate LDL receptors
Niacin	Inhibits FFA release from adipocytes
Statins (atorvastatin, cerivastatin, fluvastatin, pravastatin, simvastatin)	Inhibit cholesterol biosynthesis, upregulate LDL receptors
Combinations	As listed earlier
Triglyceride Problems	
Fibrates (e.g., clofibrate, gemfibrozil, fenofibrate)	Stimulate lipoprotein lipase activity
Niacin	As listed earlier
Fish oils	Inhibit hepatic VLDL production

FFA = Free fatty acid; LDL = low-density lipoprotein; VLDL = very-low-density lipoprotein.

DIET

Reduced fat consumption is the only treatment for patients with deficiencies of lipoprotein lipase or apo C-II. The daily fat intake is limited to 25 g by restricting all fat-enriched foods, including those made from vegetable oils. Adults with more common forms of severe hypertriglyceridemia and TG levels over 1000 mg/dL should also follow a low-fat diet to reduce TG levels to less than 500 mg/dL. Subjects with milder TG elevations benefit from a diet that is close to a fish-vegetarian diet (see Table 61–4). This very strict diet typically lowers cholesterol levels by 15% to 20% and TG levels by 30% to 40% in hypertriglyceridemics. A second major objective of diet is to reduce body fat content. Most hypertriglyceridemics show marked improvement while actively losing weight, and a significant proportion are cured after weight reduction. Finally, alcohol should be restricted to one or two servings a week; on occasion, this alone corrects the problem. If TG levels of 300 mg/dL or less are not sustained by diet, exercise programs or drugs are appropriate for many patients.

EXERCISE

TG levels are reduced after even a single exercise session, and exercise has been shown to augment lipoprotein lipase activity. The efficacy of regular aerobic exercise in patients with mild to moderate hypertriglyceridemia has been repeatedly demonstrated, and exercise has great potential in promoting weight loss. The program goal should be 45 minutes of submaximal exercise on 5 days each week. The type of aerobics, duration, and intensity should be explicitly defined by the physician to promote compliance.

DRUGS

The fibrate class of drugs (see Table 61–5) enhances lipoprotein lipase activity and may have dramatic effects in patients with severe hypertriglyceridemia who require drug treatment. Fibrates are most effective in patients with dysbetalipoproteinemia and in others with high VLDL levels reflected by high total cholesterol levels (500 to 1000 mg/dL) as well as high TG levels (1000 to 10,000 mg/dL). When hypertriglyceridemia results primarily from chylomicronemia and the cholesterol level is only moderately elevated (250 to 500 mg/dL), the fibrates are less effective than dietary fat restriction. Use of niacin in patients with moderate hypertriglyceridemia (TG levels, 500 to 1000 mg/dL) can be gratifying but requires considerable patience from both physician and patient. The starting dose is 100 mg three times daily after meals, with very slow dose escalation to 1.5 to 4.5 g/day.. Timed-release niacin preparations are also available. These have more potential to cause hepatotoxicity, and the daily dose should not exceed 1.5 to 2.0 g/day. The patient should be familiar with niacin's potential for causing hepatotoxicity, hyperuricemia, hyperglycemia, and flushing. Fish oils reduce hepatic VLDL production and are a popular but still experimental treatment for hypertriglyceridemia. The minimum effective dose is 12 to 16 g/day (e.g., 4 g with each meal and at bedtime), and TG levels are usually reduced by 40% in moderately severe hypertriglyceridemia (500 to 1500 mg/dL).

Fibrates and fish oils can increase LDL levels while lowering VLDL and chylomicron levels. On occasion, LDL levels are raised above 160 mg/dL (see Table 61–2), and this undesirable effect must be weighed against the potential gain.

Elevated LDL

POLYGENIC HYPERCHOLESTEROLEMIA

An individual's total cholesterol level is, on average, intermediate between that of his or her parents. About 60% to 70% of a patient's cholesterol or LDL level is therefore genetically determined, with the remaining contribution from age, sex, diet, and other factors. The nature of these genetic effects is not defined. Subjects in the upper range of the normal distribution have an increased CHD risk, and the upper 50% contribute about 80% of CHD cases. Those in the highest 25% are generally considered targets for diet or even drug intervention.

FAMILIAL MONOGENIC HYPERCHOLESTEROLEMIA

About 1 in 500 North Americans has a monogenic disorder producing an abnormality of the B,E receptor (see Fig. 61–1). When grown in tissue culture, the fibroblasts of affected persons exhibit approximately half the normal number of receptors. As a consequence, these persons generally have total cholesterol levels around 370 mg/dL and more than twice the average concentration of LDL. Increased LDL is manifest in the first year of life and is associated with early corneal arcus, xanthomas of the Achilles tendon and extensor tendons of the hands, and a risk for CHD that is about 25 times that in unaffected relatives. Heterozygous men have a 50% chance of myocardial infarction by 50 years of age, and the comparable risk in women is 10% to 20%. Homozygotes or those heterozygotic for two abnormal alleles (compound heterozygotes) have cholesterol levels of 650 to 1000 mg/dL severe xanthomatosis, and they typically die of cardiovascular disease before age 30.

Treatment of Hypercholesterolemia

GENERAL PRINCIPLES

The general principles in the treatment of hypercholesterolemia are the same as defined for hypertriglyceridemia and as outlined in Table 61–3.

DIET

Limitation of dietary saturated fat is central to both cholesterol- and TG-lowering diets. Carbohydrates are often substituted for the saturated fats, but high-carbohydrate diets may increase TG and reduce HDL. Monounsaturated fats are better substitutes for saturated fat. Reduction of dietary cholesterol has a small additional LDL-lowering effect. In practice, the optimal diet approaches the fish-vegetarian diet used to establish diet sensitivity (see Table 61–4). The average hypercholesterolemic lowers total cholesterol by 12% (range, 0% to 40%) on this diet. When diet responders show secondary failure, the usual cause is noncompliance. This can be identified by asking patients to complete a 7-day diet diary and reviewing the record with them. Subjects who travel extensively and eat frequently in restaurants have greatest trouble with diet prescriptions. When large populations have been studied, results with most cholesterol-lowering diets have been disappointing, with mean total cholesterol reductions in the range of 5%.

EXERCISE

Although trained endurance athletes have LDL levels about 10% lower than those of controls, endurance training is generally not effective in reducing LDL concentrations. As noted previously, exercise effects in hypertriglyceridemia are much more substantial.

DRUGS

Several considerations govern choice of drugs for hypercholesterolemics not controlled by diet. The drugs are usually prescribed for years to decades, and most are moderately expensive. The risk-benefit profile must be carefully assessed because any significant morbid or mortal effects can offset the modest potential gains. Annoying side effects limit compliance with some agents. Only a few drugs have been shown to prolong life.

The resins (see Table 61–5) are safe and effective and are the only agents extensively evaluated in children. The starting dose is 2 scoops or unit dose packets before supper; this dose is enough in many patients with mild hypercholesterolemia, and more than 6 unit doses a day is rarely worth the cost and inconvenience. A large bowl of wheat or corn bran cereal can prevent constipation during resin use, but some patients still feel bloated. Resins are contraindicated in the hypertriglyceridemias, and TG levels should be reduced to less than 300 mg/dL before resins are used in patients with mixed or combined hyperlipidemia.

Niacin is useful in patients with LDL elevations, and the same precautions that were noted for niacin use in hypertriglyceridemia apply. The drug can cause fatty liver and cirrhosis, and its long-term safety is not established. The statins (see Table 61–5) are a category of drugs that competitively inhibit HMG-CoA reductase, the rate-limiting enzyme in cholesterol biosynthesis. This inhibition induces an increase in hepatic B,E receptors, and LDL levels typically are lowered by 25% to 50%.

Reductase inhibitors are appropriate for hypercholesterolemic patients of any age who have established CHD and for other adults with moderately severe hypercholesterolemia (LDL level, >190 mg/dL). These drugs are expensive but well tolerated, and the compliance rate is excellent. Use in combination with niacin, fibrates, or cyclosporine may cause myositis and even rhabdomyolysis. The reductase inhibitors occupy a unique position in primary and secondary CHD intervention. They have been shown both to prevent cardiac end points (myocardial infarction and coronary revascularization) and to prolong life in many patient populations (Table 61–6). Preliminary evidence suggests that they may be safe in children, but more data are needed.

The fibrates are not approved for simple hypercholesterolemia. They typically lower LDL levels by only 8% to 10% but may produce dramatic results in some patients. Many patients, particularly those who have heterozygotic familial hypercholesterolemia, require two or three drugs to achieve adequate control. Resins plus niacin plus lovastatin or resins plus fibrates have been widely used. Resins or reductase inhibitors plus fish oils are also effective in patients with mixed hyperlipidemia. Familial monogenic hypercholesterolemia homozygotes are poorly responsive to diet and drugs and are considered candidates for liver transplantation. Finally, estrogen replacement therapy after the menopause can significantly lower LDL levels while increasing HDL.

Lipids and Vascular Disease

Intervention studies in the 1990s showed that cholesterol reduction by means of diet, drugs, or surgery reduces the risk of development or progression of CHD. In general, a 1% fall in LDL-cholesterol has been associated with approximately a 2% reduction in disease end points. Arteriographic studies have shown small but definite regressions of arterial lesions. With use of the more powerful reductase inhibitors, LDL-cholesterol levels have been reduced by up to 35%, and death rates in men with coronary heart disease have been reduced by 30%. A wide spectrum of patient populations, including women and the elderly, has benefited from statins in primary and secondary heart disease intervention trials (Table 61–6). These impressive results notwithstanding, it is noteworthy that even statins fail to prevent recurring coronary events or death in the majority of patients.

There is still considerable debate about the cost effectiveness of screening the general population for lipid disorders and treating individuals without vascular disease who are found to have cholesterol elevations. According to the reference ranges established by the National Cholesterol Education Program, 27% of adult Americans would be classified as having "high cholesterol" and another 30% as having "borderline high" values. Indeed, almost half of all postmenopausal women have total and LDL-cholesterol levels over 240 mg/dL and 160 mg/dL, respectively. It has been estimated that about 100,000 apparently healthy people must be

TABLE 61-6 Populations in Which Treatment with Statins Has Reduced Coronary Events

Middle-aged hypercholesterolemic men without known CHD
Middle-aged men with average cholesterol levels, below-average HDL levels, and no known CHD
Middle-aged hypercholesterolemic men and women with known CHD
Diabetic men and women with CHD
Older men (≥60 years) with CHD
Men and women with coronary bypass grafts

CHD = Coronary heart disease.

treated annually to prevent 70 deaths from heart disease.

Nevertheless, there exists general agreement that eating less saturated fat and cholesterol and adopting diet and exercise habits to reduce obesity benefits the health of most people. Preliminary data suggest a significant fall in American cholesterol levels during the 1990s, and vascular disease rates have been falling since the early 1970s. These public health effects probably have a much greater impact than medical intervention approaches.

REFERENCES

Scriver CR, Beaudet AL, Sly WS, et al (eds): The Metabolic and Molecular Bases of Inherited Disease, 7th ed. New York: McGraw-Hill, 1995.

Summary of the Second Report of the National Cholesterol Education Program (NCEP) Expert Panel on Detection, Evaluation and Treatment of High Blood Cholesterol in Adults (Adult Treatment Panel II). JAMA 1993; 264:3015–3023.

Witzum JL: Drugs used in the treatment of hyperlipoproteinemias. *In* Hardman JG, Limbird LE, Molinoff PB, et al (eds): The Pharmacological Basis of Therapeutics, 9th ed. New York: McGraw-Hill, 1996, pp 875–897.

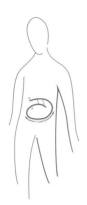

62

DISORDERS OF METALS AND METALLOPROTEINS

Peter N. Herbert

Wilson's Disease

Wilson's disease, or hepatolenticular degeneration, is an autosomal recessive disorder affecting 1 to 3 per 100,000 population. It is caused by defective hepatic excretion of copper. The consequence is copper-induced injury to many organs, particularly the liver and brain.

NORMAL COPPER METABOLISM

Copper is an essential trace element. Organ meats (particularly liver), nuts, seafood, and seeds are rich dietary sources. People ingest about 1 to 3 mg/day, and the normal adult body contains 100 to 150 mg of copper. Unlike iron, copper absorption does not appear to be tightly regulated. Copper absorption can be reduced by zinc. Zinc induces production of the cysteine-rich protein metallothioneine, which retains copper in intestinal mucosal cells. Copper so bound is poorly absorbed and is lost when the cells slough. Albumin and other proteins transport copper from the mucosal cell to the liver, which takes up most absorbed copper. Copper may be stored in the liver, bound in part to metallothioneine; it may be secreted into plasma bound to ceruloplasmin, which transports 80% of plasma copper; or it may be excreted in bile, perhaps bound to ceruloplasmin fragments. Copper is essential for several enzyme systems, including superoxide dismutase, which detoxifies free radicals. Large doses of copper consumed accidentally or intentionally can cause severe hemolysis and acute liver and kidney failure.

PATHOGENESIS

The genetic defect accounting for defective copper excretion in Wilson's disease has been localized to chromosome 13, and the product of the 7.5-kb gene is a copper-transporting ATP-ase. It is highly expressed in the liver and brain. Many mutations affect the gene, and most affected patients are compound heterozygotes. Copper incorporation into ceruloplasmin is decreased, biliary copper excretion is low, copper slowly accumulates in the liver, and eventually copper spills over into plasma. Signs and symptoms of organ dysfunction do not appear before age 6 years, but two thirds of patients have hepatic and/or brain dysfunction between ages 8 and 20 years. Delay of symptoms to age 60 years has been described.

Organ dysfunction appears to result from copper-induced hepatic inflammation and destruction or from abnormal release of hepatic copper into the circulation, with toxic effects in many other organs. Presenting features of copper-induced liver disease may resemble those of acute viral hepatitis, chronic active hepatitis, or postnecrotic cirrhosis. When copper release from the liver is abrupt and massive, transient Coombs-negative *hemolytic anemia* is produced. Prolonged increased release of copper not bound to ceruloplasmin causes destruction of the basal ganglion and, in some cases, the cerebral cortex. Prominent symptoms include tremor, muscular rigidity, and dystonic postures. Kidney damage may present as *nephrolithiasis* when renal tubular dysfunction causes hypercalcuria, and some patients develop *Fanconi's syndrome*, with aminoaciduria, glucosuria, and rickets. Copper deposits at the periphery of the cornea produce the almost diagnostic yellow-brown to green deposits called *Kayser-Fleischer rings*.

DIAGNOSIS

No laboratory test is diagnostic, but complementary results on two or more tests (Table 62–1) are helpful. Liver biopsy specimens should be assayed for copper content, which is higher in early disease and less elevated in late disease. High hepatic levels do occur in some other liver diseases such as primary biliary cirrhosis. Ceruloplasmin levels are low in 95% of cases, but low levels are not the *cause* of Wilson's disease. Confusion may arise because ceruloplasmin is an acute phase

TABLE 62-1   Diagnostic Copper Testing in Wilson's Disease

Test	Levels in Healthy Persons	Levels in Wilson's Disease
Liver copper content (μgCu/g dry weight)	10–50	100–2000
Serum ceruloplasmin (mg/dL)	20–45	0–20
Serum copper (μg/dL)	70–160	25–70
Urinary copper (μg/day)	3–35	100–1000

reactant that is also increased in pregnancy and by estrogens; under such circumstances, apparently normal ceruloplasmin levels may be seen in Wilson's disease. Total serum copper levels may be low but may overlap the normal range. Urinary copper excretion is almost always high, a finding reflecting an ancillary route of excretion. Ultimately, the combination of laboratory tests with a consistent clinical presentation yields a secure diagnosis.

TREATMENT

Low-copper diets are recommended. Zinc acetate or sulfate (150 mg/day) stimulates metallothioneine synthesis. This protein in intestinal mucosal cells reduces absorption of both dietary copper and copper in the enterohepatic circulation. Urinary excretion can be increased by chelation therapy with penicillamine (1 to 3 g/day orally) or with trientine in patients who cannot tolerate penicillamine. Initial urine copper excretion should be 1 to 5 mg/day. Up to 30% of patients have difficulty in taking penicillamine, and 5% to 10% develop severe side effects of the drug such as rash, fever, lymphadenopathy, cytopenia, lupus erythematosus, Goodpasture's syndrome, and nephrotic syndrome. Liver failure has been successfully treated with liver transplantation. Neurologic symptoms often do not improve with therapy.

Hemochromatosis

Hemochromatosis is a disorder characterized by excessive body iron storage causing multiorgan dysfunction. The condition may result from ingestion of excessive iron or multiple transfusions. This section, however, deals with *hereditary hemochromatosis*. This autosomal recessive disorder is carried by 5% to 10% of whites, and 1 in every 200 to 400 patients is homozygotic. Hemochromatosis is only one tenth as common in blacks and is rare in Asians.

NORMAL IRON METABOLISM

The body of a physiologically normal man contains about 4 g of iron. More than half is contained in hemoglobin, and about 15% is in myoglobin, heme enzymes, and nonheme enzymes. Reserve iron is normally about 1 g. Most (70%) is stored in *ferritin*, a readily available storage form, and the remainder is stored in *hemosiderin*, a product of lysosomal enzyme degradation of ferritin.

Men lose about 1 mg of iron daily, mostly from the gastrointestinal tract. Women lose more, about 1.4 mg daily, because of menstruation. An additional 1000 mg of iron is needed for each pregnancy. Western diets contain about 6 mg iron per 1000 kcal, and absorption takes place in the duodenum and upper jejunum. We normally absorb the 1.0 to 1.4 mg/day that is lost and can increase absorption when needed to about 3 to 4 mg/day with an unsupplemented diet. How the intestinal mucosal cell determines whether to transport iron into the mesenteric circulation or to store it as ferritin, ultimately to be excreted when the cell turns over, is not known. Perhaps the mucosal cell responds to the availability of circulating iron bound to transferrin.

Iron transport in the circulation is on *transferrin*, a large liver protein the synthesis of which is stimulated by iron deficiency. Transferrin synthesis is reduced by cytokines released under conditions of cell death, inflammation, or malignancy. When iron stores are normal, the plasma iron concentration is at least 50 μg/dL, and transferrin is 20% to 40% saturated (Table 62–2). Transferrin releases its iron only after binding to specific receptors on proliferating, differentiating, or heme-synthesizing cells. Nearly 1 million such receptors are present on the normoblast, whereas the mature red blood cell has none.

PATHOGENESIS OF HEREDITARY HEMOCHROMATOSIS

The gene for hemochromatosis, on chromosome 6, is called *HFE*, and it encodes a protein that is a member of the major histocompatibility complex class I–like family. When this cell membrane protein is "knocked out" in mice, they develop hemochromatosis. *HFE* in the membrane associates noncovalently with circulating β_2-microglobulin. β_2-Microglobulin knockout mice also develop hemochromatosis. Ultimately, *HFE* interacts with the transferrin receptor and reduces its affinity for diferric transferrin. More than 90% of patients with hereditary hemochromatosis have a missense mutation in the *HFE* gene, and in more than 80%, this is a Cys-282-Tyr mutation. Investigators do not yet know how reduced transferrin receptor affinity for transferrin, caused by *HFE*, leads to the iron overload of hemochromatosis.

TABLE 62-2 **Iron Indices in Healthy Persons and in Patients with Symptomatic Hemochromatosis**

Index	Levels in Healthy Persons	Levels in Hemochromatosis
Plasma iron (μg/dL)	50–150	180–300
Total iron binding capacity (μg/dL)	250–375	200–300
Percent transferrin saturation	20–40	80–100
Serum ferritin (ng/mL)	10–200	900–6000
Urinary iron after 0.5 g desferrioxamine	0–2	9–23
Liver iron (μg/100 mg dry weight)	30–140	600–1800

Affected homozygotes absorb about 3 mg, which is two to three times the normal amount of iron each day, and this condition can increase body stores by about 7 g each decade. Most patients are 40 to 60 years old before symptoms occur after the accumulation of 20 to 40 g of surplus iron. Homozygotes are, of course, equally represented in men and women, but men are 10 times more likely to develop organ dysfunction, perhaps because of the absence of menses and greater alcohol consumption.

Alcohol can mobilize iron stored in tissue ferritin, and this iron is capable of generating free (hydroxyl and ferryl) radicals that can cause lipid peroxidation and cell injury. Moreover, even without parenchymal cell damage, tissue iron, like alcohol, directly stimulates collagen production and fibrosis. A liver that is fibrotic from virtually any cause can give rise to hepatocellular carcinoma.

CLINICAL FEATURES AND PATHOLOGY

Children may be affected, but most symptomatic patients are more than 40 years old. Lethargy and weakness, common nonspecific constitutional complaints, are present in more than 80%. The skin has a fivefold increase in iron content and may be bronzed to slate gray from excessive melanin and hemosiderin pigmentation. The liver can be enlarged and firm, and elevated transaminases are characteristic in the early clinical stages. In the absence of alcoholism, fibrosis does not occur until iron content exceeds 2.2% of the liver's dry weight. Biopsy shows considerable hemosiderin in hepatocytes and bile duct epithelium and a diagnostic absence of iron loading in Kupffer cells. Signs of *cirrhosis* may appear in patients with advanced disease, but severe portal hypertension and ascites are less common than in alcoholic cirrhosis.

Hemosiderin deposits can be seen in the pancreatic islets with iron localized to the insulin-producing β cells. α Cells and exocrine cells are spared. *Insulinopenia* usually causes diabetes mellitus in advanced hereditary hemochromatosis, but patients may also have insulin resistance secondary to hepatic cirrhosis. *Gonadal atrophy* is common in men and women and results from pituitary hypogonadotropism. Symptoms include low libido, amenorrhea, impotence, and scant axillary and pubic hair. In contrast to patients with alcoholic cirrhosis, excessive estrogen production and gynecomastia are rare.

Cardiac abnormalities may cause the first overt symptoms. Hemosiderin accumulates in both myocardial fibers and interstitial cells, with less involvement of conducting tissue and the sinoatrial node. Necrosis of myocardial cells and fibrosis can occur. The predominant clinical presentation is dilated cardiomyopathy, often with ventricular ectopy. Finally, *arthralgias* and signs of degenerative joint disease are found in 45% of patients. Chondrocalcinosis and, occasionally, pseudogout can occur. The mechanism is unknown, although investigators have speculated that iron inhibits pyrophosphatase and thereby fosters the formation of pyrophosphate crystals.

DIAGNOSIS

The cost effectiveness of population screening for hemochromatosis is still debated. Initial testing should consist of serum iron and iron-binding capacity with calculation of the percentage of transferrin saturation (see Table 62–2). Values in the 45% to 54% range should lead to repeat testing in 2 years, and values $\geq$55% should prompt testing of serum ferritin and liver function tests. If the alanine aminotransferase level is abnormal or if the ferritin level is more than twice the upper normal limit, a liver biopsy is indicated to define the degree of iron overload and to detect cirrhosis. Alternatively, the patient may be tested for Cys-282-Tyr homozygosity in the *HFE* gene.

TREATMENT AND PROGNOSIS

Alcohol consumption should be limited in patients without cirrhosis and interdicted in those with cirrhosis. Patients should avoid eating raw shellfish from warm coastal waters because bacteremia with *Vibrio vulnificus* is often fatal in hemochromatosis. Vitamin C and iron supplements should not be used without medical indications.

Initial iron depletion is accomplished by removing 500 mL of blood once or twice a week until microcytic anemia develops or until the transferrin saturation and serum ferritin levels fall to less than the lower normal limits. Each unit of blood removes only 200 to 250 mg of iron, so at least 2 to 3 years of weekly phlebotomies are required. Lifelong maintenance phlebotomy, every 2 to 6 months, is then initiated using the serum ferritin level to guide therapy.

Early detection and treatment prevent the morbid consequences of hemochromatosis. Untreated, symptomatic patients have a 5-year survival rate of 20%. Even in patients with cirrhosis, phlebotomy can increase the 10-year survival rate to 75%. Cardiac failure often improves, but it can worsen despite iron depletion. Hypogonadism is not corrected by phlebotomy, and diabetes may improve but rarely disappears.

Porphyrias

Porphyrias are caused by partial deficiency of one of the eight enzymes involved in heme production (Fig. 62–1). Different forms of porphyria are associated with seven of the eight enzymes. Heme-containing proteins are made in all tissues, but bone marrow and liver produce the most heme.

The porphyrias are usefully grouped as *hepatic porphyrias* or *bone marrow porphyrias,* depending on the organ accounting for overproduction of heme synthesis intermediates (Table 62–3). The liver normally makes about 15% of the body heme, but external forces may increase hepatic heme synthesis 10-fold, and all the hepatic porphyrias are "inducible." Bone marrow makes

more than 80% of the body heme, but heme synthesis in bone marrow is not similarly inducible. The hepatic porphyrias may cause both neurotoxicity and photosensitivity, whereas the bone marrow porphyrias cause photosensitivity without neurotoxicity. This section describes the three most common varieties of porphyria and illustrates the cardinal biochemical and clinical features of these disorders.

ACUTE INTERMITTENT PORPHYRIA

Acute intermittent porphyria (AIP) is an autosomal dominant disorder, and the activity of the involved enzyme, porphobilinogen (PBG) deaminase (see Fig. 62–1), is almost always 50% or less of normal. Most patients (~90%) with the heritable disorder do not develop symptoms of porphyria. Attacks are precipitated in the minority by external stimuli to hepatic heme synthesis, particularly drugs that induce the mitochondrial cytochrome P-450.

The flux of intermediates through the heme synthetic pathway is usually at a level in which enzyme substrates are efficiently processed despite reduced enzyme activity. The rate-limiting step, controlling the stream of intermediates in hepatic heme biosynthesis, is the inducible enzyme δ-aminolevulinic acid (ALA) synthase (see Fig. 62–1). In all the forms of porphyria, including AIP, this enzyme functions normally. When defects occur beyond ALA production, ALA synthase may be induced

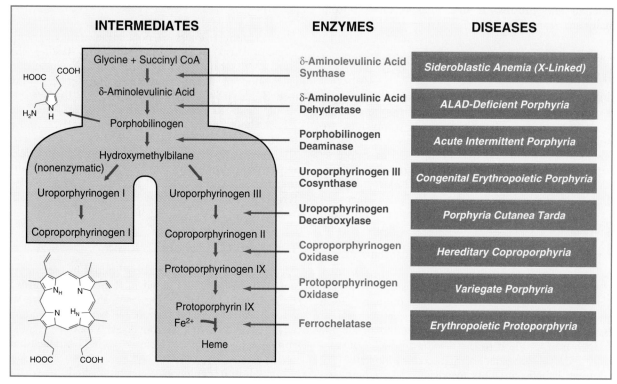

FIGURE 62–1 The heme biosynthetic pathway and the major diseases of porphyrin metabolism. The initial and last three enzymes *(in red)* are mitochondrial and the other four *(in blue)* are cytosolic. X-linked sideroblastic anemia is not classically considered a porphyria. (From Anderson KE: The porphyrias. *In* Goldman L, Bennett JC [eds]: Cecil Textbook of Medicine, 21st ed. Philadelphia: WB Saunders, 2000, p 1124.)

TABLE 62-3 **Porphyrias Grouped by Organ Source of Excess Heme Precursors**

Organ Source	Porphyria	Prevalence	Neurologic Symptoms	Skin Photosensitivity	Drug Inducible
Liver	ALA dehydratase porphyria	Very rare	+	−	+
	Acute intermittent porphyria	5–10/100,000	+	−	+
	Porphyria cutanea tarda	Uncertain, but most common porphyria	+	+	+
	Hereditary coporphyria	Rare	+	+	+
	Variegate porphyria	Not rare	+	+	+
Bone Marrow	Congenital erythropoietic porphyria	Rare	−	+	−
	Erythropoietic protoporphyria	Several hundred known worldwide	−	+	−

ALA = δ-aminolevulinic acid.

and ALA may be overproduced, processes that drive the subsequent series of reactions. In AIP, the defect is at the third enzymatic step (see Fig. 62–1), so both ALA and PBG accumulate (see Table 62–3).

The symptoms of AIP are believed to be largely, if not exclusively, the result of central or peripheral nervous system dysfunction. Two unproven theories of causation exist. One holds that ALA itself is neurotoxic. A second theory suggests that restricted hepatic heme production affects the metabolism of a critical neurotransmitter.

The symptoms of AIP can be dramatic. Abdominal pain, sometimes prompting unwarranted surgical exploration, is found in more than 90% of patients with acute attacks. In patients with accompanying nausea, vomiting, and altered bowel function, primary gastrointestinal disease is usually suspected. Sympathetic nervous system symptoms of tachycardia and hypertension may be pronounced. Hypertension can become sustained. Neuropathy, occurring in more than 60% of cases, may present as muscle weakness, even involving the cranial nerves, with respiratory paralysis and death. Prominent mental symptoms such as anxiety, paranoia, and depression may be mistaken for evidence of a primary affective disorder. Seizures, particularly in patients with hypomagnesemia or the syndrome of inappropriate antidiuretic hormone and hyponatremia, are not uncommon.

AIP is rare before puberty, and sex hormones may precipitate attacks. Many drugs can do likewise, most notably barbiturates, carbamazepine, and sulfonamides. Fasting and calorically restricted diets have precipitated attacks. In some cases, stress, infectious and other illnesses, and even surgery under local anesthesia have caused attacks. The diagnosis is made by demonstrating increased ALA and PBG in urine or decreased PBG deaminase in red blood cells.

Treatment of AIP is largely preventive. Patients must avoid alcohol, offending drugs, hypocaloric diets, and other precipitating factors. Narcotic analgesics are safe and effective during attacks, and a regimen of at least 300 g/day of dietary carbohydrate has traditionally been provided. Intravenous infusions of *hemin*, a heme derivative processed from red blood cells, inhibit ALA syn-

thase and reduce ALA and PBG production. This treatment, used for almost two decades, probably has modest efficacy. β-Adrenergic receptor blockers are effective in treating hypertension and tachycardia.

PORPHYRIA CUTANEA TARDA

Several thousand cases of *porphyria cutanea tarda* (PCT) have been identified, but accurate prevalence figures are not available. The affected enzyme is uroporphyrinogen decarboxylase (see Fig. 62–1). The major porphyrins accumulating in plasma are uroporphyrin, which is behind the partial enzymatic block, and 7-carboxylate porphyrin, the first product of the enzyme's sequential action on uroporphyrin. Uroporphyrinogen and 7-carboxylate porphyrin cause the photosensitivity in PCT.

Photosensitivity of the skin is seen in all porphyrias, except those with blocks before porphyrin production: namely, AIP and ALA dehydratase deficiency (see Fig. 62–1). Most porphyrins absorb light at a 400-nm wavelength and then release energy-generating oxygen-derived free radicals that are particularly damaging to lipid membranes.

PCT usually begins in adulthood with damage to light-exposed skin: fragility, vesicles, bullae, hyperpigmentation, and hypertrichosis are common. In patients with familial disease, the factors inducing heme synthesis are those discussed for AIP. However, uroporphyrinogen decarboxylase deficiency and PCT are usually acquired, and the acquired disease is far more common than the inherited forms. Moderate to severe alcoholism, estrogen in oral contraceptives, and hormone supplements are implicated in most cases currently recognized. Three other associations are particularly noteworthy. Most patients have evidence of iron overload and at least mild hemochromatosis. Chronic hepatitis C is found in many patients. In addition, some patients with acquired immunodeficiency syndrome have manifested PCT.

As with AIP, prevention of attacks is the focal point of management of PCT. Environmental toxins such as chlorinated hydrocarbons, alcohol, estrogen, and other drugs (Table 62–4) should be identified. Phlebotomy for hemochromatosis is effective treatment for PCT and is widely used, as described earlier. Chloroquine has been used in patients with refractory cases.

ERYTHROPOIETIC PROTOPORPHYRIA

Erythropoietic protoporphyria has been described in more than 300 patients worldwide. Unlike PCT, it typically is manifest in childhood. The deficient enzyme, ferrochelatase, is at the eighth and final step in heme

TABLE 62–4 Some Drugs Precipitating Attacks of Acute Intermittent Porphyria

Barbiturates
Carbamazepine
Chlorpropamide
Chlordiazepoxide
Danazol
Dapsone
Ergot preparations
Estrogens
Ethanol
Glutethimide
Griseofulvin
Meprobamate
Oral contraceptives
Phenytoin
Progestins
Pyrazinamide
Sulfonamide antibiotics
Theophylline
Tolbutamide
Valproic acid

biosynthesis and incorporates ferrous ion in protoporphyrin to produce heme. Because the enzyme block in erythropoietic protoporphyria is so late, massive amounts of protoporphyrin accumulate in erythrocytes, plasma, and feces. Protoporphyrin is not found in urine because it is not water soluble.

Cutaneous damage in erythropoietic protoporphyria occurs as described for PCT. Vesicles and bullae are less common. Redness and edema, resembling angioneurotic edema, can occur after a few minutes in the sun. Sun avoidance and highly protective sunscreens (sun protection factor 26 or higher) are the primary approach to management. β-Carotene may also offer some photoprotection. Anemia, which would occur if heme production were severely limited, is not common.

REFERENCES

Anderson KE: The porphyrias. *In* Goldman L, Bennett JC (eds): Cecil Textbook of Medicine, 21st ed. Philadelphia: WB Saunders, 2000, pp 1123–1130.

Bothwell TH, Charlton RW, Motulsky AG: Hemochromatosis. *In* Scriver CR, Beaudet AL, Sly WS, et al (eds): The Metabolic and Molecular Bases of Inherited Disease, 7th ed. New York: McGraw-Hill, 1995, pp 2237–2270.

Danks DM: Disorders of copper transport. *In* Scriver CR, Beaudet AL, Sly WS, et al (eds): The Metabolic and Molecular Bases of Inherited Disease, 7th ed. New York: McGraw-Hill, 1995, pp 2211–2236.

Gahl WA: Wilson's disease. *In* Goldman L, Bennett JC (eds): Cecil Textbook of Medicine, 21st ed. Philadelphia: WB Saunders, 2000, pp 1130–1132.

Kappas A, Sassa S, Galbraith RA, et al: The porphyrias. *In* Scriver CR, Beaudet AL, Sly WS, et al (eds): The Metabolic and Molecular Bases of Inherited Disease, 7th ed. New York: McGraw-Hill, 1995, pp 2103–2160.

Mendlein J, Cogswell ME, McDonnell SM, et al (eds): Iron overload, public health and genetics. Ann Intern Med 1998; 129:921–996.

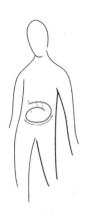

63

INHERITED DISORDERS OF CONNECTIVE TISSUE

Peter N. Herbert

Extracellular proteins and proteoglycans provide the structural framework of all organs. The building materials involved are collagens, elastins, glycoproteins other than collagen (e.g., fibronectin, fibrillin), and proteins containing glycosaminoglycan side chains (proteoglycans). Much of what is known of these critical building materials comes from investigations of humans with mutations in whom defects are manifest.

The genetically transmitted disorders in this chapter are characterized by structural changes in skin, bone, eyes, and the genitourinary, cardiovascular, and gastrointestinal systems. Selected for discussion are four disorders encountered in adult medicine that involve the fibrillar components of connective tissue. Two of these involve collagens, one involves fibrillin, and the last involves elastic tissue. Not discussed are disorders of glycosaminoglycan metabolism, the lysosomal storage mucopolysaccharidoses. These are primarily diseases of children.

Collagen Disorders

Collagens are the most abundant body proteins, accounting for more than 25% of the total. There are 18 known types of collagen and 28 collagen-encoding genes dispersed among at least 12 chromosomes. All collagens are composed of three polypeptide chains, called α chains, wound around each other in a ropelike manner. Formation of the collagen triple helix depends on repeating Gly-X-Y triplets in which X and Y are predominantly prolyl and hydroxyprolyl residues.

Disorders of collagens may result from the structural genes themselves or from enzymes involved in the posttranslational processing of collagens. Disorders are grouped into syndromes defined by their clinical states rather than by the specific protein affected. Osteogenesis imperfecta includes many collagen defects primarily affecting bone, and Ehlers-Danlos syndrome includes those with more prominent skin, joint, and blood vessel problems. However, there is considerable overlap of clinical findings as well as of molecular pathology. Abnormalities of type I collagen, for example, can cause both osteogenesis imperfecta and Ehlers-Danlos–type syndromes.

OSTEOGENESIS IMPERFECTA

All the autosomal dominant forms of osteogenesis imperfecta involve either the α_1 or α_2 chains of type I collagen (Table 63–1). This is the quantitatively major collagen in the human body and the major protein in bone. In some forms of osteogenesis imperfecta, only reduced amounts of normal collagen are secreted into the extracellular matrix, whereas in others, abnormal collagen is elaborated.

One variant of osteogenesis imperfecta is lethal in the perinatal period. Patients with the most common form, osteogenesis imperfecta type I, are of almost average stature, have blue sclerae, and come to medical attention for orthopedic problems related to brittle, osteoporotic bones. Hearing loss, often progressive, is caused by fractured and fused bones in the middle ear. Treatment remains based on symptoms, with orthopedic correction of deformities and intramedullary rodding of brittle bones.

EHLERS-DANLOS SYNDROME

There are a number of variants of Ehlers-Danlos syndrome and they have been reclassified to capture the principal features of each type (see Table 63–1). All are caused by abnormalities either in collagen synthesis or in the enzymes involved in posttranslational processing of collagen. Known variants involve types I, III, and V collagen.

The skin of a patient with Ehlers-Danlos syndrome is collagen poor and proportionately elastin rich. Skin may be pulled far away from underlying structures, promptly

TABLE 63-1   Heritable Disorders of Connective Tissue Fibrillar Proteins

Disorder	Incidence Per 100,000 Births	Genetic Abnormality	Major Clinical Manifestations
Abnormalities of Fibrous Proteins			
Osteogenesis imperfecta	~5	Mutations alter ability of α_1 or α_2 chains of type I collagen to be secreted, to form fibrils, or to be mineralized	Blue sclerae; thin, easily fractured bones; short stature; defective teeth and hearing loss common
Ehlers-Danlos syndrome	~20		
Classical type		α_1 and α_2 chains of type V collagen	Hyperextensible skin and joints
Hypermobility type		Unknown	Same as in classical type
Vascular type		α_1 chain of type III collagen	Thin, translucent skin; typical facies; arterial, intestinal, and uterine rupture; easy bruising
Kyphoscoliosis type		Lysyl hydroxyl deficiency	Severe muscle hypotaxia at birth; progressive scoliosis; rupture of ocular globe
Arthrocholasia type		Processing of α_1 and α_2 chains of type I collagen	Recurrent joint subluxations; congenital hip displacement
Dermatosparaxis type		N-terminal peptidase of type I collagen	Severe skin fragility; sagging redundant skin
Others			
Marfan's syndrome	~10	Abnormal synthesis, secretion, or accumulation of fibrillin I, a major microfibril component of elastic tissue and the zonular fibrils of the lens	Tall stature, long fingers and toes (arachnodactyly), long arms and legs (dolichostenomelia); inward displacement of sternum (pectus excavatum); dislocation of lens (ectopia lentis); lax joints; aortic dilatation, dissection, and rupture
Pseudoxanthoma elasticum	~0.6	Unknown; causes increased calcification and disruption of elastin	Redundant, lax, inelastic skin on face, neck, axilla, abdomen, and groin; hypertension; coronary and cerebral artery occlusion; gastrointestinal and urinary tract bleeding

returning to its original position upon release. Minor trauma may cause gaping wounds. Small and large joints may permit circus-like contortions, but joints are also vulnerable to sprains, subluxations, and dislocations. More serious orthopedic problems include congenital hip dislocation, severe kyphoscoliosis, tendon and muscle rupture, and clubfoot.

Many patients with Ehlers-Danlos syndrome have inguinal, hiatal, and umbilical hernias as well as gastrointestinal or genitourinary diverticula. Those with defective type III collagen, a major collagen in blood vessels and the uterus, have the vascular variant and may have arterial, intestinal, or uterine rupture. Therapy is directed at symptoms, inasmuch as correction of the connective tissue defects is not currently possible.

Marfan's Syndrome

Marfan's syndrome, long incorrectly thought secondary to a collagen abnormality, is caused by abnormalities of the ubiquitous extracellular protein fibrillin I. This cysteine-rich, 350-kd protein forms disulfide bonded aggregates and, with other proteins, generates microfibrils that are abundant in the periosteum, aorta, muscles, and tendons. Microfibrils appear to form the skeleton on which elastin disposition takes place in the skin, media of the aorta, and other tissues.

Marfan's syndrome is inherited in an autosomal dominant pattern, and 15% to 30% of cases represent new mutations. About 100 single-gene mutations in the fibrillin I gene have already been defined in Marfan's syndrome and related connective tissue diseases. There is considerable clinical heterogeneity (see Table 63–1). Typical patients have tall stature, lens dislocation, pectus deformities, and cardiovascular abnormalities. Tall stature does not distinguish Marfan's syndrome, but arm span greater than height (dolichostenomelia) is more specific. Pectus excavatum occurs more commonly than pectus carinatum, and elements of both may be present. Upward dislocation of the lens is probably present at birth in 50% to 80% of cases and generally is not progressive. Joint laxity and arachnodactyly (spider fingers) have little diagnostic specificity.

Progressive dilation of the ascending aorta usually

begins in the 20s, leading to aortic valve incompetence and aortic valve dissection. This complication limited life expectancy to 40 to 50 years in the past. Prophylactic β-adrenergic blockade slows the process. Prophylactic repair or replacement of the aortic root when its diameter reaches 55 mm can generally prevent cardiovascular catastrophe. Median life expectancy in Marfan's syndrome may now exceed 70 years.

Fibrillin I mutations account for a variety of other syndromes sharing features of Marfan's syndrome. These include dominant ectopia lentis, mitral valve prolapse with skeletal features, and familial ascending aortic aneurysm without typical ocular and skeletal features. Mutations responsible for these disorders are found throughout the fibrillin I gene and it is difficult to relate localization to phenotypic expression.

Pseudoxanthoma Elasticum

Pseudoxanthoma elasticum occasionally shows a dominant inheritance pattern, but in most families it is an autosomal recessive disorder. The candidate gene was localized to the short arm of chromosome 16 (16p13.1), and gene identification will soon be possible. Pseudoxanthoma elasticum is characterized by calcium deposition on elastic fibers, which are fragmented and clumped. The disorder may be caused by defects in elastic fiber posttranslational processing or by a component of the extracellular matrix closely linked to elastic fibers.

The skin, eyes, and arteries are affected in pseudoxanthoma elasticum. Skin in the neck, face, axillae, and inguinal folds has a cobblestone appearance as a result of coalescence of slightly raised yellow papules. Skin changes may occur as early as the midteens, and skin may become lax and redundant. Reddish-brown angioid streaks, representing fracture of Bruch's elastic membrane, may be seen on fundoscopic examination, and blindness may follow hemorrhage and neovascularization. Recurrent gastrointestinal hemorrhage, often from stomach arteries, is not uncommon. Most devastating is vascular disease, which may occur in the 20s. Abnormalities include hypertension, peripheral vascular disease with claudication or stroke, coronary artery disease, and congestive heart failure from subendocardial fibrosis and diastolic dysfunction. As in the other connective tissue diseases, treatment is directed at symptom relief through conventional approaches.

REFERENCES

Beighton P, De Paepe A, Steinmann B, et al: Ehlers-Danlos syndromes: Revised nosology, Villefranche, 1997. Am J Med Genet 1998; 77:31–37.

Byers PH: Disorders of collagen biosynthesis and structure. In Scriver CR, Beaudet AL, Sly WS, et al (eds): The Metabolic and Molecular Bases of Inherited Disease, 7th ed. New York: McGraw-Hill, 1995.

Ramirez F, Godfrey M, Lee B, et al: Marfan syndrome and related disorders. In Scriver CR, Beaudet AL, Sly WS, et al (eds): The Metabolic and Molecular Bases of Inherited Disease, 7th ed. New York: McGraw-Hill, 1995.

Royce PM, Steinmann B (eds): Connective tissue and heritable disorders: Molecular, genetic and medical aspects. New York: Wiley-Liss, 1993.

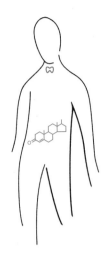

Endocrine Disease

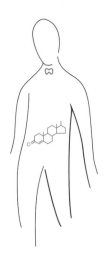

64

HYPOTHALAMIC-PITUITARY AXIS

Vivien Herman-Bonert

Anatomy

The pituitary gland, weighing 500 to 900 mg, lies at the base of the skull in the sella turcica, within the sphenoid bone. The cavernous sinus, which contains the carotid arteries and cranial nerves III, IV, and VI, borders laterally on the pituitary gland. The optic chiasm courses over the superior aspect, separated from the gland by the diaphragma sella of the dura, and the roof of the sphenoid sinus forms the floor of the sella turcica. Two thirds of the pituitary gland is composed of the anterior lobe, and one third, of the posterior lobe.

The anterior pituitary gland receives a rich vascular supply, largely from the median eminence of the hypothalamus via a hypothalamic-pituitary portal circulation. Hypothalamic stimulatory and inhibitory hormones are transported via the hypothalamic-pituitary portal circulation directly to specific cells of the anterior pituitary gland, where they regulate synthesis and secretion of pituitary trophic hormones (Fig. 64–1).

Each of the anterior pituitary hormones, adrenocorticotropic hormone (ACTH), growth hormone (GH), prolactin (PRL), and thyroid-stimulating hormone (TSH) are secreted by a specific pituitary cell type. Luteinizing hormone (LH) and follicle-stimulating hormone (FSH) are secreted by the same cell. GH, PRL, and ACTH are polypeptide hormones, whereas FSH, LH, and TSH are glycoproteins that share the same α subunit, but each has a distinctive β subunit. Arginine vasopressin (AVP), also known as antidiuretic hormone (ADH), is synthesized in the supraoptic and paraventricular nuclei of the hypothalamus and transported through long axons into the posterior lobe of the pituitary gland (Table 64–1).

Anterior Pituitary Hormone Physiology and Testing

GROWTH HORMONE

GH is a 191–amino acid peptide with a molecular weight of 22,000 d. Secretion is stimulated by the 40- and 44–amino acid hypothalamic growth hormone–releasing hormone (GHRH) and inhibited by the hypo-thalamic tetradecapeptide somatostatin. These hypothalamic factors bind to pituitary somatotroph cells and regulate GH secretion. GH binds to receptors in the liver and induces insulin-like growth factor I (IGF-I), which circulates in the blood bound to binding proteins (BPs), the most important of which is IGF-BP3. IGF-I mediates most of the growth-promoting effects of GH. GH also affects carbohydrate metabolism.

Evaluation of GH Reserve

Provocative tests that stimulate the somatotroph are necessary to assess GH deficiency, because basal GH levels are frequently very low even in normal persons. Insulin-induced hypoglycemia (insulin tolerance test) is the most reliable stimulus of GH hypersecretion. Insulin (0.05 to 0.15 U/kg) is administered intravenously to reduce the patient's blood glucose levels to 50% of initial blood glucose or to 40 mg/dL with serial sampling of serum GH and glucose. A normal response is a peak GH level in excess of 5 ng/mL at 60 minutes. Arginine infusion over 30 minutes has a peak GH stimulatory effect 1 hour after administration. L-dopa, a precursor of dopamine and norepinephrine, also stimulates GH secretion from the pituitary somatotroph. Clonidine and

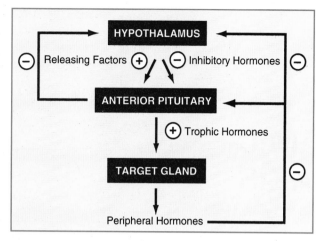

FIGURE 64–1 Feedback control of the hypothalamic-pituitary-target gland axis.

propranolol are alternate orally administered agents used to assess GH reserve. Arginine, L-dopa, clonidine, and propranolol are safer in older patients or patients with central nervous system disorders than is insulin-induced hypoglycemia. Multiple tests are performed to diagnose GH deficiency in a single patient, because only 90% of normal persons respond adequately to any single test. IGF-I and IGF-BP3 levels can be used as a screening test for GH deficiency, because IGF-BP3 levels are regulated by GH; GH deficiency is indicated by low IGF-I and IGF-BP3 levels. Low IGF-I and IGF-BP3 levels are an indication to perform provocative testing of GH secretion.

Tests for GH Hypersecretion

GH is secreted in a pulsatile manner, and the measurement of random GH levels is of no value. Moreover, cirrhosis, starvation, anxiety, type 1 diabetes mellitus, and acute illness can be associated with GH hypersecretion. However, measurement of IGF-I levels is a useful indicator of GH hypersecretion, because this level does not fluctuate throughout the day. IGF-I levels are elevated in almost all patients with GH hypersecretion. A simple and specific dynamic test for GH hypersecretion is the administration of oral glucose, in which 100 g of glucose administered orally suppresses GH levels to less than 1 ng/mL after 120 minutes in healthy volunteers. In acromegaly, GH levels may increase, remain unchanged, or decrease (however, not below 1 ng/mL) after an oral glucose load. IGF-I and oral glucose suppression tests are the cornerstones of the laboratory confirmation of GH hypersecretion in patients with acromegaly (see later discussion). Twenty to 50 percent of acromegalic patients show a paradoxical increase in GH secretion after administration of thyrotropin-releasing hormone (TRH).

PROLACTIN

PRL, a 198–amino acid, 22,000-d polypeptide, is synthesized and secreted by pituitary lactotrophs. PRL secretion is under predominantly inhibitory control by hypothalamic dopamine. TRH and vasoactive intestinal polypeptide are PRL-releasing factors. PRL secretion is episodic. Estrogens increase basal and stimulated PRL secretion; glucocorticoids and TSH blunt TRH-induced PRL secretion. PRL levels increase during pregnancy,

TABLE 64–1 Pituitary-Target Organ Hormone Axis

Hypothalamic Hormone	Pituitary Target Cell	Pituitary Hormone Affected	Peripheral Target Gland	Peripheral Hormone Affected
Stimulatory				
Anterior Lobe of Pituitary Gland				
Thyrotropin-releasing hormone (TRH)	Thyrotroph	Thyroid-stimulating hormone (TSH)	Thyroid gland	Thyroxine (T_4) Triiodothyronine (T_3)
	Lactotroph	Prolactin	Breast	
Growth hormone-releasing hormone (GHRH)	Somatotroph	Growth hormone (GH)	Liver	Insulin-like growth factor-I (IGF-I)
Gonadotropin-releasing hormone (GnRH)	Gonadotroph	Luteinizing hormone (LH)	Ovary Testis	Progesterone Testosterone
		Follicle-stimulating hormone (FSH)	Ovary Testis	Estradiol Inhibin
Corticotropin-releasing hormone	Corticotroph	Adrenocorticotrophic hormone (ACTH)	Adrenal gland	Cortisol
Posterior Lobe of Pituitary Gland				
Vasopressin			Kidney	
Oxytocin			Uterus, breast	
Inhibitory				
Somatostatin	Somatotroph	GH		
	Thyrotroph	TSH		

enhancing breast development. After childbirth, PRL stimulates milk production. However, elevated PRL levels are not needed to maintain lactation, and basal PRL secretion falls as the infant's suckling reflex maintains lactation.

Evaluation of PRL Hypersecretion

Basal PRL levels are used in the assessment of hyperprolactinemia. Basal PRL levels greater than 200 ng/mL are highly suggestive of PRL-secreting adenomas (see the later section on prolactinoma).

THYROID-STIMULATING HORMONE

TSH, a 28,000-d glycoprotein hormone, is synthesized and secreted by the pituitary thyrotroph cells; TSH secretion is stimulated by the hypothalamic tripeptide TRH. The inhibitory effect of hypothalamic somatostatin augments the negative feedback inhibition of TSH secretion by peripheral thyroid hormones. TSH attaches to receptors on the thyroid gland and activates adenylyl cyclase, stimulating iodine uptake and the synthesis and release of the thyroid hormones thyroxine (T_4) and triiodothyronine (T_3). T_4 and T_3 in turn exert negative feedback inhibition on pituitary TSH and hypothalamic TRH secretion.

Evaluation of TSH Secretion

TSH is measured by ultrasensitive assays (immunoradiometric assays), which can accurately distinguish low, normal, and high TSH levels. The ultrasensitive TSH assay has largely replaced the need for any further tests. A suppressed TSH level indicates central (secondary) hypothyroidism and an elevated level, primary hypothyroidism.

ADRENOCORTICOTROPIC HORMONE

ACTH, a 39–amino acid peptide, is synthesized as part of a larger 241–amino acid precursor molecule, proopiomelanocortin, which is subsequently enzymatically cleaved into β-lipotropin (β-LPH), ACTH, joining peptide, and an NH_2 terminal peptide in the anterior lobe of the pituitary gland. ACTH is then cleaved into α-melanocyte-stimulating hormone (N-acetyl ACTH [1–13] NH_2 [α-MSH]) and corticotropin-like peptide (ACTH [18–39]), whereas β-LPH is split into LPH and β-endorphin.

Hypothalamic corticotropin-releasing hormone (CRH) and to a lesser extent, ADH, stimulates ACTH secretion by pituitary corticotroph cells. ACTH stimulates cortisol synthesis and secretion from the adrenal gland. Cortisol exerts a negative feedback on ACTH and CRH secretion. ACTH is secreted in pulses and is under circadian control, reaching maximal levels in the last hours before awakening, followed by a steady decline to a nadir in the evening. Both psychological and physical stress increase ACTH and cortisol secretion, whereas glucocorticoids inhibit ACTH secretion as well as CRH and ADH synthesis and release. ACTH also maintains adrenal size by increasing protein synthesis.

Evaluation of ACTH Secretion

Excess ACTH secretion results in Cushing's syndrome, which may be caused by a pituitary adenoma (Cushing's disease) or by ectopic ACTH secretion (see Chapter 66). ACTH deficiency results in adrenocortical insufficiency, with decreased secretion of cortisol and adrenal androgens. Aldosterone secretion is largely regulated by the renin-angiotensin axis; therefore, aldosterone secretion remains intact.

Basal ACTH Levels. Random basal ACTH measurements are unreliable because of the short plasma half-life and pulsatile secretion of the hormone. Interpretation of plasma ACTH levels requires concomitant assessment of plasma cortisol levels. Because ACTH regulates cortisol secretion, plasma cortisol levels better reflect hypothalamic-pituitary-adrenal function. An 8 a.m. cortisol level higher than 10 μg/dL effectively rules out adrenal insufficiency but cannot be used to assess adrenal reserve. Simultaneously measured ACTH levels can be used to differentiate primary from secondary adrenal insufficiency. Plasma ACTH levels are normal to high in adrenal insufficiency because of a primary adrenal disorder and are low to absent in adrenal insufficiency secondary to hypothalamic-pituitary hypofunction. ACTH levels are also useful in establishing the etiology of Cushing's syndrome (see Chapter 66).

Evaluation of ACTH Reserve. To assess the adequacy of ACTH reserve under conditions of stress, provocative testing is performed. If compromised adrenal function is suspected, these tests are potentially hazardous, and patients should be closely monitored by a physician. Prolonged ACTH deficiency results in adrenal atrophy. Thus, adrenal cortisol reserve can be measured as an indirect test of pituitary ACTH status. Two hundred fifty micrograms of cosyntropin (Cortrosyn; synthetic ACTH [1–24] administered intravenously or intramuscularly results in an increment of 7 μg/dL or more in serum cortisol, or peak levels of more than 20 μg/dL, within 60 minutes in normal persons. An inadequate response implies either impaired pituitary ACTH secretion or primary adrenal failure.

The insulin-induced hypoglycemia test just described stimulates the hypothalamic-pituitary-adrenal axis. A peak cortisol level of at least 18 μg/dL, or doubling of the baseline cortisol 30 to 45 minutes after the onset of hypoglycemia, confirms normal ACTH reserve. Insulin-induced hypoglycemia is the most reliable test of the ACTH secretory response to stress. The test is contraindicated in elderly patients and in patients with cerebrovascular disorders, seizure disorders, or cardiovascular disease. A physician should always be in attendance during testing. Ovine CRF (1 μg/kg, intravenously) directly stimulates pituitary corticotrophs to secrete ACTH, with a peak response within 15 minutes and subsequent peak cortisol response at 30 to 60 minutes. Patients with adrenal insufficiency secondary to hypopituitarism have no ACTH response to CRF; hypothalamic dysfunction results in a delayed peak. Patients with pituitary corticotroph cell adenomas often show an exaggerated ACTH response to CRF, whereas ectopic ACTH-secreting tumors do not cause a further increase in ACTH levels.

Evaluation of ACTH Hypersecretion. Pituitary corticotroph adenomas in Cushing's disease or ectopic ACTH-secreting tumors result in ACTH hypersecretion and hypercortisolism. The diagnosis is discussed in Chapter 66.

GONADOTROPINS (LH AND FSH)

Gonadotroph secretion is regulated by hypothalamic gonadotropin-releasing hormone (GnRH), a 10–amino acid peptide secreted in a pulsatile manner, and feedback inhibition is regulated by gonadal steroids (estrogen and testosterone) and peptides (inhibin and activin). Basal LH and FSH are secreted in a pulsatile manner, concordantly with the pulsatile release of GnRH. GnRH release determines the onset of puberty and generates the midcycle gonadotropin surges necessary for ovulation. Gonadal steroids exert both positive and negative feedback effects on gonadotroph secretion. In addition, the gonadal polypeptide inhibin, produced by ovarian granulosa cells and testicular Sertoli cells, negatively inhibits FSH secretion, whereas activins stimulate FSH secretion. LH and FSH bind to receptors in the ovaries and testes and stimulate sex steroid secretion (mainly by LH) as well as gametogenesis (mainly by FSH). LH stimulates gonadal steroid secretion by testicular Leydig cells and by the ovarian follicles. In women, the ovulatory LH surge results in rupture of the follicle and then luteinization. FSH stimulates Sertoli cell spermatogenesis in men and follicular development in women.

Evaluation of Hypothalamic-Pituitary-Gonadal Axis

LH and FSH levels vary with age and with the menstrual cycle in women. Prepubertal gonadotropin levels are low, and postmenopausal women have elevated levels. Male FSH and LH levels are pulsatile but fluctuate less than those in women. During the follicular phase of the menstrual cycle, LH levels rise steadily, with a midcycle spike that stimulates ovulation. FSH rises during the early follicular phase, falls in the late follicular phase, and peaks at midcycle, concurrently with the LH surge. Both LH and FSH levels fall after ovulation. LH and FSH levels in men are measured by three pooled samples drawn 20 minutes apart, which compensates for the normal pulsatile secretion.

Gonadotropin and sex steroid estimation in women are more complex. However, women with regular menstrual cycles and a documented normal luteal phase serum progesterone concentration are unlikely to have significant gonadotropin dysfunction. In amenorrheic women, measurement of serum LH, FSH, estradiol, PRL, and human chorionic gonadotropin (hCG) can differentiate among (1) primary ovarian failure with elevated FSH and LH levels and normal PRL levels; (2) hyperprolactinemia with elevated PRL and normal/low follicular phase LH, FSH, and estradiol levels; and (3) pregnancy with a positive hCG, normal to high PRL, normal to high LH, and high estradiol.

Gonadotropin deficiency is best diagnosed by concurrent measurement of serum gonadotropins and gonadal steroid concentrations. Low or normal FSH and LH levels in the presence of a low testosterone level (in men) or a low estradiol level (in women) confirms the diagnosis. Low levels of gonadal steroids in the presence of elevated gonadotropin levels suggest primary gonadal failure.

Neuroradiologic Evaluation of the Pituitary Gland

Clinical features suggesting hypothalamic-pituitary dysfunction necessitate neuroradiologic assessment of the hypothalamus and pituitary gland to confirm the existence and extent of lesions. Endocrine evaluation should precede imaging studies, because about 10% of the normal population harbor nonfunctional asymptomatic pituitary microadenomas that are detectable by magnetic resonance imaging (MRI).

MRI is the imaging procedure of choice for hypothalamic-pituitary lesions. Lesions as small as 3 to 5 mm in diameter can be detected by MRI performed in both sagittal and coronal planes at 1.5- to 2-mm intervals. The contrast agent gadolinium is used to help differentiate small pituitary lesions from normal anterior pituitary tissue.

Microadenomas are defined as pituitary lesions less than 10 mm in diameter. Lesions less than 5 mm in diameter may not be detected by MRI and do not alter the normal pituitary contour, whereas lesions more than 5 mm in diameter may cause deviation of the pituitary stalk and convexity of the superior pituitary margin.

Macroadenomas are pituitary lesions more than 10 mm in diameter. They are easily differentiated from normal surrounding pituitary tissue by MRI. They may cause marked deviation of the pituitary stalk to the opposite side. Adenomas exceeding 15 mm frequently have suprasellar extension with compression and displacement of the optic chiasm. MRI may also show lateral extension of large adenomas into the cavernous sinus.

Empty sella syndrome, the commonest cause of an enlarged sella, is caused by herniation of the arachnoid membrane through an incompetent diaphragm sella, either after pituitary surgery or radiation, or is caused by a primary congenital defect.

Pituitary and Hypothalamic Disorders

Pituitary adenomas associated with hormonal hypersecretion are the most common pituitary lesions. The earliest clinical manifestations are usually the characteristic signs and symptoms caused by the hormone hypersecretion. Subsequently, if the tumor is a macroadenoma, local manifestations of tumor enlargement develop; these include headache, visual abnormalities (visual field defects and diplopia), sellar enlargement, and hypopituitarism. Visual loss can occur with hypothalamic or pituitary lesions and manifests typically as a bitemporal hemianopia. Neuro-ophthalmologic evaluation, including visual field assessment, should be performed. Visual field defects may be the presenting feature of nonsecretory pituitary tumors. Extension of large tumors laterally into the cavernous sinus can compress the third, fourth, or sixth cranial nerves and lead to diplopia or abnormalities of extraocular eye muscle movements. Hypopituitarism should be ruled out in these patients, and serum PRL level should be measured.

HYPOTHALAMIC DYSFUNCTION

In children and young adults, craniopharyngioma is the most frequent cause of hypothalamic dysfunction. Primary central nervous system tumors, pinealomas, and dermoid and epidermoid tumors also cause hypothalamic dysfunction in adulthood. Clinical manifestations of tumors that can cause hypothalamic dysfunction include visual loss, symptoms of raised intracranial pressure (headache and vomiting), hypopituitarism (including growth failure), and diabetes insipidus. Hypothalamic disturbances include disorders of thirst (leading to dehydration or to polydipsia and polyuria), appetite (with resultant hyperphagia and obesity), temperature regulation, behavior, and consciousness (with resultant somnolence and emotional lability). Diabetes insipidus is a common manifestation of hypothalamic lesions but rarely occurs with primary pituitary lesions. Diagnosis is confirmed by MRI. Because hypopituitarism occurs frequently with hypothalamic lesions, anterior pituitary function should be completely assessed.

Craniopharyngioma is treated by surgical resection and then radiotherapy. Biopsy of other types of hypothalamic tumors is usually required for histologic diagnosis before surgical resection, because some, such as dysgerminoma, may be radiosensitive.

HYPOPITUITARISM

Hypopituitarism results from diminished secretion of one or more pituitary hormones. The syndrome results either from anterior pituitary gland destruction or from pituitary gland dysfunction secondary to deficient hypothalamic stimulatory/inhibitory factors that normally regulate pituitary function. Hypopituitarism can be caused by congenital or acquired lesions (Table 64–2). Pituitary insufficiency is usually a slow, insidious disorder. Pituitary lesions may result in single or multiple hormone losses.

GH Deficiency

GH deficiency during infancy and childhood manifests as growth retardation, short stature, and fasting hypoglycemia. A syndrome of adult GH deficiency may manifest as increased abdominal adiposity, reduced strength and exercise capacity, decreased lean body mass and increased fat mass, and impaired psychosocial well-being. Adult GH deficiency is frequently accompanied by other symptoms of panhypopituitarism.

TABLE 64–2 Etiology of Hypopituitarism

Type of Disorder	Cause
Congenital	Septo-optic dysplasia
	Prader-Willi syndrome
	Laurence-Moon-Biedl syndrome
	Isolated anterior pituitary hormone or releasing factor deficiency
Tumors	Pituitary tumors
	Secretory adenomas
	Nonsecretory adenomas
	Hypothalamic tumors
	Craniopharyngioma
	Hamartoma
	Pinealoma
	Dermoid
	Epidermoid
	Glioma
	Lymphoma
	Meningioma
	Immunologic cancers
Infiltrative	Hemachromatosis
	Langerhans cell histiocytosis
	Sarcoidosis
	Metastatic carcinoma (breast and bronchus)
	Amyloidosis
Infectious	Tuberculosis
	Mycoses
	Syphilis
Physical trauma	Cranial trauma and hemorrhage
	Ionizing radiation
	Stalk section
	Surgery
Vascular	Postpartum pituitary necrosis (Sheehan's syndrome)
	Pituitary apoplexy
	Carotid aneurysm

TSH Deficiency

TSH deficiency causes thyroid gland involution and hypofunction. Clinical features of hypothyroidism include lethargy, constipation, cold intolerance, bradycardia, weight gain, poor appetite, dry skin, and delayed reflex relaxation time. Secondary hypothyroidism can be differentiated from primary hypothyroidism by the presence of low circulating TSH in the presence of low thyroid hormone levels.

Gonadotropin Deficiency

Central hypogonadism during childhood results in failure to enter normal puberty. Girls have delayed breast development, scant pubic and axillary hair, and primary amenorrhea. In boys, the phallus and testes remain small, and body hair is sparse. Sex steroids are required for closure of the epiphyses of the long bones; thus, in isolated gonadotropin deficiency, growth continues (as GH is intact) because there is failure of epiphyseal fusion, resulting in tall adolescents with eunuchoid proportions (upper-to-lower segment ratio less than 1). In adult women, hypogonadism manifests as breast atrophy, loss of pubic and axillary hair, and secondary amenorrhea. Hypogonadal men develop testicular atrophy, decreased libido, impotence, and loss of body hair.

ACTH Deficiency

ACTH deficiency results in adrenal failure, causing lethargy, weakness, nausea, vomiting, dehydration, orthostatic hypotension, coma, and, if untreated, death.

ADH (Vasopressin) Deficiency

Vasopressin deficiency occurs with posterior pituitary dysfunction and leads to diabetes insipidus with polyuria, polydipsia, and nocturia.

Diagnosis

The diagnosis of pituitary hormone deficiency has been discussed previously in relation to the individual hormones.

Treatment

Patients with panhypopituitarism must have adequate replacement of thyroxine, glucocorticoids, and appropriate sex steroids. Children with short stature resulting from GH deficiency should receive GH replacement therapy. The safety and efficacy of GH replacement therapy for adults who develop GH deficiency is being evaluated. Testosterone therapy in men restores libido and potency, growth of body hair, and muscle strength. Estrogen replacement therapy in females maintains secondary sex characteristics and prevents hot flashes. Human menopausal gonadotropins and hCG given intramuscularly or GnRH administered by infusion pumps may be given to induce ovulation. In patients with combined TSH and ACTH deficiency, glucocorticoids should be replaced before thyroxine, because thyroxine may aggravate adrenal insufficiency and may precipitate acute adrenal failure.

Pituitary Tumors

The pituitary comprises five cell types, each of which, either singly or in combination, can give rise to pituitary adenomas, which secrete hormones characteristic to the particular cell type. Pituitary tumors may also be "nonfunctioning"; such tumors do not secrete biologically active hormones but may secrete the α-subunit common to the glycoprotein hormones. Prolactinomas are the most common secretory pituitary tumors. Pituitary tumors are usually benign neoplasms. Isolated reports of pituitary carcinomas with distant metastases have been described.

Secretory pituitary tumors are usually diagnosed from the constellation of signs and symptoms caused by hy-

persecretion of the particular pituitary trophic hormone. GH adenomas cause acromegaly, prolactinomas cause amenorrhea and galactorrhea in women and sexual dysfunction in men, and ACTH-secreting adenomas result in Cushing's disease. Large pituitary adenomas (secretory or nonsecretory) can result in signs and symptoms caused by pressure on surrounding structures. Headache is a frequent symptom, possibly caused by pressure on the diaphragma sella. If the tumor extends into the suprasellar space, the optic chiasm may be compressed, which results in bitemporal hemianopia or a superior bitemporal defect. Lateral extension into the cavernous sinus can result in ophthalmoplegia, diplopia, or ptosis as a result of dysfunction of the third, fourth, fifth, and sixth cranial nerves. Compression of surrounding normal pituitary tissue by an enlarging tumor mass can cause hyposecretion of one or several pituitary trophic hormones, resulting in signs and symptoms of hypopituitarism. Destructive pituitary lesions result in hormone loss, which follows a particular pattern: initially GH, followed by LH and FSH, then TSH and ACTH.

PROLACTINOMAS

Of the prolactinomas, microprolactinomas are most common among women, whereas macroadenomas are seen more frequently in men. Hyperprolactinemia in women can cause hypogonadotropic hypogonadism, resulting in estrogen deficiency. Gonadotropin levels are normal, and sex steroids are decreased. PRL inhibits pulsatility in gonadotropin secretion and suppresses the midcycle LH surge with consequent anovulation. In hyperprolactinemic men, testosterone levels are usually suppressed.

Clinical Features

Regardless of the cause of hyperprolactinemia, the clinical features are the same. Prolactinomas are often recognized earlier in women who have menstrual irregularities and infertility, as opposed to men, who manifest decreased libido and impotence.

Ninety percent of hyperprolactinemic women have amenorrhea, galactorrhea, or infertility. If the prolactinoma occurs before the onset of menarche, adolescents may have primary amenorrhea. Prolactinomas account for 15% to 20% of secondary amenorrhea. Anovulation is associated with infertility. Galactorrhea may accompany, precede, or follow the menstrual irregularities, may not be clinically obvious, and may be discovered only during breast examination.

Estrogen deficiency may cause osteopenia, vaginal dryness, hot flashes, and irritability. PRL stimulates adrenal androgen production, and androgen excess can result in weight gain and hirsutism. Hyperprolactinemia may be associated with anxiety and depression.

Men usually have loss of libido and impotence as a result of hypogonadism. These symptoms are not often attributed to a prolactinoma, which results in frequent delay in diagnosis until visual impairment, headache, and hypopituitarism develop.

Diagnosis

Several physiologic conditions (pregnancy, stress, nipple stimulation), as well as certain medications (phenothiazines, methyldopa, cimetidine, metoclopramide) and pathologic states (hypothyroidism, chronic renal failure, chest wall lesions), affect PRL secretion. These conditions may be associated with mildly elevated PRL levels; however, basal PRL levels in excess of 200 ng/mL usually imply prolactinoma. The diagnosis should be confirmed by MRI.

Treatment

Medical management with a dopamine agonist, bromocriptine or cabergoline, restores gonadal function and fertility in the majority of patients. Dopamine agonists cause tumor shrinkage in a significant number of patients with macroadenomas. Trans-sphenoidal surgery is indicated in patients with visual field abnormalities or neurologic symptoms and in patients who cannot tolerate medical treatment.

ACROMEGALY AND GIGANTISM

In childhood, hypersecretion of GH leads to gigantism; in adults whose long bone epiphyses are fused, GH excess causes acromegaly with local overgrowth of bone in the acral areas. GH hypersecretion is almost always caused by a GH-secreting pituitary adenoma. Ectopic GH secretion has been described with pancreatic, breast, and lung tumors. Ectopic GHRH secretion can occur with pancreatic islet cell tumors and bronchial or intestinal carcinoids. Both ectopic GH and GHRH manifest clinically with acromegaly but are extremely rare.

Clinical Features

The clinical features of acromegaly are insidious, and it may take several years for the disfiguring features to be diagnosed. Untreated acromegaly causes increased rates of morbidity and mortality late in the course of the disorder. The most classic clinical feature is acral enlargement, manifested as widening of the hands and feet and coarsening of the facial features; frontal sinuses enlarge, leading to prominent supraorbital ridges, and the mandible grows downward and forward, resulting in prognathism and wide spacing of the teeth. Ring, glove, and shoe sizes increase as a result of soft tissue enlargement of hands and feet. The bony and soft tissue changes are accompanied by endocrine, metabolic, and systemic manifestations (Table 64–3).

Diagnosis

IGF-I mediates the classical acral changes that occur with acromegaly. IGF-I levels are elevated in virtually all acromegalic patients. Biochemical confirmation of the diagnosis is obtained by measuring GH levels 2 hours after an oral glucose load. MRI of the pituitary helps localize the tumor and assess tumor size. Ninety percent of acromegalic patients have tumors larger than 1 cm. If

TABLE 64–3 Clinical Features of Acromegaly

Change	Manifestations
Somatic Changes	
Acral changes	Enlarged hands and feet
Musculoskeletal changes	Arthralgias
	Prognathism
	Malocclusion
	Carpal tunnel syndrome
	Proximal myopathy
Skin changes	Sweating
Colon changes	Polyps
	Carcinoma
Cardiovascular symptoms	Cardiomegaly
	Hypertension
Visceromegaly	Tongue
	Thyroid
	Liver
Endocrine-Metabolic Changes	
Reproduction	Menstrual abnormalities
	Galactorrhea
	Decreased libido
Carbohydrate metabolism	Impaired glucose tolerance
	Diabetes mellitus
Lipids	Hypertriglyceridemia

no pituitary mass is detected, an extrapituitary source of ectopic GH or GHRH should be sought, through imaging studies of the chest and abdomen.

Treatment

Trans-sphenoidal microsurgery is the initial therapy of choice, resulting in rapid reduction of GH levels with a low rate of surgical morbidity. Cure rates are proportional to preoperative tumor size, with a 90% success rate for small or moderate-sized tumors (<2 cm). Radiotherapy is an effective method of reducing GH hypersecretion; however, the time until onset of its effect may be as long as 20 years, and the incidence of hypopituitarism is high. Medical management involves the use of somatostatin analogues, because bromocriptine is effective in suppressing GH in only a minority of acromegalic patients. Octreotide acetate, a long-acting somatostatin analogue, is very effective in reducing GH and IGF-I levels to normal in the majority of acromegalic patients treated; it has been reported to shrink tumors in some cases. Octreotide is administered as a subcutaneous injection, three times daily, and continuous therapy is required. Side effects include diarrhea, abdominal cramps, flatulence, and asymptomatic gallstone formation. A depot preparation administered intramuscularly once a month has been approved for the control of GH hypersecretion in acromegaly.

ACTH-SECRETING PITUITARY TUMORS

See Chapter 66.

GONADOTROPIN-SECRETING PITUITARY TUMORS

Gonadotropin-secreting pituitary tumors are rare and have been reported mainly in men. The majority of tumors are large at the time of presentation and hypersecrete only FSH. Patients usually have signs and symptoms of local pressure, such as visual impairment. Patients may also present with hypogonadism with low or normal testosterone levels or low or normal sperm counts as a result of downregulation of the pituitary-gonadal axis by the high levels of circulating gonadotropins. In rare cases, excess LH may stimulate testosterone levels.

Surgical removal of gonadotropin-secreting adenomas is the usual primary treatment. However, patients frequently require subsequent radiotherapy to adequately control LH and FSH hypersecretion.

THYROTROPIN-SECRETING PITUITARY TUMOR

This type of tumor is extremely rare, manifesting with hyperthyroidism, goiter, and inappropriately elevated TSH level in the presence of elevated thyroid hormone levels. TSH-secreting tumors are usually plurihormonal, secreting GH, PRL, and the glycoprotein hormone α-subunit, as well as TSH. Initially, tumor bulk is reduced with surgery. These tumors are often resistant to removal, which necessitates several surgical procedures or multiple doses of radiotherapy. Octreotide acetate has been found to be useful in decreasing TSH secretion in patients with these tumors and has been shown to shrink the tumor in some cases. Iodine-131 thyroid ablation or thyroid surgery may be needed to control thyrotoxicosis.

The Posterior Pituitary Gland

The posterior pituitary gland secretes ADH and oxytocin. These hormones are synthesized in the hypothalamic supraoptic and paraventricular nuclei in neuronal cell bodies that extend from the hypothalamus to the posterior pituitary. ADH, a 1084-d nonapeptide with a ring structure and disulfide linkage, helps to regulate water balance and is a potent vasoconstrictor. ADH binds to receptors on the renal tubule, increasing the water permeability of the luminal membrane of the collecting duct epithelium, thus facilitating reabsorption of water and concentration of the urine. Maximal ADH effect results in a small volume of concentrated urine with a high osmolarity (as high as 1200 mOsm/kg). Deficiency of ADH results in a large volume of very dilute urine (as low as 100 mOsm/kg). In addition to the renal tubular effects, ADH also binds to peripheral arteriolar receptors, causing vasoconstriction and resultant increase in blood pressure. However, there is a countereffect to the hypertensive effect of ADH in that ADH also causes bradycardia and inhibition of sympathetic nerve activity.

Deficiency of ADH or insensitivity of the kidneys to ADH results in diabetes insipidus, which is manifested as polyuria and polydipsia. Inappropriate secretion of ADH in excess amounts results in the syndrome of inappropriate antidiuretic hormone (SIADH) secretion and causes a hyponatremic state.

Oxytocin, a 1007-d nonapeptide that also has a ring structure and disulfide linkage, causes uterine smooth muscle contraction.

DIABETES INSIPIDUS

Diabetes insipidus can be of a central (neurogenic) origin when there is failure of the posterior lobe of the pituitary to secrete adequate amounts of ADH, or it can be of nephrogenic origin, caused by failure of the kidney to respond to adequate amounts of circulating ADH. Regardless of the cause, patients are polyuric, secreting large volumes of dilute urine. This causes cellular and extracellular dehydration, stimulating thirst, which results in polydipsia. The causes of central diabetes insipidus are entirely different from those of nephrogenic diabetes insipidus (Table 64–4). Several of the causes of hypopituitarism, especially those that involve the hypothalamus, are also causes of diabetes insipidus.

Differential Diagnosis

Diabetes insipidus (central or nephrogenic) must be distinguished from primary polydipsia, a compulsive psychoneurotic disorder manifested as a disorder of thirst, in which patients drink in excess of 5 L of water a day, resulting in decreased ADH secretion and subsequent diuresis. One possible distinguishing clinical feature is that patients with diabetes insipidus prefer cold bever-

TABLE 64–4   Causes of Diabetes Insipidus

Causes of Central Diabetes Insipidus
Idiopathic
Familial
Hypophysectomy
Infiltration of hypothalamus and posterior pituitary
Langerhans cell histiocytosis
Granulomas
Infection
Tumors (intrasellar and suprasellar)
Autoimmune
Causes of Nephrogenic Diabetes Insipidus
Idiopathic
Familial
Chronic renal disease (e.g., chronic pyelonephritis, polycystic kidney disease, or medullary cystic disease)
Hypokalemia
Hypercalcemia
Sickle cell anemia
Drugs
Lithium
Fluoride
Demeclocycline
Colchicine

ages. Several tests can be performed to confirm the diagnosis of diabetes insipidus and differentiate the syndrome from primary polydipsia. Initially, random simultaneous samples of plasma and urine for sodium and osmolarity are obtained. In diabetes insipidus (central or nephrogenic), inappropriate diuresis results in a urine osmolarity that is less than that of plasma osmolarity. Plasma osmolarity may be elevated, depending on the patient's state of hydration. However, in primary polydipsia, both plasma and urine are dilute.

The primary test used to differentiate the causes of polyuria is the water deprivation test. The patient is denied fluids for 12 to 18 hours, and body weight, blood pressure, urine volume, urine specific gravity, and plasma and urine osmolarity are measured every 2 hours. Careful supervision is required, as patients with diabetes insipidus may become rapidly dehydrated and hypotensive if denied access to water (in which case the test is stopped). A normal response is a decrease in urine output to 0.5 mL/min, as well as an increase in urine concentration to greater than that of plasma. Patients with diabetes insipidus (either central or nephrogenic) maintain a high urine output, which continues to be dilute (specific gravity, < 1.005) despite water deprivation. In patients with primary polydipsia, urine osmolarity increases to values greater than plasma osmolarity. Water deprivation is continued until the urine osmolarity plateaus (an hourly increase of < 30 mOsm/kg for three successive hours). At that point, 5 μg of ADH is administered subcutaneously, and the urine osmolarity is measured after 1 hour. In patients with complete central diabetes insipidus, urine osmolarity increases above plasma osmolarity, whereas in nephrogenic diabetes insipidus, the urine osmolarity increases less than 50% in response to ADH. Patients with partial central diabetes insipidus also show an increase in urine osmolarity, but it is less than 50%, whereas patients with primary polydipsia have increases of less than 10%. ADH levels should be measured during the water deprivation test. Patients with nephrogenic diabetes insipidus have normal or increased levels of ADH during water deprivation, in contrast to those with complete central diabetes insipidus, who have suppressed levels. Patients with partial central diabetes insipidus show a smaller than normal increase in plasma ADH during water deprivation.

Treatment

Central Diabetes Insipidus. Desmopressin acetate (DDAVP), a synthetic analogue of ADH, is usually administered intranasally or orally in the treatment of diabetes insipidus. Frequency of administration is determined by the severity of the disease. Adequacy of replacement is monitored by regular measurement of serum osmolarity and sodium.

Nephrogenic Diabetes Insipidus. As far as possible, the underlying disease process should be reversed. Specific treatment of nephrogenic diabetes insipidus aims to maintain a state of mild sodium depletion with reduction in the solute load on the kidneys and subse-

quent increased proximal tubular reabsorption. Diuretics with dietary salt restriction can be used to achieve this goal.

SIADH

The syndrome of inappropriate secretion of antidiuretic hormone is characterized by plasma ADH concentrations that are inappropriately high for plasma osmolarity, resulting in water retention and leading to hyponatremia and decreased plasma osmolarity (< 280 mOsm/kg). Urine osmolarity is inappropriately concentrated in relation to the low plasma osmolarity and is higher than the plasma osmolarity. The diagnosis can be made only in the absence of hypervolemia (nephrotic syndrome, cardiac failure, cirrhosis) and with normal renal, adrenal, and thyroid function. The clinical signs and symptoms depend on the degree of the hyponatremia and the rate of decrease of the plasma osmolarity. Headache, anorexia, vomiting, and confusion may be manifested with serum sodium levels between 115 and 120 mEq/L, whereas disorientation, stupor, coma, seizures, and focal neurologic abnormalities seldom occur until the serum sodium level is less than 110 mEq/L.

Causes

Several benign and malignant conditions are associated with SIADH (Table 64–5).

Treatment

The underlying condition associated with SIADH should be treated. Further management aims to normalize the plasma osmolarity while avoiding further expansion of the extracellular fluid. Fluid restriction is thus the cornerstone of treatment.

TABLE 64–5 Disorders Associated with Syndrome of Inappropriate Antidiuretic Hormone (SIADH) Secretion

Type of Disorder	Disorder

Pulmonary disorders	Malignant
	  Small cell carcinoma
	Benign
	  Tuberculosis
	  Pneumonia (viral, bacterial)
	  Abscess

Central nervous system disorders	Meningitis (viral, bacterial, tuberculous, fungal) Brain abscess Head trauma
Adverse drug effects	Clofibrate Chlorpropamide Cyclophosphamide Phenothiazines Carbamazepine
Tumors (ectopic production of antidiuretic hormone)	Lymphoma Sarcoma Carcinoma of duodenum or pancreas

REFERENCES

Cunnah D, Besser M: Management of prolactinomas. Clin Endocrinol 1991; 34:231.

Klibanski A, Zervas NT: Diagnosis and management of hormone-secreting pituitary adenomas. N Engl J Med 1991; 324:822.

Melmed S, Jackson I, Kleinberg D, et al: Current treatment guidelines for acromegaly. J Clin Endocrinol Met 1998; 83:2646.

Molitch ME: Gonadotroph cell pituitary adenomas. N Engl J Med 1991; 324:626.

Thorner MO, Vance ML, Horvath E, et al: The anterior pituitary. *In* Wilson J, Foster DW (eds): Williams Textbook of Endocrinology, 8th ed. Philadelphia: WB Saunders, 1992.

Vance ML: Hypopituitarism. N Engl J Med 1994; 330:1651.

65

THE THYROID GLAND

Vivien Herman-Bonert • Theodore C. Friedman

The thyroid gland secretes thyroxine (T_4) and triiodothyronine (T_3), both of which modulate energy utilization and heat production and facilitate growth. The gland consists of two lateral lobes joined by an isthmus. The weight of the adult gland is 10 to 20 g. Microscopically, the thyroid is composed of several follicles containing colloid surrounded by a single layer of thyroid epithelium. The follicular cells synthesize thyroglobulin, which is then stored as colloid. Biosynthesis of T_4 and T_3 occurs by iodination of tyrosine molecules in thyroglobulin.

Thyroid Hormone Physiology

THYROID HORMONE SYNTHESIS

Dietary iodine is essential for synthesis of thyroid hormones. Iodine after conversion to iodide in the stomach is rapidly absorbed from the gastrointestinal tract and distributed in the extracellular fluids. After active transport from the blood stream across the follicular cell basement membrane, iodide is enzymatically oxidized by thyroid peroxidase, which also mediates the iodination of the tyrosine residues in thyroglobulin to form monoiodotyrosine and diiodotyrosine. The iodotyrosine molecules couple to form thyroxine (3,5,3',5'-tetraiodothyronine) or triiodothyronine (3,5,3'-triiodothyronine). Once iodinated, thyroglobulin containing newly formed T_4 and T_3 is stored in the follicles. Secretion of free T_4 and T_3 into the circulation occurs after proteolytic digestion of thyroglobulin, which is stimulated by thyroid-stimulating hormone (TSH). Deiodination of monoiodotyrosine and diiodotyrosine by iodotyrosine deiodinase releases iodine, which then reenters the thyroid iodine pool.

THYROID HORMONE TRANSPORT

T_4 and T_3 are tightly bound to serum carrier proteins: thyroxine-binding globulin (TBG), thyroxine-binding prealbumin, and albumin. The unbound or free fractions are the biologically active fractions and represent only 0.04% of the total T_4 and 0.4% of the total T_3.

PERIPHERAL METABOLISM OF THYROID HORMONES

The normal thyroid gland secretes T_4, T_3, and reverse T_3, a biologically inactive form of T_3. Most of the circulating T_3 is derived from 5'-deiodination of circulating T_4 in the peripheral tissues. Deiodination of T_4 can occur at the outer ring (5'-deiodination), producing T_3 (3,5,3'-triiodothyronine), or at the inner ring, producing reverse T_3 (3,3,5'-triiodothyronine). T_3 is three to eight times more potent than T_4.

CONTROL OF THYROID FUNCTION

Hypothalamic thyrotropin-releasing hormone (TRH) is transported through the hypothalamic-hypophysial portal system to the thyrotrophs of the anterior pituitary gland, stimulating synthesis and release of TSH (Fig. 65–1). TSH, in turn, increases thyroidal iodide uptake and iodination of thyroglobulin, releases T_3 and T_4 from the thyroid gland by increasing hydrolysis of thyroglobulin, and stimulates thyroid cell growth. Hypersecretion of TSH results in thyroid enlargement (goiter). Circulating levels of T_4 and T_3 exert negative feedback inhibition of TRH and TSH release.

PHYSIOLOGIC EFFECTS OF THYROID HORMONES

Thyroid hormones increase basal metabolic rate by increasing oxygen consumption and heat production in several body tissues. Thyroid hormones also have specific effects on several organ systems (Table 65–1). These effects are exaggerated in hyperthyroidism and lacking in hypothyroidism, accounting for the well-recognized signs and symptoms of these two disorders.

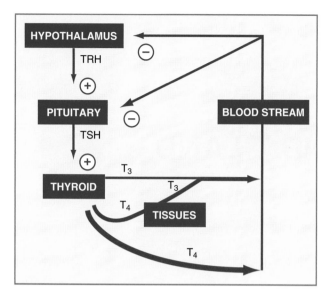

FIGURE 65–1 Hypothalamic-pituitary-thyroid axis. T_3 = Triiodothyronine; T_4 = thyroxine; TRH = thyrotropin-releasing hormone; TSH = thyroid-stimulating hormone.

Thyroid Evaluation

Thyroid gland function and structure can be evaluated by (1) serum thyroid hormone levels, (2) imaging of thyroid gland size and architecture, (3) measurement of thyroid autoantibodies, and (4) thyroid gland biopsy (by fine-needle aspiration [FNA]).

TESTS OF SERUM THYROID HORMONE LEVELS

Total serum T_4 and T_3 measure the total amount of hormone bound to thyroid-binding proteins by radioimmunoassay. Total T_4 and total T_3 levels are elevated in hyperthyroidism and low in hypothyroidism. Increase in TBG (as with pregnancy or estrogen therapy) increases the total T_4 and T_3 measured in the absence of hyperthyroidism. Similarly, T_4 and T_3 are low despite euthyroidism in conditions associated with low thyroid-binding proteins (e.g., cirrhosis or nephrotic syndrome). Thus, further tests to assess the free hormone level that reflects biologic activity must be performed. Free T_4 level can be estimated by calculating the free T_4 index or can be measured directly by dialysis.

The free thyroxine index is an indirect method of assessing free T_4. It is derived by multiplying the total T_4 by the T_3 resin uptake, which is inversely proportional to the available T_4 binding sites on TBG. Free T_4 can be measured directly by dialysis or ultrafiltration. This is more accurate and is preferred to the free thyroxine index.

Serum TSH is measured by a third-generation immunometric assay, which employs at least two different monoclonal antibodies against different regions of the TSH molecule, resulting in accurate discrimination between normal TSH levels and levels below the normal range. Thus, the TSH assay can establish the diagnoses of clinical hyperthyroidism (elevated free T_4 and suppressed TSH) and subclinical hyperthyroidism (normal free T_4 and suppressed TSH). In primary (thyroidal) hypothyroidism, serum TSH is supranormal because of diminished feedback inhibition. In secondary (pituitary) or tertiary (hypothalamic) hypothyroidism, the TSH is usually low but may be normal.

Serum thyroglobulin measurements are useful in the follow-up of patients with papillary or follicular carcinoma. After thyroidectomy and iodine 131 (^{131}I) ablation therapy, thyroglobulin levels should be less than 10 μg/L. Levels in excess of this value indicate the presence of metastatic disease.

Calcitonin measurements are invaluable in the diagnosis of medullary carcinoma of the thyroid and for following the effects of therapy for this entity.

THYROID IMAGING

Iodine 123 (^{123}I) or technetium 99m (^{99m}Tc) pertechnetate are concentrated in the gland and can be scanned with a gamma camera, yielding information about the size and shape of the gland and the location of the functional activity in the gland (thyroid scan). Functioning thyroid nodules are called "warm" or "hot" nodules; "cold" nodules are nonfunctioning. Malignancy is usually

TABLE 65–1 Physiologic Effects of Thyroid Hormone

Cardiovascular Effects
Increased heart rate and cardiac output

Gastrointestinal Effects
Increased gut motility

Skeletal Effects
Increased bone turnover and resorption

Pulmonary Effects
Maintenance of normal hypoxic and hypercapnic drive in the respiratory center

Neuromuscular Effects
Increased muscle protein turnover and increased speed of muscle contraction and relaxation

Lipids and Carbohydrate Metabolism Effects
Increased hepatic gluconeogenesis and glycogenolysis as well as intestinal glucose absorption
Increased cholesterol synthesis and degradation
Increased lipolysis

Sympathetic Nervous System Effects
Increased numbers of β-adrenergic receptors in the heart, skeletal muscle, lymphocytes, and adipose cells
Decreased cardiac α-adrenergic receptors
Increased catecholamine sensitivity

Hematopoietic Effects
Increased red blood cell 2,3-diphosphoglycerate, facilitating oxygen dissociation from hemoglobin with increased oxygen available to tissues

TABLE 65-2 Prevalence of Symptoms and Signs in Patients with Thyrotoxicosis

Symptom	Prevalence (%)
Nervousness	99
Increased sweating	91
Hypersensitivity to heat	89
Palpitation	89
Fatigue	88
Weight loss	85
Tachycardia	82
Dyspnea	75
Weakness	70
Increased appetite	65
Eye complaints	54
Swelling of legs	35
Diarrhea	23
Anorexia	9
Tachycardia	100
Goiter	100
Skin changes	97
Tremor	97
Thyroid	77
Eye signs	71
Atrial fibrillation	10
Splenomegaly	10
Gynecomastia	10
Liver palms	8

From Williams RH: Thiouracil treatment of thyrotoxicosis. J Clin Endocrinol Metab 1946; 6:1–22.

associated with a cold nodule; 16% of surgically removed cold nodules are malignant.

Thyroid ultrasound evaluation is useful in the differentiation of solid from cystic nodules. It can also guide the operator during FNA of a nodule that is difficult to palpate.

THYROID ANTIBODIES

Autoantibodies to several different antigenic components in the thyroid gland, including thyroglobulin (TgAb), thyroid peroxidase (TPO Ab, formerly called antimicrosomal antibodies), and the TSH receptor, can be measured in the serum. A strongly positive test for TgAb or TPO Ab indicates autoimmune thyroid disease. Elevated thyroid receptor-stimulating antibody occurs in Graves' disease (see later discussion).

THYROID BIOPSY

Fine-needle aspiration of a nodule to obtain cells for cytology is the best way to differentiate benign from malignant disease. FNA requires adequate tissue samples and interpretation by an experienced cytologist.

Hyperthyroidism

Thyrotoxicosis is the clinical syndrome that results from elevated circulating thyroid hormones. Clinical manifestations of thyrotoxicosis are due to the direct physiologic effects of the thyroid hormones, as well as to the increased sensitivity to catecholamines. Tachycardia, tremor, stare, sweating, and lid lag are due to catecholamine hypersensitivity.

SIGNS AND SYMPTOMS

Table 65–2 lists the signs and symptoms of hyperthyroidism with their frequency of occurrence. Thyrotoxic crisis or "thyroid storm" is a life-threatening complication of hyperthyroidism that can be precipitated by surgery, radioactive iodine therapy, or severe stress (e.g., uncontrolled diabetes mellitus, myocardial infarction, acute infection). Patients develop fever, flushing, sweating, marked tachycardia, atrial fibrillation, and cardiac failure. Marked agitation, restlessness, delirium, and coma occur frequently. Gastrointestinal manifestations may include nausea, vomiting, and diarrhea. Hyperpyrexia out of proportion to other clinical findings is the hallmark of thyroid storm.

DIFFERENTIAL DIAGNOSIS

Thyrotoxicosis usually reflects hyperactivity of the thyroid gland due to Graves' disease, toxic adenoma, multinodular goiter, or thyroiditis. However, it may be due to excessive ingestion of thyroid hormone or, rarely, thyroid hormone production from an ectopic site as seen in struma ovarii (Table 65–3 and Fig. 65–2).

Graves' Disease

Graves' disease, the most common cause of thyrotoxicosis, is an autoimmune disease, more common in women, with a peak age incidence of 20 to 40 years. One or more of the following features are present: (1) goiter; (2) thyrotoxicosis; (3) eye disease ranging from tearing to proptosis, extraocular muscle paralysis, and loss of sight as a result of optic nerve involvement; and

TABLE 65-3 Causes of Thyrotoxicosis

Common Causes
Graves' disease
Toxic adenoma (solitary)
Toxic multinodular goiter

Less Common Causes
Subacute thyroiditis (de Quervain's or granulomatous)
Hashimoto's thyroiditis with transient hyperthyroid phase
Thyrotoxicosis factitia
Postpartum (probably variant of silent thyroiditis)

Rare Causes
Struma ovarii
Metastatic thyroid carcinoma
Hydatidiform mole
Thyroid-stimulating hormone–secreting pituitary tumor
Pituitary resistance to triiodothyronine and thyroxine

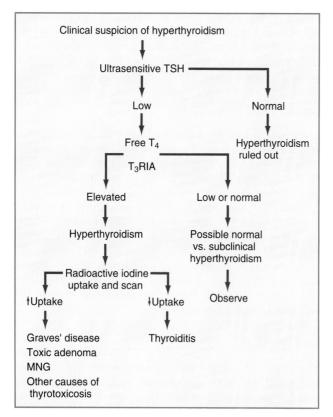

FIGURE 65-2 Algorithm for differential diagnosis of hyperthyroidism. MNG = multinodular goiter; T_3RIA = triiodothyronine radioimmunoassay; T_4 = thyroxine; TSH = thyroid-stimulating hormone.

(4) thyroid dermopathy, usually presenting as marked skin thickening without pitting in a pretibial distribution (pretibial myxedema).

PATHOGENESIS

Thyrotoxicosis in Graves' disease is due to overproduction of an antibody that binds to the TSH receptor. These thyroid-stimulating immunoglobulins increase thyroid cell growth and thyroid hormone secretion. Ophthalmopathy is due to inflammatory infiltration of the extraocular eye muscles by lymphocytes with mucopolysaccharide deposition. The inflammatory reaction that contributes to the eye signs in Graves' disease may be caused by lymphocytes sensitized to antigens common to the orbital muscles and thyroid.

CLINICAL FEATURES

The common manifestations of thyrotoxicosis (see Table 65-1) are characteristic features of younger patients with Graves' disease. In addition, patients may present with a diffuse goiter or the eye signs characteristic of Graves' disease. Older patients often do not manifest the florid clinical features of thyrotoxicosis, and the condition termed *apathetic hyperthyroidism* presents as flat affect, emotional lability, weight loss, muscle weakness,

or congestive heart failure and atrial fibrillation resistant to standard therapy.

Eye signs of Graves' disease may be a nonspecific manifestation of hyperthyroidism from any cause, ranging from lid lag due to spasm of the upper lids to the Graves' disease–specific inflammatory infiltrate of the orbital tissues leading to periorbital edema, conjunctival congestion and swelling, proptosis, extraocular muscle weakness, and/or optic nerve damage with visual impairment.

Pretibial myxedema (thyroid dermopathy) occurs in 2% to 3% of patients with Graves' disease and presents as thickening of the skin over the lower tibia without pitting. Onycholysis, characterized by separation of the fingernails from their beds, often occurs in Graves' disease.

LABORATORY FINDINGS

Elevated free T_4 and a suppressed TSH confirm the clinical diagnosis of thyrotoxicosis. Thyroid-stimulating immunoglobulin (TSH receptor antibody) is usually elevated and may be useful in patients with eye signs who do not have other characteristic clinical features. Increased uptake of ^{123}I differentiates Graves' disease from early subacute or Hashimoto's thyroiditis, in which uptake is low in the presence of hyperthyroidism. Magnetic resonance imaging or ultrasonography of the orbit usually shows orbital muscle enlargement, whether or not there are clinical signs of ophthalmopathy.

TREATMENT

Three treatment modalities are employed to control the hyperthyroidism of Graves' disease.

Antithyroid Drugs. The thiocarbamide drugs propylthiouracil, methimazole, and carbimazole block thyroid hormone synthesis by inhibiting thyroid peroxidase. Propylthiouracil also partially inhibits peripheral conversion of T_4 to T_3. Medical therapy must be administered for a prolonged period (12 to 18 months), until the disease undergoes spontaneous remission. On cessation of medication, only a small percentage of patients (20% to 30%) remain in remission, and the patients who experience relapse must then undergo definitive surgery or radioactive iodine treatment. Side effects of the thiocarbamides include pruritus and rash (about 5% of patients), cholestatic jaundice, acute arthralgias, or, rarely, agranulocytosis (0.5% of patients). Patients must be instructed to discontinue the medication and consult a physician if they develop fever or sore throat, because these may indicate agranulocytosis. At the onset of treatment, during the acute phase of thyrotoxicosis, β-adrenergic blocking drugs help alleviate tachycardia, hypertension, and atrial fibrillation. As the thyroid hormone levels return to normal, treatment with β blockers is tapered.

Radioactive Iodine. In terms of cost, efficacy, ease, and short-term side effects, radioactive iodine has benefits that exceed both surgery and antithyroid drugs. ^{131}I is the treatment of choice in adults with Graves' disease.

Patients with severe thyrotoxicosis, very large glands, or underlying heart disease should be rendered euthyroid with antithyroid medication before receiving radioactive iodine, since ^{131}I treatment can cause release into the circulation of preformed thyroid hormone from the thyroid gland; this can precipitate cardiac arrhythmias and exacerbate symptoms of thyrotoxicosis. After administration of radioactive iodine, the thyroid gland shrinks and patients become euthyroid over a period of 6 weeks to 3 months. Ten to 20 percent of patients become hypothyroid within the first year of treatment and thereafter at a rate of 3% to 5% per year. Fifty to 80 percent of patients ultimately become hypothyroid after radioactive iodine treatment. Serum TSH levels should be monitored and replacement with levothyroxine instituted if the TSH rises. Hypothyroidism may also develop after surgery or antithyroid medication, mandating lifelong follow-up in all patients with Graves' disease.

Surgery. Subtotal thyroidectomy is the treatment of choice for patients with very large glands and obstructive symptoms or multinodular glands or for patients desiring pregnancy within the next year. It is essential that the surgeon be experienced in thyroid surgery. Preoperatively, patients receive 6 weeks of treatment with antithyroid drugs so that they will be euthyroid at the time of surgery. Two weeks before surgery, oral saturated solution of potassium iodide is administered daily to decrease the vascularity of the gland. Permanent hypoparathyroidism and recurrent laryngeal nerve palsy occur in less than 2% of patients. Ten percent of patients develop recurrent thyrotoxicosis, which should be treated with radioactive iodine.

Toxic Adenoma

Solitary toxic nodules, which usually are benign, occur more frequently in older patients. Clinical manifestations are those of thyrotoxicosis. Physical examination shows a distinct solitary nodule. Laboratory investigation shows suppressed TSH and markedly elevated T_3 levels, often with only moderately elevated T_4. Thyroid scan shows a "hot nodule" of the affected lobe with complete suppression of the unaffected lobe. Solitary toxic nodules are treated with radioactive iodine. However, unilateral lobectomy, after the administration of antithyroid drugs to render the patient euthyroid, may be required for large nodules.

Toxic Multinodular Goiter

Toxic multinodular goiter occurs in older patients with long-standing multinodular goiter. Thus, the presenting clinical features are frequently tachycardia, heart failure, and arrhythmias.

Physical examination shows a multinodular goiter. The diagnosis is confirmed by laboratory features of suppressed TSH, markedly elevated T_3, moderately elevated T_4, and a thyroid scan with multiple functioning nodules. The treatment of choice is subtotal thyroidectomy. However, because these patients are frequently elderly with underlying heart disease, surgery is sometimes contraindicated. The toxic nodules are then treated with ^{131}I, but the multinodular goiter remains, with the possibility that other nodules will become toxic and require future ^{131}I treatment.

Thyroiditis

Thyroiditis may be classified as acute, subacute, or chronic. Although thyroiditis may eventually result in clinical hypothyroidism, the initial presentation is often that of hyperthyroidism due to acute release of T_4 and T_3. Hyperthyroidism due to thyroiditis can be readily differentiated from other causes of hyperthyroidism by suppressed uptake of the radioactive iodine on thyroid scan.

Acute suppurative thyroiditis, a rare complication of septicemia, presents as high fever, redness of the overlying skin, and thyroid gland tenderness; it may be confused with subacute thyroiditis. If blood cultures are negative, needle aspiration should identify the organism. Intensive antibiotic treatment and, occasionally, incision and drainage are required.

SUBACUTE THYROIDITIS

Subacute thyroiditis (de Quervain's thyroiditis or granulomatous thyroiditis) is an acute inflammatory disorder of the thyroid gland, probably secondary to viral infection, which resolves completely in 90% of cases. Subacute thyroiditis presents as fever and anterior neck pain. The patient may have symptoms and signs of hyperthyroidism. The classic feature on physical examination is an exquisitely tender thyroid gland. Laboratory findings vary with the course of the disease. Initially, the patient may be symptomatically thyrotoxic with elevated serum T_4, depressed serum TSH, and very low radioactive iodine uptake on scan. Subsequently, the thyroid status will fluctuate through euthyroid and hypothyroid phases and may return to euthyroidism. Increase in radioactive iodine uptake on the scan reflects recovery of the gland. Treatment usually includes nonsteroidal anti-inflammatory drugs, but a short course of prednisone may be required if pain and fever are severe. During the hypothyroid phase, replacement therapy with levothyroxine may be indicated.

Postpartum thyroiditis resembles subacute thyroiditis in its clinical course. It usually presents within the first 6 months after delivery and goes through the triphasic course of hyperthyroidism, hypothyroidism, and then euthyroidism, or it may present with only hypothyroidism. Some patients have an underlying chronic thyroiditis.

CHRONIC THYROIDITIS

Chronic thyroiditis (Hashimoto's thyroiditis, lymphocytic thyroiditis) from destruction of normal thyroidal architecture by lymphocytic infiltration results in hypothyroidism and goiter. Riedel's struma is probably a variant of Hashimoto's thyroiditis, characterized by extensive thyroid fibrosis resulting in a rock-hard thyroid mass. Hashimoto's thyroiditis is more common in women and is probably the most common cause of goiter and hypothyroidism in the United States. Occasionally, patients with Hashimoto's thyroiditis may have transient hyperthyroidism with low radioactive iodine uptake, owing to release of T_4 and T_3 into the circulation. This can be differentiated from subacute thyroiditis, in that the gland is nontender to palpation and antithyroid antibodies are present in high titer. Early in the disease, TgAb is markedly elevated, but it may disappear later. TPO Ab also is present early and generally remains present for years. Radioactive iodine uptake may be high, normal, or low. Serum T_3 and T_4 levels are either normal or low; when low, the TSH is elevated. FNA of the thyroid shows lymphocytes and Hürthle cells (enlarged basophilic follicular cells). Hypothyroidism and marked glandular enlargement (goiter) are indications for levothyroxine therapy. Adequate doses of levothyroxine are administered to suppress TSH levels and shrink the goiter.

Thyrotoxicosis Factitia

Thyrotoxicosis factitia presents as typical features of thyrotoxicosis from ingestion of excessive amounts of thyroxine, often in an attempt to lose weight. Serum T_3 and T_4 levels are elevated, and TSH is suppressed, as is the serum thyroglobulin concentration. Radioactive iodine uptake is absent. Patients may require psychotherapy.

Rare Causes of Thyrotoxicosis

Struma ovarii occurs when an ovarian teratoma contains thyroid tissue, which secretes thyroid hormone. Diagnosis is confirmed by demonstrating uptake of radioiodine in the pelvis on body scan.

Hydatidiform mole is due to proliferation and swelling of the trophoblast during pregnancy, with excess production of chorionic gonadotropin, which has intrinsic TSH-like activity. The hyperthyroidism remits with surgical and medical treatment of the molar pregnancy.

Hypothyroidism

Hypothyroidism is a clinical syndrome due to deficiency of thyroid hormones. In infants and children, hypothyroidism causes retardation of growth and development and may result in permanent motor and mental retardation. Congenital causes of hypothyroidism include agenesis (complete absence of thyroid tissue), dysgenesis (ectopic or lingual thyroid gland), hypoplastic thyroid,

thyroid dyshormogenesis, and central hypothyroidism. Adult-onset hypothyroidism results in a slowing of metabolic processes and is reversible with treatment. Hypothyroidism (Table 65–4) is usually primary (thyroid failure), but it may be secondary (hypothalamic or pituitary deficiency) or due to resistance at the thyroid hormone receptor. In adults, autoimmune thyroiditis (Hashimoto's thyroiditis) is the most common cause of hypothyroidism. This may be isolated or part of the polyglandular failure syndrome type II (Schmidt's syndrome), which also includes insulin-dependent diabetes mellitus, pernicious anemia, vitiligo, gonadal failure, hypophysitis, celiac disease, myasthenia gravis, and primary biliary cirrhosis. Iatrogenic causes of hypothyroidism include ^{131}I therapy, thyroidectomy, and treatment with lithium or amiodarone. Iodine deficiency or excess can also cause hypothyroidism.

CLINICAL MANIFESTATIONS

The clinical presentation of hypothyroidism (Table 65–5) depends on the age of onset and severity of thyroid deficiency. Infants with congenital hypothyroidism (also called cretinism) may present with feeding problems, hypotonia, inactivity, an open posterior fontanelle, and/or edematous face and hands. Mental retarda-

TABLE 65–4 Causes of Hypothyroidism

Primary Hypothyroidism
Autoimmune
  Hashimoto's thyroiditis
  Part of polyglandular failure syndrome, type II
Iatrogenic
  ^{131}I therapy
  Thyroidectomy
Drug-induced
  Iodine deficiency
  Iodine excess
  Lithium
  Amiodarone
  Antithyroid drugs
Congenital
  Thyroid agenesis
  Thyroid dysgenesis
  Hypoplastic thyroid
  Biosynthetic defect

Secondary Hypothyroidism
Hypothalamic dysfunction
  Neoplasms
  Tuberculosis
  Sarcoidosis
  Langerhans' cell histiocytosis
  Hemochromatosis
  Radiation treatment
Pituitary dysfunction
  Neoplasms
  Pituitary surgery
  Postpartum pituitary necrosis
  Idiopathic hypopituitarism
  Glucocorticoid excess (Cushing's syndrome)
  Radiation treatment

TABLE 65–5   Clinical Features of Hypothyroidism

Children

Learning disabilities
  Mental retardation
Short stature
  Delayed bone age
  Delayed puberty

Adults

Fatigue
Cold intolerance
Weakness
Lethargy
Weight gain
Constipation
Myalgias
Arthralgias
Menstrual irregularities
Hair loss
Dry, coarse, cold skin
Coarse, thin hair
Hoarse voice
Brittle nails
Periorbital, peripheral edema
Delayed reflexes
Slow reaction time
Orange skin hue
Bradycardia
Pleural, pericardial effusions

tion, short stature, and delayed puberty occur if treatment is delayed.

Hypothyroidism in adults usually develops insidiously. Patients often have fatigue, lethargy, and gradual weight gain for years before the diagnosis is established. A delayed relaxation phase of deep tendon reflexes ("hung-up" reflexes) is a valuable clinical sign characteristic of severe hypothyroidism. Subcutaneous infiltration by mucopolysaccharides, which bind water, causes the edema (termed *myxedema*) and is responsible for the thickened features and puffy appearance of patients with severe hypothyroidism.

Severe untreated hypothyroidism can result in myxedema coma, characterized by hypothermia, extreme weakness, stupor, hypoventilation, hypoglycemia, and hyponatremia and is often precipitated by cold exposure, infection, or psychoactive drugs.

LABORATORY TESTS

Laboratory abnormalities in patients with primary hypothyroidism include elevated serum TSH and low total and free T_4. In mild hypothyroidism, a patient will have an elevated serum TSH level with a low normal serum T_4 level.

Secondary hypothyroidism is characterized by a low or low-normal morning serum TSH in the setting of hypothalamic or pituitary dysfunction. Often, the serum total and free T_4 levels are at the lower limit of normal.

Hypothyroidism is often associated with hypercholes-terolemia and elevated creatine phosphokinase MB fraction (the fraction representative of cardiac muscle). Anemia is usually normocytic, normochromic but may be macrocytic (vitamin B_{12} deficiency due to associated pernicious anemia) or microcytic (due to nutritional deficiencies or menstrual blood loss in women).

DIFFERENTIAL DIAGNOSIS

Because the initial manifestations of hypothyroidism are subtle, the early diagnosis of hypothyroidism demands a high index of suspicion in patients presenting with one or more of the signs or symptoms listed in Table 65–5. Early symptoms that are often overlooked include menstrual irregularities (usually menorrhagia), arthralgias, and myalgias.

Laboratory diagnosis may be complicated by the finding of a low total T_4 in euthyroid states associated with low TBG, such as nephrotic syndrome, cirrhosis, or TBG deficiency; in these situations TSH and free T_4 levels are normal. A low total T_4 may also be found in the "euthyroid sick syndrome," a condition occurring in acutely ill patients. In such patients, total and, occasionally, free T_4 levels are low and the serum TSH level is usually normal but may be mildly elevated. These patients should not be treated with levothyroxine replacement and may be differentiated from patients with primary hypothyroidism by absence of a goiter, negative antithyroid antibodies, and elevated serum reverse T_3 levels, as well as by clinical presentation.

TREATMENT

Hypothyroidism should be treated with synthetic levothyroxine. Although T_3 is the more bioactive thyroid hormone, peripheral tissues convert T_4 to T_3 to maintain physiologic levels of the latter. Thus, administration of levothyroxine results in bioavailable T_3 and T_4. Triiodothyronine (liothyronine; T_3) should be avoided because of its rapid absorption and disappearance from the blood stream, resulting in fluctuating blood levels. Levothyroxine has a half-life of 8 days, so it needs to be given only once a day. The average replacement dose for adults is 100 to 150 μg/day. In healthy adults, 100 μg/day is an appropriate starting dose. In elderly patients or those with cardiac disease, levothyroxine should be increased gradually, starting at 25 μg daily, increasing this dose by 25 μg every 2 weeks. The therapeutic response to levothyroxine therapy should be monitored clinically and with serum TSH levels, which should be measured 5 weeks or more after a dose adjustment. Because overtreatment may cause osteopenia, normal serum TSH levels should be sought. Patients with secondary hypothyroidism should be treated with levothyroxine until their free T_4 is in the mid-normal range. Appropriate treatment of these patients will result in suppressed serum TSH levels.

In patients with myxedema coma, 300 to 400 μg of levothyroxine is administered intravenously as a loading dose followed by 50 μg daily as well as hydrocortisone (100 mg intravenously three times a day) and intravenous fluids. The underlying precipitating event should be corrected. Respiratory assistance and treatment of hypothermia with warming blankets may be required. Although myxedema coma carries a high mortality despite appropriate treatment, many patients improve in 1 to 3 days.

Goiter

Enlargement of the thyroid gland is called goiter. Patients with goiter may be euthyroid (simple goiter), hyperthyroid (toxic nodular goiter or Graves' disease), or hypothyroid (nontoxic goiter or Hashimoto's thyroiditis). Thyroid enlargement (often focal) also may be due to a thyroid adenoma or carcinoma. In nontoxic goiter, inadequate thyroid hormone synthesis leads to TSH stimulation with resultant enlargement of the thyroid gland. Iodine deficiency (endemic goiter) was once the most common cause of nontoxic goiter; with the use of iodized salt, it is now almost nonexistent in North America.

Dietary goitrogens can cause goiter, and iodine is the most common goitrogen. Other goitrogens include lithium and vegetable products such as thioglucosides found in cabbage. Thyroid hormone biosynthetic defects can cause goiter associated with hypothyroidism or, with adequate compensation, euthyroidism.

A careful thyroid examination coupled with thyroid hormone tests can delineate the cause of the goiter. A smooth symmetric gland, often with a bruit, and hyperthyroidism is suggestive of Graves' disease. A nodular thyroid gland with hypothyroidism and positive antithyroid antibodies is consistent with Hashimoto's thyroiditis. A diffuse, smooth goiter with hypothyroidism and negative antithyroid antibodies may be indicative of iodine deficiency or a biosynthetic defect. Goiters may become very large, extend substernally, and cause dysphagia, respiratory distress, or hoarseness. An ultrasound evaluation or radioiodine scan delineates the thyroid gland, and a thyroid uptake and scan can determine the functional activity of the goiter.

Goiters, with the exception of those due to neoplasms or autonomous nodules, are treated with thyroid hormone at a dose that suppresses TSH (100 to 200 μg/day). This treatment, which will correct the hypothyroidism and may result in slow regression of the goiter, should be continued indefinitely. Long-standing goiters may not regress but usually will not grow on levothyroxine therapy. Surgery is indicated for nontoxic goiter only if obstructive symptoms develop or substantial substernal extension is present.

Solitary Thyroid Nodules

Thyroid nodules are common. They can be detected clinically in about 4% of the population and are found in about 50% of the population at autopsy. Benign thyroid nodules are usually follicular adenomas, colloid nodules, benign cysts, or nodular thyroiditis. Patients with Hashimoto's thyroiditis may have one prominent nodule on clinical examination, but thyroid ultrasound evaluation may reveal multiple nodules. Although the majority of nodules are benign, a small percentage are malignant. In addition, most thyroid cancers are of low-grade malignancy. History, physical examination, and laboratory tests can be helpful in differentiating benign from malignant lesions (Table 65–6). For example, lymph node involvement or hoarseness is strongly suggestive of a malignant tumor.

The major etiologic factor for thyroid cancer is childhood or adolescent exposure to head and neck radiation. Previously, radiation was used to treat an enlarged thymus, tonsilar disease, hemangioma, or acne. Recently, exposure to radiation from nuclear plants (e.g., Chernobyl, Ukraine) has contributed to an increased incidence of thyroid cancer. The incidence of thyroid cancer is linearly related to the radiation dose up to 1500 rads. TSH is possibly a co-carcinogen; thus, patients exposed to high-risk radiation may benefit from TSH suppression by thyroid hormone. Patients with a history of irradiation should have their thyroid carefully palpated every 2 years. In the absence of palpable disease, imaging procedures are not warranted.

The thyroid status of a patient with a thyroid nodule may dictate further evaluation. A hyperthyroid patient is most likely to have a toxic nodule or thyroiditis, whereas a hypothyroid patient probably has a prominent nodule in a gland with Hashimoto's thyroiditis. These patients are unlikely to have malignant lesions. Euthyroid patients with a solitary nodule should undergo an FNA biopsy. This is a safe procedure that has reduced the need for surgical excision. An expert cytologist can identify most benign lesions (75% of all biopsies). In addition, malignant lesions (5% of biopsies), such as papil-

TABLE 65–6 High-Risk Factors for Malignancy in a Thyroid Nodule

History
Head/neck irradiation
Exposure to nuclear radiation
Rapid growth
Recent onset
Young age
Male sex
Familial incidence (medullary)

Physical Examination
Hard consistency of nodule
Fixation of nodule
Lymphadenopathy
Vocal cord paralysis
Distant metastasis

Laboratory/Imaging
Elevated serum calcitonin
"Cold" nodule on iodine-123 scan
Solid lesion on ultrasonography

Levothyroxine Therapy
No regression

lary, anaplastic, and medullary carcinoma, can be specifically identified. Follicular neoplasms, however, cannot be diagnosed as benign or malignant by FNA; this cytology report, along with "suspicious" cytology, requires surgical excision.

In the past, thyroid scans were used to evaluate single thyroid nodules. "Hot" thyroid nodules are almost always benign. Most cancers are "cold"; but because most benign lesions are also "cold," these patients still require FNA. Thus, thyroid scans have largely been supplanted by aspiration for evaluation of thyroid nodules.

Benign thyroid nodules may be treated with levothyroxine suppression therapy with a follow-up thyroid examination in 6 months. A significant decrease in the size of the nodule occurs in 10% to 20% of the cases and may be monitored by ultrasound. Most benign lesions and some cancers remain unchanged in size. An increase in size of the nodule while on suppression therapy warrants a reevaluation.

Thyroid Carcinoma

The most common type of thyroid carcinoma is papillary carcinoma (60%). Follicular carcinoma (20%), anaplastic carcinoma (14%), medullary carcinoma (5%), and lymphoma (1%) occur less frequently. Papillary carcinoma is associated with local invasion and lymph node spread. Poor prognosis is associated with thyroid capsule invasion, size greater than 2.5 cm, age at onset older than 45 years, tall-cell variant, and lymph node involvement. Follicular carcinoma is slightly more aggressive than papillary carcinoma and can spread by local invasion of lymph nodes or hematogenously to bone, brain, or lung. Patients may present with metastases before diagnosis of the primary thyroid lesion. Anaplastic carcinoma tends to occur in older individuals (>50 years), is very aggressive, and rapidly causes pain, dysphagia, and hoarseness. Death usually occurs in the first year.

Medullary thyroid carcinoma is derived from calcitonin-producing parafollicular cells and is more malignant than papillary or follicular carcinoma. It is multifocal and spreads both locally and distally. It may be either sporadic or familial. When familial, it is inherited in an autosomal dominant pattern and is part of multiple endocrine neoplasia type 2A (medullary carcinoma of the thyroid, pheochromocytoma, and hyperparathyroidism) or multiple endocrine neoplasia type 2B (medullary carcinoma of the thyroid, mucosal neuromas, intestinal ganglioneuromas, marfanoid habitus, and pheochromocytoma). Elevated basal serum calcitonin levels confirm the diagnosis. Measurement of serum calcitonin after pentagastrin stimulation should be performed in all first-degree relatives of patients with medullary carcinoma of the thyroid. Measurements of the *RET* proto-oncogene mutations in family members of affected individuals have allowed preclinical diagnosis of this genetic disorder.

TREATMENT

Lobectomy can be performed for papillary and follicular carcinomas less than 1.5 cm. These patients require life-long levothyroxine suppressive therapy and yearly thyroid examinations. Larger papillary or follicular tumors require near-total thyroidectomy, with modified neck dissection if there is evidence of lymph node metastases. Postoperatively, triiodothyronine is administered for 3 months. The medication is stopped for 2 weeks, and the patient is scanned with 3 mCi of [131]I. If uptake occurs, the patient is treated with ^{131}I until no further uptake is observed. Sufficient levothyroxine is then administered to suppress serum TSH to undetectable levels. Frequent neck examinations for masses should be accompanied by measurement of serum thyroglobulin levels. A rise in serum thyroglobulin levels suggests recurrence of thyroid cancer. Solitary metastatic lesions that take up ^{131}I can be treated with radioactive iodine, whereas those that do not take up ^{131}I can be treated with local x-ray therapy. Medullary carcinoma of the thyroid requires total thyroidectomy with removal of the central lymph nodes in the neck. Completeness of the procedure and monitoring for recurrence is determined by measurement of serum calcitonin.

Anaplastic carcinoma is treated with isthmusectomy to confirm the diagnosis and to prevent tracheal compression, followed by palliative x-ray treatment. Thyroid lymphomas are also treated with x-ray therapy.

The prognosis for well-differentiated thyroid carcinomas is good. Age at the time of diagnosis and sex are the most important prognostic factors. Men older than 40 and women older than 50 have a higher recurrence and death rate than do younger patients. The 5-year survival rate for invasive medullary carcinoma is 50%, whereas the mean survival for anaplastic carcinoma is 6 months.

REFERENCES

Dabon-Almirante CL, Surks MI: Clinical and laboratory diagnosis of thyrotoxicosis. Endocrinol Metab Clin North Am 1998; 27:25.

Dillman WH: The thyroid. *In* Goldman L, Bennett JC (eds): Cecil Textbook of Medicine, 21st ed. Philadelphia: WB Saunders, 2000, pp 1231–1250.

Hermus AR, Huysmans DA: Treatment of benign nodular thyroid disease. N Engl J Med 1998; 338:1438.

Weetman AP, McGregor AM: Autoimmune thyroid disease: Further developments in our understanding. Endocr Rev 1994; 15:788.

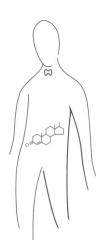

66

THE ADRENAL GLAND

Theodore C. Friedman

Physiology

The adrenal glands lie at the superior pole of each kidney and are composed of two distinct regions: the cortex and the medulla. The adrenal cortex consists of three anatomic zones: the outer *zona glomerulosa,* which secretes the mineralocorticoid aldosterone; the intermediate *zona fasciculata,* which secretes cortisol; and the inner *zona reticularis,* which secretes adrenal androgens. The adrenal medulla, lying in the center of the adrenal gland, is functionally related to the sympathetic nervous system and secretes the catecholamines epinephrine and norepinephrine in response to stress.

The synthesis of all steroid hormones begins with cholesterol and is catalyzed by a series of regulated, enzyme-mediated reactions (Fig. 66–1). Glucocorticoids affect metabolism, cardiovascular function, behavior, and the inflammatory/immune response (Table 66–1). Cortisol, the natural human glucocorticoid, is secreted by the adrenal glands in response to ultradian, circadian, and stress-induced hormonal stimulation by adrenocorticotropic hormone (ACTH). Plasma cortisol has marked circadian rhythm; levels are highest in the morning. ACTH, a 39–amino acid neuropeptide, is part of the pro-opiomelanocortin (POMC) precursor molecule, which also contains β-endorphin, β-lipotropin, corticotropin-like intermediate-lobe peptide (CLIP), and various melanocyte-stimulating hormones (MSHs). The secretion of ACTH by the pituitary gland is regulated primarily by two hypothalamic polypeptides: the 41–amino acid corticotropin-releasing hormone (CRH) and the decapeptide vasopressin. Glucocorticoids exert negative feedback upon CRH and ACTH secretion. The brain-hypothalamic-pituitary-adrenal (HPA) axis (Fig. 66–2) interacts with and influences the function of the reproductive, growth, and thyroid axes at multiple levels with major participation of glucocorticoids at all levels.

The renin-angiotensin-aldosterone system (Fig. 66–3) is the major factor controlling aldosterone secretion. Renal juxtaglomerular cells secrete renin in response to a decrease in circulating volume and/or a reduction in renal perfusion pressure. Renin is the rate-limiting enzyme that cleaves the 60-kd angiotensinogen, synthesized by the liver, to the bioinactive decapeptide, angiotensin I. Angiotensin I is rapidly converted to the octapeptide angiotensin II by angiotensin-converting enzyme (ACE) in the lungs and other tissues. Angiotensin II is a potent vasopressor and stimulates aldosterone production but does not stimulate cortisol production. Angiotensin II is the predominant regulator of aldosterone secretion, but plasma potassium concentration, sodium status, and ACTH levels also influence aldosterone secretion. ACTH also mediates the circadian rhythm of aldosterone; as a result, the plasma concentration of this hormone is highest in the morning. Aldosterone binds to the type I mineralocorticoid receptor, whereas cortisol binds to the type II glucocorticoid receptor. Binding of aldosterone to the cytosol mineralocorticoid receptor leads to Na^+ efflux into the extracellular fluid and K^+ and H^+ secretion via the sodium-potassium pump. The resultant increase in plasma Na^+ and decrease in plasma K^+ provide a feedback mechanism for suppressing renin and, subsequently, aldosterone secretion.

Approximately 5% of cortisol and 40% of aldosterone circulate in the free form; the remainder is bound to corticosteroid binding globulin and albumin.

Adrenal androgens include dehydroepiandrosterone (DHEA); its sulfate, DHEAS; and androstenedione. They are synthesized in the zona reticularis under the influence of ACTH and other adrenal androgen-stimulating factors. Although they have minimal intrinsic androgenic activity, they contribute to androgenicity by their peripheral conversion to testosterone and dihydrotestosterone. In men, excessive adrenal androgen has no clinical consequences; however in women, peripheral conversion of excess adrenal androgen secretion results in acne, hirsutism, and virilization. Because of gonadal production of androgens and estrogens and secretion of norepinephrine by sympathetic ganglia, deficiencies of adrenal androgens and catecholamines are not clinically recognized.

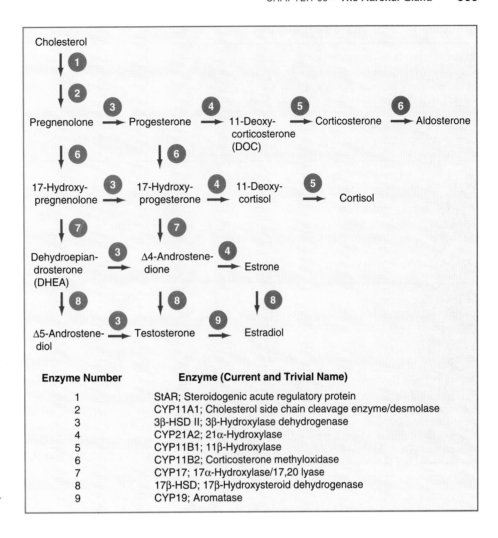

Enzyme Number	Enzyme (Current and Trivial Name)
1	StAR; Steroidogenic acute regulatory protein
2	CYP11A1; Cholesterol side chain cleavage enzyme/desmolase
3	3β-HSD II; 3β-Hydroxylase dehydrogenase
4	CYP21A2; 21α-Hydroxylase
5	CYP11B1; 11β-Hydroxylase
6	CYP11B2; Corticosterone methyloxidase
7	CYP17; 17α-Hydroxylase/17,20 lyase
8	17β-HSD; 17β-Hydroxysteroid dehydrogenase
9	CYP19; Aromatase

FIGURE 66-1 Pathways of steroid biosynthesis.

Adrenal Insufficiency

Glucocorticoid insufficiency can be either primary, resulting from the destruction or dysfunction of the adrenal cortex, or secondary, resulting from ACTH hyposecretion (Table 66–2). Autoimmune destruction of the adrenal glands (Addison's disease) is the most common cause of primary adrenal insufficiency in the industrialized world, accounting for about 65% of cases. Both glucocorticoid and mineralocorticoid secretion are diminished in this condition and, if untreated, may be fatal. Adrenal medulla function is usually spared. Approximately 70% of the patients with Addison's disease have antiadrenal antibodies.

Tuberculosis used to be the most common cause of adrenal insufficiency; however, its incidence in the industrialized world has decreased since the 1960s, and it accounts for 15% to 20% of the cases of adrenal insufficiency; calcified adrenal glands can be seen in 50% of these cases. Fungal and cytomegalovirus infections, metastatic infiltration of the adrenal glands, sarcoidosis, amyloidosis, hemochromatosis, traumatic injury to both adrenal glands, bilateral adrenal hemorrhage, and sepsis (usually meningococcemia) are rare causes of adrenal insufficiency. Many patients with human immunodefi-

ciency virus (HIV) infection have decreased adrenal reserve without overt adrenal insufficiency. Congenital causes of adrenal dysfunction include congenital adrenal hyperplasia (to be discussed), adrenal unresponsiveness to ACTH, congenital adrenal hypoplasia, and two demyelinating lipid metabolism disorders: adrenoleukodystrophy and adrenomyeloneuropathy. Iatrogenic causes of adrenal insufficiency include bilateral adrenalectomy, agents that inhibit cortisol biosynthesis (metyrapone, aminoglutethimide, trilostane, ketoconazole), adrenolytic drugs (o,p'-DDD), and the glucocorticoid antagonist RU 486.

Addison's disease may be part of two distinct autoimmune polyglandular syndromes. Type I autoimmune polyglandular syndrome, also termed autoimmune polyendocrine-candidiasis-ectodermal dystrophy (APECED) or autoimmune polyglandular failure syndrome, is characterized by the triad of hypoparathyroidism, adrenal insufficiency, and mucocutaneous candidiasis. Other, less common manifestations include hypothyroidism, gonadal failure, gastrointestinal malabsorption, insulin-dependent diabetes mellitus, alopecia areata and totalis, pernicious anemia, vitiligo, chronic active hepatitis, keratopathy, hypoplasia of dental enamel and nails, hypophysitis, asplenism, and cholelithiasis. This syndrome manifests in childhood. Type II autoimmune polyglandular syn-

TABLE 66-1   Actions of Glucocorticoids

Maintain Metabolic Homeostasis

Regulate blood glucose level, permissive effects on gluco-neogenesis, increases glycogen synthesis
Raise insulin levels, permissive effects on lipolytic hormones
Increase catabolism, decreases anabolism (except fat), inhibits growth hormone axis
Inhibit reproductive axis
Mineralocorticoid activity of cortisol

Affect Connective Tissues

Cause loss of collagen and connective tissue

Affect Calcium Homeostasis

Stimulate osteoclasts, inhibit osteoblasts
Reduce intestinal calcium absorption, stimulates parathyroid hormone release, increases urinary calcium excretion, decreases reabsorption of phosphate

Maintain Cardiovascular Function

Increase cardiac output
Increase vascular tone
Permissive effects on pressor hormones, increase sodium retention

Affect Behavior and Cognitive Function

Affect Immune System

Increase intravascular leukocyte concentration
Decreases migration of inflammatory cells to sites of injury
Suppress immune system (thymolysis, suppression of cytokines, prostanoids, kinins, serotonin, histamine, collagenase and plasminogen activator)

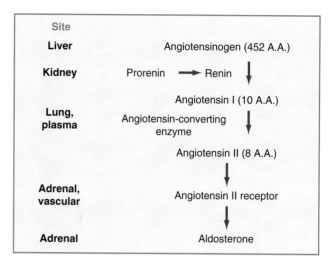

FIGURE 66-3   The renin-angiotensin-aldosterone axis. A.A. = amino acids.

drome, also called Schmidt's syndrome, is characterized by Addison's disease, autoimmune thyroid disease (Graves' disease or Hashimoto's thyroiditis), and insulin-dependent diabetes mellitus. Other associated diseases include pernicious anemia, vitiligo, gonadal failure, hypophysitis, celiac disease, myasthenia gravis, primary biliary cirrhosis, Sjögren's syndrome, lupus erythematosus,

and Parkinson's disease. This syndrome usually manifests in adults.

Adrenal insufficiency commonly manifests as weight loss, increasing fatigue, vomiting, diarrhea or anorexia, and salt craving. Muscle and joint pain, abdominal pain, and postural dizziness may also occur. Signs of increased pigmentation (initially most marked on the extensor surfaces, palmar creases, and buccal mucosa) often occur secondarily to the increased ACTH production (or other POMC-related peptides) by the pituitary gland. Laboratory abnormalities may include hyponatremia, hyperkalemia, mild metabolic acidosis, azotemia, hypercalcemia, anemia, lymphocytosis, and eosinophilia. Hypoglycemia may also occur, especially in children.

Acute adrenal insufficiency is a medical emergency, and treatment should not be delayed pending laboratory results. In a critically ill patient with hypovolemia, a plasma sample for cortisol, ACTH, and renin should be obtained, and then treatment with an intravenous bolus of 100 mg of hydrocortisone and parenteral saline administration should be initiated. A plasma cortisol concentration of more than 18 μg/dL rules out the diagnosis of adrenal crisis, whereas a value of less than 18 μg/dL in the setting of shock is consistent with adrenal insufficiency. In a patient with chronic symptoms, a 1-hour cosyntropin test should be performed. In this test, 0.25 mg ACTH$^{1-24}$ (cosyntropin) is given intravenously, and plasma cortisol is measured 0, 30, and 60 minutes later. A normal response is a plasma cortisol concentration higher than 18 μg/dL at any time during the test. A patient with a basal morning plasma cortisol concentration of less than 12 μg/dL and a stimulated cortisol concentration below 18 μg/dL probably has frank adrenal insufficiency and should receive treatment. A basal morning plasma cortisol concentration between 10 and 18 μg/dL in association with a stimulated cortisol concentration lower than 18 μg/dL probably indicates impaired adrenal reserve and a requirement for receiving cortisol replacement under stress conditions (as described later).

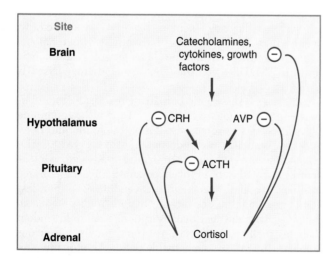

FIGURE 66-2   The brain-hypothalamic-pituitary-adrenal axis. ACTH = adrenocorticotropic hormone; AVP = arginine vasopressin; CRH = corticotropin-releasing hormone.

TABLE 66–2 **Syndromes of Adrenocortical Hypofunction**

Primary Adrenal Disorders

Combined Glucocorticoid and Mineralocorticoid Deficiency
Autoimmune
    Isolated autoimmune disease (Addison's disease)
    Polyglandular failure syndrome, type I
    Polyglandular failure syndrome, type II
Infectious
    Tuberculosis
    Fungal
    Cytomegalovirus
    Human immunodeficiency virus
Vascular
    Bilateral adrenal hemorrhage
    Sepsis
    Coagulopathy
    Thrombosis/embolism
    Adrenal infarction
Infiltration
    Metastatic carcinoma/lymphoma
    Sarcoidosis
    Amyloidosis
    Hemochromatosis
Congenital
    Congenital adrenal hyperplasia
        21α-hydroxylase deficiency
        3β-ol dehydrogenase deficiency
        20,22-desmolase deficiency
        Adrenal unresponsiveness to ACTH
        Congenital adrenal hypoplasia
        Adrenoleukodystrophy
        Adrenomyeloneuropathy
    Iatrogenic
        Bilateral adrenalectomy
        Drugs: metyrapone, aminoglutethimide, trilostane, ketoconazole, o,p'-DDD, RU 486

Mineralocorticoid Deficiency Without Glucocorticoid Deficiency
Corticosterone methyloxidase deficiency
Isolated zona glomerulosa defect
Heparin therapy
Critical illness
Converting enzyme inhibitors

Secondary Adrenal Disorders

Secondary Adrenal Insufficiency
Hypothalamic/pituitary dysfunction
Exogenous glucocorticoids
After removal of an ACTH-secreting tumor

Hyporeninemic Hypoaldosteronism
Diabetic nephropathy
Tubulointerstitial diseases
Obstructive uropathy
Autonomic neuropathy
Nonsteroidal anti-inflammatory drugs
β-adrenergic drugs

ACTH = adrenocorticotropic hormone.

Once the diagnosis of adrenal insufficiency is made, the distinction between primary and secondary adrenal insufficiency needs to be made. Secondary adrenal insufficiency results from inadequate stimulation of the adrenal cortex by ACTH. This can result from lesions anywhere along the HPA axis or occur as a sequela of prolonged suppression of the HPA axis by exogenous glucocorticoids. Secondary adrenal insufficiency manifests similarly as primary adrenal insufficiency with a few important differences: Because ACTH and other POMC-related peptides are reduced in secondary adrenal insufficiency, hyperpigmentation does not occur. In addition, because mineralocorticoid levels are normal in secondary adrenal insufficiency, symptoms of salt-craving, as well as the laboratory abnormalities of hyperkalemia and metabolic acidosis, are not present. However, hyponatremia is often seen as a result of inappropriate ADH secretion, which accompanies glucocorticoid insufficiency, resulting in impaired water excretion. Because corticotropin is the most preserved of the pituitary hormones, a patient with secondary adrenal insufficiency caused by a pituitary lesion usually has symptoms and/or laboratory abnormalities consistent with hypothyroidism, hypogonadism, or growth hormone deficiency. To distinguish primary from secondary adrenal insufficiency, a basal morning plasma ACTH value and a standing (after 2 hours) plasma renin level should be measured. A plasma ACTH value of more than 20 pg/mL (normal 5 to 30 pg/mL) is consistent with primary adrenal insufficiency, whereas a value less than 20 pg/mL probably represents secondary adrenal insufficiency. An upright plasma renin level of more than 3 ng/mL/hr is consistent with primary adrenal insufficiency, whereas a value less than 3 ng/mL/hr probably represents secondary adrenal insufficiency. The 1-hour cosyntropin test is suppressed in both secondary and primary adrenal insufficiency.

Secondary adrenal insufficiency occurs commonly after discontinuation of glucocorticoids. Alternate-day glucocorticoid treatment, if feasible, results in less suppression of the HPA axis than does daily glucocorticoid therapy. The natural history of recovery from adrenal suppression is first a gradual increase in ACTH levels, followed by the normalization of plasma cortisol levels and then normalization of the cortisol response to ACTH. Complete recovery of the HPA axis can take up to 1 year, and the rate-limiting step appears to be recovery of the CRH neurons.

TREATMENT

After stabilization of acute adrenal insufficiency, patients with Addison's disease require lifelong replacement with both glucocorticoids and mineralocorticoids. Unfortunately, most physicians overtreat patients with glucocorticoids and undertreat them with mineralocorticoids. Because overtreatment with glucocorticoids results in insidious weight gain and osteoporosis, the minimal cortisol dose tolerated without symptoms of glucocorticoid insufficiency (usually joint pain) is recommended. An initial regimen of 15 to 20 mg of hydrocortisone first thing in the morning and 5 mg of hydrocortisone at around 4 p.m. mimics the physiologic dose and is recommended. While glucocorticoid replacement is fairly uniform in most patients, mineralocorticoid replacement varies greatly. The initial dose of the synthetic mineralocorticoid fludrocortisone should be 100 μg/day and should be adjusted to keep the standing plasma renin between 1 to 3 ng/mL/hour. A standing plasma renin level higher than 3 ng/mL/hour, while the patient is taking the correct glucocorticoid dosage, is suggestive of undertreatment with fludrocortisone.

Under the stress of a minor illness (nausea, vomiting, or fever greater than 100.5°F), the hydrocortisone dose should be doubled for as short a period of time as possible. The inability to ingest hydrocortisone pills may necessitate parenteral hydrocortisone administration. Patients undergoing a major stressful event (i.e., surgery necessitating general anesthesia, or major trauma) should receive 150 to 300 mg of parenteral hydrocortisone daily (in three divided doses) with a rapid taper to normal replacement during recovery. All patients should wear a medical information bracelet and should be instructed in the use of intramuscular emergency hydrocortisone injections.

Hyporeninemic Hypoaldosteronism

Mineralocorticoid deficiency can result from decreased renin secretion by the kidneys. Resultant hypoangiotensinemia leads to hypoaldosteronism with hyperkalemia and hyperchloremic metabolic acidosis. Plasma sodium concentration is usually normal, but sodium conservation is often deficient. Plasma renin and aldosterone levels are low and unresponsive to stimuli. Diabetes mellitus and chronic tubulointerstitial diseases of the kidney are the most common underlying conditions leading to impairment of the juxtaglomerular apparatus. A subset of hyporeninemic hypoaldosteronism is caused by autonomic insufficiency. Stimuli such as upright posture or volume depletion, mediated by baroreceptors, do not cause a normal renin response. Administration of pharmacologic agents such as nonsteroidal anti-inflammatory agents, angiotensin-converting enzyme inhibitors, and β-adrenergic antagonists can also produce conditions of hypoaldosteronism. Potassium restriction, fludrocortisone, and furosemide, either singly or in combination, are effective in correcting the hyperkalemia and acidosis caused by hypoaldosteronism.

In rare cases, mineralocorticoid deficiency occurs with hyperreninism. The causes of this deficiency include a deficiency of corticosterone methyloxidase, the enzyme complex responsible for the final step of aldosterone biosynthesis, or an autoimmune-mediated destruction of the aldosterone-producing cells in the zona glomerulosa. Chronic administration of heparin and related compounds may also produce a state of hyperreninemic hypoaldosteronism.

Congenital Adrenal Hyperplasia

Congenital adrenal hyperplasia (CAH) refers to disorders of adrenal steroid biosynthesis that result in glucocorticoid and mineralocorticoid deficiencies. Because of deficient cortisol biosynthesis, a compensatory increase in ACTH occurs, inducing adrenal hyperplasia and overproduction of the steroids that precedes blockage of enzyme production (see Fig. 66–1). There are five major types of CAH, and the clinical manifestations of each disorder depend on which steroids are in excess and which are deficient. All these syndromes are transmitted in an autosomal recessive pattern. 21-Hydroxylase (CYP21) deficiency is the most common of these disorders and accounts for about 95% of the cases of CAH. In this condition, there is a failure of 21-hydroxylation of 17-hydroxyprogesterone and progesterone to 11-deoxycortisol and 11-deoxycortisone, respectively, with deficient cortisol and aldosterone production. Cortisol deficiency leads to increased ACTH release, causing overproduction of 17-hydroxyprogesterone and progesterone. Increased ACTH production also leads to increased biosynthesis of androstenedione and DHEA, which can be converted to testosterone. Patients with 21-hydroxylase deficiency can be divided into two clinical phenotypes: classic 21-hydroxylase deficiency, usually diagnosed at birth or during childhood, and late-onset 21-hydroxylase deficiency, which manifests during or after puberty. Two thirds of patients with classic 21-hydroxylase deficiency have various degrees of mineralocorticoid deficiency (salt-losing form); the remaining third are not salt-losing (simple virilizing form). Both decreased aldosterone production and increased concentrations of precursors that are mineralocorticoid antagonists, progesterone and 17-hydroxyprogesterone, contribute to salt loss in the salt-losing form, in which the enzymatic block is more severe.

The most useful measurement for the diagnosis of classic 21-hydroxylase deficiency is that of plasma 17-hydroxyprogesterone. A value greater than 200 ng/dL is consistent with the diagnosis. Late-onset 21-hydroxylase deficiency represents an allelic variant of classic 21-hydroxylase deficiency and is characterized by a mild enzymatic defect. This is the most frequent autosomal recessive disorder in humans and is present especially in Ashkenazi Jews. The syndrome usually manifests around the time of puberty with signs of virilization (hirsutism and acne) and amenorrhea or oligomenorrhea. It should be considered in women with unexplained hirsutism and menstrual abnormalities. The diagnosis is made from the finding of an elevated plasma 17-hydroxyprogesterone level (greater than 1500 ng/dL) 30 minutes after administration of 0.25 mg of synthetic ACTH (1 to 24).

The aim of treatment for classic 21-hydroxylase deficiency is to replace glucocorticoids and mineralocorticoids, suppress ACTH and androgen overproduction, and allow for normal growth and sexual maturation in children. A proposed approach to treating classic 21-hydroxylase deficiency recommends physiologic replacement with hydrocortisone and fludrocortisone in all affected patients, including those with the simple virilizing form. The deleterious effects of excess androgens can then be prevented by the use of an antiandrogen agent (flutamide) and an aromatase inhibitor (testolactone) that blocks the conversion of testosterone to estrogen. Although the traditional treatment for late-onset 21-hydroxylase deficiency is dexamethasone (0.5 mg/day), the use of an antiandrogen such as spironolactone (100 to 200 mg/day) is probably more effective and has fewer side effects. Mineralocorticoid replacement is not needed in late-onset 21-hydroxylase deficiency.

11-Hydroxylase (CYP11B1) deficiency accounts for about 5% of the cases of CAH. In this syndrome, the conversions of 11-deoxycortisol to cortisol and 11-deoxycorticosterone to corticosterone (the precursor to aldosterone) are blocked. Affected patients usually have hypertension and hypokalemia. Virilization occurs, as with 21-hydroxylase deficiency, and a late-onset form manifesting as androgen excess also occurs. The diagnosis is made from the finding of elevated plasma 11-deoxycortisol levels, either basally or after ACTH stimulation.

Rare forms of CAH are 3β-hydroxysteroid dehydrogenase (3β-HSD II), 17-hydroxylase (CYP17), and steroidogenic acute regulatory (StAR) protein deficiencies.

Syndromes of Adrenocorticoid Hyperfunction

Hypersecretion of the glucocorticoid hormone cortisol results in Cushing's syndrome, a metabolic disorder affecting carbohydrate, protein, and lipid metabolism. Hypersecretion of mineralocorticoids such as aldosterone results in a syndrome of hypertension and electrolyte disturbances.

CUSHING'S SYNDROME

Pathophysiology

Increased production of cortisol is seen in both physiologic and pathologic states (Table 66–3). Physiologic hypercortisolism occurs in stress, during the last trimester of pregnancy, and in persons who regularly perform strenuous exercise. Pathologic conditions of elevated cortisol levels include exogenous or endogenous Cushing's syndrome and several psychiatric states, including depression, alcoholism, anorexia nervosa, panic disorder, and alcohol or narcotic withdrawal.

Cushing's syndrome may be caused by exogenous ACTH or glucocorticoid administration or by endogenous overproduction of these hormones. Endogenous Cushing's syndrome is either ACTH-dependent or ACTH-independent. ACTH dependency accounts for 85% of cases and include pituitary sources of ACTH (Cushing's disease), ectopic sources of ACTH, and, in rare instances, ectopic sources of CRH. Pituitary Cushing's disease accounts for 80% of cases of ACTH-dependent Cushing's syndrome. Ectopic secretion of ACTH occurs most commonly in patients with small cell lung carcinoma. These patients are older, usually have a history of smoking and present primarily with signs and symptoms of lung cancer rather than of Cushing's syndrome. Patients with the clinical ectopic ACTH syndrome, in contrast, have mostly intrathoracic (lung and thymic) carcinoids. The remaining patients have pancreatic, adrenal, or thyroid tumors that secrete ACTH. ACTH-independent cases account for 15% of cases of

TABLE 66–3 Syndromes of Adrenocortical Hyperfunction

States of Glucocorticoid Excess

Physiologic States
Stress
Strenuous exercise
Last trimester of pregnancy

Pathologic States
Psychiatric conditions (pseudo–Cushing's disorders)
  Depression
  Alcoholism
  Anorexia nervosa
  Panic disorders
  Alcohol/drug withdrawal
ACTH-dependent states
  Pituitary adenoma (Cushing's disease)
  Ectopic ACTH syndrome
    Bronchial carcinoid
    Thymic carcinoid
    Islet cell tumor
    Small-cell lung carcinoma
  Ectopic CRH secretion
ACTH-independent states
  Adrenal adenoma
  Adrenal carcinoma
  Micronodular adrenal disease

Exogenous Sources
Glucocorticoid intake
ACTH intake

States of Mineralocorticoid Excess

Primary Aldosteronism
Aldosterone-secreting adenoma
Bilateral adrenal hyperplasia
Aldosterone-secreting carcinoma
Glucocorticoid-suppressible hyperaldosteronism

Adrenal Enzyme Deficiencies
11β-hydroxylase deficiency
17α-hydroxylase deficiency
11β-steroid dehydrogenase

Exogenous Mineralocorticoids
Licorice
Carbenoxolone
Fludrocortisone

Secondary Hyperaldosteronism
Associated with hypertension
  Accelerated hypertension
  Renovascular hypertension
  Estrogen administration
  Renin-secreting tumors
Without hypertension
  Bartter's syndrome
  Sodium-wasting nephropathy
  Renal tubular acidosis
  Diuretic/laxative abuse
  Edematous states (cirrhosis, nephrosis, congestive heart failure)

ACTH = adrenocorticotropin hormone; CRH = corticotropin-releasing hormone.

Cushing's syndrome and include adrenal adenomas, adrenal carcinomas, micronodular adrenal disease, and autonomous macronodular adrenal disease. The female-to-male ratio for noncancerous forms of Cushing's syndrome is 4:1. The median duration of symptoms before the diagnosis is made is 3 to 5 years.

Clinical Manifestations

The clinical signs, symptoms, and common laboratory findings of hypercortisolism seen in patients with Cushing's syndrome are listed in Table 66–4. Typically the obesity is centripetal, with a wasting of the arms and legs; this is distinct from the generalized weight gain seen in idiopathic obesity. Rounding of the face (so-called moon facies) and a dorsocervical fat pad ("buffalo hump") may occur in obesity that is not related to Cushing's syndrome, whereas facial plethora and supraclavicular filling are more specific for Cushing's syndrome. Patients with Cushing's syndrome may have proximal muscle weakness, so the physical finding of inability to stand up from a squat can be quite revealing. Menstrual irregularities often precede other cushingoid symptoms in affected women, whereas affected men frequently complain of poor libido and impotence. Adult-onset acne or hirsutism in women should also raise the suspicion of Cushing's syndrome. The skin striae seen in cushingoid patients are violaceous (purple or dark red), with a width of at least 1 cm. Thinning of the skin on the top of the hands is a very specific sign in younger adults with Cushing's syndrome and should always be looked for. Old pictures of patients are extremely helpful for evaluating the progression of the physical stigmata of Cushing's syndrome.

Associated laboratory findings in Cushing's syndrome include elevated plasma alkaline phosphatase levels,

granulocytosis, thrombocytosis, hypercholesterolemia, hypertriglyceridemia, and glucose intolerance/diabetes mellitus. Hypokalemic alkalosis is an infrequent finding in patients with Cushing's syndrome and usually occurs in patients with severe hypercortisolism as a result of the ectopic ACTH syndrome.

Diagnosis (Fig. 66–4)

If the history and physical examination findings are suggestive of hypercortisolism, the diagnosis of Cushing's syndrome can usually be established by collecting urine for 24 hours and measuring urinary free cortisol (UFC). UFC excretion reflects plasma unbound cortisol that is filtered and excreted by the kidney. This test is extremely sensitive for the diagnosis of Cushing's syndrome, because in 90% of affected patients, the initial UFC level is greater than 90 μg/24 hours. Patients with Cushing's disease usually have UFC levels between 300 and 1000 μg/24 hours, whereas patients with the ectopic ACTH syndrome and cortisol-secreting adrenal adenomas or carcinomas frequently have UFCs greater than 1000 μg/24 hours.

Cortisol normally is secreted in a diurnal manner; the plasma concentration is highest in the early morning (between 6 and 8 a.m.) and lowest around midnight. The normal 8 a.m. plasma cortisol level ranges between 5 and 25 μg/dL and declines throughout the day. By 11 p.m., the values are usually less than 5 μg/dL. Most patients with Cushing's syndrome lack this diurnal variation. Thus, although their morning cortisol levels may be normal, their afternoon or evening concentrations are markedly higher. Late afternoon or night values greater than 50% of the morning values are consistent with Cushing's syndrome. Measurement of random morning cortisol levels is not particularly helpful.

The overnight dexamethasone suppression test can also be used as a screening test to evaluate patients suspected of having hypercortisolism. Dexamethasone, 1 mg, is given orally at 11 p.m., and plasma cortisol is measured the following morning at 8 a.m. A morning plasma cortisol level greater than 5 μg/dL suggests hypercortisolism. This test is easy and can be performed in an outpatient setting. The test is fairly sensitive, although some pituitary adenomas are very sensitive to dexamethasone and can suppress cortisol production readily in this test. However, the test produces a significant number of false-positive results, especially in obese and depressed patients, the two patient populations in whom the differentiation from mild Cushing's syndrome may be difficult. For these reasons, collection of urine for measurement of 24-hour urinary free cortisol excretion is a better screening test.

Differential Diagnosis

Once the diagnosis of Cushing's syndrome is established, the etiology of the hypercortisolism needs to be ascertained. This is accomplished by biochemical studies, which evaluate the feedback regulation of the HPA axis; by venous sampling techniques; and by imaging procedures. Basal ACTH levels are normal or elevated in Cushing's disease and the ectopic ACTH syndrome

---

TABLE 66–4 Signs, Symptoms, and Laboratory Abnormalities of Hypercortisolism

Fat redistribution (dorsocervical and supraclavicular fat pads, temporal wasting, centripetal obesity, weight gain) (95%)
Menstrual irregularities (80% of affected women)
Thin skin/plethora (80%)
Moon facies (75%)
Increased appetite (75%)
Sleep disturbances (75%)
Hypertension (75%)
Hypercholesterolemia/hypertrigliceridemia (70%)
Altered mentation (poor concentration, decreased memory, euphoria) (70%)
Diabetes mellitus/glucose intolerance (65%)
Striae (65%)
Hirsutism (65%)
Proximal muscle weakness (60%)
Psychological disturbances (emotional lability, depression, mania, psychosis) (50%)
Decreased libido/impotence (50%)
Acne (45%)
Osteoporosis/pathologic fractures (40%)
Virilization (in women) (40%)
Easy bruisability (40%)
Poor wound healing (40%)
Edema (20%)
Increased infections (10%)
Cataracts (5%)

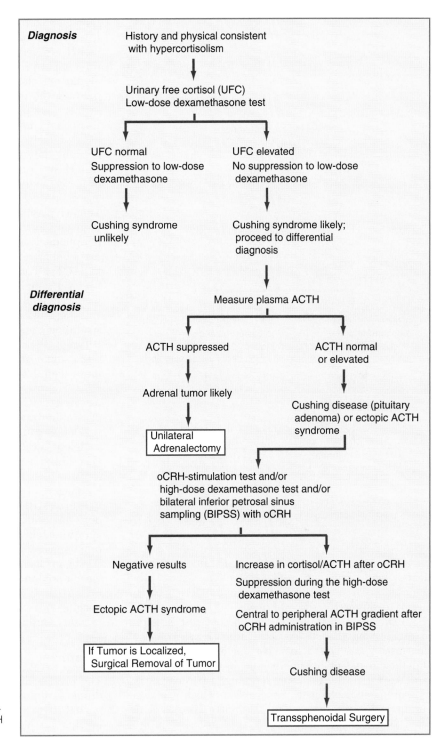

Diagnosis

History and physical consistent with hypercortisolism

↓

Urinary free cortisol (UFC)
Low-dose dexamethasone test

UFC normal
Suppression to low-dose dexamethasone

↓

Cushing syndrome unlikely

UFC elevated
No suppression to low-dose dexamethasone

↓

Cushing syndrome likely; proceed to differential diagnosis

Differential diagnosis

↓

Measure plasma ACTH

ACTH suppressed

↓

Adrenal tumor likely

↓

Unilateral Adrenalectomy

ACTH normal or elevated

↓

Cushing disease (pituitary adenoma) or ectopic ACTH syndrome

↓

oCRH-stimulation test and/or high-dose dexamethasone test and/or bilateral inferior petrosal sinus sampling (BIPSS) with oCRH

Negative results

↓

Ectopic ACTH syndrome

↓

If Tumor is Localized, Surgical Removal of Tumor

Increase in cortisol/ACTH after oCRH

Suppression during the high-dose dexamethasone test

Central to peripheral ACTH gradient after oCRH administration in BIPSS

↓

Cushing disease

↓

Transsphenoidal Surgery

FIGURE 66–4 Flow chart for evaluating a patient with suspected Cushing's syndrome. ACTH = adrenocorticotropic hormone; oCRH = ovine corticotropin–releasing hormone.

and are undetectable in primary adrenal Cushing's syndrome.

In the dexamethasone suppression test (Liddle test), 0.5 mg of dexamethasone is given orally every 6 hours for 2 days, followed by 2 mg of dexamethasone every 6 hours for another 2 days. On the second day of the high dosage of dexamethasone, urinary free cortisol is suppressed to less than 10% of that of the baseline collection in patients with pituitary adenomas but not in patients with the ectopic ACTH syndrome or adrenal cortisol-secreted tumors. Although the Liddle test is of-

ten helpful in establishing the etiology of Cushing's syndrome, it has some disadvantages. The test requires accurate measurement of urine collections, often necessitating inpatient hospitalization. In approximately 50% of patients with bronchial carcinoids causing ectopic ACTH production, cortisol secretion is suppressible by high-dose dexamethasone, which yields a false-positive result. In addition, because patients with Cushing's syndrome are often episodic secretors of corticosteroids, considerable variation in daily urinary free cortisol excretion can occur and false results can be found. There-

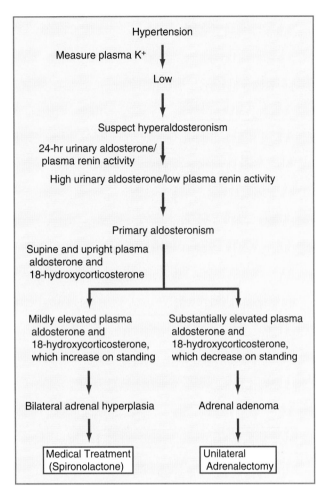

FIGURE 66–5 Flow chart for evaluating a patient with suspected primary hyperaldosteronism.

fore, the Liddle test should be used cautiously in patients who have episodic secretion, and other confirmatory tests should be performed before a patient is sent to surgery.

An overnight high-dose dexamethasone test is helpful in establishing the etiology of Cushing's syndrome. In this test, a baseline 8 a.m. cortisol level is measured, and then 8 mg of dexamethasone is given orally at 11 p.m. At 8 a.m. the following morning, a plasma cortisol measurement is obtained. Suppression, which would occur in patients with pituitary Cushing's disease, is defined as a decrease in plasma cortisol to less than 50% of the baseline level. Few patients with bronchial carcinoid have been examined, so the suppressibility of these tumors by high-dose overnight dexamethasone is not well established.

The ovine CRH (oCRH) test and bilateral simultaneous inferior petrosal sinus sampling are also used to establish the etiology of Cushing's syndrome. Corticotrophs of normal persons and of patients with pituitary Cushing's disease respond to oCRH by increasing the secretion of ACTH and, therefore, cortisol. Thus, the oCRH test cannot be used to distinguish normal persons from patients with pituitary Cushing's disease. Patients with cortisol-secreting adrenal tumors have low or undetectable concentrations of ACTH that do not re-

spond to oCRH. Patients with ectopic ACTH secretion have high basal ACTH levels that do not increase with oCRH. In patients with both the ectopic ACTH syndrome and primary adrenal hypercortisolism, cortisol levels do not change in response to oCRH. Discrepancies between the oCRH and dexamethasone tests necessitate further work-up for ascertainment of the diagnosis.

Bilateral inferior petrosal sinus sampling (BIPSS) is an extremely accurate and safe procedure for distinguishing pituitary Cushing's disease from the ectopic ACTH syndrome. Venous blood from the anterior lobe of the pituitary gland empties into the cavernous sinuses and then into the superior and inferior petrosal sinuses. Venous plasma samples for ACTH are obtained from both inferior petrosal sinuses along with a simultaneous peripheral sample both before and after intravenous bolus administration of CRH. In baseline measurements, an ACTH concentration gradient of 1.6 or more between a sample from either of the petrosal sinuses and the peripheral sample is strongly suggestive of pituitary Cushing's disease, whereas patients with ectopic ACTH syndrome or adrenal adenomas have no ACTH gradient between their petrosal and peripheral samples. After CRH administration, a central-to-peripheral gradient of more than 3.2 is consistent with pituitary Cushing's disease. The use of CRH has enabled complete distinction of pituitary Cushing's disease from nonpituitary Cushing's syndrome. An ACTH gradient ipsilateral to the side of the tumor is found in 70% to 80% of patients sampled. Although BIPSS requires a radiologist experienced in petrosal sinus sampling, it is currently available at many tertiary care facilities.

Imaging of the pituitary gland by magnetic resonance imaging (MRI) with gadolinium is the preferred procedure for localizing a pituitary adenoma. This test detects approximately 40% to 50% of pituitary ACTH-secreting tumors and can detect many pituitary tumors as small as 3 mm in diameter. About 10% of normal persons may have a nonfunctioning pituitary adenoma found on pituitary MRI. It is therefore recommended that pituitary imaging not be the sole criterion for the diagnosis of pituitary Cushing's disease.

Treatment

The preferred treatment for all forms of Cushing's syndrome is appropriate surgery. Pituitary Cushing's disease is best treated by transsphenoidal surgery. When the operation is performed by an experienced neurosurgeon, the cure rate is higher than 90%. Transsphenoidal surgery carries very low rates of morbidity and mortality. Major complications (e.g., meningitis, cerebrospinal fluid leakage, optic nerve damage, isolated thyrotropin or growth hormone deficiency) are rare. In patients with the ectopic ACTH syndrome, it is hoped that the tumor is localized by appropriate scans and then removed surgically. A unilateral adrenalectomy is the treatment of choice in patients with a cortisol-secreting adrenal adenoma. Patients with cortisol-secreting adrenal carcinomas should also be managed surgically; however, they have a poor prognosis, only 20% surviving more than 1 year after diagnosis.

Patients who have failed initial pituitary surgery or

have recurrent Cushing's disease may be treated with pituitary irradiation. Irradiation has more long-term complications than does transsphenoidal surgery and results in cure in about 60% of patients. Panhypopituitarism eventually develops in almost all these patients, and so thyroid, gonadal, and even steroid replacement may be needed. Patients with Cushing's disease who remain hypercortisolemic after pituitary surgery and irradiation or who decline irradiation should then undergo bilateral adrenalectomy. About 10% of patients with Cushing's disease who undergo bilateral adrenalectomy develop Nelson's syndrome (hyperpigmentation and an ACTH-secreting macroadenoma that often causes visual field deficits). The incidence of Nelson's syndrome is reduced if patients have undergone pituitary irradiation.

Medical treatment for hypercortisolism may be needed to prepare patients for surgery, in patients who are undergoing or have undergone pituitary irradiation and are awaiting its effects, in patients with mild Cushing's syndrome, or in patients who are not surgical candidates or who elect not to have surgery. Ketoconazole, mitotane (o,p'–DDD), metyrapone, aminoglutethimide, RU 486, and trilostane are the most commonly used agents for adrenal blockade and can be used alone or in combination.

PRIMARY MINERALOCORTICOID EXCESS

Pathophysiology

Increased mineralocorticoid activity is manifested by salt retention, hypertension, hypokalemia, and metabolic alkalosis. The causes of primary aldosteronism (see Table 66–3) are aldosterone-producing adenoma (75%), bilateral adrenal hyperplasia (25%), adrenal carcinoma (1%), or glucocorticoid-remediable hyperaldosteronism (<1%). The adrenal enzyme defects—11β-steroid dehydrogenase, 11β-hydroxylase, and 17α-hydroxylase deficiencies—and exogenous mineralocorticoid ingestion (from licorice or carbenoxolone) are also states of mineralocorticoid excess. Secondary aldosteronism (see Table 66–3) results from overactivation of the renin-angiotensin system.

Primary aldosteronism is usually recognized during evaluation of hypertension or hypokalemia and represents a potentially curable form of hypertension. Fewer than 2% of patients with hypertension have primary aldosteronism. The patients are usually between 30 and 50 years of age, and the female-to-male ratio is 2:1.

Clinical Manifestations

Hypertension, hypokalemia, and metabolic alkalosis are the main clinical manifestations of hyperaldosteronism; most of the presenting symptoms are related to hypokalemia. Symptoms in mildly hypokalemic patients are fatigue, muscle weakness, nocturia, lassitude, and headaches. If more severe hypokalemia exists, polydipsia, polyuria, paresthesias, and even intermittent paralysis and tetany can occur. Blood pressure can range from being minimally elevated to very high. Retinopathy is mild, and hemorrhages are rarely present. A positive Trousseau or Chvostek sign may occur as a result of metabolic alkalosis.

Diagnosis and Treatment

Initially, hypokalemia in the presence of hypertension must be documented (Fig. 66–5). The patient must have an adequate salt intake and discontinue diuretics before potassium measurement. If hypokalemia is found under these conditions, a 24-hour urinary aldosterone level and an upright (standing for at least 2 hours) plasma renin level should be measured. An elevated urinary aldosterone level (>15 μg/day) and a suppressed plasma renin level (<2 ng/mL/hour) suggests the diagnosis of hyperaldosteronism.

Once the diagnosis of primary aldosteronism has been demonstrated, it is important to distinguish between an aldosterone-producing adenoma and bilateral hyperplasia, because the former is treated with surgery and the latter is treated medically. In the initial test (a postural challenge), an 8 a.m. supine blood sample is drawn for plasma aldosterone, 18-hydrocorticosterone, renin, and cortisol measurement. The patient then stands for 2 hours, and an upright sample is drawn for measurement of the same hormones. A basal plasma aldosterone level of less than 20 ng/dL is usually found in patients with bilateral hyperplasia, and a value greater than 20 ng/dL suggests the diagnosis of adrenal adenoma. In bilateral hyperplasia, plasma aldosterone often increases as a result of the increase in renin in response to the upright position, whereas in adenoma, plasma aldosterone levels usually fall as a result of decreased stimulation by ACTH at 10 a.m., in comparison with 8 a.m. An 8 a.m. plasma 18-hydroxycorticosterone level of greater than 50 ng/dL that falls with upright posture occurs in most patients with an adenoma, whereas an 8 a.m. level less than 50 ng/dL that rises with the upright posture occurs in most patients with bilateral hyperplasia.

A computed tomographic (CT) scan of the adrenal glands should be performed to localize the tumor. If a discrete adenoma is seen in one adrenal gland, the contralateral gland is normal, and biochemical test results are consistent with an adenoma, the patient should undergo unilateral adrenalectomy. Patients in whom biochemical study findings are consistent with an adenoma but CT results are consistent with bilateral disease should undergo adrenal venous sampling for aldosterone and cortisol measurement. Patients in whom biochemical and localization study findings are consistent with bilateral hyperplasia should be treated medically, usually with spironolactone. Those in whom biochemical study results are consistent with bilateral hyperplasia should also be evaluated for dexamethasone-suppressible hyperaldosteronism by receiving a trial of dexamethasone, which reverses the hyperaldosteronism in this rare autosomal dominant disorder.

Hyperaldosteronism secondary to activation of the renin-angiotensin system and hypertension can occur in patients with accelerated hypertension, those with renovascular hypertension, those receiving estrogen therapy, and, rarely, in patients with renin-secreting tumors. Hyperaldosteronism without hypertension occurs in patients with Bartter's syndrome, those with sodium-wasting nephropathy, those with renal tubular acidosis, and those who abuse diuretics or laxatives.

Adrenal Medullary Hyperfunction

The adrenal medulla synthesizes the catecholamines norepinephrine, epinephrine, and dopamine from the amino acid tyrosine. Norepinephrine, the major catecholamine produced by the adrenal medulla, has predominantly α-agonist actions, causing vasoconstriction. Epinephrine acts primarily on the β receptors, having positive inotropic and chronotropic effects on the heart, causing peripheral vasodilation, and increasing plasma glucose concentrations in response to hypoglycemia. The action of circulating dopamine is unclear. Whereas norepinephrine is synthesized in the central nervous system and sympathetic postganglionic neurons, epinephrine is synthesized entirely in the adrenal medulla. The adrenal medullary contribution of norepinephrine secretion is relatively small. Bilateral adrenalectomy results in only minimal changes in circulating norepinephrine levels, although epinephrine levels are dramatically reduced. Thus, hypofunction of the adrenal medulla has little physiologic impact, whereas hypersecretion of catecholamines produces the clinical syndrome of pheochromocytoma.

PHEOCHROMOCYTOMA

Pathophysiology

Although pheochromocytomas can occur in any sympathetic ganglion in the body, more than 90% of pheochromocytomas arise from the adrenal medulla. The majority of extra-adrenal tumors occur in the mediastinum or abdomen. Bilateral adrenal pheochromocytomas occur in about 5% of the cases and may occur as part of familial syndromes. Pheochromocytoma occurs as part of multiple endocrine neoplasia type 2A or 2B. The former (Sipple's syndrome) is marked by medullary carcinoma of the thyroid, hyperparathyroidism, and pheochromocytoma; the latter is characterized by medullary carcinoma of the thyroid, mucosal neuromas, intestinal ganglioneuromas, marfanoid habitus, and pheochromocytoma. Pheochromocytomas are also associated with neurofibromatosis, cerebelloretinal hemangioblastosis (von Hippel–Lindau syndrome), and tuberous sclerosis.

Clinical Manifestations

Because the majority of pheochromocytomas secrete norepinephrine as the principal catecholamine, hypertension (often paroxysmal) is the most common finding. Other symptoms include the triad of headache, palpitations, and sweating, as well as flushing, anxiety, nausea, fatigue, weight loss, and abdominal and chest pain. These symptoms may be precipitated by emotional stress, exercise, anesthesia, abdominal pressure, or intake of tyramine-containing foods. Orthostatic hypotension can also occur. Wide fluctuations in blood pressure are characteristic, and the hypertension associated with pheochromocytoma usually does not respond to standard antihypertensive medicines.

Diagnosis and Treatment

The diagnosis of pheochromocytoma is made by demonstrating elevated urinary excretion of catecholamines or their metabolites, the metanephrines and vanillylmandelic acid, during a period of hypertension. Measurement of urinary metanephrine levels is probably the single best test, but usually urinary total catecholamines, epinephrine, norepinephrine, and vanillylmandelic acid are also measured. Measurement of plasma catecholamines is also useful. The blood sample must be drawn when the patient is hypertensive and supine and from an indwelling catheter to avoid the stress of venipuncture. A plasma norepinephrine level greater than 1500 pg/mL or an epinephrine level greater than 500 pg/mL is consistent with the diagnosis of a pheochromocytoma. If the values are only mildly elevated, a clonidine suppression test should be performed; in this test, clonidine (0.3 mg/kg) is given orally, and plasma catecholamines are measured before and 3 hours after administration. In normal persons, catecholamine levels decrease into the normal range, whereas in patients with a pheochromocytoma, levels are unchanged or increase. Once the diagnosis of pheochromocytoma is made, a CT scan of the adrenal glands should be performed. Most intra-adrenal pheochromocytomas are readily visible on this scan. If the CT scan is negative, extra-adrenal pheochromocytomas can often be localized by iodine 131–metaiodobenzylguanidine (^{131}I-MIBG), an octreotide scan, or abdominal MRI.

The treatment of pheochromocytoma is surgical if the lesion can be localized. Patients should undergo preoperative α blockade with phenoxybenzamine and α-methyl-p-tyrosine (an inhibitor of tyrosine hydroxylase, the rate-limiting enzyme in catecholamine biosynthesis) 1 to 2 weeks before surgery. β-Adrenergic antagonists should be used during surgery. Approximately 5% to 10% of pheochromocytomas are malignant. ^{131}I-MIBG or chemotherapy may be useful, but the prognosis is poor. α-Methyl-p-tyrosine may be used to decrease catecholamine secretion from the tumor.

REFERENCES

Bravo EL: Evolving concepts in the pathophysiology, diagnosis, and treatment of pheochromocytoma. Endocr Rev 15:356–368, 1994.

Cutler GB Jr, Laue L: Congenital adrenal hyperplasia due to 21-hydroxylase deficiency. N Engl J Med 323:1806–1813, 1990.

Flack MR, Oldfield EH, Cutler JGB, et al: Urine free cortisol in the high-dose dexamethasone suppression test for the differential diagnosis of the Cushing syndrome. Ann Intern Med 116:211–217, 1992.

Newell-Price J, Trainer P, Besser M, Grossman A: The diagnosis and differential diagnosis of Cushing's syndrome and pseudo-Cushing's states. Endocr Rev 19:647–672, 1998.

Orth DN: Cushing's syndrome. N Engl J Med 332:791–803, 1995.

Ross RJ, Trainer PJ: Endocrine investigation: Cushing's syndrome. Clin Endocrinol 49:153–155, 1998.

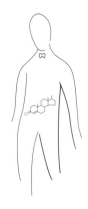

67

MALE REPRODUCTIVE ENDOCRINOLOGY

Glenn D. Braunstein

The testes are composed of Leydig (interstitial) cells that secrete testosterone and estradiol and the sperm-producing seminiferous tubules. They are regulated by the gonadotropins luteinizing hormone (LH) and folli-cle-stimulating hormone (FSH), which are secreted by the anterior pituitary under the influence of the hypothalamic decapeptide, gonadotropin-releasing hormone (GnRH) (Fig. 67–1). LH stimulates the Leydig cells to secrete testosterone, which feeds back in a negative fashion at the level of the pituitary and hypothalamus to inhibit further LH production. FSH stimulates sperm production through interaction with the Sertoli cells in the seminiferous tubules. Feedback inhibition of FSH is through gonadal steroids as well as through inhibin, a glycoprotein produced by Sertoli cells.

Biochemical evaluation of the hypothalamic-pituitary-Leydig axis is carried out by measurement of serum LH and testosterone concentrations, whereas a semen analysis and serum FSH determination provide an assessment of the hypothalamic-pituitary-seminiferous tubular axis. The ability of the pituitary to release gonadotropins can be tested dynamically through GnRH stimulation, and the ability of the testes to secrete testosterone can be evaluated through injections of human chorionic gonadotropin (hCG), a glycoprotein hormone that has biologic activity similar to that of LH.

Hypogonadism

Either testosterone deficiency or defective spermatogenesis constitutes *hypogonadism.* Often both disorders coexist. The clinical manifestations of androgen deficiency depend on the time of onset and the degree of deficiency. Because testosterone is required for wolffian duct development into the epididymis, vas deferens, seminal vesicles, and ejaculatory ducts, as well as for virilization of the external genitalia through the major intracellular testosterone metabolite, dihydrotestoster-

one, early prenatal androgen deficiency leads to the formation of ambiguous genitalia and to male pseudohermaphroditism. Androgen deficiency occurring later during gestation may result in micropenis or *cryptorchidism,* the unilateral or bilateral absence of testes in the scrotum resulting from failure of normal testicular descent. During puberty, androgens are responsible for male sexual differentiation, which includes growth of the scrotum, epididymis, vas deferens, seminal vesicles, prostate, penis, skeletal muscle, and larynx. Additionally, androgens stimulate the growth of axillary, pubic, facial, and body hair, as well as increased sebaceous gland activity, and they are responsible through conversion to estrogens for the growth and fusion of the epiphyseal cartilaginous plates seen clinically as the *pubertal growth spurt.* Thus, prepubertal androgen deficiency leads to poor muscle development, decreased strength and endurance, a high-pitched voice, sparse axillary and pubic hair, and the absence of facial and body hair. The long bones of the lower extremities and arms may continue to grow under the influence of growth hormone, a condition leading to eunuchoidal proportions in which the arm span exceeds the total height by 5 cm or more, and growth of the lower extremities is greater relative to total height. Postpubertal androgen deficiency may result in a decrease in libido, impotence, low energy, fine wrinkling around the corners of the eyes and mouth, and diminished facial and body hair.

Male hypogonadism may be classified into three categories according to the level of the defect (Table 67–1). Hypogonadism from lesions in the hypothalamus or pituitary gives rise to *secondary* or *hypogonadotropic hypogonadism,* because the low testosterone level or ineffective spermatogenesis is a result of inadequate stimulation of the testes by insufficient or inadequate concentrations of the gonadotropins. In contrast, diseases directly affecting the testes result in *primary* or *hypergonadotropic hypogonadism,* characterized by oligospermia or azoospermia and low testosterone levels but with elevations of LH and FSH because of a decrease of the negative feedback regulation on the pitui-

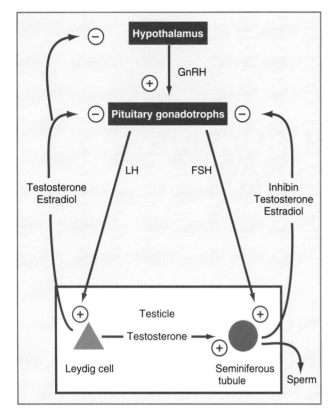

FIGURE 67–1 Regulation of the hypothalamic-pituitary-testicular axis. + = positive feedback; − = negative feedback; FSH = follicle-stimulating hormone; GnRH = gonadotropin-releasing hormone; LH = luteinizing hormone.

tary and hypothalamus by androgens and inhibin. The third category of hypogonadism results from defects in androgen action.

HYPOTHALAMIC-PITUITARY DISORDERS

Panhypopituitarism occurs congenitally from structural defects or from inadequate production or release of the hypothalamic-releasing factors. The condition may also be acquired through replacement by tumors, infarction from vascular insufficiency, infiltrative disorders, autoimmune diseases, trauma, and infections.

Kallmann's syndrome is a form of hypogonadotropic hypogonadism associated with problems in the ability to discriminate odors, either incompletely *(hyposmia)* or completely *(anosmia)*. This syndrome results from a defect in the migration of the GnRH neurons from the olfactory placode into the hypothalamus. Thus, it represents a GnRH deficiency. Patients remain prepubertal, with small, rubbery testes, and they develop eunuchoidism.

Hyperprolactinemia may result in hypogonadotropic hypogonadism because prolactin elevation inhibits normal GnRH release, decreases the effectiveness of LH at the Leydig cell level, and also inhibits some of the action of testosterone at the target organ level. Normalization of prolactin levels through withdrawal of an of-

fending drug, by surgical removal of the pituitary adenoma, or with the use of dopamine agonists reverses this form of hypogonadism.

Another form of secondary hypogonadism in male patients is caused by weight loss or systemic illness *(hypothalamic dysfunction)*. This weight loss or illness induces a defect in the hypothalamic release of GnRH and results in low gonadotropin and testosterone levels. This condition is commonly seen in patients with cancer, acquired immunodeficiency syndrome, and chronic inflammatory processes.

PRIMARY GONADAL ABNORMALITIES

The most common congenital cause of primary testicular failure is *Klinefelter's syndrome,* which occurs in approximately 1 of every 5000 live male births and is usually caused by a maternal meiotic chromosomal nondisjunction that results in an XXY genotype. At puberty, clinical findings include the following: varying degrees of hypogonadism; gynecomastia; small, firm testes measuring less than 2 cm in the longest axis (normal testes measure >3.5 cm); azoospermia; eunuchoidal skeletal proportions; and elevations of FSH and LH. Primary gonadal failure is also found in patients with another congenital condition, *myotonic dystrophy,* which is characterized by the following: progressive weakness; atrophy of the facial, neck, hand, and lower extremity muscles; frontal baldness; and myotonia.

Approximately 3% of full-term male infants have *cryptorchidism,* which spontaneously corrects during the first year of life in most of these children, so by 1 year of age, the incidence of this condition is approximately 0.75%. When the testes are maintained in the intra-abdominal position, the increased temperature leads to defective spermatogenesis and oligospermia. Leydig cell

TABLE 67–1   Classification of Male Hypogonadism

Hypothalamic-Pituitary Disorders (Secondary Hypogonadism)
Panhypopituitarism
Isolated gonadotropin deficiency
Complex congenital syndromes
Hyperprolactinemia
Hypothalamic dysfunction
Gonadal Disorders (Primary Hypogonadism)
Klinefelter's syndrome and associated chromosomal defects
Myotonic dystrophy
Cryptorchidism
Bilateral anorchia
Seminiferous tubular failure
Adult Leydig cell failure
Androgen biosynthesis enzyme deficiency
Defects in Androgen Action
Testicular feminization (complete androgen insensitivity)
Incomplete androgen insensitivity
5α-Reductase deficiency

function generally remains normal, and therefore adult testosterone levels are normal. *Bilateral anorchia,* also known as the vanishing testicle syndrome, is a rare condition in which the external genitalia are fully formed, thus indicating that ample quantities of testosterone and dihydrotestosterone were produced during early embryogenesis. However, the testicular tissue disappeared before or shortly after birth, and the result is an empty scrotum. Differentiation from cryptorchidism can be made through an hCG stimulation test. Patients with cryptorchidism have an increase in serum testosterone after an injection of hCG, whereas patients with bilateral anorchia do not.

Acquired gonadal failure has numerous causes. The adult seminiferous tubules are susceptible to a variety of injuries, and seminiferous tubular failure is found after infections such as mumps, gonococcal or lepromatous orchitis, irradiation, vascular injury, trauma, alcohol ingestion, and use of chemotherapeutic drugs, especially alkylating agents. The serum FSH concentrations may be normal or elevated, depending on the degree of damage to the seminiferous tubules. The Leydig cell compartment may also be damaged by these same conditions. In addition, some men experience a gradual decline in testicular function as they age, possibly because of microvascular insufficiency. The decreased testosterone production may be clinically manifest by lowered libido and potency, emotional lability, fatigue, and vasomotor symptoms such as hot flushes. The serum LH concentration is usually elevated in this situation.

DEFECTS IN ANDROGEN ACTION

When either testosterone or its metabolite, dihydrotestosterone, binds to the androgen receptor in target cells, the receptor is activated and binds DNA, with resulting stimulation of transcription, protein synthesis, and cell growth, which collectively constitutes androgen action. An absence of androgen receptors causes the syndrome of *testicular feminization,* a form of male pseudohermaphroditism. These genetic males have cryptorchid testes but appear to be phenotypic females. Because androgens are inactive during embryogenesis, the labial-scrotal folds fail to fuse, and a short vagina results. The fallopian tubes, uterus, and upper portion of the vagina are absent because the testes secrete müllerian duct inhibitory factor during early fetal development. At puberty, these patients have breast enlargement because the testes secrete a small amount of estradiol, and peripheral tissues convert testosterone as well as adrenal androgens to estrogens. Axillary hair and pubic hair do not grow, because androgen action is required for development. The serum testosterone concentrations are elevated as a result of continuous stimulation by LH, the concentrations of which are raised because of the inability of the testosterone to act in a negative feedback fashion at the hypothalamic level. Patients may have incomplete forms of androgen insensitivity caused by point mutations affecting the androgen receptor gene, and clinically these patients show varying degrees of male pseudohermaphroditism.

Patients who lack the 5α-reductase enzyme required to convert testosterone to dihydrotestosterone are born with a *bifid scrotum,* which reflects abnormal fusion of the labial-scrotal folds, and *hypospadias,* in which the urethral opening is in the perineal area or in the shaft of the penis. At puberty, androgen production is sufficient to partially overcome the defect; the scrotum, phallus, and muscle mass enlarge; and these patients appear to develop into physiologically normal men.

DIAGNOSIS

Figure 67–2 presents an algorithm for the laboratory evaluation of hypogonadism in a phenotypic male. Serum concentrations of LH, FSH, and testosterone should be obtained, and a semen analysis should be performed. A low testosterone level with low concentrations of gonadotropins indicates a hypothalamic-pituitary abnormality, which needs to be evaluated with serum prolactin determination and radiographic examination. Elevated concentrations of gonadotropins with a normal or low testosterone level reflect a primary testicular abnormality. If no testes are palpable in the scrotum and careful "milking" of the patient's lower abdomen does not bring retractile testes into the scrotum, then an hCG stimulation test should be performed. A rise in serum testosterone concentrations indicates the presence of functional testicular tissue, and a diagnosis of cryptorchidism can be made. An absence of a rise in testosterone levels suggests bilateral anorchia. Small, firm testes present in the scrotum are highly suggestive of Klinefelter's syndrome; this diagnosis needs to be confirmed with a chromosomal karyotype. Testes more than 3.5 cm in the longest diameter that are of normal consistency or are soft indicate postpubertal acquired primary hypogonadism. If the major abnormality is a deficient sperm count with or without an elevation of FSH, then one must differentiate between a ductal problem and acquired primary hypogonadism. When spermatozoa are present, then at least the ducts emanating from one testicle are patent; this condition indicates an acquired testicular defect. If the patient has no sperm in the ejaculate, this condition may be caused by a primary testicular problem or a ductal problem. The seminal vesicles secrete fructose into the seminal fluid. Therefore, the presence of fructose in the ejaculate should be followed by a testicular biopsy to see whether the defect results from spermatogenic failure or from obstruction of the ducts leading from the testes to the seminal vesicles. Absence of seminal fluid fructose indicates a congenital absence of the seminal vesicles and vas deferens.

MALE INFERTILITY

Infertility affects approximately 15% of couples, and male factors appear to be responsible in approximately 40% of cases. Female factors account for another 40%, whereas a couple factor is present in approximately 20% of cases. In addition to the defects in spermatogenesis that occur in patients with hypothalamic, pituitary, testicular, or androgen action disorders, hyperthyroidism, hypothyroidism, adrenal abnormalities, and systemic ill-

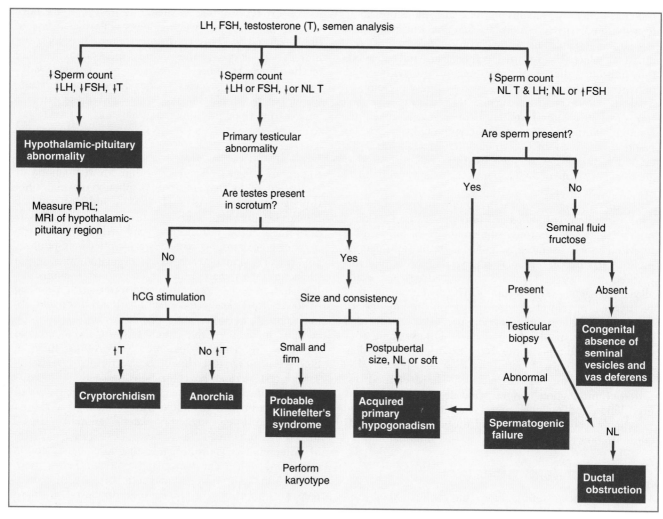

FIGURE 67–2 Laboratory evaluation of hypogonadism. FSH = follicle-stimulating hormone; hCG = human chorionic gonadotropin; LH = luteinizing hormone; MRI = magnetic resonance imaging; NL = normal; PRL = prolactin; ↑ = elevated; ↓ = decreased or low.

nesses may also result in defective spermatogenesis. Disorders of the vas deferens, seminal vesicles, and prostate may also lead to infertility, as can diseases affecting the bladder sphincter that may result in *retrograde ejaculation,* in which the sperm passes into the bladder rather than through the penis. Anatomic defects of the penis, as seen in patients with hypospadias, poor coital technique, and the presence of antisperm antibodies in the male or female genital tract also are associated with infertility.

THERAPY FOR HYPOGONADISM AND INFERTILITY

Treatment of androgen deficiency in patients who have hypothalamic-pituitary or primary testicular abnormalities is best accomplished with exogenous testosterone administration, either through intramuscular injection of intermediate-acting testosterone esters or with a transdermal testosterone patch. Testosterone therapy in-

creases libido, potency, muscle mass, strength, athletic endurance, and hair growth on the face and body. Side effects include acne, fluid retention, erythrocytosis, and, rarely, sleep apnea. This therapy is contraindicated in patients with cancer of the prostate.

If fertility is desired, patients with hypothalamic abnormalities may develop virilization and spermatogenesis with the use of GnRH given in a pulsatile fashion subcutaneously with an external pump. Direct stimulation of the testes in patients with hypothalamic or pituitary abnormalities may be accomplished with the use of exogenous gonadotropins, which increase testosterone and sperm production. If primary testicular failure is present and the patient has oligospermia, then an attempt can be made to concentrate the sperm for intrauterine insemination or in vitro fertilization. If the azoospermia is due to ductal obstruction, then repair of the obstruction may be undertaken, or aspiration of sperm from the epididymis may be accomplished for in vitro fertilization.

Erectile Dysfunction

Normal erection requires an intact central nervous system that allows psychogenic and sensory stimuli to be integrated and transmitted to the sympathetic nervous system that controls penile blood flow, patent arterial blood vessels capable of dilating and delivering blood to the penis, a normal corpora cavernosa sinus system that can become engorged with blood, an anatomically normal penis, and competence of the venous drainage system that does not leak blood from the penis during erection. The hypothalamic-pituitary-testicular axis must also be normal because testosterone is required for maintenance of normal libido and has a permissive effect in regard to erection. Thus, neurologic, vascular, urogenital, and endocrine abnormalities may result in erectile dysfunction (ED), which can span the spectrum from a total inability to obtain and maintain an erection to the ability to obtain an erection but not to maintain it long enough to complete sexual activity. *Diabetes mellitus* is one of the most common endocrine abnormalities associated with ED; at all ages, the prevalence of ED is higher in patients with diabetes than in the population at large. Numerous drugs have also been associated with ED, including antihypertensive agents, diuretics, tranquilizers, tricyclic antidepressants, H_2-receptor antagonists, antiandrogens, tobacco, alcohol, opiates, amphetamines, and cocaine.

Approximately 80% of patients with ED develop the condition because of a drug or an underlying organic illness, whereas the other 20% have a primary psychogenic cause. Organic ED generally results in a gradual and total loss of potency, with maintenance of normal libido until a secondary psychogenic decrease occurs. Conversely, patients who have psychogenic ED often have erections under some circumstances but not in others and generally have an acute onset of sexual dysfunction temporarily related to a significant life event.

Because physiologically normal men have three to five erections per night during rapid eye movement sleep, nocturnal penile tumescence monitoring allows assessment of the neurologic pathways and vascular integrity of the penis. Both arterial blood supply and penile venous competence can be assessed through Doppler ultrasonography after the intracorporeal injection of prostaglandin E_1, which induces an erection.

Psychogenic ED may be treated with behavioral therapy, which is successful in approximately half these patients. Patients who develop ED while they are taking a prescription or recreational drug that is known to be associated with ED should discontinue the drug or should have their medication switched to one that is less likely to cause the disorder.

If ED persists, if it results from an organic illness, or if it is psychogenic in origin but cannot be corrected through behavioral therapy, prostaglandin E_1 effectively induces erections in up to 80% of men. Sildenafil, which inhibits penile cyclic guanosine monophosphate breakdown and results in cavernosal smooth muscle relaxation, is effective in about 70% of men. Sildenafil, taken 60 to 90 minutes before sexual intercourse, is widely used and has largely replaced a variety of vacuum devices and penile prostheses formerly used for ED.

Gynecomastia

Gynecomastia refers to a benign enlargement of the male breast resulting from proliferation of the glandular component. This common condition is found in as many as 70% of pubertal boys and in approximately one third of adults 50 to 80 years old. Estrogens stimulate and androgens inhibit breast glandular development. Thus, gynecomastia is the result of an imbalance between estrogen and androgen action at the breast tissue level. This condition may result from an absolute increase in free estrogens, a decrease in endogenous free androgens, androgen insensitivity of the tissues, or enhanced sensitivity of the breast tissue to estrogens. Table 67–2 lists the common conditions associated with gynecomastia.

Gynecomastia must be differentiated from fatty enlargement of the breasts without glandular proliferation and other disorders of the breasts, especially breast carcinoma. *Male breast cancer* usually presents as a unilateral, eccentric, hard or firm mass that is fixed to the underlying tissues. It may be associated with skin dimpling or retraction as well as crusting of the nipple or nipple discharge. In contrast, gynecomastia occurs concentrically around the nipple and is not fixed to the underlying structures.

TABLE 67–2   Conditions Associated with Gynecomastia

Physiologic
Neonatal
Pubertal
Involutional

Pathologic
Neoplasms
  Testicular
  Adrenal
  Ectopic production of human chorionic gonadotropin
Primary gonadal failure
Secondary hypogonadism
Enzyme defects in testosterone production
Androgen insensitivity syndromes
Liver disease
Malnutrition with refeeding
Dialysis
Hyperthyroidism
Excessive extraglandular aromatase activity
Drugs
  Estrogens and estrogen agonists
  Gonadotropins
  Antiandrogens or inhibitors of androgen synthesis
  Cytotoxic agents
  Alcohol
Idiopathic

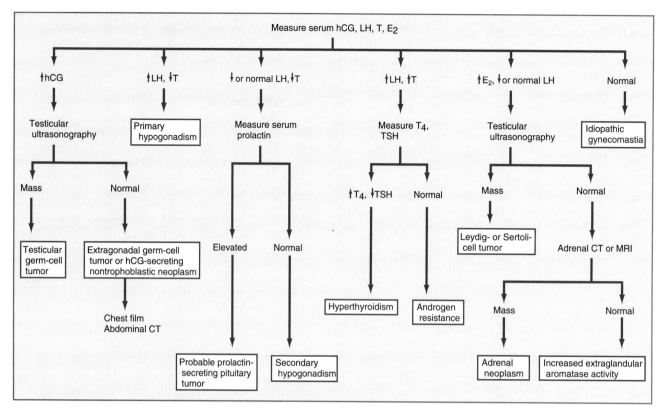

FIGURE 67–3 Diagnostic evaluation for causes of gynecomastia based on measurements of serum human chorionic gonadotropin (hCG), luteinizing hormone (LH), testosterone (T), and estradiol (E_2). CT = computed tomography; MRI = magnetic resonance imaging; T_4 = thyroxine; TSH = thyroid-stimulating hormone; ↑ = increased; ↓ = decreased. (From Braunstein GD: Gynecomastia. N Engl J Med 1993; 328:490–495. Reprinted by permission of *The New England Journal of Medicine*, Copyright 1993, Massachusetts Medical Society.)

Painful and tender gynecomastia in a pubertal male should be followed with periodic examinations, because in most patients, pubertal gynecomastia disappears within a year. Incidentially discovered, asymptomatic gynecomastia in an adult requires a careful assessment for the following: alcohol, drug, or medication use; liver, lung, or kidney dysfunction; and signs and symptoms of hypogonadism or hyperthyroidism. If these conditions are not present, then only follow-up is required. In contrast, in an adult with recent onset of progressive painful gynecomastia, thyroid, liver, and renal function should be determined. If test results are normal, then serum concentrations of hCG, LH, testosterone, and estradiol should be measured. Further evaluation should be carried out according to the scheme outlined in Figure 67–3.

Removal of the offending drug or correction of the underlying condition causing the gynecomastia may result in regression of the breast glandular tissue. If the gynecomastia persists, a trial of antiestrogens such as tamoxifen may be given for 3 months to see whether regression occurs. Gynecomastia that has been present for more than 1 year usually contains a fibrotic component that does not respond to medications. Therefore, correction usually requires surgical removal of the tissue.

Testicular Tumors

Testicular tumors represent 1% to 2% of malignant diseases in men and are the second most frequent cancer in men between the ages of 20 and 34 years. *Germ cell neoplasms* account for 95% of the tumors, whereas stromal or Leydig cell neoplasms account for the other 5%. Approximately one third to one half of germ cell tumors are seminomas, whereas the rest are composed of α-fetoprotein–secreting embryonal cell neoplasms, teratomas, or the rare hCG-secreting choriocarcinoma. These tumors generally present as a testicular enlargement, which may be associated with pain and tenderness. A few patients have gynecomastia, and fewer than 10% have symptoms of distant metastases at the time of presentation. These tumors are staged through measurements of hCG and α-fetoprotein, imaging studies, and surgery. Seminomas are radiosensitive, and orchiectomy and local radiation therapy may effect a cure. Disseminated disease is treated with both radiation therapy and chemotherapy. Patients with localized disease have a 5-year survival rate close to 100%, a rate that drops to approximately 20% in patients with widely disseminated disease. Nonseminomatous germ cell tumors are treated with surgery, radiation, and combination chemotherapy.

Aggressive therapy is associated with 5-year survival rates of between 60% and 90%.

Leydig cell tumors also present as a testicular mass and, in some patients, gynecomastia. In children, the tumors are often associated with precocious sexual development. Most are benign, and orchiectomy is curative.

Testicular tumors must be differentiated from inguinal hernias, epididymitis, orchitis, hematomas, hydrocele, and infiltrative disorders. An ultrasound evaluation enables the clinician to discriminate among many of these conditions.

Benign Prostatic Hyperplasia

Adenomatous enlargement of the prostate is present in most men older than 55 years, close to two thirds of whom have symptoms of *prostatism.* These symptoms can be divided into those related to obstruction, such as decreased force of the urine stream, urinary retention, and renal insufficiency, and those related to irritative symptoms from abnormal bladder function. The latter group includes nocturia, frequency, a sensation of incomplete voiding, urgency, and urinary incontinence. An enlarged prostate is usually found on physical examination, although significant obstructive symptoms can occur in patients with periurethral enlargement that may not be felt on digital examination of the prostate.

The mainstay of therapy for benign prostatic hyperplasia has been surgical resection of the prostate, either transurethrally or through open prostatectomy. Significant complications of surgery include incontinence, impotence, retrograde ejaculation, and bladder neck contractures. The two most commonly used medical therapies are inhibition of dihydrotestosterone production in the prostate through the use of a 5α-reductase inhibitor, finasteride, which decreases prostate volume by an average of 20% over 3 to 6 months, and the α-adrenergic blocking drugs terazosin and doxazosin, which relax the smooth muscle component of the prostate and decrease bladder outlet obstruction.

Carcinoma of the Prostate

Next to skin cancers, prostate cancers are the second most common tumors in men. Approximately 200,000 new cases are diagnosed each year, and the disease is more common among African-Americans and men with a strong family history of prostate cancer.

Early prostate cancer is asymptomatic and may be detected by routine digital examination or elevation of prostate-specific antigen (PSA), or it may be found in tissue obtained from surgery performed to relieve symptoms associated with benign prostatic hyperplasia. Because prostate cancer is so common in men in the United States, many screening strategies have been developed. Available evidence suggests that men aged 50

to 69 years derive the greatest benefit from screening, whereas men older than 69 years gain little. The probability that a man older than 50 years has prostate cancer if the PSA level is higher than 4.0 ng/mL is approximately 25%. The positive predictive value of PSA screening is increased by a digital rectal examination, which should be performed whenever a screening PSA test is obtained. A PSA level higher than 4.0 ng/mL, especially in the patient with a prostate mass detected on digital rectal examination, should lead to transrectal ultrasonography, followed in most cases by transrectal needle biopsy. Prostate cancer is staged by radiographic assessment of local disease with transrectal ultrasonography or magnetic resonance imaging, tumor marker assessment with quantitative serum PSA and acid phosphatase measurements, and bone scans for detection of bone metastases. If the disease appears to be localized to the prostate area, then staging pelvic lymphadenectomy may be performed to assess regional lymph node involvement. Locally invasive disease may cause urinary obstruction, with symptoms similar to those of benign prostatic hyperplasia, or it may obstruct the ureters and may lead to hydronephrosis and uremia. Unfortunately, many patients present with symptoms of metastatic disease, such as bone pain or pathologic fractures.

Therapeutic approaches include radical prostatectomy, radiation therapy, hormonal therapy, and chemotherapy. For a clinically unapparent, incidentally found tumor in a patient whose life expectancy is less than 10 years because of age or concurrent illness, watchful waiting alone is reasonable. For patients whose projected life expectancy is more than 10 years, watchful waiting, radical prostatectomy, and radiation therapy are current options. Radical prostatectomy, radiation therapy, or hormonal therapy is appropriate for patients whose tumors are confined to the prostate, with the choice determined by the degree of histologic differentiation of the tumor. Radiation therapy is generally used for patients with locally advanced disease that has extended outside the prostate. Patients with disseminated disease are usually treated with hormonal therapy. Because prostate cancer is androgen sensitive, hormonal therapy is directed at lowering serum testosterone levels. This end can be achieved through surgical or medical castration. Medical castration can be accomplished by giving the patient large doses of estrogen in the form of diethylstilbestrol or, more commonly, through a long-acting analogue of GnRH, which brings about down-regulation of the GnRH receptors on the pituitary gonadotrophs and leads to a lowering of LH and FSH levels and a subsequent decrease of testosterone. Some physicians prefer to perform total androgen blockade by combining a GnRH agonist with an androgen receptor antagonist, such as flutamide. However, that this combination is superior to GnRH agonist therapy alone is not clear. Chemotherapy has had limited success in patients with hormone-refractory metastatic disease. Serial PSA determinations are useful in monitoring the effects of therapy. A rising or persistently elevated level of PSA indicates the presence of residual cancer.

REFERENCES

Bagatell CJ, Bremner WJ: Androgens in men: Uses and abuses. N Engl J Med 1996; 334:707.

Braunstein GD: Testes. *In* Greenspan FS, Baxter J (eds): Basic and Clinical Endocrinology. Norwalk, CT: Appleton & Lange, 1994, pp 391–418.

Coley CM, Barry MJ, Mulley AG: ACP Clinical Guidelines. Part III: Screening for prostate cancer. Ann Intern Med 1997; 126:480–484.

Korenman SG: New insights into erectile dysfunction: A practical approach. Am J Med 1998; 105:135.

Mathur R, Braunstein GD: Gynecomastia: Pathomechanisms and treatment strategies. Horm Res 1997; 48:95.

Smyth CM, Bremner WJ: Klinefelter syndrome. Arch Intern Med 1998; 158:1309.

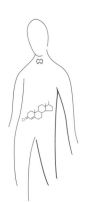

68

DIABETES MELLITUS

Philip Barnett and Glenn D. Braunstein

Definition

Diabetes mellitus comprises a heterogeneous group of metabolic diseases that are characterized by chronic hyperglycemia and disturbances in carbohydrate, lipid, and protein metabolism. These diseases result from defects in insulin secretion, insulin action, or both. Fasting or chronic hyperglycemia and postprandial hyperglycemia are mainly responsible for the acute, short-term, and late complications of this chronic disease, which affect all body organs and systems.

United States population statistics for 1997 estimated that the prevalence of diabetes in adults 20 years of age or older was similar in both sexes, and 15.7 million people had the disease (7.8%); 5.4 million of these people had undiagnosed diabetes. Diabetes, the sixth leading cause of death by disease in the United States, accounts for almost 18% of all deaths in people over 25 years of age, and it is the leading cause of end-stage renal disease (ESRD), new cases of blindness, and nontraumatic lower limb amputations. Cardiovascular disease is the major cause of diabetes-related death and is two to four times more common in patients with diabetes than in the general population. The risk of stroke is also increased. Life expectancy in middle-aged patients is reduced by 5 to 10 years. The prevalence of diabetes worldwide is reaching epidemic proportions, in large part because of increased obesity and sedentary lifestyles in both adults and children.

Diagnosis

Presentation of patients with diabetes depends on the type of diabetes and the stage of the pathologic process. Patients with *type 1 diabetes* commonly present with the classic acute symptoms of hyperglycemia: polydipsia, polyuria, weight loss, and, less frequently, polyphagia, blurred vision, and pruritus. Twenty-five percent present for the first time with diabetic ketoacidosis (DKA). In patients with *type 2 diabetes,* the disease is often present for many years (on average, 4 to 7 years) before diagnosis. The symptoms are usually less acute than in type 1 diabetes, and they may be accompanied by lethargy and fatigue in this generally older population. Chronic hyperglycemia may be associated with impairment of growth, susceptibility to infections (e.g., balanitis, vaginitis), and slow wound healing. Risk factors for type 2 diabetes are listed in Table 68–1 and include sedentary lifestyle and poor nutrition.

The criteria for diagnosing diabetes have been revised and simplified (Table 68–2). Any of the three serum glucose measurements listed in the table under diabetes mellitus may be used for diagnosis, and must be confirmed, on a subsequent day, by any one of the three. The revised diagnostic *fasting plasma glucose* (FPG) correlates with the 2-hour postload glucose cutoff point and causes fewer patients to have undiagnosed and misdiagnosed diabetes. These values identify a critical level at which the prevalence of microvascular complications increases dramatically.

Although the *oral glucose tolerance test* (OGTT) remains the standard for diagnostic purposes, measurement of FPG, which is simpler, cheaper, equally accurate, faster to perform, more reproducible, and convenient, is now recommended for routine diagnostic use. Although measurement of the *glycosylated hemoglobin* (HbA$_{1c}$) is a useful tool for monitoring glycemia and for making therapeutic decisions, it is not yet recommended for the diagnosis of diabetes. The OGTT is still used for diagnosing gestational diabetes (Table 68–3).

Some people (13.4 million, or 6.9% of the United States' population) have blood glucose levels higher than normal but do not fulfill the criteria for the diagnosis of diabetes. They are generally euglycemic and have an abnormal glucose response only when they are challenged with an OGTT. Depending on the diagnostic test used, this group or stage is referred to as either having *impaired fasting glucose* or *impaired glucose tolerance* (see Table 68–2). These persons are at increased risk of developing type 2 diabetes (7% per year) and its complications, particularly cardiovascular. The lower cutoff values for normality (previously FPG <115 mg/dL [6.4

TABLE 68–1   Criteria for Screening for Diabetes in Asymptomatic, High-Risk Persons

1. Testing for diabetes should be considered in all persons at ≥45 years and, if results are normal, should be repeated at 3-year intervals.
2. Testing should be considered at a younger age or should be carried out more frequently in individuals who
   a. Are overweight (≥20% above "ideal" body weight or a BMI ≥ 25 kg/m²*) or who have central obesity with normal BMI (22–24.9).
   b. Have a first-degree relative with diabetes (i.e., parent or sibling).
   c. Are members of a high-risk ethnic population (e.g., African-American, Hispanic-American, Native American, Asian-American, Pacific Islander).
   d. Have delivered a baby weighing >9 lb (4 kg) or with unexplained perinatal death or who have been diagnosed with gestational diabetes.
   e. Are hypertensive (≥140/90 mm Hg).
   f. Have an HDL cholesterol level ≤35 mg/dL (0.9 mmol/L) and/or a triglyceride level ≥250 mg/dL (2.82 mmol/L).
   g. On previous testing, had impaired glucose tolerance or impaired fasting glucose.

* National Institutes of Health guidelines define overweight as a BMI 25–29.9 kg/m² and obesity as a BMI ≥ 30 kg/m².
Adapted from the American Diabetes Association: Clinical practice guidelines 2000. Diabetes Care 2000; 23(Suppl 1):S4–S23.

TABLE 68–3   Screening and Diagnostic Criteria for Gestational Diabetes Mellitus

Plasma Glucose	50-g Screening Test (mg/dL)	100-g Diagnostic Test (mg/dL)
Fasting	—	95
1 h	140	180
2 h	—	155 √
3 h	—	140

From the American Diabetes Association: Clinical practice guidelines 2000. Diabetes Care 2000; 23(Suppl 1):S77–S79.

mmol/L]), and for the diagnosis of diabetes (previously FPG >140 mg/dL [7.8 mmol/L]) set new levels for earlier and more aggressive diabetes therapy, in an attempt to prevent these complications.

SCREENING FOR DIABETES IN PRESUMABLY HEALTHY PEOPLE

Screening for type 1 diabetes involves the measurement of autoantibody markers (islet cell antibody, insulin autoantibodies, glutamic acid decarboxylase, tyrosine phosphatase). Several reasons, such as lack of established cutoff values for immune markers, lack of consensus regarding effective therapy for patients with positive test results, lack of cost effectiveness, mitigate against the routine screening of both healthy children in the general population and those at high risk of developing type 1 diabetes (siblings of patients with type 1 diabetes).

Screening of certain high-risk populations for type 2 diabetes (see Table 68–1) is considered cost effective. More than one third of people with type 2 diabetes have undiagnosed disease. Because of the insidious nature of type 2 diabetes, patients have a high risk of developing complications by the time of clinical diagnosis (25% of patients with newly diagnosed type 2 diabetes have evidence of retinopathy). Early diagnosis and treatment may reduce the burden of this disease, its complications, and associated comorbidities, such as dyslipidemia, hypertension, and obesity.

Gestational diabetes mellitus refers to the presence of glucose intolerance that develops during pregnancy and returns to normal after delivery. It occurs in 2% to 5% of all pregnancies, but it may complicate as many as 14% in certain populations. If this condition is not diagnosed, or if it is left untreated, the consequences for both mother and fetus may be severe. Revised guidelines for determining who needs to be screened between 24 and 28 weeks of pregnancy for the presence of gestational diabetes include all women more than 25 years old and those younger women who fulfill one or more of the criteria in item 2, points a to d, of Table 68–1. Women at extremely high risk should be screened at their initial obstetric visit. A positive screening test, with non-FPG of 140 mg/dL (7.8 mmol/L) or more 1 hour after a 50-g glucose challenge, dictates the need for further diagnostic testing with a 3-hour, 100-g OGTT performed in the fasting state. The presence of

TABLE 68–2   Criteria for the Diagnosis of Diabetes Mellitus

	Normal	Impaired Fasting Glucose	Impaired Glucose Tolerance	Diabetes Mellitus
Fasting plasma glucose* (mg/dL)	<110 (6.1)	≥110 and <126	—	≥126 (7.0)
2-Hour postload glucose (mg/dL)†	<140 (7.8)	—	≥140 and <200	≥200 (11.1)
Random plasma glucose (mg/dL)‡	—	—	—	≥200 with symptoms

* Fasting is defined as no solid or liquid food, except water, for at least 8 hours.
† The standard oral glucose tolerance test, as described by the World Health Organization, requires a 75-g anhydrous glucose load.
‡ Random refers to any time of day, unrelated to meals.
Numbers in parentheses indicate glucose values in mmol/L.
Adapted from American Diabetes Association: Clinical practice guidelines 2000. Diabetes Care 2000; 23(Suppl 1):S4–S19.

any two of the plasma glucose values listed in Table 68–3 is diagnostic of gestational diabetes mellitus. The physician should reclassify these women 6 weeks or more post partum, using the criteria listed in Table 68–2. About 25% of lean women, and up to 50% of obese women, will go on to develop overt diabetes over a 20-year period. Pregnancy serves as a provocative test and not as a risk factor for the future development of diabetes.

Classification

Improved understanding of the origin and pathogenesis of diabetes has made it possible to revise the classification of diabetes mellitus (Table 68–4). This revision contrasts with the previous classification, which was based mainly on therapeutic requirements: insulin-dependent diabetes mellitus (IDDM) or non–insulin-dependent diabetes mellitus (NIDDM), terms that have been eliminated. Any patient with diabetes may require insulin therapy at some stage of the disease, irrespective of the classification.

TYPES 1 AND 2 DIABETES

The underlying pathologic process in most patients with *type 1 diabetes* (5% to 10% of the population with diabetes) is autoimmune destruction of the pancreatic islet β cells with absolute loss of insulin secretion. The disease has are strong human leukocyte antigen (HLA) associations and numerous antibody markers of immune destruction (Table 68–5). In few patients with type 1 diabetes, the pathogenesis remains idiopathic. Those patients with β-cell destruction or failure resulting from an identifiable nonautoimmune causes are not included in this class. *Type 2 diabetes* (90% to 95% of the population with diabetes) results from variable combinations of insulin resistance and insulin secretory defects, with one or the other abnormality predominating in different patients.

Distinguishing between type 1 and type 2 diabetes is not always a simple process. Type 2 diabetes is diagnosed in children as young as 6 years and may account for as many as 25% to 33% of all new cases of diabetes diagnosed in adolescents 9 to 19 years of age; it is often associated with an increase in weight and a parallel decrease in physical activity. These adolescents may even present in DKA, before they ultimately achieve control of their disease with diet and oral antihyperglycemic agents. Type 1 diabetes can also occur in elderly patients. This condition has sometimes been described as *latent autoimmune diabetes mellitus in adults,* and it may account for many patients who require insulin and who were previously thought to have type 2 diabetes.

Hyperglycemia, the hallmark of diabetes, changes in degree over time and reflects the severity of the underlying pathogenic process (which may progress, regress, or remain static) and its treatment, but it does not signal an alteration in the *nature* of the process.

OTHER SPECIFIC TYPES OF DIABETES

These groups together account for 1% to 2% of patients with diabetes. Inheritance of *maturity-onset diabetes of the young* is autosomal dominant, and hyperglycemia appears before the age of 25 years.

Within the small group of *genetic insulin resistance states,* impaired insulin action is the result of either a defective insulin receptor molecule (type A insulin resistance, leprechaunism, Rabson-Mendenhall syndrome) or abnormalities in postreceptor signal transduction pathways (lipoatrophic diabetes). Destruction of the pancreas results in reduced insulin secretion, with subsequent development of diabetes.

Several *insulin counterregulatory hormones* (glucagon, catecholamines, cortisol, and growth hormone) that antagonize insulin action and increase insulin resistance precipitate diabetes when they are produced in excess. *Aldosterone* in excess, through induction of hypokalemia and increased *somatostatin* production by a neoplasm, may impair insulin secretion and may cause diabetes. The hyperglycemia in these cases resolves on successful removal of the responsible tumor.

The mechanism of *drug-induced* or *chemical-induced diabetes* depends on the offending agent: β-cell destruction (the rodenticide Vacor, intravenous pentamidine, α-interferon with autoantibodies), impaired insulin action (nicotinic acid, glucocorticoids), peripheral insulin resistance and impairment of conversion of proinsulin to insulin (protease inhibitors). In some forms of immune-mediated diabetes, anti-insulin receptor antibodies may be either blocking (causing insulin resistance), or stimulating (producing hypoglycemia).

INSULIN RESISTANCE SYNDROME

Also known as the *(pluri)metabolic syndrome, Reaven's syndrome,* and *syndrome X,* this condition is not a sub-

TABLE 68–4   Etiologic Classification of Diabetes Mellitus

Type 1 diabetes
   Immune mediated
   Idiopathic
Type 2 diabetes
Other specific types
   Genetic defects of β-cell function
   Genetic defects in insulin action
   Diseases of the exocrine pancreas
   Endocrinopathies
   Drug- or chemical-induced
   Infections
   Anti-insulin receptor antibodies
   Other genetic syndromes sometimes associated with diabetes
Gestational diabetes mellitus

Adapted from the American Diabetes Association: Clinical practice guidelines 2000. Diabetes Care 2000; 23(Suppl 1):S4–S19.

TABLE 68-5 General Comparison of the Two Most Common Types of Diabetes Mellitus

	Type 1	Type 2
Previous terminology	Insulin-dependent diabetes mellitus (IDDM), type I, juvenile-onset diabetes	Non–insulin-dependent diabetes mellitus, type II, adult-onset diabetes
Age of onset	Usually <30 yr, particularly childhood and adolescence, but any age	Usually >40 yr, but any age
Genetic predisposition	Moderate; environmental factors required for expression; 35%–50% concordance in monozygotic twins; several candidate genes proposed	Strong; 60%–90% concordance in monozygotic twins; many candidate genes proposed; some genes identified in maturity-onset diabetes of the young
Human leukocyte antigen associations	Linkage to DQA and DQB, influenced by DRB(3 and 4) [DR2 protective]	None known
Other associations	Autoimmune; Graves' disease, Hashimoto's thyroiditis, vitiligo, Addison's disease, pernicious anemia	Heterogenous group, ongoing subclassification based on identification of specific pathogenic processes and genetic defects
Precipitating and risk factors	Largely unknown; microbial, chemical, dietary, other	Age, obesity (central), sedentary lifestyle, previous gestational diabetes (see Table 68–1)
Findings at diagnosis	85%–90% of patients have one and usually more autoantibodies to ICA512/IA-2/IA-2β, GAD$_{65}$, insulin (IAA)	Possibly complications (microvascular and macrovascular) caused by significant preceeding asymptomatic period
Endogenous insulin levels	Low or absent	Usually present (relative deficiency), early hyperinsulinemia
Insulin resistance	Only with hyperglycemia	Mostly present
Prolonged fast	Hyperglycemia, ketoacidosis	Euglycemia
Stress, withdrawal of insulin	Ketoacidosis	Nonketotic hyperglycemia, occasionally ketoacidosis

GAD = glutamic acid decarboxylase; IA-2/IA-2β = tyrosine phosphatases; IAA = insulin autoantibodies; ICA = islet cell antibody; ICA512 = islet cell autoantigen 512 (fragment of IA-2).

class of diabetes mellitus, but it is closely associated with it and affects at least 50 to 75 million people in the United States. It is a constellation of clinical findings and laboratory abnormalities that include glucose intolerance, insulin resistance, hyperinsulinemia (compensatory), obesity (central; abdominal or visceral), dyslipidemia (hypertriglyceridemia, increased low-density lipoprotein [LDL], and/or low high-density lipoprotein [HDL]), hypertension, elevated plasminogen activator inhibitor-1, hyperuricemia, and endothelial dysfunction. This syndrome is associated with a greatly increased risk of atherosclerotic vascular disease.

Pathogenesis

TYPE 1 DIABETES

In most patients, type 1 diabetes is an autoimmune disease in which some environmental insult (microbial, chemical, dietary) triggers an autoimmune reaction in a genetically susceptible individual (HLA-DR3 and/or HLA-DR4 is present in 90% to 95% of patients with type 1 diabetes compared with 50% to 60% in the general population). Predominantly cell mediated, destruction of the β cells of the islets of Langerhans is associated with several autoantibodies to islet cell con-

stituents (see Table 68–5). These antibodies, some of which may occur secondary to release of antigens after β-cell death, serve as markers of the immune destruction. Figure 68–1 shows how the autoimmune process may be present for several years, with competing destruction and regeneration of β cells, before the disease becomes clinically apparent. At this time, the critical mass of remaining β cells ($\sim$p10%) is unable to sustain insulin secretion at a level sufficient to maintain normal blood glucose values. After diagnosis and institution of insulin therapy, patients usually have some degree of recovery of remaining β-cell function, so exogenous insulin requirements drop to extremely low levels (the "honeymoon" period). This period usually lasts for a couple of months, but in some patients it may be as long as a year. The patient should continue exogenous insulin administration throughout this time, even at extremely low doses. At the end of this period, β-cell insulin secretion eventually fails completely, and these patients become insulin dependent, with DKA developing in the absence of insulin replacement.

TYPE 2 DIABETES

Four main elements characterize the pathophysiology of this disease: insulin resistance, β-cell dysfunction, dysregulated hepatic glucose production (HGP), and abnormal intestinal glucose absorption. In the preclinical

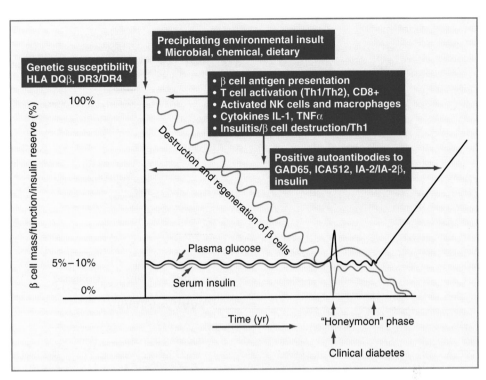

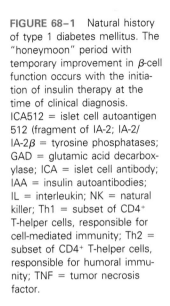

FIGURE 68-1 Natural history of type 1 diabetes mellitus. The "honeymoon" period with temporary improvement in β-cell function occurs with the initiation of insulin therapy at the time of clinical diagnosis. ICA512 = islet cell autoantigen 512 (fragment of IA-2; IA-2/IA-2β = tyrosine phosphatases; GAD = glutamic acid decarboxylase; ICA = islet cell antibody; IAA = insulin autoantibodies; IL = interleukin; NK = natural killer; Th1 = subset of CD4⁺ T-helper cells, responsible for cell-mediated immunity; Th2 = subset of CD4⁺ T-helper cells, responsible for humoral immunity; TNF = tumor necrosis factor.

phase, the pancreatic β cells compensate for a genetically predetermined peripheral *insulin resistance* (in muscle and fat) by producing more insulin (hyperinsulinemia) to maintain euglycemia. Some patients are identified at this stage while they are clinically asymptomatic. With time, the β cells gradually fail to compensate for the progressive increase in insulin resistance (stage of impaired glucose tolerance), and eventually hyperglycemia becomes clinically manifest as diabetes mellitus (Fig. 68–2). Insulin secretion is still present, but not in the hyperinsulinemic range, and the result is relative insulin deficiency. Classically, one notes early loss of the first phase of glucose-stimulated insulin secretion (peaking at 10 minutes), with subsequent gradual loss of the second phase (starting 30 minutes after glucose stimulus and peaking at 60 minutes). Other features of *β-cell dysfunction* include dysrhythmic pulsatile insulin secretion, defective glucose potentiation of nonglucose insulin secretagogues (the incretins: glucose-dependent insulinotropic polypeptide [GIP] and glucagon-like peptide-1 [GLP-1]), increased proinsulin-to-insulin ratio (from defective protease activity), accumulation of islet amyloid polypeptide, increased glucagon secretion from islet α cells, and "glucotoxicity." *Glucotoxicity* refers to the effect of chronic hyperglycemia in decreasing insulin secretion (through impaired β-cell sensitivity) and insulin activity (by increasing insulin resistance and insulin receptor tyrosine kinase activity). Glucotoxicity is a function of the duration and magnitude of the hyperglycemia and contributes to the progressive worsening of hyperglycemia. Elevated free fatty acid levels, the result of abnormal lipid metabolism in these patients, also have a toxic effect on β cells (lipo-

toxicity) and contribute further to the failure of these cells.

Before the appearance of fasting hyperglycemia, in the latter stages of hyperinsulinemia, one can usually show an *abnormality in postprandial glucose metabolism* (impaired glucose tolerance) that is not manifest clinically. The relative contributions of insulin resistance and insulin secretory defect to the pathogenesis in individual patients vary, with insulin resistance playing a dominant role in most patients who are obese (~80% to 90% in the United States) and failure of insulin secretion being more important in patients of normal weight.

The third contributing factor to hyperglycemia in type 2 diabetes is the *excessive HGP* (25% to 50% higher than normal) that results from inadequate suppression of hepatic gluconeogenesis, as a result of resistance of the liver to the inhibitory effects of insulin. Postprandial HGP is markedly increased, with a variable increase in the basal rate. Within the diabetic liver, decreased glycogen synthesis and increased fat synthesis also occur.

Hyperglycemia, with or without autonomic nerve involvement, may contribute to gastric dysmotility (symptomatic or not) and alterations in the rate of glucose absorption (usually increased), with consequent exacerbation of hyperglycemia, which results in a vicious cycle.

Amylin, a peptide hormone cosecreted with insulin from the pancreatic β cells, is thought to influence postprandial glycemic control by slowing the rate of gastric emptying and thus carbohydrate absorption and by suppressing glucagon secretion. With β-cell destruction (type 1), atrophy or "exhaustion" (type 2), the secretion of insulin and of amylin declines.

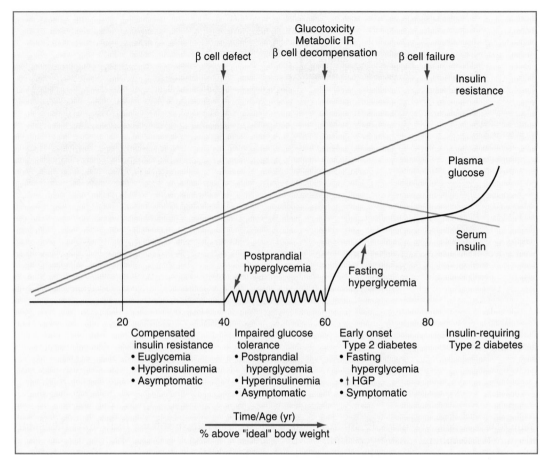

FIGURE 68–2 Natural history of type 2 diabetes mellitus. The similar numbers for age and percentage greater than "ideal" body weight are only approximate. Likewise, the age markers for the different phases of β-cell decompensation toward overt diabetes and an insulin-requiring state are approximate guides. Certain groups are more insulin sensitive and require a greater loss of β-cell function to precipitate diabetes than obese insulin-resistant people who develop diabetes after small declines in β-cell function. Use of insulin in patients with type 2 diabetes varies considerably and is not age dependent. Insulin resistance increases proportionately to adiposity, represented here by weight. HGP = hepatic glucose production; IR = insulin resistance.

Management

GOALS

The goals of management can be divided into three stages: (1) short term, involving immediate treatment to relieve symptoms such as polydipsia, polyuria, or acute infections; (2) intermediate, to return the patient to a physiologic state and a social life that are as normal as possible; and (3) long term, to prevent the development or to delay the progression of the complications of diabetes. People diagnosed with this chronic disease experience a whole range of emotions including denial, anger, guilt, and depression, and most require some form of psychological support.

The cornerstones of a comprehensive diabetes management plan include patient education, healthy nutrition, weight control, physical activity, self-monitoring of blood glucose (SMBG), and hypoglycemic agents when necessary. Patient education aims to empower patients by equipping them with the necessary knowledge about diabetes and self-management skills with which to make meaningful decisions about their health on a daily basis. Patient treatment needs to be individualized to specific medical, psychosocial, and lifestyle issues.

BLOOD GLUCOSE MONITORING

Control of blood glucose levels is the prime focus of the diabetes management plan, because hyperglycemia is a major contributor to the complications of diabetes. *SMBG* with blood glucose meters by all patients facilitates adjustments in treatment and acts as an educational tool. Ideally, during initiation or changes in therapy, SMBG should be performed while the patient is fasting, as well as preprandially, 2 hours postprandially (especially in gestational diabetes), at bedtime, and occasionally at 2 to 3 a.m., and values should be recorded.

The HbA_{1c}, by providing a measure of the average blood glucose level over the preceding 2 to 3 months, serves as an indicator of control of a patient's diabetes (Table 68–6). Caution must be exercised in using HbA_{1c} as the only gauge of diabetes control. Patients with wide fluctuations in blood glucose levels, with episodes of both marked hyperglycemia and hypoglycemia, may sometimes have normal average blood glucose levels, that is, normal HbA_{1c}. Records of SMBG are often more informative and useful for making therapeutic decisions. Measurement of serum *fructosamine* may be a useful marker for shorter-term assessment of integrated glucose concentrations (2 to 3 weeks).

STANDARDS OF CARE

Regular patient assessment includes weight, blood pressure, SMBG records, and foot examination at every office visit, with quarterly assessment of HbA_{1c}. Determination of microalbuminuria, measurement of serum creatinine levels, and a dilated retinal examination should be performed yearly. After the initial measurement of serum lipids, the frequency of reevaluation is dictated by results and treatment and should be at least yearly. Blood glucose goals for glycemic control are listed in Table 68–6. Goals for lipid levels are influenced by cardiovascular risk factors (see Chapter 9). Optimal values for patients with type 2 diabetes are as follows: LDL cholesterol, 100 mg/dL (2.6 mmol/L) or less; HDL cholesterol, more than 45 mg/dL (1.15 mmol/L) for men and 55 mg/dL (1.4 mmol/L) for women; and triglycerides, less than 200 mg/dL (2.3 mmol/L).

MEDICAL NUTRITION THERAPY

Medical nutrition therapy should be individualized to the patient's lifestyle, exercise regimen, financial resources, eating habits, and culture. General recommendations include consumption of a balanced, healthy diet, composed of the following: 10% to 20% protein, less than 30% fat (<10% saturated, <10% polyunsaturated, 10% to 15% monounsaturated), and 50% to 60% carbohydrate. Soluble fiber in the diet delays carbohydrate absorption (thus dampening the postprandial glucose peak) and improves serum lipid profiles.

Dietary adjustments are based on nutritional assessment, blood pressure, renal function, and HbA_{1c} measurements, as well as on diabetic treatment goals. The *glycemic index* refers to the increase in blood glucose level after ingestion of a particular food, expressed as a percentage of the increase after ingestion of the same amount of glucose. *Carbohydrate counting* involves using either a simple system of exchanges, or carbs (15-g carbohydrate portions), or the more precise carbohydrate gram counting. Training in nutrition self-management helps patients to make correct food choices, to plans meals and exercise, and to calculate bolus doses of insulin.

Alcohol is allowed in moderation (not more than two drinks for men, and one drink for women, per day; one alcoholic beverage is equivalent to 12 oz beer, 5 oz wine, or 1½ oz spirits) and should always be taken with food. Alcohol is not metabolized to glucose and inhibits gluconeogenesis, an effect that may result in hypoglycemia as late as 8 to 12 hours after consumption. Alcohol should not be substituted for food, but when alcohol calorie content needs to be calculated as part of a meal plan, it should be counted as fat calories (one alcoholic beverage = two fat exchanges).

WEIGHT MANAGEMENT THERAPY

Obesity is a major risk factor for type 2 diabetes and cardiovascular disease. *Healthy, reasonable, or achievable body weight* is a more realistic term than desirable or ideal body weight. A strong correlation exists between the risk of type 2 diabetes and increasing body mass index (BMI = weight (kg)/height (m^2). As little as 5% to 10% weight loss in overweight patients (BMI >25) reduces the risk of diabetes and leads to increased insulin sensitivity with improvement in glycemic control, sometimes to the extent that insulin therapy can be reduced or even stopped. This degree of weight loss also leads to significant improvements in dyslipidemia and blood pressure, as well as an increase in longevity.

EXERCISE THERAPY

As with nutrition and weight management, *exercise* is recognized as a specific therapy for patients with diabetes. Benefits include improvements in the sense of well-being, cardiovascular fitness, blood pressure, insulin sensitivity, lipid profile (consistent reduction in very LDL [VLDL]), weight reduction and maintenance, and glycemic control. Regular, moderate physical activity for at

TABLE 68–6 Blood Glucose Goals for Glycemic Control in Patients with Diabetes*

Biochemical Index	Normal	Goal	Action Suggested
Preprandial/fasting glucose (mg/dL)†	<100	80–120	<80->140
Postprandial glucose (mg/dL)†	<140	<180	>180
Bedtime glucose (mg/dL)†	<110	100–140	<100->160
HbA_{1c} (%)	<6	<7	>8

* These values are generalized to the entire population of nonpregnant adults with diabetes. Glycosylated hemoglobin (HbA_{1c}) is referenced to a nondiabetic range of 4.0%–6.0% (mean, 5.0%; SD, 0.5%).
† Measurement of capillary blood glucose. Postprandial blood glucose = 1.5–2 hours after a meal. Adapted from American Diabetes Association: Clinical practice recommendations 2000. Diabetes Care 2000; 23(Suppl 1):S23.

least 30 minutes/day (can be divided into 10-minute sessions) is recommended. Medical evaluation is advised to determine the level of fitness and appropriate exercise, based on the presence and degree of microvascular and/or cardiovascular complications. Blood glucose levels should be measured before any exercise activity is initiated. Exercise should not be undertaken in patients with FPG more than 250 mg/dL (13.8 mmol/L) with ketones, or more than 300 mg/dL (16.6 mmol/L) without ketones, because this may precipitate DKA. If FPG is less than 100 mg/dL (5.5 mmol/L), exercise may result in hypoglycemia, and carbohydrate should be consumed in advance. With the initiation of an exercise program, SMBG should be performed every 30 minutes during exercise lasting longer than 30 to 45 minutes; glucose or carbohydrate may need to be consumed, depending on glucose levels.

"TIGHT CONTROL"

With few exceptions, the aim of achieving euglycemia *tight control* in all patients with diabetes is now supported by several large studies, particularly the Diabetes Control and Complications Trial (DCCT) and the United Kingdom Prospective Diabetes Study (UKPDS). The DCCT in patients with type 1 diabetes showed that, when compared with patients receiving standard care, intensive treatment prevented or slowed the onset and/or progression of the microvascular complications of diabetes: retinopathy by 76%, neuropathy by 60%, and proteinuria by 54%. The threefold increase in the incidence of significant hypoglycemia documented in this study should not deter attempts to achieve euglycemia. The study in patients with type 2 diabetes (UKPDS) showed an overall reduction in microvascular complications of 25% with tight control. Tight glycemic control in several other studies has been associated with statistically significant reductions in cardiovascular morbidity and mortality.

All relevant studies have demonstrated a continuous association between the risk of complications and the level of glycemia, with no glycemic threshold for complications higher than the normal glucose range. Every percentage point of decrease in HbA_{1c} is associated with a 40% reduction in the risk of complications in patients with type 1 diabetes and a 35% reduction in the risk of complications in patients with type 2 diabetes. Tight control of blood pressure significantly reduces the incidence of strokes, heart failure, microvascular complications, loss of vision, and diabetes-related deaths and supports the aggressive treatment of even mild to moderate hypertension in patients with diabetes, in an attempt to reduce blood pressure to less than 130/85 mm Hg (or 125/75 mm Hg in patients with renal insufficiency and proteinuric levels exceeding 1 g/24 hours). The reduction in microvascular complications with improved blood pressure control is independent of glycemic control.

Achieving tight control through intensive therapy requires regular, close follow-up with a comprehensive diabetes health care team. In patients with type 1 disease, the use of multiple daily insulin injections or the use of a programmable insulin infusion pump (continuous subcutaneous insulin infusion) is necessary to achieve glycemic control. In patients with type 2 diabetes, exercise, medical nutrition therapy, weight reduction, and oral antihyperglycemic agents may suffice, although these patients frequently need insulin.

Tight control may be inappropriate in infants and children under 13 years of age (no long-term studies to date) and in patients with a shortened life expectancy, with severe cardiovascular disease (in whom hypoglycemia may be deleterious), with end-stage microvascular disease, with minimal complications of diabetes for 20 to 25 years, and with recurrent hypoglycemia and/or hypoglycemia unawareness.

TYPE 1 DIABETES

Patients with type 1 diabetes have an absolute requirement of *insulin* for survival. This also applies to patients with diabetes resulting from total or near-total β-cell depletion, as seen in chronic pancreatitis. Insulin is also used by patients with type 2 diabetes when combination oral agents fail to achieve glucose targets and temporarily in some patients during serious infections or surgery. Up to 58% of patients with type 2 diabetes eventually require exogenous insulin. Seventy-six percent of all patients taking insulin have type 2 diabetes. In women with gestational diabetes, when diet and exercise fail to achieve acceptable blood glucose control, insulin is required because oral antihyperglycemic agents are contraindicated in pregnancy.

Most insulin preparations are manufactured enzymatically or by recombinant DNA technology, and most are available at a concentration of 100 U/mL (U-100). Based on pharmacodynamic properties, the types of insulin currently available are rapid-acting, short-acting, intermediate-acting, and long-acting preparations (Table 68–7). Insulin therapy is usually started in the outpatient setting unless DKA is the initial presentation of type 1 diabetes. Multiple different insulin regimens exist. The regimen of bedtime insulin (NPH) and daytime sulfonylurea therapy (BIDS) has been successful in patients with type 2 diabetes as regular therapy or as a transition stage from oral antidiabetic therapy to total insulin therapy.

Standard insulin therapy consists of one to two injections per day using intermediate-acting or long-acting insulin with or without regular or lispro insulin. This approach provides simplicity, relative safety, and ease of compliance. Premixed insulins such as 70/30 (70% NPH/30% regular) or 50/50, usually administered twice daily, provide ease of use but are less likely to achieve good glycemic control. A split or mixed regimen of NPH/regular or NPH/lispro twice daily (two thirds of the calculated total daily dose before breakfast and one third before dinner; at each time two thirds NPH and one third regular or lispro) dictates regular mealtimes and insulin injections.

Intensive insulin therapy refers to multiple (three or more) daily injections, using combinations of insulins, such as regular or lispro insulins three times daily, adjusted before meals, and NPH at bedtime, or through

TABLE 68-7 Types of Insulin

Insulin Type	Generic Name	Preprandial Injection Timing* (hr)	Onset* (hr)	Peak* (hr)	Duration* (hr)	Blood Glucose (BG) Nadir* (hr)
Rapid acting	Lispro†	0–0.2	0.2–0.5	0.5–2	<5	2–4
					4–8	3–7
Short acting	Regular	0.5–(1)	0.3–1	2–6	(≤16)	(Pre–next meal)
	Lente		1–2	4–12		
Intermediate acting	NPH	0.5–(1)	1–3	6–15	16–26	6–13
Long acting	Ultralente	0.5–(1)	4–6	8–30	24–36	10–28
Mixed, short/intermediate acting	70/30					
	50/50	0.5–(1)	0.5–1	3–12	16–24	3–12

* Times depend on several factors including dose, anatomic site of injection, method (SQ, IM, IV), duration of diabetes, degree of insulin resistance, level of activity, and body temperature. Some time ranges are wide to include data from several separate studies. Preprandial injection timing depends on premeal BG values as well as insulin type. If BG is low, may need to inject insulin and eat immediately (carbohydrate portion of meal first). If BG is high, may delay meal after insulin injection and eat carbohydrate portion last.

† Insulin analogue with reversal of lysine and proline at positions 28 and 29 on the β chain.

70/30 = 70% NPH, 30% regular; 50/50 = 50% NPH, 50% regular; NPH = neutral protamine Hagedorn.

continuous subcutaneous insulin infusion. By more closely approximating normal physiologic insulin delivery, patients are able to achieve better glycemic control and increasing lifestyle flexibility. NPH should be given at least 30 minutes before a meal and can be mixed with regular insulin in the same syringe. Ultralente insulin can be given in combination with regular insulin, but it should not be mixed in the same syringe because the zinc in the ultralente insulin delays the absorption of the regular insulin.

Calculating insulin dosages is still empirical. Starting doses of insulin vary from 0.15 to 0.5 U/kg/day depending on patient size and degree of glycemia, and they may ultimately be as high as 1.5 U/kg in patients with severe insulin resistance. The calculated total daily insulin requirement is then divided according to the administration regimen chosen. In general, 40% to 50% of the total daily dose provides basal requirements, and the remainder is divided between meals in a manner proportionate to the relative carbohydrate content of the meal calculated, or using the approximate ratio of 0.8 to 1.2 U/10 g carbohydrate (slightly more at breakfast): for example, prebreakfast (rapid or regular insulin), 15% to 25%; prelunch (rapid or regular insulin), 15%; predinner (rapid or regular insulin), 15% to 20%. Requirements are increased during intercurrent illness, pregnancy, and the adolescent growth spurt. On average, insulin doses are increased every 2 to 3 days, and increments can be by as much as 10% to 20% of the total daily dose. When blood glucose values rise to more than 250 mg/dL, one should check for ketones, which are readily detected in the urine.

Elevations of FPG may be caused by several factors. The *Somogyi effect* refers to rebound hyperglycemia that follows undetected hypoglycemia, commonly "nocturnal," in the early hours of the morning. The elevated FPG in this situation is treated by decreasing the preceding evening dose of insulin and/or by altering the timing of administration (from predinner to bedtime) and/or the type of insulin used, based on the expected time to maximal effect of the insulin. This approach

causes less hypoglycemia and prevents the rebound. In the *dawn phenomenon*, the nocturnal secretion of growth hormone is responsible for a nighttime-to-morning rise in blood glucose. This condition is treated by increasing the evening dose of insulin and/or by altering the timing of administration and/or the type of insulin used. Poor insulin injection technique is an extremely common reason for increasing insulin requirements or unexplained fluctuations in blood glucose values, despite adherence to a strict exercise and nutrition program. Use of different anatomic sites for injection may be responsible for variable and erratic insulin absorption, and repeated injection into a single site leads to local "resistance" through lipohypertrophy and tissue fibrosis.

TYPE 2 DIABETES

The aim of treatment of type 2 diabetes is to reverse insulin resistance, to control intestinal glucose absorption, to normalize HGP, to improve β-cell glucose sensing and insulin secretion, and ultimately to prevent the occurrence of long-term complications. Provided pharmacologic therapy is not required immediately, all patients should be given at least a 1-month trial of diet, exercise, and weight management. If this regimen does not lead to adequate blood glucose control, the physician will need to prescribe oral antihyperglycemic agents and/or insulin. Insulin may, in fact, be needed in symptomatic patients who have type 2 diabetes with FPG values exceeding 250 mg/dL. After FPG is controlled, one may be able to substitute an oral agent. Maximal-dose sulfonylurea therapy, with doses decreasing with improved control, has been used effectively as initial treatment in patients presenting with marked hyperglycemia.

The five classes of *oral antidiabetic agents* currently available are listed in Table 68–8. The sulfonylureas and meglitinides have similar mechanisms of action and may cause hypoglycemia, hence the term *oral hypoglycemic agents*. The other classes of oral agents each target a different pathologic process and are referred to as

TABLE 68-8   Oral Antidiabetic Agents as Monotherapy

	Sulfonylureas	Biguanides	α-Glucosidase Inhibitors	Thiazolidinediones	Meglitinides
Generic name	Glimepiride, glyburide, glipizide, chlorpropamide, tolbutamide	Metformin	Acarbose, miglitol	Troglitazone, rosiglitazone, pioglitazone	Repaglinide
Mode of action	↑↑ Pancreatic insulin secretion chronically	↓↓ HGP; ↓ peripheral IR; ↓ intestinal glucose absorption	Delays PP digestion of carbohydrates and absorption of glucose	↓↓ Peripheral IR; ↑↑ glucose disposal; ↓ HGP	↑↑ Pancreatic insulin secretion acutely
Preferred patient type	Diagnosis age >30 yr, lean, diabetes < 5 yr, insulinopenic	Overweight, IR, fasting hyperglycemia, dyslipidemia	PP hyperglycemia	Overweight, IR, dyslipidemia, renal dysfunction	PP hyperglycemia, insulinopenic
Therapeutic effects					
↓ HBA$_{1c}$* (%)	1–2	1–2	0.5–1	0.8–1	1–2
↓ FPG* (mg/dL)	50–70	50–80	15–30	25–50	40–80
↓ PPG* (mg/dL)	~90	80	40–50	—	30
Insulin levels	↑	—	—	—	↑
Weight	↑	–/↓	—	–/↑	↑
Lipids	—	↓ LDL ↓↓ TG	—	↑ Large "fluffy" LDL ↓↓ TG ↑ HDL	—
Side effects	Hypoglycemia	Diarrhea, lactic acidosis	Abdominal pain, flatulence, diarrhea	Idiosyncratic hepatotoxicity with troglitazone; edema	Hypoglycemia (low-risk)
Dose(s)/day	1–3	2–3	1–3	1	1–4+
Maximum daily dose (mg)	Depends on agent	2550	150 (<60-kg bw) 300 (>60-kg bw)	Depends on agent	16
Range/dose (mg)	Depends on agent	500–1000	25–50 (<60-kg bw) 25–100 (>60-kg bw)	Depends on agent	0.5–4
Optimal administration time	~30 min premeal (some with food, others on empty stomach)	With meal	With first bite of meal	With meal (breakfast)	Preferably < 15 (0–30 min) premeals (omit if no meal)
Main site of metabolism/excretion	Hepatic/renal, fecal	Not metabolized/renal	Only 2% absorbed/fecal	Hepatic/fecal	Hepatic/fecal

* Values combined from numerous studies; values are also dose dependent.

↑ = increased; ↓ = decreased; — = unchanged; bw = body weight; FPG = fasting plasma glucose; HDL = high-density lipoprotein; HGP = hepatic glucose production; IR = insulin resistance; LDL = low-density lipoprotein; PP = postprandial; PPG = postprandial plasma glucose; TG = triglyceride.

antihyperglycemic agents. Type 2 diabetes is a progressive disease, and monotherapy is seldom successful in the long term. Combination drug therapy using submaximal doses of two or more agents, including insulin, each targeting a different metabolic abnormality, has synergistic effects that may be far greater than the effects of any agent used alone at maximal dose. The incidence and severity of adverse events are also reduced. Therapy is initiated with one class of agent, depending on the patient's characteristics and the predominant pathogenic defect (see Table 68–8), and a second agent is added if adequate glycemic control is not achieved at one-fourth to three-fourths maximal dosage. This stepped-care approach is continued until target glucose goals are achieved. Regular blood glucose estimations allow timely increases in drug dosage and the addition of other agents as necessary.

Sulfonylureas

The principal action of these drugs is to stimulate endogenous insulin secretion from the pancreatic β cells. They also increase β-cell sensitivity to glucose and exert some influence in diminishing insulin resistance. The drugs differ in potency, time of onset, duration of action, plasma protein binding, absorption characteristics, route of metabolism, and excretion. At maximal dose, they are all equally effective (except tolbutamide) in lowering blood glucose levels. Primary failure to respond to sulfonylureas occurs in 20% to 25% of patients. Secondary failure occurs at the rate of 10% to 15% per year, in part because of progressive β-cell failure and insulin resistance and in part because of poor patient compliance. Replacing one agent with another in this class is unlikely to produce a substantially different effect, and it is not recommended. The risk of hypoglycemia, the major adverse effect, increases with increasing patient age, use of a preparation with a long half-life (e.g., chlorpropamide), and renal dysfunction. Weight gain is also a recognized side effect. Characteristics of patients best suited for sulfonylureas include diagnosis at an age over 30 years and disease present for less than 5 years, residual β-cell function, relative lack of obesity, and FPG less than 300 mg/dL (see Table 68–8).

Biguanides (Metformin)

The major mechanism of action of these insulin sensitizers is in reducing HGP by inhibiting gluconeogenesis. These drugs also increase anerobic glycolysis, enhance glucose uptake and utilization by muscle, and decrease intestinal glucose absorption. In addition to their glucose-lowering effect, these drugs are associated with weight loss (5 to 10 lb), possibly related to mild nausea and anorexia, a decrease in plasma insulin levels, and significant lipid-lowering effects (decreasing total cholesterol, LDL, and triglyceride by 10% to 20%). They are well suited for use in obese, hyperlipidemic patients with type 2 diabetes. Their use in patients with impaired glucose tolerance and the metabolic syndrome as prophylaxis against development of diabetes is under investigation. Primary failure rates are approximately 12%, and secondary failure rates are between 5% and 10%.

Major adverse effects are gastrointestinal or metabolic. Gastrointestinal side effects include metallic taste, anorexia, nausea, abdominal discomfort, and diarrhea; these effects are usually mild and transient, and they improve with reduction in dose and administration with meals. The major metabolic side effect is lactic acidosis, which most often occurs in patients with renal disease (creatinine, ≥ 1.5 mg/dL in men and ≥ 1.4 mg/dL in women), low cardiac output, impaired hepatic function, or excessive alcohol intake.

α-Glucosidase Inhibitors (Acarbose, Miglitol)

Within the small bowel lumen, these agents competitively inhibit the breakdown of complex carbohydrates by antagonizing pancreatic α-amylase and the microvillar brush border α-glucosidase enzymes; thus, they delay glucose absorption and dampen the postprandial glucose and insulin peaks, with modest effect on FPG levels. When acarbose is taken with the first bite of a carbohydrate-containing meal, only 1% to 2% of the drug is absorbed. Major common side effects are gastrointestinal, including bloating, abdominal discomfort, diarrhea, and flatulence. These effects occur at the initiation of therapy and may worsen with dose increases, but they commonly disappear with continued use. The side effects can be minimized by starting with an extremely low dose (25 mg or even 12.5 mg once daily) and increasing it gradually over several weeks to a maintenance dose of 50 to 100 mg tid depending on the patient's body weight (see Table 68–8). These agents do not cause hypoglycemia when they are used alone, but hypoglycemia may occur when they are used in combination with insulin, a sulfonylurea, or a meglitinide. Oral treatment of hypoglycemia during therapy with this agent consists of administering pure glucose, fructose, or lactose (not sucrose, maltose, or starch).

Thiazolidinediones (Troglitazone, Rosiglitazone, Pioglitazone)

These agents reduce insulin resistance, improve the peripheral action of insulin, and thereby reduce hyperglycemia by increasing glucose uptake and utilization in peripheral tissues and reducing HGP. Patients have a small improvement in serum lipids (decrease in triglycerides and free fatty acids, increased HDL, and increased large "fluffy" LDL). They have little effect in the presence of euglycemia and thus tend not to produce hypoglycemia when used alone. It takes up to 3 to 4 weeks to produce a clinical effect and 10 to 12 weeks for a full effect. Troglitazone's absorption is enhanced 30% to 85% when the drug is taken with food. Troglitazone has a 25% to 53% primary failure rate. When these drugs are used in conjunction with insulin therapy, they may facilitate a reduction in insulin dose or even its discontinuation. Troglitazone is currently approved only as an adjunct in patients taking insulin or sulfonylureas with or without metformin. Rosiglitazone may be given as monotherapy or with metformin, whereas pioglitazone may be used as monotherapy or with insulin, sulfonylureas, or metformin. A major side effect of troglitazone is liver dysfunction; this appears to be idiosyncratic and, in rare instances, has resulted in fatal liver failure. Most cases of liver dysfunction have occurred within the first 6 months of therapy; generally, hepatic enzyme levels return to normal on discontinuation of the drug. Serum transaminases need to be monitored frequently in patients using this class of drugs.

Meglitinides

The only agent currently clinically available in this class is *repaglinide*. Its mechanism of action is similar to that of the sulfonylureas in stimulating insulin secretion from the pancreas. The advantages of this class over the sulfonylureas are the rapid onset and short duration of action, which suppress postprandial hyperglycemia. The drug should be taken with meals and is omitted in the absence of a meal, a feature that permits flexibility of lifestyle. The stimulation of prandial insulin secretion avoids chronic stimulation of β cells and thus leads to less between-meal and nocturnal hyperinsulinemia, which is a feature of sulfonylurea therapy. Repaglinide appears to sensitize β cells to secrete more insulin in reponse to a given glucose level, and its insulin secretagogue action is glucose dependent. For this reason, hypoglycemia is seen less often than with sulfonylureas. Clinical response to this agent is seen in about 1 week. The drug may be prescribed in the presence of renal dysfunction. Combination therapy of a sulfonylurea with repaglinide is not recommended.

Complications

ACUTE COMPLICATIONS

Hypoglycemia

See Chapter 69.

Diabetic Ketoacidosis

Although DKA develops most commonly in patients with type 1 diabetes, it can be seen in patients with type 2 diabetes, especially during acute illness. DKA is defined as being present in patients with absolute or relative insulin deficiency when the following criteria are met:

1. *Hyperglycemia:* plasma glucose levels exceeding 250 mg/dL.
2. *Ketosis:* moderate to severe ketonemia (ketone levels positive at a serum dilution of $\geq 1:2$, or serum β-hydroxybutyrate concentration >0.5 mmol/L) and moderate ketonuria (2+ to 3+ by the nitroprusside method).
3. *Acidosis:* pH of 7.3 or less and/or bicarbonate of 15 mEq/L or less.

Associated metabolic and plasma abnormalities include the following: dehydration; increased osmolality, usually less than 320 mOsm/kg; increased anion gap exceeding 12 mEq/L; increased serum amylase; elevated white blood cell count; and hypertriglyceridemia.

Precipitating factors for DKA are infection (30%), often minor (respiratory or urinary tract), new-onset diabetes (25%), problems with insulin administration (20%), and a large number of less frequent causes. Insulin deficiency and raised insulin counterregulatory hormones result in increased HGP and decreased peripheral glucose utilization and lead to hyperglycemia and hyperosmolality with consequent osmotic diuresis, electrolyte loss (Na^+, K^+, PO_4^-, Mg^{2+}, Ca^{2+}, Cl^-), and dehydration. Activation of insulin-sensitive lipase stimulates free fatty acid release from adipose tissues, which are oxidized in the liver to produce ketone bodies. Diminished peripheral utilization of ketones during insulin deficiency results in ketosis and metabolic acidosis.

DKA develops within hours to days. Because the metabolic acidosis makes the patients feel ill, they generally seek early medical attention, a feature that accounts for the lower levels of glucose and osmolality compared with hyperosmolar nonketotic syndrome (HNKS) (see Table 68–10). DKA may not always be obvious at the time of presentation because early signs and symptoms are subtle. Symptoms include nausea or vomiting, thirst or polydipsia, polyuria, abdominal pain, weakness, fatigue, and anorexia. Signs include tachycardia, orthostatic hypotension, poor skin turgor, warm or dry skin and mucous membranes, hyperventilation or Kussmaul's respiration, hypothermia or normothermia, ketones on the breath, weight loss, and altered mental status or coma.

Initial assessment includes mental status, presence of gag or cough reflex, abdominal succussion splash (requiring nasogastric tube), and urinary output. The search for a precipitating cause (e.g., infection or sepsis, myocardial infarction, pregnancy, cerebrovascular accident, trauma, psychosocial factor) is crucial, both to treat the underlying disorders and to facilitate resolution of the DKA. Baseline investigations should include the following: plasma glucose, plasma acetone, serum electrolytes, serum lipid profile, serum amylase and lipase, full blood count with differential, arterial blood gas measurement, blood cultures, culture of abscess or infected site, urine glucose and ketones, urine microscopy and culture, chest radiograph, abdominal radiograph (with abdominal pain), electrocardiogram, cardiac enzymes (if appropriate), lumbar puncture (if appropriate), serum osmolality,* and anion gap.†

Most important in the therapy of DKA is the restoration of circulating plasma volume, with maintenance of cardiac output and renal function. Intravenous fluid therapy automatically results in lowering of blood glucose by enhancing urinary glucose loss and serum dilution, it lowers osmolality and ketones, and it improve the peripheral utilization of ketones and glucose. Insulin administration facilitates the peripheral uptake of ketones and glucose, decreases the urinary glucose loss, and, most important, inhibits HGP. Electrolyte imbalances (Table 68–9) should be corrected concurrently with fluid and insulin replacement and treatment of the precipitating cause. To track the course of treatment, several parameters require regular monitoring:

1. Hourly: vital signs, mental status, fluid intake and output, plasma glucose, arterial blood gases, electrocardiogram, temperature.
2. Every 1 to 2 hours: serum electrolytes (Na^+, K^+, Cl^-, HCO_3^-).
3. Every 6 hours: serum PO_4^-, Mg^{2+}, Ca^{2+}, blood urea nitrogen, and creatinine.

When the metabolic abnormalities have been corrected, the frequency of their measurements should be reduced appropriately.

Hyperosmolar Nonketotic Syndrome

HNKS occurs almost exclusively in patients with type 2 diabetes, who are usually elderly and physically impaired, with limited access to free water. The pathogenesis of HNKS is similar to that of DKA but may be distinguished from it by the more marked hyperglycemia and the relative absence of acidosis and ketonemia and the greater degree of dehydration (Table 68–10). Free fatty acid levels are low, and the result is the absence of ketone bodies, with less nausea and vomiting. Increased lactic acid levels result from poor tissue perfusion and are more marked than in DKA. Insulin resistance is usually present, with normal or elevated levels of serum insulin. As many as 30% to 40% of patients over 65 years of age presenting with HNKS

---

* Calculation of serum osmolality: $2[Na^+(mEq/L)] + 2[K^+(mEq/L)] +$ glucose (mg/dL)/18 + BUN (mg/dL)/2.8.
† Calculation of anion gap: $Na^+ - (Cl^- + HCO_3^-)$.

TABLE 68-9 Clinical Therapeutic Guidelines for Diabetic Ketoacidosis (DKA)

Insulin Infusion Therapy

1. Start with a 10-U bolus of regular insulin IV, followed immediately by a continuous IV insulin infusion at 0.1 U/kg/hr (if weight known), otherwise 6 U/hr.
2. If glucose concentration has not decreased by 10% in 2 hr and rehydration is appropriate, double the insulin infusion rate every 2 hr. Ensure no technical causes for lack of insulin effect.
3. Glucose concentration usually returns to near normal before acidosis clears and 5% dextrose is used as rehydration fluid to support glucose levels while therapy for acidosis with IV insulin continues.

Fluid Administration

1. *Type of Fluid*
   a. If serum sodium is 135–145 mEq/L and patient has orthostatic hypotension, administer normal saline (NS).
   b. If serum sodium is 135–145 mEq/L, with no orthostatic hypotension, administer ½ NS.
   c. If serum sodium is <135 mEq/L, administer NS (irrespective of orthostasis).
   d. If serum sodium is >145 mEq/L (irrespective of orthostasis) administer ½ NS.
2. *Rate of Administration*
   a. Initial rate = "wide open." Give 1 L/hr for first 1–2 hr. Decrease rate to 250–500 mL/hr as orthostatic changes disappear.
   b. If patient is in shock, use plasma expander (albumin) and consider dopamine. Rule out myocardial infarction and sepsis.
   c. If after 2–4 hr, volume status has improved, consider changing from NS to ½ NS to prevent hypernatremia. Monitor sodium closely.
   d. Switch to 5% dextrose containing solution when plasma glucose <250 mg/dL.

Potassium Replacement

Potassium replacement should be based on q2h serum measurements, with dosing as follows:

K Level (mEq/L)	KCl Replacement dose (mEq/hr)
<3.5	10
3.6–4.0	7.5
4.1–5.0	5.0
>5.1	0

ECG changes may provide a more rapid guide to K requirements than serum values.

Bicarbonate Therapy

Exercise extreme caution and only consider using if:
1. pH < 7.0 and patient in intractable shock after adequate fluid replacement.
2. Significant cardiac dysrhythmias present.
Provide bicarbonate as follows:
1. NEVER give as an IV bolus because they may precipitate hypokalemia.
2. For pH 6.9–7.0: infuse 44 mEq $NaHCO_3$ in 1 L of 0.45% saline/5% dextrose for 1 L/hr.
3. For pH < 6.9: infuse 88 mEq $NaHCO_3$ in 1 L of 0.45% saline/5% dextrose for 1 L/hr.

Resumption of Subcutaneous (SQ) Insulin Therapy

When patients can drink and eat light foods without difficulty, convert from continuous insulin infusion to SQ (preferably at breakfast or lunch). Restart SQ insulin at ½–⅔ of maintenance dose, 30 min before the meal. Discontinue insulin infusion 30–60 min after the meal. Consider 3 or 4 times/day insulin regimen. If the patient was not previously on insulin, calculate the approximate dose based on the preceding 24-hr requirements.

TABLE 68-10 A Comparison of Diabetic Ketoacidosis and Hyperosmolar Nonketotic Syndrome

Feature	Diabetic Ketoacidosis	Hyperosmolar Nonketotic Syndrome
Age of patient	Usually <40 yr	Usually >60 yr
Duration of symptoms	Usually <2 days	Usually >5 days
Plasma glucose	Usually <600 mg/dL	Usually >600 mg/dL
Serum sodium	Normal or low (130–140 mEq/L)	Normal or high (145–155 mEq/L)
Serum potassium	Normal or high (5–6 mEq/L)	Normal (4–5 mEq/L)
Serum bicarbonate	<15 mEq/L	>15 mEq/L
Ketone bodies	Positive at ≥1:2 dilution	Negative at 1:2 dilution
pH	<7.35	>7.3
Serum osmolality	Usually <320 mOsm/kg	Usually >320 mOsm/kg
Fluid deficit	≤10% body weight	≤15% body weight
Cerebral edema	Subclinical asymptomatic, rare clinically	Very rare
Prognosis	3%–10% mortality (>20% for people >65 yr)	10%–20% mortality
Subsequent course	Insulin therapy required in most cases	Insulin therapy not usually required

may have previously undiagnosed diabetes. HNKS usually develops insidiously over days to weeks. Precipitating and/or complicating factors may include infection, intestinal obstruction, mesenteric thrombosis, pulmonary embolism, peritoneal dialysis, heat stroke, hypothermia, subdural hematoma, severe burns, and an extensive list of drugs. Some of these conditions may themselves result from the severe dehydration and poor tissue perfusion in HNKS.

Therapy of HNKS follows the same general principles as that of DKA, with particular emphasis on intravenous fluid therapy and potassium replacement. Fluid replacement should follow the same pattern as in DKA, but a greater total volume is usually required. Careful monitoring is necessary because patients often have cardiac and other comorbid conditions. Restoration of the fluid deficit should proceed more slowly than in DKA, ideally over 36 to 72 hours. Insulin therapy should only be started after rehydration is in progress. These patients may be more sensitive to insulin and may require lower doses. In view of the severe dehydration and predisposition to vascular thrombosis, these patients should receive heparin prophylaxis (5000 U heparin subcutaneously, qid).

CHRONIC COMPLICATIONS

These include microvascular complications (nephropathy, retinopathy, neuropathy) and macrovascular or cardiovascular complications (hypertension, coronary artery disease, peripheral vascular disease, cerebrovascular disease). Several different mechanisms are responsible for the development of chronic complications and include activation of the polyol pathway (with accumulation of sorbitol), formation of glycated proteins and advanced glycation end products (cross-linked glycated proteins), abnormalities in lipid metabolism, increased oxidative damage, hyperinsulinemia, hyperperfusion of certain tissues, hyperviscosity, platelet dysfunction (increased aggregation), and activation of various growth factors.

Microvascular Complications

Nephropathy. *Diabetic nephropathy* is the most common cause of ESRD in developed countries and accounts for ~30% of cases. About 20% to 30% of people with type 1 and 2 diabetes develop nephropathy, and the incidence increases with duration of disease. Fewer people with type 2 diabetes progress to ESRD than with those with type 1 disease (20% versus 75%, respectively, after 20 years). Certain ethnic and racial groups have especially high prevalence rates of severe nephropathy (Native Americans, Mexican-Americans, and African-Americans).

Initially, increased glomerular filtration rate (GFR) and renal blood flow occur in all patients and are not associated with any histologic changes. This condition progresses to glomerular hypertrophy, renal enlargement, expansion of the mesangial matrix, and thickening of the glomerular basement membrane resulting in

glomerulosclerosis. Subsequently, the GFR returns to normal, with an associated increase in intraglomerular pressure and the appearance of microalbuminuria (20 to 200 μg/min; 30 to 300 mg/24 hours), 10 to 15 years after the diagnosis of diabetes. This *incipient* or *preclinical diabetic nephropathy* is followed by a decline in GFR as the albumin excretion rate increases.

At the stage of microalbuminuria, rigorous control of blood glucose and blood pressure (using an angiotensin II–converting enzyme inhibitor), or use of angiotensin-converting enzyme inhibitors in nonhypertensive subjects, can prevent or even reverse the progression toward renal failure. Angiotensin II receptor antagonists look promising but have not been approved for this use. β Blockers and calcium channel antagonists for control of hypertension in this setting are of uncertain value.

By about 15 years after the onset of diabetes, macroalbuminuria (>200 μg/min; >300 mg/24 hours; dipstick positive) is generally present; continued blood pressure control is essential, and some dietary protein restriction (0.6 to 0.8 g/kg/day) is probably helpful, but meticulous blood glucose control is unlikely to prevent the inexorable progression of overt diabetic nephropathy to ESRD. The rate of decline in GFR, however, may be slowed, but not halted, by blood pressure and glucose control and protein restriction. Measurement of serum creatinine is an inaccurate guide to the degree of reduction in GFR. Within 5 years of the appearance of macroalbuminuria, GFR will have declined by 50% in about 50% of patients; within a further 3 to 4 years, half of these patients will have ESRD. Dialysis (hemodialysis or peritoneal dialysis) or renal transplantation is initiated when the GFR is less than 15 mL/min (serum creatinine $\pm$ 10 mg/dL or more) (see Chapter 27).

Screening for proteinuria should be performed annually in all patients, starting at the time of diagnosis in type 2 diabetes and 5 years after the diagnosis in patients with type 1 disease. The simplest method of screening for microalbuminuria is measurement of the ratio of albumin to creatinine in a random spot urine specimen. This measurement correlates closely with 24-hour urinary protein estimations. The presence of microalbuminuria increases the risk of renal disease and is also a marker for macrovascular complications.

Retinopathy. The presence and severity of *diabetic retinopathy* are related to the age at diagnosis and the duration of diabetes; 100% are affected in type 1 and 60% to 80% are affected in type 2 diabetes by 20 years. This is the most common cause of blindness between the ages of 20 to 74 years in the developed world. Approximately 25% of patients with type 2 diabetes may already have evidence of retinopathy at the time of diagnosis. The incidence of this complications is increased in Mexican-Americans and in African-Americans.

Diabetic retinopathy is a progressive condition of increasing severity accelerated by poor glycemic control. *Background,* or *nonproliferative, retinopathy* consists of increased capillary permeability, dilation of venules, and the presence of microaneurysms (focal saccular and fusiform dilatations of capillary walls as sequelae of loss of supporting pericytes and ischemic occlusion of retinal capillaries). At this stage, hemorrhages deep in the retina appear as dots, whereas more superficial nerve fiber layer hemorrhages resemble flames or blots, or they are linear. Leakage of plasma through permeable and ischemic capillary walls leads to the formation of hard exudates, as the water is reabsorbed, leaving behind deep, intraretinal yellow deposits of proteins and lipids. These deposits may be present at any stage of diabetic retinopathy. Collections of hard exudates in a circular pattern (*circinates*) reflect the presence of retinal edema that pushes these exudates peripherally. When these exudates surround the macula, they highlight macular edema (*maculopathy*), a sight-threatening condition requiring urgent attention.

Venous occlusion results in beading, reduplication, and venous loops. Intraretinal microvascular abnormalities, which are abnormal dilated capillaries within the retina, result from widespread capillary occlusion. Superficial retinal microinfarcts result in hypoxic necrosis of retinal nerve fibers and appear as white, *cotton wool spots* with irregular margins. These changes signify a worsening of the retinopathy into the *preproliferative stage*. The widespread retinal ischemia and hypoxia represented by these changes result in the release of several angiogenic growth factors and lead to the development of new vessels (*neovascularization*) on the retina, optic disc, or iris (*rubeosis iridis*). This stage is referred to as *proliferative retinopathy* and is also characterized by scarring. The new vessels are extremely fragile; they extend through the internal limiting membrane and lie between the retina and vitreous, or they attach to the vitreous and extend into it. Bleeding into the preretinal (subhyaloid) space results in a hemorrhage shaped like a boat. Hemorrhage from new vessels in the vitreous may cause sudden loss of vision. Neovascularization and fibrosis at the angle of the anterior chamber prevent normal drainage of aqueous and lead to *neovascular glaucoma* and a blind, painful eye. Shrinkage and retraction of the vitreous from the retina, which occurs with age, may result in hemorrhage from neovascularization and traction on the retina from associated fibrous tissue. Further proliferation of fibrous tissue may lead to a traction retinal detachment with visual loss, which is most marked with macular involvement.

Premature development of *senile cataracts* occurs in patients with diabetes. *"Snowflake" lens opacities* develop in younger patients, particularly during periods of poor glycemic control.

Referral to an ophthalmologist for urgent argon laser therapy is mandatory in patients with proliferative retinopathy, diabetic maculopathy, and possibly preproliferative retinopathy. This therapy can be sightsaving. *Vitrectomy* may be performed in patients with extensive, long-standing, unresolving vitreal hemorrhage or when new traction retinal detachment affects the macula or is associated with a retinal tear.

Annual dilated fundoscopic examination by an ophthalmologist should be performed in all patients with diabetes, starting 5 years after diagnosis in patients with type 1 disease. With improvement of glycemic control after initiation of insulin therapy, retinopathy may transiently worsen, before ultimately improving over a longer period.

Neuropathy

The likelihood of involvement of the nervous system by diabetes increases with the duration of the disease and is influenced by the degree of glycemic control. Any part of the peripheral or autonomic nervous system may be affected. *Peripheral polyneuropathy* occurs most commonly. This usually presents as a bilaterally symmetric, distal, primarily sensory (with or without motor), polyneuropathy, with a "glove and stocking" distribution. Pain, numbness, hyperesthesias, and paresthesias progress to sensory loss; this condition, together with loss of proprioception, leads to an abnormal gait, with repeated trauma and fractures of the tarsal bones, sometimes resulting in the development of Charcot's joints. This change leads to abnormal pressure in the feet that, together with the soft tissue atrophy related to peripheral arterial insufficiency, results in foot ulcers that may progress to osteomyelitis and gangrene. Careful, detailed, regular neurologic examination of all patients is essential, to elicit the early loss of reflexes, vibratory sensation, and light touch (using a 5.07-μg monofilament). Painful neuropathies are difficult to treat, and although they are self-limiting, they may persist for years. Improvement in glycemic control should be the primary goal. Analgesia should start with aspirin, acetaminophen, and nonsteroidal anti-inflammatory agents before one prescribes codeine and more addictive drugs such as pentazocine or narcotics. Anticonvulsants including phenytoin, carbamazepine, and gabapentin, as well as the antidepressant amitriptyline, may provide moderate relief. Burning pain may respond to the topical application of capsaicin cream. Use of plastic skin (e.g., OpSite film), transcutaneous nerve stimulation, and nerve block are sometimes effective for chronic pain.

Mononeuropathies usually present acutely, may involve any nerve in the body, and are generally self-limiting. The cranial nerves most commonly involved are the third, sixth, and fourth, in that order. *Radiculopathies* are self-limiting painful sensory syndromes of one or more spinal nerves, usually of the chest or abdomen. *Diabetic amyotrophy* causing muscle atrophy and weakness commonly involves the anterior thigh muscles and pelvic girdle, and again it may be self-limiting, resolving after several months.

Autonomic neuropathy of the sympathetic and/or parasympathetic systems has numerous presentations. Most commonly involved is the gastrointestinal tract, with gastric dysmotility, gastroparesis with delayed emptying, constipation, and diarrhea (usually nocturnal). *Gastroparesis* may respond to treatment with metoclopramide, cisapride, or erythromycin (for bacterial overgrowth). *Diarrhea* may respond to loperamide or diphenoxylate and atropine. *Orthostatic hypotension* can be treated by attention to mechanical factors (elevated head of bed), by gradual rising from a lying to standing position (including use of support stockings), and sometimes by the use of fludrocortisone. *Cardiac rhythm disturbances* can result in syncope and cardiorespiratory arrest. *Bladder involvement* may result in urinary retention or incontinence. In men, *erectile dysfunction* is multifactorial and may also be related to vascular insufficiency or venous leaks.

Diabetic Foot

Care of the feet of patients with diabetes is extremely important, to prevent foot ulcers and amputations. Risk factors include distal symmetric polyneuropathy, peripheral arterial insufficiency, areas of increased pressure, limited joint mobility and bony deformities, obesity, and chronic hyperglycemia. Patient education about foot care includes advice on daily foot inspection, appropriate footware, drying and nail cutting, and referral to a podiatrist when necessary. Early detection and treatment of blisters, ulcers, trauma, and cellulitis may prevent progression to osteomyelitis and amputation. Treatment of ulcers may include antibiotics, debridement, growth-stimulating factors, reduction of weight bearing (elevation, casting), and improvement in arterial supply (surgical, medical).

Macrovascular Complications

These complications are cardiovascular and cerebrovascular diseases including hypertension, myocardial ischemia and infarction, transient ischemic attacks and stroke, and peripheral vascular disease. The pathogenesis of *atherosclerosis* and *vascular thrombosis* in patients with diabetes is similar to that in persons without diabetes, except the process is markedly accelerated. Studies in which intensive insulin therapy is used to achieve tight glucose control demonstrate improvement in cardiovascular disease. Women with diabetes have the same risk profile as men at all ages. *Hypertension* (50% of patients with type 2 disease), dyslipidemia (40% of patients with type 2 diabetes at diagnosis), obesity, and hyperglycemia are major risk factors.

Aggressive treatment of hypertension, to less than 130/85 mm Hg, should preferably start with an angiotensin-converting enzyme inhibitor or angiotensin receptor antagonist for potential renal protection. All other classes of antihypertensive agents may be used, including selective β_1-blocking drugs, which are also used in the secondary prevention of myocardial infarction. β Blockers may increase the severity of hypoglycemia by inhibiting glycogenolysis and gluconeogenesis and may mask the warning symptoms and signs of hypoglycemia by blunting the adrenergic response to hypoglycemia. However, the potential adverse effects of β blockers in patients with diabetes have not been consistently observed in the clinical setting.

The procoagulant state of the blood in patients with diabetes is due to *platelet hypersensitivity* to the aggregating properties of thromboxane, which is synthesized in excess. Low-dose aspirin (80 to 160 mg/day) is recommended as primary prevention in patients with diabetes who are at high risk of cardiovascular disease, as well as secondary prevention in those with evidence of large vessel disease. Cessation of smoking, management of obesity and dyslipidemia, and initiation of safe exercise all decrease the risk and severity of macrovascular disease.

REFERENCES

American Diabetes Association: Clinical practice recommendations 2000. Diabetes Care 2000; 23(Suppl 1):S1–S115.

Barnett P: Diabetic ketoacidosis. *In* Mohsenifar Z, Shah PK (eds): Practical Critical Care in Cardiology. New York: Marcel Dekker, 1998, pp 389–423.

Clark CM, Lee DA: Prevention and treatment of the complications of diabetes mellitus. N Engl J Med 1995; 332:1210–1217.

Diabetes Control and Complications Trial Research Group: The effect of intensive treatment of diabetes on the development and progression of long-term complications in insulin-dependent diabetes mellitus. N Engl J Med 1993; 329:977–986.

Rosenbloom AL, Joe JR, Young RS, et al: Emerging epidemic of type 2 diabetes in youth. Diabetes Care 1999; 22:345–354.

United Kingdom Prospective Diabetes Study. Lancet 1998; 352:832–833, 837–853, 854–865.

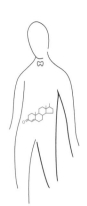

69

HYPOGLYCEMIA

Philip Barnett

Definition

Hypoglycemia is defined as a recorded blood glucose concentration lower than normal. Plasma glucose is maintained on a day-to-day basis within a narrow range of 72 to 144 mg/dL (4.0 to 8.0 mmol/L) by several hormonal and neural factors. Failure of any of these glucoregulatory mechanisms may result in hypoglycemia. Clinically significant hypoglycemia is rare and is based on the demonstration of Whipple's triad: signs and symptoms of hypoglycemia, in the presence of a low plasma glucose concentration (<45 mg/dL), that are relieved by restoration of plasma glucose to normal concentrations. Low plasma glucose values without signs and symptoms or vice versa do not constitute clinical hypoglycemia.

Physiology of Glucose Homeostasis

Normal fasting and preprandial plasma glucose values are less than 110 mg/dL (6.1 mmol/L). Postprandially, increases occur in blood glucose and insulin concentrations, influenced by meal composition, size, and time of day, that peak at 1 hour and return to normal after 3 to 4 hours. Two-hour postprandial glucose values do not exceed 140 mg/dL (7.8 mmol/L). The postprandial state comprises the first 4 to 5 hours after a meal. Insulin is the predominant hormone suppressing hepatic glucose production, promoting glycogen storage, and stimulating extrahepatic glucose utilization. The postabsorptive state begins 4 to 5 hours after a meal.

The response to low plasma glucose levels, *glucose counterregulation,* occurs on several levels. Central nervous system detection of low glucose levels stimulates the hypothalamus and pituitary to release growth hormone and adrenocorticotropin. Catecholamines, particularly epinephrine, are released from the adrenal medulla, and cortisol is released from the adrenal cortex.

Insulin secretion is reduced and glucagon secretion is augmented as a direct effect of low blood glucose concentration on pancreatic islets and in response to central neurogenic stimulation. Of the four counterregulatory hormones, glucagon, epinephrine, growth hormone, and cortisol, glucagon is the most important in the acute response to hypoglycemia. It acts rapidly to increase hepatic glucose production through *glycogenolysis,* the major source of fasting glucose, and *gluconeogenesis,* which becomes increasingly important as glycogen stores are depleted. In patients with type 1 diabetes of more than 3 to 5 years' duration, the glycogen response is lost. Epinephrine is also part of the rapid counterregulatory hormone response to hypoglycemia and plays a major role when it replaces the lost glucagon response in patients with type 1 diabetes. Epinephrine is also subsequently lost as a response to hypoglycemia 10 to 15 years after diagnosis in approximately 25% of patients with diabetes. Epinephrine inhibits insulin secretion and thereby inhibits glucose uptake by muscle. It stimulates glycogenolysis and lipolysis, and the resultant increase in free fatty acids acts as a stimulus for hepatic gluconeogenesis. Growth hormone and cortisol characterize the delayed response to hypoglycemia (2 to 3 hours) by enhancing glucagon's effect and antagonizing the action of insulin by accelerating hepatic gluconeogenesis, by suppressing muscle glucose utilization, and by stimulating lipolysis, ketogenesis, and proteolysis. With prolonged hypoglycemia, the liver itself responds through autoregulation with an increase in glucose production.

SIGNS AND SYMPTOMS OF HYPOGLYCEMIA

The various signs and symptoms of hypoglycemia appear at different glycemic thresholds, related to different mechanisms, and they can be divided into *neurogenic* (increased autonomic nervous system activity) and *neuroglycopenic* (depressed activity of the central nervous system) (Table 69–1). Signs and symptoms may vary among patients but are fairly constant for a given person. Accommodation to hypoglycemia results from a re-

TABLE 69–1 Signs and Symptoms of Hypoglycemia

Neurogenic

Sweating
Pallor
Tachycardia or hypertension
Palpitations
Tremor or shaking
Nervousness or anxiety
Irritability
Tingling, paresthesias (mouth and fingers)
Hunger
Nausea or vomiting

Neuroglycopenic

Warmth or weakness
Headache
Tiredness or drowsiness
Fainting or dizziness
Blurred vision
Mental dullness or confusion
Abnormal behavior
Amnesia
Seizures
Coma

setting of glycemic thresholds. Patients with diabetes may suffer from hypoglycemic unawareness, with serious consequences. Loss of warning symptoms and signs results from progressive loss of glucagon and epinephrine responses over time, lowering of the glycemic threshold by intensive therapy and/or hypoglycemic episodes, and autonomic dysfunction resulting from the diabetic process. The delayed counterregulatory responses of growth hormone and cortisol are usually too late to prevent neuroglycopenia.

The definition of a normal blood glucose level depends on the circumstances, the sex of the patient, and the sample tested. Glucose concentrations vary according to the sample measured; arterial, venous, or capillary blood; and whole blood versus plasma or serum. Venous plasma glucose is the usual sample measured and is approximately 15% higher than whole blood concentrations. Patients with diabetes use capillary whole blood for daily self-monitoring purposes. Some newer glucose sensing devices sample interstitial fluid. Normal plasma glucose values during a fast are different in men and women; in men, the fasting plasma glucose concentration is 55 mg/dL (3.1 mmol/L) at 24 hours and 50 mg/dL (2.8 mmol/L) at 48 and 72 hours, whereas in premenopausal women, it is as low as 35 mg/dL (1/9 mmol/L) at 24 hours without symptoms of hypoglycemia. Postprandial values have a different normal range. Exercise in healthy persons generally does not lead to a fall in glucose levels. Concern about hypoglycemia stems from the condition's possibly devastating effects on the brain. The central nervous system cannot synthesize glucose or store enough glycogen for more than a few minutes' glucose supply. The brain cannot use free fatty acids as an energy source, and ketone bodies, which are generated late, are not useful in acute hypoglycemia.

Because glucose is the predominant metabolic fuel for the central nervous system, significant hypoglycemia can cause brain dysfunction, acute and/or permanent, and if hypoglycemia is prolonged, it may result in brain death.

GLYCEMIC THRESHOLDS

Despite the ranges of normality discussed earlier, the glycemic thresholds listed in this paragraph apply to the general population. Falling plasma glucose concentrations trigger a set sequence of events. Within the physiologic plasma glucose range, a drop in glucose to a range of less than 81 to 83 mg/dL (4.5 to 4.6 mmol/L) results in decreased insulin secretion. At levels slightly lower than the normal range, 65 to 68 mg/dL (3.6 to 3.8 mmol/L), secretion of the insulin counterregulatory hormones occurs: glucagon and epinephrine at 68 mg/dL, growth hormone at 67 mg/dL, and cortisol at 58 mg/dL. The glycemic threshold for symptoms of hypoglycemia is approximately 54 mg/dL (3.0 mmol/L), and for cognitive dysfunction, it is approximately 47 mg/dL (2.6 mmol/L). These glycemic thresholds vary in response to the level of glucose control, particularly in patients with diabetes; poorly controlled diabetes with persistent hyperglycemia results in higher glucose thresholds, whereas lower glucose thresholds are reset after single or repeated hypoglycemic episodes. In some persons, major symptoms of central nervous system dysfunction may not occur until the plasma glucose concentration reaches 20 mg/dL, because these persons have a compensatory increase in cerebral blood flow.

Clinical Classification of Hypoglycemia

Hypoglycemia occurs most commonly as a side effect of the treatment of diabetes mellitus, usually associated with impairment of insulin counterregulatory responses. The incidence increases with attempts to achieve euglycemia through tight control of glucose concentrations; 65% of patients with type 1 diabetes in the Diabetes Control and Complications Trial, and 11% of patients with type 2 diabetes in the United Kingdom Prospective Diabetes Study had episodes of hypoglycemia that required assistance of a second party to administer therapy with either intramuscular or subcutaneous glucagon or intravenous glucose. Other causes of hypoglycemia in patients with diabetes include overdose of insulin or oral agents, missed or delayed meals, and uncompensated exercise (immediate and/or delayed, ≤24 hours). *Nocturnal hypoglycemia*, manifested by night sweats, snoring, vivid dreams, and deep sleep, occurs in as many as 50% of patients receiving insulin. Maximum insulin sensitivity at 2 or 3 a.m. may coincide with peak exogenous insulin action. Treatment usually includes changing the timing of intermediate-acting insulin from dinner to bedtime and/or changing the the dose. The following discussion addresses the separate causes of hypoglycemia listed in Table 69–2.

TABLE 69–2 **Clinical Classification of Hypoglycemia**

Fasting (Postabsorptive) Hypoglycemia

Drugs
  Insulin, sulfonylureas*, meglitinides*, alcohol
  β-Adrenergic antagonists (nonselective)
  Quinine, pentamidine*
  Salicylates, sulfonamides
  Others
Critical illness
  Hepatic, renal, and cardiac dysfunction
  Adrenal insufficiency†
  Sepsis or shock
  Malnutrition or anorexia nervosa
Hormone deficiencies
  Hypopituitarism (growth hormone)
  Adrenal insufficiency (cortisol)†
  Catecholamine deficiency (epinephrine)
  Glucagon deficiency
Endogenous hyperinsulinemia
  Pancreatic β-cell disorders
    Tumor (insulinoma)
    Nontumor
  β-Cell secretagogue (e.g., sulfonylurea, meglitinide)
  Autoimmune hypoglycemia
    Insulin autoantibodies
    Insulin receptor autoantibodies
    ?Islet β-cell antibodies
    Addison's disease†
  Ectopic insulin secretion (rare)
Exogenous hyperinsulinemia
Hypoglycemia of infancy and childhood
Non β-cell tumors

Reactive (Postprandial) Hypoglycemia

Alimentary hypoglycemia
Idiopathic (functional) hypoglycemia
Congenital enzyme deficiencies in adults
  Hereditary fructose intolerance
  Galactosemia

---

* Responsible for endogenous hyperinsulinemia.

† Cortisol deficiency may result from adrenal insufficiency from numerous causes, including infection, hemorrhagic destruction, and autoimmune disease.

Adapted from Cryer PE: Hypoglycemia: Pathophysiology, Diagnosis and Management. New York: Oxford University Press, 1997.

FASTING (POSTABSORPTIVE) HYPOGLYCEMIA

This condition results from an imbalance between hepatic glucose production (decreased) and peripheral glucose utilization (increased).

Drugs

Insulin, sulfonylureas, meglitinides, and alcohol are the most common causes of fasting hypoglycemia. Insulin is a well-recognized cause of hypoglycemia in the treatment of diabetes. *Factitious hypoglycemia* resulting from the covert use of insulin by persons with and without diabetes can be detected by elevated serum insulin levels in the absence of elevated C-peptide levels.

Overdosage with sulfonylureas occurs more commonly in elderly patients with long-acting first-generation agents such as chlorpropamide. This overdosage is usually inadvertent but occasionally intentional, and it may be determined by measuring serum or urine sulfonylurea levels. Because of the mechanism of sulfonylurea action, insulin and C-peptide levels are elevated. Patients with sulfonylurea-induced hypoglycemia should not be discharged from the emergency room after initial normalization of plasma glucose concentrations because hypoglycemia recurs soon afterward as a result of the long half-life of many of these agents, a half-life that may be even longer in patients with comorbid conditions such as renal dysfunction. It may take several days of continuous glucose treatment before the hypoglycemia resolves. Hypoglycemia related to meglitinide therapy or overdose would not be expected to be as severe as that caused by sulfonylureas, because of the short duration of action of this class of hypoglycemic agents.

Excessive alcohol consumption is a common cause of hypoglycemia. In patients with diabetes treated with drugs (oral agents and/or insulin), the combination with alcohol can be dangerous. Hypoglycemia may occur many hours after ingestion of alcohol ("morning after the night before"). Alcohol suppresses hepatic gluconeogenesis, and hypoglycemia occurs in malnourished patients with chronic alcoholism or after a several-day binge of alcohol consumption with little food intake (depleted hepatic glycogen reserves).

Nonselective β-adrenergic antagonists may cause hypoglycemia in patients with diabetes (especially type 1) who do not have a normal glucagon counterregulatory response and depend on the adrenergic response to hypoglycemia. β2-Adrenergic antagonists mask the adrenergic symptoms and impair recovery from hypoglycemia. These agents also reduce the glycogenolytic response to epinephrine in muscle. Low doses of β1-selective adrenergic antagonists do not produce these effects, although in high doses their selectivity is incomplete.

Pentamidine (particularly parenteral), through β-cell destruction, causes acute insulin release with hypoglycemia. After this acute phase, the destroyed β cells fail to produce insulin, and hyperglycemia results. In children, salicylates may lead to increased insulin secretion through prostaglandin inhibition. Quinine can cause excessive pancreatic insulin release.

Critical Illness

In hospitalized patients, the most common cause of hypoglycemia is use of drugs, especially insulin. Next are single or multiple organ system failures (particularly hepatic, renal, cardiac, and adrenal), malnutrition, sepsis, and shock. The mechanism of hypoglycemia in each setting is multifactorial and not always entirely clear. Disease or failure of one organ system may affect another system and so may result in hypoglycemia, such as seen in right-sided cardiac failure causing hepatic congestion. Hepatic failure results in impaired gluconeogenesis as well as an inability to store and release glycogen. Renal failure may lead to prolongation of the half-life of hypoglycemia-inducing agents (sulfonylureas, insulin). Malnutrition also plays a major role in renal failure as a cause of hypoglycemia. Insulin antibodies and hypothyroidism may also delay insulin clearance and may increase the risk of hypoglycemia. In adrenal insufficiency, lack of cortisol, which normally supports gluconeogenesis, may result in hypoglycemia. Sepsis is associated with increased glucose utilization in excess of glucose production. Severe malaria may be associated with hypoglycemia resulting from increased glucose utilization by parasitized red blood cells.

Insulinoma

This rare pancreatic β-cell tumor has an incidence of 1 in 250,000 patient years and is more common in women (60%). It occurs at all ages; the median age at diagnosis is 50 years in sporadic cases and 23 years in patients with multiple endocrine neoplasia type 1 syndrome (8% to 10% of cases). Most of these tumors are benign (90% to 95%), solitary (93%), confined to the pancreas (99%), and small (average 1 to 2 cm). Characteristically, insulinomas remain undiagnosed or misdiagnosed (20%) (as psychiatric or neurologic disorders) for several years. Long-term insulin secretion, *hyperinsulinemia*, which is not responsive to falling glucose concentrations in the fasting state, results in persistent hypoglycemia. Patients eat frequently to stave off the hypoglycemia and may gain weight (20%). Adaptation to the hypoglycemia over time results in manifestation of neuroglycopenic symptoms far more commonly than neurogenic symptoms. Most patients have fasting hypoglycemia (demonstrated by a 72-hour fast; Table 69–3), symptoms of hypoglycemia with plasma glucose less than 45 mg/dL, and inappropriately elevated serum insulin, C-peptide, and proinsulin levels (>20% of total insulin). Some patients have reactive hypoglycemia as well. A C-peptide suppression test, in which endogenous insulin and C-peptide are normally suppressed during an insulin infusion, is impaired in the presence of an insulinoma, but this test is not routinely performed.

After the biochemical diagnosis of an insulinoma, surgical resection by an experienced surgeon is generally recommended, irrespective of negative tumor localization studies. Localization of insulinomas using computed tomography, ultrasound, magnetic resonance imaging, celiac-axis angiography, or transhepatic portal venous sampling may be unsuccessful because of the generally small size of these tumors. At operation, tumors are often found by intraoperative ultrasound or palpation of the pancreas. Distal pancreatectomy is sometimes performed if no tumor is found during the surgical procedure.

In patients unwilling to undergo surgical treatment, in patients awaiting surgery, or in those in whom surgical treatment has failed, medical therapy using diazoxide (which inhibits insulin secretion) or octreotide is indicated. Other drugs that raise blood glucose levels include phenytoin, chlorpromazine, propranolol, and verapamil. Continuous subcutaneous infusion of glucagon prevents hypoglycemia. In patients with malignant insu-

TABLE 69–3 **Protocol for Performing a 72-Hour Fast**

1. Patient admitted to hospital. Start fast after evening meal at 1800 hr.
2. Blood glucose level monitored by bedside reflectance glucose meter q4h and when symptoms of hypoglycemia develop. The presence of urinary ketones confirms that the patient is fasting.
3. When symptoms of hypoglycemia develop accompanied by a blood glucose level of ≤50 mg/dL (plasma glucose of ≤45 mg/dL), draw "diagnostic labs," consisting of a fasting plasma glucose concentration, serum insulin, C-peptide and proinsulin levels, and a serum sample for sulfonylurea agents and insulin-like growth factor I (IGF-I) and IGF-11 levels (the latter three to be sent only once per fast). The fast is terminated at this time.
4. The fast is terminated when the patient has symptoms of hypoglycemia and a documented blood glucose of <50 mg/dL (or laboratory plasma glucose of <45 mg/dL) or after 72 hr. In the absence of documented hypoglycemia at the end of 72 hr, vigorous exercise for 2 hr may result in a fall in blood glucose.
5. The patient is fed a meal and is discharged from the hospital.
6. If severe, persistent hypoglycemia is documented, the patient may need to be started on medication, such as diazoxide, to prevent further episodes of hypoglycemia while the work-up is proceeding.

linoma, streptozotocin, with or without doxorubicin or fluorouracil, has been used.

Non–β-Cell Tumors

Fasting hypoglycemia may be caused by a variety of rare, non–β-cell tumors. Many (~50%) are large, slow-growing, mesenchymal tumors, often malignant. More than one third are retroperitoneal, one third intra-abdominal, and the rest intrathoracic. Epithelial tumors include heptocellular carcinomas (~25%), adrenocortical carcinomas (5% to 10%), and gastrointestinal (carcinoid) tumors (5% to 10%). Lymphomas account for 5% to 10%. In most patients, overproduction of insulin-like growth factor II (IGF-II) and, more particularly, the incompletely processed form, "big" IGF-II, is responsible for hypoglycemia, as a result of their direct insulin-like actions, as well as their suppression of glucagon and growth hormone (hence IGF-I) levels.

Diagnosis is made on the basis of hypoglycemia in a patient with a known tumor or elevated IGF-II levels. A 72-hour fast shows hypoglycemia with appropriately suppressed serum insulin, C-peptide, and proinsulin levels. Treatment involves tumor resection. If surgical treatment is not completely successful, glucocorticoids may be beneficial.

Insulin and Insulin Receptor Autoantibodies

These extremely rare conditions may be associated with other autoimmune disorders. Antibody binding to insulin may result in hypoglycemia by releasing insulin at an inappropriate time or by preventing its degradation. Receptor antibodies may cause insulin resistance or, alternatively, hypoglycemia, through insulin receptor agonist activity (with elevated C-peptide).

REACTIVE (POSTPRANDIAL) HYPOGLYCEMIA

This form of hypoglycemia typically occurs within 4 hours of food consumption; glucose levels fall more rapidly than insulin levels. Some persons with impaired glucose tolerance initially have a delayed excessive insulin response to a meal that results in reactive hypoglycemia. In all forms of fasting hypoglycemia, patients may also demonstrate reactive hypoglycemia.

Alimentary Hypoglycemia

This condition occurs in persons who have undergone gastric surgery (gastrectomy, gastrojejunostomy, pyloroplasty, gastric bypass, or vagotomy). Symptoms of hypoglycemia occur between 30 and 180 minutes after eating. Early emptying of food from the stomach into the duodenum, with its rapid absorption, together with enhanced secretion of insulinotropic incretins, leads to hyperglycemia and early marked hyperinsulinemia. As opposed to hypoglycemia, symptoms of "dumping" (<1 hour after meals) include abdominal fullness, nausea, and weakness.

Idiopathic Hypoglycemia

The existence of this overdiagnosed condition is still in dispute. In most patients, adrenergic symptoms, which are usually vague, do not occur simultaneously with biochemical hypoglycemia and are not relieved by consuming food. Occasionally, artificial testing situations (5-hour oral glucose tolerance test; 72-hour fast) may suggest the diagnosis, but these findings are not borne out after a mixed meal.

Diagnostic Work-up of Hypoglycemia

Hypoglycemia occurs most commonly in patients with drug-treated diabetes mellitus. To evaluate a patient for the presence of hypoglycemia, the clinician should document that true hypoglycemia is present. Ambulatory patients can be trained in self-monitoring of blood glucose, particularly during symptomatic episodes of hypoglycemia. If blood glucose levels are low (≤50 mg/dL) and the symptoms resolve after carbohydrate ingestion, the patient probably has true hypoglycemia. If symptoms are present without documentation of hypoglycemia, an alternate explanation must be sought. If hypoglycemia occurs in the fed state, after excluding a history of gastric surgery, the likely cause is impaired glucose tolerance

(confirmed by oral glucose tolerance test) or, in rare cases, idiopathic reactive hypoglycemia (diagnosis by exclusion). If reactive hypoglycemia is diagnosed, the patient should consult a dietitian for a diet plan designed to ameliorate these episodes (e.g., frequent low-carbohydrate meals).

Fasting hypoglycemia is more likely to be caused by an organic medical problem, although some of the underlying disorders (such as insulinoma and adrenal insufficiency) can present with both fasting and reactive hypoglycemia (see Table 69–2). When patients are hospitalized and are acutely ill, the distinction between fasting and reactive hypoglycemia is less clear; the work-up is then based on an understanding of the patient's underlying medical problems and medications and the ways in which these conditions may alter blood glucose levels.

The standard evaluation of hypoglycemia attributable to any other underlying cause includes admitting the patient to the hospital for a supervised 72-hour fast (see Table 69–3). During the fast, the patient is allowed only noncaloric, noncaffeinated beverages, except for essential medications, and should be active during the day. Approximately 75% of patients with an insulinoma develop symptomatic hypoglycemia within the first 24 hours, 10% in the next 24 hours, and only 5% in the final 24 hours. Difficulties in performing the fast arise when blood glucose levels fall to less than 50 mg/dL and the patient has no symptoms of hypoglycemia, or when the patient develops symptoms at normal blood glucose levels. In the former situation, one should continue measuring blood glucose levels, with the patient under close medical observation, until these concentrations fall to less than 50 mg/dL. In the latter instance, the fast can be continued as long as is clinically warranted to convince both patient and physician that the symptoms are not associated with hypoglycemia. Table 69–4 summarizes the expected findings in various conditions at the completion of the fast.

Treatment

The diagnosis of hypoglycemia should be considered in every unconscious patient. The initial treatment of a confused or comatose patient is to infuse a bolus of 50 mL IV of 50% glucose, preferably after a blood sample for laboratory analysis has been obtained. If hypoglycemia is documented, blood should then be tested for levels of insulin, C-peptide, cortisol, drugs, toxins, hypoglycemic agents (e.g., sulfonylurea or meglitinide), and alcohol. A portion of the sample should be kept for later analysis of proinsulin, carnitine, insulin antibodies, and lactate, if necessary.

Intravenous, intramuscular, or subcutaneous glucagon (1 mg) can be used in the absence of an intravenous glucose preparation. The bolus of glucose should be followed by the continuous infusion of 5% to 10% glucose (≤20% to 30%) at a rate sufficient to keep the plasma glucose level of more than 100 mg/dL. The re-

TABLE 69-4 **Interpretation of Results from a 72-Hour Fast**

Condition	Plasma Glucose (mg/dL)	Insulin (μU/mL)	C-Peptide (nmol/L)	Proinsulin (pmol/L)	Plasma Sulfonylurea Level	Insulin-like growth factor II
Normal*	≥45 in men ≥36 in women	<6	<0.2	<5	−	−
Insulinoma	≤45	≥6	≥0.2	≥5	−	−
Exogenous insulin	≤45	≥6[†]	<0.2	<5	−	−
Sulfonylurea agents	≤45	≥6	≥0.2	≥5	+	−
Tumor secreting IGF-II	≤45	≤6	<0.2	<5	−	+ (↓ IGF-I)

*Normal insulin, C-peptide, and proinsulin levels may be higher if blood glucose levels are not <60 mg/dL. [†] Insulin levels may be very high (>100 μU/mL) in these patients.
IGF = insulin-like growth factor; − = absent; + = present or elevated.
Adapted with permission from Service FJ: Hypoglycemic disorders. N Engl J Med 1995; 332:1144–1152.

quirement of 8 to 10 g/hour of glucose to prevent recurrent hypoglycemia suggests diminished glucose production as a cause of the hypoglycemia, with higher requirements reflecting increased peripheral glucose utilization. When the patient is capable of eating, a diet with a minimum of 300 g/day of carbohydrates should be supplied. In many situations, especially after administration of long-acting insulin or oral hypoglycemic drugs, hypoglycemia persists for an extended time. Treatment and close observation should continue during this time to prevent a relapse. Mild hypoglycemia can be managed with oral glucose tablets (4 to 5 g), fruit juice, or equivalent, followed by a snack containing carbohydrate and protein, if the patient will have to wait more than 30 minutes for the next meal.

Long-term therapy depends on the cause of the hypoglycemia. If the hypoglycemia is a secondary process (such as from hepatic or renal failure or sepsis), treatment of the underlying disorder will resolve the hypoglycemia. If the hypoglycemia results from an insulinoma, then surgical removal of the tumor is the treatment of choice.

Dietary therapy is the cornerstone of the management of all types of reactive hypoglycemia. Patients should avoid simple or refined carbohydrates. Some patients also benefit from frequent, small meals or snacks that contain a mixture of carbohydrate, fat, and protein. Restricting the daily carbohydrate intake to 35% to 40% of total calories and increasing protein intake can be helpful, if a regimen of avoidance of simple carbohydrates and eating more frequently is ineffective. Drug therapy with propantheline bromide or phenytoin may sometimes be helpful, but it should be reserved for severe cases. If the disorder results from alimentary hypoglycemia, dietary therapy is usually helpful; in refractory cases (rare), surgical treatment to slow gastric transit time may be successful.

REFERENCES

Bolli GB: Hypoglycemia in type 1 diabetic patients. *In* De Fronzo RA (ed): Current Therapy of Diabetes Mellitus. St. Louis: CV Mosby, 1998, pp 55–59.

Cryer PE: Hypoglycemia: Pathophysiology, Diagnosis and Management. New York: Oxford University Press, 1997.

Fanelli C, Pampanelli S, Epifano L: Relative roles of insulin and hypoglycaemia on induction of neuroendocrine responses to, symptoms of, and deterioration of cognitive function in hypoglycaemia in male and female humans. Diabetologia 1994; 37:797–807.

Marks V, Teale JD: Investigation of hypoglycemia. Clin Endocrinol 1996; 44:133–136.

Service FJ: Hypoglycemic disorders. N Engl J Med 1995; 332:1144–1152.

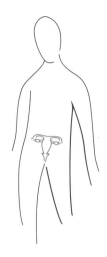

70

WOMEN'S HEALTH: GENERAL CONCEPTS

Sally L. Hodder • *Anne L. Taylor*

Women's health has traditionally been understood to mean reproductive and gynecologic health, areas in which women's health needs are easily perceived to be distinct. Examination of causes of mortality in women emphasizes the problem of equating only reproductive or gynecologic health with women's overall health. Cardiovascular disease, cancer (non–gender-specific cancer of the lung causes more deaths in women than breast cancer), cerebrovascular diseases, pneumonia, chronic lung disease, and accidental deaths are the major causes of mortality in women. Disability in women is far more likely to be caused by nongynecologic diseases such as osteoporosis and stroke than by gynecologic diseases. Female gender is a significant factor for diseases of nonreproductive organs such as the heart, bone, and brain. Consideration of the role that gender difference plays in disease processes is critical to an understanding of women's health issues. An excellent description of the necessary components of women's health (Table 70–1) has been proposed by the National Academy on Women's Health Medical Education and is useful in examining the broad spectrum of women's health.

Studies of the natural history of diseases prevalent in both men and women and clinical trials of therapeutic efficacy have been performed mainly in men. Such studies do not always reflect the full expression of the disease, nor do they provide treatment decisions that may be extrapolated to women. For example, cardiovascular disease is the number 1 cause of mortality in both men and women, but the impact of risk factors, treatment, and outcomes differ in men and women. Although investigational efforts designed to define the effects of gender on health and disease are critical for the optimal medical care of both men and women, women have historically been excluded from clinical trials because of (1) fears of harming pregnant women and fetuses, (2) anxiety about potentially confounding variables generated by hormonal cycles, and (3) increased cost engendered by necessary subgroup analysis. Therefore, data guiding optimal medical care for many illnesses are less complete for women than for men.

Gender Differences in the Epidemiology of Disease by Age Group

Although women have longer lifespans than men, they have higher rates of disability. At the extremes of age, few gender differences in causes of morbidity and mortality exist. After adolescence, significant gender differences in morbidity and mortality begin to emerge. Both men and women 20 to 39 years of age die most frequently from *accidents*, whereas *human immunodeficiency virus (HIV) infection* is the second most common cause of mortality in men and the third in women. *Breast and uterine cancers* are the second most common cause of mortality in women 20 to 39 years of age, whereas *suicide* is the third most common cause of mortality in young men. Women in this age group have serious morbidity (infertility and cervical neoplasia) related to sexually transmitted diseases and significantly greater morbidity from eating disorders.

Causes of death become more disparate for the 40- to 59-year age group. *Cancer* is the leading cause of mortality in women, with breast and lung cancer accounting for most deaths. Heart disease is the second most common cause of death in women, followed by accidents. Men in this age group are most likely to die of *heart disease* (nearly three times more deaths than among women), lung and colon cancer, and HIV infection.

In the 60- to 79-year age group, *heart disease* and *cancer* are by far the most common causes of death in both men and women; cancer (lung, breast, and colon) is relatively more common in women and heart disease more common in men. Both men and women older than 79 years of age are most likely to die of heart disease, with roughly twice as many deaths from heart disease in women in comparison with men. Cancer is the second most common cause of death for both sexes in this age group; colon cancer and lung cancer are the

607

TABLE 70-1 **Women's Health Knowledge Base**

Knowledge of those conditions unique to women (i.e., gynecologic and obstetric conditions)
Knowledge of those conditions more common in women (i.e., autoimmune diseases, depression, breast cancer)
Knowledge of those conditions with serious impact for women (e.g., osteoporosis)
Knowledge of those conditions with manifestations, risk factors, interventions, or outcomes different in women (e.g., coronary heart disease)
Knowledge of changes in women's health and wellness needs over women's lifespans (i.e., nutritional requirements, hormonal changes)

Adapted from Donoghue GD (ed): Women's Health in the Curriculum: A Resource Guide for Faculty. Philadelphia: National Academy on Women's Health Medical Education (NAWHME), 1996.

most common malignant diseases in women. *Cerebrovascular diseases* are the third most common cause of mortality in both men and women.

Women who are more than 50 years old are three times more likely than men to suffer from *osteoporosis.* Elderly women also have significantly more social isolation than men, a further contributor to poor health and functional status.

Sexually transmitted diseases are a major cause of morbidity in young women, yet two common causes of these diseases, *Neisseria gonorrhoeae* and *Chlamydia trachomatis*, are frequently asymptomatic in women while causing symptoms in men. Screening for these diseases in young women therefore becomes an effective preventive strategy. An understanding of the gender differences in epidemiology and clinical manifestations of disease is crucial to good clinical care.

Exercise Across the Feminine Life Cycle

Regular exercise (both aerobic and resistive) has salutary effects on cardiovascular health, lipid profiles, blood pressure control, maintenance of bone density, insulin and glucose metabolism, and breast cancer incidence. Although the health benefits are substantial, fewer than 10% of women 18 to 65 years of age exercise regularly and appropriately. During adolescence, approximately one third of girls are involved in organized athletics. The numbers of women involved in regular exercise activities decline further with advancing age, whereas the health benefits of exercise increase with age.

Aerobic exercise capacity is measured by maximal oxygen uptake. *Resistive capacity* is measured by the amount of weight that can be lifted under standardized conditions. Both aerobic exercise and resistive exercise are necessary for optimal health benefits. Maximal oxygen uptake is greater in men than in women, a difference attributable to higher body fat content, lower muscle mass, lower hemoglobin concentrations, and smaller

lung capacities and cardiac stroke volumes in women. Gender differences in maximal oxygen uptake decrease when comparing male and female endurance athletics as the result of changes in muscle and body fat composition of elite female athletes.

For maximal benefit, aerobic exercise should include 30 to 40 minutes of an aerobic activity at least three times weekly at 60% to 90% of the age-predicted maximal heart rate. This goal can be accomplished by running, stair climbing, use of cross country ski machines, cycling, or swimming. Although swimming is suitable for older women with musculoskeletal problems, it lacks the advantages of weight-bearing exercise on bone density. Intense aerobic exercise in young women may be associated with small size and delayed menarche. Although this effect has been observed largely in gymnasts and ballerinas, it has not been consistently noted in other competitive female athletes such as swimmers and basketball and volleyball players; this finding suggests that the observed abnormalities may reflect the relatively small size of young women who select the sport, rather than a training effect.

Strength training results in increased muscle mass, increased bone density, and improved functional capacity. Measurement of strength training includes the amount of resistance and the frequency of repetitions of each muscle motion against the resistance. Skeletal muscle enlargement resulting from resistive exercise is considerably less in women than in men.

Exercise during pregnancy is beneficial to maintain normal blood pressure, glucose tolerance, and normal weight gain. However, special considerations exist. Intense exercise should be avoided because imbalances in the distribution of blood flow to the placenta may occur. Exercise in the supine position is also to be avoided because pressure by the gravid uterus on the vena cava and aorta may cause circulatory impairment. Women who exercise regularly before pregnancy should continue to exercise during pregnancy, and they should avoid extremes of temperature and of exercise levels. Pregnant women who have not exercised before pregnancy should initiate only a low-intensity exercise regimen.

Gender and the Patient-Physician Interaction

In addition to gender-related physiologic variables, the interaction between patient and physician influences health status. Improved communication between physician and patient results in improved patient adherence to treatment plans and better outcomes. Women tend to ask more questions of and provide more information to their health care providers and exhibit more emotion than men. Women are more commonly perceived by physicians to make excessive demands on a physician's time and to lack understanding of medical terminology. Men are more likely than women to receive technically detailed information from physicians. Some physicians are more likely to ascribe a psychosomatic origin to women's complaints. Women seek more information, communication, and partnership building from their health care providers than men, actions that may be interpreted by health care providers as making excessive time demands. Concentration by the physician on efficiency may compromise a woman's ability to ask questions and to receive information; this often has a negative impact on her satisfaction with her health care.

Effective medical history taking must consider gender differences in communication style. Questions should be actively solicited from women. If the physician is unable to spend the necessary time with a patient during a busy office session, the patient may be asked to return for an additional appointment to supply additional technical information while more fully addressing the patient's concerns and questions. Ancillary personnel may provide the necessary technical information that women seek. The time taken to understand a patient's concerns and expectations greatly enhances patient adherence to treatment and follow-up.

REFERENCES

Carlson KJ, Skochelak SE: What do women want in a doctor? Communication issues between women and physicians. *In* Wallis LA (ed): Textbook of Women's Health. Philadelphia: Lippincott-Raven, 1998, pp 33–38.

Donoghue GD (ed): Women's Health in the Curriculum: A Resource Guide for Faculty. Philadelphia: National Academy on Women's Health Medical Education (NAWHME), 1996.

Johnson TL, Fee E: Women's health research: An introduction. *In* Haseltine FP (ed): Women's Health Research: A Medical and Policy Primer. Washington, DC: American Psychiatric Press, 1997, pp 3–26.

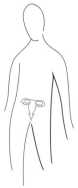

HORMONAL INFLUENCES ON WOMEN'S HEALTH

Sally L. Hodder • Anne L. Taylor

Normal Physiology

Three distinct hormonal phases occur during a woman's life. In *childhood*, estradiol levels are low, and both the hypothalamus and the pituitary are exquisitely sensitive to the inhibitory effects of circulating hormone. At *puberty*, as the hypothalamus becomes less sensitive, pulsatile gonadotropin-releasing hormone levels initiate puberty, with increased gonadotropin secretion enhancing ovarian production of estrogen. Prolactin levels rise during puberty, and the pituitary episodically releases growth hormone. With establishment of regular ovulation, women experience monthly cycles of estrogen and progesterone secretion from the ovary. Estrogen and progesterone act by binding to specific receptor proteins that subsequently bind to DNA to regulate transcription. Target tissues of steroid hormones produce a measurable response when hormone exposure occurs. In adults, both reproductive and nonreproductive tissues contain measurable levels of estrogen receptors. Nonreproductive tissue sites with detectable, active estrogen receptors include bone, arterial endothelium and smooth muscle, brain, and urethral mucosa. Estrogen plays an important role in the healthy maintenance of these and other tissues.

In the *perimenopausal period*, ovarian responsiveness to gonadotropins decreases, and levels of estrogen and progesterone fall, whereas levels of luteinizing hormone and of follicle-stimulating hormone levels increase. Various symptoms such as hot flashes, insomnia, weight gain, and anxiety may occur at this time. Ovaries in postmenopausal women continue to secrete testosterone and androstenedione. Peripheral conversion of androgens results in the low circulating levels of estrogen observed in postmenopausal women. Higher estrogen levels are observed in obese women because of the increased androgen conversion in adipose tissue; this phenomenon places obese women at increased risk for endometrial hyperplasia and carcinoma. Because women currently live approximately one third of their lives after menopause, the health consequences of endogenous estrogen loss and the potential benefits of long-term hormone replacement are critical issues in clinical medicine.

The normal menstrual cycle is a series of hormonal events that result in changes in the endometrium. The normal cycle is usually 21 to 35 days in duration and consists of three phases: the *follicular or proliferative phase*, the *ovulatory phase*, and the *luteal or secretory phase* (Fig. 71–1). During the first half of the cycle, gonadotropin-releasing hormone secreted by the hypothalamus stimulates pituitary secretion of follicle-stimulating hormone and luteinizing hormone. Circulating folllicle-stimulating hormone stimulates estrogen secretion by ovarian follicles that, in turn, prompts endometrial proliferation. During the follicular phase, one ovarian follicle becomes dominant. At midcycle, ovulation occurs when a surge in luteinizing hormone results in release of the oocyte from the dominant follicle. Remaining follicular cells form the progesterone-producing corpus luteum. If fertilization does not occur, the corpus luteum secretes progesterone only for approximately 14 days and subsequently involutes. Both estrogen and progesterone levels decrease as the corpus luteum is progressively broken down. Falling progesterone levels result in shedding of the endometrium and the onset of menstruation. A normal menstrual period lasts 7 days or less. In the perimenopausal period, cycle length may decrease because of a shortened follicular phase and decreased progesterone secretion. Cycles lasting less than 21 days are considered abnormal.

Dysmenorrhea and Premenstrual Syndrome

Dysmenorrhea is a group of symptoms most prominently manifested by pelvic pain that occur just before

610

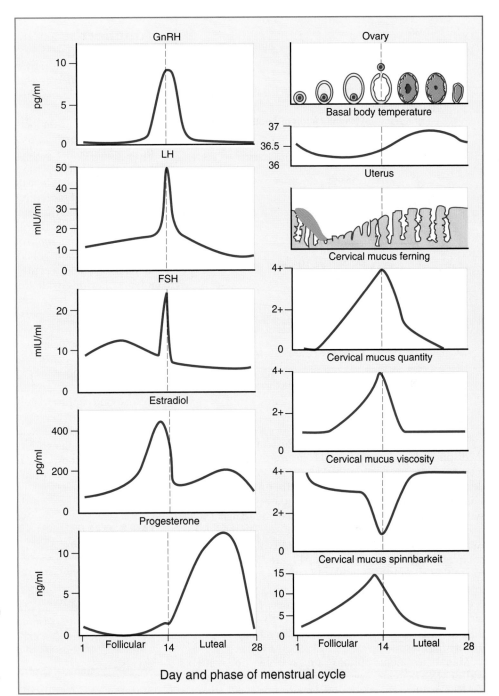

FIGURE 71–1 Schematic representation of the normal menstrual cycle. FSH = follicle-stimulating hormone; GnRH = gonadotropin-releasing hormone; LH = luteinizing hormone. (From Braunstein GD: Female reproductive disorders. *In* Hershman JD [ed]: Endocrine Pathophysiology: A Patient-Oriented Approach. Philadelphia: Lea & Febiger, 1988, p 153.)

and during menstruation. Dysmenorrhea occurring without the presence of disease is known as *primary dysmenorrhea*. The pelvic pain results from uterine contractions mediated by prostaglandins. Nonsteroidal anti-inflammatory agents that inhibit prostaglandin synthesis effectively control pelvic pain in most women. *Secondary dysmenorrhea* occurs when pelvic disorders such as *endometriosis* (the presence of endometrial tissue outside the uterus), *adenomyosis* (endometrial tissue within the uterine wall), or *fibroids* are present.

Premenstrual syndrome (PMS) is a collection of symptoms that are typically present in the 1 to 2 weeks preceding the onset of menstruation and resolve in the first 1 to 2 days of menstruation. Although most women have mild symptoms, approximately 5% to 10% have multiple symptoms that interfere with daily functioning. Symptoms are diverse and may include irritability, low self-esteem, insomnia, fatigue, lightheadedness, food cravings, thirst, breast tenderness, edema, and weight gain. Some women even report changes in cognitive function, with difficulty in concentrating and short-term memory problems. The precise cause of PMS remains unknown; however, ovulation is a prerequisite for its occurrence.

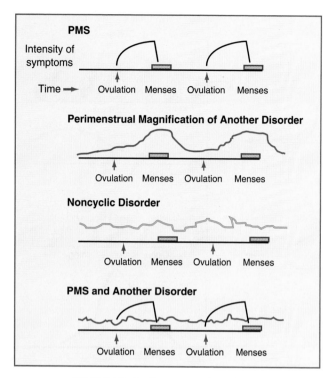

FIGURE 71-2   Premenstrual syndrome.

The challenge for physicians is to identify PMS and to distinguish it from noncyclic disorders or from perimenstrual intensification of symptoms of other disorders. Evaluation must include a thorough history of symptoms with establishment of their timing. Daily symptom charts, completed over two menstrual cycles, may be helpful to analyze different symptom patterns. As Figure 71–2 illustrates, symptoms of PMS resolve completely during menstruation. Figure 71–2 also illustrates that diagnosis may be difficult when premenstrual intensification of symptoms of an underlying disorder occurs or when PMS is superimposed on another ailment. Unless the patient's history clearly suggests PMS, the clinician must first diagnose and treat any suspected underlying disorders.

Many treatment options are available for patients with PMS. Regular exercise and dietary alterations including decreased caffeine intake and increased complex carbohydrate intake may alleviate PMS symptoms. However, few prospective, randomized clinical trials have been conducted to document benefit. Daily administration of fluoxetine, a selective serotonin reuptake inhibitor, may improve premenstrual dysphoria. Daily supplementation with 1000 mg of calcium carbonate, available without prescription, has been effective in decreasing a variety of premenstrual symptoms including dysphoria, fatigue, and back pain. Patient selection for PMS treatment should be undertaken when symptoms are severe enough to affect a woman's lifestyle and well-being. Therapy should be targeted to relief of specific symptoms. For example, selective serotonin reuptake inhibitors should be prescribed for patients in whom premenstrual dysphoria is paramount.

Amenorrhea

Amenorrhea is the absence of menstrual bleeding. *Primary amenorrhea* is the failure of menstruation to occur, whereas *secondary amenorrhea* is the cessation of menses.

Anatomic and endocrinologic disorders may result in primary amenorrhea, as outlined in Table 71–1. *Structural abnormalities* of the lower female genital tract such as vaginal aplasia or an imperforate hymen are observed in patients with normal secondary sexual development and are often associated with cyclic symptoms such as pelvic pain and PMS. *Gonadal dysgenesis* occurs in persons born with streak gonads that lack oocytes. *Turner's syndrome,* 45,X gonadal dysgenesis, is the most common gonadal disorder resulting in primary amenorrhea and occurs in 1 in 3000 to 5000 female infants. Persons with this disorder are characteristically short and may have associated somatic anomalies. Gonadal dysgenesis in persons having either a 46,XX or a 46,XY karyotype is associated with normal to tall stature without associated somatic abnormalities. Persons with *resistant ovary syndrome* have ovarian follicles present on biopsy, a 46,XX karyotype, and normal secondary sex characteristics; however, the ovary is unable to respond appropriately to gonadotropin stimulation. Primary amenorrhea may be the presenting complaint in 46,XY males with *testicular feminization* who appear as phenotypic females. Although normal breast development occurs, these persons lack pubic and axillary hair, because androgen receptors in hair follicles are absent.

TABLE 71-1   Causes of Primary Amenorrhea

Lower Tract Defects
Vaginal aplasia or atresia
Imperforate hymen

Uterine Disorders
Congenital absence of the uterus
Destruction of the endometrium

Gonadal Disorders
Gonadal dysgenesis*
17α-Hydroxylase deficiency*
Resistant ovary syndrome*
Chronic anovulation
Testicular feminization

Adrenal Disorders
Congenital adrenal hyperplasia

Thyroid Disorders
Hypothyroidism*

Pituitary-Hypothalamic Disorders
Hypopituitarism*
Prolactin-secreting pituitary tumor*
Nutritional or exercise-induced delay*
Constitutional delay*

* Associated with lack of or incomplete secondary sexual development.

Hyperthyroidism and *hypopituitarism* during adolescence may both result in sexual infantilism. *Anorexia nervosa, bulimia,* and *excessive dieting* may result in primary amenorrhea as a result of hypothalamic dysfunction. Normal menarche occurs when the nutritional abnormality is corrected. Girls such as gymnasts and ballerinas who exercise excessively and have little body fat may also have primary amenorrhea. Normal menarche follows when exercise is decreased and body fat is increased. *Constitutional delay* in the onset of menses occurs in girls with family histories of late menarche. Although some secondary sexual characteristics may be present in these girls, menses may not begin until they are >16 years of age.

A history and physical examination should be performed in all patients with primary amenorrhea. Presence of weight loss from excessive exercise, eating disorder, or systemic illness should be sought and treated if present. After these disorders have been ruled out, the diagnostic algorithm presented in Figure 71–3 should be followed. Estrogen replacement therapy should be initiated in patients with hypogonadism or untreatable hypothalamic-pituitary disorders to prevent the development of osteopenia, which occurs in women with longstanding estrogen deficiency. Thyroid replacement therapy effectively treats primary amenorrhea associated with hypothyroidism.

The many causes of secondary amenorrhea are summarized in Table 71–2; pregnancy is the most common cause. Uterine infection or surgical manipulation may result in endometrial scarring and subsequent hormonal unresponsiveness. The most common cause of ovarian-mediated secondary amenorrhea is *chronic anovulation,* formerly known as *polycystic ovary syndrome.* Although this condition is classically associated with obesity, hirsutism, and infertility, many women with chronic anovulation may have only oligomenorrhea, menses at intervals of more than 40 days, or secondary amenorrhea. *Ovarian follicle destruction* may result from chemotherapeutic agents, particularly alkylating agents and pelvic irradiation. *Ovarian tumors* are rarely associated with amenorrhea in the case of androgen-secreting tumors. *Adrenal disorders* may result in amenorrhea as the result of either androgen excess or as a late manifestation of adrenal cortical insufficiency. Secondary amenorrhea resulting from *congenital adrenal hyperplasia* may be mild or late in onset (see Chapter 66). Although both *hypothyroidism* and *hyperthyroidism* may result in amenorrhea, hyperthyroidism is a major cause of amenorrhea, whereas polymenorrhea, cycles lasting less than 21 days, is more often associated with hypothyroidism. Pituitary destruction may occur from certain disorders including tumors, infections, infiltration, and vascular and immunologically mediated destruction. *Hyperprolactinemia* interferes with normal cyclic gonadotropin release and ultimately leads to amenorrhea. *Infertility* and *galactorrhea* may or may not accompany oligoamenorrhea or amenorrhea. *Hyperprolactinemia* may be caused by a pituitary adenoma or may be drug-induced with agents such as phenothiazines, narcotics, and monoamine oxidase inhibitors. Finally, *hypothalamic dysfunction* may result from emotional stress as well as from weight loss due to eating disorders or systemic illness.

After pregnancy has been ruled out in patients presenting with amenorrhea, progesterone may be administered in an effort to determine whether appropriate estrogen priming of the endometrium is present. Failure of menstrual bleeding to occur within several weeks of progesterone administration indicates estrogen deficiency or abnormal endometrium. Estrogen administration for 1 to 2 months followed by menstrual bleeding occurs in persons with estrogen deficiency but not in those with an endometrial abnormality. Women with a suspected endometrial abnormality should be referred to a gynecologist for further work-up. An algorithm for evaluation of secondary amenorrhea is presented in Figure 71–4.

Treatment of secondary amenorrhea depends on the cause. Patients with ovarian failure resulting from underlying pituitary or hypothalamic dysfunction should be evaluated for estrogen replacement therapy. Ovarian and adrenal neoplasms should be surgically removed. Patients with chronic anovulation may be treated with progesterone every 1 to 3 months to ensure adequate shedding of the endometrium. Oral contraceptives may be used to treat hirsutism and virilization.

TABLE 71–2   Causes of Secondary Amenorrhea

Pregnancy

Uterine Disorders
Endometrial scarring
Endometrial atrophy

Ovarian Disorders
Premature menopause
    Chemotherapy or radiation
    Idiopathic or autoimmune
Ovarian tumors
Chronic anovulation

Adrenal Disorders
Late-onset congenital adrenal hyperplasia
Cushing's syndrome
Virilizing adrenal tumors
Adrenocortical insufficiency

Hypothalamic-Pituitary Disorders
Acquired hypopituitarism
Hyperprolactinemia
Drug suppression
Nutritional disorders

Extrahypothalamic Nervous System Disorders

Abnormal Uterine Bleeding

Abnormal uterine bleeding includes oligomenorrhea, characterized by menses at intervals of more than 40 days, and polymenorrhea, characterized by menses at intervals of less than 21 days. *Menorrhagia* refers to excessive bleeding (either in amount or in duration),

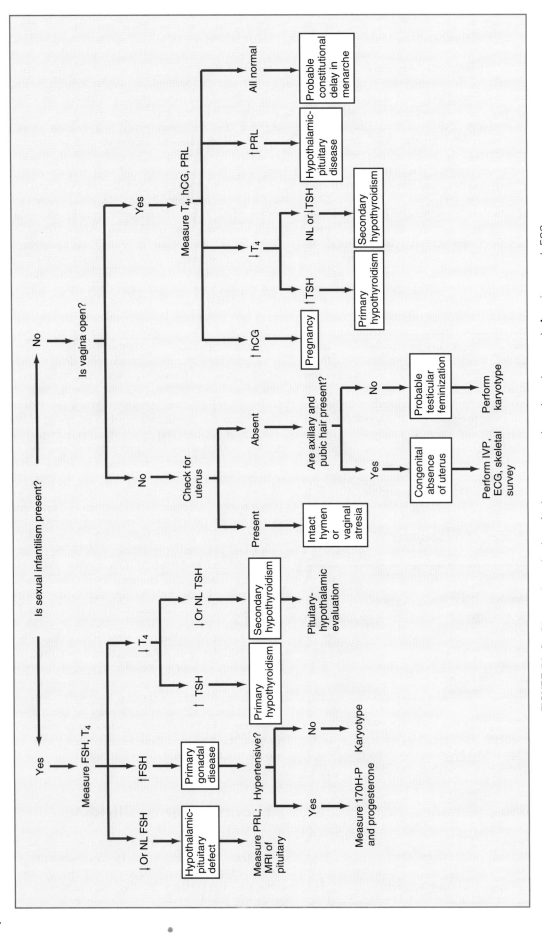

FIGURE 71–3 Diagnostic evaluation of primary amenorrhea. ↓ = decreased; ↑ = increased; ECG = electrocardiogram; FSH = follicle-stimulating hormone; hCG = human chorionic gonadotropin; IVP = intravenous pyelogram; MRI = magnetic resonance imaging; NL = normal; 17OH-P = 17 α-hydroxyprogesterone; PRL = prolactin; T₄ = thyroxine; TSH = thyroid-stimulating hormone.

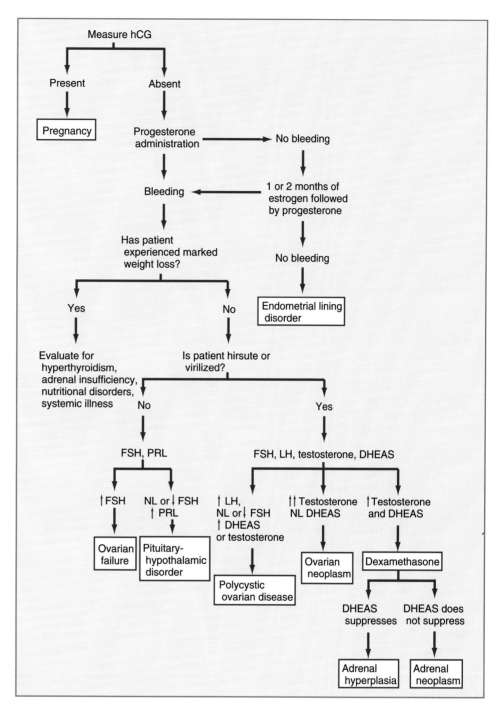

FIGURE 71-4 Evaluation of secondary amenorrhea (see text for details). ↑ = increased; ↑↑ = markedly increased; ↓ = decreased; DHEAS = dehydroepi-androsterone-sulfate; FSH = follicle-stimulating hormone; hCG = human chorionic gonadotropin; LH = luteinizing hormone; NL = normal; PRL = prolactin.

and *metrorrhagia* indicates irregular intervals between menses. Table 71–3 categorizes some of the many possible causes of abnormal bleeding. *Anovulation* is a common cause of abnormal uterine bleeding in both adolescents and perimenopausal women. In perimenopausal women, declining ovarian function may result in abnormal bleeding, and careful evaluation is essential to rule out neoplasia. In addition, pregnancy must be excluded.

Anovulatory or oligovulatory bleeding may occur as the result of hypothalamic, pituitary, ovarian, adrenal, or thyroid dysfunction. In *chronic anovulation,* the ovary secretes estrogen, but ovulation does not occur and thus progesterone is not secreted. High tonic estrogen levels are also present in the setting of estrogen-secreting ovarian tumors. Long-term endometrial exposure to estrogen without opposing progesterone may result in endometrial hyperplasia or carcinoma. Therefore, prompt and accurate diagnosis of anovulatory bleeding and appropriate treatment are crucial.

Evaluation requires a thorough history in an attempt to identify whether ovulation is occurring. Menses at regular intervals, preceded by breast tenderness or other premenstrual symptoms, usually indicate the presence of ovulation. Examination should include careful inspection for signs of androgen excess and of potentially associ-

TABLE 71–3 Abnormal Uterine Bleeding

Cause	Clinical Findings
Hormonal abnormalities	Failure to release gonadotropin-releasing hormone
	Hyperprolactinemia
	Hypothyroidism
	Waning ovarian function
	Estrogen secreting ovarian tumors
	Chronic anovulation
Structural abnormalities	Leiomyoma
	Polyps
	Uterine cancer
	Cervical cancer
	Endometritis
Bleeding diatheses	Thrombocytopenia
	Platelet dysfunction
Miscellaneous	Pregnancy

ated disorders (see Table 71–3). Pregnancy must always be excluded. Further evaluation is largely determined by the patient's age and by whether the patient's history indicates the presence or absence of ovulation. Adolescents in whom pregnancy and infection have been excluded and in whom the history suggests anovulatory bleeding may not require further invasive testing. On the other hand, perimenopausal women, who often have bleeding related to declining ovarian function, require further evaluation such as ultrasonography and endometrial biopsy to exclude uterine disease.

Treatment depends on accurate diagnosis. Adolescents may benefit from estrogen therapy to ensure adequate endometrial proliferation. Perimenopausal women with abnormal uterine bleeding not associated with neoplasia may benefit from cyclic estrogen and progesterone therapy. Removal of uterine polyps or leiomyomas, if present, may also be curative. Complete evaluation may not reveal a cause of the abnormal bleeding. In severe, refractory cases, hysterectomy or endometrial ablation may be considered.

Hirsutism

Hirsutism, the inappropriate growth of hair in women, may be androgen dependent (usually occurring in areas of the body that are sensitive to androgen such as the chin) or androgen independent (occurring over major portions of the body). Androgen-independent hirsutism may be caused by drugs such as minoxidil. Possible causes of androgen-dependent hirsutism are summarized in Table 71–4. *Chronic anovulation,* previously known as polycystic ovary syndrome, is commonly associated with hirsutism. The *HAIR-AN syndrome* includes the presence of hyperandrogenism (HA), insulin resistance (IR) caused by increased ovarian production of testosterone, and acanthosis nigricans (AN). Hirsutism from excessive adrenal androgen production in *congenital ad-*

renal hyperplasia results from increased secretion of corticotropin by the pituitary in response to deficient cortisol synthesis. Mild *21α-hydroxylase deficiency,* the most common enzyme deficiency associated with hirsutism, occurs in approximately 1% of hirsute women. *Cushing's disease* results in hirsutism from corticotropin-mediated adrenal secretion of androgens.

In addition to the history and physical examination, laboratory evaluation should include measurement of serum testosterone, dehydroepiandrostenedione, and 17-hydroxyprogesterone, as outlined in Figure 71–5.

Therapy must be tailored to the cause. Patients should be advised that medical therapy does not have an immediate effect, and a trial of 6 months must be given before decisions of therapeutic efficacy may be made. Underlying neoplasms should be surgically removed, and adrenal hyperplasia should be treated with glucocorticoids. Antiandrogen agents such as spironolactone and flutamide may be useful. Cosmetic treatments such as bleaching, waxing, and electrolysis can be important adjuncts to medical therapy.

Hormone Therapy

Hormone therapy is often used for control of conception. Hormonal contraceptives can be administered as oral medications or as injectable or implantable preparations. *Oral contraceptive agents* are the most widely used form of contraception in the industrialized world. Table 71–5 describes the benefits of oral contraceptives, whereas Table 71–6 describes contraindications to their use.

Current oral contraceptive formulations contain combinations of estrogen in doses ranging from 20 to 50 μg and progestin in varying types and dosages. Additionally,

TABLE 71–4 Causes of Androgen-Dependent Hirsutism

Ovarian Disorders

Chronic anovulation
Virilizing ovarian tumors
HAIR-AN syndrome
Hyperthecosis

Adrenal Disorders

Congenital adrenal hyperplasia
  21-Hydroxylase deficiency
  3β-Hydroxysteroid dehydrogenase deficiency
  11-Hydroxylase deficiency
Virilizing adrenal tumors

Hypothalamic-Pituitary Disorders

Acromegaly
Cushing's disease

Exogenous Androgens

Anabolic steroids
Danazol

HAIR-AN = hyperandrogenism, insulin resistance, and acanthosis nigricans.

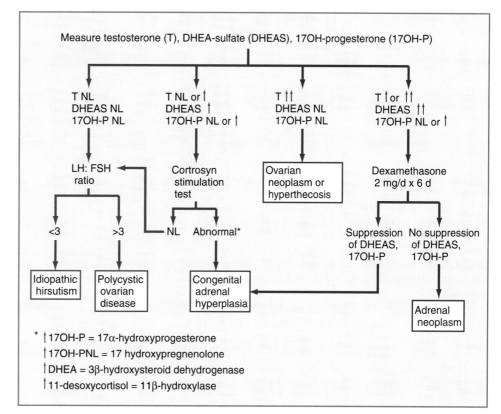

FIGURE 71–5 Laboratory evaluation of hirsutism (see text for details). ↑ = increased; ↑ ↑ = markedly increased; DHEAS = dehydroepiandrosterone; NL = normal; 17OH-P = 17α-hydroxyprogesterone.

* ↑17OH-P = 17α-hydroxyprogesterone
↑17OH-PNL = 17 hydroxypregnenolone
↑DHEA = 3β-hydroxysteroid dehydrogenase
↑11-desoxycortisol = 11β-hydroxylase

some oral contraceptives contain only progestin. When oral contraceptives are used properly, the failure rate for combination pills is 1% to 2%, and that for progestin-only pills is 4% to 9%. Injectable or implantable contraceptives such as medroxyprogesterone and levonorgestrol have a contraceptive effect that lasts for months.

Before prescribing contraceptive hormone therapy, the physician should obtain a detailed medical history, particularly with respect to past or current malignant diseases, breast disease, liver disease, thrombophlebitis, hypertension, migraine headache, stroke, diabetes, and smoking. A menstrual history should also be taken, and the presence of abnormal uterine bleeding should prompt appropriate investigation before initiation of oral contraceptive therapy. Thorough thyroid, breast, pelvic, and abdominal examinations should be performed.

TABLE 71–5   Benefits Associated with Oral Contraceptives

Reduced Pregnancy Risk
Morbidity and mortality
Ectopic pregnancy
Anemia
Spontaneous and induced abortions

Reduced Risk of Hospitalizations and Gynecologic Surgery
Pelvic inflammatory disease, salpingitis, infertility
Ovarian cancer
Functional ovarian cysts
Uterine fibroids
Endometrial cancer
Abnormal bleeding

Other Benefits
Reduced dysmenorrhea
Fewer mood swings and less premenstrual syndrome
Increased bone mass
Less rheumatoid arthritis
Less benign breast disease

From: Shoupe D: Contraception—Conception control. *In* Wallis LA (ed): Textbook of Women's Health. Philadelphia: Lippincott-Raven, 1998.

TABLE 71–6   Contraindications to Oral Contraceptive Use

Age >35 yr and smoker or hypertensive
Current or past history of cerebral vascular or systemic vascular disease
Marked impairment of liver function
Current or past history of thromboembolic disorders
Known or suspected carcinoma of the breast
Known or suspected estrogen-dependent neoplasia
Undiagnosed abnormal genital bleeding
Pregnancy
Severe hyperlipidemia
Severe migraine headaches with localizing signs
Uncontrolled hypertension
Symptomatic gallbladder disease
Uncontrolled diabetes mellitus
Sickle cell disease

From Shoupe D: Contraception—Conception control. *In* Wallis LA (ed): Textbook of Women's Health. Philadelphia: Lippincott-Raven, 1998.

When considering prescription of oral contraceptive agents in women >35 years old, the physician must review several issues. The combination of oral contraceptives and smoking increases the risk of myocardial infarction by 20-fold because of the interaction of the procoagulant effects of oral contraceptives and abnormal endothelial function induced by cigarette smoking. Oral contraceptives have not been associated with increases in the incidence of breast cancer. Decreases in malignant tumors of the ovary and endometrium are seen in oral contraceptive users. Perimenopausal women taking oral contraceptives have less bone loss than those women receiving replacement estrogen therapy.

Estrogen replacement therapy, commonly known as *hormone replacement therapy,* is given for many reasons (Table 71–7). At the time of natural menopause, hormone replacement therapy may be administered for short-term amelioration of menopausal symptoms or for longer-term prevention of osteoporosis or coronary artery disease.

Although estrogen therapy has many beneficial effects in women with estrogen-deficient states, unopposed estrogen use stimulates the endometrium and may result in uterine hyperplasia or, rarely, carcinoma. Therefore, postmenopausal women with intact uteri who receive hormone replacement therapy require progestins in either a cycled fashion or as a small daily dose. Progestins have opposing effects to estrogen on high-density lipo-

TABLE 71–8 Contraindications to Hormone Replacement Therapy

Absolute Contraindications	Relative Contraindications
Presence or history of breast cancer	Family history of breast cancer
Breast mass, unevaluated	History of thromboembolism
Presence of noneradicated endometrial cancer	Enlarging or excessively bleeding fibroids
Active thromboembolic disease	Severe endometriosis, untreated
Acute and chronic liver disease	
Unexplained vaginal bleeding	
Pregnancy	

From Wallis LA, Barbo DM: Hormone replacement therapy (HRT). *In* Wallis LA (ed): Textbook of Women's Health. Philadelphia: Lippincott-Raven, 1998.

protein cholesterol and have vasoconstrictor effects on vasomotor function. Therefore, progestins are not indicated in women who have had hysterectomies. Long-term hormone replacement therapy (>5 to 10 years) is associated with small but significant increases in the incidence of breast cancer (1.3 to 1.5 risk ratio), a risk that is not affected by the use of progestins. The effect of hormone replacement therapy on ovarian cancer risk is unclear. Contraindications to hormone replacement therapy are shown in Table 71–8.

In the postmenopausal woman, the benefit of estrogen on bone, cardiovascular, and brain tissue must be weighed against its neoplastic stimulatory efforts on the endometrium. Therefore, enormous interest has been shown in identifying compounds with the beneficial effects of estrogen but without negative side effects. Tissue-selective estrogen receptor modulators are a group of compounds that bind to estrogen receptors and may act as either agonists or antagonists. The two best characterized agents in this class are raloxifene and tamoxifen. Both act as estrogen agonists in bone tissue and prevent remodeling, and both agents lower total cholesterol levels. Both tamoxifen and raloxifene act as estrogen antagonists in breast tissue and thus retard the growth of estrogen-dependent tumors. The two compounds have opposite effects, however, on uterine tissue; tamoxifen acts as a partial agonist and stimulating endometrial tissue, whereas raloxifene acts as an estrogen antagonist and suppresses endometrial proliferation. Raloxifene is used to prevent osteoporosis in high-risk postmenopausal women, whereas tamoxifen is used as adjunctive treatment in estrogen receptor–positive breast cancer as well as for prevention of breast cancer. Development of tissue-selective estrogen receptor modulators with few agonist effects on reproductive tissue but with potent agonist effects in nonreproductive tissue may represent an important therapeutic strategy to improve the health and functional capacity of postmenopausal women.

TABLE 71–7 Indications for Estrogen Administration

Absence of or Premature Halt in Ovarian Function
Ovarian agenesis
Premature menopause, spontaneous
Induced cessation of menses
    Oophorectomy
    Radiation
    Chemotherapy
Excessive exercise amenorrhea
Anorexia nervosa or bulimia
Postpartum depression

Symptoms at Menopause
Vasomotor
Urogenital
Skin and mucous membranes
Musculoskeletal
Psychological
Higher integrative functions
Insomnia
Fatigue

Urogenital Atrophy
Dryness
Dyspareunia
Dysuria and frequency
Urge incontinence
Stress incontinence
Bleeding

From Wallis LA, Barbo DM: Hormone replacement therapy (HRT). *In* Wallis LA (ed): Textbook of Women's Health. Philadelphia: Lippincott-Raven, 1998.

REFERENCES

Couchman GM, Hammond CB: Physiology of reproduction. *In* Scott JR (ed): Danforth's Obstetrics and Gynecology, 8th ed. Philadelphia: Lippincott Williams & Wilkins, 1999, pp 47–64.

Johnson SR: Premenstrual syndrome. *In* Wallis LA (ed): Textbook of Women's Health. Philadelphia: Lippincott-Raven, 1998, pp 691–697.

Levine DW, Hillard PJ: The menstrual cycle and abnormal uterine bleeding. *In* Wallis LA (ed): Textbook of Women's Health. Philadelphia: Lippincott-Raven, 1998, pp 601–610.

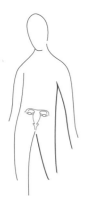

72

DISEASES COMMON IN WOMEN

Sally L. Hodder • Anne L. Taylor

Cardiovascular Diseases

Cardiovascular diseases kill more women annually than all forms of cancer, chronic lung disease, pneumonia, and diabetes, but the prevalence and consequences of heart disease in women are often underestimated. It is widely believed that male gender is associated with susceptibility to cardiovascular morbidity and mortality and female gender is associated with protection from cardiovascular disease. These generalizations are true for men and women in early adulthood, but they become progressively less relevant with each decade of life. By the seventh and eighth decades of life, heart disease is almost equally prevalent in men and women. Significant differences exist between men and women with respect to the impact of risk factors in the development of coronary atherosclerosis, the presentation and clinical features of coronary heart disease, and the morbidity and mortality of coronary events. Women develop the disease approximately 10 years later than men; however, when women suffer a myocardial infarction, their outcome is substantially poorer than that of their male counterparts. Women presenting with myocardial infarction are less likely to be managed aggressively by their physicians. Comparison of women by ethnicity shows that cardiovascular mortality in African-American women is 34% higher than in white women.

Risk factors for coronary heart disease in women are generally the same as those in men (see Chapter 7). However, the *impact* of many risk factors differs between men and women. For example, diabetes mellitus increases the risk of developing coronary heart disease by threefold to sevenfold in women compared with twofold to threefold in men. A low high-density lipoprotein cholesterol level is a stronger predictor of coronary heart disease in women than in men, and an elevated triglyceride level may also be a more important risk factor in women. Hypertension has an equal effect on coronary disease risk in men and women, and control of hypertension results in equivalent reductions in coronary heart disease risk in men and women. Overall, however, there is less available evidence that modification of risk factors in women results in a reduced risk of coronary heart disease. Reduction of cholesterol in women with established coronary heart disease has substantial secondary preventive effects; however, women with hypercholesterolemia are less often treated than men with this disorder. Cigarette smoking, an especially important risk factor for women taking oral contraceptives, has been increasing at higher rates among young women than among young men. The effects of psychosocial factors such as depression (five times more common in women), social and economic support (diminished in older women), and gender-specific responses to stress all require further study.

Most existing data suggest that the risk of coronary heart disease is significantly reduced in women who take postmenopausal hormone replacement therapy. The cardioprotective biologic effects of estrogen (Table 72–1) include regulation of endothelial production of nitric oxide, elevation in high-density lipoprotein cholesterol, reduction in low-density lipoprotein cholesterol and fibrinogen, and smooth muscle antiproliferative and antioxidant effects. However, the epidemiologic data that guide usage of estrogens for prevention of coronary heart disease have significant limitations, with differences in risk profiles and health behaviors between the estrogen users and nonusers. One large clinical trial (Heart and Estrogen/Progestin Replacement Study [HERS]) in women with established coronary artery disease failed to show a difference in mortality or myocardial infarction rates between treated and untreated groups. Further randomized clinical trials are needed to understand the utility of estrogen for prevention of coronary artery disease.

Significant differences exist between men and women in the clinical presentation of coronary artery disease. Myocardial infarction is more often the initial presentation in men, whereas angina is more frequently the initial presentation in women. Women with established

TABLE 72–1   Estrogen Effect on Cardiovascular Risk Factors

Risk Factor	Change
Lipid effects:	
Low-density lipoprotein	↓
High-density lipoprotein	↑
Triglycerides	↑
Lipoprotein (a)	↓
Endothelial effects	
Endothelin (vasoconstrictor)	↓
EDRF (vasodilation)	↑
Other effects	
Oxidation of low-density lipoprotein	↓
Cell proliferation	↓

EDRF = endothelium-dependent relaxing factor.
From Wallis LA, Barbo DM: Hormone replacement therapy (HRT). *In* Wallis LA (ed); Textbook of Women's Health. Philadelphia: Lippincott, Williams & Wilkins, 1998.

coronary heart disease have significantly higher short- and long-term mortality rates after myocardial infarction. After myocardial infarction, women are twice as likely as men to have congestive heart failure, recurrent angina, and recurrent infarction. Factors possibly related to the poorer outcome of women include older age at presentation and higher prevalence rates of diabetes and hypertension. Treatment patterns for men and women also differ, with women significantly less likely to receive aggressive management that includes cardiac catheterization and revascularization procedures. Significant differences in physician interpretation of a patient's symptoms and the patient's assessment of risk of symptoms may also contribute to gender differences in outcomes.

Stroke is the third leading cause of death in the United States and the most important cause of severe disability in the United States. Although men have a higher prevalence of stroke, women have higher mortality rates due to stroke. African-American women have an increased prevalence of stroke when compared with white women. Of the recognized risk factors for stroke in both men and women, hypertension and diabetes mellitus are more prevalent in women. The incidence of stroke is not affected by hormone replacement therapy, although mortality may be reduced by hormone replacement therapy.

Osteoporosis

Osteoporosis is a preventable and treatable disease, yet many women are unaware that they have osteoporosis until sustaining an often life-threatening fracture. Postmenopausal white women are most often affected by osteoporosis. Approximately 15% of American women older than the age of 49 have osteoporosis, whereas another 40% to 50% have low bone mass. In the United States, there are approximately 5 million women with osteoporosis and 15 million with low bone mass. This compares with 1.5 million men older than age 49 with

osteoporosis and 6.5 million men with low bone mass. In 1995 more than $13 billion was spent on osteoporosis-associated fractures, with 80% of this money used to treat women. Estrogen receptors are present in bone tissue, and estrogen production at menarche, in addition to weight-bearing activities, is critical to achieving maximal adult bone density. Loss of estrogen at menopause results in a decline in new bone synthesis. In addition to gender and race, conditions associated with secondary amenorrhea, including eating disorders, are major risk factors for the development of osteoporosis. The National Osteoporosis Foundation has defined the following as major risk factors for fracture development in women: low body weight (<58 kg), current smoker, and first-degree relative with or personal history of low-trauma fracture (see Chapter 76).

Osteoporosis has been defined as a bone mineral density 2.5 standard deviations below the mean peak value in young adults. Individuals with a bone mineral density between 1.0 and 2.49 standard deviations below the mean are defined as being osteopenic or having low bone mass. Techniques to evaluate bone marrow density are described in Chapter 76. Because therapeutic interventions for osteoporosis usually have their maximal effect on the spine, bone mineral density of the spine is clinically used to assess response to therapy.

Because therapy is very effective in fracture prevention in postmenopausal women, primary care should include an assessment of a woman's risk for development of osteoporosis. Measurement of bone mineral density is indicated in all women with risk factors (see Table 76–2) as well as in women with osteopenia, height loss, or spinal deformity noted on radiographs of the spine.

Treatment and prevention of osteoporosis require maintenance of sufficient calcium and vitamin D intake throughout life as well as regular weight-bearing exercise. Vitamin D should be supplemented in individuals, particularly the elderly, at risk for vitamin D deficiency. Current and future therapies for osteoporosis in women are presented in Table 72–2. Estrogen-replacement therapy is the most effective available agent for the prevention and treatment of osteoporosis in postmenopausal women. Estrogens act to inhibit bone reabsorption. Estrogen-replacement therapy is most effective if begun within 5 years of menopause. Conjugated estrogens, micronized estradiol, and transdermal estrogen are effective in reducing spine and femoral neck bone loss. Progestin therapy should be used with estrogen-replacement therapy to decrease the risk of endometrial hyperplasia and carcinoma induced by unopposed estrogen acting on the uterus. Raloxifene, a selective estrogen-receptor modulator, prevents bone loss in the spine and hip, but to a lesser extent than estrogen-replacement therapy or alendronate. The attractive aspect of raloxifene is that the endometrium is not stimulated. Therefore, addition of cyclic progestin is unnecessary, making raloxifene an acceptable agent to some women who do not wish to use cyclic estrogen and progestin replacement therapy.

The roles of biphosphonate compounds and calcitonin in preventing bone loss are described in Chapter 76.

In patients with osteoporosis, fracture risk should be

TABLE 72–2 **Current and Future Therapies for Osteoporosis and Osteoporosis Prevention in Women**

Drug	Dose	Side Effects
Conjugated estrogens	0.625 mg/day	Breast tenderness/enlargement Vaginal candidiasis Thromboembolic disease Nausea/vomiting
Micronized estradiol	0.5 mg/day	Same as above
Transdermal estradiol	0.05–0.1 mg/day‡	Same as above *plus* skin irritation at the application site
Raloxifene*	60 mg/day	Thromboembolic disease
Alendronate	5 mg/day	Esophagitis
	10 mg/day	Esophageal hemorrhage
Calcium	1000–1500 mg/day	
Vitamin D	400–800 IU/day	
Calcitonin-salmon	200 IU/day	Nausea, flushing, diarrhea
Sodium-fluoride†	50–75 mg/day	Gastric irritation Stress fractures
Parathyroid hormone†	400 IU/day	

*Approved by the U.S. Food and Drug Administration (FDA) for prevention only.
†Not FDA approved.
‡Transdermal patch replaced twice weekly.
Caution: estrogens should be cycled with progestins in women and intact uteri.

minimized. Efforts should be made to eliminate modifiable risk factors such as smoking and excess alcohol use. Strategies to prevent falls should include limiting sedative drugs and promotion of exercise. Heavy lifting should be avoided.

Finally, realistic therapeutic goals should be established. Effective therapy will halve the fracture risk but not eliminate it. Patients presenting with a new fracture should be given appropriate analgesia, and the physician should discuss the importance of continuing osteoporosis therapy.

Breast Cancer and Benign Breast Disease

Breast cancer is the most common malignancy in women, accounting for approximately 30% of cancers in women and for more than 40,000 deaths annually. Risk factors for development of breast cancer are found in Table 69–1 in the 4th edition of this book. Fifteen percent of breast cancers are diagnosed in women younger than the age of 40. By the time a woman is 80 years of age, she has a 1 in 10 probability of developing breast cancer. Certain inherited mutations in *BRCA-1* and *BRCA-2* genes are associated with an increased incidence of breast cancer.

The role of ovarian hormones in the development of breast cancer is incompletely understood. Tamoxifen, an estrogen antagonist in breast tissue, reduces the incidence of breast cancer in the contralateral breast of women with estrogen-receptor–positive tumors. Tamoxifen may also, however, act as an estrogen agonist in endometrial tissue, explaining the observed increased incidence of endometrial cancer in patients on tamoxifen.

Although genetic screening and possible hormone manipulation remain promising strategies to decrease the incidence of breast cancer, breast cancer screening is the best current strategy to decrease breast cancer mortality. Mammography is more sensitive than breast examination to detect small cancers; however, mammograms fail to detect 10% to 15% of breast cancers. Breast cancer mortality is significantly reduced in women older than the age of 50 in whom yearly mammography and breast examination is performed. Although there is debate on the appropriate screening procedures for women aged 40 to 49, the American Cancer Society recommends that women aged 40 to 49 should receive screening mammograms. Monthly breast self-examination as well as yearly clinical breast examination by a physician are important screening strategies.

It is important to evaluate aggressively breast complaints in women to avoid delays in the diagnosis of breast cancer. The incidence of breast cancer as the underlying etiology of a breast mass increases with increasing age. Breast masses in adolescents are commonly due to fibroadenomas. Ten percent of breast masses are malignant in women aged 25 to 40, whereas 35% are malignant in the 35- to 55-year age group, and 85% of breast masses in women older than the age of 55 are due to carcinoma. Fibroadenomas constitute 25% of breast masses in women aged 25 to 40 and 10% in women aged 35 to 55. Fibrocystic breast disease accounts for 55% of breast masses in the 25- to 40-year age group and 30% in the 35- to 55-year age group. Cystic masses are easily distinguished from solid masses with fine-needle aspiration. Cysts that yield bloody fluid or fail to resolve completely with aspiration should be further evaluated with biopsy. Presence of breast erythema or skin dimpling requires biopsy to rule out carcinoma even if breast examination and mammogram fail to show a defined mass. Paget's carcinoma should be considered in cases of nipple scaling and ruled out by punch biopsy. Staging and treatment strategies are discussed in Chapter 56.

Breast pain is a common complaint. An associated breast mass must be thoroughly evaluated to exclude the presence of breast cancer. Dietary modulation to decrease caffeine ingestion may be beneficial in some patients with breast pain. Although oral contraceptive agents do not appear to cause breast pain, hormone replacement therapy may do so. Estrogen dose alteration may be helpful.

Cancer of the Cervix, Uterus, and Ovary

Malignancies of the female reproductive tract affect approximately 70,000 Americans yearly with more than 20,000 deaths per year attributable to cancers of the ovary, uterus, and cervix.

The incidence and mortality due to cervical cancer have markedly decreased in the United States over the past 30 years. This decrease is largely due to the broad use of Papanicolaou (Pap) smears. A single negative Pap smear decreases the risk of cervical cancer by 45%, whereas nine negative Pap smears decrease the risk by 99%. Current recommendations for the performance of Pap smears specify that an initial smear should be performed at age 18, or at the time an adolescent becomes sexually active. Three annual Pap smears should be performed, with subsequent frequency determined by the presence of risk factors. The majority of cervical carcinomas are squamous cell, with approximately 90% of these tumors containing human papillomavirus (HPV) DNA. More than 90% of cervical intraepithelial lesions believed to be precursors of cervical carcinoma also contain HPV DNA, suggesting a role for this virus in oncogenic transformation. About 25 HPV types infect the human anogenital tract. Some HPV types are associated with low-grade squamous intraepithelial lesions, whereas other specific types, most often type 16 or 18, are associated with high-grade intraepithelial lesions and squamous cell carcinomas. Viral integration of types 16 and 18 results in overexpression of certain viral proteins; these proteins subsequently bind and inactivate cellular proteins that suppress cellular proliferation, resulting in a selective advantage for HPV-infected cells. Information on staging, treatment, and prognosis of cervical cancer is found in Chapter 56.

Endometrial carcinoma accounts for 7% of all malignancies in women in the United States. Unlike cervical carcinoma, endometrial cancer has been increasing in the United States, probably owing to the presence of an aging population. Most are adenocarcinomas, although a small percentage of these tumors are sarcomas. There are currently no accepted methods to screen for endometrial cancer; Pap smears are not a sensitive method for detection. However, the presence of atypical endometrial cells in the Pap smear in a premenopausal woman or of any endometrial cells in a postmenopausal woman should prompt further evaluation to exclude the presence of endometrial neoplasia. The most common presenting symptom is abnormal uterine bleeding. Any uterine bleeding in a postmenopausal woman or change in bleeding pattern in a woman on hormone replacement therapy is indication for thorough evaluation that includes an endometrial biopsy.

Ovarian carcinoma occurs in approximately 1 in 70 women in the United States. Unlike carcinoma of the cervix, there are no effective screening methods. Unlike endometrial carcinomas, which may present at an early stage with abnormal bleeding, ovarian carcinomas are frequently asymptomatic until the disease has progressed to an advanced stage (see Chapter 56).

Sexually Transmitted Diseases and Pelvic Inflammatory Disease

The health impact of sexually transmitted diseases (STDs) is disproportionately borne by women. Women are more easily infected than men by most STDs. Diagnosis is more difficult in women because the acute infection may be asymptomatic, and serious sequelae such as pelvic inflammatory disease (PID), infertility, perinatal and neonatal morbidity and mortality, and cervical carcinoma may result. Anyone engaging in sexual intercourse is at risk for acquiring an STD. For treatable infections such as chlamydia, gonorrhea, or syphilis, it is crucial to treat all sexual contacts of infected individuals. Clinics providing care solely to women should either alter their normal daily operation and treat male contacts or make arrangements for the appropriate treatment of male sexual partners. Chapter 107 provides specific treatment recommendations of infection with individual pathogens.

Screening strategies for some organisms are effective in detecting the presence of infection in largely asymptomatic populations. Because 75% of women with *Chlamydia trachomatis* infections are asymptomatic and 20% to 40% of infected women may develop PID, screening for *C. trachomatis* is an important strategy to control morbidity. Adolescents are at particular risk, because it is estimated that 1 in 10 are infected with this organism. Frequent screening for *C. trachomatis* is recommended for sexually active adolescents and for women aged 20 to 24, particularly if the woman does not use barrier contraceptives or has new or multiple sexual partners. Treatment of infected pregnant women prevents transmission of *C. trachomatis* to infants at delivery. Individuals treated for chlamydia should be advised to abstain from sexual intercourse for 7 days after a single-dose regimen or until a 7-day regimen is completed.

With infection by *Neisseria gonorrhoeae*, a large proportion of women are also asymptomatic and 10% to 40% of untreated women develop PID. Although less common than *C. trachomatis*, gonorrhea rates have increased in adolescents in many geographic regions. Therefore, screening is an important strategy for control of this infection. All women at high risk for STDs should be screened periodically. Women at especially high risk include but are not limited to the following groups: (1) sexually active adolescents, (2) women with a past history of gonorrhea, (3) prostitutes, and (4) homeless women.

Syphilis is a curable disease that increased dramatically among women of all ages from 1985 to 1990. Female adolescents had twice the rate of syphilis as their male counterparts for the year 1993. African-American women have rates of syphilis seven times that observed in the female population as a whole. Congenital syphilis is a catastrophic neonatal infection that is largely preventable, yet in 1993 there were 3000 reported cases in the United States. Serologic screening of all pregnant women should be performed. However, because one third of women giving birth to infants with congenital syphilis have no prenatal care, and one half of mothers of infected infants will have had a negative serologic test in the first trimester of pregnancy, repeat serologic testing at delivery is indicated in high-risk patients. All infants whose mothers test positive for syphilis should be treated, as should sexual contacts of the mother.

Human immunodeficiency virus (HIV) screening should be routinely offered to all pregnant women, because many HIV-infected women are asymptomatic, and appropriate treatment of the HIV-infected mother reduces maternal-infant HIV transmission by at least 67% (see Chapter 108). Counseling about the risk posed by heterosexual contact, particularly with partners who use intravenous drugs, as well as the protective effect of condoms, should be a normal part of routine health care for both men and women.

PID is a spectrum of upper genital tract inflammatory disorders that can include any combination of endometritis, salpingitis, tubo-ovarian abscess, and pelvic peritonitis. Sexually transmitted infectious organisms are implicated in most cases. Adolescents are at greater risk than women of other ages. Other recognized risk factors include multiple sexual partners and new sexual partners within the past 30 days. PID is the leading cause of preventable infertility. A single episode of PID results in infertility in 13% of affected women. Infertility rates skyrocket with subsequent PID episodes, with approximately 30% of women becoming infertile after two PID episodes and 50% to 75% becoming infertile after three or more episodes. Subsequent ectopic pregnancy, the leading cause of pregnancy-related deaths in African-American women, is a major complication.

Diagnosis of PID is made difficult by the diversity of signs and symptoms that may be present. Many patients may be asymptomatic; two thirds of patients with laparoscopic evidence of old PID cannot recall a past history of the disease. Moreover, some women may have very mild symptoms, such as a vaginal discharge and dyspareunia. Although laparoscopy may be used to diagnose salpingitis, it is not readily available for use in most acute cases. The diagnosis of PID is therefore based on clinical findings, but no single historical, physical, or

TABLE 72–3 **Treatment Regimens for Pelvic Inflammatory Disease**

Intravenous Regimens

Cefotetan, 2 g q12h, or cefoxitin, 2 g q6h, + doxycycline, 100 mg q12h

Clindamycin, 900 mg q8h, + gentamicin, 2 mg/kg loading dose followed by 1.5 mg/kg q8h*

Other Regimens

Ceftriaxone, 250 mg IM (single dose), or cefoxitin, 2 g IM (single dose), with probenecid, 1 g, + doxycycline, 100 mg bid for 14 days

*Although single daily dose gentamicin has not been evaluated for the treatment of pelvic inflammatory disease, it is efficacious in other analogous situations.

From Centers for Disease Control and Prevention: 1998 Guidelines for treatment of sexually transmitted diseases. MMWR Morbid Mortal Wkly Rep 1998; 47(RR-1).

laboratory finding is both sensitive and specific for the PID. Empirical treatment for PID should be initiated in any patient at risk for PID in whom all of the following criteria are present and for which no other diagnosis is identified: (1) lower abdominal tenderness, (2) adnexal tenderness, and (3) cervical motion tenderness. Further support for the diagnosis is provided by abnormal cervical discharge and documentation of infection with *N. gonorrhoeae* or *C. trachomatis*. Definitive criteria for diagnosing PID include (1) histopathologic evidence of endometritis on endometrial biopsy, (2) thickened fluid-filled fallopian tubes with or without free pelvic fluid or tubo-ovarian abscess demonstrated by abdominal imaging, and (3) laparoscopic abnormalities consistent with PID. A low threshold for consideration of this diagnosis and for initiating empirical treatment in women presenting with atypical symptoms is needed.

Table 72–3 presents treatment regimens recommended by the Centers for Disease Control and Prevention. There are no currently available data comparing the efficacy of either parenteral with oral treatment reg-

TABLE 72–4 **Criteria for Hospitalization of Persons with PID**

Surgical emergencies such as appendicitis cannot be excluded.

The patient is pregnant.

The patient does not respond clinically to oral antimicrobial therapy.

The patient is unable to follow or tolerate an outpatient oral regimen.

The patient has severe illness, nausea and vomiting, or high fever.

The patient has a tubo-ovarian abscess.

The patient is immunodeficient (i.e., has human immunodeficiency virus infection with low CD4 counts, is taking immunosuppressive therapy, or has another disease).

From Centers for Disease Control and Prevention: 1998 Guidelines for treatment of sexually transmitted diseases. MMWR Morbid Mortal Wkly Rep 1998; 47(RR-1).

imens or inpatient and ambulatory treatment settings. Table 72–4 contains currently recommended criteria for hospitalization of patients with PID. Patients should show marked clinical improvement within 3 days after treatment is initiated. Patients who remain febrile or fail to show diminished abdominal, adnexal, and cervical motion tenderness usually require additional diagnostic studies or surgical intervention. Sexual partners of PID patients should be evaluated for STDs and treated for *C. trachomatis* and *N. gonorrhoeae* infection even if evidence is not found by diagnostic studies.

Urinary Incontinence

Incontinence, an involuntary loss of urine, occurs when bladder pressure exceeds urethral pressure. It may be further categorized as stress incontinence (related to position changes or Valsalva's maneuver when coughing or sneezing), urge incontinence (loss of urine with urgency to urinate), overflow incontinence (pressure in maximally distended bladder is relieved by flow of urine out of bladder), and functional incontinence (loss of urine due to extrinsic factors, such as stroke or immobility). Incontinence is common in women; in fact, the incidence may approach 25% in postmenopausal women. This contrasts to its uncommon occurrence in men. The normal female urethra has many folds that result in a mucosal seal. Urethral mucosa cells possess estrogen receptors, and estrogen is necessary for maintenance of a highly functional urethral mucosa. In the perimenopausal period, stress incontinence may occur due to a loss of the elasticity and tone of the urethral epithelium. In addition to mucosal abnormalities due to hypoestrogen states, bladder outlet dysfunction may also result from presence of cystourethrocele (relaxation of the bladder and urethra into the vagina), weakness of the external sphincteric mechanism (e.g., pudendal nerve damage), and bladder neck incompetence (usually due to a previous invasive procedure such as urethropexy).

Evaluation of women with incontinence should include a history that clearly characterizes the type of incontinence as well as its frequency. Current medications, coexistent medical problems (e.g., diabetes mellitus or primary neurologic disease), and current hormonal status are also important components of the history. Physical examination should include a complete pelvic examination with careful observation of vaginal and urethral mucosa. In addition, a complete neurologic examination should be performed. Rectal examination that specifically assesses resting anal sphincter tone, presence or absence of rectocele, presence of an anal wink, and ability to voluntarily contract sphincters is also required. Further evaluation should include urinalysis and cultures to rule out urinary tract infection and determination of postvoid residual urine volume. Referral to a urologist or urogynecologist for performance of urodynamics is indicated in patients with previous pelvic surgery, nocturnal enuresis, continuous incontinence, increased postvoid residuals, or history or signs of neurologic disease. Experts disagree on whether urodynamic evaluation is required before surgery for all women with stress incontinence without other symptoms or signs.

Treatment depends on the etiology of the incontinence. Many medical treatments are available. Hormone replacement therapy is often helpful in postmenopausal women with incontinence. Other medical therapies are listed in Table 72–5. In addition to pharmacologic therapy, pelvic muscle exercises may improve pelvic floor muscle strength. Regular voiding without waiting for the urinary urge may also be helpful. Surgery may be indicated when more conservative therapies fail.

Domestic Violence

Violence against women is a major health care issue. In the United States, domestic violence is the leading cause of injury to women aged 15 to 44. It is estimated that 2 to 4 million women in the United States are physically abused every year and that violence may occur in up to one of every four families. Domestic violence occurs across all cultural, ethnic, and socioeconomic boundaries. Frequent physician visits for multiple

TABLE 72–5 **Treatment of Urinary Incontinence**

Medication	Indication	Starting Dosage
Oxybutynin chloride	Urgency incontinence Frequency/urgency	2.5 mg one to three times daily
Hyoscyamine sulfate	Urgency incontinence Frequency/urgency	½ (0.375 mg pill) one to two times daily
Propantheline bromide	Urgency incontinence Frequency/urgency	15 mg one to three times daily
Imipramine hydrochloride	Urgency incontinence Mixed incontinence	10 mg one to three times daily
Pseudoephedrine*	Stress incontinence	30 mg one to three times daily
Phenylpropanolamine*	Stress incontinence	50 mg one to three times daily

*These medications are best administered in sustained-release formulas as in Rondec TR, Enlex LA, or Ornade.
From Bavendan TG: Urinary Tract Health and Disorders of Women. *In* Wallis LA (ed): Textbook of Women's Health. Philadelphia: Lippincott-Raven, 1998.

complaints may be an indication that a woman is a victim of violence, inasmuch as women often complain of multiple somatic illnesses rather than the abuse. In families where women are victims of violence, children are also frequently assaulted. Thus, it is imperative for physicians to identify patients who are victims of domestic violence.

Domestic violence encompasses violence not only in marital relationships but also in other significant relationships such as dating and cohabitation. Although all female patients should be asked about the possibility of physical, sexual, and emotional abuse, few primary care physicians consistently attempt to elicit such information. Although it is often emotionally difficult and embarrassing for an abused woman to reveal information about her past or current history of abuse, abused women are likely to respond honestly to personal history questions when alone with their physicians.

Illness associated with domestic violence may present in a variety of health care settings and in numerous physical and psychological ways. The emergency department is often utilized by women victims of domestic abuse. Multiple fractures, vulvar and rectal scarring, or suicide attempts often signify presence of domestic violence. Despite risk of serious injury or death, women with a history of domestic violence often present to primary care physicians with other somatic complaints. Sensitive screening of women for a history of family violence is essential. Treatment of domestic violence includes immediate assessment and management of injuries. Provision for emotional and psychological support as well as counseling regarding safe havens for the patient and her children are essential elements in managing victims of domestic violence.

Disorders of Cognition and Affect

The incidence and patterns of cognition and affective disorders are different in men and women. Depression, anxiety, and seasonal affective disorders are two to three times more common in women than men. Although the incidence of schizophrenia is equal in men and women, the onset is approximately 5 years later in women and may be exacerbated during low estrogen states. Bipolar disorder is equally prevalent in men and women, but women have more depressive episodes and more rapid cycling of moods. In addition, drug-induced and hyper-thyroid-induced rapid cycling is much more prominent in women.

The greater prevalence of depression and anxiety may, in part, be mediated by hormonal effects on neurotransmitter activity. Estrogen produces antidopaminergic and serotonin-enhancing effects, whereas progesterone metabolites affect γ-aminobutyric acid receptors.

Mood and psychologic state change with hormonal fluctuations of the reproductive cycle. Premenstrual dysphoric disorder occurs during the luteal phase of the menstrual cycle and abates within 1 to 2 days of menstruation. Oral contraceptives may precipitate recurrences of depression in women with a history of depression. The risk of psychosis or other major psychiatric illness is low during pregnancy but high in the postpartum period. Approximately 10% of women develop significant postpartum depression, with a peak incidence 4 to 5 months after delivery. Postpartum depression has been associated with emotional and intellectual deficits in children; thus, recognition and appropriate treatment may benefit both mothers and children. Whereas estrogen treatment has been associated with relief of postpartum depression, it may induce rapid cycling of bipolar disorder.

At menopause, a variety of neurophysiologic and cognitive changes occur. Women with a history of previous reproductive cycle–related mood disorders appear to have an increased risk for perimenopausal depression.

In elderly populations, the incidence of Alzheimer's dementia is 2.7-fold higher in women, whereas the incidence of multi-infarct dementia is the same in the two sexes. Epidemiologic data suggest that estrogen replacement therapy may retard or prevent the development of Alzheimer's dementia, and clinical trials are being performed to study this issue.

REFERENCES

Bavendam TG: Urinary tract health and disorders of women. *In* Wallis LA (ed): Textbook of Women's Health. Philadelphia: Lippincott-Raven, 1998, pp 421–432.

Centers for Disease Control and Prevention: 1998 guidelines for treatment of sexually transmitted diseases. MMWR Morbid Mortal Wkly Rep 1998; 47(RR-1).

Eastell R: Treatment of postmenopausal osteoporosis. N Engl J Med 1998; 338:736–746.

Haskell SG, Richardson ED, Horwitz RI: The effect of estrogen replacement therapy on cognitive function in women: A critical review of the literature. J Clin Epidemiol 1997; 50:1249–1264.

Mosca L, Manson J, Sutherland S, et al: Cardiovascular disease in women: A statement for healthcare professionals from the American Heart Association. Circulation 1997; 96:2468–2482.

Wallis LA, Barbo DM: Hormone replacement therapy (HRT). *In* Wallis LA (ed): Textbook of Women's Health. Philadelphia: Lippincott-Raven, 1998, pp 731–746.

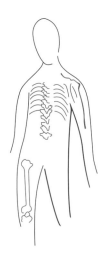

Diseases of Bone and Bone Mineral Metabolism

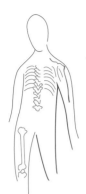

73

NORMAL PHYSIOLOGY OF BONE AND BONE MINERALS

F. Richard Bringhurst

Bone Structure and Metabolism

Bone is one of the largest organs in the body. It is superbly designed to carry out several vital functions: (1) providing shape and support for the body; (2) protecting the hematopoietic system and the structures within the cranium, pelvis, and thorax; (3) allowing for movement by providing levers, articulations, and points of attachment for muscles; and (4) serving as a reservoir for essential ions such as calcium, phosphorus, magnesium, and sodium.

TYPES OF BONE

The skeleton is composed of two main types of bone. *Cortical bone,* sometimes called compact bone, is arranged as circumferential lamellae in the subperiosteal and endosteal layers and as concentric lamellae around a central vascular supply (referred to as *osteons* or *haversian systems*) between these two surfaces (Fig. 73–1). Cortical bone constitutes roughly 80% of the adult skeleton and predominates in the shafts of the long bones. *Trabecular bone,* sometimes called spongy or cancellous bone, is arranged in microscopically parallel lamellae. An interconnected, open meshwork of thin plates, trabecular bone predominates in the vertebral bodies, ribs, pelvis, and ends of the long bones and is more metabolically active than cortical bone. The structures of cortical and trabecular bone are optimized to resist bending or torsional versus compressive stresses, respectively.

COMPOSITION OF BONE

Cellular Components

Bone is composed of cellular and noncellular components. The three most specialized cell types necessary for the metabolic activities of bone are osteoblasts, osteoclasts, and osteocytes. *Osteoblasts* are derived from pluripotential bone marrow stem cells that are capable of differentiation into fibroblastic, adipocytic, or chondrocytic/osteoblastic lineages. A critical signal for osteoblastic differentiation is provided by expression of the transcription factor cbfa-1. When dormant osteoblasts ("bone-lining cells") on the bone surface are activated to mature osteoblasts, they synthesize uncalcified bone matrix, or *osteoid,* and then promote its subsequent mineralization. Osteoblasts express specific receptors for parathyroid hormone (PTH), 1,25-dihydroxyvitamin D (1,25-[OH]$_2$D), insulin-like growth factor I, insulin, interleukin-1, interleukin-6, interleukin-11, thyroid hormones, estrogens, androgens, and glucocorticoids.

Osteoclasts are derived from hematopoetic precursors of the monocyte and macrophage lineage that fuse to form multinucleated giant cells capable of attaching to mineralized bone by specific signals *(RGD sequences)* present within exposed bone matrix proteins. By creating a localized acidic environment under the ruffled border of the cell, osteoclasts can dissolve the bone mineral and can provide an ideal environment for proteolytic enzymes to degrade the bone matrix. Osteoclasts and their progenitors appear to lack receptors for PTH, various cytokines, vitamin D, and other hormones that regulate osteoclastogenesis. Osteoclast formation proceeds through intimate cell-to-cell contact with neighboring marrow stromal or osteoblastic cells, which respond to osteoclast-inducing hormones and cytokines by increasing their expression of membrane-bound monocyte colony–stimulating factor and osteoclast differentiation factor, molecules for which specific receptors exist on the surface of osteoclast precursors. Mature osteoclasts also express calcitonin receptors, which inhibit their function. In addition, osteoclast activity is stimulated by interleukin-1, prostaglandin E$_2$, and tumor necrosis factor. When osteoclasts excavate an area of bone,

629

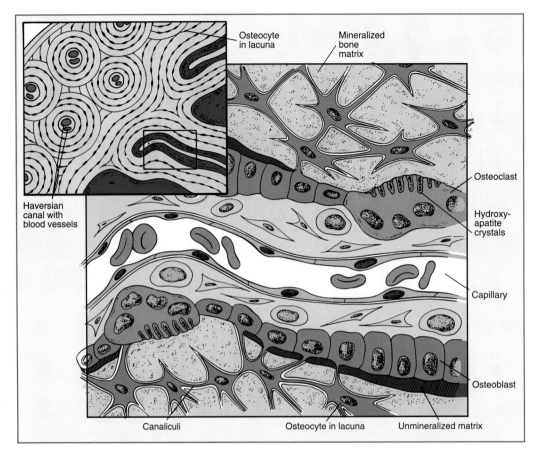

FIGURE 73–1 The most active bone remodeling occurs around the haversian canals, through which capillaries run. Osteoclasts and osteoblasts in all stages of development are found in greatest density in these areas. The *larger-scale inset drawing* depicts the syncytium-like layer of osteoblasts, connected with lacunar osteocytes through canaliculi, across which substances are exchanged between the modified bone interstitial fluid and the systemic extracellular fluid (ECF). (From Levine MM, Kleeman CR: Hypercalcemia: Pathophysiology and treatment. Hosp Pract 1987; 22:93; © 1987, The McGraw-Hill Companies. Illustration by Robert Margulies.)

membrane-embedded proteins, such as transforming growth factor-β, are released to signal local activation of osteoblasts, which then lay down new bone and attempt to repair the defect. This dynamic remodeling process occurs throughout the skeleton and provides the opportunity for regional changes in bone mass.

Osteocytes are terminally differentiated osteoblasts that maintain cell-to-cell contact by extended processes that traverse microscopic tunnels *(canaliculi)* within the mineralized bone. Osteocytes may play an important role in transducing responses to deformation and mechanical stress in bone.

Noncellular Components

The noncellular components of bone include the organic matrix and the inorganic matrix, which comprise roughly one third and two thirds, respectively, of total bone mass. *Type I collagen,* the most abundant structural protein in bone, makes up 90% of the organic matrix. Other proteins in bone include small amounts of other collagens and a host of noncollagenous proteins, including osteonectin, osteocalcin, osteopontin, fibronectin,

thrombospondin, bone sialoprotein, proteoglycans, and serum proteins. The inorganic matrix of bone is largely composed of *hydroxyapatite,* a mineral with the formula $Ca_{10}(PO_4)_6(OH)_2$. Its crystals are laid down on the collagen fibrils and the glycoproteins and proteoglycans *(ground substance)* between collagen fibrils. Other cations, notably magnesium and sodium, as well as calcium phosphates and many trace minerals, also are incorporated within the bone mineral phase and may be liberated when bone is resorbed by osteoclasts.

Calcium Metabolism

Total-body calcium in physiologically normal adults is about 1 to 2 kg. Ninety-nine percent of this calcium resides within the skeleton, 1% is in the extracellular fluid, and 0.1% is free intracellularly within the cytosol. Calcium has two important physiologic roles. In bone, calcium salts are essential for maintaining the structural integrity of the skeleton. In the extracellular fluid and the cytosol, calcium is essential for a variety of biochemical and cellular processes. Calcium also acts as an intracellular second messenger for many hormones, paracrine factors, and neurotransmitters.

EXTRACELLULAR CALCIUM

Calcium circulates in the plasma in three forms (Fig. 73–2): (1) ionized calcium (approximately 50%); (2) protein-bound calcium (approximately 40%); and (3) calcium that is complexed, mainly to bicarbonate, citrate, and phosphate (about 10%). The free or ionized fraction of blood calcium is physiologically the most important. Albumin accounts for most of the protein binding of calcium; globulins account for the remainder. Acidosis decreases binding of calcium to albumin and thereby increases ionized calcium, whereas alkalosis produces the converse situation. Changes in the concentration of serum proteins, especially albumin, therefore may affect the measurement of the total blood calcium independently of the ionized fraction. The impact of altered albumin concentrations may be approximately assessed by use of the following formula:

Corrected total calcium concentration (mg/dL)
= measured total calcium concentration (mg/dL)
+ 0.8 [4 − measured albumin concentration (g/dL)]

The ionized calcium concentration is physiologically controlled and is directly relevant to both neuromuscular function and activation of the calcium sensor in parathyroid glands and elsewhere. Thus, direct measurement of ionized calcium should be performed in situations such as critical illness, in which accurate knowledge of blood calcium is important and abnormal serum protein concentrations or acid-base disturbances may have altered the relation between total and ionized calcium.

INTRACELLULAR CALCIUM

The normal cytosolic calcium concentration is about 0.1 μM, or 1/10,000 of extracellular levels. This low concentration, which is stringently maintained by a system of active transport pumps on the inner and plasma membranes of cells, is needed to generate rapid cytosolic calcium transients critical for muscle contraction, neuromuscular transmission, and hormone or receptor signaling.

CALCIUM BALANCE

The level of ionized calcium in the extracellular fluid is homeostatically maintained by an effective balance of calcium absorption, calcium excretion, bone formation, and bone destruction. The principal sites of this regulation are the epithelia of the proximal small intestine and the renal tubules, although bone cells may cause large internal fluxes of calcium into and out of the skeleton. These calcium fluxes are controlled mainly by PTH and 1,25-(OH)₂D.

CALCIUM ABSORPTION

The normal dietary intake of healthy adults varies greatly. The average diet of an adult in the United States contains approximately 400 to 1000 mg of calcium, mostly derived from dairy products. On average, adults require daily calcium intakes of more than 400 mg to balance obligate losses in urine, feces, and sweat. The efficiency of intestinal calcium absorption is ad-

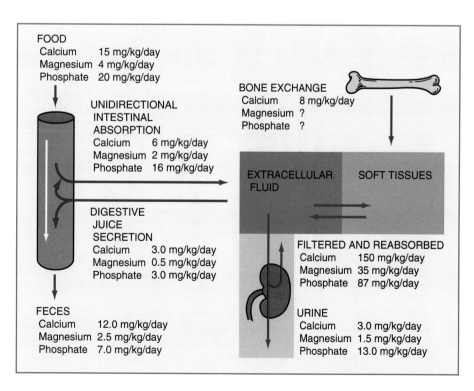

FIGURE 73–2 Typical mineral fluxes in adults. (Modified from Aurbach GD, Marx SJ, Spiegel AM: Parathyroid hormone, calcitonin, and the calciferols. *In* Wilson JD, Foster DW [eds]: Williams Textbook of Endocrinology, 7th ed. Philadelphia: WB Saunders, 1985, p 1144.)

justed in response to intake across the range of 10% to 70% of the ingested calcium. Calcium absorption occurs principally in the duodenum and the jejunum by an active process that involves buffered transcellular movement and extrusion into the blood against a steep electrochemical gradient. Several components of this process are strongly stimulated by 1,25-$(OH)_2D$, the main regulator of active intestinal calcium transport. Synthesis of 1,25-$(OH)_2D$ by the renal tubules is activated by PTH when dietary calcium availability is reduced. Thus, calcium absorptive efficiency is influenced by dietary intake (at low calcium intakes, fractional calcium absorption is greater than at high calcium intakes), as well as by age (calcium absorption declines with advancing age) and certain underlying medical conditions such as intestinal malabsorption and absorptive idiopathic hypercalciuria.

CALCIUM EXCRETION

Calcium is lost in urine, feces, and, to a minor extent, sweat. Fecal calcium excretion consists of both the fraction of the ingested calcium that was not absorbed and the calcium that is secreted into the gastrointestinal tract as part of biliary, pancreatic, and gastric juices. Secretion in gastric juices accounts for an obligate fecal loss of roughly 100 mg/day.

The other major route of calcium excretion is the kidneys. The glomeruli filter approximately 7 to 10 g of calcium each day, 98% of which is normally reabsorbed. The principal sites of renal calcium reabsorption are the proximal tubule, the ascending limb of the loop of Henle, and the distal tubules. The amount of calcium excreted in the urine of physiologically normal persons is usually between 100 and 300 mg/day. Excretion of more than 4 mg/kg/day is abnormal and usually reflects increased delivery of calcium to the kidney from the gut or the bone. Reabsorption of renal tubular calcium is enhanced by PTH, acting at the distal convoluted tubule. Calcium excretion is promoted by hypercalcemia or hypermagnesemia, both of which activate the calcium-sensing receptor in Henle's loop to inhibit calcium (and magnesium) reabsorption there, and by increased delivery of sodium to the distal tubule, which causes chloride channels to be flooded and blocks the small but critical fraction of calcium reabsorption that occurs in this nephron segment. Thiazide diuretics, which directly inhibit distal tubular chloride channels, promote distal tubular calcium reabsorption and reduce calcium excretion. Renal calcium excretion also is increased by PTH deficiency; increased bone calcium release in metabolic acidosis; high dietary protein intake; or severe, chronic phosphate depletion.

Phosphorus Metabolism

Phosphate is necessary for a variety of structural and metabolic functions. Total-body phosphate is approximately 1000 g, of which 85% is present as hydroxyapatite in the mineral phase of bone and 10% is intracellu-

lar. Extracellular phosphorus exists largely as inorganic phosphate ions. Intracellularly, phosphorous is a key constituent of a broad range of molecules, including DNA and RNA, membrane phospholipids, carbohydrate intermediates, and proteins. The attachment and removal of phosphate groups to and from proteins, performed by various kinases and phosphatases, respectively, play critical roles in regulating cellular metabolism and function. High-energy phosphoester bonds present in molecules such as ATP and creatine phosphate serve as reservoirs of metabolic energy that drive cellular metabolism, ion transport, muscle contraction, protein synthesis, and cell replication. Phosphate deficiency therefore may profoundly impair function in a broad range of tissues.

NORMAL PLASMA PHOSPHORUS

Normal plasma inorganic phosphate concentration is 0.8 to 1.4 mmol/L (2.5 to 4.5 mg/dL). This is conventionally expressed as elemental phosphorus because the distribution of phosphorus among its various protonated forms (mainly $H_2PO_2^-$ and HPO_4^{2-}) varies with pH. In contrast to calcium, inorganic phosphorus is 85% free and only 15% protein bound. Of the non–protein-bound component, some is complexed to sodium, calcium, and magnesium. Inorganic phosphate entry into cells, which occurs against an electrochemical gradient and thus is energy dependent, is mediated by specific sodium-phosphate cotransporters. The extracellular concentration of inorganic phosphate seems less tightly regulated than those of calcium or magnesium and may vary by 30% to 50% during the course of the day, particularly in response to meals. Serum inorganic phosphate levels are influenced by age (higher in children and postmenopausal women), diet (levels decrease after carbohydrate ingestion), pH, and several hormones, including PTH, 1,25-$(OH)_2D$, insulin, and growth hormone.

ABSORPTION OF DIETARY PHOSPHATE

The average diet in the United States contains approximately 600 to 1600 mg/day of phosphorus, 60% to 80% of which is absorbed by passive transport in response to the phosphate concentration within the intestinal lumen. Phosphorus absorption therefore is directly proportional to dietary phosphorus intake. Active transport of phosphate also can occur and is stimulated by 1,25-$(OH)_2D$. The composition of foods is such that selective deprivation of dietary phosphate hardly ever occurs. Starvation causes loss of body phosphate from both bone and cellular sources and thus produces progressive phosphate depletion but not hypoposphatemia. In rare cases, selective phosphate depletion follows consumption of large amounts of antacids containing aluminum hydroxide, which binds phosphate and prevents its absorption.

EXCRETION OF PHOSPHATE

Most plasma phosphate is filtered by the glomerulus, after which 80% to 90% is actively reabsorbed, mostly in the proximal tubule. Proximal tubular reabsorption results from the action of an apical membrane sodium phosphate cotransporter, the expression or activity of which is increased by phosphate depletion, hypoparathyroidism, volume contraction, growth hormone, and hypocalcemia. Conversely, urinary phosphate excretion is increased by PTH, PTH-related protein, phosphate loading, volume expansion, hypercalcemia, systemic acidosis, hypokalemia, hypomagnesemia, glucocorticoids, calcitonin, carbonic anhydrase inhibitors, thiazides, and furosemide. Abundant clinical and experimental evidence points to the existence of a circulating phosphaturic hormone, which is presumed to be secreted in response to increased phosphate availability. Although not yet chemically identified or cloned, this hormone already has been named *phosphatonin* and has been implicated as the humoral mediator responsible for the syndrome of *oncogenic osteomalacia* (see Chapter 75).

HYPOPHOSPHATEMIA

Causes of hypophosphatemia are listed in Table 73–1. Hypophosphatemia does not necessarily indicate a depletion of total-body inorganic phosphate, because only 1% of total-body phosphate exists in the extracellular fluid compartment, and relatively small changes in trans-

TABLE 73–1 Causes of Hypophosphatemia

Increased Urinary Losses
Hyperparathyroidism
Humoral hypercalcemia of malignancy
Oncogenic osteomalacia
Extracellular fluid volume expansion
Diabetes mellitus
Acquired renal tubular defects (hypokalemia, hypomagnesemia)
X-linked hypophosphatemic rickets (vitamin D–resistant rickets)
Alcohol abuse
Renal tubular acidosis
Hypothyroidism
Drugs: diuretics, glucocorticoids, calcitonin, bicarbonate
Decreased Intestinal Absorption
Vitamin D deficiency
Malabsorption syndromes
Antacid abuse
Alcohol abuse
Shifts into Cells
Carbohydrate administration
Acute alkalosis
Nutritional recovery syndrome
Acute gout
Salicylate poisoning
Gram-negative bacteremia
Sequela of hypothermia

Adapted from Favus MJ (ed): Primer on the Metabolic Bone Diseases and Disorders of Mineral Metabolism. Kelseyville, CA: American Society for Bone and Mineral Research, 1990.

TABLE 73–2 Consequences of Severe Hypophosphatemia

Acute
Hematologic
Red cell dysfunction and hemolysis
Leukocyte dysfunction
Platelet dysfunction
Muscle
Weakness
Rhabdomyolysis
Respiratory failure
Myocardial dysfunction
Kidney
Increased 25-OH-D 1α-hydroxylase activity
Increased calcium, bicarbonate, and magnesium excretion
Metabolic acidosis
Reduced formation of 2,3-diphosphoglycerate with impaired tissue oxygen delivery
Central nervous system dysfunction
Chronic
Osteomalacia or rickets

Adapted from Smith LH Jr: Phosphorus deficiency and hypophosphatemia. *In* Wyngaarden JB, Smith LH Jr, Bennett JC (eds): Cecil Textbook of Medicine, 19th ed. Philadelphia: WB Saunders, 1992, p 1137.

cellular movements of phosphate can dramatically affect serum phosphate concentrations. Conversely, significant phosphate depletion may coexist with normal serum inorganic phosphate levels, especially if renal clearance is impaired. The pathogenesis and differential diagnosis of hypophosphatemia are discussed in Chapter 75.

Symptoms of hypophosphatemia usually do not occur until serum inorganic phosphate levels fall to less than 1 to 1.5 mg/dL. The short-term effects, listed in Table 73–2, relate mainly to a generalized reduction in intracellular high-energy phosphate availability and of the activity of energy-requiring cellular processes. In erythrocytes, phosphate depletion lowers 2,3-diphosphoglycerate and thus can impair tissue oxygen delivery. Hemolytic anemia and dysfunction of leukocytes and platelets can occur with severe hypophosphatemia (i.e., <1.0 mg/dL). In muscle, phosphate depletion may produce myalgias and weakness, including cardiac and respiratory muscle weakness, and may lead to rhabdomyolysis if the depletion is severe. Phosphate depletion increases urinary excretion of calcium, bicarbonate, and magnesium and increases synthesis of 1,25-$(OH)_2$D. Central nervous system impairment ranges from irritability, fatigue, and weakness to encephalopathy and coma. The consequences of long-term phosphate depletion include osteomalacia and rickets (see Chapter 75).

The metabolic abnormalities associated with phosphate depletion are rapidly reversible by correcting the underlying disorder or adding phosphate therapy, although the bone abnormalities may require months or years of replacement therapy. Milk contains approximately 1000 mg/L of phosphorus and is, like meats and most other dietary staples, an excellent source of phosphorus. Alternatively, or in addition, sodium and potassium phosphate tablets (which contain 250 mg of inorganic phosphate) can be given in amounts of 1.5 to 3 g/day in divided doses. Diarrhea, nausea, and bloating are common side effects of oral phosphate therapy, especially at higher doses. In rare circumstances, such as in patients with profound neurologic disturbances, respiratory muscle weakness, ventricular dysfunction, or hemolysis, administration of intravenous phosphate may be warranted.

HYPERPHOSPHATEMIA

Causes of hyperphosphatemia are listed in Table 73–3. Most commonly, hyperphosphatemia results from renal insufficiency (acute or chronic), although it also may be seen in hypoparathyroidism, acromegaly, rhabdomyolysis, acute tumor lysis, hemolytic anemia, vitamin D intoxication, or sodium etidronate administration. In growing children, fasting serum inorganic phosphate is higher than in healthy adults. In chronic renal insufficiency, normal serum inorganic phosphate levels are maintained by decreased renal phosphate reabsorption until the glomerular filtration rate falls to less than 20 to 25 mL/min. The most important acute effects of hyperphosphatemia are hypocalcemia and tetany (see Chapter 74). Hyperphosphatemia lowers serum calcium levels acutely by complexing with calcium and chronically by inhibiting the activity of renal 1α-hydroxylase, thereby diminishing synthesis of $1,25\text{-}(OH)_2D$. Severe hyperphosphatemia also may cause metastatic calcifications, particularly in patients with normal or elevated serum calcium levels. Treatment of hyperphosphatemia generally requires restricting dietary phosphorus and administering phosphate binders such as aluminum hydroxide or calcium carbonate. Phosphate is efficiently removed by dialysis in renal failure. Because of the risk of aluminum toxicity with long-term aluminum therapy, calcium salts have become the first-line therapy for chronic hyperphosphatemia in renal failure.

Magnesium Metabolism

In the adult, magnesium constitutes about 0.35 g/kg of body weight. Slightly more than half of total-body magnesium is in bone, and most of the remainder is localized in the intracellular compartment. Magnesium is the second most abundant intracellular cation, after potassium, and is the major intracellular divalent cation. Approximately 60% of intracellular magnesium resides in mitochondria, and only about 5% to 10% is free in the cytosol. Magnesium plays an important structural role in bone crystals and is a cofactor in many vital enzymatic reactions.

Physiologically normal adults require about 0.15 to 0.18 mmol/kg/day of magnesium to maintain a positive balance. The average diet contains about 7 to 30 mmol (168 to 720 mg) of magnesium per day, derived mainly from meats and green vegetables. About 40% of ingested magnesium is absorbed in the intestine; the amount varies directly with dietary intake. Magnesium metabolism bears some relation to that of calcium: (1) absorption of both is stimulated by $1,25(OH)_2D$–dependent (but distinct) active transport mechanisms in the small intestine; (2) renal excretion of both ions is promoted by binding to the calcium-sensing receptor; (3) both hypercalcemia and hypermagnesemia suppress PTH secretion by binding to calcium-sensing receptors on parathyroid cells; and (4) magnesium is necessary for the release of PTH and for its action on target tissues.

Magnesium availability usually is assessed by measuring its serum concentration, even though this value does not parallel tissue or intracellular magnesium concentrations closely. In the plasma, magnesium circulates at a level of 0.75 to 1.05 mmol/L (1.8 to 2.5 mg/dL), of which approximately 30% is protein bound and the remainder is ionized. The extent of body stores of magnesium can be assessed more reliably by measuring basal urinary magnesium excretion (in the absence of tubular magnesium wasting) or the percentage of an intravenous load of magnesium that is excreted in the urine (the Thoren test). Retention of more than 25% to 50% is presumed to reflect depleted stores.

The kidney is the main site of magnesium excretion, with less than 2% of endogenous magnesium appearing in the feces. About 2% to 10% of the filtered load of magnesium is normally excreted in the urine; the remainder is reabsorbed, primarily in the thick limb of the ascending loop of Henle. Urinary magnesium excretion increases with the inhibition of proximal tubular reabsorption by osmotic diuretics or with extracellular fluid volume expansion. Some drugs, notably furosemide and cisplatin, inhibit magnesium reabsorption in the loop of

---

TABLE 73–3 Causes of Hypophosphatemia

Decreased Renal Phosphate Excretion

Renal failure (acute or chronic)
Hypoparathyroidism
Pseudohypoparathyroidism
Acromegaly
Etidronate
Tumoral calcinosis

Increased Phosphate Entry into Extracellular Fluid

Excess phosphate administration (intravenous, oral, or rectal)
Transcellular shifts
  Rhabdomyolysis
  Acute tumor lysis
  Hemolytic anemia
  Acidosis
  Catabolic states
  Infections
  Hyperthermia
  Fulminant hepatitis
Vitamin D intoxication

Adapted from Favus MJ (ed): Primer on Metabolic Bone Diseases and Disorders of Mineral Metabolism. Kelseyville, CA: American Society for Bone and Mineral Research, 1990.

Henle. PTH and aldosterone both decrease renal magnesium reabsorption. When dietary magnesium is severely restricted, urinary losses should fall to less than 1 mEq/day.

HYPOMAGNESEMIA

Magnesium deficiency usually occurs in association with more generalized nutritional and metabolic abnormalities. It can result from decreased absorption, increased renal or intestinal losses, or redistribution of magnesium into bone or soft tissues. The most common causes of hypomagnesemia are listed in Table 73–4. Clinically, magnesium deficiency is most often encountered in patients with alcoholism (poor dietary intake, vomiting, diminished absorption, and/or increased renal excretion), those with diabetes, patients with malabsorption, and during prolonged intravenous fluid therapy. Significant depletion of magnesium may result in the abnormalities listed in Table 73–5. Most often, the clinical presentation of hypomagnesemia results from symptoms from the associated hypocalcemia (caused by interference with the secretion and action of PTH) and hypokalemia (caused by an inability of the kidney to preserve potassium). Other clinical manifestations of hypomagnesemia include neuromuscular hyperexcitability and electrocar-

TABLE 73–4   Causes of Hypomagnesemia

Decreased Absorption
Poor dietary intake
Malabsorption syndromes
Extensive bowel resection
Ethanol effect on absorption

Increased Gastrointestinal Losses
Acute and chronic diarrhea
Intestinal and biliary fistulas
Vomiting or nasogastric suction

Increased Renal Losses
Chronic intravenous fluid therapy
Chronic renal disease (tubular, glomerular, interstitial)
Osmotic diuresis
Diabetes mellitus
Hypercalcemia
Phosphate depletion
Metabolic acidosis
Primary aldosteronism
Drugs
    Diuretics (furosemide, ethacrynic acid)
    Aminoglycosides
    Cisplatin
    Cyclosporine
    Amphotericin B
    Ethanol

Internal Redistribution
Acute pancreatitis
Hungry bone syndrome

Adapted from Smith LH Jr: Disorders of magnesium metabolism. *In* Wyngaarden JB, Smith LH Jr, Bennett JC (eds): Cecil Textbook of Medicine, 19th ed. Philadelphia: WB Saunders, 1992, p 1139.

TABLE 73–5   Consequences of Magnesium Deficiency

Neuromuscular
Lethargy, weakness, fatigue, decreased mentation
Neuromuscular irritability (partly from associated hypocalcemia)

Gastrointestinal
Anorexia, nausea, vomiting
Paralytic ileus

Cardiovascular
Prolongation of PR and QT intervals
Tachyarrhythmias
Increased sensitivity to digitalis

Metabolic
Hypocalcemia (from decreased parathyroid hormone secretion and action)
Hypokalemia (from renal potassium wasting)

Adapted from Smith LH Jr: Disorders of magnesium metabolism. *In* Wyngaarden JB, Smith LH Jr, Bennett JC (eds): Cecil Textbook of Medicine, 19th ed. Philadelphia: WB Saunders, 1992, p 1139.

diographic abnormalities such as prolongation of the PR and QT intervals and arrhythmias.

Treatment of magnesium deficiency is rarely an emergency, except when the patient has paralysis or tetany. A common approach is to administer 2 g of $MgSO_4$ (16 mEq Mg) IM q8h as a 50% solution. Because these injections can be painful, however, it often is preferable to administer 48 mEq/day IV (preferably as $MgCl_2$ to prevent binding of calcium by sulfate) by continuous infusion. Either regimen usually produces a normal or slightly elevated serum magnesium level. Because a normal serum level frequently does not indicate repletion of total-body magnesium stores, however, therapy should be continued for several days, during which time associated abnormalities such as hypocalcemia and hypokalemia should correct themselves. In patients with chronic magnesium loss, magnesium oxide can be given orally in a dose of 300 mg/day of elemental magnesium in divided doses. The most common side effect of oral replacement therapy is diarrhea. Caution should be exercised when magnesium is administered to patients with renal insufficiency, to prevent hypermagnesemia.

HYPERMAGNESEMIA

Hypermagnesemia almost always occurs in the setting of renal insufficiency. In such patients, excessive use of magnesium-containing antacids and cathartics or parenteral magnesium may produce hypermagnesemia. Magnesium administration is standard therapy for preeclampsia and may cause intoxication in both the mother and the neonate. Modest elevations of serum magnesium levels are seen in patients with familial hypocalciuric hypercalcemia, lithium ingestion, and volume depletion.

Neuromuscular symptoms are the most common presenting manifestations of hypermagnesemia. Somnolence may be seen at magnesium concentrations of 3 mEq/L; the deep tendon reflexes generally disappear at serum concentrations of 4 to 7 mEq/L; and respiratory depression and apnea occur at higher concentrations. Moderate hypermagnesemia may result in hypotension. At concentrations of more than 5 mEq/L, electrocardiographic abnormalities such as prolonged PR and QT intervals and increased QRS duration may occur, and at extremely high levels (>15 mEq/L), patients may experience complete heart block or cardiac arrest. In most circumstances, the only treatment needed is to discontinue magnesium administration. In patients with renal failure, dialysis against a low-magnesium bath lowers magnesium levels. In emergencies, calcium can be given in a dose of 100 to 200 mg IV over 5 to 10 minutes to antagonize the toxic effects of magnesium.

Vitamin D

In terms of its availability, metabolism, and mechanism of action, vitamin D is more properly a steroid hormone than a vitamin. Although a dietary necessity for vitamins exists, no dietary source of vitamin D is needed when exposure to sunlight is sufficient. Like other steroid hormones, vitamin D undergoes several chemical transformations to achieve a fully biologically active form. The close regulation of the final step, renal synthesis of 1,25-$(OH)_2D$, is typical of hormones. Finally, like other steroid hormones, vitamin D exerts its biologic effects by binding to specific, high-affinity receptors in target tissues.

SYNTHESIS

The active form of vitamin D is synthesized in three sequential steps in the skin, liver, and kidneys (Fig. 73–3). In the skin, ultraviolet light converts 7-dehydrocholesterol to previtamin D_3, which is then slowly converted nonenzymatically to vitamin D_3 (cholecalciferol). Vitamin D_3, bound to a specific vitamin D–binding protein (DBP), is then transported to the liver, where it is enzymatically hydroxylated to 25-hydroxyvitamin D (calcifidiol or 25-OH-D). This activation step, catalyzed by a cytochrome P-450 mixed-function oxidase in hepatocytes, is not under tight homeostatic regulation. Although 25-OH-D is only weakly biologically active, its circulating level furnishes a good index of the bioavailability of vitamin D because it has a long serum half-life (2 to 3 weeks). Then, 25-OH-D, bound to DBP, is transported to the kidney and other organs, where it is either hydroxylated at the 1 position to produce 1,25-dihydroxycholecalciferol (calcitriol or 1,25-$[OH]_2D$), the most biologically active form of vitamin D, or in other positions to produce a variety of other steroids. Renal 1α-hydroxylation is under tight metabolic control and is increased by PTH, hypophosphatemia, hypocalcemia, growth hormone, insulin, estrogens, prolactin, and low levels of 1,25-$(OH)_2D$. Conversely, renal synthesis of

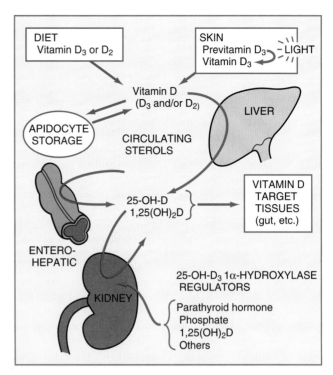

FIGURE 73–3 The vitamin D endocrine system. Vitamin D_2 (from diet) and vitamin D_3 (from diet or from conversion of 7-dihydrocholesterol in skin) are progressively hydroxylated in liver and kidney to produce 1,25-$(OH)_2D$ (calcitrol). (From Marx SJ: Mineral and bone homeostasis. *In* Wyngaarden JB, Smith LH Jr, Bennett JC [eds]: Cecil Textbook of Medicine, 19th ed. Philadelphia: WB Saunders, 1992, p 1402.)

1,25-$(OH)_2D$ is diminished by hypercalcemia, hyperphosphatemia, high levels of 1,25-$(OH)_2D$, low levels of PTH, and severe renal disease, as well as in many elderly people.

ABSORPTION

The dietary source of vitamin D is either vitamin D_2 (*ergocalciferol*), formed from irradiation of ergosterol (a plant sterol), or vitamin D_3. Ergocalciferol differs from cholecalciferol in the structure of its side chain but is equal in potency, undergoes the same biotransformations, and is measured by the same commonly employed competitive protein-binding assays.

Although the minimal dietary requirement for vitamin D is difficult to establish, the suggested daily intake in the United States ranges from 5 μg (200 IU) to 15 μg (600 IU) for adults 19 to 50 years of age or older than 70 years, respectively. Many experts, however, recommend that all adults ingest 20 μg (800 IU) of vitamin D daily. Because vitamin D is a fat-soluble vitamin, chronic malabsorption of fat without adequate exposure to ultraviolet light can lead to hypovitaminosis D.

FUNCTION

Vitamin D acts with PTH to maintain the level of ionized calcium and phosphate in extracellular fluid by actions on the intestine, bone, and, to a lesser extent, the kidney. Vitamin D, in the form of 1,25-(OH)$_2$D, enhances the intestinal absorption of calcium, magnesium, and phosphate by upregulating the transcription of specific genes, such as that for the calcium-binding protein *calbindin,* whose protein products facilitate active transport of these ions. By ensuring adequate availability of calcium and phosphate in the extracellular fluid, vitamin D supports the mineralization of cartilage matrix during endochondral bone formation and of bone matrix (*osteoid*). Although 1,25-(OH)$_2$D exerts direct effects on osteoblasts, including regulation of alkaline phosphatase and osteocalcin synthesis, experiments with animals that lack the nuclear vitamin D receptor have shown that vitamin D is not necessary for mineralization of bone matrix (as long as extracellular mineral ion concentrations can be maintained by other means). In addition, 1,25-(OH)$_2$D acts directly on bone marrow stromal cells to increase bone resorption through increased generation and activation of osteoclasts. Vitamin D also may enhance renal tubular reabsorption of calcium. Active vitamin D metabolites exert direct inhibitory genomic effects on the parathyroid glands that reduce the transcription of the PTH gene and thereby limit further stimulation by PTH of renal 1,25-(OH)$_2$D synthesis. Vitamin D also may play an important role in regulating the differentiation and proliferation of other cell types not directly involved in bone or mineral metabolism, including lymphocytes and keratinocytes.

DIAGNOSIS OF VITAMIN D DEFICIENCY

Vitamin D deficiency generally is indicated by a low serum level of 25-OH-D. This condition may be caused by dietary deficiency, malabsorption, or sunlight deprivation, but it also can result from long-term exposure to drugs, such as phenobarbital or carbamazepine, that increase hepatic metabolism and clearance of 25-OH-D. In many patients with low levels of 25-OH-D, serum 1,25-(OH)$_2$D levels actually may be normal or increased, particularly if serum PTH levels are high. Other findings that support the diagnosis of vitamin D deficiency include mild hypocalcemia, hypophosphatemia, secondary hyperparathyroidism, and decreased urinary calcium excretion. Deficiency of 1,25-(OH)$_2$D secretion, despite normal levels of 25-OH-D substrate, is seen most often in patients with severe renal disease, but it also occurs in patients with hypoparathyroidism or with inherited or acquired defects in 1α-hydroxylation of 25-OH-D (see Chapter 75). In rare cases, resistance to 1,25-(OH)$_2$D occurs because of mutations in the vitamin D receptor gene. Such patients have biochemical and clinical features of vitamin D deficiency but have elevated blood levels of 1,25-(OH)$_2$D. Many of these patients also have defects in hair and tooth development.

HYPERVITAMINOSIS D

Hypervitaminosis D occurs from the excessive ingestion of vitamin D or one of its active metabolites or from the abnormal conversion of 25-OH-D to 1,25-(OH)$_2$D at sites not subject to normal metabolic regulation. The latter occurs in granulomatous diseases such as sarcoidosis and tuberculosis and in certain T-cell lymphomas in which the 1α-hydroxylase is pathologically expressed in the abnormal tissue. Clinically, hypervitaminosis D presents with hypercalcemia, hyperphosphatemia, and/or metastatic calcification. The hypercalcemia results from both vitamin D's effect on calcium absorption and its osteolytic effects. Hyperphosphatemia results from increased intestinal phosphate absorption, increased bone resorption, and decreased renal clearance of phosphate by parathyroid suppression. Vitamin D intoxication caused by ingesting ergocalciferol can persist for several weeks after discontinuing therapy, whereas the effects of intoxication with calcitriol generally subside in several days. Treatment of vitamin D intoxication involves discontinuing vitamin D, vigorous hydration to reduce urinary calcium and phosphate concentrations, and, in some patients, the addition of corticosteroids. Other therapies for acute hypercalcemia, such as intravenous bisphosphonates or calcitonin (see Chapter 74), seldom are required.

HYPOVITAMINOSIS D

The clinical picture of hypovitaminosis D is that of hypocalcemia (see Chapter 74), osteomalacia (see Chapter 75), or rickets (see Chapter 75).

Calcitonin

Calcitonin is a 32–amino acid peptide that is secreted by the parafollicular C cells of the thyroid gland. Its secretion is regulated acutely by the serum calcium concentration (when the blood calcium level rises, calcitonin secretion increases). The main biologic effect of calcitonin is to inhibit osteoclastic bone resorption.

HYPOCALCITONINEMIA

Patients with calcitonin deficiency do not have any recognized abnormalities. Patients who have undergone total thyroidectomy, for example, maintain normal blood calcium and phosphate concentrations, do not require calcitonin replacement, and do not have a greater incidence of osteoporosis.

HYPERCALCITONINEMIA

Elevated serum calcitonin concentrations are seen in patients with medullary carcinoma of the thyroid gland, with a malignant tumor of the calcitonin-producing C cells, and with many other neoplasms in which calcitonin may be expressed ectopically. Despite high calcitonin levels, these patients do not have bone disease or metabolic disorders of calcium or inorganic phosphate. Early stages of medullary thyroid carcinoma may be detected by measuring the calcitonin response to intravenous calcium or pentagastrin administration.

REFERENCES

Bringhurst FR: Calcium and phosphate distribution, turnover, and metabolic actions. *In* DeGroot LJ (ed): Endocrinology. Philadelphia: WB Saunders, 1995, pp 1015–1043.

Favus MJ (ed): Primer on the Metabolic Bone Diseases and Disorders of Mineral Metabolism, 2nd ed. New York: Raven Press, 1993.

Holick MF: Vitamin D: Photobiology, metabolism, and clinical applications. *In* DeGroot LJ (ed): Endocrinology. Philadelphia: WB Saunders, 1995, pp 990–1014.

Levi M, Cronin RE, Knochel JP: Disorders of phosphate and magnesium metabolism. *In* Coe FL, Favus MJ (eds): Disorders of Bone and Mineral Metabolism. New York: Raven Press, 1992, pp 587–610.

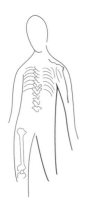

THE PARATHYROID GLANDS, HYPERCALCEMIA, AND HYPOCALCEMIA

Joel S. Finkelstein

Normal Physiology

The four parathyroid glands are found in close association with the thyroid gland. Occasionally, one of the glands may be in an aberrant location, usually in the superior mediastinum. Each normal gland weighs approximately 25 mg.

SECRETION OF PARATHYROID HORMONE

Parathyroid hormone (PTH) is an 84-amino acid, single-chain polypeptide with a molecular weight of 9500. PTH is initially synthesized as a larger precursor molecule, pre-pro-PTH, consisting of 115 amino acids. This precursor is rapidly converted within the glands to an intermediate form of 90 amino acids termed *pro-PTH*, which is subsequently converted to the 84-amino acid hormone. The biologic activity of PTH resides in the first 34 residues. PTH is secreted primarily as the intact molecule, although C-terminal fragments are also released from the parathyroid glands. After release into the circulation, the intact hormone is rapidly cleaved, primarily in the liver and kidney, to smaller biologically inactive midregion and carboxy-terminal fragments. Consequently, most of the circulating immunoactive PTH is composed of C-terminal fragments. Biologically active amino-terminal fragments seem not to circulate. Intact PTH has a plasma half-life of 2 to 4 minutes.

PTH secretion is controlled primarily by the serum ionized calcium level. When the ionized calcium level falls, PTH secretion is stimulated; when the ionized calcium level rises, the secretion of PTH is suppressed. Calcium regulates PTH secretion by interacting with calcium-sensing receptors in the membranes of parathyroid cells. The other major regulator of PTH is calcitriol

(1,25-dihydroxyvitamin D, or 1,25-[OH]$_2$D), which inhibits PTH synthesis. Chronic hypocalcemia and calcitriol deficiency lead to parathyroid hyperplasia.

ACTIONS OF PARATHYROID HORMONE

The main function of PTH is to defend against hypocalcemia (Fig. 74–1). PTH acts by binding to specific receptors on the membrane of PTH-responsive cells, such as osteoblasts and renal tubular cells. *Signal transduction* occurs by activation of membrane-bound adenylate cyclase with the subsequent intracellular release of cyclic adenosine monophosphate (cAMP) or by activation of phospholipase C. Products of phospholipase C activation increase intracellular ionized calcium concentrations and activate protein kinase C. The major actions of PTH are as follows:

1. Stimulation of bone resorption by osteoclasts and consequent release of calcium and phosphate into the extracellular fluid. The mechanism by which PTH works on bone is not well understood. PTH receptors have not been demonstrated on osteoclasts, so the bone-resorbing effect of PTH appears to be indirect. In contrast, osteoblasts do contain PTH receptors. In response to PTH, cells of the osteoblast lineage increase production of RANK ligand (also called *osteoclast-differentiating factor*), a tumor necrosis factor–like protein that stimulates osteoclastic bone resorption. The action of PTH on bone is partially impaired in patients with deficiencies of calcitriol or intracellular magnesium.
2. Stimulation of renal tubular reabsorption of calcium and magnesium.
3. Inhibition of the renal tubular reabsorption of phosphate and bicarbonate that enhances urinary

639

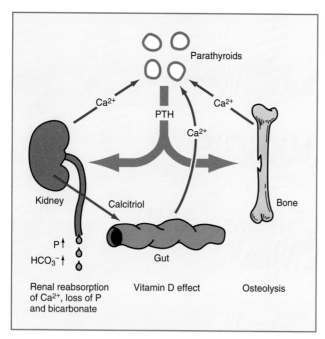

FIGURE 74–1 Actions of parathyroid hormone (PTH) in calcium homeostasis.

loss of these substances. This action helps to eliminate the phosphate released from bone, which could otherwise tend to reduce ionized calcium levels. A mild metabolic acidosis from the bicarbonate loss occurs with PTH excess.

4. Stimulation of synthesis of the active form of vitamin D, 1,25-$(OH)_2$D, from 25-hydroxyvitamin D through activation of the specific 1α-hydroxylase in the kidney. By virtue of its effect on 1,25-$(OH)_2$D synthesis, PTH indirectly enhances the intestinal absorption of calcium.

MEASUREMENT OF PARATHYROID HORMONE

The circulating level of PTH can be measured directly by radioimmunoassay. In the past, the antibodies used to measure PTH were multivalent and heterogeneous, and they recognized fragments of the PTH molecule that were often biologically inert. This problem was particularly noteworthy in patients with renal failure because the kidney normally clears the biologically inert C-terminal fragments of PTH. The development of double-antibody assays (immunoradiometric and immunochemiluminometric assays) allowed measurement of intact, biologically active PTH and thereby helped to differentiate more clearly hypercalcemic disorders that are mediated by PTH from those that are not mediated by PTH.

Hypercalcemia

Hypercalcemia is a common clinical disorder that may develop in the setting of a serious underlying illness or often is detected by routine laboratory testing in patients without any obvious illness. Primary hyperparathyroidism is the most common cause of hypercalcemia in the general population, although malignant disease remains the most common cause of hypercalcemia among hospitalized patients.

CLINICAL MANIFESTATIONS

The clinical manifestations of hypercalcemia are summarized in Table 74–1. In general, the severity of the symptoms tends to parallel the level of ionized calcium in extracellular fluid, but wide variations can occur. The severity of the symptoms may also depend on the rate of rise of the serum calcium level. Nausea, vomiting, and polyuria, all consequences of hypercalcemia, can produce dehydration and thereby can decrease renal calcium clearance and worsen hypercalcemia.

TABLE 74–1 Signs and Symptoms of Primary Hyperparathyroidism

Related to Hypercalcemia
Central nervous system
Lethargy
Drowsiness
Depression
Impaired ability to concentrate
Confusion
Stupor
Coma
Neuromuscular
Proximal muscle weakness
Hyporeflexia
Gastrointestinal
Nausea
Vomiting
Anorexia
Constipation
Peptic ulcer disease (?)
Pancreatitis
Renal
Polyuria
Polydipsia
Decreased concentrating ability
Impaired renal function
Nephrocalcinosis
Nephrolithiasis
Cardiovascular
Hypertension
Short QT internal
Bradycardia
Increased sensitivity to digitalis
Related to Hypercalciuria
Nephrolithiasis
Related to Effect of Parathyroid Hormone on Bone and Joints
Arthralgias
Bone pain
Bone cysts
Gout
Pseudogout

DIFFERENTIAL DIAGNOSIS

Causes of hypercalcemia are listed in Table 74–2. More than 90% of patients with hypercalcemia have either primary hyperparathyroidism or a malignant disease. Using modern immunoradiometric or chemiluminometric assays, the distinction between these two disorders can almost always be made on the basis of the serum PTH level, which is elevated or inappropriately normal in patients with primary hyperparathyroidism and suppressed in patients with hypercalcemia associated with malignant disease.

PRIMARY HYPERPARATHYROIDISM

In *primary hyperparathyroidism*, PTH is secreted inappropriately despite an elevation in the ionized calcium level in the extracellular fluid. Although PTH secretion is partially autonomous, negative feedback regulation can be demonstrated (although with an altered set point) because PTH can be partially suppressed by calcium. The peak incidence of primary hyperparathyroidism occurs in the third to fifth decade, and the condition is more common in women than in men. It is estimated that the annual incidence of primary hyperparathyroidism is estimated to be 1 in 1000 men over 60 years of age and 2 in 1000 women over 60 years of age. Most patients are identified by multiphasic screening while they are still asymptomatic.

Etiology

Approximately 85% of patients with primary hyperparathyroidism have enlargement of a single parathyroid gland (*parathyroid adenoma*). Most parathyroid adeno-

TABLE 74–2 Differential Diagnosis of Hypercalcemia

Primary hyperparathyroidism
Malignant disease
  Osteolytic metastases (e.g., breast cancer)
  Humoral hypercalcemia of malignancy (e.g., lung, head and neck, esophagus, renal cell, ovary, multiple myeloma)
  Production of 1,25-$(OH)_2D$ (e.g., lymphoma)
Sarcoidosis, tuberculosis, and other granulomatous diseases
Thyrotoxicosis
Drug-induced
  Vitamin D intoxication
  Vitamin A intoxication
  Thiazide diuretics
  Lithium
  Tamoxifen
  Theophylline
Immobilization (in setting of high bone turnover)
Milk-alkali syndrome
Familial hypocalciuric hypercalcemia
Adrenal insufficiency
Acute and chronic renal failure
Pheochromocytoma
Acromegaly
Jansen-type metaphyseal chondrodysplasia

mas result from the clonal expansion of a single cell. Expression of the calcium-sensing receptor protein is reduced in parathyroid adenomas, although somatic mutations in the gene have not been reported with these tumors. Tumor-specific genetic defects have been characterized in a small number of sporadic parathyroid adenomas including (1) a pericentric inversion on chromosome 11 that results in a relocation of *PRAD1* (parathyroid adenoma 1 or cyclin D1) proto-oncogene next to the 5′-PTH gene-promoter sequences with consequent increased expression of cyclin D1 and (2) deletions in the retinoblastoma (*Rb*) gene, particularly in parathyroid carcinomas. Most (and perhaps all) parathyroid adenomas contain chromosomes with multiple gene deletions. These are particularly common in chromosome 11q13, the location of the *MEN1* gene.

Most of the remaining 15% of patients have hyperplasia of all four parathyroid glands, though the enlargement is often asymmetric, so some glands may grossly resemble adenomas, whereas others appear indistinguishable from normal parathyroid glands. In some patients, hyperparathyroidism occurs as part of a familial disorder without other endocrinologic abnormalities. In others, it occurs as part of *multiple endocrine neoplasia type I* (Wermer's syndrome, characterized by hyperparathyroidism, pancreatic islet cell tumors, and pituitary tumors) or *multiple endocrine neoplasia type II* (Sipple's syndrome, characterized by hyperparathyroidism, medullary carcinoma of the thyroid, and pheochromocytoma. Patients with the *familial hyperparathyroidism–jaw tumor syndrome* have defects on chromosome 1. Most patients with familial forms of hyperparathyroidism have parathyroid hyperplasia, and the disorder is inherited in an autosomal dominant fashion.

Parathyroid carcinoma is a rare cause of primary hyperparathyroidism. Parathyroid carcinoma tends to grow slowly and to spread locally, although it occasionally metastasizes to lungs, liver, or bone. Long-term survival is common. Although serum calcium and PTH levels are usually higher in patients with parathyroid carcinoma than in other patients with primary hyperparathyroidism, the disorder may be clinically indistinguishable from other forms of primary hyperparathyroidism and difficult to diagnose at the time of initial surgery.

Approximately 10% to 20% of patients taking *lithium* develop primary hyperparathyroidism. Lithium shifts the set point of the calcium-PTH response curve to the right and leads to parathyroid hyperplasia or, less often, adenoma. Hypercalcemia can disappear with the cessation of lithium therapy.

Symptoms and Signs

With the widespread use of multiphasic chemistry screening, most patients with primary hyperparathyroidism are asymptomatic at presentation or present with vague symptoms such as fatigue, weakness, arthralgias, or mental disturbances (see Table 74–1). Although symptoms are usually mild, they may worsen with intercurrent illnesses and may lead to severe alterations in mental status. On rare occasions, patients may present with life-threatening hypercalcemia and severe symptoms, so-called *acute primary hyperparathyroidism* or *parathyroid crisis.* Approximately 10% to 15% of patients with primary hyperparathyroidism develop *kidney stones,* usually composed of calcium oxalate or calcium phosphate, in contrast to a prevalence of 60% to 70% many years ago before the advent of routine chemistry screening. Other complications of hyperparathyroidism include pancreatitis, chondrocalcinosis, calcific periarthritis, and, perhaps, peptic ulcer disease.

Laboratory and Radiologic Manifestations

Serum calcium levels are continuously or intermittently elevated and serum phosphorus levels tend to be low in primary hyperparathyroidism. Occasionally, however, the total serum calcium concentration is in the upper normal range but with an elevated ionized calcium level. The serum calcium level may also be normal in the setting of concomitant vitamin D deficiency. In these patients, frank hypercalcemia can develop with correction of the vitamin D deficiency. Serum alkaline phosphatase concentrations are usually normal but may be elevated, especially in patients with osteitis fibrosa cystica. Urinary calcium levels may be normal or elevated. Elevated urinary calcium levels help to distinguish patients with primary hyperparathyroidism from those with familial hypocalciuric hypercalcemia (see later). Mild hyperchloremic acidosis is sometimes present. Serum PTH levels are frankly elevated in most patients; about 10% of patients have PTH levels that are in the "normal" range but inappropriately high for the level of serum calcium. Serum $1,25\text{-}(OH)_2D$ levels may be high-normal or even elevated because of the stimulatory effect of PTH on renal 1α-hydroxylase activity.

Most patients with primary hyperparathyroidism show no radiographic evidence of bone disease. The classic radiographic finding of osteitis fibrosa cystica is uncommon today. The most common radiographic finding in patients with primary hyperparathyroidism is *osteopenia.* Occasionally, radiographs may show subperiosteal bone resorption of the distal phalanges (Fig. 74–2), resorption of the distal end of the clavicle, or a "salt-and-pepper" appearance of the skull. Bone densitometry measurements often indicate a disproportionate loss of cortical bone. Radiographic or ultrasound examination of the kidneys may show renal stones or diffuse deposition of calcium in the renal parenchyma *(nephrocalcinosis).*

Evaluation and Diagnosis

The diagnosis of primary hyperparathyroidism is based on the presence of hypercalcemia with an elevated or inappropriately normal PTH level. With immunoradiometric and immunochemiluminometric assays, distinguishing primary hyperparathyroidism from non–PTH-mediated causes of hypercalcemia is rarely a problem (Fig. 74–3). A 24-hour urine specimen should be collected to help rule out familial hypocalciuric hypercalcemia (see later). Most of the other causes of hypercalcemia listed in Table 74–2 can be readily identified by other clinical manifestations or by laboratory studies.

The diagnosis of hyperparathyroidism can be

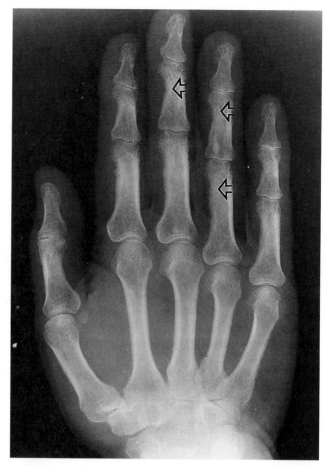

FIGURE 74–2   Subperiosteal bone resorption in the phalanges of a patient with primary hyperparathyroidism.

strengthened by radiologic evidence of subperiosteal bone resorption. Parathyroid ultrasonography is usually reserved to assist the surgeon before neck exploration once the diagnosis of primary hyperparathyroidism has been established biochemically, although the need for ultrasonography in uncomplicated cases is controversial. Many masses identified by ultrasound examination of the neck are discovered to be thyroid nodules, lymph nodes, or asymmetric parathyroid hyperplasia. A nodule felt in the neck is more likely to be a thyroid nodule than a parathyroid adenoma.

Indications for Treatment

The treatment of choice for symptomatic patients with primary hyperparathyroidism is surgical removal of the abnormal gland or glands. A panel of experts from a National Institutes of Health consensus conference suggested the following guidelines, which are arbitrary, for surgical treatment of patients with asymptomatic primary hyperparathyroidism:

1. A markedly elevated serum calcium level (i.e., 1.0 to 1.6 mg/dL higher than the upper limit of normal).
2. A history of prior life-threatening hypercalcemia.

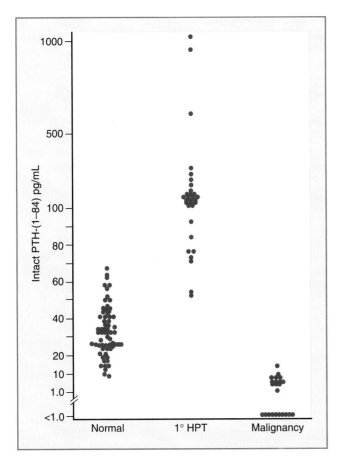

FIGURE 74–3   Intact parathyroid hormone (PTH) 1–84 levels measured by immunoradiometric assay in sera from 72 normal individuals, 37 patients with surgically proven hyperparathyroidism (HPT), and 24 patients with hypercalcemia associated with malignancy. (From Nussbaum SR, Zahradnik RJ, Lavigne JR, et al: Highly sensitive two-site immunoradiometric assay of parathyrin, and its clinical utility in evaluating patients with hypercalcemia. Clin Chem 1987; 33:1364; with permission.)

3. Kidney stone or stones detected by abdominal radiography.
4. Creatinine clearance reduced by more than 30% compared with age-matched normal subjects.
5. Marked hypercalciuria (>400 mg/24 hours).
6. Substantially reduced bone density, particularly if more than 2 standard deviations below age-matched and sex-matched control subjects.
7. Patients in whom medical surveillance is neither desirable nor suitable:
   a. Patients who request surgical treatment.
   b. Patients for whom consistent follow-up is deemed unlikely.
   c. Patients for whom coexistent illness complicates medical management.
   d. Patients 50 years old or younger.

Among those patients in whom medical surveillance is recommended, the National Institutes of Health consensus panel recommended that patients be seen at least twice each year until the stability of the preceding parameters is established. At each visit, the patient should be queried carefully with respect to potential symptoms of hypercalcemia, and blood pressure, serum calcium, and creatinine clearance should be measured. Abdominal radiographs, a 24-hour urinary calcium determination, and a bone density measurement of the proximal radius should be performed annually. Adequate hydration should be encouraged. Thiazide diuretics should be avoided because they may worsen hypercalcemia. Dietary intake of calcium should be moderate because severe restriction may stimulate PTH secretion further. Oral phosphate administration may be beneficial if severe hypophosphatemia is present, but it requires close attention to avoid hyperphosphatemia. In postmenopausal women, estrogen replacement therapy prevents bone loss and may lower serum calcium levels modestly.

HYPERCALCEMIA OF MALIGNANCY

Hypercalcemia of malignancy occurs in 10% to 20% of patients with cancer during the course of their illness. Hypercalcemia usually occurs late in the course of malignant disease, and survival is often limited to weeks or months after it develops. Malignant disease is rarely the cause of unexplained hypercalcemia. Hypercalcemia is most frequently seen in patients with squamous carcinomas of the lung or head and neck, breast cancer, renal cell cancer, and hematologic malignant diseases such as multiple myeloma or lymphoma. In patients with T-cell lymphomas associated with the human T-cell lymphotrophic virus-I, the incidence of hypercalcemia approaches 100%. The three major mechanisms that produce hypercalcemia in patients with malignant diseases are localized bone destruction by osteolytic metastases, tumor production of PTR-like protein (PTHrP), and tumor production of calcitriol.

Localized Bone Destruction as a Cause

Extensive *localized bone destruction* is often an important cause of hypercalcemia in patients with multiple myeloma, breast cancer, or lymphomas. In these patients, tumor metastases may release bone-resorbing cytokines directly into the skeleton or may stimulate host mononuclear cells to elaborate mediators that stimulate nearby osteoclasts to resorb bone. *Lymphotoxin*, a member of the same family of immune cell products as tumor necrosis factor and interleukin-1, is the major bone-resorbing factor produced by cultured human myeloma cells. Breast cancer cells can produce prostaglandin E2, whereas lymphocytes in lymphomas can elaborate interleukin-1α and interleukin-1β, tumor necrosis factor, and 1,25-(OH)$_2$D, all of which are potent stimulators of osteoclastic bone resorption. Even in patients with these malignant diseases, however, humoral mechanisms may contribute to hypercalcemia, as evidenced by the diffuse osteoporosis often seen in patients with multiple myeloma, by the occurrence of hypercalcemia in some patients with breast cancer in the absence of detectable skeletal metastases, and by the enhanced intestinal absorption of calcium in patients with lymphomas that produce 1,25-(OH)$_2$D.

Parathyroid Hormone–Related Protein as a Cause

In most patients with malignancy-associated hypercalcemia, the primary mechanism of hypercalcemia is increased osteoclastic bone resorption resulting from production of PTHrP. This syndrome is frequently referred to as *humoral hypercalcemia of malignancy*. The syndrome is most common in patients with squamous cell carcinomas of the lung, esophagus, or head and neck, but it is also seen in patients with renal, bladder, ovarian, breast, and other carcinomas. PTHrP is a 141-amino acid protein in which 9 of the first 13 amino acids are identical to those of PTH. As with PTH, PTHrP's full biologic activity on mineral ion homeostasis resides in its first 34 amino acids. PTH and PTHrP bind to the same receptors on bone and kidney, and both peptides increase bone resorption, renal calcium reabsorption, urinary phosphate excretion, and nephrogenous cAMP excretion. Although PTHrP stimulates 1,25-$(OH)_2D$ production, 1,25-$(OH)_2D$ levels are typically normal in patients with humoral hypercalcemia of malignancy for reasons that are unclear. Immunoassays for PTH do not detect PTHrP. Assays are now available to assess PTHrP levels directly. PTHrP has been identified in many normal tissues including keratinocytes, breast, nerve cells, and placenta, and it has a variety of paracrine roles in these tissues.

Calcitriol as a Cause

Tumor production of *calcitriol* is the cause of hypercalcemia in most patients with Hodgkin's disease and in about one third of patients with non-Hodgkin's lymphoma. Hypercalcemia induced by calcitriol usually responds to glucocorticoid therapy.

OTHER CAUSES OF HYPERCALCEMIA

Familial hypocalciuric hypercalcemia (also known as familial benign hypercalcemia) is a rare genetic disorder, transmitted as an autosomal dominant trait. It is caused by inactivating mutations of the calcium-sensing receptor gene, so a higher than normal serum calcium level is required to suppress PTH release, and renal tubules conserve calcium inappropriately. Affected heterozygotes typically present with modest hypercalcemia and relative hypocalciuria. Patients are usually asymptomatic, and the condition is detected as a result of screening after a member of the kindred has been identified or in the evaluation of patients initially thought to have asymptomatic primary hyperparathyroidism. Hypercalcemia has been detected in family members as early as the first months of life. Immunoactive PTH levels are usually normal but may be mildly elevated, thus causing confusion with primary hyperparathyroidism. Serum magnesium levels are usually high-normal or frankly elevated. Because parathyroid surgery fails to cure the hypercalcemia unless total parathyroidectomy is performed, surgical treatment is usually contraindicated in patients with familial hypocalciuric hypercalcemia. To screen for this disorder, urinary calcium excretion should be deter-

mined in patients with asymptomatic hypercalcemia, and serum calcium levels should be measured in the relatives of patients with hypocalciuria. The diagnosis should be suspected in hypercalcemic patients with normal or elevated PTH levels who present at a young age, who have a family history of hypercalcemia or milial hypocalciuric hypercalcemia, who have hypermagnesemia, and/or who have a urinary calcium excretion of less than 100 mg/24 hours despite a normal creatinine clearance. Homozygous inactivating mutations of the calcium-sensing receptor gene lead to severe neonatal hypercalcemia.

Hypercalcemia resulting from *vitamin D intoxication* can be caused by excessive vitamin D ingestion or endogenous overproduction of 1,25-$(OH)_2D$. The latter occurs in some patients with granulomatous diseases (e.g., sarcoidosis or tuberculosis) or malignant lymphomas resulting from extrarenal 25-(OH)D 1α-hydroxylase activity. In patients with vitamin D intoxication, hypercalcemia is caused by both increased intestinal calcium absorption and increased bone resorption.

As a result of high bone turnover, hypercalcemia occasionally occurs in patients with *hyperthyroidism*. Immobilization regularly leads to accelerated bone turnover and hypercalciuria and can produce hypercalcemia in patients whose underlying rate of bone turnover is high, as is seen in young people, patients with primary or secondary hyperparathyroidism, and patients with Paget's disease.

The *milk-alkali syndrome* is becoming more common because of the increasing use of calcium carbonate to treat osteoporosis, dyspepsia, and the hyperphosphatemia of chronic renal failure. The milk-alkali syndrome appears to begin with the development of hypercalcemia caused by ingestion of large amounts of calcium in susceptible persons. Hypercalcemia lowers the glomerular filtration rate and thereby limits calcium excretion. Increased alkali intake, a fall in the glomerular filtration rate, and hypercalcemia lead to metabolic alkalosis, which stimulates renal calcium reabsorption and worsens the hypercalcemia. Other uncommon causes of hypercalcemia include adrenal insufficiency, pheochromocytoma (from PTHrP production or concurrent multiple endocrine neoplasia type II), acromegaly (from calcitriol production or concurrent multiple endocrine neoplasia type I), vitamin A intoxication, theophylline toxicity, the diuretic phase of acute tubular necrosis (particularly in patients with rhabdomyolysis), Jansen-type metaphyseal chondrodysplasia (from constitutive activation of the PTH-PTHrP receptor gene), and the use of thiazide diuretics, particularly in patients who have some degree of underlying parathyroid autonomy or who are taking large doses of calcium.

TREATMENT OF HYPERCALCEMIA

Whenever possible, the treatment of hypercalcemia should be directed toward reversal of the underlying pathogenetic abnormality. For example, severe or symptomatic primary hyperparathyroidism is usually treated surgically. Successful treatment of malignant disease may reverse or diminish its associated hypercalcemia, at least temporarily. The slight hypercalcemia found in patients with hyperthyroidism or with adrenal insufficiency is readily reversible by the treatment of the underlying disorder.

In patients with severe hypercalcemia ($\geq$13 to 14 mg/dL) or who are symptomatic, medical treatment is indicated. The following approaches may be used in sequence or concurrently if indicated by the severity of the hypercalcemia. The mainstays of therapy for most patients are hydration with isotonic saline solution and intravenous pamidronate.

Hydration. Dehydration frequently accompanies severe hypercalcemia. Restoration of intravascular volume may significantly reduce hypercalcemia. Inhibiting sodium reabsorption in the proximal tubule and in the loop of Henle reduces passive transport of calcium and increases urinary calcium excretion. Volume expansion with isotonic saline inhibits sodium reabsorption and increases calcium excretion. Caution must be exercised in administering large volumes of saline, particularly in elderly patients and in patients with cardiac or renal disease.

Bisphosphonates. Bisphosphonates are structural analogues of pyrophosphate that inhibit osteoclast-mediated bone resorption. Two bisphosphonates are available for the treatment of hypercalcemia in the United States: ethane hydroxy 1,1-diphosphonic acid (etidronate disodium, EHDP, Didronel) and aminohydroxypropylidene bisphosphonate (APD, pamidronate). Etridonate is administered as a daily IV infusion for 3 days at a dose of 7.5 mg/kg/day. It is rarely used today. Pamidronate is the mainstay of therapy for patients with malignancy-associated hypercalcemia, but it is also effective in patients with hyperparathyroidism and vitamin D intoxication. It is administered in a dose of 30 to 90 mg IV over 4 to 24 hours. Fever is an occasional side effect of pamidronate therapy. The maximum hypocalcemic effect is seen in 1 to 2 days, and serum calcium levels generally remain in the normal range for weeks to months.

Furosemide (or Ethacrynic Acid). Loop diuretics facilitate sodium and calcium excretion. They should not be administered, however, until intravascular volume has been restored with saline administration. Otherwise, further dehydration and worsening hypercalcemia may ensue. Because patients given these diuretics also lose potassium and magnesium, serum levels of these substances must be monitored closely during intensive treatment and losses replaced. Thiazide diuretics should be avoided because they decrease renal calcium excretion and may worsen hypercalcemia.

Glucocorticoids. High doses of glucocorticoids (prednisone, 50 to 100 mg/day, or the equivalent of another agent) may lower serum calcium levels, especially in patients with sarcoidosis, vitamin D intoxication, multiple myeloma, or other hematologic malignant diseases.

Calcitonin. Calcitonin inhibits osteoclastic bone resorption and increases urinary calcium excretion. When administered subcutaneously or IM in a dose of 2 to 4 IU/kg every 6 to 12 hours, it decreases the release of calcium from bone. Calcitonin therapy usually lowers serum calcium concentrations by 1 to 2 mg/dL within 2 to 3 hours. Tachyphylaxis generally develops in several days, however, with a rebound in serum calcium levels. Thus, calcitonin is most useful as an adjunctive therapeutic agent (together with isotonic saline and pamidronate) in patients with severe hypercalcemia.

Dialysis. On rare occasions, such as in patients with acute hypercalcemia and renal insufficiency, hemodialysis against a low-calcium or zero-calcium bath or peritoneal dialysis may be required for the treatment of hypercalcemia.

Calcium Receptor Mimetics. Agents that bind to the calcium receptor and suppress release of PTH are in development. These drugs may become useful medical therapies for patients with PTH-mediated hypercalcemia.

Others. Mithramycin, gallium nitrate, and phosphate administration are other forms of therapy for hypercalcemia. They are rarely used in current practice.

Hypocalcemia

Hypocalcemia is an abnormal reduction in serum ionized calcium concentration. A reduction in the total serum calcium concentration, as may occur in patients with hypoalbuminemia, does not necessarily reflect a reduction in ionized calcium (see Chapter 75).

ETIOLOGY AND PATHOGENESIS

Causes of hypocalcemia are summarized in Table 74–3. Most causes of hypocalcemia result from a deficiency in the production, secretion, or action of PTH or 1,25-(OH)$_2$D. Hypocalcemia occasionally results from hyperphosphatemia or malabsorption of calcium.

Hypoparathyroidism

The causes of *hypoparathyroidism* range from surgical removal of the parathyroid glands to resistance to the action of PTH at the tissue level. Patients with hypoparathyroidism have reduced mobilization of calcium from bone, reduced renal reabsorption of calcium, reduced renal clearance of inorganic phosphate, and decreased intestinal calcium absorption resulting from reduced synthesis of 1,25-(OH)$_2$D. The results are hypocalcemia and hyperphosphatemia. Hypoparathyroidism can result from autoimmune destruction of the parathyroid glands either as a sporadic disorder or as part of an inherited syndrome associated with mucocutaneous candidiasis and other hormone deficiencies (*autoimmune polyglandular failure syndrome type I*). Many of these patients have antibodies directed against the calcium-sensing receptor. Hypoparathyroidism after neck surgery may reflect removal of the parathyroid glands or disruption of their blood supply.

Hypomagnesemia induces a functional state of hypoparathyroidism resulting from a combination of impaired

TABLE 74–3 Causes of Hypocalcemia

Hypoparathyroidism
  Postsurgical
  Hypomagnesemia
  Autoimmune polyglandular failure syndrome type I
  Activating mutations of the calcium-sensing receptor gene
  Sequela of neck irradiation
  Infiltrative (e.g., hemochromatosis, granulomatous diseases)
  DiGeorge's syndrome
  Idiopathic
Parathyroid hormone resistance
  Pseudohypoparathyroidism
  Hypomagnesemia
Vitamin D deficiency
  Decreased dietary intake
  Lack of sunlight exposure
  Intestinal malabsorption
  Sequela of gastrectomy
  Anticonvulsant therapy
  Vitamin D–dependent rickets type I
Vitamin D resistance
  Vitamin D–dependent rickets type II
Chronic renal failure
Hyperphosphatemia
  Renal failure
  Tumor lysis syndrome
  Rhabdomyolysis
  Excessive phosphate administration
Hungry bone syndrome
Osteoblastic metastases (e.g., prostate cancer)
Acute pancreatitis
Multiple citrated blood transfusions
Gram-negative sepsis
Medications
  Bisphosphonates
  Calcitonin
  Mithramycin
  Foscarnet

PTH secretion and end-organ resistance to the effects of PTH. Impairment of PTH secretion and action rarely occurs until the serum magnesium concentration falls to less than 1 mg/dL (0.8 mEq/L).

The causes of hypoparathyroidism are listed in Table 74–4. Less common causes of hypoparathyroidism include granulomatous or malignant infiltration of the parathyroid glands, iron overload of the parathyroid glands, DiGeorge's syndrome (congenital abnormality representing absence of the embryologic formation of the parathyroid glands and the thymus with severe immunodeficiency), and neck irradiation.

In some patients with hypoparathyroidism, no cause can be determined. Many patients with so-called "idiopathic" hypoparathyroidism appear actually to harbor activating mutations of the calcium-sensing receptor gene. The disorder has an autosomal dominant mode of inheritance. Before therapy, serum calcium levels are decreased, and serum PTH levels are low or inappropriately normal. With therapy, PTH levels become suppressed, and marked hypercalciuria is common. Mu-

tations in the signal peptide sequence of pre-pro-PTH that prevent its processing to PTH also cause autosomal dominant hypoparathyroidism.

Pseudohypoparathyroidism

In contrast to patients with hypoparathyroidism in whom PTH levels are inappropriately low for the degree of hypocalcemia, PTH levels are elevated in patients with *pseudohypoparathyroidism* (PHP) resulting from end-organ resistance to PTH action. Most patients with PHP have hyperphosphatemia and low serum calcitriol levels. Studies have demonstrated that PHP represents a group of disorders, which share resistance to PTH action but have variable biochemical abnormalities, end-organ responses to exogenous PTH, and molecular defects in PTH action. Patients with PHP type Ia have a deficient urinary cAMP response to PTH administration. These patients also have a more generalized abnormality impairing cAMP production in other tissues and often have a group of somatic abnormalities referred to as *Albright's hereditary osteodystrophy* (short stature, round face, subcutaneous ossifications, short metacarpals and metatarsals, obesity, and basal ganglia calcifications). The molecular defect in patients with PHP Ia is reduced activity of the α stimulatory subunit of the guanine nucleotide-binding protein that couples PTH to adenyl cyclase ($G_s\alpha$).

Some patients exhibit the somatic abnormalities of Albright's hereditary osteodystrophy and low $G_s\alpha$ activity but have a normal serum calcium level and a normal response of urinary cAMP to exogenous PTH. This variant is called *pseudo-PHP*. Pseudo-PHP is genetically related to PHP. Expression of PTH resistance in families may require maternal transmission of the mutated Gsα

TABLE 74–4 Signs and Symptoms of Hypocalcemia

Neuromuscular Irritability
Paresthesias: circumoral, fingers, and toes
Carpal-pedal spasm: positive Chvostek's or Trousseau's sign
Laryngospasm
Bronchospasm
Blepharospasm
Tetany

Central Nervous System
Seizures
Electroencephalographic abnormalities
Increased intracranial pressure with papilledema
Extrapyramidal disturbances

Cardiovascular
Prolonged QT interval
Heart block
Congestive heart failure

Other
Abnormalities of teeth, fingernails, skin, and hair
Lenticular cataracts

gene. Patients with PHP type Ib have normal $G_s\alpha$ activity and biochemical abnormalities similar to those seen in PHP Ia, but they lack the Albright's hereditary osteodystrophy phenotype. A defect in the expression of PTH receptor mRNA may be at fault. Intriguingly, the gene for familial PHP type Ib is closely linked to the $G_s\alpha$ gene. Patients with PHP type II have a reduced phosphaturic increase to exogenous PTH despite a normal response in urinary cAMP excretion, a finding suggesting a defect in the ability of cAMP to initiate the metabolic events typical of PTH action. PHP type II does not appear to have a genetic basis.

Vitamin D Deficiency and Resistance

Hypocalcemia can also result from *vitamin D deficiency, abnormalities in vitamin D metabolism,* or *resistance to the actions of vitamin D.* In these patients, normal or low levels of serum inorganic phosphate and elevated serum PTH concentrations usually accompany hypocalcemia. The causes of vitamin D deficiency and resistance are discussed in Chapter 75.

Chronic Renal Failure

Chronic renal failure is the most common cause of hypocalcemia. The hypocalcemia results from hyperphosphatemia, reduced $1,25-(OH)_2D$ production, and impaired sensitivity of the skeleton to PTH action. Patients develop secondary hyperparathyroidism and parathyroid gland hyperplasia. In patients with long-standing secondary hyperparathyroidism, autonomous parathyroid function and hypercalcemia can occur ("tertiary hyperparathyroidism").

Other Causes

Other causes of hypocalcemia include the following: hyperphosphatemia resulting from renal failure, phosphate administration, rhabdomyolysis, malignant hyperthermia, or acute tumor lysis; acute pancreatitis, possibly because of chelation of calcium by free fatty acids; osteoblastic metastases, such as in prostate cancer; citrate administration in patients receiving multiple blood transfusions; EDTA administration in persons receiving large doses of certain iodinated x-ray contrast media; foscarnet administration (by complexing with calcium); gram-negative sepsis; and medications that inhibit bone resorption such as bisphosphonates, calcitonin, and mithramycin. Transient hypocalcemia frequently occurs after surgical removal of solitary parathyroid adenomas because of rapid movement of calcium and phosphate into bones ("hungry bone syndrome").

SIGNS AND SYMPTOMS

Hypocalcemia is often asymptomatic. Symptoms depend on the level of blood calcium, the duration of hypocalcemia, and the rate at which hypocalcemia develops (see Table 74–4). The most frequent symptoms of hypocalcemia result from neuromuscular irritability, including paresthesias of the hands, feet, and circumoral region and muscle cramps. Severe hypocalcemia can produce bronchospasm, laryngeal stridor, diplopia, blepharospasm, and seizures. Other central nervous system manifestations include electroencephalographic abnormalities, increased intracranial pressure with papilledema, myelopathy, and extrapyramidal disturbances caused by calcification of the basal ganglia. Cardiac manifestations of hypocalcemia include prolongation of the QT interval and, rarely, congestive heart failure. Physical examination may reveal a positive Chvostek sign (twitching of the facial muscles after tapping of the facial nerve) and a positive Trousseau sign (carpal spasm after inflation of the blood pressure cuff for 2 minutes above the systolic blood pressure). Cataracts, basal ganglia signs, and abnormalities of the teeth, hair, skin, and fingernails are occasionally seen.

LABORATORY AND RADIOLOGIC MANIFESTATIONS

Hyperphosphatemia and serum PTH levels that are either undetectable or inappropriately low for the levels of serum calcium characterize hypocalcemia resulting from hypoparathyroidism. In PHP, PTH levels are high because of end-organ resistance to PTH. The diagnosis of PHP may require determination of the urinary cAMP and phosphaturic responses to exogenous PTH infusion (the Ellsworth-Howard test). In patients with other causes of hypocalcemia, such as malabsorption or vitamin D deficiency, serum inorganic phosphate levels are generally low or normal and serum PTH levels are increased. A notable exception is chronic renal failure, which is characterized by secondary hyperparathyroidism and hyperphosphatemia. In patients with hereditary PHP, calcifications in the basal ganglia as well as short fourth and fifth metacarpals and metatarsals can be seen on radiographs.

TREATMENT

The mainstays of therapy for hypocalcemia are calcium and vitamin D. Patients with acute symptomatic hypocalcemia may require intravenous administration of calcium salt solutions. In such situations, one ampule of 10% calcium gluconate, which contains approximately 90 mg of elemental calcium, can be infused over 5 to 10 minutes. Less acute administration of intravenous calcium gluconate can be achieved by mixing calcium gluconate with dextrose and infusing 500 to 1000 mg of calcium over 24 hours with close monitoring of the blood calcium level. If hypomagnesemia is present, it should be corrected (see Chapter 73).

The management of chronic hypocalcemia depends on its underlying origin. Most patients require treatment with a combination of oral calcium and one of several vitamin D preparations. In mild vitamin D deficiency, one or two multivitamins, each containing 400 IU of vitamin D, together with 800 to 1200 mg of oral calcium may be sufficient. Patients with hypoparathyroidism typically require high doses of vitamin D (e.g., vitamin D_2, 25,000 to 100,000 U/day) or 1,25-$(OH)_2D$ (0.25 to 2.0 μg/day) plus oral calcium in amounts sufficient to maintain serum calcium levels in the low-normal range. Urinary calcium excretion should be monitored closely. Compared with vitamin D_2, 1,25-$(OH)_2D$ has the advantages of more rapid onset of action and short half-life, but it is more expensive. If patients are hyperphosphatemic, administration of aluminum-containing antacids may occasionally be necessary. Hypercalciuria, largely caused by the absence of PTH-induced renal calcium reabsorption, can be controlled by thiazide diuretics, which may also help to maintain normocalcemia. Thiazide therapy is usually not needed, however. In patients with chronic renal failure, hyperphosphatemia should be controlled with oral calcium supplements alone, if possible, to avoid metabolic bone disease from aluminum toxicity.

REFERENCES

Bilezkian JP: Management of acute hypercalcemia. N Engl J Med 1992; 326:1196–1203.

Broadus AE, Mangin M, Ikeda K, et al: Humoral hypercalcemia of malignancy: Identification of a novel parathyroid hormone–like peptide. N Engl J Med 1988; 319:556–563.

Fitzpatrick LA, Arnold A: Hypoparathyroidism. *In* DeGroot LJ (ed): Endocrinology, 3rd ed. Philadelphia: WB Saunders, 1995, p 1123.

Mundy GR: Hypercalcemia of malignancy revisited. J Clin Invest 1988; 82:1–6.

Pearce SHS, Williamson C, Kifor O, et al: A familial syndrome of hypocalcemia with hypercalciuria due to mutations in the calcium-sensing receptor. N Engl J Med 1996; 335:1115–1122.

Pollak MR, Brown EM, Chou YH, et al: Mutations in the Ca^{2+}-sensing receptor gene causes familial hypocalciuric hypercalcemia and neonatal severe hyperparathyroidism. Cell 1993; 75:1297–1303.

Potts JT Jr (ed): Proceedings of the NIH Consensus Development Conference on Diagnosis and Management of Asymptomatic Primary Hyperparathyroidism. J Bone Miner Res 1991; 6(Suppl 2):S1–S166.

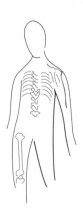

75

OSTEOMALACIA AND RICKETS

F. Richard Bringhurst

Osteomalacia and rickets are disorders of skeletal calcification. *Osteomalacia* is a failure to mineralize the newly formed organic matrix of bone *(osteoid)*. In children, osteomalacia is accompanied by defective mineralization of cartilage matrix within the zone of provisional calcification that is required for normal skeletal growth at the open epiphyses.

Pathogenesis

In forming new bone, osteoblasts lay down osteoid in an appositional fashion. The osteoid matrix, composed mainly of type I collagen, subsequently becomes mineralized by deposition of inorganic salts, principally calcium phosphate (as hydroxyapatite). The delay between matrix deposition and mineralization is such that a thin "seam" of unmineralized osteoid, perhaps 5 to 10 μm thick, normally exists on the surface of newly formed bone. *Matrix mineralization* is an active process, mediated by osteoblasts, that requires (1) adequate concentrations of both calcium and phosphate ions in the extracellular fluid, (2) an appropriate pH level (approximately 7.6), (3) bone matrix that is normal in composition and rate of synthesis, and (4) control of inhibitors of mineralization. Defects in any of these steps can lead to osteomalacia.

An analogous process is mediated by hypertrophic chondrocytes in the most proximal portion of the epiphyseal growth plate. Proper mineralization of the cartilage matrix, composed mainly of type X collagen, is essential for mechanical stability of the growth plate and for the timely vascular invasion and remodeling required for formation of the primary spongiosa of the lengthening bone. Defective cartilage mineralization therefore slows growth and leads to deformity of the epiphyses and metaphyses of bones that develop through the endochondral sequence, including the long bones of the extremities.

Specific Causes

Causes of osteomalacia and rickets are listed in Table 75–1. The major categories of diseases that produce osteomalacia or rickets are as follows: vitamin D deficiency, from decreased intake or absorption or cutaneous synthesis, accelerated clearance, impaired activation to 1,25-dihydroxyvitamin D (1,25-[OH]$_2$D), or peripheral resistance to 1,25-(OH)$_2$D action; chronic hypophosphatemia and/or hypocalcemia; systemic acidosis; and inhibitors of mineralization.

VITAMIN D DEFICIENCY OR RESISTANCE

As can be seen in Figure 73–3, formation of biologically active 1,25-(OH)$_2$D in the kidney requires adequate circulating precursor (25-OH-D), which is generated by hepatic 25-hydroxylation of vitamin D obtained either from the diet or by cutaneous synthesis using energy from ultraviolet rays of sunlight. Disorders that interfere with any of these steps can lead to vitamin D deficiency and osteomalacia or rickets.

Osteomalacia caused by *vitamin D deficiency* is relatively common in elderly people, many of whom have little exposure to sun and eat diets deficient in milk, eggs, and fish liver oils. *Intestinal malabsorption* is another common cause of vitamin D deficiency, especially in those with pancreatobiliary disease, sprue, or regional ileitis from Crohn's disease who cannot properly absorb dietary fats. Such patients frequently malabsorb calcium as well, because of complexing of calcium by free fatty acids in the gut lumen.

Hepatic metabolism and biliary excretion of vitamin D metabolites may be accelerated by certain *drugs*, notably isoniazid, rifampin, and certain anticonvulsants, including phenobarbital and carbamazepine. Because the vitamin D–binding protein, to which circulating vitamin D and its metabolites are bound, normally is extensively filtered at the glomerulus and subsequently is reabsor-

TABLE 75–1   Causes of Osteomalacia and/or Rickets

Vitamin D Deficiency or Resistance

Lack of vitamin D
  Dietary deficiency, sunlight deprivation
  Malabsorption (pancreatic insufficiency, sprue, inflammatory bowel disease, sequela of gastrectomy, intestinal bypass or resection)
Increased clearance of vitamin D or its metabolites
  Drugs (isoniazid, rifampin, phenobarbital, carbamazepine)
  Nephrotic syndrome
  Chronic ambulatory peritoneal dialysis
Defective activation of vitamin D
  Renal insufficiency
  Hypoparathyroidism
  Hepatic cirrhosis
  Mutant 1α-hydroxylase gene (VDDR-I)
Tissue resistance to 1,25-(OH)$_2$D
  Vitamin D receptor mutations (VDDR-II)
  Drugs (ketoconazole, phenytoin)

Chronic Hypophosphatemia

X-linked hypophosphatemic rickets (VDRR)
Other genetic renal phosphate-wasting syndromes (autosomal dominant hypophosphatemic rickets, autosomal recessive hypophosphatemic rickets, hereditary hypophosphatemic rickets with hypercalciuria, Dent's disease)
Fanconi's syndromes
Oncogenic osteomalacia
Aluminum hydroxide anatacid abuse

Systemic Acidosis

Distal renal tubular acidosis
Proximal renal tubular acidosis
Ureterosigmoidostomy, ileal loop
Carbonic anhydrase inhibitors

Calcium Malabsorption and Chronic Hypocalcemia Inhibitors of Mineralization

Sodium fluoride
Bisphosphonates (especially etidronate)
Aluminum

Miscellaneous

Hypophosphatasia

VDDR = vitamin D–dependent rickets; VDRR = vitamin D–resistant rickets.

bed by the renal tubules, excessive losses of vitamin D commonly occur in patients with *nephrotic syndrome.* Vitamin D metabolites also may be lost during continuous ambulatory peritoneal dialysis.

Hepatic conversion of vitamin D to 25-OH-D nor-mally is highly efficient and is rarely affected by liver disease, although patients with end-stage liver disease occasionally may have impaired 25-hydroxylase activity. The major cause of defective vitamin D activation is *chronic renal failure,* in which impaired activity of the renal 25-OH-D 1α-hydroxylase occurs, despite secondary hyperparathyroidism, resulting from a loss of functioning renal mass and progressive hyperphosphatemia.

Children with *vitamin D–dependent rickets type I* have a genetic defect in the activity of renal 1α-hydroxylase, despite normal or high levels of 25-OH-D, that leads to hypocalcemia, low levels of 1,25-(OH)$_2$D, appropriately elevated serum parathyroid hormone (PTH), and hypophosphatemia (Table 75–2). These children are treated effectively with physiologic replacement doses of 1,25-(OH)$_2$D.

Hereditary resistance to 1,25-(OH)$_2$D, often called *vitamin D–dependent rickets type II,* is a rare disorder caused by any of a large number of loss-of-function mutations within the vitamin D receptor gene. These defects include the following: (1) a failure of 1,25-(OH)$_2$D to bind to its receptor, either because of a gene deletion or because of a mutation in the receptor's hormone-binding domain; (2) an inadequate number of receptors per cell; (3) a defect in the localization of the hormone-receptor complex to the nucleus; or (4) decreased binding by the hormone-receptor complex to DNA, as a result of mutations in the DNA-binding domain of the receptor. Biochemical abnormalities are similar to those in patients with vitamin D–dependent rickets type I, except serum concentrations of 1,25-(OH)$_2$D are markedly elevated (see Table 75–2). Depending on the nature and severity of the receptor defect, treatment with large doses of 1,25-(OH)$_2$D$_3$ may be helpful.

CHRONIC HYPOPHOSPHATEMIA

The causes of *chronic hypophosphatemia* are summarized in Table 75–1. The dietary content of phosphorous is so high (and intestinal absorption so efficient) that inadequate intake of phosphate hardly ever occurs. The only exception to this is the syndrome, now mainly historical with the advent of nonprescription histamine blockers, of excessive intake of aluminum-containing antacids (aluminum binds phosphate and prevents phosphate absorption). Hypophosphatemia, often severe, is common among hospitalized and other acutely ill patients, but in this setting it usually is caused by transient intracellular shifts associated with respiratory alkalosis, rapid correction of metabolic acidosis, catecholamine ex-

TABLE 75–2   Typical Laboratory Findings in Rickets

	Calcium	Phosphate	25-OH-D	1,25-(OH)$_2$D	iPTH
VDDR-I	D	D	N or I	D	I
VDDR-II	D	D	N or I	I	I
VDRR	N	D	N	N or D	N

D = Decreased; I = increased; iPTH = immunoreactive parathyroid hormone; N = normal; VDDR = vitamin D–dependent rickets; VDRR = vitamin D–resistant rickets.

cess, or therapy of hyperglycemia, and it does not persist long enough to cause defective bone mineralization.

Hypophosphatemia and phosphate depletion of sufficient chronicity to interfere with skeletal mineralization in a clinically evident manner therefore nearly always can be traced to ongoing renal losses. Most often, this condition occurs in the setting of secondary hyperparathyroidism caused by an abnormality in the vitamin D axis, as described earlier.

The most common cause of primary chronic renal tubular phosphate wasting is the disorder X-linked hypophosphatemic rickets. Affected children harbor a loss-of-function mutation in the gene on the X chromosome that encodes *PHEX*, a putative cell-surface peptidase expressed in bone and certain other tissues (but not kidney) that normally must function in some way to limit renal phosphate excretion. Perhaps this enzyme inactivates the putative phosphaturic hormone, termed *phosphatonin*, which has been functionally identified as a tumor product in the disorder oncogenic osteomalacia (see later). The *PHEX* mutation causes defective renal tubular phosphate reabsorption (from underexpression of the sodium-phosphate cotransporter, NaPi-2), hypophosphatemia, and a defect in 1α-hydroxylation of vitamin D manifested as inappropriately normal blood 1,25-$(OH)_2D$ concentrations, low-normal serum and urinary calcium levels, and high-normal or slightly elevated serum PTH (Fig. 75–1; also see Table 75–2). Interestingly, no clear gene-dose effect is noted, and heterozygous females may be as severely affected as hemizygous males. Childhood rickets and growth retardation in X-

linked hypophosphatemic rickets are supplanted by osteomalacia and bone pain in adults.

Certain rare genetic disorders that impair renal phosphate reabsorption also have been described, including autosomal dominant and recessive forms of hypophosphatemic rickets, hereditary hypophosphatemic rickets with hypercalciuria, and Dent's disease. Hereditary and acquired proximal tubulopathies (Fanconi's syndromes) often produce both chronic hypophosphatemia and acidosis, which may combine to produce particularly severe osteomalacia. In rare cases, adult-onset osteomalacia may appear together with all the biochemical abnormalities typical of X-linked hypophosphatemic rickets (hypophosphatemia, borderline hypocalcemia or hypocalciuria, inappropriately normal blood 1,25-$[OH]_2D$ levels, and normal or high serum PTH) in patients with certain mesenchymal tumors that usually are benign (e.g., hemangiopericytomas, giant cell tumors of bone) but can be malignant (i.e., lung or prostate cancers). In these patients, said to have *oncogenic osteomalacia*, the biochemical abnormalities are rapidly reversed and the osteomalacia is cured if the offending neoplasm can be identified and excised. This clinical evidence of a humoral phosphaturic factor has been corroborated in laboratory studies of these tumors and of their secreted bioactive phosphaturic product, phosphatonin, which is presumed to be an unidentified phosphate-regulating hormone.

PURE CALCIUM MALABSORPTION

Malabsorption of calcium, independent of alterations in vitamin D metabolism, may be a primary or contributing factor in the development of osteomalacia in patients who have undergone partial gastrectomy, intestinal resection, or bypass or who have generalized intestinal diseases such as regional enteritis or sprue. In these patients, serum calcium levels are usually normal or slightly low, serum inorganic phosphate levels are low, 25-OH-D levels are normal or low, 1,25-$(OH)_2D$ levels are normal or increased, and serum immunoreactive PTH (iPTH) concentrations are elevated.

SYSTEMIC ACIDOSIS

Acidosis increases resorption of bone, mainly through stimulated osteoclastic activity but possibly also by direct physicochemical dissolution of bone mineral to buffer retained hydrogen ions. A decrease in systemic pH also may inhibit mineralization by lowering the pH to less than the critical level needed for normal mineralization at sites of matrix calcification. Conditions that produce chronic acidosis and are associated with rickets and/or osteomalacia include proximal and distal renal tubular acidosis, ureterosigmoidostomy, and Fanconi's syndrome.

INHIBITORS OF MINERALIZATION

Aluminum-containing antacids or dialysis fluids high in aluminum in patients with chronic renal failure (rarely seen now) may inhibit mineralization, as may sodium

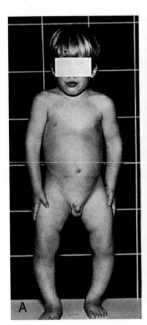
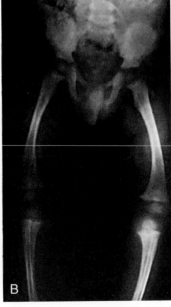

FIGURE 75–1 The clinical *(A)* and radiographic *(B)* appearance of a young boy with X-linked hypophosphatemic rickets. Note the striking bowing of the legs, apparent in both femora and tibiae, with flaring of the ends of the bones at the knee. (Courtesy of Dr. Sara B. Arnaud. From Bikle DB: Osteomalacia and rickets. *In* Wyngaarden JB, Smith LH Jr, Bennett JB [eds]: Cecil Textbook of Medicine, 19th ed. Philadelphia: WB Saunders, 1992, p 1408.)

fluoride and high cumulative doses of bisphosphonates (best described with etidronate disodium).

Clinical Manifestations

The clinical features of rickets are mainly related to skeletal pain and deformity, fracture of the abnormal bone, slippage of epiphyses, and disturbances in growth. Affected children may be listless, weak, and hypotonic, particularly when vitamin D deficiency is also present. Dental eruption is delayed, and enamel defects, another reflection of impaired mineralization, are common. The epiphyses are enlarged, as are the costochondral junctions, the latter producing the classic *rachitic rosary*. Depending on the underlying cause, the child also may have symptoms of hypocalcemia, often presenting as seizures. If the condition is treated appropriately before the child is 4 years old, the permanence of the skeletal deformities usually can be minimized. In vitamin D–dependent rickets type II, associated ectodermal dysplasia, dental abnormalities, and abnormal facies typically lead to early recognition and diagnosis.

In adults, osteomalacia is often difficult to diagnose on clinical grounds alone. Diffuse skeletal pain, often prominent around the hips, and proximal muscle weakness are the most common complaints. Physical examination may reveal a waddling gait, muscle weakness, bone tenderness, and hypotonia with preservation of brisk reflexes.

Laboratory and Radiographic Features

The laboratory findings depend on the specific cause of the mineralization defect, as reviewed earlier. The most typical findings are slight hypocalcemia, more profound hypophosphatemia, elevated serum alkaline phosphatase, low-normal urinary calcium excretion, and an elevated level of serum iPTH. Although some of these values may be normal, it is unusual for all of them to be normal in a patient with osteomalacia. Serum levels of 25-OH-D often are depressed. Serum $1,25\text{-}(OH)_2D$ levels may be elevated, despite low 25-OH-D levels, in vitamin D–deficient patients with secondary hyperparathyroidism. More often, however, serum $1,25\text{-}(OH)_2D$ levels are (inappropriately) normal or, particularly in pa-

tients with renal disease, frankly low. Bone mineral density may be decreased, normal, or even increased, depending on the cause of the mineralization defect. A comparison of the typical laboratory features of osteomalacia, primary hyperparathyroidism, and osteoporosis is given in Table 75–3.

The radiographic findings in osteomalacia are usually nonspecific and show only diffuse osteopenia. Trabeculae are poorly defined, the corticomedullary junction is blurred, and the cortices are thinned. The only specific radiographic manifestation is the *pseudofracture*, or Looser's zone. Classically, pseudofractures are bilateral, symmetric, and oriented perpendicular to the surface of the bone (Fig. 75–2). They are most common on the concave surfaces of the proximal femur, femoral neck, pubic and ischial rami, pelvis, ribs, and axillary margins of the scapula.

In rickets, the most characteristic alterations occur at the epiphyseal growth plate, which is widened and irregularly calcified. Enlargement of the growth plate leads to flaring, cupping, and fraying of the metaphyses (see Fig. 75–1). Bowing of long bones, scoliosis, a bell-shaped thorax, basilar invagination of the skull, and acetabular protrusion all may occur in rachitic bones.

Diagnosis

In osteomalacia and rickets, mineralization of osteoid (and of cartilage in rickets) does not keep pace with formation of osteoid. The diagnosis of rickets is usually apparent on clinical and radiographic grounds, whereas the diagnosis of osteomalacia is best established by iliac crest bone biopsy after double tetracycline labeling. In patients with osteomalacia, osteoid seams are wider than normal and cover a greater extent of bone surface. The rate of bone formation is depressed. A mean osteoid seam width of more than 15 μm and a mineralization lag time of more than 100 days are generally considered appropriate kinetic criteria to diagnose osteomalacia; however, some experts also require an absolute increase in the total osteoid volume and an increased number of osteoid lamellae.

Treatment

Because the causes of osteomalacia and of rickets are diverse, generalizing treatment is difficult. Most patients

TABLE 75–3 **Typical Laboratory Findings in Serum in Metabolic Bone Diseases**

	Calcium	Phosphate	Alkaline Phosphatase	iPTH
Osteomalacia	N or D	D	I	I
Primary hyperparathyroidism	I	D	I	I
Osteoporosis	N	N	N	N

D = Decreased; I = increased; iPTH = immunoreactive parathyroid hormone; N = normal.

require calcium and vitamin D therapy, and some require large supplements of phosphate. In patients with intestinal malabsorption, doses of vitamin D may have to be increased (≤50,000 to 100,000 U/week) beyond the level of 800 to 1000 U/day that usually is adequate

for uncomplicated vitamin D deficiency. Intramuscular vitamin D may be needed in some patients with severe fat malabsorption. In patients with vitamin D deficiency, administering vitamin D leads to rapid healing of bone with an associated large requirement for both calcium and phosphate. Therefore, providing calcium supplements as well as vitamin D (usual diets generally provide adequate phosphate in this setting) is essential. Normalization of serum alkaline phosphatase and iPTH levels may take several months, and bone healing may continue for a year or more. The clinician should monitor the success of therapy and should verify that the patient's serum calcium, phosphate, and 25-OH-D levels have normalized and that calcium availability is adequate, as reflected by a urinary calcium excretion of at least 100 mg/day.

In patients with severe hypophosphatemia, as in X-linked hypophosphatemic rickets, oral phosphate therapy is associated with a rapid rise in serum inorganic phosphate levels, which may suppress serum calcium levels, reduce excretion of urinary calcium, and transiently elevate serum iPTH. Combined therapy with $1,25\text{-}(OH)_2D_3$ and phosphate accelerates healing of the bone disease and allows use of lower doses of oral phosphate supplements in patients with X-linked hypophosphatemic rickets. In some patients, calcium supplements (separated from the phosphate supplements) may be needed, although urinary calcium excretion must be carefully monitored to minimize the risk of nephrocalcinosis. Addition of thiazide diuretics may prove useful in reducing urinary calcium excretion in this setting.

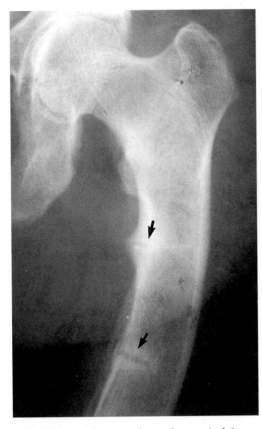

FiGURE 75–2 Pseudofractures (Looser's zones) of the medial aspect of the femur of a patient with osteomalacia. (Courtesy of Dr. Daniel Rosenthal.)

REFERENCES

Favus MJ (ed): Primer on the Metabolic Bone Diseases and Disorders of Mineral Metabolism, 2nd ed. New York: Raven Press, 1993.
Goldring SR, Krane SM, Avioli LV: Disorders of calcification: Osteomalacia and rickets. *In* DeGroot LJ (ed): Endocrinology, 3rd ed. Philadelphia: WB Saunders, 1995, pp 1204–1227.

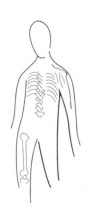

76

OSTEOPOROSIS

Joel S. Finkelstein

General Considerations

Osteoporosis, the most common type of metabolic bone disease, is characterized by a parallel reduction in bone mineral and bone matrix such that bone is decreased in amount but is of normal composition. Osteoporosis affects 20 million Americans and leads to approximately 1.3 million fractures in the United States each year, including 250,000 hip fractures. During their lifetimes, women lose about 50% of their trabecular bone and 30% of their cortical bone, and 30% of all postmenopausal white women eventually have osteoporotic fractures. By extreme old age, one third of all women and one sixth of all men will have a hip fracture. The annual cost of health care and of lost productivity resulting from osteoporosis is estimated to be nearly $14 billion in the United States.

Etiology and Pathogenesis

At any time, bone density depends on both the peak bone density achieved during development and the subsequent adult bone loss (Fig. 76–1). Thus, osteopenia can result from either deficient pubertal bone accretion or accelerated adult bone loss, or both.

DETERMINANTS OF PEAK BONE DENSITY

Bone density increases dramatically during puberty in response to gonadal steroids and eventually reaches values in young adults that are nearly double those of children. Other factors that influence peak bone density are listed in Table 76–1. The impact of genetic factors on bone density has been demonstrated in several ways. For example, bone density is lower in the daughters of women with osteoporosis than in the daughters of women without osteoporosis. Moreover, the concordance of bone density is much higher among monozygotic twins than dizygotic twins. Several genes, including the vitamin D receptor gene, the genes encoding type I procollagen, and the estrogen receptor gene, have been implicated in the pathogenesis of osteoporosis, but no conclusive genetic linkages have been demonstrated.

Men have higher bone density than women, and African-Americans have higher bone density than whites. Men with histories of constitutionally delayed puberty have decreased peak bone density, a finding that may be important in the pathogenesis of osteoporosis in some men. Similar findings have been reported in women with delayed menarche. Studies in identical twins suggest that moderate calcium supplementation can enhance prepubertal bone accretion. Associations between peak bone density and physical activity have also been reported.

PHYSIOLOGIC CAUSES OF ADULT BONE LOSS

After peak bone density is reached, bone density remains stable for years and then declines. Considerable evidence suggests that bone loss begins before menses cease in women and in the third to fifth decade in men. In women, once menopause is established, the rate of bone loss is accelerated severalfold. During the first 5 to 10 years of menopause, trabecular bone is lost faster than cortical bone, with rates of approximately 2% to 4% and 1% to 2% per year, respectively. A woman can lose 10% to 15% of her cortical bone and 25% to 30% of her trabecular bone during this time; this loss can be prevented by estrogen replacement therapy. Furthermore, rates of bone loss vary considerably among women. A subset of women in whom osteopenia is more severe than expected for their age is said to have *type I* or *postmenopausal osteoporosis* (Fig. 76–2). Clinically, type I osteoporosis often presents with vertebral crush fractures or Colles' fractures. The mechanism whereby estrogen deficiency leads to bone loss is still not established. Evidence suggests that estrogen deficiency increases local production of bone-resorbing cytokines such as interleukin-1, interleukin-6, and tumor necrosis factor, and estrogen administration stimulates

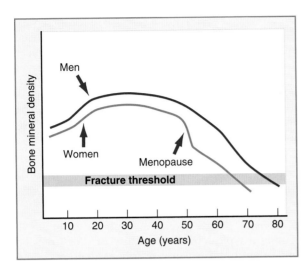

FIGURE 76–1 Cortical bone mineral density versus age in men and women. Women have lower peak cortical bone density than men and experience a period of rapid bone loss during menopause, so they reach the fracture threshold (the level of bone density at which the risk of developing osteoporotic fractures begins to increase) earlier than do men.

production of osteoprotegerin, a soluble member of the tumor necrosis factor receptor family that may inhibit bone resorption. Because estrogen also increases local production of growth factors that stimulate bone formation such as insulin-like growth factor I and transforming growth factor-β, estrogen deficiency may diminish bone formation. Estrogen deficiency increases the skeleton's sensitivity to the resorptive effects of parathyroid hormone. Estrogen deficiency therefore leads to a small increase in serum calcium levels. According to one hypothesis, increased calcium levels suppress parathyroid hormone secretion and thereby decrease renal 1,25-dihydroxyvitamin D (1,25-[OH]$_2$D) formation, which then limits intestinal calcium absorption (see Fig. 76–2). Finally, the discovery of estrogen receptors on osteoblasts suggests that estrogen deficiency may also alter bone formation directly.

Once the period of rapid postmenopausal bone loss ends, bone loss continues at a more gradual rate throughout life. The osteopenia that results from normal aging, which occurs in both women and men, has been termed *type II* or *senile osteoporosis* (Fig. 76–3). Because type II osteoporosis is associated with a more

TABLE 76–1   Factors That May Affect Peak Bone Mass

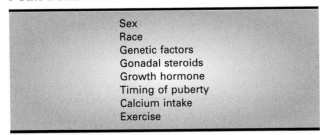

Sex
Race
Genetic factors
Gonadal steroids
Growth hormone
Timing of puberty
Calcium intake
Exercise

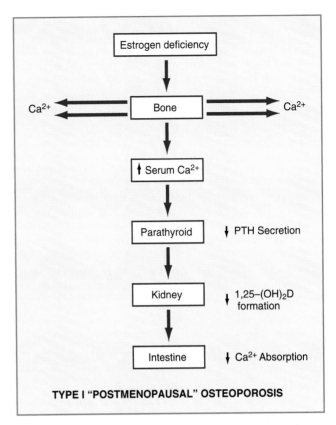

FIGURE 76–2 Physiologic alterations in women with type I ("postmenopausal") osteoporosis. PTH = parathyroid hormone.

balanced decrease in cortical and trabecular bone mass, fractures of the hip, pelvis, wrist, proximal humerus, proximal tibia, and vertebral bodies all occur commonly. Factors that may be important in the pathogenesis of type II osteoporosis include the following: (1) a primary defect in the ability of the kidney to make 1,25-(OH)$_2$D

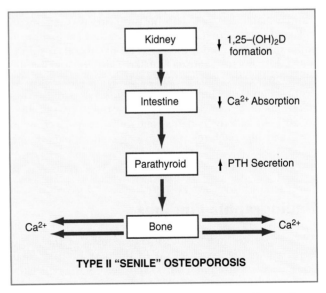

FIGURE 76–3 Physiologic alterations in women with type II ("senile") osteoporosis. PTH = parathyroid hormone.

and/or decreased intestinal sensitivity to 1,25-(OH)$_2$D, a change that leads to diminished calcium absorption and mild secondary hyperparathyroidism; and (2) a decrease in osteoblastic bone formation with aging. Finally, the distinctions between type I and type II osteoporosis are often arbitrary, and these syndromes may overlap.

SECONDARY CAUSES OF ADULT BONE LOSS

Many of the disorders that can lead to osteoporosis independent of the normal effects of menopause in women and of aging in both women and men are listed in Table 76–2. These conditions should be considered when one evaluates patients with osteoporosis and include endogenous and exogenous glucocorticoid excess, hypogonadism, hyperthyroidism, hyperparathyroidism, vitamin D deficiency, gastrointestinal diseases, bone marrow disorders, immobilization, connective tissue diseases, and use of certain drugs.

Clinical Manifestations

Osteoporosis is asymptomatic unless it results in a fracture, usually a vertebral compression fracture or a fracture of the wrist, hip, rib, pelvis, or humerus. Vertebral compression fractures often occur with minimal stress, such as when sneezing, bending, or lifting a light object. The middle and lower thoracic and upper lumbar regions are most frequently involved. Back pain usually begins acutely, often radiates laterally to the flanks and anteriorly, and then subsides gradually over several weeks. Patients with multiple fractures that result in spinal deformity may have a chronic backache that is made worse by standing. Such patients lose height and may develop the characteristic dorsal kyphosis and cervical lordosis known as the *dowager's hump*. In some patients, vertebral collapse can occur slowly and without symptoms. Hip fractures are of the femoral neck and intertrochanteric types. Hip fractures are associated with falls and occur either as a result of modest trauma or, in some instances, before the fall. The likelihood of suffering a hip fracture during a fall is also related to the direction of the fall, so fractures are more likely to occur when the patient falls to the side. Secondary complications of hip fractures carry a mortality rate of 15% to 20% in elderly patients, and 30% of patients who have had hip fractures require long-term nursing home care.

Radiographic Findings

A characteristic radiograph of osteoporosis of the spine is shown in Figure 76–4. With the loss of trabecular bone in the vertebral bodies, the vertebral end plates appear to be accentuated. Vertebral deformity may take the form of *collapse* (reduction in both anterior and posterior height), *anterior wedging* (reduction in anterior height), or the so-called *codfish deformity* (caused by weakening of the subchondral plates and expansion of the intervertebral discs). Protrusion of the intervertebral discs in the vertebral bodies produces *Schmorl's nodules*. In the absence of fractures, radiographs are insensitive indicators of bone loss because a substantial reduction in bone mass is required before bone loss is visible radiographically.

Diagnosis

The diagnosis of osteopenia can be made by either documenting a typical fragility fracture or measuring bone mineral density, in which case a bone density value less than the lower limit of normal for sex-matched young adults establishes the diagnosis. The World Health Organization's nomenclature uses the term *osteopenia* to refer to a condition in which bone mineral density is between 1 and 2.5 standard deviations less than peak bone mass and the term *osteoporosis* to refer to a condition in which bone mineral density is more than 2.5 standard deviations less than peak bone mass. Although this terminology may have clinical utility, *osteopenia* is actually a generic term that refers to decreased bone mass, regardless of the severity or the histopathologic features. A true diagnosis of osteoporosis requires a histomorphometric analysis of bone because some persons with low bone mineral density have osteomalacia.

Several techniques are available for measuring bone mineral density in the axial and appendicular skeleton (Table 76–3). Large, prospective studies have demonstrated that bone density measurements of the distal and proximal radius, os calcis, proximal femur, or spine can predict the development of the major types of osteoporotic fractures, including hip fractures. Regardless of the anatomic site measured, the risk of future osteoporotic fractures is increased by 50% to 100% for every 1 standard deviation that bone density is decreased. Measurement of bone density at a specific skeletal site, however, predicts fractures at that site better than when bone density is measured at a different site. Of the available techniques, quantitative computed tomography (QCT) of the spine is the most sensitive method for diagnosing osteopenia because it measures trabecular bone within the vertebral bodies exclusively. Because the expense and radiation dose of QCT are high and its reproducibility is relatively poor, it is not an ideal technique when repeat measurements aimed at detecting small changes in bone density are needed. Single photon absorptiometry of the proximal forearm has good precision and low radiation exposure, but it is relatively insensitive for detecting osteopenia because it measures cortical bone, which is lost more slowly than trabecular bone in early menopause. Dual photon absorptiometry, the first technique available for measuring bone density in the spine and hip, is limited by poor reproducibility, long examination times, and artifacts caused by vascular calcifications and changes in the radioactive source. For

TABLE 76–2 Secondary Causes of Osteoporosis

Endocrine Diseases

Female hypogonadism
  Hyperprolactinemia
  Hypothalamic amenorrhea
  Anorexia nervosa
  Premature and primary ovarian failure
Male hypogonadism
  Primary gonadal failure (e.g., Klinefelter's syndrome)
  Secondary gonadal failure (e.g., idiopathic hypogonadotropic hypogonadism)
  Delayed puberty
Hyperthyroidism
Hyperparathyroidism
Hypercortisolism
Growth hormone deficiency

Gastrointestinal Diseases

Subtotal gastrectomy
Malabsorption syndromes
Chronic obstructive jaundice
Primary biliary cirrhosis and other cirrhoses
Alactasia

Bone Marrow Disorders

Multiple myeloma
Lymphoma
Leukemia
Hemolytic anemias
Systemic mastocytosis
Disseminated carcinoma

Connective Tissue Diseases

Osteogenesis imperfecta
Ehlers-Danlos syndrome
Marfan's syndrome
Homocystinuria

Drugs

Alcohol
Heparin
Glucocorticoids
Thyroxine
Anticonvulsants
Gonadotropin-releasing hormone agonists
Cyclosporine
Chemotherapy

Miscellaneous Causes

Immobilization
Rheumatoid arthritis

terior and lateral projections. Lateral spine DXA is more sensitive than anteroposterior spine DXA for detecting osteoporosis, although its reproducibility is slightly worse.

Secondary causes of osteoporosis should be sought in patients with an established diagnosis of osteoporosis, particularly when bone density is significantly lower than that of age-matched and sex-matched persons. A history and physical examination that focus on the factors that may affect peak bone mass (see Table 76–1) and secondary causes of osteoporosis (see Table 76–2) combined with selected laboratory tests are sufficient in most patients. Levels of serum calcium, inorganic phosphate, and alkaline phosphatase are usually normal in patients with osteoporosis, although the alkaline phosphatase may be elevated transiently after a fracture. Other routine chemistry studies can help to exclude renal or hepatic diseases, and a complete blood count may help to uncover a hematologic or myeloproliferative disorder. Because multiple myeloma can mimic involutional osteoporosis, the diagnosis should be considered in an evaluation of patients with osteoporosis, particularly those with severe disease. Measuring serum parathyroid hormone and 25-OH vitamin D levels is recommended to exclude hyperparathyroidism and vitamin D deficiency. The serum thyroid-stimulating hormone level

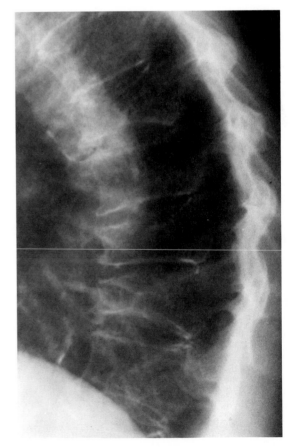

FIGURE 76–4 Radiograph showing radiolucency, compression fractures, and kyphosis in the spine of a patient with osteoporosis.

most patients, dual energy x-ray absorptiometry (DXA) of the lumbar spine or hip is the method of choice for measuring bone mineral density. Because DXA scans of the spine in the anteroposterior projection include both the trabecular-rich vertebral bodies and the cortical-rich posterior spinal elements, DXA is not as sensitive as QCT for detecting early trabecular bone loss. Its far greater precision, low radiation dose, rapid examination time, and lower cost, however, make DXA preferable to QCT in most situations. Newer DXA scanners can measure spinal bone mineral density in both the anteropos-

TABLE 76-3   Techniques for Measuring Bone Mineral Density*

Sites Measured	Precision (%)	Accuracy (%)	Scan Time (min)	Radiation Dose (mrem)
Quantitative computed tomography (QCT)	2–10	5–20	10–15	100–1000
Lumbar spine				
Proximal radius				
Distal radius				
Single photon absorptiometry (SPA)	1–3	4–6	3–5	10–20
Proximal radius				
Distal radius				
Calcaneus				
Dual photon absorptiometry (DPA)	2–6	4–10	20–40	10–15
Lumbar spine anteroposterior				
Lumbar spine lateral				
Proximal femur				
Total body				
Dual energy x-ray absorptiometry (DXA)	1–2	3–5	2–8	1–3
Lumbar spine anteroposterior				
Lumbar spine lateral				
Proximal radius				
Distal radius				
Proximal femur				
Total body				

*For SPA, numbers refer to measurements of the proximal radius. For QCT, numbers refer to measurements of the lumbar spine. For DPA and DXA, numbers refer to anteroposterior measurements of the lumbar spine.

should be checked when thyrotoxicosis is suspected. In men with unexplained osteoporosis, the serum testosterone level should be measured. The clinical utility of measuring biochemical markers of bone formation (serum osteocalcin, bone-specific alkaline phosphatase, or type I procollagen carboxy-terminal propeptide) and bone resorption (urine hydroxyproline, urine pyridinoline cross-links, or urine cross-linked N-telopeptides of type I collagen) has not been established. These markers may possibly help to predict rates of bone loss or the response to therapy, and bone turnover measurements may be useful in some subjects with unexplained osteoporosis. Finally, in selected patients, iliac crest bone biopsy after double tetracycline labeling may be useful, particularly for distinguishing osteoporosis from osteomalacia.

Treatment

Reversal of established osteoporosis is not possible. Early intervention, however, can prevent osteoporosis in most people, and later intervention can halt the progression of osteoporosis once it has developed. If a secondary cause of osteoporosis is present, specific treatment should be aimed at correcting the underlying disorder. During the acute phase of vertebral compression, attention is directed toward relieving pain with analgesics, muscle relaxants, heat, massage, and/or rest. Many patients with discomfort related to osteoporotic fractures or deformity benefit from a well-designed program of physical therapy. Some patients appear to benefit from a

corset or an orthopedic back brace. Both weight-bearing and non–weight-bearing exercises appear to have beneficial effects on bone mass. For most patients, exercises to strengthen the abdominal and back muscles are appropriate, and referral to a physical therapist with expertise in treating osteoporotic patients is often helpful. Precautions to prevent falls should be taken. Pharmacologic therapy is aimed at preventing further bone loss and decreasing the likelihood of future fracture.

CALCIUM

Both dietary calcium intake and fractional intestinal calcium absorption decrease with age. Most postmenopausal women consume less than 500 mg/day of calcium, far below the United States recommended dietary allowance of 1000 to 1500 mg. Calcium appears to retard, but not arrest, cortical bone loss from the forearm in women who are within the first several years of menopause. Most studies have failed to demonstrate a protective effect of calcium on spinal bone loss in early menopausal women. Calcium therapy appears to be more effective in arresting bone loss in late menopausal women, although some studies indicate that administering calcium does not halt their bone loss completely. Most experts recommend that postmenopausal women consume between 1000 and 1500 mg/day of calcium, either in their diet or from supplements. Because calcium may enhance peak bone mass, the recommended dietary allowance of calcium for adolescents and young adults in the United States is 1200 to 1500 mg/day. Most calcium supplements should be taken with meals, although calcium citrate may be taken when the stomach is empty. Clinically important differences among various forms of calcium supplementation are difficult to demonstrate.

VITAMIN D AND ITS METABOLITES

Vitamin D is important for absorption of calcium from the gastrointestinal tract. Although vitamin D deficiency is common, it is rarely diagnosed. One study reported that more than half of medical inpatients have hypovitaminosis D. Because of low vitamin D intake, insufficient exposure to sunlight, and reduced ability to synthesize vitamin D in the skin, elderly people are particular risk for vitamin D deficiency. Vitamin D deficiency may lead to secondary hyperparathyroidism and accelerated bone loss.

Small doses of vitamin D (800 IU/day) plus calcium reduce the incidence of hip fractures and other nonspinal fractures in elderly men and women. Because toxicity from such doses of vitamin D has not been reported, this therapy can be recommended to virtually all postmenopausal women. The current recommended daily intake of vitamin D is 200 IU for adults 19 to 50 years old, 400 IU for adults 51 to 70 years old, and 600 IU for adults older than 70 years. Some experts, however, recommend that all adults consume 800 IU of vitamin D each day.

The use of 1,25-$(OH)_2$D as a therapy for postmenopausal osteoporosis is more controversial. Although investigators have reported that a regimen of 0.5 μg/day of 1,25-$(OH)_2$D plus calcium administration preserves spinal bone mass and decreases the rate of fractures, whether 1,25-$(OH)_2$D therapy is superior to treatment with physiologic doses of vitamin D is unclear. Because the therapeutic index of 1,25-$(OH)_2$D therapy is small, the use of this agent should probably be reserved for patients who are not candidates for other forms of pharmacologic therapy.

ESTROGEN

Both oral and transdermal estrogen replacement therapies prevent bone loss in estrogen-deficient women, regardless of when therapy is begun. Although case-control studies suggest that estrogen therapy significantly reduces the risk of forearm, vertebral, pelvic, and hip fractures in postmenopausal women, a large, randomized controlled trial failed to demonstrate a significant reduction in clinical fractures in postmenopausal women receiving hormone replacement therapy. The minimally effective doses of estrogen to prevent bone loss are 0.625 mg/day of conjugated estrogens, 2 mg/day of estradiol, 25 μg/day of ethinyl estradiol, or 50 μg/day of transdermal estrogen, although some studies have shown that lower doses of conjugated estrogens (0.3 mg/day) prevent bone loss when they are combined with sufficient calcium intake. The appropriate duration of estrogen replacement therapy has not been established.

The decision to prescribe estrogen is influenced by several factors and should be individualized. In some women, estrogen is prescribed to alleviate menopausal symptoms. In others, the prospect of adhering to a treatment program that will produce cyclic menstruation is unacceptable. When given without concomitant progestin, estrogen replacement therapy increases the risk of endometrial carcinoma. Thus, in women whose uterus is intact, estrogen replacement therapy should be combined with a progestin, administered either cyclically (5 to 10 mg of medroxyprogesterone acetate for 12 to 14 days each month) or continuously (2.5 mg/day of medroxyprogesterone acetate). The latter regimen often eliminates menstrual bleeding after an initial period of 3 to 6 months, during which irregular bleeding may occur. In women who have had a hysterectomy, unopposed estrogen should be given daily. Estrogen therapy is generally contraindicated in women with a history of endometrial cancer. Hormone replacement therapy increases the risk of venous thromboembolic events.

The relationship between estrogen replacement therapy and breast cancer or cardiovascular disease has been the subject of many case-control and cohort studies, yet it remains unclear. Some studies suggested that postmenopausal estrogen use, particularly when continued for more than 5 to 10 years, is associated with an increased risk of breast cancer, although other studies failed to detect such a relationship. Numerous case-control and cohort studies have reported that estrogen replacement therapy decreases the risk of major coronary disease by approximately 40% to 50%. The potential for bias because of patient selection or uneven diagnostic surveillance in these nonrandomized studies cannot be excluded, however. In fact, the first large, randomized controlled trial to assess the effects of estrogen-progestin replacement therapy on the occurrence of nonfatal myocardial infarction or cardiovascular death in postmenopausal women with established coronary disease failed to detect any overall difference between treated and untreated women. Results from the Women's Health Initiative should establish whether hormone replacement therapy alters the incidence of cardiovascular events in women who do not have preexisting coronary artery disease.

BISPHOSPHONATES

Bisphosphonates inhibit osteoclastic bone resorption and are an important form of therapy for osteoporosis. Until the 1990s, the only bisphosphonate available for oral administration in the United States was etidronate, although it is not approved by the Food and Drug Administration for treating osteoporosis. Prospective studies demonstrated that cyclic etidronate increases spinal bone mineral density slightly and decreases the incidence of vertebral fractures in late menopausal women when it is given for 2 to 3 years. The effect on fracture rate of continuing etidronate therapy for more than 2 to 3 years is unclear. Etidronate also prevents bone loss in early menopausal women. The most common dose of etidronate is 400 mg/day for the first 2 weeks of every 3-month period. To ensure adequate absorption, the drug must be taken on an empty stomach.

Alendronate, a second-generation bisphosphonate that is much more potent than etidronate, is approved by the United States Food and Drug Administration for both prevention and treatment of postmenopausal osteoporosis. In women with preexisting vertebral fractures, alendronate therapy increases bone density of the spine and hip and reduces the risk of spinal and nonspinal fractures. Alendronate also reduces the risk of spinal fractures in women who do not have preexisting vertebral fractures. The recommended dose of alendronate is 10 mg/day in women with established osteoporosis and 5 mg/day for prevention of osteoporosis. Alendronate must be taken with 8 oz of water after an overnight fast, and patients should remain upright and fasting at least 30 minutes after its ingestion. Esophagitis is a potentially serious side effect.

SELECTIVE ESTROGEN RECEPTOR MODULATORS

All currently available estrogen receptor antagonists have some intrinsic estrogen-like activity and thus have been called *selective estrogen receptor modulators* (SERMs). Tamoxifen, the first selective estrogen receptor modulator in widespread clinical use, prevents spinal bone loss, lowers serum cholesterol levels, and blocks the effects of estrogen on the breast in postmenopausal women, but it induces endometrial hyperplasia. Another selective estrogen receptor modulator, raloxifene, prevents postmenopausal bone loss and lowers low-density lipoprotein cholesterol levels without any effect on the endometrium or breast in early postmenopausal women. In women with established postmenopausal osteoporosis, raloxifene reduces the risk of spinal fractures and also appears to reduce the incidence of estrogen receptor–positive cases of breast cancer. Like hormone replacement therapy, raloxifene increases the risk of venous thromboembolic events. Raloxifene is approved by the Food and Drug Administration for prevention of osteoporosis and is under investigation for treatment of established osteoporosis and prevention of breast cancer.

The molecular basis for the differential effects of raloxifene on estrogen-responsive tissues is reasonably well understood. Both estrogen and raloxifene bind to the same site of the estrogen receptor. When estrogen binds to its receptor, the complex assumes a conformation that allows binding of specific coactivator proteins. When raloxifene binds to the estrogen receptor, however, the receptor folds in such a way that prevents binding of these proteins and may recruit binding of additional corepressor proteins. Differential expression of these coactivator and corepressor proteins in tissues may be involved in the tissue-specific effects of raloxifene and estrogen.

CALCITONIN

Calcitonin is a 32-amino acid peptide produced by the thyroid C cells. Osteoclasts have calcitonin receptors, and calcitonin inhibits bone resorption. The effects of calcitonin on bone loss in early postmenopausal women have been inconsistent. In late postmenopausal women, calcitonin appears to prevent spinal bone loss, although appendicular bone loss continues. The effect of calcitonin therapy on the rate of osteoporotic fractures has not

been well studied, although one study suggests that it may slightly reduce the risk of vertebral fractures. Calcitonin is approved by the Food and Drug Administration for treatment of women with established postmenopausal osteoporosis and is available for both parenteral and intranasal use. The recommended dose is 100 IU subcutaneously or 200 IU intranasally each day, given with adequate calcium and vitamin D. Side effects such as nausea and flushing are common in patients treated with parenteral calcitonin, but they are rare with subcutaneous calcitonin administration. In occasional patients, calcitonin may have an analgesic effect. Thus, it may be particularly useful in patients with osteoporosis who have chronic pain related to fractures or skeletal deformity.

FUTURE THERAPIES

Several therapeutic agents are currently in clinical trials. Sodium fluoride is well known to increase spinal bone density. A traditional formulation of sodium fluoride therapy, however, failed to reduce the risk of vertebral fractures and actually increased the incidence of fractures of the appendicular skeleton. Lower doses of a slow-release formulation of sodium fluoride may increase spinal bone density without accelerating cortical bone loss and appears to reduce the incidence of spinal fractures.

Parathyroid hormone, when given intermittently in low doses, is a potent stimulator of osteoblastic bone formation. One study demonstrated that parathyroid hormone prevents bone loss in young women with severe estrogen deficiency. Parathyroid hormone also increases bone density in women with postmenopausal osteoporosis who are receiving estrogen. Other bone anabolic agents are currently being investigated.

Glucocorticoid-Induced Bone Loss

Bone loss is a common complication of glucocorticoid excess. The most important adverse effects of glucocorticoids on bone metabolism appear to be suppressed osteoblast activity and a vitamin D–independent inhibition of intestinal calcium absorption. Enhanced osteoclastic activity may also be important. The ability of glucocorticoids to suppress bone formation appears to be mediated, at least in part, by suppression of local secretion of insulin-like growth factor I in bone and by accelerated osteoblast apoptosis.

The predominant effect of administering glucocorticoids on the skeleton is a loss of trabecular bone, although cortical bone mass also decreases. Bone loss is fastest in the first 6 to 12 months of therapy, but accelerated bone loss appears to persist as long as therapy is continued.

If the physician anticipates that glucocorticoid therapy will be maintained for several months or longer, treatment to prevent bone loss should be strongly considered, particularly in estrogen-deficient women and when a high dosage of glucocorticoids is used. Several small studies showed that calcitonin therapy prevents spinal bone loss in patients receiving long-term glucocorticoid therapy. One controlled study demonstrated that a regimen of 0.5 to 1.0 μg of calcitriol plus 1000 mg/day of calcium prevents spinal bone loss for at least 1 year in patients who are starting treatment with glucocorticoids. Because of the potential for hypercalciuria and/or hypercalcemia, however, patients receiving calcitriol therapy require careful monitoring. Calcitriol therapy seems most logical in patients with low urinary calcium excretion, a finding suggesting poor intestinal absorption of calcium, and it should be avoided in patients with hypercalciuria. Large, randomized controlled trials have demonstrated that bisphosphonate therapy (etidronate, alendronate, or risedronate) prevents bone loss from the spine and hip in patients receiving glucocorticoid therapy and may reduce the risk of spinal fractures. Alendronate, at a dose of 5 mg/day, is approved for treatment of glucocorticoid-induced osteoporosis, al-though a higher dose (10 mg/day) may be required in estrogen-deficient women. Physiologic vitamin D replacement (400 IU/day), can be safely recommended in all patients receiving glucocorticoids, and calcium supplementation (1000 mg/day) should be added unless urinary calcium excretion is excessive. In patients with hypercalciuria, addition of a thiazide diuretic may be useful.

REFERENCES

American College of Rheumatology Task Force on Osteoporosis Guidelines: Recommendations for the prevention and treatment of glucocorticoid-induced osteoporosis. Arthritis Rheum 1996; 39:1791–1801.

Christiansen CC (ed): Consensus Development Conference on Osteoporosis. Am J Med 1993; 95(Suppl 5A):1S–78S.

Eastell R: Treatment of postmenopausal osteoporosis. N Engl J Med 1998; 338:736–746.

Johnston CC, Slemenda CW, Melton LJ III: Clinical use of bone densitometry. N Engl J Med 1991; 324:1105–1109.

Neer RM: Osteoporosis. *In* DeGroot LJ (ed): Endocrinology, 3rd ed. Philadelphia: WB Saunders, 1995, pp 1228–1258.

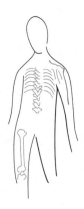

77

PAGET'S DISEASE OF BONE

Margaret P. Seton

Paget's disease is a chronic disorder of bone that may be monostotic or polyostotic. The disease was described in 1876 by Sir James Paget, who called the disease *osteitis deformans*. He attributed the pathologic changes and gradual deformation in bone to an inflammatory condition. Paget's disease is characterized by intense osteoclastic bone resorption followed by increased osteoblastic activity, resulting in deposition of woven bone. It is commonly asymptomatic, detected incidentally on radiographs or after finding an elevated serum alkaline phosphatase level. It may, however, result in pain, gross skeletal deformity, fracture, or neurologic compression syndromes.

Incidence and Prevalence

After osteoporosis, Paget's disease is the second most common bone disease; it is estimated to affect more than 3% of persons over 40 years of age in the United States. Its prevalence varies with geographic location; it is more common in the United States, Great Britain, France, Germany, and Australia, and it occurs infrequently in Scandinavia, the Middle East, and Asia.

Etiology

The cause of Paget's disease is still unknown. Some evidence, such as the finding of particles that resemble paramyxovirus nucleocapsids in the osteoclasts of pagetic bone, suggests that Paget's disease is a late complication of a viral infection. Immunohistologic data have suggested a role for measles, respiratory syncytial virus, and canine distemper virus. In situ hybridization studies have reported measles or canine distemper virus transcripts in pagetic osteoclasts. No intact virus has been isolated from pagetic bone, however, and controversy about the role of a viral infection continues. Other findings suggest a genetic predisposition to Paget's disease. Ethnic and geographic clustering of patients with Paget's disease is noted, and 15% to 30% of affected patients have a family history of the disorder. Genetic analyses of multiple affected kindreds support an autosomal dominant pattern of inheritance. Genetic studies have shown a linkage with chromosome markers on 18q21–22 in some families, markers that are consistently identified in a kindred of persons in Northern Ireland with *familial expansile osteolysis*. This osteolytic bone disease shares some marked similarities to Paget's disease, including autosomal dominant transmission and accelerated bone resorption.

Pathology and Pathophysiology

In areas of pagetic bone, osteoclasts are increased in number and size and contain multiple pleomorphic nuclei, increased rough endoplasmic reticulum, and organelles. Osteoblast activity remains coupled to osteoclastic bone resorption, so both bone resorption and formation are increased. The resultant bone is woven in appearance and is structurally abnormal, however. Vascularity of the abnormal bone is increased, and peritrabecular fibrosis may replace the normal cellular marrow. Eventually, the processes of resorption and formation may slow, leaving sclerotic, pagetic bone.

Increased bone resorption may result from local stimulation of osteoclast proliferation and activation by cytokines such as interleukin-6 (IL-6). Pagetic osteoclasts have receptors for IL-6 and also produce IL-6. IL-6 is detectable in marrow plasma and serum from patients with Paget's disease but not in healthy people.

Clinical Picture

Most patients with Paget's disease are asymptomatic and have only one or a few affected skeletal sites (Table 77–

TABLE 77-1   Clinical Manifestations of Paget's Disease

Musculoskeletal pain
Degenerative arthritis in joints near affected areas
Headache
Skeletal deformity
Pathologic fractures
Enlarged skull
Erythema and warmth over pagetic bones
Hearing loss
Platybasia with or without basilar invagination
Neurologic compression syndromes
Angioid streaks in retina
Increased cardiac output; rarely congestive heart failure
Bone tumors
   Osteogenic sarcoma
   Fibrosarcoma
   Chrondrosarcoma
   Reparative granuloma
   Giant cell tumor
Laboratory abnormalities
   Increased serum alkaline phosphatase (bone fraction)
   Increased urinary hydroxyproline
   Hypercalciuria and hypercalcemia during immobilization
   Hyperuricemia
   Characteristic radiographs
   Increased uptake on bone scan

1). The most commonly affected sites include the pelvis, femur, spine, skull, and tibia; involvement of the hands or feet is rare. Back pain, headache, and pain in the hips and legs are common complaints in those with symptoms. Arthritis is often found in joints near areas involved with Paget's disease, particularly when subchondral bone is affected or when the integrity of the joint is compromised by enlarged, distorted bones. The patient may have deformity of the skull or other affected bones. Pathologic fractures may occur, but small fissure fractures along the convex surface of long bones are more common. Spinal cord or nerve root compression with associated radicular pain and weakness may result from expanding pagetic bone. When the skull is involved, hearing is commonly affected. Other cranial nerve palsies are seen less frequently. Softening of the base of the skull may produce flattening (*platybasia*) with the development of basilar invagination and may lead to neurologic compression syndromes. Once areas of pagetic involvement have been identified, the disease does not usually involve new bone sites, although local extension may occur along affected areas.

Associated Conditions

Secondary arthritis is a common and often debilitating complication of periarticular Paget's disease. *Hyperuricemia* and *gout* may occur with increased frequency in affected persons. *Secondary hyperparathyroidism* has been noted in 15% to 20% of patients with Paget's disease. The occurrence of primary hyperparathyroidism in patients with Paget's disease is currently believed to be a clinical coincidence.

The most serious complication of Paget's disease is *sarcomatous degeneration,* which occurs most commonly in the setting of severe polyostotic disease and may be heralded by a sudden increase in pain, a soft tissue mass, or a pathologic fracture. Most tumors are osteogenic sarcomas, although fibrosarcomas and chondrosarcomas are also seen. Benign giant cell tumors, most often affecting the skull, are also seen in bone affected by Paget's disease.

Laboratory Assessment

Biochemical markers of bone formation, such as serum alkaline phosphatase, and bone resorption, such as urinary excretion of hydroxyproline, are usually increased in patients with active disease. Serum bone-specific alkaline phosphatase activity and urinary excretion of pyridinoline and cross-linked *N*-telopeptides of type I collagen may be more sensitive markers for assessing disease activity in patients with low levels of disease activity. The serum concentration of osteocalcin, another marker of bone formation, is often in the normal range and is not a clinically useful marker of disease activity.

A *bone scan* is the most useful test. *Radiographs* of affected areas confirm the presence of Paget's disease and are useful for monitoring disease progression as well as for evaluating complications. Early in the course of the disease, osteolysis may be seen as *osteoporosis circumscripta* in the skull or pelvis (Fig. 77–1A) or as an advancing "blade of grass" in long bones (see Fig. 77–1B). Later, in the mixed phase of the disease, expanded bones with cortical thickening, coarse trabecular markings, and both lytic and sclerotic areas are seen on radiographs (see Fig. 77–1C). In the late stages of the disease, when bone turnover is quiescent, sclerotic bone predominates (see Fig. 77–1D). Bone biopsy is rarely needed to diagnose Paget's disease and should be avoided in weight-bearing areas.

Treatment

The two major goals of therapy are to relieve symptoms and to prevent complications. Treatment is indicated in the following situations: for patients with symptoms that cannot be managed with salicylates or nonsteroidal anti-inflammatory drugs; when the disease involves a weight-bearing bone, the spine, the skull, or bone near a major joint; or when bone deformity, hearing loss, neurologic impairment, or high-output congestive heart failure is present. Treatment may be indicated during periods of immobilization to prevent accelerated bone loss and hypercalciuria. Persons who are asymptomatic or who have minimal symptoms can often be managed with salicylates or nonsteroidal anti-inflammatory drugs. Antiresorptive agents such as calcitonin or the bisphosphonates form the mainstay of therapy and have replaced the

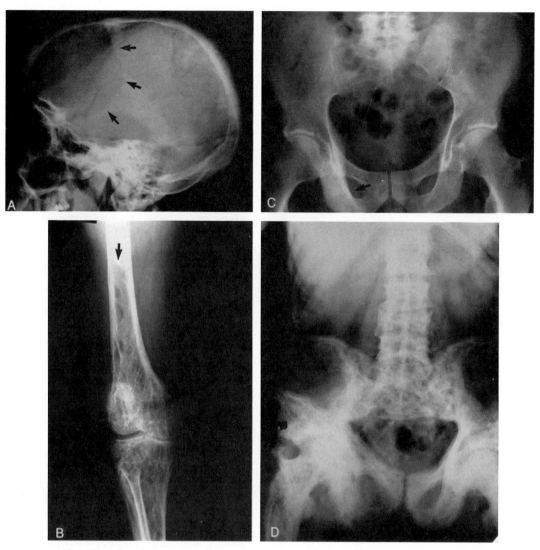

FIGURE 77–1   Typical radiographic abnormalities in patients with Paget's disease. *A,* Osteoporosis circumscripta of the skull. *B,* Lytic lesions in the femur with the characteristic "blade of grass" or "flame-like" lesion. *C,* Blastic involvement of the right ischial ramus of the pelvis with thickening of the medial cortex. *D,* Mixed lytic and blastic disease involving entire pelvis along with L4 and L5 and both femoral heads. (Courtesy of Dr. Daniel Rosenthal.)

use of cytotoxic agents such as plicamycin. Calcitonin, in addition to its antiresorptive action, may have a significant analgesic effect in some persons. The usual dose of calcitonin is 50 to 100 U/day by subcutaneous injection. Side effects include nausea and flushing, which usually resolve with continued use. The incidence of side effects can be minimized by gradually increasing the dose and administering the drug before bedtime. Calcitonin therapy can be used to decrease blood flow to pagetic bone preoperatively. Intranasal calcitonin is not approved by the United States Food and Drug Administration for treatment of Paget's disease.

Bisphosphonates are also useful for the treatment of Paget's disease. Previously, etidronate disodium was the only bisphosphonate available. Although effective, its use was limited by a tendency to induce abnormal mineralization when it was given at high doses or for more than 6 months at a time. The recommended dose is 5 mg/kg/day for 6 months, followed by 6 months without treatment. Its use is contraindicated in patients with lytic disease in weight-bearing bones. Etidronate is rarely used in the United States today.

The introduction of second-generation bisphosphonates represents a significant advance in the treatment of Paget's disease. These agents may induce a biochemical remission in patients who respond incompletely to treatment with etidronate or calcitonin. Furthermore, these drugs do not produce mineralization defects at the recommended doses. Parenteral pamidronate, an aminobisphosphonate, often reduces serum alkaline phosphatase and urinary hydroxyproline excretion into the normal range for 1 year or longer. In patients with mild disease, a single infusion of 30 to 60 mg may be sufficient to induce a biochemical remission of Paget's disease. Patients with more severe disease often require two or three weekly or biweekly infusions of 60 to 90 mg.

Cumulative doses of 240 to 480 mg may be required in some patients. Alendronate, another aminobisphosphonate, normalizes markers of bone turnover in most patients with Paget's disease when given in an oral dose of 40 mg/day for 6 months. Fewer than 10% of patients treated with alendronate have a biochemical recurrence within 12 months. More recently, two additional bisphosphonates, tiludronate and risedronate, have been approved for treatment of Paget's disease. The recommended dosage of tiludronate is 400 mg/day for 3 months, and the recommended dosage of risedronate is 30 mg/day for 2 months. As with pamidronate and alendronate, many patients treated with tiludronate or risedronate remain in biochemical remission for many months, or even years, after therapy is discontinued. Some evidence indicates that patients who have an in-complete biochemical response to one bisphosphonate may respond to a different agent. When treating patients with bisphosphonates, the clinician should ensure that the patient maintains adequate calcium (at least 1 g/day) and vitamin D (800 IU/day) intake, to prevent the development of secondary hyperparathyroidism.

REFERENCES

Delmas PD, Meunier PJ: The management of Paget's disease of bone. N Engl J Med 1997; 336:558–566.

Singer FR, Wallach S (eds): Paget's Disease of Bone: Clinical Assessment, Present and Future Therapy. New York: Elsevier, 1991.

Siris ES: Paget's disease of bone. *In* Favus MJ (ed): Primer on the Metabolic Bone Diseases and Disorders of Mineral Metabolism, 3rd ed. New York: Raven Press, 1996, pp 409–419.

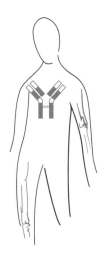

Musculoskeletal and Connective Tissue Disease

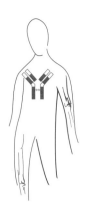

78

APPROACH TO THE PATIENT WITH RHEUMATIC DISEASE

Joseph H. Korn

The rheumatic diseases encompass a range of musculo-skeletal and systemic disorders that share the clinical involvement of joints and periarticular tissues. The causes of arthritis range from local trauma to infection, gout, osteoarthritis, and autoimmune connective tissue diseases, such as rheumatoid arthritis and systemic lupus erythematosus (SLE). Distinguishing localized from systemic processes, executing logical diagnostic procedures, and embarking on appropriate therapeutic courses depend on careful clinical evaluation. As in other areas, history and physical examination are paramount, and laboratory tests are more confirmatory than diagnostic. The "connective tissue screen" is done at the bedside and not in the laboratory. The practice of either including or excluding connective tissue disease based on laboratory panels is unreliable and therefore is unwise.

Musculoskeletal History and Examination

Features in the medical history that are useful in distinguishing different types of arthritis are listed in Tables 78–1 and 78–2. Appreciating the demographics of different illnesses provides useful information for diagnostic evaluation. Spondyloarthropathies present predominantly in young men, SLE in young women, gout in middle-aged men and postmenopausal women, and osteoarthritis in the elderly. Asymmetric pain and swelling in the knees have different connotations in a 70-year-old patient than in a 20-year-old patient. The patient's history provides the basis for distinction of inflammatory versus noninflammatory arthropathies. *Inflammatory arthritis* is characterized by pain at rest, morning stiffness, and improvement with activity. In *osteoarthritis* and *nonarthritic musculoskeletal problems,* pain is generally not present at rest and is precipitated by activity. Occa-sionally, however, osteoarthritic joints are stiff and are initially improved with activity. *Gout* is abrupt in onset, *septic arthritis* is less so, and most other disorders are slow and insidious. Patterns of joint involvement—symmetry, migratory features, large versus small joints, and locations characteristic of specific diseases—are also key items in the patient's history. Constitutional features such as fatigue, weight loss, and fever are seen in systemic autoimmune disease and infection but not in other localized conditions.

On physical examination, one should carefully assess active and passive range of motion in all joints and evaluate for the presence of tenderness, swelling, deformity, and joint effusions (Fig. 78–1). Patients are frequently unaware of detectable joint abnormalities, including deformity and effusion, and the presence of either is a sign of joint disease. Reported pain may be referred from another site, and this feature can be elucidated by examination. Thus, pain in the knee is often a sign of hip disease and may be reproduced on examination of the hip. The presence of palpable synovitis, thickening of the synovial membrane, is helpful in diagnosing inflammatory arthritis such as rheumatoid arthritis. Different diseases have distinctive patterns of joint involvement providing critical diagnostic information. Prominent disease of distal interphalangeal joints is seen in psoriasis and in inflammatory osteoarthritis. Wrist involvement and metacarpophalangeal involvement are almost universal in rheumatoid arthritis but rare in osteoarthritis. Examination of the axial skeleton may reveal diminished lumbar flexion, decreased rotational motion of the spine, and decreased chest expansion, features of ankylosing spondylitis and other spondyloarthropathies.

Rheumatic diseases may involve any organ system, and a full physical examination should be performed on all patients. One should look for fundoscopic changes (SLE), uveitis (spondyloarthropathy, juvenile arthritis), conjunctivitis (Reiter's syndrome), oral and other mu-

TABLE 78–1 Clinical Features Helpful in Evaluation of Arthritis

Age, gender, ethnicity, family history
Pattern of joint involvement
 Monoarticular, oligoarticular, polyarticular
 Large versus small joints
 Symmetry
Insidious versus rapid onset
Inflammatory versus noninflammatory pain (e.g., morning stiffness, gelling, night pain)
Presence of constitutional symptoms and signs (e.g., fever, fatigue, weight loss)
Presence of synovitis, bursitis, tendinitis
Involvement of other organ systems (e.g., rash, mucous membrane lesions, nail lesions)
Presence of arthritis-associated diseases (e.g., psoriasis, inflammatory bowel disease)
Anemia, proteinuria, azotemia
Presence of erosive joint disease

cous membrane ulcers (Reiter's syndrome, SLE, Behçet's syndrome), lymphadenopathy (SLE, Sjögren's syndrome), and cutaneous lesions (psoriasis, scleroderma, SLE, vasculitides). Lesions of psoriasis in the scalp, umbilicus, and anal crease, thickening of the skin on the fingers in scleroderma, and mucous membrane ulcers are often overlooked. The lung examination may show evidence of interstitial fibrosis (scleroderma, SLE, rheumatoid arthritis, myositis), and the cardiac evaluation may reveal aortic insufficiency (SLE, Reiter's syndrome, ankylosing spondylitis), pulmonary hypertension (systemic sclerosis), or evidence of cardiomyopathy (systemic sclerosis, myositis, amyloidosis). Pleural and pericardial rubs may be present in SLE, rheumatoid arthritis, and scleroderma. Hepatosplenomegaly (SLE, rheumatoid arthritis) and abdominal distention (scleroderma) are also valuable clinical clues. Muscular examination may reveal weakness from myositis, neuropathy (vasculitis, SLE), or myopathy (steroid myopathy). A complete neurologic examination is critical and may reveal carpal tunnel syndrome, peripheral neuropathy such as mononeuritis multiplex (an asymmetric sensory and/or motor neuropathy seen in many vasculitides), and central nervous system disease (SLE, vasculitis).

At the initial evaluation, one important question is whether diagnosis and treatment of the patient's problem require urgent attention. Infectious processes obviously belong in this category. The presence of acute joint inflammation, fever, and systemic signs such as chills, night sweats, and leukocytosis all provide supporting evidence for infection. Gouty arthritis may share some or even all of these clinical features, but it tends to be more abrupt in onset. Inflammation extending beyond the margins of the joint is characteristic of septic arthritis and is otherwise seen only in crystal disease and rheumatoid arthritis. Nonarticular processes may mimic infectious arthritis: cellulitis, septic bursitis, tenosynovitis, and phlebitis. Analysis of synovial fluid is the key to diagnosis.

Acute nerve entrapment or spinal cord compression, tendon rupture, and fractures may all occur in the absence of obvious trauma. Spinal cord compression may be the result of a herniated disc or vertebral subluxation. Tendon rupture may occur in inflammatory arthritis, particularly in the wrist in rheumatoid arthritis. Pelvic and other "insufficiency" fractures may be seen in patients with osteoporosis or osteomalacia. Careful musculoskeletal and neurologic examinations help in the detection of these disorders, each of which requires urgent treatment.

TABLE 78–2 Differentiating Features of Common Arthritides

Disease	Demographics	Joints Involved	Special Features	Laboratory Findings
Gout	Men, postmenopausal women	Monoarticular or oligoarticular	Podagra, rapid onset of attack, polyarticular gout, tophi	SF: crystals, high WBC, >80% PMN
Septic arthritis	Any age	Usually large joints	Fever, chills	SF: high WBC, >90% PMN, culture
Osteoarthritis	Increases with age	Weight-bearing, hands		Noninflammatory SF
Rheumatoid arthritis	Any age, predominantly women ages 20–50 yr	Symmetric, small joints	Rheumatoid nodules, extra-articular disease	SF: high WBC, >70% PMN
Reiter's syndrome	Young males	Oligoarticular, asymmetric	Urethritis, conjunctivitis, skin and mucous membranes	SF: moderate WBC, >50% PMN
Spondyloarthropathy	Young to middle-aged males	Axial skeleton, pelvis (sacroiliac joints)	Uveitis, aortic insufficiency, enthesopathy	
Systemic lupus erythematosus	Females in childbearing years	Hands, knees	Nonerosive joint disease, autoantibodies, multiorgan disease	SF: low-moderate WBC, mostly mononuclear; almost 100% have antinuclear antibodies

PMN = neutrophils; SF = synovial fluid; WBC = white blood cells.

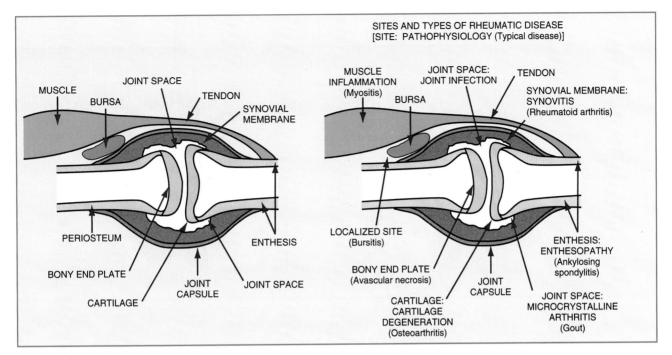

FIGURE 78–1　Anatomic structures of the musculoskeletal system *(left).* Location of musculoskeletal disease processes *(right).* (From Bennett JC, Plum F [eds]: Cecil Textbook of Medicine, 20th ed. Philadelphia: WB Saunders, 1996, p 1440.)

In systemic rheumatic diseases, the onset is usually more insidious, and the clinical course is prolonged. Treatment is usually less urgent and can be safely deferred, particularly if the diagnosis is uncertain. However, in some disorders, potential threats to life or the possibility of serious and/or irreversible organ damage may exist. In SLE and systemic vasculitis, patients may have central or peripheral nervous system disease, including brain and peripheral nerve infarcts, glomerulonephritis, inflammatory or hemorrhagic lung disease, coronary artery involvement, intestinal infarcts, and digital infarcts. Threatened digital loss may also be seen in scleroderma and Raynaud's disease. *Renal crisis* may occur in scleroderma, with vasculopathy leading to renal infarcts, azotemia, microangiopathy, and severe hypertension. Urgent therapy to ameliorate or prevent damage may be indicated in these disorders. In giant cell arteritis, acute blindness is a potential complication, and the diagnosis requires urgent therapy even before confirmatory biopsy. Acute inflammatory myositis should be promptly treated because it may progress rapidly to involvement of respiratory musculature. In some cases, major organ involvement may be occult; when systemic disease is suspected, the patient's lung and kidneys should be carefully evaluated.

Laboratory Testing

As noted earlier, *synovial fluid analysis* is an important part of the evaluation of arthritis (Table 78–3); it helps to distinguish inflammatory from noninflammatory arthritis and can be diagnostic of infectious arthritis or crystal disease. Aspiration and analysis of fluid before therapy are critical to appropriate decision making.

Although autoantibodies are often considered the hallmark of rheumatic diseases, their diagnostic utility in individual patients is actually much less than commonly believed. Although almost 100% of patients with SLE have antinuclear antibodies, as do most patients with scleroderma and autoimmune myositis, the proportion of patients with positive tests in other rheumatic diseases is much lower. Conversely, 15% to 25% of healthy persons have antinuclear antibodies when commercial test kits are used, sometimes in titers as high as 1:320. Elderly persons and patients with nonrheumatic systemic diseases such as malignant disease and nonrheumatic autoimmune disease such as thyroiditis or hypothyroidism have even higher frequencies. Other specific autoantibodies may be more useful and are discussed in subsequent chapters. *Rheumatoid factor* is found in approximately 80% to 90% of patients with rheumatoid arthritis but also in a variety of other rheumatic diseases, in chronic infection, in neoplasia, and in almost any state that can cause chronic hyperglobulinemia. Neither a positive test nor a negative test result is diagnostic, and results should be interpreted only in clinical context.

Tests for acute phase proteins, C-reactive protein, and erythrocyte sedimentation rate are nonspecific, but positive results suggest the presence of inflammatory disease. In some cases, such as in patients with giant cell arteritis and polymyalgia rheumatica, these tests may be useful both in diagnosis and in following the course of disease and therapy. The presence of anemia

TABLE 78-3   Classification of Synovial Effusions by Synovial White Cell Count

Group	Diagnosis (Examples)	Appearance	Synovial Fluid White Cell Count/mm³*	Polymorphonuclear Cells (%)
Normal		Clear, pale yellow	0–200	<10
I. Noninflammatory	Osteoarthritis Trauma	Clear to slightly turbid	50–2000 (600)	<30
II. Mildly inflammatory	Systemic lupus erythematosus	Clear to slightly turbid	100–9000 (3000)	<20
III. Severely inflammatory (noninfectious)	Gout	Turbid	2000–160,000 (21,000)	~70
	Pseudogout	Turbid	500–75,000 (14,000)	~70
	Rheumatoid arthritis	Turbid	2000–80,000 (19,000)	~70
IV. Severely inflammatory (infectious)	Bacterial infections	Very turbid	5000–250,000 (80,000)	~90
	Tuberculosis	Turbid	2500–100,000 (20,000)	~60

*Mean values in parentheses.

may suggest chronic disease or hemolytic anemia; leukopenia, especially lymphopenia, suggests SLE, and thrombocytosis indicates active inflammation. Leukocytosis may also reflect inflammation or infection; corticosteroid therapy also elevates the white blood cell count, often dramatically. Urinalysis should always be performed in patients with systemic disease, and one should look for proteinuria, red blood cells, and casts as evidence of occult renal disease.

Radiographic Studies

Radiographic evaluation often shows changes characteristic of particular diseases. In rheumatoid arthritis, patients have classically erosive disease of the small joints of the wrists, the ulnar styloid, the metacarpophalangeal and proximal interphalangeal joints, and the small joints in the foot. The erosions are bland and nonreactive. In contrast, erosive psoriatic arthritis has sclerotic reaction, and the patient may have characteristic telescoping of joints, so-called *pencil-in-cup lesions*. Large erosions with overhanging sclerotic margins and even juxtaarticular tophi may be seen in gout. In ankylosing spondylitis, sacroiliitis is seen on pelvic films and has high diagnostic specificity; *syndesmophytes* (calcification of the outer rim of the annulus fibrosis), bridging osteophytes, calcification of spinal ligaments, and, in late stages, a typical bamboo spine are seen on lumbar and chest radiographs. Joint space narrowing, bony spurs, and sclerosis are seen in osteoarthritis. *Chondrocalcinosis* is a common finding and may be asymptomatic or may lead to crystal arthritis.

In acute arthritis, radiographs are much less helpful because bony changes take time to develop; only in septic joint disease does one see destruction early. Magnetic resonance imaging is the procedure of choice for evaluating early avascular necrosis of bone, especially the hips, as well as suspected meniscal or rotator cuff disease. Ultrasound may be used to detect synovial cysts, especially Baker's cysts of the knee.

In many instances, diagnosis can be made with certainty only by pathologic examination of tissue. Muscle biopsy may be necessary to establish a diagnosis of inflammatory muscle disease, and nerve biopsy may be needed to detect vasculitis. Skin biopsy may both establish the diagnosis of vasculitis and differentiate among different types. Renal biopsy is often needed for diagnosis as well as for treatment decisions and prognosis.

In summary, the evaluation of arthritis begins with a careful assessment of the location and pattern of joint involvement, the differentiation of inflammatory from mechanical and other causes, and the consideration of nonarticular systemic features. The patient's age and gender, family history, medication history, and the presence of other medical conditions are also important, often key, features. Laboratory and radiographic studies, in particular synovial fluid analysis, provide confirmatory, and sometimes diagnostic, information.

REFERENCES

Felson DT: Epidemiology of the rheumatic diseases. *In* Koopman WJ (ed): Arthritis and Allied Conditions, 13th ed. Baltimore: Williams & Wilkins, 1997, p 3.

Gordon DA: Approach to the patient with musculoskeletal disease. *In* Goldman L, Bennett JC (eds): Cecil Textbook of Medicine, 21st ed. Philadelphia: WB Saunders, 2000, pp 1472–1475.

Sergent JS: Approach to the patient with pain in more than one joint. *In* Kelley WN, Harris ED Jr, Ruddy S, et al (eds): Textbook of Rheumatology, 5th ed. Philadelphia: WB Saunders, 1997, p 381.

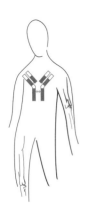

79

RHEUMATOID ARTHRITIS

Joseph H. Korn

Rheumatoid arthritis (RA) is a systemic disease characterized by inflammatory polyarthritis, involving small and large joints, and constitutional features. It is the prototypic inflammatory arthritis with characteristic clinical features such as morning stiffness, improvement of symptoms with activity, and gelling. Most patients have progression to some level of destruction of bone and cartilage as well as involvement of tendon sheaths; in many patients, this process leads to deformity and significant loss of function. Extra-articular manifestations, including vasculitis, are common, may involve almost any organ system, and may be serious.

Epidemiology and Genetics

RA is among the most common autoimmune diseases, with a prevalence of approximately 1% among the general population. Prevalence is similar in the United States, Europe, and Africa but somewhat lower in Asian populations. It has a female-to-male ratio of 3:1, and onset is most common in the third through fifth decades of life. Human leukocyte antigen (HLA)–DR4 is a genetic risk factor, and persons who are DR4-positive appear to have more serious, seropositive (rheumatoid factor–positive) disease. Specific DR4 amino acid sequences in the DR-β molecule antigen binding site are associated with disease susceptibility. The underlying cause of the disease—that is, the trigger in the susceptible host—is unknown.

Pathology

The hallmark of joint involvement is the *synovial pannus,* a proliferative synovium infiltrated with mononuclear cells, particularly monocytes and T lymphocytes. The pannus "invades" at the bone-cartilage-synovial interface with progressive destruction of the bone and cartilage. This process is evident radiographically as marginal bony erosions. In other tissues, as well as in

the synovium, *rheumatoid nodules* may be seen. These are large granulomas with areas of central necrosis, surrounding mononuclear cells, and an outer layer of palisading histiocytes. *Lymphoid aggregates* may be extensive and may assume the appearance of lymphoid follicles.

Pathophysiology

In a joint affected by RA, two related processes are noted (Table 79–1). Symptoms of joint pain and swelling are secondary to an inflammatory process in the synovial space and joint fluid. This inflammation is a result of polymorphonuclear cell chemotaxis and activation, release of prostanoids (prostaglandins and leukotrienes), and concomitant generation of reactive oxygen species, including free radicals, superoxide anion, peroxynitrite, and peroxy and hydroperoxy acids. Polymorphonuclear cell enzymes, including matrix metalloproteinases such as collagenase, stromelysin and gelatinases, and cathepsins promote superficial cartilage erosions. Much more important to the destruction of cartilage and bone is the process occurring in the synovial tissue. There, proliferative synovial cells are activated by lymphocytes and monocytes to (1) elaborate matrix metalloproteinases that directly degrade cartilage and bone matrix and (2) to release proinflammatory prostanoids (Fig. 79–1). The monocyte products interleukin-1 (IL-1) and tumor necrosis factor-α (TNF-α) are central to this process. TNF-α is particularly key in activation of matrix metalloproteinases and IL-1 in stimulating prostaglandin E$_2$ (PGE$_2$). In addition, TNF-α, IL-1, and lymphotoxin are osteoclast-activating factors; osteoclasts are the central cell in resorption of calcified matrix. The activated pannus of proliferating synovial tissue invades the cartilage and bone and behaves like a locally invasive tumor. Other cytokines such as IL-6, induced by IL-1 and TNF-α, as well as IL-1 itself, play a role in the systemic features of disease, including fever, myalgia, weight loss, and induction of acute phase proteins. B cells and plasma cells in the synovium synthesize rheumatoid fac-

TABLE 79–1   Pathogenesis of Rheumatoid Arthritis

Tissue Phase

Immune cell localization to synovial tissue
T- and B-cell and monocyte recruitment
  T-cell activation and proliferation and cytokine release
  B-cell elaboration of rheumatoid factor and other antibodies
  Monocyte elaboration of inflammatory cytokines: IL-1, TNF-α, IL-6
Synovial cell proliferation and activation by IL-1 and TNF-α
  Release of inflammatory eicosanoids (PGE₂)
  Synthesis of collagenase and other matrix metalloproteinases
  Erosions of bone and cartilage
Osteoclast and chondrocyte activation
  Release of proteases
  Resorption of bone and cartilage

Fluid Phase

Immune complexes in synovial fluid
Complement activation and release of C3a, C5a
Neutrophil recruitment and activation
  Release of prostaglandins, leukotrienes, and reactive oxygen species
  Release of lysosomal enzymes
Vasodilatation, development of joint effusions, pain, and swelling
Superficial cartilage erosions

IL-1 = interleukin-1; IL-6 = interleukin-6; PGE₂ = prostaglandin E₂; TNF-α = tumor necrosis factor-α.

tor, an IgM antibody directed to IgG, as well as other antibodies, including antibodies to matrix degradation products. These enter the synovial fluid and, as complexes, play a role in complement activation as well as in polymorphonuclear cell activation and chemotaxis.

Clinical Features

RA is a symmetric polyarthritis involving, typically, the small joints of the hands and feet, the wrists, and the ankles. Other joints frequently involved include the cervical spine, the shoulders, the elbows, the hips, and the knees. Any diarthrodial (synovial) joint may be involved, including the apophyseal, temporomandibular, and cricoarytenoid joints. Involved joints are swollen, warm, and tender, and they may have effusions. The synovium, normally a few cell layers thick, becomes palpable on examination (*synovitis*). Prolonged *morning stiffness*, usually lasting more than 1 hour, and often many hours, is a classic feature in RA as well as in other inflammatory arthropathies. Morning is the worst time of day for patients, and their symptoms are generally improved with moderate activity (Table 79–2).

Over time, RA progresses to joint destruction and deformity. Erosive lesions of bone and cartilage are radiographically and pathologically visible at the margins of bone and cartilage, the site of synovial attachment. *Tenosynovitis*, inflammation of tendon sheaths, leads to tendon malalignment, stretching, and/or shortening. Among common deformities are ulnar deviation at the

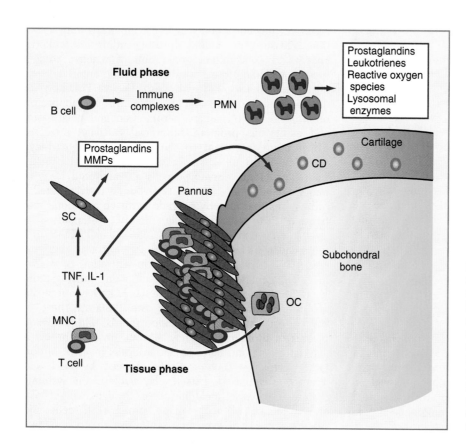

FIGURE 79–1 Pathogenetic events in rheumatoid arthritis. The proliferative synovial pannus invades at the bone-cartilage interface. Interleukin 1 (IL-1) and tumor necrosis factor-α (TNF-α) activate synovial cells (SC) to produce prostaglandins and matrix metalloproteinases (MMPs). In the synovial fluid, polymorphonuclear leukocytes (PMN), activated by immune complexes and complement, produce mediators of inflammation and destruction. CD = chondrocyte; MNC = mononuclear cell; OC = osteoclast.

TABLE 79-2 Clinical Characteristics of Rheumatoid Arthritis

Articular
Morning stiffness, "gelling"
Symmetric joint swelling
Predilection for wrists, proximal interphalangeal, metacarpophalangeal, and metatarsophalangeal joints
Erosions of bone and cartilage
Joint subluxation and ulnar deviation
Inflammatory joint fluid
Carpal tunnel syndrome
Baker's cyst

Nonarticular
Rheumatoid nodules: subcutaneous, pulmonary, scleral
Vasculitis, especially skin, peripheral nerves, and bowel
Pleuropericarditis
Scleritis and episcleritis
Leg ulcers
Felty's syndrome

metacarpophalangeal joints and volar subluxation at these joints, volar subluxation at the wrists, and flexion and extension contractures in the proximal and distal interphalangeal joints of the fingers that lead to characteristic *swan-neck deformity* (flexion contracture at the distal interphalangeal [DIP] joint and hyperextension at the proximal interphalangeal joint) or *boutonnière deformity* (flexion contracture at the proximal interphalangeal joint and hyperextension at the DIP joint). Erosions of the ulnar styloid can lead to sharp bony prominences and rupture of extensor tendons. Synovitis at the wrists can lead to median nerve compression and carpal tunnel syndrome. Cervical spine disease may lead to C1–C2 subluxation and spinal cord compression; caution should be taken in moving the neck when the patient is being anesthetized for a surgical procedure. The degree of subluxation can be monitored by looking at the distance between C1 and the odontoid in flexion-extension films. If spinal cord compression does occur, emergency surgical intervention should be undertaken. Rupture of synovial fluid from the knee into the calf (Baker's cyst) may mimic thrombophlebitis or, occasionally, cellulitis.

The clinical course and severity of the arthritis are variable. Some patients have mild, slowly progressive disease with few deformities and little bony destructive change. At the opposite extreme are patients who have a rapidly progressive course that, untreated, leads to crippling and deforming arthritis. Most patients fall in between, with various levels of disability; some have a waxing and waning course over a period of years with acute episodes of single or multiple joint exacerbations.

RA is a systemic disease with constitutional symptoms: morning stiffness, fatigue, low-grade fever, weight loss, myalgia, and anemia. In addition, specific organs other than the musculoskeletal system may be involved (see Table 79–2). Grossly palpable subcutaneous *rheumatoid nodules* are often seen at the elbow, along other extensor tendon surfaces, and less commonly in the lungs, pleura, pericardium, sclerae, and other sites, including, in rare cases, the heart. The occurrence of

multiple pulmonary nodules in patients with RA and pneumoconiosis is known as *Caplan's syndrome*. Pleuritis, pericarditis, and interstitial lung fibrosis occur in a few patients; pericarditis can be severe and life-threatening, and acute interstitial lung disease can be associated with pulmonary hemorrhage. Vasculitis, associated with circulating complexes of IgG and rheumatoid factor, leads to cutaneous lesions, including ulcers and skin necrosis, mononeuritis multiplex, and intestinal infarction. *Sjögren's syndrome* (sicca complex) is often present. *Felty's syndrome* (splenomegaly, leukopenia, and recurrent pulmonary infections) is a rare complication and is often accompanied by leg ulcers and vasculitis. Even in patients without vasculitis, pulmonary, or pleuropericardial disease, the mortality rate in RA is increased by a variety of causes, including side effects of therapy and infection.

Diagnosis

RA is a clinical diagnosis. Symmetric synovitis of small joints—that is, warm, swollen joints with synovial hypertrophy, morning stiffness, and fatigue—is the classic presenting symptom. About 20% to 30% of patients present with monoarticular disease, usually in the knee. In such patients, the diagnosis cannot be made until the disease evolves. *Systemic lupus erythematosus* can have a similar clinical presentation and may be difficult to differentiate unless other features are present. In rare cases, *Lyme disease* is polyarticular and symmetric in onset. *Viral arthritis* is best distinguished by its limited course. In the older patient, polymyalgia rheumatica, hypothyroidism, and paraneoplastic syndromes, including hypertrophic osteoarthropathy, should be considered.

Examination of joint fluid is the most helpful laboratory procedure. The fluid is inflammatory, with more than 10,000 white blood cells and a predominance of polymorphonuclear leukocytes, typically 80% or more. Rheumatoid factor, an IgM antibody directed to IgG, is found in 80% to 90% of patients with RA. The presence of rheumatoid factor is neither necessary nor sufficient for diagnosis. Other disorders, such as lupus, may be associated with a positive rheumatoid factor, and 10% to 20% of patients with RA are seronegative. Seropositive patients are more likely to have severe erosive disease, to have nodules, and to have other extra-articular features. Antinuclear antibodies are common but not diagnostically helpful.

Treatment

The goals of treatment are to control pain, to preserve maximal function, and to prevent deformity and destruction. *Nonsteroidal anti-inflammatory drugs* (NSAIDs) are useful in controlling pain and inflammation and may thus improve daily function; however, they do not affect the underlying disease process, particularly erosion and joint destruction. These agents function largely by inhibiting prostaglandin synthesis, an effect mediated by inhibiting the enzyme cyclooxygenase (COX). Aspirin and other nonselective NSAIDs such as ibuprofen and indomethacin inhibit both cyclooxygenases, COX-1 and COX-2, whereas the newest selective NSAIDs have marked preferential inhibition of COX-2 (see later discussion).

Anti-inflammatory doses used in RA are substantially greater than analgesic or antipyretic doses, 12 to 16 aspirin/day or 2400 to 3200 mg ibuprofen/day. Although NSAIDs are generally safe, gastrointestinal toxicity, especially bleeding and ulcer perforation, inhibitory effects on platelet function, and decreases in renal blood flow are serious toxicities in some patients. Given the large number of treated patients, even a small proportion amounts to large numbers of serious and even fatal complications of therapy. The foregoing side effects are a direct consequence of inhibition of prostaglandin synthesis. The constitutive production of PGE_2 in the gastric mucosa and in the kidney and of thromboxane A_2 in platelets uses the enzyme COX-1, whereas the cytokine-induced production of PGE_2 in synovial cells and the production of PGE_2 by activated leukocytes use COX-2. As mentioned, the newest NSAIDs have marked selectivity for COX-2 and may thus avoid most of the classic NSAID toxicity.

A second class of drugs has been called *disease-modifying antirheumatic drugs* (DMARDs) or *slow-acting antirheumatic drugs* (SAARDs) (Table 79–3). As the latter name suggests, the effects of these drugs are not manifest until weeks or even months after therapy is initiated. Previously, many of these drugs were given only late in the course of disease and/or only to patients with the most advanced cases. Recognition of the extent

of disability resulting from RA and evidence that many of these agents inhibit the progression of erosive disease have led to earlier and more widespread use of these agents.

Methotrexate, hydroxychloroquine (and chloroquine), gold salts, oral gold, sulfasalazine, azathioprine, D-penicillamine, cyclosporine, and cyclophosphamide are all DMARDs. Methotrexate is probably the most widely used because of high efficacy, relatively low toxicity, ease of administration and, among this group, most rapid onset of action, as early as 4 weeks. This drug has hematologic, pulmonary, and hepatic side effects, the last of which are characterized by a small risk of cirrhosis, as well as a high potential for teratogenicity. Among the oldest of these drugs is gold salts. Given as weekly injections, gold thiomalate or thioglucose is effective in controlling disease in many patients; a few patients go into true and complete remission. However, many patients experience side effects including bone marrow suppression, glomerulonephritis, and rash. Responses are typically seen only after 2 to 6 months of treatment. Oral gold appears less effective and may work by different mechanisms. Hydroxychloroquine is lowest in toxicity but appears also to be less effective for severe disease; it has a slow onset of action. Cyclophosphamide, azathioprine, and cyclosporine are immunosuppressive drugs that are effective agents in treating RA. In addition to the risk of both common and unusual infections, cyclophosphamide carries a risk of bladder and late lymphoid malignant disease; the latter risk may also be present with azathioprine. Combinations of agents may be effective in some patients in whom single agents fail.

Two newer agents have been approved. *Leflunomide* is an inhibitor of pyrimidine biosynthesis. Its toxicity profile and efficacy appear similar to those of methotrexate. *Etanercept* is a soluble TNF-α–receptor–IgG Fc fragment molecule; it inhibits the action of TNF-α and in trials appears exceptionally effective at least in the short term. Some concern exists about potentiated risk for serious infection. Other biologic inhibitors of TNF-α and IL-1 may soon be available, including the IL-1 receptor antagonist, anti–TNF-α antibodies, and other TNF-α receptor preparations; an antibody to TNF is already available for Crohn's disease. In addition, recombinant forms of natural anti-inflammatory cytokines are undergoing clinical trials.

Corticosteroids should be used sparingly, in low doses, and optimally for short periods. Although they are useful for brief exacerbations of the disease, or to bide time while waiting for DMARDs to work, some patients require more prolonged use for control of disease activity. Prednisone, in doses as low as 5 mg/day, has dramatic effects usually within 1 to 2 days. As a consequence, experience has shown that it is much easier to start than to stop taking corticosteroids. The long-term side effects of steroids, particularly in a disease marked by relative immobility, can be devastating and include osteoporosis and pathologic fractures, as well as avascular necrosis of bone. Supplemental calcium, vitamin D, and bisphosphonates should be added in patients who receive long-term therapy. Intra-articular steroids are useful in exacerbations involving only a few

TABLE 79–3 Treatment of Rheumatoid Arthritis

Nonsteroidal Anti-Inflammatory Drugs
Aspirin
Nonacetylated salicylates
Nonsalicylate nonselective prostaglandin inhibitors
Selective cyclooxygenase-2 inhibitors

Slow-Acting Antirheumatic Drugs
Azathioprine
Cyclosporine
D-Penicillamine
Hydroxychloroquine
Injectable gold salts
Leflunomide
Methotrexate
Oral gold
Minocycline
Sulfasalazine

Biologic Agents
Etanercept (soluble TNF-receptor)
Anti-TNF antibody
Interleukin-1 receptor antagonist protein*
Anti-inflammatory cytokines*

*Not approved for RA or in development
TNF = tumor necrosis factor.

joints. Efficacy is high, and these agents have almost no side effects.

Joint replacement surgery plays an important role in patients who have had severe destructive joint disease, particularly in the knee and hip. Early reconstructive surgery in the hand and foot can improve function and sometimes can prevent deformity and tendon rupture.

Physical therapy and *occupational therapy* play an important role in many patients. Physical therapy improves muscle strength and conditioning and maintains joint mobility. Splints for the wrists, used at night, may help to prevent deformity. Various appliances are available that help to protect joints and to make daily activities easier. These range from Velcro "buttons," to special grips for keys and writing implements, to raised chairs and toilet seats.

Prognosis

Available data suggest that 50% of patients are disabled in terms of work within 5 years, and the overall mortality rate is increased, at least in patients with severe RA. Increased mortality is related to infection, pulmonary and renal disease, and gastrointestinal bleeding, some of this no doubt a result of therapeutic interventions. Early and aggressive use of DMARDs has been beneficial, and most patients respond well to therapy. Studies have shown that DMARDs retard the development of erosive joint disease, control symptoms, and improve functional capacity. Some of the newer DMARDs have shown dramatic results, at least in the short term. Whether long-term rates of improvement with these agents, used either alone or as part of combination therapy, will be as impressive is not yet clear.

In summary, considerable strides have been made in understanding the pathogenesis and clinical outcomes of RA. Although the underlying cause of RA is unknown, advances in cell biology, immunology, and molecular biology have led to dramatic alterations in therapies available to treat this disease. Molecular modeling has led to the development of a newer class of COX-2–selective prostaglandin inhibitors. The development of novel effective biologic agents and the earlier introduction of aggressive therapy should prevent joint deformity and destruction and should improve short-term and long-term outcomes. Assessment of efficacy in long-term studies and evaluation of long-term risks and toxicities will determine whether these drugs become the new paradigms for treatment of RA.

REFERENCES

Arnett FC: Rheumatoid arthritis. *In* Goldman L, Bennett JC (eds): Cecil Textbook of Medicine, 21st ed. Philadelphia: WB Saunders, 2000, pp 1492–1499.

Harris ED Jr: Clinical Features of Rheumatoid Arthritis. *In* Kelley WN, Harris ED Jr, Ruddy S, et al (eds): Textbook of Rheumatology, 5th ed. Philadelphia: WB Saunders, 1997, p 898.

Jain R, Lipsky PE: Treatment of rheumatoid arthritis. Med Clin North Am 1997; 81:57.

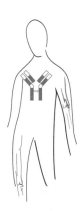

80

SPONDYLOARTHROPATHIES

Peter A. Merkel

The *seronegative spondyloarthropathies* are a related group of inflammatory disorders with clinical features unique among rheumatic diseases. The four types of spondyloarthropathies in adults are ankylosing spondylitis, reactive arthritis (Reiter's disease), enteropathic arthritis (inflammatory bowel disease), and psoriatic arthritis. The peripheral arthropathies associated with either inflammatory bowel disease or psoriasis are not always associated with spondylitis and can also be considered separate entities. In addition is a juvenile form of spondyloarthropathy similar to ankylosing spondylitis that generally persists into adulthood. The cardinal features of the spondyloarthropathies are inflammation of the sacroiliac joints *(sacroiliitis)*, spine *(spondylitis)*, tendon insertion sites *(enthesitis)*, and anterior chamber of the eye *(uveitis)*. Other manifestations are present within each type. Because these diseases are so similar, they are best described first by highlighting the features common to all types of spondyloarthropathy and then by mentioning the unique manifestations of each type.

Epidemiology

Ankylosing spondylitis is much more common among adolescent boys and young men, but this finding may reflect underdiagnosis in women, in whom disease manifestations may be milder than in men. *Reactive arthritis* is more common among men when it follows genitourinary *Chlamydia trachomatis* infection, but the gender distribution is even found among postdysentery cases. *Inflammatory arthritis* including spondylitis affects approximately 5% to 8% of patients with psoriasis and 10% to 25% of patients with ulcerative colitis or Crohn's disease. The gender ratio is also apparent among patients with spondylitis associated with psoriasis and inflammatory bowel disease, in which patients commonly present in young or middle adulthood.

Pathogenesis

Among the most fascinating aspects of the spondyloarthropathies are their strong associations with HLA-B27, a specific allele of the B locus of the human leukocyte antigen (HLA) encoding class I major histocompatibility complex genes. The frequency of HLA-B27 among whites is approximately 6% to 8%. However, up to 90% of white patients with ankylosing spondylitis and 80% of white patients with Reiter's syndrome or juvenile spondyloarthropathy are HLA-B27 positive; these percentages are even higher among those patients with uveitis. The rate of HLA-B27 positivity among patients with inflammatory bowel disease or psoriasis and peripheral arthritis is not increased unless spondylitis is present, in which case the frequency of HLA-B27 is 50%. The frequency of HLA-B27 varies widely among other ethnic groups, but it is associated with spondyloarthropathy in many groups. Furthermore, other major histocompatibility complex antigens have been associated with spondylitis among HLA-B27–negative patients; these class I antigens are cross-reactive with HLA-B27. Rodents transgenic for HLA-B27 develop inflammatory abnormalities strikingly similar to those seen in B27-associated human diseases.

In addition to the strong genetic links to the spondyloarthropathies, important associations exist between specific bacterial agents and disease pathogenesis. Reactive arthritis can be induced by genitourinary infection with *Chlamydia trachomatis* or diarrheal illness with *Shigella, Salmonella, Campylobacter,* and *Yersinia* species, as well as *Klebsiella pneumoniae* infection. These infections appear to trigger an inflammatory response, possibly as a result of persistence of bacterial antigens. However, no one theory of pathogenesis of spondyloarthropathies explains the clinical spectrum of these disorders, and more research is clearly needed to solidify an understanding of their origin.

Clinical Features

COMMON CLINICAL FEATURES AMONG THE SPONDYLOARTHROPATHIES

As mentioned earlier, the spondyloarthropathies have considerable clinical overlap with one another and are most easily considered as a group of related disorders. Table 80–1 outlines the clinical features of these disorders. Because of the delay in presentation of different clinical manifestations of these chronic diseases, the condition in some patients appears to "evolve" from one type of spondyloarthropathy to another. For example, a patient initially diagnosed with ankylosing spondylitis may subsequently develop inflammatory bowel disease or psoriasis. For this reason, clinicians need to be attuned to possible extra-articular manifestations of disease in patients with spondyloarthropathies.

The spondyloarthropathies are not associated with positive tests for rheumatoid factor, antinuclear antibodies, or any other autoimmune serologies. A family history of spondylitis may be present.

Sacroiliitis and *spondylitis* are the hallmarks of the spondyloarthropathies and are not seen in any other rheumatic diseases. Sacroiliitis may present in a subtle fashion with low back or gluteal area pain, but it can also cause severe pain. Patients generally have significant morning stiffness, sometimes of many hours' duration, and pain after periods of inactivity. Sacroiliitis may mimic sciatica with radiating pain into the gluteal and posterior thigh areas. Spondylitis may occur at any area of the spine, but it often progresses first in the lumbar spine and subsequently in the cervical and thoracic regions. The sacroiliac joints and the spine become painful and stiff with increasingly reduced range of motion as bony fusion occurs over time. Involvement of the spine and costovertebral joints may result in restrictive lung physiology. Fusion on the spine increases the risk of vertebral fractures in patients with spondyloarthropathies and, depending on the angle of fusion, may cause significant kyphosis and reduced line of sight. When bony fusion is complete, the pain may be significantly reduced.

Enthesitis may occur in many different anatomic locations. These include spinous processes, costosternal junctions, ischial tuberosities, plantar aponeuroses, and Achilles tendons.

The *peripheral arthritis* of the spondyloarthropathies, when it occurs, begins as an episodic, asymmetric, oligoarticular process often involving the lower extremities. The arthritis can progress and may become chronic and disabling. A unique feature of spondyloarthropathies is the appearance of fusiform swelling of an entire finger or toe, referred to as *dactylitis* or *sausage digits*.

Uveitis, inflammatory disease of the anterior chamber of the eye, is a common extra-articular manifestation of the spondyloarthropathies, especially among HLA-B27–positive patients. Bouts of uveitis are usually monocular, acute in onset, painful, and accompanied by eye redness and blurred vision. Recurrent attacks are common. Uveitis may be serious and may lead to blindness. Anterior uveitis may be the presenting symptom of spondyloarthropathy; thus, all patients with anterior uveitis should be screened for signs and symptoms of these disorders.

Spondyloarthropathies may occasionally involve other organ systems and may cause significant morbidity and mortality. Aortitis, especially occurring in the ascending segment, can result in aortic insufficiency from aortic root dilitation, aortic dissection, and cardiac conduction system abnormalities. Pulmonary fibrosis of the apical regions can occur, often in an insidious fashion. Spinal cord compression can result from atlantoaxial joint subluxation, cauda equina syndrome, or vertebral fractures. In rare cases, long-standing spondyloarthropathy is associated with secondary amyloidosis.

TABLE 80–1   Comparison of the Spondyloarthropathies

	Ankylosing Spondylitis	Posturethral Reactive Arthritis	Postdysenteric Reactive Arthritis	Enteropathic Arthritis	Psoriatic Arthritis
Sacroiliitis	+++++	+++	++	+	++
Spondylitis	++++	+++	++	++	++
Peripheral arthritis	+	++++	++++	+++	++++
Articular course	Chronic	Acute or chronic	Acute > chronic	Acute or chronic	Chronic
HLA-B27	95%	60%	30%	20%	20%
Enthesopathy	++	++++	+++	++	++
Common extra-articular manifestations	Eye Heart	Eye GU Oral/GI Heart	GU Eye	GI Eye	Skin Eye
Other names	Bekhterev's arthritis, Marie-Strümpell disease	Reiter's syndrome, SARA, NGU, chlamydial arthritis	Reiter's syndrome	Crohn's disease, ulcerative colitis	

GI = Gastrointestinal; GU = genitourinary; HLA = human leukocyte antigen; NGU = nongonococcal urethritis; SARA = sexually acquired reactive arthritis.
From Cush JJ, Lipsky PE: The spondyloarthropathies. *In* Goldman L, Bennett JC (eds): Cecil Textbook of Medicine, 21st ed. Philadelphia: WB Saunders, 2000.

SPECIFIC CLINICAL FEATURES OF THE SPONDYLOARTHROPATHIES

Reactive (Reiter's) Arthritis

Among the unique clinical features of reactive (Reiter's) arthritis are *urethritis*, *conjunctivitis*, and certain dermatologic problems. The urethritis may be secondary to the chlamydial infection that triggers the disease, or it may be a sterile inflammatory discharge also seen in diarrhea-associated disease. Conjunctivitis may be mild in reactive arthritis and is distinct from uveitis. *Keratoderma blennorrhagicum* is a distinct papulosquamous rash usual found on the palms or soles. *Circinate balanitis* is a rash that may appear on the penile glans or shaft of men with reactive arthritis. Nonpitting *nail thickening* as well as *oral ulcers* may also occur in patients with reactive arthritis. These lesions can be confused with similar findings in patients with psoriasis and inflammatory bowel disease, respectively.

Psoriatic Arthritis

Five identifiable clinical patterns of psoriatic arthritis are recognized: (1) *distal interphalangeal joint involvement with nail pitting;* (2) *asymmetric oligoarthropathy* of both large and small joints; (3) *arthritis mutilans,* severe, destructive arthritis; (4) *symmetric polyarthritis,* identical to rheumatoid arthritis; and (5) *spondyloarthropathy.* These patterns are not exclusionary, and clinical overlap is significant. Spondylitis or sacroiliitis may occur along with any of the other four patterns. The prevalence of HLA-B27 is increased among the patients with spondylitis or sacroiliitis, but not among patients with the other patterns. Little or no temporal association exists between the skin disease and the arthritis in psoriasis, and either can precede the other by many years.

Enteropathic Arthritis (Inflammatory Bowel Disease)

The inflammatory bowel diseases, Crohn's disease and ulcerative colitis (see also Chapter 36), are frequently associated with both spondyloarthropathy and peripheral arthritis. The peripheral arthritis is typically nonerosive and oligoarticular.

Radiographic Features

The radiographic features of the spondyloarthropathies are highly specific and, in the correct clinical setting, virtually diagnostic of these diseases. These changes progress over many years of illness. Sacroiliitis is usually the earliest radiographic sign of the spondyloarthropathies and results in sclerosis and erosions of the sacroiliac joints with eventual bony fusion (Fig. 80–1A). Bony erosions and osteitis may occur at sites of enthesitis. Many different radiographic changes occur secondary to chronic spinal inflammation, including ossification of the annulus fibrosus, calcification of spinal ligaments, bony sclerosis and "squaring" of vertebral bodies, and ankylosis of apophyseal joints. These changes can lead to ver-

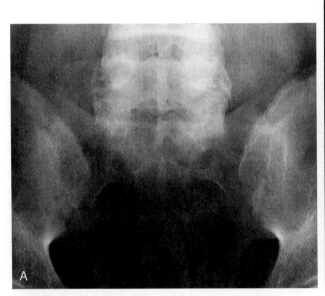
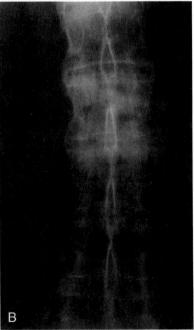

FIGURE 80–1 *A,* Bilaterally symmetric sacroiliitis in ankylosing spondylitis. *B,* Lumbar spondylitis in ankylosing spondylitis with symmetric, marginal bridging syndesmophytes and calcification of the spinal ligament. (From Cush JJ, Lipsky PE: The spondyloarthropathies. *In* Goldman L, Bennett JC [eds]: Cecil Textbook of Medicine, 21st ed. Philadelphia: WB Saunders, 2000, pp 1499–1507.)

tebral fusion and a *bamboo spine* appearance (Fig. 80–1*B*).

Treatment

No cure has yet been found for any of the spondyloarthropathies, but effective treatment for many of the manifestations is available. *Patient education* regarding their disease is essential and allows for identification of affected family members and earlier presentation of urgent clinical features, such as uveitis. *Physical therapy* including a daily stretching program, postural adjustments, and strengthening can be useful in maintaining proper bony alignment, in reducing deformities, and in maximizing function. Selective use of *orthopedic surgery* may be highly effective in correcting significant spinal deformities or instability.

The most important medical therapy for patients with symptomatic spondylitis and sacroiliitis consists of *nonsteroidal anti-inflammatory drugs* (NSAIDs). NSAIDs can provide significant relief of spinal pain and stiffness, and many patients take these drugs continuously for years. No clear evidence indicates that systemic glucocorticoids benefit patients with spondyloarthropathies, and these agents are generally avoided. *Intra-articular glucocorticoid injection* into sacroiliac or other involved joints may provide temporary relief. Similarly, the role and efficacy of immunosuppressive agents in the treatment of the axial manifestations of the spondyloarthropathies have not been established. In contrast, the peripheral arthritis of spondyloarthropathies has been shown in clinical trials to improve with *sulfasalazine*. *Methotrexate* is also regularly used for the peripheral arthritis, but no large clinical trials have been performed with this agent in these diseases.

Flares of *uveitis* require care by an ophthalmologist experienced in treating inflammatory eye diseases. Topical or intraocular glucocorticoids may suffice, but systemic therapy with glucocorticoids or immunosuppressive medications may be necessary to control the inflammation and to prevent permanent visual loss.

Specific types of spondyloarthropathy may require different therapies, including that for the underlying associated disease. Evaluation and treatment for *Chlamydia trachomatis* and associated sexually transmitted diseases in patients with reactive arthritis and their sex partners are essential. Aggressive medical therapy for the more disabling and destructive forms of psoriatic arthritis is often prescribed in a manner similar to that used for patients with rheumatoid arthritis. Immunosuppressive therapy for the skin disease may also help the arthritis of patients with psoriasis. Treatments for the gastrointestinal manifestations of inflammatory bowel disease may also be beneficial for the rheumatic symptoms.

REFERENCES

Arnett FC: Seronegative spondyloarthropathies: B. Reactive arthritis (Reiter's syndrome) and enteropathic arthritis. *In* Klippel JH (ed): Primer of the Rheumatic Diseases, 11th ed. Atlanta: Arthritis Foundation, 1997, pp 184–188.

Boumpas DT, Tassiulas IO: Psoriatic arthritis. *In* Klippel JH (ed): Primer of the Rheumatic Diseases, 11th ed. Atlanta: Arthritis Foundation, 1997, pp 175–179.

Cush JJ, Lipsky PE: The spondyloarthropathies. *In* Goldman L, Bennett JC (eds): Cecil Textbook of Medicine, 21st ed. Philadelphia: WB Saunders, 2000, pp 1499–1507.

Inman RD: Seronegative spondyloarthropathies: D. Treatment. *In* Klippel JH (ed): Primer of the Rheumatic Diseases, 11th ed. Atlanta: Arthritis Foundation, 1997, pp 193–195.

Khan MA: Seronegative spondyloarthropathies: C. Ankylosing spondylitis. *In* Klippel JH (ed): Primer of the Rheumatic Diseases, 11th ed. Atlanta: Arthritis Foundation, 1997, pp 189–193.

Taurag JD: Seronegative spondyloarthropathies: A. Epidemiology, pathology, and pathogenesis. *In* Klippel JH (ed): Primer of the Rheumatic Diseases, 11th ed. Atlanta: Arthritis Foundation, 1997, pp 180–183.

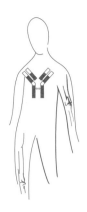

81

SYSTEMIC LUPUS ERYTHEMATOSUS

Peter A. Merkel

Systemic lupus erythematosus (SLE, lupus) is a multisystem autoimmune disorder of unknown cause and is strongly associated with various autoantibodies. The clinical course of SLE is characterized by periods of both active disease and remission, with manifestations ranging from mild dermatologic and joint symptoms to life-threatening internal organ failure and cytopenias. The diagnosis is based on a combination of clinical and laboratory findings, and certain clinical subsets have been identified.

SLE can occur at any age, including in children and the elderly, can strike both genders, and is found in all ethnic and racial groups. However, it is much more common among women and is both more common and often more severe among blacks and Hispanics. The most common age at first presentation is in the second, third, or fourth decade.

Pathogenesis

Although the origin of SLE is not yet known, increasing evidence indicates that it is caused, or at least influenced, by a combination of genetic, immunologic, hormonal, and possibly environmental factors. Both large population studies and animal models of SLE have increased the understanding of disease pathogenesis. The genetic contribution to SLE has been demonstrated in studies of specific ethnicities, families, twin cohorts, and other groups. Certain genes related to the human leukocyte antigen system, various other immune markers, and specific proteins have all been considered possible candidate genes associated with SLE. Many different immune abnormalities have been noted in patients with SLE, a finding implicating dysregulation of both the humoral and cellular immune systems in the pathogenesis of the disease. The established roles of immune complex formation and abnormalities in the complement system in certain manifestations of SLE also support an immunologic origin for SLE. Hormonal influences on SLE are indicated by the striking differences in disease prevalence between men and women, as well as the variances in disease activity with pregnancy and other physiologic states of sex hormonal changes. Finally, various environmental agents, including microorganisms, are suspected of influencing lupus activity and possibly explaining observed geographic clustering of cases.

Clinical Manifestations

Virtually any organ system may be involved in SLE, often in multiple ways. Table 81–1 outlines many, but not all, of the clinical manifestations of SLE. The prognosis for patients with SLE ranges from chronic, smoldering disease with relatively minor problems to rapidly progressive, life-threatening illness and early mortality. Among the manifestations that result in critical illness in patients with SLE are lupus nephritis, lupus cerebritis, pulmonary hemorrhage, and small vessel vasculitis of major organs such as the mesentery or brain. *Lupus nephritis* refers to a spectrum of glomerulopathies that range from minor focal scarring to diffuse proliferative destruction of glomeruli with active inflammation and immune complex deposition. Both the renal disorder and the clinical syndromes are usually classified according to the World Health Organization classification system for renal disease in SLE. This system includes six classes of disorder ranging from normal tissue (class I) to advanced sclerosing glomerulonephritis (class VI). Class V refers to diffuse membranous glomerulopathy, a distinct nephritic syndrome that can be present either in isolation or in conjunction with the other classes. *Lupus cerebritis* is a vague term encompassing a variety of central neurologic deficits, including psychosis, seizures, or coma. The more subtle cognitive and psychological manifestations of SLE are areas of active current clinical research and should not be overlooked when physicians

TABLE 81-1 Clinical Manifestations of Systemic Lupus Erythematosus

Systemic and Miscellaneous	**Hematologic**
Fever	Hemolytic anemia*
Malaise/fatigue	Nonhemolytic anemia
Lymphadenopathy	Leukopenia*
Recurrent spontaneous abor-	Lymphopenia*
tions	Thrombocytopenia*
Premature fetal delivery	**Musculoskeletal**
Vascular	Arthritis*
Raynaud's phenomenon	Arthralgias
Arterial or venous thrombosis	Avascular necrosis
Vasculitis (almost any loca-	Myositis
tion)	**Neurologic**
Livedo reticularis	Psychosis*
Dermatologic	Seizures*
Malar (butterfly) rash*	Depression
Discoid lesions*	Cognitive impairment
Photosensitivity*	Headache
Oral, genital, nasal ulcers*	Cerebritis
Maculopapular rash	Transverse myelitis
Panniculitis	Peripheral neuropathy
Alopecia	Episcleritis or scleritis
Subacute cutaneous lupus	**Cardiac**
Urticaria	Pericarditis*
Renal	Myositis
Cellular casts or glomerulone-	Libman-Sacks endocarditis
phritis*	**Pulmonary**
Proteinuria or membranous	Pleuritis*
nephropathy or nephrotic	Alveolar hemorrhage
syndrome*	Pulmonary hypertension
Gastrointestinal	Shrinking lung syndrome
Pancreatitis	Interstitial lung disease
Lupus enteropathy	Pulmonary emboli
Peritoneal serositis	
Hepatitis/hepatomegaly	
Serologic Abnormalities	
Autoantibodies*	
Hypocomplementemia	
Elevated acute phase reac-	
tants	

*An item in the American College of Rheumatology diagnostic criteria.

treat patients. Lupus nephritis, cerebritis, and vasculitis can all develop insidiously and may be in advanced stages by the time they become clinically apparent. *Pulmonary hemorrhage* is a rare and potentially catastrophic manifestation of SLE that may result in fulminant hemoptysis and respiratory failure. The *arthritis* of lupus is usually nonerosive, but it can result in significant joint laxity and disability. The *skin manifestations* of SLE are protean and can cause permanent scarring and disfigurement that can be personally devastating to patients. Common cutaneous features of SLE include the classic malar *(butterfly)* rash, discoid lesions, alopecia, photosensitivity, and urticaria.

Pregnancy presents unique problems for patients with SLE. Women with SLE may have severe disease flares during pregnancy. Similarly, underlying organ damage or medications for SLE can cause or worsen maternal pregnancy-related complications. The rate of spontaneous abortions and fetal prematurity is significantly higher among pregnant women with SLE, and many of these miscarriages are associated with antiphospholipid antibodies (see Chapter 82).

Various *autoantibodies* are found in patients with SLE and are the hallmark laboratory features of the disease. Table 81-2 outlines many of the autoantibodies found in SLE. Virtually all patients with SLE (99%) test positive for antinuclear antibodies when a sensitive assay is used. Although many of the specific antigens to which these antinuclear antibodies are directed have been determined, and are useful both diagnostically and clinically in SLE, some antibodies are also seen in other autoimmune diseases. Antibodies to double-stranded DNA and the Smith (Sm) antigen are highly specific for lupus, whereas antibodies to Ro and La antigens are also commonly found in patients with rheumatoid arthritis and are especially common in patients with Sjögren's syndrome. Certain antibodies are associated with specific clinical manifestations of disease. For example, many patients with lupus nephritis have anti–double-stranded DNA antibodies. The relationship between antibodies to ribosomal P or neuronal antigens and lupus cerebritis is still under investigation. Autoantibodies alone are not diagnostic for any autoimmune disease but must be interpreted in the clinical context.

SLE is a clinical diagnosis; no one test or feature is fully diagnostic of the disease. Furthermore, many patients' clinical syndromes "evolve" over time, and only after several years are they recognized as having SLE. To classify patients with SLE more accurately and reproducibly for research purposes, an internationally accepted set of diagnostic criteria was developed (Table 81-3). By design, the diagnostic specificity of these criteria is high, to ensure that all subjects enrolled in research studies truly have SLE. However, although these criteria are valuable for practicing clinicians, patients may have clinical lupus without meeting the criteria. More than half of the manifestations listed in Table 81-1 are not part of the criteria.

Patients with SLE may manifest all the features of the *antiphospholipid antibody syndrome*, including multiple thromboses, thrombocytopenia, and recurrent spontaneous miscarriages. See Chapter 82 for details on the antiphospholipid antibody syndrome.

Patients with SLE may also have *secondary Sjögren's syndrome* and may have xerophthalmia, xerosis, and other clinical features of this disease. See Chapter 85 for details on Sjögren's syndrome.

Clinical Subsets

OVERLAP SYNDROME

Some patients with symptoms consistent with autoimmune disease do not readily fit one diagnosis and have clinical and laboratory features of two or more specific diseases such as SLE, rheumatoid arthritis, Sjögren's

TABLE 81–2 **Autoantibodies in Patients with Systemic Lupus Erythematosus (SLE)***

Test	Sensitivity (%)	Specificity (%)	Predictive Value (%)
ANA	99	80	15–35
dsDNA	70	95	95
ssDNA	80	50	50
Histone	30–80	Moderate	Moderate
Nucleoprotein	58	Moderate	Moderate
Sm	25	99	97
RNP (U1-RNP)	50	87–94	46–85
Ro (SS-A)	25–35		
La (SS-B)	15		
PCNA	5	95	95

*Cytoplasm: mitochondria, lysosomes, microsomes, ribosomes. RNA: dsRNA, ssRNA, rRNA. Cell membranes: red blood cells, white blood (T and B) cells, platelets, brain. Other: clotting factors (APL), thyroid, rheumatoid factors, BFP-STS. In SLE, anti-DNA and anti-Sm are associated with renal disease, anti-RNP with Raynaud's, and anti-Ro with photosensitivity. Anti-RNP is seen in SLE, rheumatoid arthritis, scleroderma, Sjögren's syndrome, and mixed connective tissue disorders. Anti-Ro (SS-A) is seen in SLE, Sjögren's syndrome, primary photosensitivity, and primary biliary cirrhosis. Anti-La (SS-B) is seen in SLE and Sjögren's syndrome.
ANA = antinuclear antibodies; PCNA = proliferating cell nuclear antigen; RNP = ribonuclear protein.
From Schur PH: System lupus erythematosus. *In* Bennett JC, Plum F (eds): Cecil Textbook of Medicine, 21st ed. Philadelphia: WB Saunders, 2000, p 1511.

syndrome, or scleroderma. Such patients may be considered to have an *overlap syndrome.* Patients with overlap disease are often followed for development of new features of the "parent" disorders.

DRUG-INDUCED LUPUS ERYTHEMATOSUS

Certain medications may induce a lupus-like syndrome referred to as *drug-induced lupus erythematosus (DILE).* DILE is generally a milder form of SLE with arthritis, serositis, and constitutional symptoms common, whereas renal or central nervous system involvement is rare. The most common and well-studied medications associated with DILE are procainamide and hydralazine, but many other drugs have been implicated, including anticonvulsants, β blockers, and antimicrobials; new drugs continue to be implicated in DILE. Although these drugs may induce antinuclear antibodies in some patients, only a subset of those patients will actually develop clinical DILE. Although antibodies to histones are found in up to 90% of patients with DILE, only rarely are patients found to have antibodies to double-stranded DNA or other lupus-related antigens. DILE is reversible on drug discontinuation.

NEONATAL LUPUS ERYTHEMATOSUS

Neonatal lupus erythematosus is a rare disorder that exclusively affects some children born to mothers with maternal anti-Ro or anti-La antibodies. These antibodies pass through the placenta and are involved in disease causation. Manifestations include transient rashes, thrombocytopenia, hemolytic anemia, and, the most serious problem, permanent complete heart block. Although the dermatologic and hematologic problems are transient and readily treatable, the conduction system abnormalities are often permanent and are associated with high intrauterine and peripartum mortality. Fewer than 5% of children born to Ro-positive and/or La-positive women will have neonatal lupus erythematosus. The mothers of affected children do not necessarily have SLE or another autoimmune disease themselves. However, some of these women who have no obvious signs or symptoms of SLE present years later with a more definable autoimmune disease.

Treatment

No cure for lupus has yet been found, and treatment is aimed at reducing inflammation, suppressing the immune system, and closely following patients clinically to identify disease features as early as possible. Treatment with glucocorticoids and immunosuppressive agents has reduced both the morbidity and the mortality of patients with SLE, although these treatments themselves are associated with extensive toxicity. Many cases of SLE are mild and remain so for the life of the patient. Thus, the physician must weigh carefully the benefits of therapy against the known risks of treatment, especially long-term therapy.

Patient education and *prophylactic measures* to prevent disease flares are central to the care of patients with lupus. Sunscreens and protective clothing are effective in avoiding photosensitivity reactions. The use of estrogen-containing oral contraceptives is controversial in SLE, but many centers avoid these medications because of evidence that they are associated with an increase in lupus activity. The use of low-dose estrogen replacement therapy for postmenopausal women with SLE is not controversial and is encouraged to protect

TABLE 81–3   Criteria for Classification of Systemic Lupus Erythematosus*

Criterion	Definition
1. Malar rash	Fixed erythema, flat or raised, over the malar eminences, tending to spare the nasolabial folds
2. Discoid rash	Erythematous raised patches with adherent keratotic scaling and follicular plugging; atrophic scarring may occur in older lesions
3. Photosensitivity	Skin rash as a result of unusual reaction to sunlight by patient history or physician observation
4. Oral ulcers	Oral or nasopharyngeal ulceration, usually painless, observed by a physician
5. Arthritis	Nonerosive arthritis involving two or more peripheral joints, characterized by tenderness, swelling, or effusion
6. Serositis	a. Pleuritis: convincing history of pleuritic pain or rub heard by a physician or evidence of pleural effusion OR b. Pericarditis: documented by electrocardiogram or rub or evidence of pericardial effusion
7. Renal disorder	a. Persistent proteinuria >0.5 g/day or >3+ if quantitation not performed OR b. Cellular casts: may be red cell, hemoglobin, granular, tubular, or mixed
8. Neurologic disorder	a. Seizures: in the absence of offending drugs or known metabolic derangements, e.g., uremia, ketoacidosis, or electrolyte imbalance OR b. Psychosis: in the absence of offending drugs or known metabolic derangements, e.g., uremia, ketoacidosis, or electrolyte imbalance
9. Hematologic disorder	a. Hemolytic anemia: with reticulocytosis OR b. Leukopenia: <4000/mm³ total on two or more occasions c. Lymphopenia: <1500/mm³ on two or more occasions OR d. Thrombocytopenia: <100,000/mm³ in the absence of offending drugs
10. Immunologic disorder	a. Anti-DNA: antibody to native DNA in abnormal titer OR b. Anti-Sm: presence of antibody to Sm nuclear antigen OR c. Positive finding of antiphospholipid antibodies based on (1) an abnormal serum level of IgG or IgM anticardiolipin antibodies, (2) a positive test result for lupus anticoagulant using a standard method, or (3) a false-positive serologic test for syphilis known to be positive for at least 6 months and confirmed by *Treponema pallidum* immobilization or fluorescent treponemal antibody absorption test
11. Antinuclear antibody	An abnormal titer of antinuclear antibody by immunofluorescence or an equivalent assay at any point in time and in the absence of drugs known to be associated with "drug-induced lupus" syndrome

*The classification is based on 11 criteria. For the purpose of identifying patients in clinical studies, a person shall be said to have systemic lupus erythematosus if any 4 or more of the 11 criteria are present, serially or simultaneously, during any interval of observation.

Adapted from Schur PH: Systemic lupus erythematosus. *In* Bennett JC, Plum F (eds): Cecil Textbook of Medicine, 20th ed. Philadelphia: WB Saunders, 1996; and Hochberg MC for the Diagnostic and Therapeutic Criteria Committee of the American College of Rheumatology: Updating the American College of Rheumatology Revised Criteria for the Classification of Systemic Lupus Erythematosus. Arthritis Rheum 1997; 40:1725.

patients from osteoporosis and possibly heart disease. Protective or warm clothing and avoidance of vasoconstrictive drugs are helpful in treating Raynaud's phenomenon in SLE, and these patients may also benefit from vasodilator therapy. Psychological support is essential for patients with SLE because this chronic disease may cause depression and anxiety in many patients. Routine immunizations, such as for influenza and pneumococcus, are recommended in all patients.

Although nonsteroidal anti-inflammatory medications

are used for mild arthralgias, *glucocorticoids* remain the main anti-inflammatory agents for SLE. Glucocorticoids are used for almost all manifestations of lupus in doses ranging from extremely small alternate-day doses to huge pulsed intravenous doses. Although glucocorticoids are often effective for lupus, the chronic nature of the disease may lead to prolonged use of these medications and extensive toxicity, including obesity, diabetes mellitus, accelerated atherosclerosis, osteoporosis, avascular necrosis, cataracts, glaucoma, and increased risk of infections. To avoid such toxicities, different immunomodulating agents are used to provide a steroid-sparing effect. In addition, some manifestations, such as nephritis and severe vasculitis, are only partially responsive to glucocorticoids and require other immunosuppressive agents for greater disease control.

Antimalarial medications have been found to be effective agents in SLE and are an important part of treatment for many patients. Hydroxychloroquine and chloroquine are especially effective for the fevers, arthritis, and mucocutaneous manifestations of SLE. Many patients take one of these drugs on a long-term basis because investigators have demonstrated that patients who discontinue the medications, even if they are asymptomatic at the time, experience significantly more flares than patients who continue the medications. Although retinal toxicity is not common, it is dose dependent; the extent of routine ophthalmologic screening required for patients taking these drugs is controversial, but it is at most biannually.

Azathioprine is an immunosuppressive agent prescribed in patients with lupus either when glucocorticoids alone are not fully effective or to allow for a reduction in glucocorticoid dosage. Toxicities of azathioprine include leukopenia, anemia, and an increased risk of infection. An area of ongoing controversy is whether prolonged use of this drug poses an increased risk of hematologic malignant disease.

Cyclophosphamide is the most potent immunosuppressive agent used to treat SLE. However, because this drug is extremely toxic, especially with long-term use, it is usually reserved for the most severe disease manifestations of lupus. In a series of studies, mostly conducted at the National Institutes of Health, cyclophosphamide by monthly intravenous administration was effective in reducing the rate of progression of lupus nephritis to end-stage renal disease. Patients with severe lupus cerebritis or small vessel necrotizing vasculitis are often treated with cyclophosphamide, although extensive trials or even case series demonstrating the efficacy of this approach are lacking. Acute toxicities of cyclophosphamide include pancytopenia, alopecia, mucositis, and hemorrhagic cystitis. Long-term use of cyclophosphamide may lead to transitional cell carcinoma, hematologic malignant disease, sterility, premature menopause, and opportunistic infections.

Many other treatments have been suggested for SLE, most of which try to manipulate the immune response in some manner. *Intravenous immunoglobulin* is effective for the thrombocytopenia of SLE but is less well established for other indications. Trials of *plasmapheresis* in lupus nephritis have failed to demonstrate any efficacy, although this therapy continues to be studied for this indication. *Methotrexate* is increasingly prescribed for patients with lupus, especially for treatment of arthritis, although no clinical trials have been performed for this medication in SLE. Investigators have shown long-standing interest in hormonal therapy for SLE, but no consistent effect of such agents has been demonstrated. Great potential and optimism exist for "biologic" immunomodulating agents produced by the biotechnology industry to provide new, effective treatments for SLE.

REFERENCES

Gladman DD, Urowitz MB: Systemic lupus erythematosus: B. Clinical and laboratory features. *In* Klippel JH (ed): Primer of the Rheumatic Diseases, 11th ed. Atlanta: Arthritis Foundation, 1997, pp 251–257.

Hochberg MC for the Diagnostic and Therapeutic Criteria Committee of the American College of Rheumatology: Updating the American College of Rheumatology Revised Criteria for the Classification of Systemic Lupus Erythematosus. Arthritis Rheum 1997; 40:1725.

Klippel JH: Systemic lupus erythematosus: C. Treatment. *In* Klippel JH (ed): Primer of the Rheumatic Diseases, 11th ed. Atlanta: Arthritis Foundation, 1997, pp 258–262.

Pisetsky DS: Systemic lupus erythematosus: A. Epidemiology, pathology, and pathogenesis. *In* Klippel JH (ed): Primer of the Rheumatic Diseases, 11th ed. Atlanta: Arthritis Foundation, 1997, pp 246–251.

Schur PH: Systemic lupus erythematosus. *In* Goldman L, Bennett JC (eds): Cecil Textbook of Medicine, 21st ed. Philadelphia: WB Saunders, 2000, pp 1509–1517.

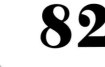

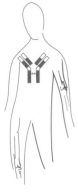

ANTIPHOSPHOLIPID ANTIBODY SYNDROME

Peter A. Merkel

Antiphospholipid antibody syndrome (APS) is a disorder characterized by any or all of the following three manifestations in the setting of positive tests for antiphospholipid antibodies: (1) recurrent arterial and/or venous thromboses, (2) thrombocytopenia, or (3) recurrent spontaneous abortions. Because APS is a relatively newly described syndrome, the full clinical spectrum is still being defined, and well-accepted diagnostic criteria do not yet exist.

APS is considered *secondary* if it occurs in conjunction with systemic lupus erythematosus (SLE) or another autoimmune disease and *primary* if it occurs in isolation. The discovery of *antiphospholipid antibodies* and of their clinical associations has improved the understanding of the clinical spectrum of SLE because each manifestation of APS can be seen in SLE (see also Chapter 81). The false-positive test results for syphilis found in many patients with SLE are actually caused by antiphospholipid antibodies. In recognition of the importance of these antibodies, the American College of Rheumatology revised the diagnostic criteria for SLE in 1997 to include antiphospholipid antibodies.

Etiology

Animal studies suggest that antiphospholipid antibodies are directly pathogenic, but the exact mechanism of action is not known. The likely existence of other cofactors for the development of APS could explain why only a subset of people who produce antiphospholipid antibodies goes on to present with manifestations of APS. Among the more thoroughly studied cofactors for APS is β_2-glycoprotein.

Clinical Features

The clinical features of APS are outlined in Table 82–1. The list of clinical associations with APS continues to grow, but only the original three cardinal manifestations of thrombosis, thrombocytopenia, and recurrent spontaneous abortions are universally accepted as part of APS. The association of APS with SLE and the varied sequelae of arterial thromboses, such as strokes, make the assignment of disorders to APS difficult. The term *catastrophic APS* has been coined to describe patients who present with multiple thromboses, positive antiphospholipid antibodies, and often life-threatening illness.

Diagnosis

The diagnosis of APS is made by combining clinical features with laboratory evidence of antiphospholipid antibodies. No internationally accepted diagnostic criteria exist for APS; however, most authorities agree that the diagnosis should not be made unless at least one of the major features of APS is present, the patient repeatedly tests positive for either anticardiolipin antibodies or the lupus anticoagulant, and alternative diagnoses have been eliminated. Patients with APS should be screened for possible concomitant SLE or other autoimmune diseases.

Laboratory testing for antiphospholipid antibodies is complex and can be confusing or misunderstood. Although several types of antiphospholipid antibodies are recognized, the two that are used clinically to establish the diagnosis are *anticardiolipin antibodies* and the *lu-*

TABLE 82–1 Clinical Features of Antiphospholipid Antibody Syndrome

Definite Features
Arterial thrombosis
Venous thrombosis
Thrombocytopenia
Recurrent pregnancy loss
Possible Features
Hemolytic anemia
Livedo reticularis
Leg ulcers
Chorea
Transverse myelitis
Vasculitis
Cardiac valvular abnormalities

pus anticoagulant. The lupus anticoagulant is a misnomer that reflects the early observation that it can result in a prolonged partial thromboplastin time. Various methods are used to test for the lupus anticoagulant. The partial thromboplastin time test is *not* a screening test for the lupus anticoagulant. When patients are screened for APS, they should be tested for both anticardiolipin antibodies and the lupus anticoagulant. Furthermore, patients with APS should demonstrate repeatedly positive results for these tests.

Treatment

Currently, neither a cure for APS nor a single treatment for all its manifestations exists. Rather, treatment is specific to each aspect of APS. For patients with demonstrated hypercoagulability, indefinite anticoagulation is usually prescribed as prophylaxis against recurrence. Warfarin is the usual drug of choice, with the international normalized ratio (INR) often kept in the upper range for anticoagulation (i.e., INR = 3.0 to 4.5). Heparin is also an effective anticoagulant for patients with APS.

The thrombocytopenia of APS often does not need treatment, but it usually responds to glucocorticoids. Intravenous immunoglobulin, danazol, splenectomy, and immunosuppressive agents have also been used for this indication. The approach to treatment of thrombocytopenia in APS is similar to that of idiopathic thrombocytopenic purpura.

The rate of recurrent pregnancy loss in APS has been shown to be markedly reduced after treatment with low-dose aspirin in combination with either heparin or glucocorticoids, with heparin usually the favored option. Although immunosuppression with cyclophosphamide and plasmapheresis has been used for thrombosis in APS and in catastrophic APS, no consensus exists on the utility of such regimens.

REFERENCES

Harris EN: Antiphospholipid syndrome. *In* Klippel JH (ed): Primer of the Rheumatic Diseases, 11th ed. Atlanta: Arthritis Foundation, 1997, pp 313–315.

Hochberg MC for the Diagnostic and Therapeutic Criteria Committee of the American College of Rheumatology: Updating the American College of Rheumatology Revised Criteria for the Classification of Systemic Lupus Erythematosus. Arthritis Rheum 1997; 40: 1725.

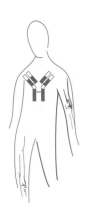

83

SYSTEMIC SCLEROSIS (SCLERODERMA)

Joseph H. Korn

Systemic sclerosis (SSc) is a disease characterized by cutaneous and visceral fibrosis, vascular dysfunction, most prominently Raynaud's phenomenon, and immune activation. The term *scleroderma* (thick skin) highlights the most obvious feature of the disorder and is often used synonymously. However, although cutaneous changes can be widespread and disabling, visceral and vascular manifestations are, in most cases, more serious and are the major cause of mortality. These features include inflammatory interstitial lung disease leading to fibrosis, myocardial fibrosis and conduction abnormalities, pulmonary hypertension, renovascular disease, intestinal hypomotility and severe gastroesophageal reflux, and digital ischemia, infection, and infarction.

Epidemiology and Genetics

SSc has an annual incidence of 10 to 20 per million and a prevalence that is approximately 10-fold greater. The disease is three- to fourfold more common in women. Onset before the third decade is unusual, and incidence rises slowly through the fourth through seventh decades of life. Familial occurrence is unusual, and twin studies suggest a mixture of genetic and environmental factors. However, multiple different autoimmune rheumatic diseases may occur in the same family, such as an index case with SSc, a mother with systemic lupus erythematosus (SLE), and an aunt with rheumatoid arthritis.

Pathology and Pathophysiology

The pathogenesis of scleroderma has three noteworthy aspects: (1) a metabolic defect in fibroblast metabolism leading to overproduction of collagen and other matrix proteins, (2) vascular injury and obliteration, and (3) immune cell activation and autoimmunity (Fig. 83-1). Pathologic examination reflects these processes. In the skin, one sees a marked increase in connective tissue matrix with replacement of subcutaneous fat and secondary skin appendages such as hair follicles and sweat and sebaceous glands. The patient has infiltrates of activated mononuclear cells, T lymphocytes, and monocytes in the dermis. Blood vessels in the skin, kidney, heart, and elsewhere demonstrate endothelial cell and smooth muscle cell proliferation leading to intimal occlusion, medial thinning, and perivascular cuffing with connective tissue. No vasculitis exists per se, that is, inflammation within the blood vessel wall, and the process has been called *vasculopathy*. In the blood, there is evidence of immune activation, with increased levels of circulating cytokines and T-cell receptor molecules. Finally, autoantibodies are directed at nuclear antigens, including species of antinuclear antibodies that show high specificity for SSc (see later discussion) but with a role in pathogenesis that is not established.

The relationship among vascular, connective tissue, and immune events is unclear. Although immune cells can stimulate fibrosis, fibroblasts from scleroderma-involved skin display abnormalities in connective tissue metabolism even ex vivo, a property that does not depend on continued immune stimulation. The origin of vascular injury is unclear but may include T-cell factors and free radicals. Vascular injury and tissue hypoxia, in turn, may contribute to fibrosis.

Clinical Features

The two distinct subsets of SSc are limited cutaneous (lcSSc) and diffuse cutaneous (dcSSc). Although these entities are identified based on the extent of cutaneous involvement, classification also implies patterns of visceral disease (Table 83-1). Patients with lcSSc, also

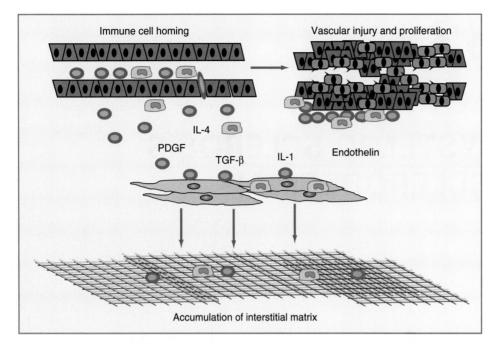

FIGURE 83–1 Pathogenetic processes in systemic sclerosis. Vascular injury leads to intimal proliferation of both endothelial cells (*in red*) and smooth muscle cells (*in blue*). Fibroblasts are activated to deposit increased amounts of interstitial matrix. IL = interleukin; PDGF = platelet-derived growth factor; TGFβ = transforming growth factor-β.

called *limited scleroderma*, have skin thickening limited to the distal extremities, usually just the fingers and toes, and the face. Dermal fibrosis is accompanied by loss of subcutaneous fat and atrophy of the overlying epidermis. The result is thickened skin tightly tethered to the underlying fascia. The skin thickening leads to loss of joint mobility and the development of contractures, as well as decreased pliability of skin in other locations. Replacement of secondary skin structures with fibrosis leads to loss of hair and sweat glands; the dry skin is prone to fissures and infection.

Raynaud's phenomenon is a triphasic vascular response to cold exposure consisting of pallor, cyanosis, and reactive hyperemia. It is present in more than 90% of patients and may precede other manifestations by years. Raynaud's phenomenon may be severe enough to cause digital ulcerations, ischemia, and infarction. Other vascular features include telangiectasia of the face,

TABLE 83–1 **Clinical Features of Systemic Sclerosis**

	Diffuse Scleroderma	Limited Scleroderma
Skin induration	Widespread: extremities, trunk, face	Fingers, toes, face
Raynaud's	80%–90%; ischemia, digital ulcers	95%–100%; ischemia, digital ulcers
Telangiectasia	Common	May be extensive
Calcinosis	Common	Common
Esophageal hypomotility and reflux	80%–90%, may be severe; strictures	90%, may be severe
Malabsorption, intestinal hypomotility	Common, may be severe	Less common, not usually severe
Interstitial lung disease	Common, major cause of death	Uncommon, rarely severe
Pulmonary hypertension	Secondary to pulmonary fibrosis; primary type uncommon	3%–5%; "primary type"
Cardiac fibrosis, cardiomyopathy	Common	Secondary to pulmonary hypertension
Renal disease	Vasculopathy, renal infarcts	None
Myositis	May be severe	None
Tendon friction rubs	Common	None
Antinuclear antibodies	Common	Common
	30%–40% antitopoisomerase I	50% anticentromere
	5%–10% anticentromere antibodies to RNA polymerase	10% antitopoisomerase

hands, and chest, intestinal telangiectasia that may cause bleeding, and dilated nail fold capillaries. Esophageal hypomotility may lead to dysphagia, and decreased lower esophageal sphincter pressure causes severe gastroesophageal reflux with resultant heartburn and even esophageal ulcers and stricture. The acronym *CREST* (cutaneous calcinosis, Raynaud's phenomenon, esophageal dysmotility, sclerodactyly, and telangiectasia) has been used to describe this subgroup and highlights the cardinal clinical manifestations. Pulmonary hypertension is a late complication, seriously affecting 3% to 5% of patients with lcSSc, and resembles primary pulmonary hypertension; obliterative disease of the pulmonary vascular tree occurs, with interstitial lung disease. The onset is insidious, and patients may have few symptoms until vascular disease is well advanced.

Patients with *diffuse skin disease* (dcSSc) generally experience rapid and progressive symmetric induration of the skin of the extremities, face, and trunk. Visceral organ involvement is common, with renovascular disease, interstitial inflammatory lung disease, and cardiac involvement the most serious. Renal involvement commonly presents as severe hypertension, often abrupt in onset, with proteinuria, microangiopathy, and rapidly progressive renal insufficiency; it has been termed *scleroderma renal crisis*. If it is left untreated, rapidly progressive renal failure with renal infarcts is the predictable outcome. Interstitial lung disease is common and presents as nonproductive cough, dyspnea, or fatigue. Cardiac disease is secondary to vascular occlusion and microinfarcts; arrhythmias and cardiomyopathy with congestive heart failure may develop. Pleuritis and pericardial effusions, sometimes large, may be seen.

Intestinal involvement includes the esophageal manifestations seen in lcSSC but is more extensive, and hypomotility often affects the length of the intestinal tract. Diarrhea and malabsorption are common and result from bacterial overgrowth and deconjugation of bile acids. Abdominal bloating and constipation may be a direct result of hypomotility. With advanced hypomotility and intestinal fibrosis, progressive weight loss and inanition may occur. Colonic involvement includes herniation of mucosa through an atrophic muscular layer with colonic sacculations and severe dilatation, which may be mistaken for toxic megacolon. Musculoskeletal manifestations include inflammatory myositis, tendinitis, and polyarthritis resembling rheumatoid arthritis but without erosive arthropathy. Fatigue and malaise are common symptoms.

Diagnosis and Differential Diagnosis

SSc is a clinical diagnosis suggested by the presence of Raynaud's phenomenon, esophageal reflux, and sclerodactyly. Raynaud's phenomenon is a common condition affecting 5% to 10% of the adult population and is much more common in women. Although most cases are idiopathic, defined causes include exposure to vibrating instruments such as jackhammers and chain saws, certain drugs such as β blockers and ergots, and blood disorders such as cryoglobulinemia and hyperviscosity syndrome. Raynaud's phenomenon is also seen in other connective tissue diseases such as dermatomyositis, SLE, and rheumatoid arthritis. The presence of other clinical features of SSc, such as severe heartburn or telangiectasia and the presence of antinuclear antibodies, particularly specific antibodies in high titer, indicate the risk of developing scleroderma. However, antinuclear antibodies are not specific for scleroderma or other autoimmune diseases, and some patients with SSc do not have autoantibodies.

At presentation, the distinction between lcSSc and dcSSc is not always obvious because many clinical features are common to both subsets. Clues that suggest the development of diffuse SSc include palpable or audible tendon friction rubs resulting from fibrosis around tendons, puffiness and swelling of the hands, and tightness of the skin proximal to the hands. Most patients have antinuclear antibodies. Of patients with dcSSc, 30% to 50% have antibodies to *topoisomerase I* (also called Scl-70); this subgroup and patients with antibodies to RNA polymerases are at higher risk of renal and lung disease. Fifty percent of patients with lcSSC have anticentromere antibodies, and these patients appear to be at higher risk of pulmonary hypertension.

A small subset of patients with dcSSc have vascular and visceral manifestations of the disease but without the dermal manifestation of skin thickening; the term *scleroderma sine scleroderma* has been used to describe these patients. In addition, some patients have overlapping features of multiple connective tissue diseases including scleroderma, SLE, dermatomyositis, and rheumatoid arthritis. Although some investigators have used the term *mixed connective tissue disease* to describe these patients, *undifferentiated connective tissue disease* is a better term: Many of these patients, with time, develop a more classic picture of a single entity, most commonly SSc or SLE. Others patients continue to have this overlap syndrome.

Other entities that may resemble SSc include diffuse morphea, scleroderma, eosinophilic fasciitis and eosinophilia myalgia syndrome, and certain environmental or drug-induced scleroderma syndromes (Table 83–2). *Morphea* is a form of localized scleroderma, occurring more commonly in children. Patients have inflammatory skin infiltrates and dermal fibrosis and atrophy, but no Raynaud's or systemic manifestations. This condition can occur as a single lesion, multiple lesions, or in linear form. The linear form may affect large body parts and often involves tissues down to fascia and muscle. Contractures and deformity may result.

Treatment

No single treatment exists for SSc. However, therapy directed at specific organ involvement is often effective

TABLE 83–2 **Scleroderma-like Syndromes**

	Distinguishing Features
Other Diseases	
Morphea	Patchy or linear distribution
Eosinophilic fasciitis	Sparing of hands, biopsy shows involvement extending to fascia and muscle
Scleredema (of Buschke)	Prominent involvement of neck, shoulders, and upper arms; hands spared; association with diabetes
Scleromyxedema	Association with gammopathy; skin lichenoid and thickened but not tethered; may have Raynaud's phenomenon
Graft-versus-host disease	Skin changes similar to scleroderma; vasculopathy
Environmental Agents and Drugs	
Bleomycin	Skin and lung fibrosis similar to scleroderma
L-Tryptophan	Eosinophilia-myalgia; from contaminant or metabolite
	Fever, eosinophilia, neurologic manifestations, pulmonary hypertension
Organic solvents	Trichloroethylene and others implicated
	Clinically indistinguishable from idiopathic systemic sclerosis
Pentazocine	Localized lesions at injection sites
Toxic oil syndrome	Contaminated rapeseed oil (Spanish epidemic 1981)
	Similar to eosinophilia myalgia syndrome
Vinyl chloride disease	Vascular lesions, acro-osteolysis, sclerodactyly
	No visceral disease

(Table 83–3), and the need for treatment is sometimes urgent. No agent has been proven to retard or reverse skin disease, although some studies suggest that methotrexate and cyclophosphamide may be effective, particularly before marked fibrosis occurs. Several agents that inhibit collagen synthesis or promote its breakdown are under investigation. Prevention of digital ulcers by avoiding skin trauma, and prompt treatment of ulcers when they do occur, may prevent progression to severe infection and/or amputation. Various vasodilating agents are effective in improving symptoms of Raynaud's phenomenon and may also be effective in preventing the development of digital ulcers or in promoting their healing. Calcium channel blockers are most widely used, but drugs such as nitroglycerin ointment or patches and doxazosin or prazosin are also appropriate.

New hypertension in the setting of scleroderma is a manifestation of renal crisis. Regular blood pressure monitoring allows early treatment before renal damage is extensive. Renal crisis is an emergency and should be aggressively treated with angiotensin-converting enzyme inhibitors, preferably in an inpatient setting, until the patient's blood pressure is controlled. The availability of angiotensin-converting enzyme inhibitors has dramatically altered the course and outcome of renal crisis in SSc. Occasionally, renal "crisis" with proteinuria and microangiopathy occurs without hypertension.

Early recognition of inflammatory interstitial lung dis-

TABLE 83–3 **Therapeutic Approaches to Systemic Sclerosis**

Manifestation	Pathophysiology	Treatment
Raynaud's phenomenon	Vascular hyperreactivity	Calcium channel blockers; smoking cessation; direct vasodilators
	Vascular obliteration	
Digital ulcers	Ischemia, infection	Antibiotics; treat Raynaud's phenomenon
Swollen puffy hands	Vascular leak, inflammation	Short-term, low-dose corticosteroids
Esophageal reflux	Loss of lower esophageal sphincter function; ischemic damage to myenteric plexus	Proton pump inhibitors; H_2 blockers; promotility agents: cisapride, metaclopramide
Intestinal hypomotility	Ischemic damage to myenteric plexus; intestinal fibrosis	Promotility agents
Malabsorption	Bacterial overgrowth	Antibiotics
Interstitial lung disease	Inflammation; fibrosis	Cyclophosphamide, corticosteroids
Cardiac arrhythmia	Myocardial ischemia and fibrosis	Antiarrhythmic agents
Renal crisis	Vasculopathy	Angiotensin-converting enzyme inhibitors; angiotensin II–receptor antagonists
Myositis	Inflammatory damage	Corticosteroids; methotrexate
Skin thickening	Fibroblast (defect); inflammation leading to fibrosis	Drugs under investigation
		? Methotrexate

ease is important if treatment is to prevent progression to distortion of lung architecture and irreversible fibrosis. Diagnosis is best made by high-resolution computed tomography and bronchoalveolar lavage or biopsy; evaluation with these modalities should be done before prominent symptoms are present. Cyclophosphamide therapy appears to be effective in treating inflammatory lung disease and in arresting the decline in lung function.

Gastrointestinal reflux disease, which may progress to stricture, is best treated with proton pump inhibitors. Diarrhea and malabsorption are usually responsive to antibiotics that suppress bacterial overgrowth. Several drugs may help with intestinal motility. Joint manifestations often respond to nonsteroidal anti-inflammatory drugs, but occasionally short courses of corticosteroids are needed; caution should be exercised with corticosteroids because these agents have been implicated in precipitating renal crisis. Joint symptoms may result from scarring and inflammation around tendons. Mild asymptomatic elevations of muscle enzymes do not require treatment, but inflammatory myositis should be treated with corticosteroids and/or methotrexate. A summary of therapeutic approaches is given in Table 83–3.

Prognosis

Survival in scleroderma improved dramatically in the 1990s. This may be attributed to early aggressive treatment of renal disease, early recognition and treatment of pulmonary interstitial disease, better therapies for infection and gastrointestinal involvement, and attention to nutritional needs. Overall survival is approximately 70% at 10 years; patients with lcSSc have better survival rates unless pulmonary hypertension is present.

REFERENCES

Gulin J, Korn JH: Systemic sclerosis: Challenges in diagnosis and management. J Musculoskeletal Med 1999; 16:288.

Medsger TA Jr: Systemic sclerosis (scleroderma): Clinical aspects. *In* Koopman WJ (ed): Arthritis and Allied Conditions, 13th ed. Baltimore: Williams & Wilkins, 1997, p 1433.

Medsger TA Jr, Steen VD: Classification, prognosis. *In* Clements PJ, Furst DE (eds): Systemic Sclerosis. Baltimore: Williams & Wilkins, 1996, p 51.

Wigley FM: Systemic sclerosis (scleroderma). *In* Goldman L, Bennett JC (eds): Cecil Textbook of Medicine, 21st ed. Philadelphia: WB Saunders, 2000, pp 1517–1522.

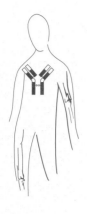

84

IDIOPATHIC INFLAMMATORY MYOPATHIES

Robert W. Simms

The idiopathic inflammatory myopathies (IIMs) include polymyositis, dermatomyositis, myositis associated with malignancy, myositis associated with other connective tissue disease, and inclusion body myositis. These conditions have in common the clinical features of progressive symmetric proximal weakness, elevation of muscle enzymes, muscle histologic features demonstrating mononuclear inflammatory cell infiltrates and muscle fiber necrosis, and characteristic electromyographic abnormalities. The IIMs differ in their association with extramuscular manifestations and with certain autoantibody profiles (Tables 84–1 and 84–2).

The IIMs as a group and individually are relatively rare conditions, with estimated prevalence rates of between 2 and 10 per million and incidence rates between 0.5 and 8.4 cases per million. The male-to-female ratio is approximately 2:1 for polymyositis and dermatomyositis. Inclusion body myositis predominates in men. The age distribution of IIMs is bimodal, with a peak between ages 10 and 15 years in children with dermatomyositis and another peak between ages 40 and 60 years. Both myositis associated with malignancy and inclusion body myositis are more common after the age of 50 years.

Pathology and Pathophysiology

The hallmark of the IIMs is inflammatory infiltrate within muscle tissue. The infiltrate is primarily lymphocytic, but macrophages, plasma cells, and sometimes eosinophils, basophils, and neutrophils are present. In polymyositis, the infiltrate typically clusters in the endomysial area around muscle fibers, whereas in dermatomyositis, the infiltrate predominates in the perimysial area around the fascicles and small blood vessels. Perifascicular atrophy occurs more frequently in dermato-

myositis. Necrotizing vasculitis is uncommon. Inclusion body myositis is characterized by the presence of intracellular vacuoles, which under electron microscopy appear as intracytoplasmic, intranuclear tubular, or filamentous inclusions.

The association of IIMs with other autoimmune disorders (including Hashimoto's thyroiditis, myasthenia gravis, primary biliary cirrhosis, and connective tissue diseases), in some cases with autoantibodies (see Table 84–2) and the response to corticosteroids, suggests an autoimmune pathogenesis. This hypothesis is also supported by the identification of T cells cytotoxic to muscle in biopsy specimens and in peripheral blood of patients with polymyositis and dermatomyositis. Autoimmunity is also suggested by the finding of immunoglobulin deposition and complement components in the capillaries and small arterioles in dermatomyositis. Inclusion body myositis probably represents a special case, given its distinctive pathologic features, because amyloid deposits have been identified in the vacuoles that characterize this condition.

Clinical Presentation

Patients with IIM typically present with insidious proximal muscle weakness; in rare cases, the presentation is more fulminant, with both proximal and distal muscle weakness. An indolent onset over years with both proximal and distal involvement suggests inclusion body myositis. The symmetric proximal muscle weakness often impairs specific tasks such as getting up from a sitting position, getting out of a car, and reaching overhead or combing the hair, and it should be distinguished from conditions that produce a generalized fatigue or loss of energy that rarely interferes with these functions. Approximately one third of patients with poly-

TABLE 84–1 Classification of the Idiopathic Inflammatory Myopathies

Primary idiopathic polymyositis
Primary idiopathic dermatomyositis
Polymyositis or dermatomyositis associated with malignancy
Juvenile dermatomyositis (or polymyositis)
Overlap syndrome of polymyositis or dermatomyositis with another autoimmune rheumatic disease
Inclusion body myositis

myositis have upper esophageal involvement, which produces dysphagia and, occasionally, aspiration of oral contents. Myalgia occurs in approximately one half of patients, but it is generally mild, although it may cause confusion with polymyalgia rheumatica among older patients.

The assessment of muscle strength should include active resistive testing; the physician should keep in mind that this testing should also be supplemented by asking the patient to perform specific tasks such as getting up from a low chair without using the arms, raising the arms over the head, and lifting the head from the examining table when in the supine position. The examiner should be aware that assessment of motor power may be confounded by the fatigue or pain of arthritis or myalgia.

In dermatomyositis, a characteristic skin eruption occurs, usually preceding the development of myositis. In rare cases, patients have the classic skin manifestations without the myositis (*dermatomyositis sine myositis* or *amyopathic dermatomyositis*). The rash has several distinctive varieties: Gottron's lesions, the erythematous or poikilodermatous rash, and the heliotrope rash. *Gottron's papules* consist of erythematous, sometimes scaly papules, plaques, or macules (Gottron's sign) over the metacarpophalangeal and proximal interphalangeal

joints. The *poikilodermatous eruption* of dermatomyositis consists of an erythematous or violaceous rash on the face, trunk, neck, extremities, or scalp. Occasionally, it has a characteristic distribution in the shape of a V on the anterior chest, or the so-called *shawl sign* (back of neck, upper torso, and shoulders). The *heliotrope (lilaccolored) rash* occurs in 30% to 60% of patients with dermatomyositis and is located characteristically on the upper eyelids, but it may be difficult to detect in dark-skinned patients.

Various nonmuscular and nondermatologic manifestations of the IIM may occur (Table 84–3). Pulmonary involvement in polymyositis and dermatomyositis may take several forms, including respiratory muscle weakness, interstitial lung disease, pulmonary hypertension, pulmonary vasculitis, and aspiration pneumonia. Respiratory muscle involvement may include the chest wall musculature and the diaphragm and is clinically significant in approximately 5% of patients. Respiratory failure necessitating ventilatory assistance is fortunately rare. Esophageal and tongue involvement appears to be a risk factor for this complication. Interstitial lung disease occurs in approximately 10% to 30% of patients with either polymyositis or dermatomyositis and in the case of polymyositis is frequently associated with the presence of antisynthetase (Jo-1) antibodies, fever, Raynaud's phenomenon, and arthritis (*the antisynthetase syndrome*) (see Table 84–2). Curiously, the severity of the interstitial lung disease may be independent of the severity of myositis.

Cardiac involvement in IIM may include conduction blocks, arrhythmias, and myocarditis; appears to be more common than previously estimated (up to 70% in one series); and, as in interstitial lung disease, may be independent of the severity of myositis. Dysphagia, the result of myositis of striated muscle in the upper one third of the esophagus, occurs in up to 30% of patients with IIM. Less common involvement includes cricophar-

TABLE 84–2 Myositis Syndromes and Associated Autoantibodies

Autoantibody	Clinical Features	Treatment Response
Anti-Jo 1 (also known as antisynthetase)*	Polymyositis or dermatomyositis Acute interstitial lung disease Fever Arthritis Raynaud's phenomenon	Moderate with persistent disease
Anti-SRP†	Polymyositis Abrupt onset Severe weakness Palpitations	Poor
Anti-Mi2‡	Dermatomyositis V sign and shawl sign Cuticular overgrowth	Good

* Anti-Jo 1 is the most common myositis-specific autoantibody. It is known as *antisynthetase* because the putative antibody target is an RNA synthetase. The prevalence of anti-Jo 1 is approximately 20%. Other antisynthetase antibodies include anti–PL-7, anti-PL-12, anti-EJ, and anti-OJ, each of which has a prevalence of less than 3%.
† Its prevalence is approximately 5%.
‡ The prevalence of anti-Mi2 is approximately 10%.
SRP = signal recognition particle.

TABLE 84-3 Extramuscular Manifestations of Polymyositis and Dermatomyositis

Pulmonary
Respiratory muscle weakness
Aspiration
Interstitial lung disease
Pulmonary hypertension
Pulmonary vasculitis
Cardiac
Heart block
Arrythmias
Cardiomyopathy
Gastrointestinal
Esophageal dysmotility
Stomach, small or large bowel dysmotility
Arthritis
Nonerosive, symmetric, small joint

yngeal muscle dysfunction and, in children with dermatomyositis, intestinal vasculitis.

The relationship of IIM with malignant disease has been clarified by population-based studies showing a modest increase in risk (approximate twofold relative risk) within 1 to 2 years of the diagnosis of dermatomyositis and possibly polymyositis. The malignancies associated with dermatomyositis include those that occur most commonly in the general population. They include cancers of the lung, breast, colon, prostate, and ovary. Experts recommend a thorough history, examination, and screening rectal examination; Papanicolaou's stain in women; urinalysis; blood chemistry studies; chest radiograph; and prostate-specific antigen measurement in men. Serial gynecologic examinations, transvaginal ultrasonography, and serial CA-125 determinations to screen fully for ovarian cancer in women with recently diagnosed dermatomyositis may also be reasonable.

Diagnosis

The diagnosis of IIM is suspected by the typical history and physical examination. Muscle enzymes such as creatine phosphokinase and aldolase are markedly elevated. The diagnosis is confirmed by muscle biopsy, ideally an open biopsy to allow the optimal assessment of muscle architecture, although needle biopsy may be adequate for the diagnosis of polymyositis or dermatomyositis in many cases. The ideal muscle to sample for biopsy is one that is involved but not atrophic. Most commonly, the quadriceps or deltoid muscle is examined by biopsy. Electron microscopy is helpful to establish the diagnosis of inclusion body myositis, and special stains to identify excess glycogen or lipid are useful to exclude metabolic myopathies. With the possible exception of Jo-1 antibodies and the identification of the antisynthetase syndrome

(see Table 84–2), the role of myositis-specific antibodies remains limited because they lack sensitivity, and not all are commercially available.

Electromyography alone cannot enable one to establish the diagnosis, but it can indicate muscle involvement in patients with dermatologic or nonmuscular features. Typical electromyographic features are listed in Table 84–4. Magnetic resonance imaging is increasingly used to identify sites of muscle involvement, but it is rarely diagnostic. This technique may be most useful for monitoring the course of IIM.

Differential Diagnosis

Many different conditions should be considered in the differential diagnosis of myositis (Table 84–5). These include other myopathies (infectious myositis, drug-induced disorders, muscular dystrophies, metabolic myopathies, and endocrine disorders) and/or neurologic conditions (e.g., myasthenia gravis, Guillain-Barré syndrome).

Treatment

The mainstay of treatment for the IIMs consists of the corticosteroids. Initially, prednisone is begun at a high dose (e.g., 60 mg/day) until the creatine phosphokinase level has returned to normal or muscle strength has markedly improved. Occasionally, extremely high doses of intravenous corticosteroids are used for severely ill patients. Subsequently, corticosteroids are gradually tapered, depending on the clinical response. Approximately one third to one fourth of patients require additional immunosuppressive agents such as methotrexate or azathioprine because of steroid resistance, intolerable side effects, or inability to taper corticosteroids without inducing a flareup in disease. Cyclophosphamide and cyclosporine have proved effective in steroid-resistant cases; however, their toxicity limits widespread use. Clinical trials have established the efficacy and low tox-

TABLE 84-4 Typical Electromyographic Features of Polymyositis and Dermatomyositis

Low-amplitude, short-duration motor unit action potentials
Typical myopathic pattern
Polyphasic potentials
Resulting from asynchronous firing of fibers
Increased insertional activity and fibrillation
Attributed to damage to nerve endings or motor end plates
Complex repetitive discharges
Thought to be the result of inflammatory damage to the sarcolemma

TABLE 84-5 **Differential Diagnosis of Idiopathic Inflammatory Myositis**

Infectious	**Metabolic Myopathies**
Viral myositis:	Myophosphorylase deficiency (McArdle's disease)
Retroviruses (HIV, HTLV-I)	
Enteroviruses (echovirus, Coxsackievirus)	Phosphofructokinase deficiency
Other viruses (influenza, hepatitis A and B,	Myoadenylate deaminase deficiency
Epstein-Barr virus)	Acid maltase deficiency
Bacterial: pyomyositis	Lipid storage diseases
Parasites: trichinosis, cysticercosis	Acute rhabdomyolysis
Fungi: candidiasis	
	Drug-Induced Myopathies
Idiopathic	Alcohol
Granulomatous myositis (sarcoid, giant cell)	D-Penicillamine
Eosinophilic myositis	Zidovudine
Eosinophilia-myalgia syndrome	Colchicine
	Chloroquine, hydroxychloroquine
Endocrine/Metabolic Disorders	Lipid-lowering agents
Hypothyroidism	Cyclosporine
Hyperthyroidism	Cocaine, heroin, barbiturates
Hypercortisolism	Corticosteroids
Hyperparathyroidism	
Hypoparathyroidism	**Neurologic disorders**
Hypocalcemia	Muscular dystrophies
Hypokalemia	Congenital myopathies
	Motor neuron disease
	Guillain-Barré syndrome
	Myasthenia gravis

HIV = human immunodeficiency virus; HTLV-I = human T-cell lymphotropic virus–I.

icity of intravenous gammaglobulin in dermatomyositis. This therapy appears to work by blocking deposition of activated complement fragments and thereby protecting muscle capillaries from complement-mediated injury. Although intravenous gammaglobulin is attractive because of its low toxicity, its long-term efficacy is unknown, and its long-term use is limited by its expense.

REFERENCES

Medsger TA, Oddis CV: Inflammatory muscle disease: Clinical features. In Klippel JH, Dieppe PA (eds): Rheumatology, 2nd ed. London: CV Mosby, 1998, pp 7.13.1–7.13.13.
Wortmann RL: Idiopathic inflammatory myopathies. In Goldman L, Bennett JC (eds): Cecil Textbook of Medicine, 21st ed. Philadelphia: WB Saunders, 2000, pp 1534–1538.

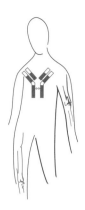

85

SJÖGREN'S SYNDROME

Peter A. Merkel

Sjögren's syndrome is a chronic immune-mediated, inflammatory disorder of exocrine gland dysfunction and other systemic features. The most common manifestations include inflammation and destruction of the lacrimal and salivary glands, leading to dry eyes (keratoconjunctivitis sicca or xerophthalmia) and dry mouth (xerostomia). Sjögren's syndrome is associated with various autoantibodies and systemic clinical features, including interstitial lung disease, vasculitis, and lymphoma.

Patients are considered to have *secondary* Sjögren's syndrome if they also have another immunologic disorder, such as systemic lupus erythematosus, rheumatoid arthritis, systemic sclerosis (scleroderma), and primary biliary cirrhosis, and to have *primary* Sjögren's syndrome if no underlying immunologic disorder is present. Although more common among women, Sjögren's syndrome does affect men and is found among people of all ages, races, and ethnicities.

Clinical Features

The clinical features of Sjögren's syndrome can be divided into those associated with exocrine gland dysfunction (Table 85–1) and those associated with extraglandular manifestations (Table 85–2). Dry eyes and mouth are by far the most common problems and are very troubling to patients. Many of the extraglandular manifestations, although often rare, can be life- or organ-threatening. For patients with secondary Sjögren's syndrome, it can be difficult to differentiate signs and symptoms of Sjögren's syndrome from those of the underlying disorder.

The clinical association with Sjögren's syndrome of most concern is a marked increase in the prevalence of lymphoma. These lymphomas (usually B cell types) may involve malignant transformation of clinically involved exocrine glands or involve sites not clinically apparent, such as cervical lymph nodes. It is prudent to have a low threshold to consider the diagnosis of lymphoma in patients with Sjögren's syndrome who present with new

masses, constitutional features, or persistent glandular swelling that is either resistant to treatment or changes in character.

Diagnosis

There have been a number of different diagnostic criteria proposed for Sjögren's syndrome without consensus on any one set. Common to each set of criteria is the requirement to demonstrate the following: (1) subjective and objective evidence of both keratoconjunctivitis sicca and xerostomia; (2) presence of at least one of the following four autoantibodies: antinuclear antibodies, rheumatoid factor, anti-Ro antibodies, or anti-La antibodies (these latter two are also known as SS-A and SS-B antibodies, respectively, so named for Sjögren's syn-

TABLE 85–1 Clinical Features of Sjögren's Syndrome Associated with Exocrine Gland Dysfunction

Problems Secondary to Lacrimal Gland Dysfunction
Dry, irritated eyes with foreign-body sensation
Corneal abrasions
Erythematous eyes

Problems Secondary to Salivary Gland Dysfunction
Dry mouth
Oral sores
Dental caries
Lingual and labial fissures
Dysphagia
Gastroesophageal reflux
Parotid and/or submandibular gland swelling

Problems Secondary to Other Exocrine Dysfunction
Dyspareunia
Pancreatic malabsorption
Pancreatitis

TABLE 85-2 Extraglandular Clinical Features of Sjögren's Syndrome

Skin and Mucous Membranes

Xerosis

Lower extremity purpura, associated with hyperglobulinemia and/or leukocytoclastic vasculitis on biopsy

Photosensitive lesions, indistinguishable from that of sub-acute cutaneous lupus erythematosus

Pulmonary

Chronic bronchitis secondary to dryness of the tracheobronchial tree

Lymphocytic interstitial pneumonitis, interstitial pulmonary fibrosis, chronic obstructive lung disease, bronchiolitis obliterans organizing pneumonia, pseudolymphoma with intrapulmonary nodules

Musculoskeletal

Polymyositis

Polyarthralgias, polyarthritis

Renal

Tubulointerstitial nephritis, type 1 renal tubular acidosis

Central Nervous System

Focal defects including multiple sclerosis, stroke

Diffuse deficits including dementia, cognitive dysfunction

Spinal cord involvement including transverse myelitis

Peripheral Nervous System

Peripheral sensorimotor neuropathy

Reticuloendothelial System

Splenomegaly

Lymphadenopathy and development of pseudolymphoma

Liver

Hepatomegaly

Primary biliary cirrhosis

Vascular

Raynaud's phenomenon

Small vessel vasculitis, with either a mononuclear perivascular infiltrate or leukocytoclastic changes on biopsy

Endocrine

Hypothyroidism due to Hashimoto's thyroiditis

Other autoimmune endocrinopathies

From Hochberg MC: Sjögren's syndrome. *In* Bennett JC, Plum F (eds): Cecil Textbook of Medicine, 20th ed. Philadelphia, WB Saunders, 1996, p 1488.

drome); and (3) exclusion of underlying diseases that may mimic Sjögren's syndrome. Biopsy specimens from salivary glands, which are easily obtainable from the lower lip, may demonstrate characteristic findings of focal lymphocytic infiltration of predominantly CD4 T cells. These histologic features imply that cell-mediated processes are essential in the pathogenesis of Sjögren's syndrome.

Keratoconjunctivitis sicca can be objectively documented by either measuring decreased tear production with Schirmer's filter paper test (<5 mm of wetting in 5 minutes after placement in the lower eyelid) or viewing corneal abrasions by rose bengal staining and slit lamp examination. Reduced salivary production can be demonstrated by provocative sialometry.

The differential diagnosis of Sjögren's syndrome includes a wide variety of infectious and infiltrative diseases that may cause keratoconjunctivitis sicca symptoms and/or lacrimal and salivary gland enlargement. Human immunodeficiency virus causes diffuse infiltrative lymphadenopathy syndrome, which closely mimics Sjögren's syndrome. Diffuse infiltrative lymphadenopathy syndrome, however, involves predominantly CD8 T cells. Additional infections to consider in patients with keratoconjunctivitis sicca symptoms include hepatitis B and C, human T cell leukemia virus, syphilis, infection with mycobacteria, and others. Infiltrative diseases may involve lacrimal and salivary glands and present in a fashion similar to Sjögren's syndrome. These infiltrative diseases include sarcoidosis, the amyloidoses, hemochromatosis, and others. Diseases that result in abnormal neural input to exocrine glands, such as multiple sclerosis, must also be considered in a patient with keratoconjunctivitis sicca symptoms.

Many drugs from various pharmaceutical classes have anticholinergic properties that result in clinically significant symptoms of dry eyes and mouth and mimic Sjögren's syndrome. Such medication classes include antidepressants, decongestants, and antihypertensives. The list of medications with anticholinergic side effects is quite long, and all medications, including over-the-counter products, should be carefully reviewed in any patient presenting with signs or symptoms of Sjögren's syndrome.

TABLE 85-3 Treatments for Sjögren's Syndrome

Local Treatment of Exocrine Dysfunction

Xerophthalmia

Artificial tears

Eyeglasses/goggles

Punctal occlusion by means of plugs or electrocautery

Xerostomia

Artificial saliva

Fluoride treatments/good dental care

Avoid glucose lozenges/candies

Dyspareunia

Vaginal lubricants

Systemic Treatment of Exocrine Dysfunction

Pilocarpine

When possible, avoid or discontinue medications with anticholinergic effects

Treatment of Systemic Manifestations

Nonsteroidal anti-inflammatory drugs

Antimalarial agents: hydroxychloroquine or chloroquine

Glucocorticoids

Immunosuppressive agents

Treatment

Treatment of Sjögren's syndrome consists of either local measures to counter the exocrine deficiencies or systemic therapy to counter the exocrine and inflammatory disease. Treatment options are outlined in Table 85–3. Patient education is important, and some measures outlined can be considered prophylactic.

REFERENCES

Hochberg MC: Sjögren's syndrome. *In* Goldman L, Bennett JC (eds): Cecil Textbook of Medicine, 21st ed. Philadelphia: WB Saunders, 2000, pp 1522–1524.

Fox RI: Sjögren's syndrome. *In* Klippel JH (ed): Primer of the Rheumatic Diseases, 11th ed. Atlanta: The Arthritis Foundation, 1997, pp 283–288.

86

VASCULITIDES

Peter A. Merkel

The vasculitides constitute a spectrum of diseases involving inflammation and necrosis of blood vessels with resulting ischemia of those tissues supplied by the affected vessels. Vasculitis can involve virtually any organ system, although each specific syndrome has unique aspects. These are rare diseases with clinical presentations that vary considerably, often leading to delay in diagnosis. Because these disorders can often be life and organ threatening, it is imperative for physicians to have some familiarity with these diseases. There are many types of vasculitis and a number of clinical features common to them. In this chapter the similarities among the vasculitides are emphasized, and then some of the specific syndromes are briefly outlined.

Classification

Because of the wide variation in clinical presentation, anatomic involvement, and overlapping features, both the classification and the diagnosis of these disorders are difficult. Multiple classification systems have been proposed, including those that sort the diseases by vessel size, by pathologic lesion, by autoantibodies, or by associated conditions. Table 86–1 outlines the vasculitides as classified by the size of involved vessels. This is only a partial list of vasculitic syndromes, and there is considerable overlap among the categories, especially between the small and medium artery diseases.

The ability of clinicians and researchers to agree on definitions of vasculitides is important for conducting clinical research, deciding on treatment protocols, and determining patients' prognoses.

Pathogenesis

The clinical manifestations of vasculitis result from disruption of blood flow in vessels with resulting ischemia. Inflammation and necrosis of blood vessel walls can cause leakage, stenosis, or total obliteration of the vessel. Stenosis may also be the result of the fibrosis and remodeling that often follow the inflammatory stage of vasculitis. The extent and nature of the damage vary with vessel caliber, thickness, and location.

A number of vasculitides involve inflammatory disease of nonvascular structures, and these may be the most serious aspect of a specific patient's disease. For example, patients with Wegener's granulomatosis often have destruction of the sinuses and trachea, retro-orbital lesions, and pulmonary nodules. Neural involvement in vasculitis may result from vascular insufficiency or from the direct destruction of neural tissue by inflammation.

The etiology and pathogenesis of most vasculitides are still unknown. However, there is a great deal of evidence for multiple mechanisms for tissue destruction in these diseases. It is likely that not only do different vasculitis syndromes have different causes but also that more than one triggering process or pathologic mechanism is involved even within one type of vasculitis. There is evidence that each of the following pathogenic processes is important: immune complex deposition and humoral immune responses, T cell–mediated cellular immunity, autoantibodies, cytokine activation, and toxins.

Infectious causes for a number of the vasculitides have often been proposed, given the geographic variations in prevalence and presence of granulomas in some types. Proposed etiologic agents include bacteria, mycobacteria, and viruses. There is now clear evidence that hepatitis C virus is the cause of most cases of mixed cryoglobulinemic vasculitis. Hepatitis B and C infections have also long been associated with polyarteritis nodosa but are clearly not involved in all cases.

A wide variety of drugs have been implicated as causative agents for vasculitis. Drugs from most pharmaceutical classes as well as herbal supplements have been linked to leukocytoclastic vasculitis, although definitive proof from large studies or drug rechallenges is lacking for most agents. Systemic vasculitis has also been linked to a variety of agents, including sympathomimetics, illegal drugs of abuse, hematopoietic growth factors, and many commonly used drugs.

TABLE 86–1 Classification of the Vasculitides

Large Vessel Vasculitides

Takayasu's arteritis

Giant cell arteritis/polymyalgia rheumatica

Aortitis associated with an underlying inflammatory disease such as spondyloarthropathy, relapsing polychondritis, or retroperitoneal fibrosis

Medium Vessel Vasculitides

Polyarteritis nodosa

Churg-Strauss syndrome

Kawasaki disease

Small Vessel Vasculitides

Wegener's granulomatosis

Henoch-Schönlein purpura

Leukocytoclastic vasculitis

Microscopic polyangiitis

Cryoglobulinemic vasculitis

Primary angiitis of the central nervous system

Vasculitis associated with connective tissue diseases

Clinical Features

The clinical manifestations of vasculitis vary widely among the different types of vasculitis as well as among different patients with the same type. Table 86–2 outlines many of the clinical manifestations that may be seen in patients with vasculitis. However, no one type of vasculitis involves all of these features. Which features are present often depends on the vessel size involved in that specific type of vasculitis. For example, the large vessel vasculitides may involve aortic aneurysmal dilatation, but they are not associated with purpura, as seen in small and some medium vessel diseases. Furthermore, some organ systems can be involved in different ways in the different types of vasculitis. Renal insufficiency, for example, may be seen with involvement of the renal arteries in polyarteritis nodosa as well as by glomerulonephritis in Wegener's granulomatosis. The features of specific vasculitides are described later in this chapter.

Although vasculitides are rare diseases, the appearance of some of the listed features should always be seen as clinical "red flags" and warrant investigation for vasculitis. Among these features are unexplained hemoptysis, glomerulonephritis, palpable purpura, and mononeuritis multiplex. Some patients with vasculitis may have a chronic smoldering clinical course, whereas other patients may present with fulminant disease such as rapidly progressive renal failure or massive pulmonary hemorrhage. Vasculitis may also present as unexplained multisystemic disease.

The morbidity and mortality rates of vasculitis are variable. Although treatments continue to improve the course of patients with these diseases, the toxic effects of the anti-inflammatory and immunosuppressive agents used are also severe. Some forms of vasculitis are self-limited, but some are rapidly progressive if not treated. With some types of vasculitis, patients are prone to relapse even after long periods of inactive disease.

Specific Types of Vasculitis

A complete description of all of the vasculitides is beyond the scope of this book, but brief reviews of the most common types follow. Whereas many of the clinical features of vasculitis were just outlined, each type has its own unique features as well as pattern of disease presentation. When possible, it is quite useful to establish accurately not only that a vasculitis is present but also which type it is. The clinical patterns of different types of vasculitis allow clinicians to anticipate clinical problems and conduct appropriate testing to prevent more widespread damage. Many of the treatment protocols used vary with the type of vasculitis.

GIANT CELL ARTERITIS/POLYMYALGIA RHEUMATICA

Giant cell arteritis (GCA), also known as temporal arteritis or cranial arteritis, is the most common type of systemic vasculitis. GCA is a large vessel vasculitis that especially involves branches of the carotid artery. GCA affects patients older than age 50 years and has a female predominance. The most common clinical signs of GCA include headaches, which are often continuous and poorly responsive to analgesics; scalp tenderness; visual disturbance; jaw claudication; malaise; and arthralgias. The most dreaded complication of GCA is monocular

TABLE 86–2 Clinical Features of Vasculitis

Constitutional Symptoms	Gastrointestinal
Fevers	Bowel ischemia/infarction
Weight loss	
Fatigue	**Renal**
	Glomerulonephritis
Skin	Nephrotic syndrome
Purpura	Renovascular involvement
Livido reticularis	Hypertension
Digital infarction	
	Neurologic
Musculoskeletal	Mononeuritis multiplex
Arthralgia	Visual disturbance
Arthritis	Stroke
	Lightheadedness
Cardiovascular	
Pulselessness/bruits common in large vessel disease	**Laboratory Abnormalities**
	Anemia
	Eosinophilia
Claudication	Elevated acute phase reactants
Aneurysms	Renal insufficiency
	Active urinary sediment
Pulmonary	
Alveolar hemorrhage	
Nodules	

blindness, which is almost never reversible. Most patients with GCA (90%) have an elevated erythrocyte sedimentation rate. Anemia and fever are common and may be the presenting features. Any elderly patient with new onset of headaches or visual changes should be investigated for possible GCA. Rarely, other branches of the aorta or the aorta itself are involved in GCA.

Diagnosis of GCA is confirmed by biopsy of a segment of either or both temporal arteries. Characteristic findings include inflammation and destruction of the internal elastic lamina, often with giant cells present. The pathologic changes may skip segments, necessitating examination of multiple levels.

Polymyalgia rheumatica (PMR) is the name given to the symptom complex that includes pain and stiffness, often profound, of the shoulder and hip girdles and proximal extremities. Occasionally, true synovitis may be seen. PMR occurs in the same population as GCA and is also typically associated with an elevated erythrocyte sedimentation rate and anemia. Diagnosis is made on clinical grounds and rapid response to glucocorticoid treatment. Differentiating PMR from early elderly-onset rheumatoid arthritis can often be difficult.

PMR and GCA are likely part of the same disease spectrum. Both diseases may present in a very indolent fashion or with a fulminant course. Many patients with GCA will have PMR symptoms either at diagnosis or on tapering of glucocorticoids. Similarly, patients who present with PMR symptoms alone may progress to frank arteritis. All patients with PMR must be regularly questioned and examined for signs and symptoms of GCA.

Treatment of GCA always involves high-dose glucocorticoids with tapering over 6 to 12 months. PMR is treated with much lower dosages of glucocorticoids. A rapid response to glucocorticoids, usually within 1 to 2 days, is the norm for both GCA and PMR. Although the toxic effects from glucocorticoids may be considerable, the outcome for patients with GCA or PMR is excellent. It is rare for visual loss to occur while patients are on glucocorticoid therapy, but relapses can occur either during glucocorticoid tapering or months to years after cessation of treatment.

TAKAYASU'S ARTERITIS

Takayasu's arteritis is a large vessel vasculitis that predominantly affects young women but can be seen in either men or women up to age 50 years. Also known as "pulseless disease," Takayasu's arteritis results in stenosis of the aorta and its main branches, including involvement of the cerebral, brachiocephalic, renal, mesenteric, femoral, and coronary arteries. Stenoses of the proximal aorta and its branches are the most common. Frequent presenting symptoms include limb claudication, lightheadedness, and constitutional findings such as malaise, fever, or arthralgias. Patients may also be asymptomatic with even extremely tight stenoses. Delay in diagnosis, sometimes for many years, is common. The clinical course is quite variable, with long periods of active and inactive disease alternating within a single patient.

Diagnosis is usually made by conventional angiography. Treatment involves chronic glucocorticoids, with some patients shown to benefit from use of the immunosuppressive agents methotrexate or cyclophosphamide. Although collateral vessels often develop around sites of stenosis, vascular surgery and angioplasty play important roles in maintaining proper blood flow to vital organs.

POLYARTERITIS NODOSA

Polyarteritis nodosa (PAN) is a medium vessel inflammatory vasculitis involving segmental necrotizing lesions, often at arterial branch points, leading to stenoses, aneurysms, thromboses, infarction, or hemorrhage. Virtually any organ system can be affected, but the more commonly involved ones include renal, gastrointestinal, and peripheral nervous systems. Elevated levels of acute-phase reactants are common. There is a well-established association between infection with both hepatitis B and C viruses and PAN, although not all patients are infected with one of these viruses. Diagnosis is usually established by either biopsy or angiography. Because the disease may often be undetected or present only after a major ischemic event has occurred, examination of surgical specimens may lead to its diagnosis.

Treatment of PAN is based on glucocorticoid therapy, with other immunosuppressive agents used in more severe cases. The use of antiviral therapy in patients with positive serologic studies for hepatitis B or C has gained favor, and early reports of this approach are encouraging.

CHURG-STRAUSS SYNDROME

Churg-Strauss syndrome (CSS), also known as allergic granulomatosis and angiitis, is a medium- and small-vessel vasculitis that has a number of extravascular manifestations that distinguish it from other vasculitides. The classic presentation of CSS is that of a middle-aged person with chronic asthma who develops pulmonary infiltrates, vasculitis, and eosinophilia. The vasculitis commonly involves the skin, peripheral nerves, and gastrointestinal system, but other organs may be affected. Biopsy specimens often show microgranulomas and eosinophilic deposits. The lung infiltrates may be patchy and are extremely responsive to glucocorticoids. There have been some recent case reports of CSS occurring after initiation of treatment with leukotriene inhibitors for asthma. Diagnosis can be made on clinical grounds when most of the manifestations are present, but tissue biopsy is often necessary. Eosinophilia is present in almost all patients at diagnosis but resolves rapidly on administration of glucocorticoids. Antineutrophil cytoplasmic autoantibodies (ANCA) are positive in many patients with CSS, usually of the P-ANCA/anti-MPO type (see later).

Treatment is based on glucocorticoids, but other immunosuppressive agents are sometimes used in an attempt to allow for successful tapering of glucocorticoids. The prognosis is fairly good for patients with CSS, but relapsing disease is common.

WEGENER'S GRANULOMATOSIS

Wegener's granulomatosis (WG) is a small-to-medium vessel vasculitis with many extravascular manifestations. Although any anatomic area can be affected by WG, the three most common sites of involvement are the sinuses and upper airway, the lungs, and the kidneys. Patients may only be diagnosed after months or even years of subtle symptoms. However, WG can also present with fulminant alveolar hemorrhage and/or rapidly progressive glomerulonephritis, both of which account for much of the mortality in the disease. Destruction of the nasal and sinus tissues may result in facial deformities. Inflammatory pseudotumors may form anywhere but are common in the lung and retro-orbital spaces. Skin, peripheral nerve, and eye involvement is common.

Diagnosis is usually based on tissue biopsy. Tests for ANCA (see later) are positive in 90% of patients with renal involvement and 70% of patients without renal disease at presentation. Most positive ANCA are of the C-ANCA/anti-PR3 type, but P-ANCA/MPO positivity is also seen.

The mortality of untreated WG approaches 100%. Treatment with glucocorticoids is helpful in stabilizing the acute inflammatory process but is almost always inadequate. Thus, patients are treated with a combination of glucocorticoids and immunosuppressive agents, especially cyclophosphamide or methotrexate. Relapse is common, even many years after remission of disease.

HENOCH-SCHÖNLEIN PURPURA

Henoch-Schönlein purpura (HSP) is a small vessel vasculitis most commonly affecting children and young adults, although it can present at any age. The classic clinical triad of palpable purpura, arthritis, and abdominal pain occurs in 80% of patients. Fever and glomerulonephritis are also common manifestations. Immunoglobulin and complement deposition can be seen in affected tissues, and serum IgA levels are often elevated. IgA deposition in glomerular lesions is characteristic. Diagnosis is usually made on clinical and laboratory grounds. Although HSP can occasionally result in bowel perforation or significant renal disease, the majority of patients have no long-term sequelae. Although most cases remit within weeks of presentation, remission in the subsequent few months is common. Treatment of HSP is usually supportive, with nonsteroidal anti-inflammatory agents used for arthralgias and arthritis. Glucocorticoids are sometimes used in more symptomatic patients. The treatment of those patients who develop chronic renal disease is controversial, but it may involve glucocorticoids and immunosuppressive agents.

LEUKOCYTOCLASTIC VASCULITIS

Leukocytoclastic vasculitis (LCV) is more a sign of disease than a unique vasculitis. LCV refers to inflammation and fibrinoid necrosis of vessel walls and deposition of cellular debris in the surrounding tissue of the skin.

The clinical sign of LCV is palpable purpura that can be seen in most of the medium and small vessel vasculitides.

LCV may be the only obvious sign of a systemic vasculitis; thus, all patients with LCV must be evaluated extensively for more diffuse disease as well as various infectious diseases. When an isolated finding, LCV is often a manifestation of a drug reaction. Most classes of drugs have been implicated in causing LCV, although proper evidence of causality is often lacking. It is prudent to discontinue any nonessential medication, especially those recently instituted, in patients with newly diagnosed LCV.

Therapy for LCV is directed at the underlying vasculitis or other disease. In cases of presumed drug-induced LCV, drug discontinuation may be sufficient or a short course of glucocorticoids may be given.

Diagnosis

The diagnosis of vasculitis is made by combining the clinical presentation with laboratory, radiographic, or pathologic data. The "gold standard" for the diagnosis of any vasculitis remains tissue biopsy. Commonly sampled sites include skin, peripheral nerves, lungs, sinuses, kidneys, and temporal arteries. Because the inflammation and necrosis of vasculitis often involve skip lesions, multiple sections from various tissue levels, especially vessels, are sampled from the biopsy material. It is important to understand that the diagnosis of vasculitis may come from tissue abnormalities that do *not* involve vascular inflammation per se. For example, a biopsy from a pulmonary nodule in a patient with Wegener's granulomatosis may show granulomas with palisading histiocytes and giant cells but no vascular inflammation or destruction, yet such a biopsy would still be diagnostic for Wegener's granulomatosis.

Angiography can be very useful in diagnosing vasculitis or in evaluating the extent of disease. Vasculitis may cause stenoses, tapering, microaneurysms, and other abnormalities that alter flow. However, only those syndromes involving medium or large arteries will show abnormalities on traditional angiography. Magnetic resonance arteriography is evolving into an increasingly useful tool for studying vascular disease, with the resolution of images rapidly improving. However, both catheter-based and magnetic resonance arteriography can be misleading for the diagnosis of vasculitis because vasospasm, atherosclerosis, noninflammatory endothelial diseases, emboli, or thrombi may all cause abnormalities on angiography. Current angiographic techniques cannot detect small vessel vasculitis.

Certain laboratory studies are useful in diagnosing vasculitis. Urinalysis may show red blood cell casts, providing strong evidence of glomerulonephritis, a common aspect of vasculitis. ANCA, which are discussed in detail later, may be extremely useful in the evaluation of certain types of vasculitis. Other laboratory abnormalities, such as eosinophilia and elevated acute-phase reactants,

TABLE 86–3 Mimickers of Vasculitis

Infection
Meningococcemia
Sepsis
Syphilis

Neoplasms
Kaposi's sarcoma
Lymphoma

Emboli
Cardiac emboli
Cholesterol emboli

Thrombosis
Cerebral artery
Renal vein

Vasoconstriction
Drugs (e.g., cocaine, vasopressors)
Blood (e.g., subarachnoid hemorrhage)

Fibrosis
Radiation
Previously healed or resolving vasculitis

Atherosclerosis
Carotid disease and strokes
Peripheral vascular disease

Congenital Abnormalities/Anatomic Variants
Fibromuscular dysplasia (e.g., renal arteries)
Ehlers-Danlos syndrome
Aneurysms

Miscellaneous Disorders
Amyloidosis
Sarcoidosis
Calciphylaxis

may be suggestive of and consistent with vasculitis but are never diagnostic alone.

A variety of pathologic processes may mimic the clinical presentation of vasculitis, leading to misdiagnosis. Table 86–3 outlines some of these processes and provides specific examples. Given that vasculitis is a rare diagnosis and that the treatment often involves significant toxic effects, it is imperative that clinicians conduct a thorough evaluation to exclude other diagnoses.

Autoantibodies and Vasculitis

The discovery of the association between ANCA and the spectrum of vasculitis that includes Wegener's granulomatosis, microscopic polyangiitis, and the Churg-Strauss syndrome (allergic granulomatous vasculitis) has been an important advance in the diagnosis of these diseases. ANCA are detected by both immunofluorescence and enzyme-linked immunosorbent assay. Antibodies to proteinase 3 (PR3) produce the cytoplasmic immunofluorescence pattern (C-ANCA), and antibodies to myeloperoxidase (MPO) produce the perinuclear immunofluorescence pattern (P-ANCA). The combination of positive ANCA by immunofluorescence and enzyme-linked immunosorbent assay provides the most specificity and, in some clinical settings, may allow for the diagnosis of vasculitis to be made. ANCA positivity and frank vasculitis are increasingly being reported in response to exposure to certain medications, including hydralazine, propylthiouracil, and others. Although there are some reports linking ANCA to the pathogenesis of certain vasculitides, more research is needed to establish firmly the roles of these antibodies, if any, in the pathogenesis of these diseases.

Treatment

Treatment of specific vasculitides is described earlier, but some general comments apply to most types of vasculitis. These diseases are serious and often life-threatening and almost always require medical therapy. Although glucocorticoids and various immunosuppressive agents are mainstays for the treatment of vasculitides, very few large, controlled trials have been conducted in these disorders, and much of the treatment approach is based on expert anecdotal opinion. Cyclophosphamide, despite its serious acute and chronic toxic effects, remains the most widely used agent for serious life-threatening disease. In some cases of drug-induced disease, drug discontinuation alone may result in complete remission of active vasculitis.

Some measures can be taken to lessen toxic effects of therapy for vasculitis. Patients who will be treated with an extended course of glucocorticoids should all be evaluated for osteoporosis, with prophylactic therapy initiated early in the treatment. The teratogenicity of methotrexate, cyclophosphamide, and other immunosuppressive drugs must be taken into account when treating women of childbearing years. Infection during immunosuppression is a major cause of morbidity and mortality, and routine or opportunistic infections must be considered when patients have new clinical findings. It is now the standard of care to prescribe prophylaxis, usually with trimethoprim-sulfamethoxazole, for *Pneumocystis carinii* pneumonia in patients receiving glucocorticoids and an immunosuppressive agent. Antivirals and newer immunomodulating agents are being developed and will be investigated for the treatment of systemic vasculitis.

One of the most common treatment errors is the tendency toward overtreatment. Overtreatment may involve either unnecessarily high doses of glucocorticoids or extremely extended courses of medication. The cumulative toxic effects of glucocorticoids must be balanced against the risk of irreversible disease recurrence in patients under regular medical supervision. The treatment of vasculitis should be managed by physicians experienced in both the clinical course of these rare diseases and the use of immunosuppressive therapies.

REFERENCES

Cupps TR: Vasculitis: A. Epidemiology, pathology, and pathogenesis. *In* Klippel JH (ed): Primer of the Rheumatic Diseases, 11th ed. Atlanta: The Arthritis Foundation, 1997, pp 289–293.

Hoffman GS: Vasculitis: C. Treatment. *In* Klippel JH (ed): Primer of the Rheumatic Diseases, 11th ed. Atlanta: The Arthritis Foundation, 1997, pp 300–304.

Hunder GC: Vasculitis: B. Clinical and laboratory features. *In* Klippel JH (ed): Primer of the Rheumatic Diseases, 11th ed. Atlanta: The Arthritis Foundation, 1997, pp 293–300.

Rosenwasser LJ: The vasculitic syndromes. *In* Goldman L, Bennett JC (eds): Cecil Textbook of Medicine, 21st ed. Philadelphia: WB Saunders, 2000, pp 1524–1527.

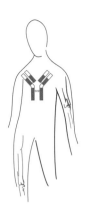

87

CRYSTAL ARTHROPATHIES

Joseph H. Korn

Gout

Gout is a metabolic disorder first described by Hippocrates approximately 2500 years ago. Its clinical manifestations include acute and chronic arthritis, deposits of uric acid in and around joints and skin (tophi), renal stones, and, in most patients, hyperuricemia. Uric acid is the metabolic breakdown product of purine metabolism. Accumulation of uric acid can be a result of a primary defect in purine/uric acid metabolism leading to overproduction of uric acid and/or a result of a primary defect in renal clearance. Alternatively, secondary or acquired abnormalities of uric acid production or excretion can lead to uric acid accumulation and clinical manifestations of gout.

EPIDEMIOLOGY

Gout is principally a disease of men and, to a lesser extent, postmenopausal women. The prevalence of gout is directly related to the degree of hyperuricemia. Uric acid levels, which are low in childhood, increase at puberty, the rise approximately twofold greater in males than in females. Levels in men and women increase with age, with a sharper increase in women after menopause, but a substantial difference between men and women is maintained. Overall, gout occurs in 2% to 3% of the adult male population. The prevalence is age dependent: 0.24% younger than age 44, 3.4% in the 45- to 64-year age group, and rising to 5% in those older than age 65. In individuals with normal uric acid levels, the risk is less than 1%, rising to 20% to 30% in those with uric acid levels 2 to 3 mg/dL above normal. It appears that for a given uric acid level, the risk for women of developing gout is similar; however, because of lower uric acid levels, the prevalence of gout is much lower in women than in men and gout is rarely noted before menopause. Age-specific prevalence rates in women are less than 0.1% when it occurs in women younger than age 44, 1.4% from ages 45 to 64, and 1.9% in those older than age 65.

URIC ACID METABOLISM

Uric acid is the breakdown product of the purines adenine and guanine. The low solubility of uric acid, which at neutral pH is largely in the form of monosodium urate, combined with uric acid excretion that normally just keeps pace with production, allows for accumulation of crystals of monosodium urate in the body in susceptible individuals. Total-body uric acid stores are approximately 1800 mg, and turnover is high, about one third daily. Two thirds of daily input comes from de novo purine synthesis and one third from dietary sources. Excretion is two thirds renal, with the balance largely eliminated in the gastrointestinal tract.

Purine biosynthetic pathways have three basic features: (1) de novo synthesis driven by phosphoribosylpyrophosphate (PRPP) and glutamine, (2) purine interconversion (e.g., adenylic acid—inosinic acid—guanylic acid) and (3) reutilization pathways whereby the intermediate breakdown products adenine, guanine, and hypoxanthine are recaptured by reaction with PRPP rather than undergoing further degradation to xanthine and uric acid. Recapture is catalyzed by the enzyme hypoxanthine-guanine phosphoribosyl transferase (HGPRTase). Abnormalities of this enzyme lead to overaccumulation of PRPP and drive purine synthesis, resulting in increased serum levels of uric acid. Severe homozygous deficiency of HGPRTase results in the self-mutilation disease Lesch-Nyhan syndrome. Some glycogen storage diseases and abnormalities of pentose shunt metabolism can also lead to uric acid overproduction.

Overall, 10% to 20% of patients with primary gout have increased uric acid production, of which less than 2% is due to a defined enzyme deficiency. Diseases with increased cell turnover such as leukemias and lymphomas, disorders of hematopoiesis (i.e., sickle cell disease, thalassemia), and widespread psoriasis can lead to uric acid overproduction and secondary gout (Table 87–1). Clinically, the most important stimulus to uric acid production is alcohol, which can increase de novo synthesis dramatically.

In the kidney, uric acid is filtered at the glomerulus, essentially completely reabsorbed in the proximal tu-

TABLE 87-1   Causes of Hyperuricemia

Decreased Urate Excretion	Increased Urate Production
Impaired renal function	Ethanol
Dehydration	Myeloproliferative diseases
Acidosis	Ineffective erythropoiesis (sickle cell, thalassemia)
Low dose salicylates	Widespread psoriasis
Diuretics	Cytotoxic drugs
Pyrazinamide	Glycogen storage diseases
Cyclosporine	G6PD deficiency
Levodopa	HGPRTase deficiency
Ethambutol	Increased PRPP synthetase activity
Nicotinic acid	
Hypothyroidism	

G6PD = glucose-6-phosphate dehydrogenase; HGPRTase = hypoxanthine-guanine phosphoribosyl transferase; PRPP = phosphoribosyl pyrophosphate.

bule, and then actively secreted and reabsorbed in the distal tubule and collecting tubule. More than two thirds of individuals with primary gout, and up to 90% in some series, have normal production of uric acid but have a primary and specific defect in uric acid clearance; that is, a higher serum uric acid level is needed to excrete the same amount of uric acid. Secondary gout may result from any disorder leading to decreased renal function; from decreased urine flow and acidosis, which favor urate reabsorption; or from drugs that compete for organic acid transport. Diuretics (including thiazides and furosemide), aspirin (which at low doses preferentially inhibits urate secretion), dehydration, and acidosis all lead to decreased urate clearance. Lead nephropathy has been long associated with gout (saturnine gout); as a

tubular toxin, lead has disproportionate effects on urate clearance.

PATHOGENESIS OF ACUTE ARTHRITIS

When there is an imbalance between uric acid production and excretion, uric acid accumulates at various sites as both microscopic deposits and grossly visible deposits called tophi. Intra-articular and periarticular urate crystals are important in the pathogenesis of acute attacks of gout. Attacks of gout are thought to result from either local trauma leading to shedding of crystals from local deposits or de novo precipitation of microcrystals (Fig. 87–1). Trauma to the first metatarsophalangeal joint from walking may underlie its predominant involvement.

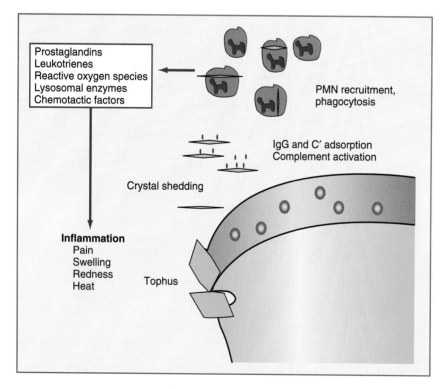

Prostaglandins
Leukotrienes
Reactive oxygen species
Lysosomal enzymes
Chemotactic factors

PMN recruitment, phagocytosis

IgG and C' adsorption
Complement activation

Crystal shedding

Inflammation
Pain
Swelling
Redness
Heat

Tophus

FIGURE 87–1   Pathogenesis of acute gout. Shedding of crystals leads to leukocyte activation and release of inflammatory mediators.

Increased uric acid synthesis and increased serum levels may also precipitate attacks. For example, dehydration, acidosis, alcohol ingestion, and extensive cell death from chemotherapy all lead to temporary rises in uric acid levels in the blood. Rapid lowering of uric acid levels, with allopurinol, for example, sometimes leads to partial solubilization and breakdown of tophi and crystal shedding. Newly formed or shed uric acid crystals in the synovial fluid or interstitium may activate complement, leading to polymorphonuclear leukocyte (PMN) chemotaxis and crystal phagocytosis. PMN activation leads to release of inflammatory mediators, including prostaglandins, leukotrienes, and reactive oxygen species, as well as further PMN accumulation. The latter is mediated by chemotactic leukotrienes (LTB4) and chemokines, such as interleukin-8, facilitated by increased vascular permeability from the actions of these mediators.

CLINICAL PRESENTATION

Acute gouty arthritis is characterized by a rapid crescendo onset. Typically, the patient goes to sleep without symptoms and is awakened by severe pain, erythema, and swelling in the affected joint. The first metatarsophalangeal joint is the most commonly involved, and this involvement is termed *podagra*. Pain and inflammation extend to the skin, which is often very erythematous and warm. As described by Sydenham in the 1800s, there is an inability to "bear the weight of bedclothes," and the patient frequently cannot put on a sock or cover the foot with a sheet. Any joint may be involved in acute gout, but the foot, ankle, and knee, followed by small joints of the hands, the wrists, and the elbows, follow the toe in frequency; involvement of the hips, shoulders, and apophyseal joints is unusual. The predominant involvement of lower extremity joints may be due to hydrostatic factors. During the day, with the legs in the dependent position, there is transudation of plasma into the interstitial space; at night, water is more quickly reabsorbed than uric acid, leading to higher concentrations of uric acid in the interstitial fluid and precipitation of crystals. The lower temperature in joints may also contribute to urate precipitation.

On examination, the affected joint is warm or hot, and any motion is resisted. The overlying skin is red to violaceous and extraordinarily tender; inflammation commonly extends beyond the confines of the joint. For example, when the great toe is involved, inflammation and erythema may extend to the midfoot or proximally. Occasionally two or more joints are simultaneously involved. A similar process may occur in bursae, particularly the olecranon, and may cause confusion with septic bursitis. At times the process may be both more subdued and widespread, leading to chronic polyarthritis, which may clinically masquerade as rheumatoid arthritis or other inflammatory arthritides.

When there is significant uric acid accumulation in the body, visible tophi may be present. These are most commonly seen adjacent to joints near articular surfaces, in bursae, and on extensor surfaces of tendons and, less commonly, on cartilaginous structures such as the pinnae of the ear. In severe cases there may be deposition in soft tissues, including the renal interstitium, where higher concentrations of uric acid are achieved. Individuals who overproduce and overexcrete uric acid are at risk for the development of renal stones; in general, those with greater than 700 mg/day of uric acid in the urine are at risk. Stones may be composed of uric acid, or uric acid may form a nidus for calcium and other stones.

DIAGNOSIS

The acute onset of inflammatory monoarthritis in a joint of the lower extremity, particularly in middle-aged and older men, is likely to be gout, particularly when the first metatarsophalangeal joint is affected. The differential diagnosis includes septic arthritis, pseudogout (calcium pyrophosphate deposition disease), reactive arthritis/Reiter's syndrome, monoarticular presentation of rheumatoid arthritis or other inflammatory arthritides, Lyme disease, viral arthritis, and sarcoid. Infectious arthritis is obviously the most important and usually the most difficult to differentiate at presentation. Low-grade fever is common in acute gout, and occasionally the patient's temperature may reach 39°C (102.2°F). The patient with septic joint disease usually has a more insidious onset than a patient with gout, is more systemically ill, has chills and sweats accompanying the fever, and has peripheral leukocytosis and toxic granulation of peripheral blood PMNs.

The joint fluid in gout is inflammatory, with more than 10,000 white blood cells (sometimes >50,000) and more than 90% PMNs. Polarized light microscopic examination of synovial fluid is the key to diagnosis. Intracellular, needle-shaped, negatively birefringent crystals are both pathognomonic for and essential to the definitive diagnosis of acute gouty arthritis: viewed under polarized light with a red compensator, urate crystals are yellow when parallel to the compensator axis and blue when perpendicular. Crystals may range in length from 1 to 2 μm to 15 to 20 μm, sometimes appearing like a lance that has pierced the neutrophil. Extracellular crystals, when typical in size and shape, are helpful but not diagnostic of acute gouty arthritis. Urate crystals may also be seen in the white "cheesy" or toothpaste-like material obtained from tophaceous deposits and occasionally from a joint into which a tophus has ruptured.

In 5% to 10% of cases of gouty arthritis, crystals are not seen in the affected joint; occasionally, crystals may be found in an asymptomatic joint. In other instances, particularly in small joints such as the metatarsophalangeal, synovial fluid may be difficult to aspirate. In a patient with known gout, a presumptive diagnosis is reasonable unless clinical features suggest septic joint disease. Serum uric acid is not helpful; many patients have normal levels at the time of an acute attack, and 15% never have levels outside the normal range, at least with routine testing. Furthermore, elevated uric acid levels are found in a high proportion of the nongouty population. Radiographs may show tophi or typical "rat bite" marginal joint erosions with sclerotic borders and overhanging edges characteristic of gout. Mild peripheral blood leukocytosis, elevated erythrocyte sedimentation rate, and increased acute-phase proteins may be seen but are not diagnostically useful.

CHRONIC POLYARTICULAR GOUT

Gout may manifest as chronic polyarthritis with or without acute attacks of arthritis. Patients often have multiple juxta-articular tophi and develop destructive, erosive joint disease. Occasionally, polyarticular gout may look like rheumatoid arthritis, and tophi may be mistaken for rheumatoid nodules. Radiographs in gout typically show sclerotic changes at erosive borders, in contrast to the nonreactive margins in rheumatoid arthritis. Examination of synovial fluid is diagnostic, and every rheumatoid arthritis patient should have synovial fluid examined for crystals at least once.

TREATMENT

Acute Arthritis

A variety of treatments are effective for acute gouty arthritis (Table 87–2). Joint drainage per se has a therapeutic effect in removing degenerating PMN and in relieving joint distention. Intra-articular corticosteroids have rapid onset of action and are almost free of side effects; they may be instilled at the time of joint aspiration if the diagnosis of gout is fairly certain. Oral prednisone, in a tapering course starting at 30 to 40 mg/day, may be used; however, in patients with underlying diabetes or diabetic susceptibility, hyperglycemia may be triggered. Nonsteroidal anti-inflammatory drugs are highly effective when adequate anti-inflammatory doses are used. Indomethacin has been the traditional agent in doses of 150 to 200 mg/day for the first 2 to 3 days. Colchicine prevents release of PMN chemotactic factor(s) and inhibits phospholipase activation, which is needed for prostaglandin synthesis. It is particularly effective early in the attack, resulting in rapid resolution of symptoms, and is much less effective after 24 hours. Colchicine should be given as 1.2 mg orally initially, followed by up to two additional 0.6-mg doses at 2-hour intervals. The practice of using hourly doses until abdominal cramps or diarrhea supervene is to be discouraged, and caution should be used when there is hepatic or renal insufficiency. Intravenous colchicine is effective and rapid in onset, but a few cases of fatal arrhythmia have been reported and its use has been largely abandoned. Parenteral adrenocorticotropic hormone and parenteral glucocorticoids are both effective treatments but more costly. It is reasonable to treat patients who have had acute gout with colchicine prophylaxis for several weeks to prevent recurrent attacks (see later).

INTERCRITICAL GOUT

After a single attack of gout, the physician must decide whether to recommend long-term therapy. A substantial number of patients will have rare attacks, even untreated, and there is little rationale for lifelong therapy. In patients who have tophi, polyarticular disease, or renal stones, long-term treatment is clearly indicated. Patients with very high serum uric acid levels or whose first attack occurs at a young age are at greatest risk of frequent attacks and of developing chronic gouty arthritis, tophaceous gout, and/or destructive joint disease. After a first attack, after the acute period is over, serum and 24-hour urinary excretion of uric acid should be evaluated. Unless the serum urate is markedly deviated from normal, it is reasonable to observe the patient. If patients have frequent recurrent attacks, prophylactic treatment is advised (Table 87–3). In older patients with mild gout and occasional attacks, prophylaxis with colchicine alone may be sufficient. In patients with frequent attacks, or when colchicine alone is ineffective, treatment directed at uric acid is indicated. Probenecid inhibits urate reabsorption in the distal tubule and promotes excretion. Its uricosuric effect depends on normal or near-normal renal function. Probenecid is particularly useful in patients with impaired urate clearance, that is, increased serum levels and low-to-normal daily excretion. In patients who are overproducers of uric acid, or when there are tissue stores of uric acid (i.e., tophi), there may be a sustained increase in uric acid excretion to a level where there is risk of renal stones.

Allopurinol inhibits xanthine oxidase, the enzyme that catalyzes the formation of xanthine from hypoxanthine and uric acid from xanthine. It is effective in lowering uric acid levels whether due to impaired clearance or overproduction. Allopurinol, although generally safe, has greater toxicity than probenecid and has been associated with hepatitis and severe skin reactions. If allopurinol or probenecid are used, colchicine prophylaxis should be initiated at the same time and continued for several

TABLE 87–2 Treatment of Acute Gout

Drug	Route	Dose (day 1)	Side Effects
Colchicine	PO	1.2–2.4 mg	Diarrhea, cramps
Methylprednisolone	Intra-articularly	10–80 mg	Cost
Prednisone	PO	30–40 mg	Increased blood sugar
			Mask infection
Adrenocorticotropic hormone	IM	40–80 units	Cost
NSAIDS	PO	Anti-inflammatory doses (e.g., indomethacin, 150–200 mg; naproxen, 1500 mg)	Gastritis, bleeding, renal insufficiency

IM = intramuscularly; PO = orally.

TABLE 87–3 Treatment of Intercritical Gout

Drug	Dose	Mechanism of Action	Side Effects
Colchicine	0.6–1.2 mg/day	Prophylaxis for attacks No effect on uric acid	Very safe, rare myopathy
Probenecid	1–1.5 g/day	Uricosuric No anti-inflammatory activity	Very safe
Allopurinol	300–600 mg/day	Inhibits uric acid synthesis No anti-inflammatory activity	Dermatitis, hepatitis, marrow failure

months. Initiation of allopurinol, in particular, can precipitate gouty attacks; presumably, the rapid lowering of uric acid mobilizes tissue deposits and facilitates shedding of preformed crystals. Neither allopurinol nor probenecid should be started in the setting of an acute attack.

Dietary purines account for a relatively small proportion of daily uric acid turnover. Anchovies, sweetbreads, organ meats, and cellular leafy vegetables such as spinach are particularly high in purines. Other than avoiding ethanol and perhaps anchovies, there is little rationale and little clinical effect from drastic dietary alterations.

Patients with chronic arthritis should have pharmacologic therapy directed at lowering serum uric acid. In addition, chronic use of nonsteroidal agents (other than aspirin) may be required for control of chronic pain and inflammation. Occasionally, surgical removal of tophi may be beneficial, particularly in locations where they become irritated, inflamed, or infected.

Asymptomatic Hyperuricemia

There is little rationale in treating asymptomatic elevations of uric acid, particularly if they are due to treatment with diuretics. In patients who are to receive chemotherapy, short-term prophylaxis with allopurinol may prevent both gout and renotubular precipitation of uric acid.

Calcium Pyrophosphate Deposition Disease

Calcium pyrophosphate deposition disease (CPPD) is due to deposition of crystals of calcium pyrophosphate in articular cartilage and fibrocartilage. Such deposits are common and increase in incidence with advancing age, affecting over 30% of individuals older than the age of 80. In most individuals, these are an asymptomatic radiographic finding termed *chondrocalcinosis*. The menisci of the knee, the triangular fibrocartilage of the wrist, and the symphysis pubis are most commonly affected. Articular cartilage may be involved anywhere, but the knee, wrist, and ankle are the sites most commonly involved. Acute gout-like attacks of arthritis may result when crystals shed from such deposits; hence, the disease is often called pseudogout. Occasionally, particularly in middle-aged women, a chronic polyarthritis resembling rheumatoid arthritis may occur, involving especially the wrists and fingers. Acute hemorrhagic arthritis has also been reported.

CPPD is increased in patients with diabetes, hyperparathyroidism, gout, and hemochromatosis, among other disorders. In patients with hemochromatosis, CPPD occurs at an earlier age, may be the presenting clinical finding, and characteristically involves the second and third metacarpophalangeal joints, areas usually not involved in idiopathic CPPD.

DIAGNOSIS AND TREATMENT

The diagnosis of acute CPPD arthropathy or pseudogout is made by the finding of intracellular, positively birefringent, rhomboid-shaped crystals in synovial fluid aspirates. Crystals may be small and fragmented and are less easily found than urate crystals. Chondrocalcinosis on a radiograph suggests, but does not establish, the diagnosis of acute pseudogout. Acute attacks of CPPD are effectively treated with nonsteroidal anti-inflammatory drugs or with intra-articular corticosteroids.

Other Crystal Disorders

Hydroxyapatite crystals are composed of basic calcium phosphates and deposit at soft tissue sites, particularly tendons and bursae. Calcific tendonitis, especially in the supraspinatus tendon and subacromial bursae, is one manifestation. Oxalate crystals may deposit in cartilage and intervertebral discs.

REFERENCES

Hershfield MS: Gout and uric acid metabolism. *In* Goldman L, Bennett JC (eds): Cecil Textbook of Medicine, 21st ed. Philadelphia: WB Saunders, 2000, pp 1541–1548.

Kelley WN, Wortmann RL: Gout and hyperuricemia. *In* Kelley WN, Harris ED Jr, Ruddy S, Sledge CB (eds): Textbook of Rheumatology, 5th ed. Philadelphia: WB Saunders, 1997, p 1313.

Ryan LM, McCarty DJ: Calcium pyrophosphate crystal deposition disease, pseudogout and articular chondrocalcinosis. *In* Koopman WJ (ed): Arthritis and Allied Conditions, 13th ed. Baltimore: Williams & Wilkins, 1997, p 2103.

Schumacher HR Jr: Crystal deposition arthropathies. *In* Goldman L, Bennett JC (eds): Cecil Textbook of Medicine, 21st ed. Philadelphia: WB Saunders, 2000, pp 1548–1550.

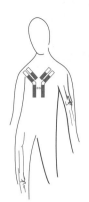

88

OSTEOARTHRITIS

Robert W. Simms

Osteoarthritis (OA) is the most common joint disorder, occurring in 60% to 90% of individuals older than the age of 65. OA is the most common cause of long-term disability in most populations. It has a large economic impact as the result of both direct medical costs (cost of physician visits, laboratory tests, medications, operations) and indirect costs (lost wages, home care, lost wage-earning opportunities). OA is an increasingly important public health problem whose impact will increase as the population ages.

Pathology

Also known as degenerative arthritis, OA is characterized by the progressive loss of articular cartilage with associated remodeling of subchondral bone. OA, however, is a complex disorder with one or more identifiable risk factors, which range from biomechanical, metabolic, and inflammatory processes to age, gender, and genetic factors. OA may result from a variety of biomechanical insults, including repetitive or isolated joint trauma. Certain occupations that pose repeated joint stress (such as knee OA in dock workers and finger OA in assembly line workers) predispose to early OA. Gender and race also figure prominently as risk factors for OA. Whereas OA is equally prevalent in men and women younger than age 45, it is more common among women after age 55. Nodal OA, involving the distal and proximal interphalangeal joints, is much more common in women and tends to affect female first-degree relatives. Knee OA is more common among African-American women than whites. Certain metabolic disorders such as hemochromatosis and ochronosis are also associated with OA. Mutations in the genes encoding types II, IX, and X collagen have been identified in several kinships, resulting in abnormal collagen and premature OA. Inflammatory joint disease such as rheumatoid arthritis may result in cartilage degradation and biomechanical factors that lead to secondary OA. The destruction of articular cartilage is therefore best viewed as the final product of a variety of possible etiologic factors.

OA is classified into two basic forms: primary and secondary (Table 88–1). Primary OA is the idiopathic variety, which may be localized or generalized. Secondary OA is the result of a range of conditions, including congenital and developmental disorders, other bone and joint disorders, and endocrine, neurologic, and miscellaneous causes.

The earliest finding in OA is fibrillation of the most superficial layer of the articular cartilage. With time, the disruption of the articular surface becomes deeper with extension of the fibrillations to subchondral bone, fragmentation of cartilage with release into the joint, matrix degradation, and, eventually, complete loss of cartilage, leaving only exposed bone. Early in this process the cartilage matrix undergoes significant change with increased water and decreased proteoglycan content. This is in contrast to dehydration of cartilage, which occurs with aging. The "tidemark" zone, separating the calcified cartilage from the radial zone, becomes invaded with capillaries. Chondrocytes initially are metabolically active and release a variety of cytokines and metalloproteinases, contributing to matrix degradation, which in the later stages results in penetration of fissures to subchondral bone, as well as release of fibrillated cartilage into the joint space. An imbalance between tissue inhibitors of metalloproteinases and the production of metalloproteinases may be operative in OA. Subchondral bone increases in density, and cystlike bone cavities containing myxoid, fibrous, or cartilaginous tissue occur. Osteophytes, bony proliferations at the margin of joints at the site of bone-cartilage interface, may also form at capsule insertions. Osteophytes contribute to joint motion restriction and are thought to be the result of new bone formation in response to the degeneration of articular cartilage, but the precise mechanism for their production remains unknown.

A variety of crystals have been identified in synovial fluid and other tissues from osteoarthritic joints, most notably calcium pyrophosphate dihydrate and apatite. Although these crystals clearly have potent inflammatory potential, their role in the pathogenesis of OA remains uncertain. Frequently, these crystals are asymptomatic and do not correlate with extent or severity of disease.

TABLE 88-1   Classification of Osteoarthritis

Idiopathic	Secondary
Localized	**Post-traumatic**
Hands	Congenital or developmental disorders
Feet	
Knee	Localized
Medial compartment	Generalized
Lateral compartment	Bone dysplasias
Patellofemoral compartment	Metabolic diseases (e.g., hemochromatosis, ochronosis)
Hip	**Calcium Deposition Disease**
Spine	Calcium pyrophosphate deposition disease
Generalized	Apatite arthropathy
Small joint (peripheral) and spine	**Other**
Large joint and spine	Inflammatory joint diseases
Mixed and spine	Rheumatoid arthritis, septic arthritis
	Neuropathic arthropathy
	Avascular necrosis

The diversity of risk factors predisposing to OA suggests that a wide variety of insults to articular cartilage, including biomechanical trauma and chronic articular inflammation as well as genetic and metabolic factors, can contribute to or trigger the cascade of events that result in the characteristic pathologic features of OA described earlier (Fig. 88–1). At some point, the cartilage degradative process becomes irreversible, perhaps the result of an imbalance of regulatory molecules such as tissue inhibitors of metalloproteinases. With progressive changes in articular cartilage, joint mechanics become altered, in turn perpetuating the degradative process.

Clinical Features and Diagnosis

Pain is the characteristic feature of OA. Pain is typically deep aching discomfort, slow in onset, initially aggravated with activity, improved with rest, and localized to the involved joint. Occasionally, pain is referred to a distant site, for example, pain originating in the hip may be referred to the anterior thigh or knee. The pain associated with OA may result from venous engorgement of subchondral bone, periarticular tissues, or synovitis. With progressive disease and complete loss of cartilage, pain may occur at rest. Stiffness, particularly after prolonged inactivity, is characteristic but is not as prolonged as that associated with rheumatoid arthritis, usually lasting for 20 or 30 minutes. Exacerbation of symptoms with weather change is a common feature reported by patients with OA. Examination reveals joint line ten-

derness and bony enlargement of the joint with or without effusion. Crepitation on motion and limitation of joint motion are additional characteristic features.

Several subtypes of generalized OA have been identified. The nodal form of OA, involving primarily the distal interphalangeal joints, is most common in middle-aged women, typically with a strong family history among female first-degree relatives. Erosive, inflammatory OA is associated with prominent erosive, destructive changes, especially in the finger joints, and may suggest rheumatoid arthritis, although systemic inflammatory signs and other typical features of rheumatoid arthritis (nodules, proliferative synovitis, extra-articular features, rheumatoid factor) are absent.

The diagnosis of OA is based on the history, physical examination, and characteristic radiographic features. The physician must distinguish OA from inflammatory joint diseases such as rheumatoid arthritis and identify those patients who have the secondary form of OA. Distinguishing OA from inflammatory joint diseases involves identifying the characteristic pattern of joint involvement and the nature of the individual joint deformity. Joints involved in OA include the distal interphalangeal joints, proximal interphalangeal joints, first carpometacarpal joints, facet joints of the cervical and lumbar spine, hips, knees, and first metatarsophalangeal joints. Involvement of the wrist, elbows, shoulders, and ankles is uncommon, except in the case of trauma, congenital disease, or endocrine/metabolic disease. Joint deformity associated with OA is characteristic in several locations: Heberden's and Bouchard's nodes in the hands and, depending on the compartment of the knee, valgus or varus deformity. Inflammatory signs such as joint warmth, synovial thickening, and fusiform deformity are generally not seen in OA, but effusions, particularly of the knee, are common. The radiographic features of OA include subchondral sclerosis, joint space narrowing, subchondral cysts, and osteophytes.

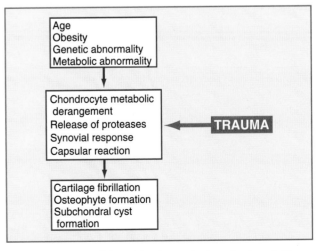

FIGURE 88–1   Scheme for the production of osteoarthritis.

Treatment

The natural history of OA is quite variable, with periods of relative stability interspersed with rapid deterioration or even improvement. The management of OA should therefore be tailored to the individual patient and may include a variety of modalities, such as education, physical measures, pharmacologic therapies, and surgical approaches. Education includes advice on joint protection, exercise, and appropriate use of pharmacologic therapies. Physical modalities encompass strengthening exercises, for example, isometric quadriceps strengthening for knee OA and grip strengthening for small-joint hand OA. The physical therapist can play an important role in both education and monitoring of specific exercises. Weight loss may retard knee OA progression in obese patients. The use of assistive devices such as a cane provides important joint protection for patients with advanced knee or hip OA. Neoprene knee braces have been shown to be beneficial, perhaps by improving proprioception. Orthotics to provide cushioning and heel wedges to counteract valgus or varus deformities of the knee may provide significant symptomatic improvement. Spinal orthoses may provide benefit to patients with significant cervical or lumbar OA. Local applications such as heat and ultrasound may provide short-term benefit.

Pharmacologic therapy for OA provides symptomatic relief but has not been shown to successfully alter the course of the disease. Although the optimal pharmacologic treatment approach remains undefined, an individualized regimen accounting for potential toxicities and patient comorbidities appears to be the most rational approach. The available pharmacologic therapies include simple analgesics, nonsteroidal anti-inflammatory drugs (NSAIDs, including the newer COX-2 selective agents), intra-articular corticosteroids, "chondroprotective" agents, and antidepressants. Simple analgesics are useful and generally well tolerated in mild to moderate OA; stronger narcotic agents may be indicated in more severe disease. The use of NSAIDs has been controversial in OA, largely because of the debate over risks and benefits. NSAIDs clearly provide analgesic benefit, but their anti-inflammatory effect has little application in OA, a predominantly noninflammatory condition. Furthermore, the potential toxicity of NSAIDs, particularly affecting the gastrointestinal tract, has created concern and calls to limit their use in OA. Agents that limit the gastrointestinal toxicity of NSAIDs, such as misoprostol and omeprazole used in combination with NSAIDs, have become popular. The newer COX-2 selective agents such as celecoxib and rofecoxib appear to have reduced gastrointestinal toxicity compared with a few selected NSAIDs, but they appear to offer no advantage in terms of efficacy (pain relief or improved function) in OA. Intra-articular therapies such as corticosteroids and synthetic hyaluronate appear to provide modest symptomatic benefit, especially in the knee. "Chondroprotective" agents such as chondroitin sulfate and glucosamine (key constituents of glycosaminoglycans) have been shown in short-term European clinical trials to be of modest symptomatic benefit in OA, although there is no evidence that these agents (which are currently classified as nutritional supplements in the United States) actually repair or retard cartilage degradation.

Surgical management of OA includes total joint replacement as well as intra-articular debridement and lavage. Total joint replacement in the hip and knee are extremely effective in relieving pain and improving function. Because the resultant artificial joints have limited life spans, however, their use is restricted to patients with end-stage OA of the hip or the knee. The roles of intra-articular lavage and joint debridement remain controversial; some studies show little long-term benefit.

REFERENCES

Kuettner KE, Thomar EJMA: Cartilage integrity and homeostasis. *In* Klippel JH (ed): Rheumatology, 2nd ed. London: CV Mosby, 1998, pp 8.6.1–8.6.13.

Schnitzer TJ: Osteoarthritis (degenerative joint disease). *In* Goldman L, Bennett JC (eds): Cecil Textbook of Medicine, 21st ed. Philadelphia: WB Saunders, 2000, pp 1550–1554.

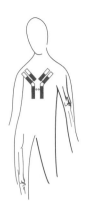

89

NONARTICULAR SOFT TISSUE DISORDERS

Robert W. Simms

The nonarticular soft tissue disorders account for the majority of musculoskeletal complaints in the general population. These disorders include a large number of anatomically localized conditions (bursitis and tendinitis), as well as a more generalized pain disorder, namely, fibromyalgia syndrome. The majority of these nonarticular soft tissue conditions include common syndromes in which the etiology and pathogenesis are poorly understood. Thus, the nonarticular soft tissue syndromes are generally best classified according to the anatomic region involved, for example, as "shoulder pain." Once the region is defined, an attempt is made to identify the structure at fault, such as supraspinatus tendon, bicipital tendon, subacromial bursa, or others. In the case of back pain, precise anatomic delineation of the structure involved (e.g., intervertebral disc, facet joint, ligaments, or paraspinal muscle) is frequently impossible. Precise data on prevalence or incidence of most nonarticular soft tissue syndromes are not available, but these conditions account for up to approximately 30% of all outpatient visits.

Etiology and Pathogenesis

The precise pathophysiology of most cases of nonarticular soft tissue disorders remains unknown, although in many cases predisposing factors can be identified, such as "overuse" or repetitive activities (e.g., tennis elbow or lateral epicondylitis) or biomechanical factors (e.g., leg-length discrepancy in trochanteric bursitis). The term *tendinitis* implies that there is an inflammatory process present in the involved tendon sheath; however, small tendon tears, periostitis, or even nerve entrapment have been postulated as potential mechanisms. Similarly, although bursitis implies bursal inflammation, demonstrable inflammation is difficult to find. In some cases, for example, in acute bursitis of the olecranon or prepatel-

lar bursa, the mechanism is an acute inflammatory response to sodium urate crystals deposited in the soft tissue, an extra-articular manifestation of gout. The favorable response of tendinitis and bursitis syndromes to anti-inflammatory agents, including corticosteroids, supports the view that at least one component of these syndromes is the result of an inflammatory process. In myofascial pain syndrome the causes are even more obscure. Frequently, overuse and trauma are cited as etiologic factors; however, many cases lack antedating mechanical factors. In the case of fibromyalgia syndrome, which is characterized by pain, muscle spasm, and tender points in muscle or tendon structures, depression may be a predisposing factor.

Classification of Bursae

Many of the soft tissue rheumatic syndromes involve bursae. Bursae are closed sacs lined with mesenchymal cells that are similar to synovial cells, which are strategically located to facilitate tissue gliding. Most bursae develop concurrently with synovial joints during embryogenesis, although new ones can develop in response to mechanical stress or inflammation (e.g., iliopsoas bursa, trochanteric bursa, semimembranous bursa). In general, bursae do not communicate with joints; an exception is the semimembranous or popliteal bursa in the knee that communicates with the anterior knee in approximately 40% of individuals. The subacromial or subdeltoid bursa communicates with the glenohumeral joint only if there is a complete tear of the rotator cuff tendon. Bursae are divided anatomically into the *superficial* bursae (e.g., suprapatellar, olecranon) and the *deep* bursae (e.g., subacromial, iliopsoas, trochanteric). Although most forms of bursitis involve isolated, local conditions, some may be the result of systemic conditions such as gout.

TABLE 89–1 Differentiating Nonarticular Soft Tissue Disorders from Articular Disease

	Nonarticular Soft Tissue Disorders	Articular Disease
Limitation of motion	Active > passive	Active = passive
Crepitus of articular surfaces (structural damage)	0	+/−
Tenderness		
Synovial (fusiform)	0	+
Local	+	0
Swelling		
Synovial (fusiform)	0	+
Local	+/−	0

Diagnosis of Nonarticular Soft Tissue Disorders

Tendinitis, bursitis, and myofascial disorders should be distinguished from articular disorders. In most cases, this can be accomplished by a careful examination of the involved structure (Table 89–1). General principles of the musculoskeletal examination are as follows:

1. Observation: If deformity or soft tissue swelling is present, is it fusiform (surrounding the entire joint in a symmetric fashion) or is it localized? Nonarticular disorders are distinguished from articular disorders by local rather than fusiform deformity.
2. Palpation: Is tenderness localized or in a fusiform distribution? Is an effusion present? Nonarticular disorders are distinguished from articular disorders by local, not fusiform or joint-line, tenderness. The presence of an effusion almost always indicates an articular disorder.
3. Assessing range of motion: The musculoskeletal examination includes the assessment of both *active* (the patient attempts to move the symptomatic structure) and *passive* (the examiner moves the symptomatic structure) range of motion.

Articular disorders are generally characterized by equal impairment of both active and passive movement (due to the mechanical limitation of joint motion resulting from proliferation of the synovial membrane, the presence of an effusion, or derangement of intra-articular structures). Nonarticular disorders are characterized by impairment of active movement to a much greater degree than passive movement.

Bursitis

CLINICAL PRESENTATION

Septic Bursitis

Superficial forms of bursitis, particularly olecranon bursitis and prepatellar and occasionally infrapatellar bursitis, are more frequently infected or involved with crystal deposition than deep bursae. Presumably, this is the result of direct extension of organisms through subcutaneous tissues. Most commonly, *Staphylococcus aureus* is isolated from infected superficial bursae. Infectious bursitis should be suspected with surrounding cellulitis, ery-

TABLE 89–2 Bursitis Syndromes

Location	Symptom	Finding
Subacromial	Shoulder pain	Tender subacromial space
Olecranon	Elbow pain	Tender olecranon swelling
Iliopectineal	Groin pain	Tender inguinal region
Trochanteric	Lateral hip pain	Tender at greater trochanter
Prepatellar	Anterior knee pain	Tender swelling over patella
Infrapatellar	Anterior knee pain	Tender swelling lateral or medial to patellar tendon
Anserine	Medial knee pain	Tender medioproximal tibia (below joint line of knee)
Ischiogluteal	Buttock pain	Tender ischial spine (at gluteal fold)
Retrocalcaneal	Heel pain	Tender swelling between Achilles tendon insertion and calcaneus
Calcaneal	Heel pain	Tender central heel pad

thema, fever, and peripheral leukocytosis. Definitive diagnosis and especially exclusion of infectious bursitis of subcutaneous bursae generally require aspiration of the distended bursa. The bursal fluid should be sent for cell count, culture, and examinination for crystals.

Nonseptic Bursitis

Nonseptic bursitis frequently presents as "overuse" conditions, which are associated with sudden or unaccustomed repetitive activity of the associated extremity. The two most common types of bursitis are subacromial and trochanteric bursitis (Table 89–2). Subacromial bursitis is the most common overall cause of shoulder pain and presents as pain over the lateral upper arm or deltoid muscle that is exacerbated with abduction of the arm. It is the result of compression of the inflamed rotator cuff tendon between the acromion and the humeral head. Because the rotator cuff forms the floor of the subacromial bursa, bursitis in this location actually results from tendinitis of the rotator cuff. Occasionally, subacromial bursitis or rotator cuff tendinitis results from osteophyte compression of the rotator cuff tendon originating from the acromioclavicular joint. The differential diagnosis includes tears of the rotator cuff, intra-articular pathology of the glenohumeral joint, bicipital tendinitis, cervical radiculopathy, and referred pain from the chest.

Trochanteric bursitis is the result of inflammation at the insertion of the gluteal muscles at the greater trochanter and produces lateral thigh pain, which is often worse when lying on the affected side. Women seem to be more prone to develop this condition, perhaps because of increased traction of the gluteal muscles due to the relatively broader pelvis. Other potential risk factors include local trauma, overuse activities such as jogging, and leg-length discrepancies (primarily on the side with the longer leg). These factors are thought to lead to increased tension of the gluteus maximus on the iliotibial band and produce bursal inflammation. The differential diagnosis of trochanteric bursitis includes lumbar radiculopathy (particularly of the L1 and L2 nerve roots), meralgia paraesthetica (entrapment of the lateral cutaneous nerve of the thigh as it passes under the inguinal ligament), true hip joint disease, and intra-abdominal pathology.

TREATMENT

Septic bursitis is treated with the combination of serial aspiration of the infected bursa and antibiotics, initially directed against *Staphylococcus aureus* and then adjusted depending on the results of bursal fluid cultures. The approach to nonseptic bursitis should include rest, local heat, and, unless contraindicated (peptic ulcer disease, renal disease, advanced age), nonsteroidal anti-inflammatory drugs (NSAIDs). Usually, the most effective approach is a local injection of corticosteroid. Superficial bursae with obvious swelling should be aspirated first, before corticosteroid is injected. For deep bursae such as the subacromial or trochanteric bursae, aspiration yields little if any fluid and direct injection of corticoste-

roid without attempted aspiration is most comfortable for the patient. Caution is advised in attempted aspiration or injection of the iliopsoas bursa, the ischiogluteal bursa, and the gastrocnemius-semimembranosus bursa (Baker's cyst). These bursae lie close to important neural and/or vascular structures, and aspiration should only be attempted by those with extensive experience.

Tendinitis

CLINICAL PRESENTATION

Most tendinitis syndromes are the result of inflammation in the tendon sheath. Overuse with microscopic tearing of the tendon is the most common risk factor for tendinitis, but tendon compression by an osteophyte may occur, for example, in the rotator cuff tendon compressed by an osteophyte originating from the acromioclavicular joint.

One of the most common forms of tendinitis is lateral epicondylitis, also known as "tennis elbow" (Table 89–3). This is a common overuse syndrome among tennis players, but it can be seen in many other settings requiring repetitive extension of the forearm (e.g., painting overhead). The diagnosis is confirmed by exclusion of elbow joint pathology and the finding of local tenderness at the lateral epicondyle, which is typically exacerbated by forearm extension against resistance. Achilles tendinitis and peroneal and posterior tibial tendinitis may occur in the setting of an underlying seronegative arthropathy such as Reiter's syndrome or psoriatic arthritis.

TREATMENT

Therapy for tendinitis is similar to that of bursitis, with the use of NSAIDs, local heat, and corticosteroid injection. Rest, physical therapy, occupational therapy, and occasionally ergonomic modification are useful adjuncts. The goal of corticosteroid injection in tendinitis is to infiltrate the tendon sheath rather than the tendon itself, because direct injection into a tendon may result in rupture of the tendon. Attempted corticosteroid injection of the Achilles tendon should be avoided because of the propensity of this tendon to rupture.

Fibromyalgia Syndrome

Fibromyalgia syndrome, formerly known as fibrositis, is a controversial chronic pain condition characterized by increased tenderness at muscle and tendon insertions; it is therefore considered a form of soft tissue rheumatism. Although it has been the subject of only recent investigation, descriptions of the syndrome exist far back in the medical literature. Controversy persists, however, because of the lack of objective diagnostic or pathologic findings.

TABLE 89-3 Tendinitis Syndromes

Location	Symptom	Finding
Extensor pollicis brevis and abductor pollicis longus (DeQuervain's tenosynovitis)	Wrist pain	Pain on ulnar deviation of the wrist, with the thumb grasped by the remaining four fingers (Finkelstein's test)
Flexor tendons of fingers	Triggering or locking of fingers in flexion	Tender nodule on flexor tendon On palm over metacarpal joint
Medial epicondyle	Elbow pain	Tenderness of medial epicondyle
Lateral epicondyle	Elbow pain	Tenderness of lateral epicondyle
Bicipital tendon	Shoulder pain	Tenderness along bicipital groove
Patellar	Knee pain	Tenderness at insertion of patellar tendon
Achilles	Heel pain	Tender Achilles tendon
Tibialis posterior	Medial ankle pain	Tenderness under medial malleolus with resisted inversion of the ankle
Peroneal	Lateral mid-foot or ankle pain	Tenderness under lateral malleolus with passive inversion

PATHOPHYSIOLOGY

Investigators have examined diverse mechanisms in fibromyalgia syndrome, including studies of muscle, sleep physiology, neurohormonal function, and psychological status. Although the pathophysiology remains unknown, an increasing body of literature points to central (central nervous system) rather than peripheral (muscle) mechanisms. Muscle tissue has been a focus of investigation for many years. Initial studies, including histologic and histochemical studies, suggested a possible metabolic myopathy; however, carefully controlled studies indicate that these abnormalities were simply the result of deconditioning. Sleep studies suggested that disruption of deep sleep (stage IV) by so-called alpha-intrusion (the normal awake electroencephalographic pattern) may play a causal role, but this was later found in other disorders, more likely indicating effect rather than cause. Several studies have suggested that subtle hypothalamic-pituitary-adrenal axis hypofunction may occur in fibromyalgia syndrome, although it remains uncertain whether these changes are constitutive or are the result of fibromyalgia. Fibromyalgia has long been linked to psychological disturbance. Most studies have confirmed high lifetime rates of major depression, which range from 34% to 71%. High lifetime rates of migraine, irritable bowel syndrome, and panic disorder have also been associated with fibromyalgia syndrome, suggesting that fibromyalgia may be part of an "affective spectrum" group of disorders.

CLINICAL PRESENTATION AND DIFFERENTIAL DIAGNOSIS

The clinical presentation of fibromyalgia syndrome is generally that of the insidious onset of chronic, diffuse, poorly localized musculoskeletal pain, typically accompanied by fatigue and sleep disturbance. The physical examination shows a normal musculoskeletal examination, with no deformity or synovitis; however, there is widespread tenderness especially at tendon insertion sites (indicating a general reduction in pain threshold). The American College of Rheumatology has published the results of a multicenter study to identify clinical classification criteria for fibromyalgia syndrome, which were shown to have high sensitivity and specificity (Table 89–4). These criteria have facilitated population-based studies, which suggest that fibromyalgia syndrome affects approximately 2% of the population and up to 7% of women. Approximately 10% of surveyed patients are disabled to varying degrees by their symptoms; therefore, the economic impact is large. The prevalence of fibromyalgia appears to be similar in most ethnic and racial groups.

Approximately one third of the patients identify antecedent trauma as a precipitant for their symptoms, one third of patients describe a viral prodrome, and one third have no clear precipitant. A variety of less typical presentations have been described, including a predominantly neuropathic presentation with paresthesias (numbness and tingling) in a nondermatomal distribution, an arthralgic rather than myalgic presentation, and an axial skeletal presentation (resembling degenerative disc disease). Many patients may have undergone inva-

TABLE 89-4 ACR Classification Criteria for Fibromyalgia Syndrome

For classification purposes, patients are said to have fibromyalgia if both criteria are satisfied.
1. *History of chronic, widespread pain:* Pain is considered widespread when present above and below the waist on both sides of the body. *Chronic* is defined as greater than 3 months in duration.
2. *Pain in 11 of 18 tender points on digital palpation:* Occiput, low cervical, trapezius, supraspinatus, second rib, lateral epicondyle, gluteal, greater trochanter, knee

sive diagnostic tests and in some cases inappropriate procedures such as carpal tunnel release or cervical or lumbar laminectomies.

Conditions that should be considered in the differential diagnosis of fibromyalgia syndrome include polymyalgia rheumatica, hypothyroidism, polymyositis, and early systemic lupus erythematosus or rheumatoid arthritis. In general, however, symptoms present for many months or years without evidence of other signs or symptoms of an underlying connective tissue disease, making other possible diagnoses unlikely. Laboratory and radiographic studies are usually normal in patients with fibromyalgia syndrome. Exclusion of other conditions, such as osteoarthritis, rheumatoid arthritis, or systemic lupus erythematosus, by radiography, erythrocyte sedimentation rate, assays for rheumatoid factor or antinuclear antibody, and other tests is no longer considered a necessary preliminary to the diagnosis of fibromyalgia syndrome, which should be diagnosed on the basis of positive criteria.

TREATMENT

The treatment of fibromyalgia includes reassurance that the condition is not a progressive, crippling, or life-threatening entity. A combination of treatment options including medication and physical measures is helpful in most patients. Medication shown to be helpful in short-term, double-blind, placebo-controlled trials includes amitriptyline and cyclobenzaprine. Low doses of these medications (e.g., 10 to 30 mg of amitriptyline, 10 to 30 mg of cyclobenzaprine) are moderately effective and generally well tolerated. Studies have also shown that newer antidepressants of the specific serotonin reuptake inhibitor class are also effective, particularly in combination with low doses of tricyclic antidepressants. Patients should also be encouraged to take an active role in the management of their condition. They should, if possible, begin a progressive, low-level aerobic exercise program to improve muscular fitness and sense of well-being. A combination approach is effective in most patients in alleviating symptoms, although a small minority of patients require more intensive treatment strategies, such as psychiatric or pain center referral.

REFERENCES

Ball EV: Non-articular rheumatism. *In* Goldman L, Bennett JC (eds): Cecil Textbook of Medicine, 21st ed. Philadelphia: WB Saunders, 2000, pp 1559–1560.

Simms RW: Fibromyalgia syndrome: Current concepts in pathophysiology, clinical features and management. Arthritis Care Res 1996; 9: 315–328.

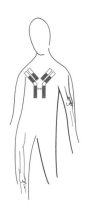

90

RHEUMATIC MANIFESTATIONS OF SYSTEMIC DISORDERS

Robert W. Simms

A large number of systemic disorders have musculoskeletal manifestations. These are frequently the presenting manifestations and may provide clues to the initial and perhaps earlier diagnosis and treatment (Table 90–1).

Rheumatic Syndromes Associated with Malignancy

HYPERTROPHIC OSTEOARTHROPATHY

Hypertrophic osteoarthropathy (HOA) is a form of long bone periostitis associated with clubbing of the fingers and toes. Approximately 90% of cases are associated with lung cancer. Other disorders associated with HOA include cystic fibrosis, pulmonary fibrosis, chronic pulmonary infections, pulmonary arteriovenous fistulas, mesothelioma, congenital heart disease, cirrhosis, and inflammatory bowel disease. Isolated digital clubbing (a bulbous deformity of the distal digits with loss of the normal angle between the nail and the nail bed) is associated with pleuropulmonary disease in approximately 80% of cases, but only a small minority of patients turn out to have cancer. Chronic digital clubbing does not appear to lead to the development of HOA. The most common long bones involved in HOA are the distal femur, tibia, and radius. The pathogenesis is unknown, and its understanding is complicated by the diversity of conditions associated with HOA. Increased blood flow on the bones and in adjacent connective tissue is a uniform finding, perhaps the result of humoral or neural mechanisms.

HOA typically produces bone and joint pain with swelling that results from periarticular periostitis. Joints appear swollen, but there is no proliferative synovium or inflammation, and joint fluid is noninflammatory. Radiographic features include periostitis with periosteal new bone formation, especially along the distal and/or proximal fourths of long bones, and are diagnostic. Treatment of the underlying disorder ameliorates HOA.

LEUKEMIA AND LYMPHOMA

Leukemia may simulate various rheumatic syndromes by producing synovitis or bone pain resulting from direct invasion of the synovium or marrow expansion. Approximately 6% of adult patients with leukemia present with rheumatic manifestations, which precede the diagnosis of leukemia by an average of 3 months. The most common presentation is an asymmetric, large joint oligoarthritis, often accompanied by low back pain. In children, up to 60% with acute leukemia present with either monoarthritis or polyarthritis. Although lymphoma is frequently associated with bone lesions, arthritis is a rare presentation. The combination of nocturnal bone pain, hematologic abnormalities, and radiographic features such as periosteal elevation should suggest the possibility of leukemia. Treatment of the leukemia usually results in resolution of the musculoskeletal manifestations.

CARCINOMATOUS POLYARTHRITIS

In rare cases, metastatic or occult carcinoma may be associated with polyarthritis, which is not the result of direct infiltration of the synovium by tumor. The peak age at onset is in the 60s, and there is no gender predisposition. Nonintrathoracic malignancies predominate. The differential diagnosis includes HOA, rheumatoid arthritis, and polymyalgia rheumatica. Treatment of the underlying malignancy produces resolution of the arthritis.

Malignant Disorders

Hypertrophic osteoarthropathy
Lymphoma
Leukemia
Carcinoma polyarthritis

Hematologic Disorders

Hemophilia
Sickle cell disease
Thalassemia
Multiple myeloma
Amyloidosis

Gastrointestinal Disorders

Spondyloarthropathies
Whipple's disease
Hemochromatosis
Primary biliary cirrhosis

Endocrinopathies

Diabetes
Hypothyroidism
Hyperthyroidism
Hyperparathyroidism

Other

Sarcoidosis

Hematologic Disorders

HEMOPHILIA

Hemarthrosis is the most common bleeding complication of either hemophilia A (factor VIII deficiency) or hemophilia B (factor IX deficiency) and occurs in up to two thirds of patients. It may occur spontaneously or as the result of minor trauma, and its frequency and age at onset are determined by the level of factor deficiency. Acute, painful swelling of the knees, elbows, and ankles is the most common presentation. A chronic arthropathy with persistent synovitis may also occur, perhaps as a result of excessive iron deposition in synovial membrane and cartilage. Radiographic findings are those of degenerative joint disease with joint space narrowing, subchondral sclerosis, and cyst formation. Treatment consists of prompt administration of factor VIII or IX concentrate or recombinant forms, intra-articular corticosteroid injections, local ice application, rest, and later physical therapy. Aspiration is indicated only if concomitant sepsis is suspected or if the joint is unusually tense, and only after factor VIII replacement. There is no evidence to suggest that prophylaxis of acute hemarthrosis may reduce the incidence of chronic synovitis and future joint damage.

SICKLE CELL DISEASE

Of the sickle cell hemoglobinopathies, sickle cell anemia (SS), sickle β-thalassemia, S-thalassemia sickle C disease (SC), and sickle D disease (SD) all produce musculoskeletal complications, which include painful crises, arthropathy, dactylitis, osteonecrosis, osteomyelitis, and gout. Sickle cell crises are the most common musculoskeletal features, producing pain in the chest, back, and joints. Involvement of joints may produce a painful arthritis, typically of the large joints. The mechanism of the arthropathy is thought to be the result of articular reaction to juxta-articular bone infarction or infarction of the synovial membrane. The synovial fluid is typically noninflammatory. Dactylitis resulting from vaso-occlusion in bone may occur in young children, producing acute, painful, nonpitting edema of the hands and feet. Osteonecrosis of the femoral head or shoulder may also result from repeated crises and is most common in SS disease. An increased incidence of septic arthritis and osteomyelitis has been associated with sickle cell disease; *Salmonella* is the bacterial species most frequently isolated in the case of osteomyelitis.

Gout presumably resulting from the increased marrow turnover and urate production is an uncommon complication of sickle cell disease.

THALASSEMIA

β-Thalassemia major (also known as Cooley's anemia) is one of the most severe forms of congenital hemolytic anemia and may produce musculoskeletal manifestations from significant expansion of the erythroid bone marrow. These include osteoporosis, pathologic fractures, and epiphyseal deformities. Thalassemia minor has been associated with a noninflammatory arthritis, perhaps also the result of articular reaction to chronic marrow expansion.

MULTIPLE MYELOMA AND AMYLOIDOSIS

Multiple myeloma is one of the most common plasma cell dyscrasias and is frequently accompanied by musculoskeletal manifestations, which include bone pain resulting from lytic bone lesions, pathologic fractures, and osteoporosis. The diagnosis of multiple myeloma should be suspected in any of these clinical settings and is confirmed with the finding of a monoclonal gammopathy and sheets of immature/neoplastic plasma cells on bone marrow biopsy. Amyloidosis of the primary (AL) type accompanies approximately 15% of cases of myeloma. Alternatively, primary amyloidosis occurs without marked plasma cell proliferation on bone marrow biopsy, but patients have evidence of a plasma cell dyscrasia by virtue of the presence of a serum monoclonal gammopathy. Infrequently, amyloid joint infiltration produces a symmetric, small joint polyarthritis simulating rheumatoid arthritis. Occasionally, marked infiltration of the shoulder joints with amyloid deposits produces an anterior glenohumeral soft tissue deformity known as the "shoulder pad" sign. The diagnosis of this form of amyloidosis is the most easily established with the abdominal fat pad aspirate with the demonstration of apple-green birefringent fluorescence on Congo red staining. Optimal treatment of AL amyloidosis now consists of high-dose chemotherapy with stem cell transplantation.

There are three other principal systemic forms of amyloidosis: secondary (AA amyloidosis), heredofamilial (FAP amyloidosis), and β_2-microglobulin–associated (β_2M amyloidosis). Secondary amyloidosis is a rare complication of chronic inflammatory conditions such as rheumatoid arthritis, inflammatory bowel disease, or familial Mediterranean fever. Certain chronic infections such as leprosy, tuberculosis, and osteomyelitis are also associated with this form of amyloidosis. The amyloid fibrils are derived from the acute phase reactant, serum amyloid A protein. The disease usually presents as proteinuria or gastrointestinal symptoms because of infiltration of the kidney or gastrointestinal tract. The diagnosis generally requires organ biopsy, because the sensitivity of the abdominal fat pad aspirate is considerably lower in AA amyloidosis than in the AL form. Treatment consists of controlling the underlying disorder producing the chronic inflammatory process.

Heredofamilial amyloidosis is the least common form of amyloidosis. It is a rare autosomal dominant disease that is the result of single point mutations in the gene coding for transthyretin, a thyroid transport protein. Transthyretin is synthesized principally in the liver. Amyloid fibrils in this disease are composed of fragments of mutant transthyretin that have a propensity to form amyloid fibrils. The condition typically presents as an axonal and/or autonomic neuropathy late in life. Abdominal fat aspiration has high sensitivity in the diagnosis of this type of amyloidosis. Studies suggest that the optimal treatment is orthotopic liver transplantation, which prevents further production of the mutant transthyretin.

β_2-Microglobulin–associated amyloidosis occurs almost exclusively in patients on long-standing hemodialysis. This disease typically presents with carpal tunnel syndrome and flexor tendon deposits in the hands or in the rotator cuff. Cystic bone deposits in the carpal bones, hips, shoulders, and cervical spine have also been described. The pathogenesis of β_2-microglobulin–associated amyloidosis is not completely understood but may in part be the result of altered proteolysis of β_2-microglobulin in long-standing hemodialysis. Treatment includes physical measures such as splinting for carpal tunnel syndrome and physical therapy for shoulder involvement. Anti-inflammatory agents may provide additional symptomatic relief. Surgical removal of carpal or shoulder deposits may be required. Renal transplantation may be the most effective way to halt progression.

Gastrointestinal Diseases

WHIPPLE'S DISEASE

Whipple's disease is a rare, multisystemic disease of late-middle-aged to elderly men and is characterized by the presence of fever, abdominal pain, steatorrhea with weight loss, lymphadenopathy, and arthritis, the last of which is now known to result from infection with *Tropheryma whippleii*. Polyserositis, arterial hypotension, hyperpigmentation, and various central nervous system

manifestations, such as personality changes, memory loss, dementia, and spastic paraparesis, may also occur. The organism's DNA can be detected in duodenal biopsy specimens. Biopsy has long been used to detect this unculturable organism in histiocytes of the lamina propria, which show intracytoplasmic inclusions of irregular granular material that is positive on periodic acid–Schiff staining. This last finding is not specific for Whipple's disease, and therefore polymerase chain reaction to detect the organism's DNA is now the preferred technique for diagnosis.

The arthritis of Whipple's disease occurs in 60% to 90% of patients and is the most common prodrome. Classically, the arthritis is an intermittent migratory oligoarthritis lasting from a few hours to days, with spontaneous remission. Some patients have only arthralgia, whereas others have a florid polyarthritis. Synovial fluid findings are typically inflammatory, with a high percentage of mononuclear cells. Treatment consists of antibiotic therapy with tetracycline, which results in complete resolution within 1 week to 1 month.

HEMOCHROMATOSIS

Hereditary hemochromatosis is an autosomal recessive disorder associated with increased iron absorption and deposition that, via hemosiderin, eventually produces multiorgan damage. Hemochromatosis is among the most common genetic diseases among Europeans, with a homozygous prevalence of 0.3% to 0.5% and a heterozygote frequency of 6.7% to 10%. Ninety percent of white hereditary hemochromatosis patients are homozygous for the same mutation (C282Y) in the *HFE* gene. HFE protein forms complexes with the transferrin receptor, which is important in iron transport, and mutations in *HFE* decrease its affinity for the receptor, impairing iron transport and resulting in iron overload.

The classic clinical features of hemochromatosis include hepatic cirrhosis, cardiomyopathy, diabetes mellitus, pituitary dysfunction, skin pigmentation, and sicca syndrome. Symmetric arthropathy of the second and third metacarpal joints is a disabling complication that occurs in approximately 50% of patients. Radiographic manifestations are similar to those of osteoarthritis (see Chapter 88) and often include the presence of chondrocalcinosis. Occasionally, superimposed attacks of pseudogout dominate the clinical picture. Osteoarthritis-like disease occurring in a middle-aged man with involvement of the metacarpophalangeal joints should indicate the possibility of hemochromatosis. Formerly, the diagnosis was suggested by high serum levels of iron, ferritin, and transferrin and confirmed by liver biopsy. Currently, the diagnosis may be established with identification of the mutated gene sequence in DNA obtained from peripheral blood.

PRIMARY BILIARY CIRRHOSIS

Primary biliary cirrhosis is an inflammatory disease of the intrahepatic bile ducts that is frequently associated with other disorders presumed to be autoimmune, including limited scleroderma (see Chapter 83), rheumatoid arthritis (see Chapter 79), Sjögren's syndrome (see

Chapter 85), autoimmune thyroiditis, and renotubular acidosis. Ninety percent of patients have detectable IgG antimitochondrial antibodies, which are rare in other forms of liver disease. Up to 50% of patients with primary biliary cirrhosis have secondary Sjögren's syndrome, which represents the most common rheumatic disorder associated with primary biliary cirrhosis. Other musculoskeletal complications include (1) osteomalacia caused by reduced vitamin D absorption and (2) accelerated osteoporosis. The diagnosis of primary biliary cirrhosis should be suspected in a patient with unexplained pruritus or elevation of serum alkaline phosphatase levels. A positive antimitochondrial antibody test provides strong evidence, which should then be confirmed with a liver biopsy.

Endocrine Disorders

DIABETES

There are many musculoskeletal complications of diabetes (Table 90–2). One of the most common complications is the so-called diabetic "stiff-hand syndrome," which is characterized by waxy thickening of the skin in long-standing type I or II diabetes. Occasionally, it may be present before the onset of overt diabetes and may create confusion because of the similar appearance to scleroderma-like sclerodactyly. These changes are thought to be the result of excess sugar alcohols, such as sorbitol, producing excess water content in the skin and leading to increased stiffness. Joint contractures, flexor tendon contractures (including Dupuytren's), and thickening produce a condition known as diabetic cheiroarthropathy, or the syndrome of limited joint mobility, and appear to be related to the duration of diabetes. Although it is most common in the fingers, limited mobility may also occur in the shoulders.

Charcot or neuropathic arthropathy may occur with any neuropathy, but it is most commonly associated with diabetes. Tarsal and tarsometatarsal joints are most commonly involved, and trauma together with diminished pain perception, proprioception, and position sense are major factors in the genesis of this arthropathy. The most common presentation is swelling of the foot with little or no pain. Characteristic radiographic features include the so-called sucked-candy appearance. Treatment consists of non–weight bearing, which results in ankylosis of the affected joints.

HYPOTHYROIDISM

Almost one third of patients with frank hypothyroidism present with objective musculoskeletal findings. A rheumatoid arthritis–like presentation involving especially the large joints is characteristic. Wrists, metacarpophalangeal joints, and proximal interphalangeal joints may also be involved. Joint pain, stiffness, and detectable synovial thickening are present. Synovial fluid is generally noninflammatory. Pseudogout may also be a presenting manifestation of hypothyroidism. Myopathy, especially proximal, is common in hypothyroidism and is

TABLE 90–2 Musculoskeletal Manifestations of Endocrine Disease

Endocrine Disease	Musculoskeletal Manifestation
Diabetes mellitus	Carpal tunnel syndrome
	Charcot arthropathy
	Adhesive capsulitis
	Syndrome of limited joint mobility (cheiroarthropathy)
	Diabetic amyotrophy
	Diabetic muscle infarction
Hypothyroidism	Proximal myopathy
	Arthralgias
	Joint effusions
	Carpal tunnel syndrome
	Chondrocalcinosis
Hyperthyroidism	Myopathy
	Osteoporosis
	Thyroid acropachy
Hyperparathyroidism	Myopathy
	Arthralgias
	Erosive arthritis
	Chondrocalcinosis
Hypoparathyroidism	Muscle cramps
	Soft tissue calcifications
	Spondyloarthropathy
Acromegaly	Carpal tunnel syndrome
	Myopathy
	Raynaud's phenomenon
	Back pain
	Premature osteoarthritis
Cushing's syndrome	Myopathy
	Osteoporosis
	Avascular necrosis

often associated with elevation of creatine phosphokinase levels. Muscle biopsy specimens show atrophy of type II fibers but no inflammation. Thyroid replacement results in gradual improvement of both the arthropathy and myopathy of hypothyroidism.

HYPERTHYROIDISM

Four principal rheumatic manifestations occur in thyrotoxicosis: proximal myopathy, shoulder periarthritis, thyroid acropachy (thickened skin with periosteal new bone formation), and osteoporosis. Myopathy is common, occurring in 70% of hyperthyroid patients, but it is seldom a presenting manifestation. Periarthritis of the shoulder (especially bilateral) occurs in up to 10% of patients. Thyroid acropachy consists of clubbing and soft tissue swelling of the hands and feet. Radiographs show periosteal new bone formation, which is best seen on the radial aspect of the second and third metacarpals. Osteoporosis is produced by increased bone turnover, which accompanies the hyperthyroid state.

HYPERPARATHYROIDISM

Musculoskeletal manifestations are common in hyperparathyroidism and are the initial manifestations in up to 15% of patients. Pseudogout is the most common rheumatic complication, occurring in up to 10% of patients with hyperparathyroidism, although radiographic chondrocalcinosis is seen in up to 40%. A rheumatoid arthritis–like disorder has also been described with involvement of the knees, wrists, hands, and shoulders, showing radiographic erosions. In contrast to rheumatoid arthritis, however, synovial proliferation is absent, the joint space is preserved, and erosions are characteristically on the ulnar side, as opposed to rheumatoid arthritis, in which the erosions are typically on the radial side.

Secondary hyperparathyroidism is common in patients with chronic renal failure and is a component of renal osteodystrophy. Musculoskeletal features are similar to those described earlier.

Sarcoidosis

Sarcoidosis is a multisystemic inflammatory disorder manifested by formation of noncaseating granulomas. It may be associated with both acute and chronic rheumatic manifestations. The acute syndrome is known as Löfgren's syndrome and consists of the classic triad of hilar adenopathy, erythema nodosum, and arthritis. It occurs in approximately 15% of those presenting with sarcoidosis. The arthritis is usually symmetric and migratory, frequently involving the ankles, although it may be difficult to distinguish from erythema nodosum and periarthritis of the ankle. Joint effusions are typically noninflammatory. The arthritis is nondeforming, nonerosive, and self-limited, usually not lasting more than 3 to 4 months. The nonarticular manifestations of Löfgren's syndrome also have an excellent prognosis.

Chronic arthropathy involving the knees, ankles, wrists, and elbows occurs less frequently and is generally associated with active multisystemic disease. Synovial thickening and effusions are common; a synovial biopsy specimen may show the typical noncaseating granulomas. Treatment of acute sarcoid arthropathy includes the use of nonsteroidal anti-inflammatory drugs or, occasionally, a short course of corticosteroids. Treatment of the chronic arthropathy is dependent on the severity of the extra-articular manifestations that usually accompany it. Corticosteroids are generally needed to control the systemic disease.

REFERENCES

Ball EV: Systemic diseases in which arthritis is a feature. *In* Goldman L, Bennett JC (eds): Cecil Textbook of Medicine, 21st ed. Philadelphia: WB Saunders, 2000, pp 1556–1558.

Simms RW: Arthropathies associated with hematologic and malignant disorders. *In* Klippel JH (ed): Primer on the Rheumatic Diseases, 11th ed. Atlanta: Arthritis Foundation, 1997, pp 337–338.

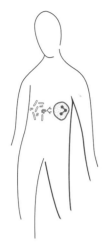

SECTION XV

Infectious Disease

91

ORGANISMS THAT INFECT HUMANS

Michael M. Lederman

Of diseases afflicting humans, most that are curable and preventable are caused by infectious agents. The infectious diseases that capture the attention of physicians and the public periodically shift—for example, from syphilis to tuberculosis to acquired immunodeficiency syndrome (AIDS)—but the challenges of dealing with these processes endure. To the student, an understanding of infectious diseases offers insights into medicine as a whole. Osler's adage (with updating) remains relevant: "He [or she] who knows syphilis [AIDS], knows medicine."

Viruses

Viruses produce a wide variety of clinical illnesses. A virus consists of either DNA or RNA (in rare cases, both) wrapped within a protein nucleocapsid. The nucleocapsid may be covered by an envelope composed of glycoproteins and lipids. Viral genes can code for only a limited number of proteins, and viruses possess no metabolic machinery. They are entirely dependent on host cells for protein synthesis and replication and are therefore obligate intracellular parasites. Some viruses are dependent on other viruses to produce active infection. Such is the case with the delta agent, which produces disease only in the presence of hepatitis B infection. All must attach to receptors on the host cell and achieve entry into the cell through mechanisms that include receptor-mediated endocytosis, fusion, and pinocytosis. Once within the cells, the virus uncoats, allowing its nucleic acid to utilize host cellular machinery to reproduce (productive infection) or to integrate into the host cell (latent infection). Some viruses, such as influenza virus, cause disease by lysis of infected cells. Others, such as hepatitis B virus, do not directly cause cell destruction but may involve the host immune responses in the pathogenesis of disease. Still others, such as the human T lymphotropic virus type I, promote neoplastic transformation of infected cells.

Viruses have developed several mechanisms for evading host defense mechanisms. By multiplying within host cells, viruses can avoid neutralizing antibodies and other extracellular host defenses. Some viruses can spread to uninfected cells by intercellular bridges. Others, especially the herpes group and human immunodeficiency virus, are capable of persisting without multiplication in a metabolically inactive form within host cells for prolonged periods (latency). The influenza virus is capable of extensive gene rearrangements, resulting in significant changes in surface antigen structure. This allows new strains to evade host antibody responses directed at earlier strains.

Some viruses, as they exit the host cell during productive infection, may carry antigens of host cell origin, thus providing another potential mechanism for evading host defenses. Others, such as the human immunodeficiency virus, induce profound immune dysfunction and thus paralyze host defenses.

Chlamydiae

Chlamydiae are also obligate intracellular parasites, but, unlike viruses, they always contain both DNA and RNA, divide by binary fission (rather than multiplying by assembly), can synthesize proteins, and contain ribosomes. They are unable to synthesize adenosine triphosphate and thus depend on energy from the host cell to survive. The three chlamydial species known to cause disease in humans are *Chlamydia trachomatis*, *Chlamydia pneumoniae*, and *Chlamydia psittaci*. *C. trachomatis* causes trachoma, the major cause of blindness in the developing world, and a variety of sexually transmitted genitourinary disorders, including urethritis, salpingitis, and lymphogranuloma venereum. *C. pneumoniae* is a common cause of atypical pneumonia, bronchitis, and sinusitis. *C. psittaci*, the cause of a common infectious disease of birds, can produce a serious systemic illness with prominent pulmonary manifestations in humans. Chlamydiae are susceptible to tetracyclines and the macrolide antibiotics.

Rickettsiae

Rickettsiae are also small bacterial organisms that, like chlamydiae, are obligate intracellular parasites. Rickettsiae are primarily animal pathogens that generally produce disease in humans through the bite of an insect vector, such as a tick, flea, louse, or mite. Most of these organisms specifically infect vascular endothelial cells. With the exception of Q fever and human ehrlichiosis, rash caused by vasculitis is a prominent manifestation of these often disabling febrile illnesses. These organisms are susceptible to tetracyclines and chloramphenicol.

Mycoplasmas

Mycoplasmas are the smallest free-living organisms. In contrast to viruses, chlamydiae, and rickettsiae, mycoplasmas can grow on cell-free media and produce disease without intracellular penetration. Like other bacteria, these organisms have a membrane, but, unlike other bacteria, they have no cell walls. Thus, antibiotics that are active against bacterial cell walls have no effect on mycoplasmas. Four major species of mycoplasma may cause disease in humans. *Mycoplasma pneumoniae* is an agent of pharyngitis and pneumonia, whereas *M. hominis* and *Ureaplasma urealyticum* are agents of genitourinary disease. *M. fermentans* is an unusual cause of disseminated disease in healthy people but may cause fulminant disease in immunosuppressed patients. Mycoplasmas are sensitive to erythromycin, tetracycline, or both.

Bacteria

Bacteria are a tremendously varied group of organisms that are generally capable of cell-free growth, although some produce disease as intracellular parasites. There are numerous ways of classifying bacteria, including morphology, ability to retain certain dyes, growth in different physical conditions, ability to metabolize various substrates, and antibiotic sensitivities. Although combinations of these methods are used to identify bacteria in clinical bacteriology laboratories, relatedness for taxonomic purposes is established by DNA homology.

SPIROCHETES

Spirochetes are slender, motile, spiral-shaped organisms that are not readily seen under the microscope unless stained with silver or viewed under darkfield illumination. Many of these organisms cannot yet be cultured on artificial media or in cell culture. Four genera of spirochetes cause disease in humans. *Treponema* species include the pathogens of syphilis and the nonvenereal, endemic, syphilis-like illnesses of yaws, pinta, and bejel. The illnesses caused by these organisms are chronic and characterized by prolonged latency in the host. Penicillin is active against *Treponema*. *Leptospira* species are the causative agents of leptospirosis, an acute or subacute febrile illness occasionally resulting in aseptic meningitis, jaundice, and (in rare cases) renal insufficiency. *Borrelia* species are arthropod-borne spirochetes that are the causative agents of Lyme disease (see Chapter 95) and relapsing fever. During afebrile periods in relapsing fever, these organisms reside within host cells and emerge with modified cell surface antigens. These modifications may permit the bacterium to evade host immune responses and produce relapsing fever and recurrent bacteremia. *Spirillum minus* is one of the causative agents of rat-bite fever.

ANAEROBIC BACTERIA

Anaerobes are organisms that cannot grow in atmospheric oxygen tensions. Some are killed by very low oxygen concentrations, whereas others are relatively aerotolerant. As a general rule, anaerobes that are pathogens for humans are not as sensitive to oxygen as nonpathogens. Anaerobic bacteria are primarily commensals. They inhabit the skin, gut, and mucosal surfaces of all healthy individuals. In fact, the presence of anaerobes may inhibit colonization of the gut by virulent, potentially pathogenic bacteria. Anaerobic infections generally occur in two circumstances:

1. Contamination of otherwise sterile sites with anaerobe-laden contents. Examples include (a) aspiration of oral anaerobes into the bronchial tree, producing anaerobic necrotizing pneumonia; (b) peritonitis and intra-abdominal abscesses after bowel perforation; (c) fasciitis and osteomyelitis after odontogenic infections or oral surgery; and (d) some instances of pelvic inflammatory disease.
2. Infections of tissue with lowered redox potential as the result of a compromised vascular supply. Examples include (a) foot infections in diabetic patients, in whom vascular disease may produce poor tissue oxygenation; and (b) infections of pressure sores, in which fecal anaerobic flora gain access to tissue whose vascular supply is compromised by pressure.

The pathogenesis of anaerobic infections—that is, soilage by a complex flora—generally results in polymicrobial infections. Thus, the demonstration of one anaerobe in an infected site generally implies the presence of others. Often, facultative organisms (organisms capable of anaerobic and aerobic growths) coexist with anaerobes. Certain anaerobes, such as *Clostridium*, produce toxins that cause well-defined systemic illnesses such as food poisoning, tetanus, and botulism. Other toxins may play a role in soft tissue infections (cellulitis, fasciitis, and myonecrosis) occasionally produced by *Clostridium* species. *Bacteroides fragilis*, the most numerous bacterial pathogen in the normal human colon, has a polysaccharide capsule that inhibits phagocytosis and promotes abscess formation. Clues to the presence of anaerobic infection include (1) a foul odor (the diagnosis of anaerobic pneumonia can, on occasion, be made from across the room); (2) the presence of gas, which may be seen radiographically or manifested by crepitus on examination (not all gas-forming infections are anaerobic, however); and (3) the presence of mixed gram-positive and gram-negative flora on a Gram stain of purulent exudate, especially when there is little or no growth on plates cultured aerobically. Many pathogenic anaerobes are sensitive to penicillin. Exceptions are strains of *Bacteroides fragilis* (usually sensitive to metronidazole, clindamycin, or ampicillin/sulbactam) and *Clostridium difficile,* which is almost always sensitive to metronidazole and vancomycin. Strains of *Fusobacterium* may also be relatively resistant to penicillin. As a general rule, infections caused by anaerobes originating from sites above the diaphragm are more often (but not always) penicillin sensitive, whereas infections below the diaphragm are often caused by penicillin-resistant organisms, notably *Bacteroides fragilis.*

GRAM-NEGATIVE BACTERIA

The cell walls of these bacteria, which appear pink on a properly prepared Gram stain, contain lipopolysaccharide, a potent inducer of cytokines such as tumor necrosis factor, and are associated with fever and septic shock. These organisms cause a wide variety of illnesses. Gram-negative bacteria are the most common cause of cystitis and pyelonephritis. *Haemophilus* species are common pathogens of the respiratory tract and cause otitis media, sinusitis, tracheobronchitis, and pneumonia. Lower respiratory tract infections with these organisms are particularly common in adults with chronic obstructive pulmonary disease. *Haemophilus* can be an important cause of meningitis, particularly in children. Except for *Haemophilus* species, gram-negative bacteria are uncommon causes of community-acquired pneumonia but are common causes of nosocomial pneumonia.

Except for the peculiar risk of *Pseudomonas* infection in intravenous drug users, gram-negative organisms are rare causes of endocarditis on natural heart valves but are occasional pathogens on prosthetic valves. The Enterobacteriaceae include *Escherichia coli, Klebsiella, Enterobacter, Serratia, Salmonella, Shigella,* and *Proteus.* These are large gram-negative rods. Except for the occasional presence of a clear space surrounding some *Klebsiella* (representing a large capsule), these organisms are not readily distinguished from each other on Gram's stain. The Enterobacteriaceae can be thought of as gut-related or genitourinary pathogens. *Salmonella,* a relatively common cause of enteritis, may occasionally infect atherosclerotic plaques or aneurysms. *Shigella* is an agent of bacterial dysentery. *Proteus* species, which split urea, are the agents associated with staghorn calculi of the urinary collecting system. Increasingly, gram-negative bacteria that are often resistant to multiple antibiotics are important causes of nosocomial infection.

Gram-negative cocci that cause disease in humans include *Neisseria* and *Moraxella* species. These kidney bean–shaped diplococci are not distinguishable from one another on Gram's stain. *Neisseria meningitidis* is an important cause of meningitis, and *Neisseria gonorrhoeae* causes gonorrhea. *Moraxella catarrhalis,* which is part of the normal oral flora, is a cause of lower respiratory tract infection.

GRAM-POSITIVE BACTERIA

Although these organisms (which appear deep purple on Gram's stain) lack endotoxin, infections with gram-positive bacteria also produce fever and cannot be reliably distinguished on clinical grounds from infections caused by gram-negative bacteria.

GRAM-POSITIVE RODS

Infections caused by gram-positive rods are relatively uncommon outside certain specific settings. Diphtheria is rare, but other corynebacteria produce infections in the immunocompromised host and on prosthetic valves and shunts. Because corynebacteria are regular skin colonizers, they often contaminate blood cultures; in the appropriate setting, however, they must be considered potential pathogens. *Listeria monocytogenes* resembles *Corynebacterium* on initial isolation, and this foodborne pathogen is an increasingly important cause of meningitis and bacteremia in the immunocompromised patient. *Bacillus cereus* is a recognized cause of food poisoning. Serious infections with this and other *Bacillus* species occur among intravenous drug users. Infections with *Clostridia* species were discussed previously.

GRAM-POSITIVE COCCI

Staphylococcus aureus is a common pathogen that can infect any organ system. It is a common cause of bacteremia and sepsis. The organism often colonizes the anterior nares, particularly among insulin-treated diabetics, hemodialysis patients, and intravenous drug users; these populations therefore have a greater frequency of infections with this organism. Hospital workers colonized with *S. aureus* have been responsible for hospital epidemics of staphylococcal disease.

Generally protected by an antiphagocytic polysaccharide capsule, staphylococci also possess catalase, which inactivates hydrogen peroxide—a mediator of bacterial killing by neutrophils. Staphylococci tend to form abscesses; the low pH within an abscess cavity also limits the effectiveness of host defense cells. Staphylococci elaborate several toxins that mediate specific manifestations of disease. A staphylococcal enterotoxin is responsible for staphylococcal food poisoning. Staphylococcal toxins also mediate the scalded skin syndrome and the multisystem manifestations of toxic shock syndrome. Most staphylococci are penicillinase producing, and an increasing proportion are resistant to penicillinase-resistant penicillin analogues. Although referred to as methicillin-resistant *S. aureus* (MRSA), they are resistant to all beta-lactams. Vancomycin remains active against most strains. Some staphylococci are "tolerant" to cell wall–active antibiotics such as penicillins or vancomycin; such organisms are inhibited but not killed by these agents. The clinical significance of tolerance is not certain.

Other staphylococci are distinguished from *S. aureus* primarily by their inability to produce coagulase. Some of these coagulase-negative staphylococci produce urinary tract infection (*S. saprophyticus*). Another, *S. epidermidis*, is part of the normal skin flora and an increasingly important cause of infection on foreign bodies such as prosthetic heart valves, ventriculoatrial shunts, and intravascular catheters. Like *Corynebacterium, S. epidermidis* may be a contaminant of blood cultures but in the appropriate setting should be considered a potential pathogen. *S. saprophyticus* is sensitive to a variety of antibiotics used in the treatment of urinary tract infection; *S. epidermidis* is usually resistant to all beta-lactams but sensitive to vancomycin.

Streptococci are classified into groups according to the presence of serologically defined carbohydrate capsules (Lancefield typing). Group A streptococci produce skin infections and pharyngitis. These organisms are also associated with the immunologically mediated poststreptococcal disorders—glomerulonephritis and acute rheumatic fever. Group D streptococci include enterococci, which are unique among the streptococci in their uniform resistance to penicillin. Recently, strains of enterococci that are also resistant to vancomycin have emerged; infections with these multidrug-resistant organisms have not responded well to available therapies, and nosocomial spread of these organisms is a growing problem in many hospitals.

Streptococci are further classified according to the pattern of hemolysis on blood agar—α for incomplete hemolysis (producing a green discoloration on the agar), β for complete hemolysis, and γ for nonhemolytic strains. An important α-hemolytic strain is *S. pneumoniae* (pneumococcus), the most common cause of bacterial pneumonia and an important cause of meningitis and otitis media. Penicillin resistance in pneumococcal isolates is an increasingly important problem. These organisms remain susceptible to vancomycin, although recently some strains that are tolerant to vancomycin have been identified. A heterogeneous group of streptococci, often improperly referred to as viridans streptococci (these organisms may show α- or γ-hemolysis), includes several species of streptococcus that are common oral or gut flora and are important agents of bacterial endocarditis, abscesses, and odontogenic infections.

MYCOBACTERIA

Mycobacteria are a group of rod-shaped bacilli that stain weakly gram positive. These organisms are rich in lipid content and are recognized in tissue specimens by their ability to retain dye after washing with acid alcohol (acid fast). These bacteria are generally slow-growing (some require up to 6 weeks to demonstrate growth on solid media), obligate aerobes. They generally produce chronic disease and survive for years as intracellular parasites of mononuclear phagocytes. Some escape intracellular killing mechanisms by blocking phagosome/lysosome fusion or by disrupting the phagosome. Almost all provoke cell-mediated immune responses in the host,

and clinical disease expression may be related in large part to the nature of the host immune response. Tuberculosis is caused by *Mycobacterium tuberculosis*. Other mycobacteria (nontuberculous mycobacteria) can cause diseases resembling tuberculosis. Certain rapid-growing mycobacteria cause infections after surgery or implantations of prostheses, and *M. avium complex* (MAC) is an important cause of disseminated infection among patients with AIDS. MAC is frequently resistant to drugs usually used in the treatment of tuberculosis. Leprosy is a mycobacterial disease of skin and peripheral nerves caused by the noncultivatable *M. leprae*.

ACTINOMYCETALES

Nocardia and *Actinomyces* are weakly gram-positive filamentous bacteria. *Nocardia* is acid fast and aerobic; *Actinomyces* is anaerobic and not acid fast. *Actinomyces* inhabits the mouth, gut, and vagina and produces cervicofacial osteomyelitis and abscess, pneumonia with empyema, and intra-abdominal and pelvic abscess, the last often associated with intrauterine contraceptive devices. *Nocardia* most commonly produces pneumonia and brain abscess. Approximately half of patients with *Nocardia* infection have underlying impairments in cell-mediated immunity. Infections with either of these organisms require long-term treatment. *Actinomyces* is relatively sensitive to many antibiotics; penicillin is the treatment of choice. *Nocardia* infections are treated with high doses of sulfonamides.

Fungi

Fungi are larger than bacteria. Unlike bacteria, they have rigid cell walls that contain chitin as well as polysaccharides. They grow and proliferate by budding, by elongation of hyphal forms, and/or by spore formation. Except for *Candida* and related species, fungi are rarely visible on Gram-stained preparations but can be stained with Gomori's methenamine silver stain or calcofluor white. They are also resistant to potassium hydroxide and can often be seen on wet mounts of scrapings or secretions to which several drops of a 10% solution of potassium hydroxide have been added. Fungi are resistant to antibiotics used in the treatment of bacterial infections and must be treated with drugs active against their unusual cell wall. Most fungi can exist in a yeast form (round to ovoid cells that may reproduce by budding) and a mold form, a complex of tubular structures (hyphae) that grow by branching or extension.

Candida species are oval yeasts that often colonize the mouth, gastrointestinal tract, and vagina of healthy individuals. They may produce disease by overgrowth and/or invasion. *Candida* stomatitis (thrush) often occurs in individuals who are receiving antibiotic or corticosteroid therapy or who have impairments of cell-mediated immunity. Vulvovaginitis caused by *Candida* may occur in these same settings but is also seen among women with diabetes mellitus or with no apparent predisposing factors. *Candida* can also colonize and infect the urinary tract, particularly in the presence of an indwelling urinary catheter. Occasionally, *Candida* species may gain entry into the blood stream and produce sepsis. This most frequently occurs in the setting of neutropenia after chemotherapy, where the portal of entry is the gastrointestinal tract, or in individuals receiving intravenous feedings, in whom the catheter is the source of the infection. Mucosal candidiasis can be treated with topical (clotrimazole) or systemic (fluconazole) imidazole drugs; systemic candidiasis is generally treated with parenteral amphotericin B or imidazoles.

Histoplasma capsulatum is a fungus endemic to the Ohio and Mississippi River valleys and produces a mild febrile syndrome in most individuals and a self-limited pneumonia in some. Occasionally, patients develop potentially fatal disseminated disease. Some individuals with chronic pulmonary disease may develop chronic pneumonia as a result of this yeast. Systemic or progressive disease is treated with parenteral amphotericin B or itraconazole.

Coccidioides immitis is endemic in the southwestern United States and, like *H. capsulatum*, produces a self-limited respiratory infection or pneumonia in most infected individuals. Immunocompromised individuals are at greatest risk for fatal systemic dissemination. Fluconazole or amphotericin B is used for progressive or extrapulmonary disease.

Cryptococcus neoformans is a yeast with a large polysaccharide capsule. It produces a self-limited or chronic pneumonia, but the most common clinical manifestation of infection with this fungus is a chronic meningitis. Although patients with impairment in cell-mediated immunity are at risk for cryptococcal meningitis, some patients with this syndrome have no identifiable immunodeficiency. Treatment is with amphotericin B combined with flucytosine. Long-term oral fluconazole therapy is effective in preventing relapse in persons with AIDS.

Blastomyces dermatitidis is a yeast also endemic in the Ohio and Mississippi River basins. Acute self-limited pulmonary infection is followed in rare instances by disseminated disease. Skin disease is most common, but bones and the genitourinary tract may be involved as well. Amphotericin B is used for treating systemic disease.

Aspergillus is a mold that produces several different clinical illnesses in humans. Acute bronchopulmonary aspergillosis is an IgE-mediated hypersensitivity to *Aspergillus* colonization of the respiratory tract. This condition produces wheezing and fleeting pulmonary infiltrates in patients with asthma. Occasionally, *Aspergillus* will colonize a preexistent pulmonary cavity and produce a mycetoma or fungus ball. Hemoptysis is the most serious complication of such infection. Invasive pulmonary aspergillosis is rarely a chronic illness of marginally compromised hosts; more often, it is a cause of acute, life-threatening pneumonia in patients with neutropenia or in recipients of organ transplants. Amphotericin B is the drug of choice for invasive aspergillosis.

The zygomycetes (Mucorales) are molds with ribbon-shaped hyphae that produce disease in patients with poorly controlled diabetes mellitus or hematologic malignancy or in recipients of organ transplantation. Invasive disease of the palate and nasal sinuses, which may extend intracranially, is the most common presentation, but pneumonia may be seen as well. These infections are generally treated with surgical excision plus amphotericin B.

Pneumocystis carinii was once thought to be a protozoan; genetic analyses have classified *P. carinii* as a fungus. This organism causes life-threatening pneumonia in patients with impaired cell-mediated immunity; it is the most common major opportunistic pathogen in persons with AIDS (see Chapter 108).

Protozoans

The protozoal pathogens listed in Table 91–1 are all important causes of disease within the United States. Infections caused by these organisms are diagnosed as

TABLE 91–1 **Some Protozoal Diseases of Humans**

Protozoan	Clinical Illness	Transmission	Diagnosis
Plasmodium	Malaria: fever, hemolysis	Mosquito, transfusion	Peripheral blood smear
Babesia microti	Fever, hemolysis	Tick, transfusion	Peripheral blood smear
Trichomonas vaginalis	Vaginitis	Sexual contact	Vaginal smear
*Toxoplasma gondii**	Fever, lymph node enlargement; encephalitis, brain abscess in compromised host	Raw meat, cat feces	Serologies, tissue biopsy
Entamoeba histolytica	Colitis, hepatic abscess	Fecal-oral	Stool smear, serologies
Giardia lamblia	Diarrhea, malabsorption	Fecal-oral	Stool smear, small bowel aspirate
*Cryptosporidium**	Diarrhea	?Fecal-oral	Sugar flotation, acid-fast stain of stool, biopsy
*Isospora belli**	Diarrhea, malabsorption	?Fecal-oral	Wet mount or acid-fast stain of stool
*Microsporidium**	Diarrhea, malabsorption, dissemination	?Fecal-oral	Small bowel biopsy, Electron microscopy

* Important opportunistic pathogens in persons with acquired immunodeficiency syndrome (see Chapter 108).

indicated in Table 91–1 and are discussed in the relevant disease-oriented chapters.

Helminths

Diseases caused by helminths are among the most prevalent diseases in the developing world but are uncommon causes of illness in North America. In contrast to the pathogens discussed previously, helminths are multicellular parasites. Helminth diseases found in the United States include ascariasis (maldigestion, obstruction), hookworm (intestinal blood loss), enterobiasis (pinworm, anal pruritus), and strongyloidiasis (gastroen-

teritis, dissemination in the immunocompromised host). It is important to recognize the risk of other helminthic diseases in travelers returning from endemic regions (see Chapter 110).

REFERENCES

Bruckner DA, Colonna P: Nomenclature for aerobic and facultative bacteria. Clin Infect Dis 1993; 16:598–605.

Summanen P: Microbiology terminology update: Clinically significant anaerobic gram-positive and gram-negative bacteria (excluding spirochetes). Clin Infect Dis 1993; 16:606–612.

Tyler KL, Dermody TS: Introduction to viruses and viral diseases. *In* Mandell GL, Bennett JC, Dolin R (eds): Principles and Practice of Infectious Diseases, 5th ed. New York: Churchill Livingstone, 2000, pp 1314–1325.

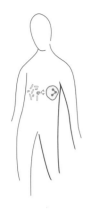

92

HOST DEFENSES AGAINST INFECTION

Robert A. Salata

Infectious agents and hosts are engaged in a complex struggle that has evolved over eons. The pathogenic and evasive mechanisms of microbes are countered by multiple and overlapping host immune and nonspecific defense mechanisms. In some cases, the pathogen "wins," with destruction of the host; in others, the host immune response prevails, with eradication of the parasite. Often, there occurs a standoff characterized by latent infection or symbiosis; pathogens capable of a latent phase have the capacity to reactivate as the host ages or as its immune response deteriorates because of superimposed diseases.

A few general statements are germane with regard to the roles of the components of the host defense network in the response to infectious diseases. The skin and mucosal surfaces represent the primary interface with the external world and its microbial flora. At these sites, anatomic barriers, the nonspecific inflammatory response, secretory IgA, products of effector cells, and the normal microbial flora defend against the development of invasive disease. Neutrophils are the critical effector cells in defense against infection with organisms constituting the normal microbial flora, such as Enterobacteriaceae, *Staphylococcus aureus*, *Candida*, and *Aspergillus*. Once local barriers are breached, the specific immune response, often acting in concert with nonspecific effector mechanisms, is required to control the infection.

The elements of the host response that are critical in combating many of the more common infectious agents are known. *Antibody*, which is the product of the interactions of B cells, antigen, and T-helper cells, is critical for defense against encapsulated pathogenic bacteria such as *Streptococcus pneumoniae*, *Haemophilus influenzae*, *Neisseria meningitidis*, and *Salmonella* species. The cellular immune response—specifically T-cell–dependent macrophage activation—is the critical effector arm against organisms capable of evading destruction by the effector cell and replicating intracellularly. An example of such an organism is *Mycobacterium tuberculosis*. Antiviral immunity is more difficult to characterize and varies with the agent in question. Neutralizing antibody provides sufficient protection against viruses with an extracellular phase (such as rubella). Protective mechanisms operant against viruses with a latent intracellular phase in the host, such as the herpesviruses, are chiefly provided by T cells. In this case, cytotoxic T lymphocytes (CTLs) often must destroy the infected host cells to expose the virus to neutralizing factors in the external milieu (antibody, complement).

In this chapter, local barriers to infection are discussed first. Thereafter, the interaction of the components of the immune system is presented, followed by discussion of nonspecific effector mechanisms. Finally, host defenses against representative infectious agents are discussed.

Local Barriers to Infection

Both nonspecific and specific host defense mechanisms contribute to the prevention of infectious diseases. Because few microorganisms can penetrate intact skin, the integument and the mucous membranes provide vital mechanical barriers to infection. The indigenous flora of these surfaces, particularly anaerobic bacteria, prevent colonization with virulent organisms by competing for nutrients and receptor sites on host cells and by producing factors, termed *bacteriocins,* that are toxic to other bacteria. The local milieu, chiefly the pH and redox potential, provides an additional barrier to colonization and infection with certain pathogenic organisms. Gastric acid reduces bacterial counts by 10-fold to 10,000-fold. The normal flow of mucus and other secretions helps to eliminate microorganisms from mucosal surfaces. The mucociliary blanket, for example, transports organisms away from the lungs. In addition, locally produced and active antimicrobial substances prevent infection. Factors contributing to protection of the urinary tract include pH, bladder flushing, prostatic secretions, hypertonicity of the renal medulla, and length of the urethra.

In the vagina, estrogens promote the growth of acidogenic bacteria, which produce an environment unfavorable to most pathogens. Lactoperoxidase, lysozyme, and lactoferrin in salivary and vaginal secretions and milk have microbicidal activity. Secretory IgA has a particularly important role in this respect because it opsonizes organisms and thereby blocks their ability to adhere to epithelial surfaces and to colonize the mucosa.

Components of the Immune System

The principal cells of the immune system are bone marrow–derived (B) and thymus-dependent (T) lymphocytes and mononuclear phagocytes. These cells are organized as a recirculating pool of lymphocytes and monocytes, bone marrow cells, and organized lymphoid tissue (lymph nodes, spleen, Peyer's patches, and the thymus).

The primary function of the immune system is to destroy foreign organisms and to clear foreign antigens without damaging host tissues. Immunity is also important in maintaining certain infectious agents in a latent stage and in destroying virally infected cells or cells that have undergone malignant transformation. The immune response is characterized by three features: immunologic memory, specificity, and systemic action. The functional organization of the immune response can be considered in six sequential steps: encounter, recognition, activation of lymphocytes, deployment, discrimination, and regulation.

ENCOUNTER

Microbes and soluble antigens encounter antigen-presenting cells (APCs) in the tissues and are ingested and catabolized. Monocytes, macrophages, dendritic cells,

and Langerhans cells are examples of APCs. The physical form of the antigen and the site of exposure or breaching of tissue determine which type of APC is relevant. Particulates are more readily ingested by active phagocytes such as macrophages; dendritic cells may be critical to the handling of soluble protein antigens. The gastrointestinal and respiratory tracts, which are important sites for interface of the immune system with the environment, possess well-differentiated APCs in submucosal areas. Some microbes elicit a neutrophilic inflammatory response and are phagocytosed and degraded by neutrophils, thereby bypassing traditional APCs and eliciting inflammation but little detectable immune response. Nonetheless, acute infection almost invariably produces an antibody response and memory for the same, presumably as a result of the processing of soluble microbial products. The disposition of soluble antigen is determined by the likelihood of uptake by APCs; an aggregated form of antigen or antigen bound by specific antibody in immune complexes favors uptake by APCs. After ingestion by APCs, the foreign antigen is degraded in acidic vesicles and is reprocessed to the surface of the cell, where, in close approximation, or bound to determinants encoded by the class II major histocompatibility complex (MHC), it is accessible to lymphocytes. APCs also produce cytokines such as interleukins (e.g., IL-1 and IL-6), which amplify immune induction.

RECOGNITION

The immune system has the capability of responding to an almost infinite number of antigens. B cells and T cells appear to use similar mechanisms to generate and express the diversity required for such a broad range of specific antigenic responses.

Five classes of antibodies (isotypes) are recognized (Table 92–1). An *IgG antibody* (Fig. 92–1) consists of two light (kappa or lambda) chains and two heavy chains. Each antibody has constant regions, which are

TABLE 92-1 Properties of Human Immunoglobulins

	IgG	IgA	IgM	IgD	IgE
H chain class	γ	α	μ	δ	ε
Molecular weight (approximate)	150,000	170,000	900,000	180,000	190,000
Complement fixation (classic)	++	0	++++	0	0
Opsonic activity (for binding)	++++	++	0	0	0
Reaginic activity	0	0	0	0	++++
Serum concentration (approximate mg/dL)	1500	150–350	100–150	2	2
Serum half-life (days)	23	6	5	3	2.5
Major functions	Recall response; opsonization; transplacental immunity	Secretory immunity	Primary response; complement fixation	?	Allergy; anthelmintic immunity

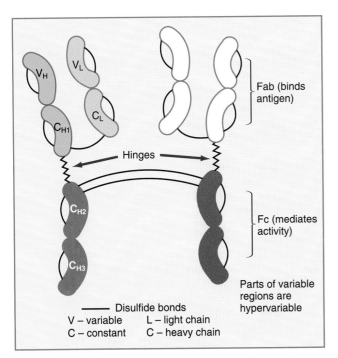

FIGURE 92–1 Diagram of the overall structure of immunoglobulin G, which is the basic structural pattern for all immunoglobulins (see text), drawn to highlight the various reactive areas and to emphasize the globular domain features of the immunoglobulin molecule. (From Bennett JC, Plum F [eds]: Cecil Textbook of Medicine, 20th ed. Philadelphia: WB Saunders, 1995, p 1394.)

identical in structure to all antibodies of that class, and distinctive antigen recognition sites whose structures are variable. An IgG_1 molecule has two such antigen-combining sites. The antigen-combining sites of antibody molecules recognize the three-dimensional structure of an antigen and bind to an antigen in a lock-and-key manner through multiple weak, noncovalent interactions. The variable regions consist of the approximately 110 N-terminal amino acids of each chain. Three short, hypervariable regions are present in each of the light and heavy chains. The six hypervariable regions form the combining site.

The generation of antibody diversity is understood at the molecular level. The variable portion of the heavy chain is encoded by three different genes: V, D, and J; investigators have identified 500 to 1000 different V genes, 10 D genes, and 4 J genes. The variable portions of the light chains are encoded by V and J genes; investigators have identified 200 possible V genes and 6 J genes. During the differentiation of B cells, somatic translocations randomly select the V, D, and J heavy chain genes and the V and J light chain genes that will be transcribed in that cell. The diversity achieved by these means is enormous. Somatic mutations in B cells allow the possibility of improving the fit between antibody and antigen; repeated or sustained exposure to antigen selects B cells capable of producing antibody with the highest binding affinity. These circulate as *memory cells*.

T lymphocytes can be divided into two subpopula-

tions based on the polypeptide chains constituting the antigen receptor. The $\alpha\beta$ *T cells*, constituting the larger population (~95%), possess a receptor comprising a heterodimer of α and β polypeptide chains. The variable portion of the $\alpha\beta$ T cell receptor is composed of the approximately 100 N-terminal amino acids. The generation of diversity is by translocation of V, D, and J genes, as is the case for B lymphocytes. The T-cell receptor is directed at the foreign antigen associated with MHC determinants. $\alpha\beta$ T cells can be divided by their surface expression of glycoproteins into CD4 and CD8 subpopulations. CD4 and CD8 cells also differ in their genetic restriction and function. Class I MHC products are recognized by CD8 suppressor T cells/ CTLs, and class II products are recognized by CD4 helper T cells. The T-cell receptor recognizes linear peptides of 5 to 20 amino acids in length. The second subpopulation of T lymphocytes, $\gamma\delta$ *T cells*, constitutes approximately 5% of circulating and lymphoid T cells; their T-cell receptor contains a heterodimer of γ and δ chains. Activation of $\gamma\delta$ T cells does not require recognition of either the class I or class II MHC products on APCs.

ACTIVATION OF LYMPHOCYTES

The initial physical apposition of T cells and APCs is stabilized by interactions of so-called *accessory molecules* on T cells with their respective ligands on APCs. Accessory molecules are usually members of the immunoglobulin or integrin gene family. For example, leukocyte functional antigen-1 on the T cell binds to intercellular adhesion molecule-1 on the APCs, and CD2 on the T cell binds with leukocyte functional antigen-3 on APCs. These reciprocal interactions facilitate the initial cell contact and are reinforced during the process of activation. CD4 helper T cells are activated when the T-cell receptors are occupied and are effectively cross-linked by the antigen–class II MHC complex on the surface of an APC (Fig. 92–2). Activation of the T cell is promoted by IL-1 and IL-6 released as a consequence of the cellular interactions. The helper T cell enlarges, secretes a variety of lymphokines, and divides to form a clone. The antigen molecule may also form a bridge between T cells and B cells and may thus permit the targeted delivery of B-cell growth and differentiation factors from T cell to B cell. The B cell, which is activated by a combination of signals provided by binding of antigen and by T cells, enlarges, divides, and differentiates into an antibody-producing cell. T-cell products also promote an isotype switch from IgM to production of IgG, IgA, or IgE.

The initial exposure of humans to microbial antigens leads to the proliferation of B cells that recognize the antigen and differentiate into antibody-forming plasma cells. T-cell help is required for responses to most antigens, although bacterial polysaccharides may directly elicit antibody production. After the first exposure to an antigen, IgM is the main antibody class or isotype produced. An isotype switch then occurs such that IgG predominates. On any repeated exposure to the antigen, production of IgG antibody is accelerated, and antibody

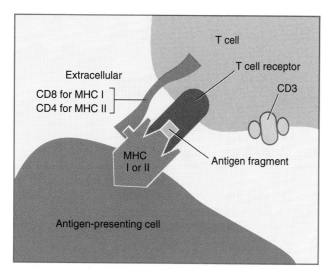

FIGURE 92-2 The molecular events in antigen presentation. Shown are the interactions among the various molecules, including the major histocompatibility complex (MHC), the T-cell receptor, the CD8 or CD4 molecules, and the CD3 complex. (Redrawn from Bennett JC: Introduction to diseases of the immune system. *In* Wyngaarden JB, Smith LH Jr, Bennett JC [eds]: Cecil Textbook of Medicine, 19th ed. Philadelphia: WB Saunders, 1992, p 1440.)

is produced in high titer and with high avidity for the antigen. *Secretory IgA* is found in tears, saliva, and bronchial, nasal, vaginal, prostatic, and intestinal secretions. Its primary role is to prevent organisms and antigens from attaching to and breaching mucosal barriers.

IgM accounts for 10% of normal immunoglobulins and is the antibody isotype most efficient at complement fixation. Both IgM and IgG can neutralize the infectivity of viruses and can lyse bacteria through complement fixation. Mononuclear phagocytes, neutrophils, and some lymphocytes possess surface receptors for the Fc fragment of IgG and/or the third component of complement. Therefore, IgG antibody or complement can bind to and opsonize bacteria and can facilitate their phagocytosis (Fig. 92-3), and IgG antibody can arm host effector cells for preferential destruction of selected targets by the process of antibody-dependent cell-mediated cytotoxicity (ADCC).

APCs and CD4 cells acting in concert are required for activation of CD8 cells for cytotoxic and suppressor cell activity. The activated CD4 cell also secretes certain factors important in hematopoiesis, mobilization of bone marrow precursor cells, chemotaxis of mononuclear and other cells to areas of inflammation, and expression of the cellular immune response.

In experimental studies, helper T lymphocytes can be divided into two subpopulations. The *Th1 subset* secretes IL-2, IL-12, and interferon-γ and is more effective at stimulating cellular immune responses. For example, interferon-γ activates macrophages to destroy certain facultative intracellular pathogens. In contrast, *Th2 cells* secrete cytokines that favor B-cell growth and differentiation (IL-4, IL-5, IL-6, IL-9, IL-10, and IL-13). Further distinctions concerning the heterogeneity of CD4 cells in humans are not nearly so clear.

Special consideration is warranted concerning cyto-

toxic mechanisms that destroy parasitized host cells. Certain viruses usurp the machinery of cells that they infect and replicate intracellularly, where they are inaccessible to antibody and complement. The only effective host response requires destruction of the parasitized host cell. This is usually accomplished by class I MHC–restricted CD8 cells that target on virally encoded proteins expressed on the host cell surface. Antibody to the viral products can also bind to the host cell surface and can render it susceptible to destruction by Fc receptor–bearing effector cells in the process of ADCC. Class II MHC–restricted cytotoxicity mediated by CD4 lymphocytes can be called into play when host cells are heavily parasitized with certain organisms such as mycobacteria or after ingestion and presentation of viral or other microbial products by APCs. The relative roles of class II as opposed to class I MHC–restricted cytotoxicity and ADCC in the destruction of parasitized host cells vary with the infectious agent. Once the host cell is destroyed, however, the microbe is susceptible to antibody, complement, or attack of other phagocytes and T lymphocytes.

DEPLOYMENT

The mobility of lymphocytes is central to the memory and systemic function of the immune response. Some progenies of activated B and T cells return to the resting stage and leave the peripheral lymphoid tissue to traffic as memory cells in the recirculating pool. These lymphocytes perfuse the tissues of the body and can reenter the lymph nodes. Reinfection or reexposure to

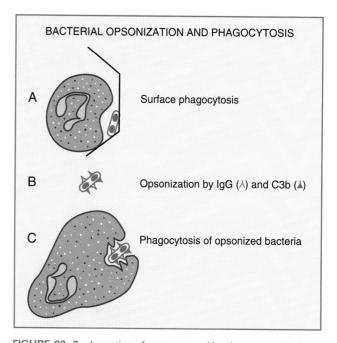

FIGURE 92-3 Ingestion of pneumococci by the neutrophil. In the absence of opsonins, the slippery pneumococcus must be forced against an alveolar surface to be ingested, the inefficient process of surface phagocytosis. Bacteria are opsonized by C3b and immunoglobulin G, which interact with receptors on the neutrophil and thereby facilitate phagocytosis.

an antigen at any site can lead to activation of memory lymphocytes.

The events thus far discussed are required for activation of antigen-specific lymphocytes. Neither antibody nor activated lymphocytes can directly destroy pathogenic organisms. Rather, they act in concert with antigen-nonspecific components of the immune response, including phagocytes and the complement and other molecular systems, to destroy pathogenic microbes. For example, one of the key cytokines produced by activated CD4 cells is interferon-γ; this interferon activates mononuclear phagocytes and thus renders them capable of killing intracellular parasites and tumors.

DISCRIMINATION

Tolerance of self-antigens prevents autoimmune disease. Several mechanisms contribute to tolerance. Early in ontogeny, exposure to antigen leads to refractoriness to that antigen. This process has been termed *clonal anergy*. Suppressor T cells are activated when soluble antigen is injected intravenously without adjuvant; this maneuver resembles exposure to most self-antigens. Moreover, self-antigens are not presented to reactive CD4 cells in combination with class II MHC determinants, so immune induction fails to occur. The breakdown of tolerance and autoimmune disease may result from a combination of factors: tissue damage exposing new antigens to the immune system and genetic factors that regulate the response to self-antigens and determine end-organ susceptibility to damage. Cross-reactivity exists between bacterial and mammalian cellular products. In persons expressing an autoimmune diathesis, whether on a genetic basis or some other basis, bacterial infection may trigger autoimmune tissue damage.

REGULATION

The immune response must be appropriate to the challenging event; too weak a response may permit unchecked infection, whereas too strong a response may damage tissue. Regulatory mechanisms amplify or mute an immune response and may be specific or nonspecific.

Antigen itself regulates the immune response. As antigen is cleared, a process enhanced by specific antibody, only lymphocytes bearing the highest-affinity receptors are activated. Once antigen is cleared entirely, the immune response diminishes, although memory cells continue to provide surveillance for reexposure to the antigen. Antibody has an additional role in immunoregulation, because immune complexes may directly modulate the response of specific lymphocytes. Antibody may also be directed at the antigen-combining site of antibody itself. Production of *anti-idiotypic antibodies* is stimulated by the immune response and may suppress further production of the relevant antibody.

Activation of the immune response also induces cellular regulatory mechanisms. For example, the activated CD4 cell is an important stimulus for induction of suppression by CD8 cells and mononuclear phagocytes. Cytokines that may mediate suppression of CD4 cell responses include IL-4, IL-10, transforming growth factor-β, and the IL-1 receptor antagonist.

Nonspecific Effector Mechanisms

COMPLEMENT

Complement activity results from the sequential interaction of a large number (25 are recognized) of plasma and cell membrane interactive proteins. The *classic complement pathway* is activated by antibody-coated targets or antigen-antibody complexes. The *alternative pathway* is activated by bacterial polysaccharides. Complement binds to bacteria and facilitates their attachment by C3b receptors on phagocytes, thus constituting the *heat-labile opsonic system* (see Fig. 92–3); it directly damages certain bacteria and viruses, and it induces inflammation through chemotactically active fragments. The classic complement pathway is the major effector mechanism for antibody-mediated immune responses. The Fc receptor of antigen-activated antibody molecules binds and activates C1. The alternative pathway is activated in the absence of antibody by constituents of the microbial surface, including polysaccharides, and generates C3 convertase, which catalyzes proteolysis of C3. Both classic and alternative pathways converge and form the membrane attack complex involving C5 to C9. This complex produces pores in the membrane of microbes and subjects them to osmotic lysis.

The complement system has several other notable biologic functions. C3b or iC3b deposited on the surface of microbes binds to complement receptors (CR1, CR3, and CR4) on neutrophils and macrophages and promotes phagocytosis. C5a is a chemotaxin for neutrophils and activates oxidative burst activity. C5a and C3a also stimulate histamine release from mast cells and thus promote inflammation. Finally, C3b furthers clearance of immune complexes by linking them to CR1 on the erythrocyte surface.

NEUTROPHILS

Neutrophils respond rapidly to chemotaxins and are the primary effector cells of the acute inflammatory response. They are activated by cytokines, including interferon-γ and tumor necrosis factor; this activation enhances neutrophil adhesion to vascular endothelium near the sites of infection, the first step in local accumulation. The cytokines also activate oxidative metabolism. In turn, stimulated neutrophils have been shown to secrete immunoregulatory cytokines IL-12 and IL-10. Neutrophils ingest antibody and complement-opsonized bacteria and destroy so-called "extracellular" bacteria by exposing them to toxic oxygen metabolites in the presence of myeloperoxidase and halide. Neutrophils also possess potent antibacterial peptides termed *defensins*.

MONONUCLEAR PHAGOCYTES

Macrophages differ from other phagocytic cells in that they have immunoregulatory and secretory properties in addition to their role as effector cells of cell-mediated immunity. Macrophages ingest and kill extracellular bacteria directly and in antibody-dependent reactions. Facultative intracellular pathogens have evolved various means for escaping intracellular destruction. These include disruption and escape from the phagosome, as well as blockage of phagosome-lysosome fusion. The process of activation of macrophages by T cells and their products overcomes the evasive mechanisms to destroy the organism. The macrophage activation factor varies according to the microbe in question. For many microbes, including *Toxoplasma gondii* as an example, it is interferon-γ. Data suggest that tumor necrosis factor may have a critical role in activating the killing of *M. tuberculosis*.

NATURAL KILLER CELLS

Natural killer (NK) cells are large lymphocytes with cytoplasmic granules, sometimes referred to as large granular lymphocytes. They lack specific antigen receptors but can kill certain tumor cells or normal cells infected by a virus. NK cells are neither T cells nor B cells, although they express the CD2 molecule and a low-affinity receptor for the Fc portion of IgG (CD16). They can acquire additional specificity by virtue of FcR-dependent attachment to IgG antibody–coated targets and can thereby serve as effector cells of ADCC. They produce and respond to cytokines, which modulate their functions. The mediators of target lysis include porins and other granule contents.

γδ T CELLS

γδ T cells have excited interest as a potential intermediary between nonspecific inflammatory cells and specific immune effector cells. They constitute approximately 5% of T cells in circulation and in lymphoid organs. γδ T cells are not class I or class II MHC restricted and appear to target broadly cross-reactive human serum proteins (HSPs). Therefore, they may function in the initial or innate response to microbes and possibly in the pathogenesis of autoimmune diseases. γδ T cells express cytokines and possess cytotoxic function. Their relative role in infection and immunity awaits definition. Integration of the various host defense mechanisms is apparent as one examines resistance to specific representative infectious agents.

Resistance to Extracellular Bacteria: Encapsulated Organisms

STREPTOCOCCUS PNEUMONIAE

The type-specific polysaccharide capsule is a major virulence factor because of its antiphagocytic properties. Antibody to the polysaccharide is itself capable of preventing pneumococcal disease, as reflected by experimental studies and the efficacy of pneumococcal polysaccharide vaccines.

In the absence of immunity, pneumococci reaching the alveoli are not effectively contained by the host. Their phagocytosis by neutrophils is inefficient, because organisms must be trapped against a surface to be ingested (*surface phagocytosis;* see Fig. 92–3). The pneumococcus does, however, elicit a neutrophilic inflammatory response. The organism activates complement by the alternative pathway and interactions of C-reactive protein in serum with pneumococcal C-polysaccharide. Activated complement fragments (C3a, C5a, C567) and bacterial oligopeptides are chemotactic for neutrophils. Opsonic complement fragments (C3b) coating pneumococci favor their attachment to neutrophils but are less effective in promoting phagocytosis and killing than is specific antibody. Clinical observations also directly support the primal role of antibody in immunity. The development of specific antibody on days 5 to 9 of untreated pneumococcal pneumonia produces a clinical "crisis," with dramatic resolution of symptoms. Opsonization of *S. pneumoniae* by type-specific antipolysaccharide antibody promotes ingestion and oxidative burst activity, with destruction of the organism.

NEISSERIA MENINGITIDIS

Capsular polysaccharide also represents an important virulence factor for meningococci. In addition, pathogenic *Neisseria* species produce an IgA protease that dissociates the Fc fragment from the Fab portion of secretory and serum IgA and thus interferes with effector properties of the antibody molecule. Antibody-dependent, complement-mediated bacterial killing is the most critical host defense against meningococci. In illustration of this principle, the age-specific incidence of meningococcal meningitis during the first 12 years of life is inversely proportional to the age-related frequency of serum bactericidal antibody directed against capsular and cell wall bacterial antigens. Therefore, the presence of bactericidal antibody is associated with protection against the meningococcus. In epidemic situations, 40% of persons who become colonized with the epidemic strain but who lack bactericidal antibodies develop disease. Protective serum antibody is elicited by colonization with the following: (1) nonencapsulated and encapsulated strains of meningococci of low virulence, which elicit antibodies cross-reactive with virulent strains; and (2) *Escherichia coli* and *Bacillus* species with cross-reacting capsular polysaccharides. The lack of bactericidal activity in the serum of adolescents and adults manifesting susceptibility to *N. meningitidis* may be due to blocking IgA antibody. Susceptibility of patients lacking C6, C7, or C8 to meningococcal infection provides important evidence that the dominant protective mechanism against this organism involves complement-mediated bacteriolysis. Evaluation of persons who develop meningococcal disease in a nonepidemic setting sometimes reveals underlying abnormalities of the complement system.

Resistance to Obligate Intracellular Parasites: Viruses

Host antiviral defense is characterized by overlap and redundancy, which allow a rapid and effective response to most viral agents. The key element of the response varies with the virus, the site, and the timing. Initially, infection is limited at the local site by type I interferons, which increase the resistance of neighboring cells to spread of the infection. Complement directly neutralizes some enveloped viruses. NK cells destroy infected cells, a process enhanced by the interferons. As specific antibody is produced, IgA neutralizes the virus at mucosal surfaces; IgG neutralizes a virus that has spread systemically to extracellular sites and allows uptake and destruction by FcR-bearing effector cells through antibody (ADCC). Later, effector cells, or CTLs, are expanded and activated to lyse host cells expressing viral antigens in the context of MHC products. CTLs disrupt parasitized cells and expose viruses to extracellular neutralization and clearance mechanisms.

The host thus directs several defenses against viral infection. The same humoral and cellular mechanisms that destroy bacteria clear extracellular viruses. The host immune response is also effective against intracellular replicative stages of viruses and may destroy infected host cells that express viral antigens on their surfaces. Clinical and experimental observations indicate the respective roles of humoral and cellular immunity in resisting certain viruses. In Hodgkin's disease, in advanced human immunodeficiency virus infection, and in T-lymphocyte–deficient experimental models, selective defects in cellular immunity lead to reactivation of certain latent Herpesviridae: herpes simplex, varicella-zoster, and cytomegalovirus. The prominent role for cellular immunity against these agents is biologically advantageous because virions spread intercellularly through desmosomes or intercellular bridges; viruses thereby avoid exposure to the antibody-rich extracellular milieu. Destruction of virus-infected cells by specific CTLs becomes an essential first step in host defense by allowing extracellular mechanisms to mop up free viral particles.

In contrast, antibody-dependent and complement-dependent mechanisms assume major importance against viruses that themselves lyse host cells and spread by extracellular means; for these agents, passive transfer of antibody confers protection. Nevertheless, the absence of greatly increased susceptibility of hypogammaglobulinemic patients to measles and influenza implies the continued contribution of cellular immunity in protection against these agents and indicates important overlap in antiviral host effector mechanisms. The major antiviral defenses include humoral mechanisms, cellular immunity, and interferons.

HUMORAL DEFENSES

Complement-Independent Neutralization

Specific IgG, IgM, and IgA neutralize infectivity of viruses. The respective antibodies first combine with proteins of the virus coat. Resulting conformational changes may prevent adsorption of viruses to cells and cellular penetration; sometimes, antibody coating of an extracellular virus interferes with subsequent intracellular events, such as uncoating. Alternatively, antibody may physically aggregate viral particles.

IgA is the key defender against viral infections that begin on or are confined to respiratory epithelium. For infections such as poliomyelitis, measles, and rubella, which begin on a mucosal surface and then disseminate hematogenously, local IgA antibody prevents infection, whereas serum IgG antibody prevents disease.

Complement-Facilitated Neutralization

Complement neutralizes some enveloped viruses by direct or antibody-dependent steric changes or aggregation. Infected host cells expressing surface virus antigens are also susceptible to lysis by mechanisms involving the alternate complement pathway and are further enhanced by antibody.

Opsonization of extracellular viruses by complement and IgG antibody facilitates phagocytosis by neutrophils and macrophages. This process destroys some viruses (enteroviruses) but aids cellular penetration and replication of others (arboviruses).

Enzyme Inhibition

Antibody may interfere with release of progeny influenza virus by blocking viral neuraminidase. Replication is thereby limited, although the virion is not neutralized.

CELLULAR IMMUNITY

Cellular Cytotoxicity

These defenses are of chief relevance for viruses that spread by intercellular means.

Cytotoxic T Lymphocytes. These cells appear early in viral infection and are specific for viral antigens expressed on the surface of parasitized cells. Most are CD8 cells that effect class I MHC–restricted killing. Class II MHC–restricted killing by CD4 cells is also important in the immune response to certain viruses. CD4 cells also promote differentiation and activation of CD8 and CTLs.

Antibody-Dependent Cell-Mediated Cytotoxicity. Virus-infected cells that display surface viral antigens are opsonized by IgG antibodies and are lysed by ADCC. The effector cells are lymphocytes (killer cells), macrophages, and neutrophils; all bear surface Fc receptors.

Natural Killer Cells. NK cells spontaneously lyse virally infected cells; this effector mechanism is activated by interferon-γ and IL-2.

Interferons

The antiviral action of interferons provides a major host defense against viruses. Interferons are a family of proteins produced by lymphocytes, fibroblasts, epithelial cells, and macrophages early in the course of viral infection, before specific antibody develops. Exposure of cells to interferon induces their synthesis of proteins that, in turn, selectively inhibit the production of viral proteins. The immunoregulatory effects of interferon-γ may also contribute indirectly to antiviral immunity by activating effector cells.

Type I interferons consist of two serologically distinct families of proteins. *Interferon-γ* is produced by mononuclear phagocytes, and *interferon-β* is produced by fibroblasts; other cells can also secrete these factors in response to viral infection. Viral infection induces type I interferon, which protects uninfected neighboring cells by inducing synthesis of enzymes that interfere with replication of viral RNA or DNA. Type I interferons have two other functions that promote viral defense: they promote the lytic potential of NK cells, and they increase target expression of class I MHC molecules; the result is increased target susceptibility to lysis by CTLs. Interferon-γ is a type II interferon with prominent immunoregulatory activity produced by activated T lymphocytes.

Resistance to Facultative Intracellular Parasites: *Mycobacterium tuberculosis*

Activation of host phagocytes provides the critical defense mechanism against *M. tuberculosis*. Primary infection progresses locally in the nonhypersensitive host, because ingested organisms persist and multiply within mononuclear phagocytes. The bacteria escape intracellular digestion by virtue of constituents (sulfatides, suramin, poly-D-glutamic acid) that inhibit phagolysosomal fusion. Antibody-coated mycobacteria do not evade phagolysosomal fusion but nonetheless resist degradation, probably because of shielding provided by their rich lipid content. The development of cellular immunity leads to T-lymphocyte–dependent macrophage activation and to the killing of the intracellular tubercle bacillus organism. The lesions of primary tuberculosis regress. However, latent foci persist, and delayed reactivation remains a threat throughout the lifetime of the host.

REFERENCES

Abbas AK, Lichtman AH, Pober JS: Cellular and Molecular Immunology. Philadelphia: WB Saunders, 1991.

Anderson G, Moore NC, Owen JJT, et al: Cellular interactions in thymocyte development. Annu Rev Immunol 1996; 14:73–99.

Biron CA: Cytokines in the generation of immune responses to, and resolution of, virus infections. Curr Opin Immunol 1994; 6:530–538.

Holland SM, Gallin JI: Evaluation of the patient with suspected immunodeficiency. *In* Mandel GL, Bennett JE, Dolin R (eds): Principles and Practices of Infectious Diseases, 4th ed. New York: Churchill Livingstone, 1995, pp 1490–1580.

Nossal GJV: Current concepts: Immunology. The basic components of the immune system. N Engl J Med 1987; 316:1320.

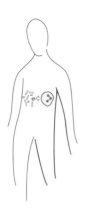

93

LABORATORY DIAGNOSIS OF INFECTIOUS DISEASES

Michael M. Lederman

Five basic laboratory techniques can be used in the diagnosis of infectious diseases: (1) direct visualization of the organism; (2) detection of microbial antigen; (3) a search for "clues" produced by the host response to specific microorganisms; (4) detection of specific microbial nucleotide sequences; and (5) isolation of the organism in culture. Each technique has its use and its pitfalls. The laboratory can usually provide the clinician with prompt, accurate, and, if used judiciously, inexpensive diagnosis.

Diagnosis by Direct Visualization of the Organism

In many infectious diseases, pathogenic organisms can be directly visualized by microscopic examination of readily available tissue fluids. With the use of Gram's or acid-fast stains, bacteria, mycobacteria, and *Candida* can be readily identified. An India ink preparation can often identify *Cryptococcus*, and potassium hydroxide (KOH) preparations can occasionally identify other fungal pathogens.

Because Gram's and acid-fast stains are now generally performed by laboratory technicians, a description of their techniques is not provided in this text. The following three diagnostic procedures are described, however, because they continue to provide simple, inexpensive approaches to bedside diagnosis of clinically important infections.

INDIA INK PREPARATION

A drop of centrifuged cerebrospinal fluid (CSF) is placed on a microscope slide next to a drop of artist's India ink. A coverslip is placed over the drops, and the area of mixing of CSF and India ink is examined at 100× magnification. Cryptococci are identified by their large capsules, which exclude the India ink (Fig. 93–1).

KOH PREPARATION

A drop of sputum, a skin scraping, or a smear of vaginal or oral exudate is placed on a slide together with 1 drop of 5% to 40% KOH. A coverslip is placed on the specimen, and the slide is heated for 2 to 5 seconds above a flame. The condenser of the microscope is lowered, and the specimen is examined at 100× magnification when searching for elastin fibers (whose presence in sputum suggests a necrotizing pneumonia) or 400× when looking for fungal forms. The KOH will partially dissolve host cells and bacteria, sparing fungi and elastin fibers.

TZANCK'S PREPARATION

A vesicle suspected of harboring herpesvirus (zoster or simplex) is unroofed with a scalpel, and the base is gently scraped. The scrapings are placed on a glass slide, air dried, and stained with Wright's stain, Giemsa's stain, or a rapid stain such as methylene blue. The slide is then examined at low (100×) power for the presence of multinucleated giant cells; their characteristic appearance is then confirmed at high (400×) power. Although this direct bedside technique identifies the host response to infection (see later) and not the organism itself, demonstration of giant cells is diagnostic for herpesvirus infection.

Other techniques can be used, but they require more sophisticated techniques. Silver staining using the Gomori methenamine technique can identify most fungi, including *Pneumocystis carinii*. Experienced pathologists can also identify *P. carinii* on Giemsa-stained specimens of induced sputum. Immunofluorescence techniques rapidly identify pathogens such as *Legionella pneumophila* and *Bordetella pertussis*. Immunofluorescence can also be used to identify cells infected with influenza virus, respiratory syncytial virus, and adenovirus in respiratory sections. Darkfield microscopy can identify *Treponema pallidum*, and electron microscopy can often detect viral particles in infected cells.

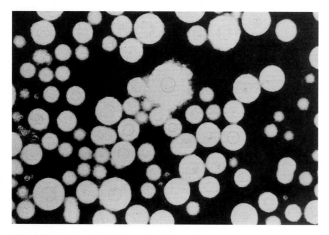

FIGURE 93–1   India ink preparation of cerebrospinal fluid revealing encapsulated cryptococci. Note the large capsules surrounding the smaller organisms.

Diagnosis by Detection of Microbial Antigens

Certain pathogens can be detected by examination of specimens for microbial antigens (Table 93–1). These studies can be performed rapidly—often within 1 hour. The diagnosis of meningitis caused by *Streptococcus pneumoniae*, some strains of *Haemophilus influenzae*, and *Neisseria meningitidis* can be made rapidly by detection of specific polysaccharide antigen in the CSF using latex agglutination. Although these diagnoses can also be made by Gram's stain or India ink preparation, antigen detection is especially helpful when attempts at direct visualization of the pathogen are not diagnostic (e.g., in the patient with partially treated bacterial meningitis). Immunofluorescence techniques using antibodies directed against the organisms identify pathogens such as *Legionella pneumophila* and *Bordetella pertussis* in respiratory secretions. Immunofluorescence can also be used to identify cells infected with influenza virus, respiratory syncytial virus, and adenovirus. The demonstration of hepatitis B surface antigen in blood establishes the presence of infection by this virus.

Diagnosis by Examination of Host Immune or Inflammatory Responses

Histopathologic examination of sampled or excised tissue often shows patterns of the host inflammatory response that can narrow down diagnostic possibilities. As a general rule, a polymorphonuclear leukocytic infiltrate suggests an acute bacterial process. A lymphocytic infiltrate suggests a more chronic process and is characteristically seen in viral, mycobacterial, and fungal infections. Eosinophilia suggests helminthic infestations. Granuloma formation points to mycobacterial and certain fungal infections. Some diseases, such as syphilis (obliterative endarteritis), cat-scratch disease (mixed granulomatous, suppurative, and lymphoid hyperplastic changes), and lymphogranuloma venereum (stellate abscesses), have fairly characteristic histologic features. Several viral infections produce characteristic changes in host cells, which are detectable by cytologic examination. Skin or respiratory infection with herpesviruses, or pneumonia caused by cytomegalovirus or measles virus, for example, can be diagnosed with reasonable accuracy by cytologic examination (e.g., Tzanck's preparation for herpesvirus infection).

Similarly, examination of infected fluids such as CSF will provide clues to etiology. Bacterial infections generally provoke a polymorphonuclear leukocytosis with elevated protein and depressed glucose concentrations. Viral infections most often provoke a lymphocytic pleocytosis; protein elevations are less marked, and glucose levels are usually normal.

Host cell–mediated immune responses can be used to help make certain diagnoses. A positive skin test for delayed-type hypersensitivity to mycobacterial or fungal antigens indicates active or previous infection with these agents. A negative skin test may be seen despite active infection in individuals with depression of cell-mediated immunity (anergy). Therefore, control skin tests using commonly encountered antigens (e.g., *Candida*, mumps, *Trichophyton*) are often applied to ascertain if the patient can mount a delayed-type hypersensitivity response. Occasionally, the response to disease-related antigens is depressed selectively.

Host humoral responses may be used to diagnose

TABLE 93–1   **Diseases Often Diagnosed by Detection of Microbial Antigens**

Disease	Assay	Agent Detected
Meningitis	Latex agglutination	*Streptococcus pneumoniae, Haemophilus influenzae, Neisseria meningitidis, Cryptococcus*
Respiratory tract infection	Immunofluorescence Enzyme immunoassay	*Bordetella pertussis, Legionella pneumophila,* influenza virus, respiratory syncytial virus, adenovirus
Genitourinary tract infection	Enzyme immunoassay	*Chlamydia* species, herpes simplex viruses 1 and 2
Hepatitis B	Radioimmunoassay	Hepatitis B surface antigen

certain infections, particularly those caused by organisms whose cultivation is difficult (e.g., *Ehrlichia chafeensis*) or hazardous to laboratory personnel (e.g., *Francisella tularensis*). In general, two sera are obtained at intervals of at least 2 weeks. A fourfold or greater rise (or fall) in antibody titer generally suggests a recent infection. Antibodies of the IgM class also suggest recent infection.

Assays that Detect Microbial Nucleotide Sequences

Detection of microbial nucleotide sequences can provide a sensitive and specific means of identification of pathogens in clinical specimens. These genetic molecular diagnostic techniques can provide rapid speciation of slow-growing microbial isolates. In addition, these techniques can also provide rapid quantitation of pathogens that can establish the prognosis and also determine the effectiveness of modes of therapy. Finally, genetic analyses can identify genetic markers of antimicrobial resistance that can guide the selection of therapy.

The exquisite sensitivity and specificity of these techniques are consequences of the specificity of DNA base pairing and the dramatic amplifications of signals that can be provided by techniques such as the quantitative polymerase chain reaction (PCR), nucleic acid sequence–based amplification (NASBA), and branched-chain signal amplification (bDNA) analyses.

The sensitivity of these techniques has revolutionized laboratory diagnostics. For example, most standard techniques for detection of microbial antigens cannot reliably detect fewer than 100,000 molecules in clinical samples. In contrast, the genetic techniques discussed earlier are being used now to routinely identify as few as 20 to 50 molecules in clinical samples and can be modified to have even greater sensitivity.

Clinical Applications of Molecular Diagnostics

Speciation. The slow replication of mycobacteria limits rapid speciation of these organisms after their identification in clinical samples. In certain clinical settings, such as those that may occur in persons with human immunodeficiency virus (HIV) infection, the distinction between nontuberculous mycobacteria and *Mycobacterium tuberculosis* may be particularly important. Genetic probes that distinguish among these organisms can provide rapid speciation after only limited growth.

Diagnosis of Infection. In acute HIV infection, detection of genomic HIV-1 RNA in plasma can provide diagnosis of this syndrome weeks before the development of diagnostic HIV-specific antibodies (see Chapter 108). Detection of herpes simplex virus sequences within cerebrospinal fluid (CSF) can provide a sensitive and specific diagnosis of herpes simplex encephalitis. Similar assays have been used for diagnosis of cytomega-

lovirus infection, syphilis of the central nervous system, and *Bartonella henselae* infection. It is anticipated that numerous infectious diseases will soon be diagnosed with great sensitivity by means of this technique. The exquisite sensitivity of this technique may, however, yield false-positive results unless the assays are carefully standardized and performed with great care.

Quantification of Microbial Infection. Molecular diagnostic assays have been refined and standardized to permit reliable quantification of microbial genomic sequences in clinical samples. These quantitative assays have provided evidence that the magnitude of microbial replication is predictive of disease outcome in both HIV infection and hepatitis C infection. Moreover, sequential application of these techniques to clinical samples can monitor the activity of therapy against these viral infections.

Detecting Genetic Markers for Antimicrobial Resistance. Microbial resistance to therapeutic interventions is an increasing problem in infectious diseases. When genetic sequences that confer resistance to therapies are known, assays to detect them can be applied rapidly to clinical samples, providing information that can be used to select treatment regimens. Direct analysis of plasma HIV sequences has provided genetic information that can predict the failure of specific modes of therapy; application of this information to the selection of treatment regimens can enhance the likelihood that treatment will be effective.

Diagnosis by Isolation of the Organism in Culture

Isolation of a single microbe from an infected site is generally considered evidence that the infection is caused by this organism. However, information obtained from the culture must be interpreted according to the clinical setting. For example, cultures obtained from ordinarily contaminated sites (e.g., vagina, pharynx) may be overgrown with nonpathogenic commensals, and fastidious organisms such as *Neisseria gonorrhoeae* are difficult to recognize unless cultured on medium that selects for their growth. Similarly, cultures of expectorated "sputum" may also be uninterpretable if heavily contaminated with saliva. The culture of an organism from an ordinarily sterile site is reasonable evidence for infection with that organism. On the other hand, the failure to culture an organism may simply result from inadequate culture conditions (e.g., "sterile" pus from a brain abscess cultured only on aerobic media). Most brain abscesses are caused by anaerobic bacteria that do not grow under aerobic conditions. Thus, when submitting samples for culture, the physician must alert the laboratory to likely pathogens.

Gram's stains of specimens submitted for culture are often invaluable aids to the interpretation of culture results. A Gram stain of "sputum" will readily detect contamination by saliva if squamous epithelial cells are seen. On the other hand, a Gram stain revealing bacteria despite negative cultures suggests infection by fastidious organisms. The presence of an organism in high density and within neutrophils also suggests that the corresponding bacterial isolate is causing disease rather than colonizing the patient or contaminating the specimen. Gram's staining of the initial clinical specimen may also help determine the relative importance of different isolates when cultures show mixed flora.

Viral Isolation

Because all viral pathogens that can be cultured require eukaryotic cells in which to grow, virus isolation is expensive and often laborious. Throat washings, rectal swabs, or cultures of infected sites should be transported immediately to the laboratory or, if this is not possible, placed in virus transport medium and refrigerated overnight until they can be cultured in the laboratory. Certain viruses such as human immunodeficiency virus and cytomegalovirus are often cultivated from whole blood samples. Notifying the laboratory of the suspected pathogens allows selection of the best cell lines or systems for culture. The clinician must be aware of the viruses that the hospital's laboratory can isolate. A fourfold rise in titer of antibody to the isolated virus suggests that it is causing disease rather than simply colonizing the area sampled.

Isolation of *Rickettsia*, *Chlamydia*, and *Mycoplasma*

Rickettsiae are cultivated primarily in reference laboratories. Diagnosis of rickettsial illness is generally made on clinical grounds and confirmed serologically. Although chlamydiae can be propagated in cell cultures used in most hospital virology laboratories, chlamydial infection is most often diagnosed through antigen detection techniques. Mycoplasmas will grow on selective media; the prolonged period of incubation required results with little advantage over serologic diagnosis.

Bacterial Isolation

Isolation of common bacterial pathogens is achieved readily by most hospital laboratories. Specimens should be carried promptly to the laboratory. In instances in which likely isolates may be fastidious (e.g., bacterial meningitis) and laboratories are closed, the specimen should be placed directly onto the culture medium, with careful attention to sterile techniques.

Isolation of anaerobic bacteria is often critically important for clinical diagnosis. When anaerobes are suspected, the specimen, if pus or liquid, can be drawn into a syringe, the air expelled, and the syringe capped before transport to the laboratory. Otherwise, specimens must be taken immediately to the laboratory or placed in an anaerobic transport medium appropriate for survival of pathogens. Because of contamination by oral anaerobes, sputum should not be cultured anaerobically unless the sample was obtained by transtracheal or percutaneous lung aspiration.

Isolation of Fungi and Mycobacteria

Specimens for fungal and mycobacterial culture must be processed and cultured by the microbiology laboratory. Although some fungi and rapid-growing mycobacteria grow readily on standard agars used for routine isolation of bacteria, others, such as *Mycobacterium tuberculosis* and *Histoplasma capsulatum*, must be cultured on special media for as long as several weeks.

REFERENCE

Gill VJ, Fedorko DP, Witebsky FG: The clinician and the microbiology laboratory. *In* Mandell GL, Bennett JC, Dolin R (eds): Principles and Practice of Infectious Diseases, 5th ed. New York: Churchill Livingstone, 2000, pp 184–222.

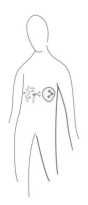

94

ANTIMICROBIAL THERAPY

Michael M. Lederman

The most dramatic advance in medical practice in the 20th century was the development of antimicrobial therapy. Antimicrobials are agents that interfere with microbial metabolism, resulting in inhibition of growth or death of bacteria, viruses, fungi, protozoa, or helminths. Some, like penicillin, are natural products of other microbes. Others, such as sulfa drugs, are chemical agents synthesized in the laboratory. Still others are semisynthetic, with chemical modifications of naturally occurring substances that result in enhanced activity (e.g., nafcillin) and/or diminished toxic effects.

The most effective antimicrobials are characterized by their relatively selective activity against microbes. Some, such as penicillins and amphotericin B, interfere with the synthesis of microbial cell walls that are absent in human cells. Others, such as trimethoprim and sulfa drugs, inhibit obligate microbial synthesis of essential nucleic acid intermediates, pathways not required by human cells. Still others, such as acyclovir, an antiviral agent, are relatively inactive until metabolized by pathogen-derived enzymes. The newly developed antiretroviral agents selectively inhibit viral enzymes that are essential for replication. Antimicrobial agents, although relatively selective in activity against microbes, have variable degrees of toxicity for human cells. Thus, monitoring for toxicity during antimicrobial therapy is important.

The Pathogen

If the pathogen has been clearly identified (see Chapter 93), a drug with a narrow spectrum of activity (i.e., highly selective for the particular pathogen) is usually the most reasonable choice. If the pathogen responsible for the patient's illness has not been identified, then the physician must choose a drug or combination of drugs active against the most likely pathogens in the specific setting. In either instance, the physician must be guided by patterns of antimicrobial resistance common in the community and in the specific hospital. Some pathogens (e.g., group A streptococci) are almost always sensitive to narrow-spectrum antimicrobials such as penicillin. Other pathogens, such as staphylococci, are variably resistant to penicillins but almost always susceptible to vancomycin. Resistance patterns, particularly among hospital-acquired bacteria, may vary widely and are important in devising antimicrobial strategies. Broad-spectrum antimicrobial coverage for all febrile patients ("shotgunning") must not be substituted for carefully evaluating the clinical problem and pinpointing therapy directed toward the most likely pathogen or pathogens. Widespread use of broad-spectrum antimicrobials almost invariably leads to emergence of resistant strains. On the other hand, the more sick a patient appears and the less certain the physician is of the responsible pathogen, the more important initial, empirical, broad-spectrum coverage becomes. Initial empirical treatment is also frequently indicated in the immunocompromised febrile patient (e.g., the patient with severe neutropenia secondary to chemotherapy). Once the pathogen is isolated and its antimicrobial sensitivities are known, empirical therapy must be scaled down to a definitive regimen with optimal activity against the specific microorganism.

Site of Infection

The location of the infection is also important in determining the selection and dosage of an antimicrobial. Deep-seated infections and bacteremic infections generally require higher doses of antimicrobials than, for example, superficial infections of the skin, upper respiratory tract, or lower urinary tract. Penetration of antimicrobials into sites such as the meninges, eye, and prostate is quite variable. Thus, treatment of infections at these sites involves selection of an antimicrobial agent that penetrates these tissues in concentrations sufficient to inhibit or kill the pathogen. The meninges are relatively resistant to penetration by most antimicrobials; inflammation renders the meninges somewhat more permeable. Therefore, high doses of antibiotics are the rule when treating meningitis. Bacterial infections of certain sites such as the heart valves or meninges must be treated with antibiotics that kill the microbe (bactericidal) as opposed to simply inhibiting its growth (bacteriostatic). This is so because local host defenses at these sites are inadequate to rid the host of infecting organisms. Infections involving foreign bodies may be impossible to eradicate without removing the foreign material.

Antimicrobials alone are often insufficient in the treatment of large abscesses. Although many drugs achieve reasonable concentrations in abscess walls, the low pH antagonizes the activity of some drugs (e.g., aminoglycosides), and some drugs bind to and are inactivated by white blood cells or their products. The large number of organisms, their depressed metabolism in this unfavorable milieu, and the frequent polymicrobial nature of certain abscesses increase the likelihood that some organisms present may be resistant to antimicrobial therapy. Most extracranial abscesses should be drained whenever anatomically possible.

Characteristics of the Antimicrobial

The physician must know the pharmacokinetics of the drug (i.e., its absorption, its penetration into various sites, its metabolism and excretion) and its toxic effects, as well as its spectrum of antimicrobial activity, before selecting it for use (Table 94–1).

DISTRIBUTION AND EXCRETION

Lipid-soluble drugs, such as chloramphenicol and rifampin, penetrate most membranes, including the meninges, more readily than do more ionized compounds, such as the aminoglycosides. Understanding a drug's distribution, rate and site of metabolism, and route of excretion is essential in selecting the appropriate drug and dose. Drugs excreted unchanged in the urine may be particularly good for the treatment of lower urinary tract infection or for the treatment of systemic infection in the presence of renal insufficiency. Some antimicrobials are metabolized in the liver and must be adjusted appropriately in the presence of hepatic dysfunction.

ACTIVITY OF THE DRUG

The physician must understand the spectrum of activity of the drug against microbial isolates, the mechanism of activity of the agent, and whether it is bactericidal or bacteriostatic in achievable concentrations. As a general rule, cell wall–active drugs are likely to be bactericidal. Bactericidal drugs are necessary for treatment of infections sequestered from effective host inflammatory responses such as meningitis and endocarditis. With the exception of aminoglycosides and certain azalide and macrolide antibiotics, agents inhibiting protein synthesis at ribosomal sites are generally bacteriostatic.

TOXIC EFFECTS OF THE DRUG

The physician must have a thorough understanding of the contraindications of the drug, as well as the major toxic effects and their general frequencies. This will help in evaluating the risks of treatment and will also assist in advising the patient about possible adverse reactions. History of drug hypersensitivity must be sought before prescribing any antimicrobials. The presence or absence of previous reactions to penicillin should be documented for every patient. Patients with a history suggestive of immediate hypersensitivity to penicillin, such as hives, wheezing, hypotension, laryngospasm, or angioedema at any site, must be considered at risk for anaphylaxis. These patients should not receive penicillins or related drugs (cephalosporins or imipenem) if adequate alternatives are available. The major and minor determinants of penicillin allergy (breakdown products that bind to serum proteins to form haptens) can be used to detect most persons at risk for serious immediate hypersensitivity. If skin test reactivity to these determinants is present and there are no reasonable alternatives to therapy with penicillin or a related compound, these patients may be desensitized to penicillin using a graduated protocol of intracutaneous penicillin administration. Desensitization should be done only in consultation with an experienced allergist. Patients with a history of an uncomplicated morbilliform or delayed rash after penicillin therapy are not likely to be at risk for immediate hypersensitivity and may be treated with cephalosporins, for which the risk of cross-hypersensitivity to penicillins is likely to be in the range of 5%. Evidence suggests that cross-hypersensitivity to aztreonam is less common.

Route of Administration

Oral administration of antimicrobials can often prevent the morbidity and expense associated with parenteral (intravenous or intramuscular) administration. Although some antimicrobials (e.g., amoxicillin and the fluoroquinolones) are very well absorbed after oral administration, most patients hospitalized with severe infections should be treated, at least initially, with intravenous antibiotics. Gut absorption of antimicrobials can be unpredictable, and the intravenous route often permits administration of greater amounts of drug than can be tolerated orally. Intramuscular administration of some antimicrobials can result in excellent drug absorption but should be avoided in the presence of hypotension (erratic absorption) and coagulation disorders (hematomas). Repeated intramuscular injections are uncomfortable and can also result in the formation of sterile abscesses (e.g., pentamidine).

Duration of Therapy

Antimicrobial therapy should be initiated as part of a treatment plan of defined duration. In some settings, the duration of optimal antimicrobial therapy is established (e.g., 10 days but not 7 days of oral penicillin will prevent rheumatic fever after streptococcal pharyngitis); in many others, the duration of treatment is empirical

TABLE 94–1   Characteristics of Commonly Used Antimicrobial Agents

Drug Class	Site of Action	Excretion/Metabolism	Uses/Activity
Antibacterials			
β-Lactams			
Penicillins	Cell wall	Renal	Streptococci, *Neisseria*, oral anaerobes
β-Lactamase–resistant penicillins (e.g., nafcillin)	Cell wall	Renal and/or hepatic	Methicillin-sensitive staphylococci
Amino penicillins (e.g., ampicillin)	Cell wall	Renal	Gram-positive organisms, not staphylococci, some gram-negative organisms
Extended-spectrum penicillins (e.g., mezlocillin)	Cell wall	Renal	Broad-spectrum gram-positive organisms; gram-negative organisms, including *Pseudomonas,* not *Staphylococcus*
β-Lactamase inhibitors (e.g., clavulanic acid)	Inactivates β-lactamase	Renal/metabolic	Used with ampicillin, piperacillin, or ticarcillin, expands activity to include anaerobes, many gram-negative organisms, and methicillin-sensitive staphylococci
*Cephalosporins**	Cell wall		
First generation (e.g., cefazolin)		Renal	Broad spectrum
Second generation (e.g., cefuroxime)		Renal	Some with anaerobic activity (e.g., cefoxitin)
Third generation (e.g., ceftriaxone)		Renal or hepatic	Some active against *Pseudomonas* (e.g., ceftazidime)
Monobactams			
Aztreonam	Cell wall	Renal	Aerobic gram-negative bacilli
Carbapenems			
Imipenem/cilastatin	Cell wall	Renal	Very broad-spectrum, some enterococci, and methicillin-sensitive staphylococci
Vancomycin	Cell wall	Renal	Coagulase-positive and coagulase-negative staphylococci, other gram-positive bacteria
Sulfonamides/trimethoprim	Inhibit nucleic acid synthesis	Renal	Gram-negative bacilli, *Salmonella, Pneumocystis carinii, Nocardia*
Fluoroquinolones	DNA gyrase	Some hepatic metabolism	Broad spectrum, including *Legionella,* newer agents also active vs. streptococci or anaerobes
Metronidazole	DNA disruption	Hepatic metabolism	Anaerobes, *Clostridium difficile,* amebas, *Trichomonas*
Rifampin	Transcription	Hepatic metabolism/renal	*Mycobacterium tuberculosis;* meningococcal and *Haemophilus influenzae* prophylaxis
Aminoglycosides	Ribosome	Renal	Gram-negative bacilli; no activity in anaerobic conditions
Chloramphenicol	Ribosome	Hepatic metabolism/renal	Broad spectrum; especially useful for *Salmonella,* anaerobes, *Rickettsia*
Clindamycin	Ribosome	Hepatic metabolism/renal	Anaerobes; gram-positive cocci
Tetracyclines	Ribosome	Renal/hepatic metabolism	Broad spectrum; especially useful for spirochetes, *Rickettsia*

Table continued on following page

TABLE 94–1   Characteristics of Commonly Used Antimicrobial Agents
Continued

Drug Class	Site of Action	Excretion/Metabolism	Uses/Activity
Macrolides/Azalides			
Erythromycin	Ribosome	Hepatic	Gram-positive cocci, *Legionella*, *Mycoplasma*
Azithromycin Clarithromycin	Ribosome	Hepatic	High intracellular levels have enhanced activity against mycobacteria, *Toxoplasma*
Antifungals			
Polyenes			
Amphotericin B	Binds membrane ergosterol	?	Most fungi
Flucytosine	Blocks DNA synthesis	Renal	Candidiasis; *Cryptococcus* with amphotericin B
Azoles	Block ergosterol biosynthesis	Renal	
Ketoconazole		Hepatic	Mucosal candidiasis, pulmonary histoplasmosis (nonmeningeal)
Itraconazole		Hepatic	Histoplasmosis, blastomycosis
Fluconazole		Renal	Candidiasis, cryptococcosis, coccidioidomycosis
Antivirals			
Acyclovir	DNA polymerase	Renal	Herpes simplex, including encephalitis; herpes zoster in immunosuppressed hosts
Famciclovir	DNA polymerase		Herpes simplex, zoster
Ganciclovir	DNA polymerase	Renal	Cytomegalovirus, herpesviruses
Foscarnet	DNA polymerase	Renal	Cytomegalovirus, herpesviruses, ?HIV
Cidofovir	DNA polymerase	Renal	Cytomegalovirus, herpesviruses
Amantadine/rimantadine	?Uncoating	Renal	Influenza A treatment and prophylaxis
Zanamavir	Neuraminidase	Renal	Influenza A and B
Oseltamavir	Neuraminidase	Renal	Influenza A and B
Ribavirin	?RNA synthesis	Hepatic/renal	RSV, Hepatitis C (together with interferon-α)
Interferon-α	Immunomodulator		Hepatitis B, C ?HIV
Antiretrovirals			
Nucleoside reverse transcriptase inhibitors†	Reverse transcriptase	Renal and/or hepatic	HIV-1
Non-nucleoside reverse transcriptase inhibitors‡	Reverse transcriptase	Hepatic	HIV-1
Protease inhibitors§	HIV-1 protease	Hepatic	HIV-1

* As a rule, first-generation cephalosporins have better activity against gram-positive cocci and minimal CNS penetration. Second-generation cephalosporins have somewhat better activity against gram-negative bacteria and may penetrate the CNS. Third-generation cephalosporins have the broadest activity against gram-negative bacteria and generally penetrate the CNS, but they are relatively less active against gram-positive cocci.

† These include zidovudine, stavudine, didanosine, zalcitabine, lamivudine, abavavir.

‡ These include efavirenz, nevirapine, delavirdine.

§ These include indinavir, nelfinavir, ritonavir, saquinavir, amprenavir.

CNS = central nervous system; HIV = human immunodeficiency virus; RSV = respiratory syncytial virus.

and sometimes can be based on the clinical and bacteriologic course. Blood stream infections without endocarditis or other focal infections can generally be treated for 10 to 14 days. Pneumococcal pneumonia can be effectively treated in 7 to 10 days. The duration of therapy for endocarditis is largely dictated by the characteristics of the culpable microorganism but generally is at least 4 weeks.

Combinations

Combinations of antimicrobials are indicated in serious infection when they provide more effective activity against a pathogen than any single agent. In some instances, combinations of drugs are used to prevent the emergence of resistance (e.g., infections due to *Mycobacterium tuberculosis*). In others, combinations are used because they provide synergistic action against the pathogen (e.g., penicillin, a cell wall–active antibiotic, facilitates uptake of aminoglycosides by enterococci). In still other instances, drug combinations are used in empirical therapies to cover a wide spectrum of potential pathogens when the causative agent is unidentified or when infection is likely to be due to a mixture of organisms (e.g., fecal soilage of the peritoneum). The use of more than one drug increases the likelihood of toxic effects, increases costs, and often increases the risk of superinfection.

Monitoring of Antimicrobial Therapy

The physician and patient should be alert to potential toxic effects and should be prepared to halt the drug in the event of serious toxic effects. For some antimicrobials, such as aminoglycosides, the ratio of effective to toxic drug levels is low. Thus, serum levels of the drug must be monitored to ensure appropriate dosing. For certain infections (e.g., infective endocarditis due to relatively resistant organisms), monitoring of antimicrobial activity in serum shortly after (peak) and just before (trough) drug administration may help guide antimicrobial choices and usage. Although these techniques are not well standardized, clinicians often adjust drugs and doses to maintain serum bactericidal titers of at least 1:8 in treating certain forms of endocarditis (e.g., enterococcal) in which the antimicrobial resistance pattern of the microorganism may be quite variable.

Antiviral Agents

As obligate intracellular pathogens, viruses depend on interactions with host cellular machinery for completion of the life cycle. Thus, many potential antiviral treatment strategies are limited by toxic effects on host cells. Specificity for viruses or virus-infected cells can be obtained by interfering with the function of unique viral elements (e.g., the M2 protein of influenza virus that is the target of amantadine and rimantadine) or by developing drugs such as acyclovir that must be processed by viral enzymes (in this instance, phosphorylated by herpesvirus thymidine kinase) before becoming active. In contrast to antibacterial drugs, however, antiviral agents generally have a limited spectrum of activity, with each agent useful against a small number of viruses. In the 1990s there was a dramatic increase in the numbers and types of drugs effective in the treatment of viral infections. This has been particularly striking in the field of antiretroviral therapies (see Chapter 108). Additional developments in therapies for other viruses (e.g., hepatitis B and hepatitis C viruses) are anticipated.

Antifungal Agents

A number of drugs are useful in the treatment of fungal diseases. Most target the ergosterol-containing cell membrane either by inhibiting ergosterol synthesis (azoles) or by aggregating in proximity to ergosterol and increasing membrane permeability (polyenes). Flucytosine inhibits fungal DNA synthesis. Increasing resistance to azoles and flucytosine among clinically relevant fungal isolates limits the utility of these agents in patients requiring chronic therapy.

Antimicrobial Resistance Testing

As treatment options expand, the emergence of antimicrobial resistance to therapies is predictable. Thus, physicians must be prepared to evaluate the resistance patterns of specific microbial isolates. Resistance testing is now routinely provided for bacterial pathogens and is increasingly used in the design of antiretroviral treatment strategies (see Chapter 108). Certain resistance assays are not yet fully standardized, and all require some level of expertise to facilitate their interpretation. Thus, interpretation of resistance assay results to guide treatment decisions, whether for serious bacterial, fungal, or viral infections, should generally involve discussion with an expert in infectious diseases.

REFERENCES

Hayden FG: Antiviral drugs other than antiretrovirals. *In* Mandell GL, Bennett JE, Dolin R (eds): Principles and Practice of Infectious Diseases, 5th ed. New York: Churchill Livingstone, 2000, pp 460–490.

Karchmer AW: Antibacterial therapy. *In* Goldman L, Bennett JC (eds): Cecil Textbook of Medicine, 21st ed. Philadelphia: WB Saunders, 2000, pp 1591–1603.

Opal SM, Mayer KH, Medeiros AA: Mechanisms of bacterial antibiotic resistance. *In* Mandell GL, Bennett JE, Dolin R (eds): Principles and Practice of Infectious Diseases, 5th ed. New York: Churchill Livingstone, 2000, pp 236–252.

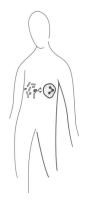

95

FEVER AND FEBRILE SYNDROMES

Robert A. Salata

Regulation of Body Temperature

Although "normal" body temperature ranges vary considerably, oral temperature readings in excess of 37.8°C (100.2°F) are generally abnormal. In healthy humans, core body temperature is maintained within a narrow range, so that for each individual, daily temperature variations greater than 1°C to 1.5°C are distinctly unusual. This homeostasis is controlled by hypothalamic nuclei that establish set points for body temperature. Homeostasis is effected by a complex balance between heat-generating and heat-conserving mechanisms that raise body temperature, on the one hand, and mechanisms that dissipate heat and lower body temperature, on the other. Heat is regularly generated as a by-product of obligate energy utilization (e.g., cellular metabolism, myocardial contraction, breathing). When an increase in body temperature is needed, shivering—nondirected muscular contraction—generates large amounts of heat. Peripheral vessels constrict to diminish heat lost to the environment. At the same time, the person feels cold; this heat preference promotes heat-conserving behavior, such as wrapping up in a blanket.

Obligate heat loss to the environment occurs through the skin and by evaporation of water through sweat and respiration. When the body must cool down, heat loss is promoted. Vasodilation flushes the skin capillaries, temporarily raising skin temperature but ultimately lowering core body temperature by increasing heat loss through the skin to the cooler environment. Sweating promotes rapid heat loss through evaporation, and at the same time the subject feels warm and sheds blankets or initiates other activities to promote heat loss.

Fever and Hyperthermia

Fever is an elevated body temperature that is mediated by an increase in the hypothalamic heat-regulating set point. Thus, although fever may be precipitated by exogenous substances such as bacterial products, the increase in body temperature is achieved through physiologic mechanisms. In contrast, hyperthermia is an increase in body temperature that overrides or bypasses the normal homeostatic mechanisms. As a general rule, body temperatures in excess of 41°C (105.8°F) are rarely physiologically mediated and suggest hyperthermia. Hyperthermia may be seen after vigorous exercise, in patients with heat stroke, as a heritable reaction to anesthetics (malignant hyperthermia), as a response to phenothiazines (neuroleptic malignant syndrome), and occasionally in patients with central nervous system disorders such as paraplegia (see also Chapter 113). Some patients with severe dermatoses are also unable to dissipate heat and therefore experience hyperthermia.

Fever is usually a physiologic response to infection or inflammation. Monocytes or tissue macrophages are activated by various stimuli to liberate various cytokines with pyrogenic activity (Fig. 95–1). Interleukin-1 is also an essential cofactor in initiation of the immune response. Another pyrogenic cytokine, tumor necrosis factor-α, or cachectin, activates lipoprotein lipase and may also play a role in immune cytolysis. Another cytokine, tumor necrosis factor-β, or lymphotoxin, has similar properties. A fourth, interferon-alfa, has antiviral activity (see Chapter 92). Interleukin-6, a cytokine that potentiates B-cell immunoglobulin synthesis, also has pyrogenic activity. Endogenous pyrogens activate the anterior preoptic nuclei of the hypothalamus to raise the set

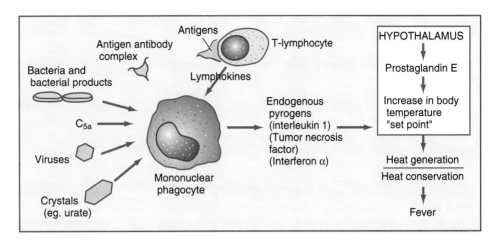

FIGURE 95–1 Pathogenesis of fever.

point for body temperature. Infection by all types of microorganisms can be associated with fever. Tissue injury with resulting inflammation, as seen in myocardial or pulmonary infarction or after trauma, can produce fever. Certain malignancies such as lymphoma and leukemia, renal cell carcinoma, and hepatic carcinoma are also associated with fever. In some instances, this is related to liberation of endogenous pyrogen by monocytes in the inflammatory response surrounding the tumor; in other cases, the malignant cell may release an endogenous pyrogen. Many immunologically mediated disorders, such as connective tissue diseases, serum sickness, and some drug reactions, are characterized by fever. In most cases of drug-induced fevers, the mechanisms of fever are unknown. Virtually any disorder associated with an inflammatory response (e.g., gouty arthritis) can be associated with fever. Certain endocrine disorders such as thyrotoxicosis, adrenal insufficiency, and pheochromocytoma can also produce fever.

The association of fever with infections or inflammatory disorders raises the question of whether fever is beneficial to the host. For example, interleukin-1 (an endogenous pyrogen) is critical for initiation of the immune response, certain in vitro immune responses are marginally enhanced by elevated temperatures, and some infectious organisms prefer cooler temperatures. It is not certain, however, that fever is helpful to humans in any infectious disease, with the possible exception of neurosyphilis. Fever is deleterious in certain situations. Among individuals with underlying brain disease and even in healthy elderly persons, fever can produce disorientation and confusion. Fever and associated tachycardia may compromise patients, especially the elderly, with significant cardiopulmonary disease. In young children, fever can result in seizures. Fever should be controlled if the patient is particularly uncomfortable or whenever it poses a specific risk to the patient. Fever in children with a history of febrile seizures and in patients with severe congestive heart failure or recent myocardial infarction should be treated with antipyretics, such as salicylates or acetaminophen. Acetaminophen or nonsteroidal anti-inflammatory drugs (NSAIDs) are indicated

for children because of the causative role of salicylates in Reye's syndrome.

Heat stroke almost always results from prolonged exposure to high environmental temperature and humidity, usually associated in otherwise healthy individuals with strenuous exercise. It is characterized by a body temperature greater than 40.6°C (105°F) and is associated with altered sensorium or coma and with cessation of sweating. Rapid cooling is critical to the patient's survival. Covering the patient with cold (11°C), wet compresses until core temperature reaches 39°C is the most effective initial therapeutic approach and should be followed by intravenous infusions of fluids appropriate to correct the antecedent fluid and electrolyte losses.

FEVER PATTERNS

The normal diurnal variation in body temperature results in a peak temperature in the late afternoon or early evening. This variation often persists when patients have fever. In certain instances, fever patterns may be helpful in suggesting the cause of fever. Rigors—true shaking chills—often herald a bacterial process (especially blood stream infection), although they may occur in cases of viral infection, as well as in drug or transfusion reactions. Hectic fevers, which are characterized by wide swings in temperature, may indicate the presence of an abscess, disseminated tuberculosis, or collagen vascular diseases. Patients with malaria may have a relapsing fever with episodes of shaking chills and high fever, which are separated by 1 to 3 days of normal body temperature and relative well-being. Patients with tuberculosis may be relatively comfortable and unaware of a markedly elevated body temperature. Patients with uremia, diabetic ketoacidosis, or hepatic failure generally have a lower body temperature; thus, normal temperature readings in these settings may indicate infection. Similarly, elderly patients with infection often fail to mount a febrile response and may present instead with loss of appetite, confusion, or even hypotension without fever. The administration of anti-inflammatory drugs (aspirin, NSAIDs, corticosteroids) also blunts or ablates the febrile response.

Acute Febrile Syndromes

Fever is one of the most common complaints that bring patients to a physician. The challenge is in discerning the few individuals who require specific therapy from among the many with self-limited benign illness. The approach is simplified by considering patients in three groups: (1) those with fever without localizing symptoms and signs, (2) those with fever and rash, and (3) those with fever and lymphadenopathy. This chapter deals only with fever caused by microbial agents. Clearly, autoimmune, neoplastic, and other disease processes may cause fever as well.

FEVER ONLY

Most patients with fever as their sole complaint defervesce spontaneously or present with localizing clinical or laboratory findings within 2 to 3 weeks of onset of illness (Table 95–1). Beyond 3 weeks, the patient can be considered to have a fever of unexplained origin (FUO),

TABLE 95–1   Infections Presenting with Fever as Sole or Dominant Feature

Infectious Agent	Epidemiology/Exposure History	Distinctive Clinical and Laboratory Findings	Diagnosis
Viral			
Rhinovirus, adenovirus, para-influenza virus, enterovirus, echovirus	None (adenovirus in epidemics) Summer, epidemic	Often URI symptoms Occasionally, aseptic meningitis, rash, pleurodynia, herpangina	Throat and rectal cultures, serologies
Influenza	Winter, epidemic	Headache, myalgias, arthralgias	Throat cultures, serologies
EBV, CMV	See text		
Colorado tick fever	Southwest, northwest, tick exposure	Biphasic illness, leukopenia	Blood, CSF cultures, erythrocyte-associated viral antigen (indirect immunofluorescence)
Bacterial			
Staphylococcus aureus	IV drug users, patients with IV plastic cannulas, hemodialysis, dermatitis	Must exclude endocarditis	Blood cultures
Listeria monocytogenes	Depressed cell-mediated immunity	One half have meningitis	Blood, CSF cultures
Salmonella typhi, S. paratyphi	Food or water contaminated by carrier or patient	Headache, myalgias, diarrhea or constipation, transient rose spots	Early blood, bone marrow cultures; late stool culture
Streptococci	Valvular heart disease	Low-grade fever, fatigue, anemia	Blood cultures
Post–Animal Exposure			
Coxiella burnetii (Q fever)	Infected livestock	Retrobulbar headache, occasionally pneumonitis, hepatitis, culture-negative endocarditis	Serologies
Leptospira interrogans	Water contaminated by urine from dogs, cats, rodents, small mammals	Headache, myalgias, conjunctival suffusion Biphasic illness Aseptic meningitis	Serologies
Brucella species	Exposure to cattle or contaminated dairy products	Occasionally epididymitis	Blood cultures, serologies
Ehrlichia chaffeensis	South and southeast; deer or dog tick exposure	Acute onset of headache, fever, myalgias; leukopenia and thrombocytopenia	PCR, serologies
Granulomatous Infection			
Mycobacterium tuberculosis	Exposure to patient with tuberculosis, known positive tuberculin skin test	Back pain suggests vertebral infection; sterile pyuria or hematuria suggests renal infection	Liver, bone marrow histology, cultures
Histoplasma capsulatum	Mississippi and Ohio River valleys	Pneumonitis, oropharyngeal lesions	Serologies; histology and cultures on liver, bone marrow, oral lesions

CMV = Cytomegalovirus; CSF = cerebrospinal fluid; EBV = Epstein-Barr virus; IV = intravenous; PCR = polymerase chain reaction; URI = upper respiratory infection.

a designation with its own circumscribed group of management considerations, as discussed later.

Viral Infections

In young, healthy individuals, acute febrile illnesses generally represent viral infections. The causative agent is rarely established, largely because establishing the precise diagnosis seldom has major therapeutic implications. Rhinovirus, parainfluenza, or adenovirus infections are usually, but not invariably, associated with symptoms of coryza or upper respiratory tract infection (rhinorrhea, sore throat, cough, hoarseness). Enterovirus and echovirus infections occur predominantly in summer, usually in an epidemic setting. Undifferentiated febrile syndromes account for the majority of enteroviral infections, but the etiology is more likely to be established definitively when a macular rash, aseptic meningitis, or a characteristic syndrome such as herpangina (vesicular pharyngitis caused by coxsackievirus A) or acute pleurodynia (fever, chest wall pain, and tenderness caused by coxsackievirus B) is present. Serologic surveys also indicate that many arthropod-borne viruses (California encephalitis virus; eastern, western, and Venezuelan equine encephalitis; St. Louis encephalitis) usually produce mild, self-limited febrile illnesses. Influenza causes sore throat, cough, myalgias, arthralgias, and headache in addition to fever; it most often occurs in an epidemic pattern during the winter months. It is unusual, however, for fever to persist beyond 5 days in uncomplicated influenza.

The mononucleosis syndromes caused by Epstein-Barr virus, primary HIV infection (see Chapter 110), cytomegalovirus, and (in rare cases) *Toxoplasma gondii* may present in a typhoidal manner—that is, with fever but little or no lymphadenopathy. Diagnosis and management are discussed later in the section "Generalized Lymphadenopathy," the more typical presentation of these processes.

The syndromes just described are, with the exception of acute HIV infection, self-limited and untreatable. The impetus for establishing a specific diagnosis, therefore, is small. The differentiation between viral and other causes of febrile illnesses is, on the other hand, of critical importance. Viral cultures of the throat and rectum and virus-specific antibodies in acute and convalescent serum samples may allow retrospective diagnosis of viral etiology. Usually, however, the fever is gone long before results of serologies become available.

Bacterial Infections

Bacterial disease may cause septicemia, which dominates the clinical presentation (see Chapter 96). *Staphylococcus aureus* frequently causes sepsis, sometimes without an obvious primary site of infection. Fever may be the predominant clinical manifestation of the illness. *S. aureus* sepsis should be considered in patients undergoing intravenous therapy with a plastic cannula, hemodialysis patients, intravenous drug users, and patients with severe chronic dermatoses. In the patient with *S. aureus* bacteremia, the question of whether intravascular infec-

tion exists is key in determining the length of therapy. The following are more typical of endocarditis: community-acquired infection, long duration of symptoms, absence of removable focus of infection (e.g., intravenous cannula, soft tissue abscess), metastatic sites of infection (e.g., septic pulmonary emboli, arthritis, meningitis), younger age, history of injection drug use, and new heart murmur. *Listeria monocytogenes* septicemia is seen predominantly in patients with depressed cell-mediated immunity. Up to one half of patients with *Listeria* sepsis have meningitis. Occasionally, a relatively indolent clinical syndrome belies the bacterial etiology of *S. aureus* and *L. monocytogenes* bacteremia.

Enteric fevers may also present in a subacute fashion despite the presence of bacteremia. The major species producing this syndrome are *Salmonella typhi*, which has a human reservoir, and *Salmonella paratyphi* A, B, and C. The paratyphoid strains also have their major reservoir in humans but produce less severe disease than *S. typhi*, which is acquired by ingestion of food or water contaminated with fecal material from a chronic carrier or a patient with typhoid fever. A large number of bacteria (10^6 to 10^8) must be ingested to cause disease in the normal host. Major host risk factors are achlorhydria, malnutrition, malignancy (particularly lymphomas), sickle cell anemia, and other defects in cellular and humoral immunity. *S. typhi* penetrates the gut wall and enters the lymphoid follicles (Peyer's patches), where it multiplies within mononuclear phagocytes and produces local ulceration. Primary bacteremia occurs with spread to the reticuloendothelial system (liver, spleen, and bone marrow). After further multiplication at those sites, secondary bacteremia occurs and can localize to lesions such as tumors, aneurysms, and bone infarcts. Infection of the gallbladder, particularly in the presence of gallstones, leads to a chronic carrier state. Approximately 2 weeks after exposure, patients develop prolonged fever with chills, headache, and myalgias. Diarrhea or constipation may be present but usually does not dominate the clinical picture. Occasionally, crops of rose spots (2- to 4-mm erythematous maculopapular lesions) appear on the upper abdomen but are evanescent. If left untreated, typhoid fever usually resolves in about 1 month. However, complication rates are high because of bowel perforation, metastatic infection, and general debility of patients. *S. typhi* may be isolated from blood or stool to confirm the diagnosis. Typhoid fever should be treated with third-generation cephalosporins or fluoroquinolones. Bactericidal agents become the drug of choice in patients with endocarditis, infected aneurysms, and sickle cell anemia; in patients with sickle cell anemia the dose-related bone marrow suppression by chloramphenicol is unacceptable.

Localized bacterial infection can be clinically occult and present as an undifferentiated febrile syndrome. Intra-abdominal abscess, vertebral osteomyelitis, streptococcal pharyngitis, urinary tract infection, infective endocarditis, and early pneumonia may all cause fever with surprisingly few clinical clues to the location of the infection. Therefore, urinalysis, throat and blood cultures, and chest radiography should be performed in the febrile patient presenting with features suggestive of a bacterial infection.

Febrile Syndromes Associated with Animal Exposure

Q fever, brucellosis, and leptospirosis are diseases associated with exposure to fluids from infected animals and may have similar clinical presentations.

Q Fever. Q fever is an underrecognized cause of acute febrile illness. Humans are infected by inhalation of aerosolized particles or by contact with placental and amniotic fluids from infected animals. The source of animal exposure may go unnoticed. For example, in an outbreak of Q fever at the University of Colorado Medical School, 70% of infected individuals lacked direct exposure to infected sheep.

Q fever characteristically begins explosively with severe, often retrobulbar headache, high fever, chills, and myalgias. Pneumonitis and hepatitis may occur but are seldom severe. Diagnosis is usually based on a fourfold rise in titer of complement-fixing antibodies. If not treated, Q fever lasts 2 to 14 days. *Coxiella burnetii* is sensitive to tetracycline, which should be used in its treatment (2 g/day orally for 14 days). Q fever may cause endocarditis, apparently as a form of reactivation of infection. The occurrence of hepatomegaly and thrombocytopenia in a patient with apparently culture-negative endocarditis may be a clue to this diagnosis.

Leptospirosis. Humans are infected with *Leptospira interrogans* by exposure to urine from infected dogs, cats, wild mammals, and rodents. Exposure on the farm, in the slaughterhouse, on camping trips, or during swims in contaminated water is frequent. After an incubation period of about 1 week, patients develop chills, high fever, headache, and myalgias. The illness often pursues a biphasic course. During the second phase of illness, fever is less prominent, but headache and myalgias are excruciating and nausea, vomiting, and abdominal pain become prominent complaints. Aseptic meningitis is the most important manifestation of the second or immune phase of the illness. Suffusion of the bulbar conjunctivae, with visible corkscrew vessels surrounding the limbus, is a useful early sign of leptospirosis. Lymphadenopathy, hepatomegaly, and splenomegaly may occur. Leptospirosis may also pursue a more severe clinical course characterized by renal and hepatic dysfunction and hemorrhagic diathesis (Weil's syndrome). Darkfield examination will reveal leptospires in body fluids. The diagnosis is made by a fourfold rise in indirect hemagglutination antibody titer. Early antibiotic treatment shortens the duration of fever and may reduce complications. However, to be effective, antibiotics must be initiated presumptively, before serologic confirmation. Penicillin G, 2.4 to 3.6 million U/day, or tetracycline, 2.0 g/day given orally, is effective therapy.

Brucellosis. *Brucella* species infect the genitourinary tract of cattle (*Brucella abortus*), pigs (*Brucella suis*), and goats (*Brucella melitensis*). Humans are exposed occupationally or by ingestion of unpasteurized dairy products. Acute disease is characterized by chills, fever, headache, and arthralgias and sometimes by lymphadenopathy, hepatomegaly, and splenomegaly. During the

associated bacteremia, any organ may be seeded. Epididymo-orchitis and vertebral or sacroiliac involvement are characteristic localized findings. With or without antibiotic treatment of acute infection, brucellosis may relapse or enter a chronic phase. *Brucella* species can be isolated from blood or other normally sterile fluids. However, the organism requires special media and conditions for growth. Otherwise, diagnosis must be made serologically. Treatment consists of doxycycline, 100 mg twice daily, and rifampin, 600 mg/day given orally for 21 days. Trimethoprim, 480 mg/day, with sulfamethoxazole, 2400 mg/day given orally, is an acceptable alternative regimen (especially in children), but relapses may be more frequent.

Cat-Scratch Disease. Tender enlargement of a regional lymph node, sometimes associated with low-grade fever, is a major manifestation of this illness, caused by a small bacillus, *Bartonella henselae*. This infection is discussed in detail later.

Granulomatous Infection

Tuberculosis. Extrapulmonary and miliary tuberculosis may present as febrile syndromes. In disseminated tuberculosis, initial chest radiographs may be normal and tuberculin skin tests are often nonreactive. This is particularly true in elderly patients. Protracted fevers of uncertain origin should always suggest this possibility. Liver biopsy and bone marrow biopsy have a high yield in miliary disease. Genitourinary and vertebral tuberculosis may present as unexplained fever. However, careful history, urinalysis, intravenous pyelography, and radiographs of the spine should reveal the site of tissue involvement. Extrapulmonary tuberculosis should be treated for the first 2 months with isoniazid, 300 mg orally; rifampin, 600 mg orally; ethambutol, 15 mg/kg/day; and pyrazinamide, 15 to 30 mg/kg (maximum, 2 g/day), given orally. Thereafter, isoniazid and rifampin are continued for 7 months (longer in cases of skeletal tuberculosis). The ethambutol can be discontinued once the organism is shown to be sensitive to isoniazid. Corticosteroids may be a useful adjunctive measure in the patient with severe systemic toxicity or central nervous system involvement (see Chapter 97). The dosage of corticosteroids should be tapered as soon as the patient shows symptomatic improvement.

Histoplasmosis. Most individuals living in endemic areas in the Mississippi and Ohio River valleys have a subclinical, self-limited febrile illness as a manifestation of acute pulmonary histoplasmosis. Although patients may complain of chest pain or cough, physical examination of the chest is usually unremarkable despite radiographic findings of infiltrates and mediastinal and hilar adenopathy. Therefore, in the absence of chest radiographs, the lower respiratory tract component of the illness is easily overlooked. A complement fixation titer of at least 1:32 or a fourfold rise in titer is suggestive of the diagnosis of acute histoplasmosis. Although spontaneous resolution of symptoms is the norm, unusually prolonged illness (more than 2 to 3 weeks) may require antifungal treatment with amphotericin B or itraconazole.

Progressive disseminated histoplasmosis may occur as a consequence of reactivation of latent infection in immunosuppressed individuals (e.g., acquired immunodeficiency syndrome [AIDS]) or may reflect an uncontained or poorly contained primary infection. The febrile illness in such patients is protracted. Oropharyngeal nodules and ulcerative lesions are commonly found in disseminated histoplasmosis. Biopsy of such lesions permits rapid diagnosis. Serologic studies are less helpful in disseminated histoplasmosis, because they are positive in fewer than one half of cases; cultures and methenamine silver stains of bone marrow biopsy specimens, however, should establish the diagnosis. In AIDS patients, *Histoplasma* urine antigen detection is a sensitive predictor of disseminated infection. Disseminated histoplasmosis is treated with amphotericin B, 0.5 to 0.6 mg/kg/day administered intravenously for a total dose of 2 to 3 g. Itraconazole, 400 to 600 mg/day for 6 to 12 months, appears to be an effective alternative for patients who are unable to tolerate amphotericin B and who do not have meningeal disease.

Other Granulomatous Infections. Malaria produces febrile paroxysms that in some cases occur every 48 (*Plasmodium vivax*) to 72 (*P. malariae*) hours. The diagnosis should be suspected in travelers who have returned from endemic areas, intravenous drug users, and recipients of blood transfusions. *P. falciparum* causes a high level of parasitemia and is associated with a high mortality rate unless recognized and treated promptly. Daily fever often occurs in this form of malaria. Although *P. vivax* and *P. malariae* may cause relapsing infection long after primary infection, because of latent extraerythrocytic infection, the course is milder. Demonstration of parasites in blood smears establishes the diagnosis of malaria.

Many, if not most, infectious diseases may present as fever as an early finding, with subclinical or eventual clinical involvement of specific organ systems. Examples include cryptococcosis, coccidioidomycosis, psittacosis, infection with *Legionella* species, and *Mycoplasma pneumoniae* infections. Pulmonary involvement by these infectious agents often produces few signs on physical examination; chest radiographs often reveal more prominent abnormalities than are suspected clinically.

FEVER AND RASH

Some of the febrile syndromes already discussed may occasionally be associated with a rash (Table 95–2). This section, however, considers diseases in which rash is a prominent feature of the presentation. The most life-threatening infections associated with fever and rash include meningococcemia, staphylococcal bacteremia, and Rocky Mountain spotted fever (RMSF).

Bacterial Diseases

Petechial lesions, purpura, and ecthyma gangrenosum are lesions associated with bacteremia (see Chapter 96).

TABLE 95–2   Differential Diagnosis of Infectious Agents Producing Fever and Rash

Maculopapular Erythematous
Enterovirus
EBV, CMV, *Toxoplasma gondii*
Acute HIV infection
Colorado tick fever virus
Salmonella typhi
Leptospira interrogans
Measles virus
Rubella virus
Hepatitis B virus
Treponema pallidum
Parvovirus B19
Human herpesvirus 6

Vesicular
Varicella-zoster
Herpes simplex virus
Coxsackievirus A
Vibrio vulnificus

Cutaneous Petechiae
Neisseria gonorrhoeae
Neisseria meningitidis
Rickettsia rickettsii (Rocky Mountain spotted fever)
Rickettsia typhi (murine typhus)
Ehrlichia chaffeensis
Echoviruses
Viridans streptococci (endocarditis)

Diffuse Erythroderma
Group A streptococci (scarlet fever, toxic shock syndrome)
Staphylococcus aureus (toxic shock syndrome)

Distinctive Rash
Ecthyma gangrenosum—*Pseudomonas aeruginosa*
Erythema chronicum migrans—Lyme disease

Mucous Membrane Lesions
Vesicular pharyngitis—Coxsackievirus A
Palatal petechiae—rubella, EBV, scarlet fever (group A streptococci)
Erythema—toxic shock syndrome (*Staphylococcus aureus* and group A streptococci)
Oral ulceronodular lesion—*Histoplasma capsulatum*
Koplik's spots—measles virus

CMV = Cytomegalovirus; EBV = Epstein-Barr virus; HIV = human immunodeficiency virus.

Disseminated gonococcemia causes sparse vesiculopustular, hemorrhagic, or necrotic lesions on an erythematous base, typically on the extremities and particularly their dorsal surfaces (see Chapter 107). Meningococcemia is also an important cause of fever and a petechial rash that may be sparse.

Bacterial toxins produce characteristic clinical syndromes. Pharyngitis or other infections with an erythrogenic toxin-producing *Streptococcus* may lead to scarlet fever. Diffuse erythema begins on the upper part of the chest and spreads rapidly, although sparing palms and soles. Small red petechial lesions are found on the palate, and the skin has a sandpaper texture caused by occlusion of the sweat glands. The tongue at first shows a yellowish coating and then becomes beefy red. The rash of scarlet fever heals with desquamation. *Corynebacterium haemolyticum* also produces pharyngitis and rash.

Toxic shock syndrome (TSS) was first recognized as a distinct entity in 1978 and became epidemic in 1980 and 1981, probably because of the marketing of hyperabsorbable tampons. *S. aureus* strains producing toxic shock syndrome toxin (TSST-1) or other closely related exotoxins cause the syndrome. TSST-1 is a potent stimulus of interleukin-1 production by mononuclear phagocytes and enhances the effects of endotoxin; these properties may be important in the pathogenesis of this syndrome. Most cases have occurred in 15- to 25-year-old girls and women using tampons. Other settings include prolonged use of contraceptive diaphragms, vaginal or cesarean deliveries, and nasal surgery. TSS in men is usually caused by superficial staphylococcal infections and abscesses. Patients with TSS develop the abrupt onset of high fever (temperature >40°C [104°F]), hypotension, nausea and vomiting, severe watery diarrhea, and myalgias, followed in severe cases by confusion and oliguria. Characteristically, diffuse erythroderma (a sunburn-like rash) with erythematous mucosal surfaces is apparent. Later, intense scaling and desquamation of the skin, particularly of the palms and soles, occurs. Laboratory abnormalities include elevated liver and muscle enzyme levels, thrombocytopenia, and hypocalcemia. Diagnosis is based on the clinical findings and requires specific exclusion of RMSF, meningococcemia, leptospirosis, and measles. Management of the patient consists of restoring an adequate circulatory blood volume by administration of intravenous fluids, removal of tampons if present, and treatment of the staphylococcal infection with nafcillin, 12 g/day intravenously. Vancomycin is the alternative therapy for nafcillin-resistant staphylococci. Patients must be advised against using tampons in the future, because TSS often recurs within 4 months of the initial episode if tampon use continues.

A streptococcal toxic shock–like syndrome associated with scarlet fever toxin A may also occur as a complication of group A streptococcal soft tissue infections and occasionally after cases of influenza. Major manifestations include cellulitis and/or fasciitis with septicemia, shock, acute respiratory distress syndrome, renal failure, hypocalcemia, and thrombocytopenia. Treatment consists of high-dose penicillin and supportive measures. The mortality remains high (>30%) with optimal current therapy.

Viral Infections

The rashes associated with viral infections may be so typical as to establish unequivocally the cause of the febrile syndrome (Table 95–3). Varicella-zoster requires special consideration because of the availability of effective antiviral drugs. In the normal host, neither chickenpox nor herpes zoster confined within specific dermatomes requires treatment with antiviral agents. Ophthalmic zoster demands antiviral treatment, because it is associated with potentially severe complications, including orbital compression syndromes and intracranial extension. Acyclovir is also effective in decreasing the severity of chickenpox in immunocompromised children and in limiting the extradermatomal spread of zoster in immunocompromised adults.

Rickettsial Diseases

In the United States, three rickettsial diseases are endemic: RMSF, Q fever, and murine typhus. Rash is not a characteristic of Q fever. RMSF is a misnomer, because most cases occur in the southeastern United States. The causative organism, *Rickettsia rickettsii*, is transmitted from dogs (or small wild animals) to ticks to humans. Infection occurs primarily during warmer months, the periods of greatest tick activity. About two thirds of patients cite a history of tick exposure. After 2 to 14 days, there is the fulminant onset of severe frontal headache, chills, fever, myalgias, conjunctivitis, and, in one fourth, cough and shortness of breath. At this point, the diagnosis may be particularly obscure. Rash characteristically begins on the third to fifth day of illness as 1- to 4-mm erythematous macules on hands, wrists, feet, and ankles. Palms and soles may be involved. The rash may be transient, but it usually spreads to the trunk and may become petechial. Intravascular coagulopathy develops in some severely ill patients. Diagnosis and institution of appropriate therapy should be based on the clinical findings. The specific complement fixation test shows a rise in titers and allows retrospective confirmation of the diagnosis. Treatment is with doxycycline, 100 mg twice daily given orally or parenterally, or tetracycline, 25 to 50 mg/kg/day for 7 days, administered orally.

Human Ehrlichiosis

Human ehrlichiosis is an acute, febrile illness caused most frequently by *Ehrlichia chaffeensis* (human monocytic ehrlichiosis [HME]) or other *Ehrlichia* species causing human granulocytic ehrlichiosis (HGE). *E. chaffeensis*, like *R. rickettsii*, is transmitted by woodland exposure to deer or dog ticks and causes illness with peak incidence in the summer months. Since first recognized in 1986, cases of HME have been identified in 21 contiguous southeastern states from Maryland to Texas. The illness characteristically begins with fever, chills, headache, and myalgias, with a maculopapular rash occurring in fewer than a third of cases. Although there is a wide spectrum of illness, roughly half of clinically recognized cases are associated with pulmonary infiltrates; acute respiratory distress syndrome, often associated with renal failure, may develop, most often in elderly patients. In untreated patients, the mortality rate may exceed 10% in hospitalized cases.

HGE peaks in July and occurs in areas where infected *Ixodes* ticks are found. Nine percent of patients have concurrent Lyme disease or babesiosis. This implies that these diseases are likely transmitted by the same tick vector. HGE usually presents as a nonspecific flulike illness with fever, chills, malaise, headache, nau-

TABLE 95-3   Fever and Rash in Viral Infection

Acute HIV infection	Maculopapular truncal rash may occur as early manifestation of infection.	Associated fever, sore throat, and lymph node enlargement may persist for 2 or more weeks.
Coxsackievirus/echovirus	Maculopapular "*rubelliform*": 1–3 mm, faint pink, begins on face, spreading to chest and extremities. "*Herpetiform*": vesicular stomatitis with peripheral exanthem (papules and clear vesicles on an erythematous base), including palms and soles (hand, foot, and mouth disease).	Summertime, no itching or lymphadenopathy; multiple cases in household or community-wide epidemic; mostly diseases of children.
Measles	Erythematous, maculopapular rash begins on upper face and spreads down to involve extremities, including palms and soles; Koplik's spots are bluish-gray specks on a red base found on buccal mucosa near second molars; atypical measles occurs in individuals who receive killed vaccine, then are exposed to measles; the rash begins peripherally and is urticarial, vesicular, or hemorrhagic.	Incubation period, 10–14 days; first, severe upper respiratory symptoms, coryza, cough, conjunctivitis; then Koplik's spots, then rash.
Rubella	Maculopapular rash beginning on face and moving downward; petechiae on soft palate.	Incubation, 12–35 days; adenopathy: posterior auricular, posterior cervical, and suboccipital.
Varicella	Generalized vesicular eruption; lesions in different stages from erythematous macules to vesicles to crusted; spreads from trunk centrifugally. Zoster—see text.	Incubation, 14–15 days; late winter, early spring.
Herpes simplex virus	Oral primary: small vesicles on pharynx, oral mucosa, which ulcerate; painful and tender. Recurrent: vermillion border, one or few lesions. Genital: see Chapter 107.	Incubation, 2–12 days.
Hepatitis B	Prodrome in one fifth: erythematous maculopapular rash, urticaria.	Arthralgias, arthritis; abnormal liver function tests; hepatitis B antigenemia.
EBV	Erythematous, maculopapular rash on trunk and proximal extremities; occasionally urticarial or hemorrhagic.	Transiently occurs in 5–10% of patients during first week of illness.

EBV = Epstein-Barr virus; HIV = human immunodeficiency virus.

sea and vomiting, leukopenia, and thrombocytopenia. Elderly patients tend to have more severe disease.

Presumptive diagnosis of HME and HGE is made on clinical grounds in patients with acute febrile illnesses, which are generally associated with decreasing leukocyte and platelet counts, after tick exposure. Peripheral blood smears may show intracellular organisms called morulae in infected leukocytes. Serodiagnosis is sensitive but helpful only in retrospective confirmation of diagnosis. Treatment with tetracycline, 500 mg four times a day for 7 days, is effective in decreasing both duration and severity of illness.

Major clinical distinctions between human ehrlichiosis and RMSF include the earlier, more frequent, and more severe cutaneous manifestations of RMSF and the more common pulmonary manifestations and the characteristically decreasing leukocyte counts in ehrlichiosis.

Lyme Disease

Lyme disease is a common, multisystem spirochetal infection caused by *Borrelia burgdorferi* and transmitted by the tick *Ixodes dammini*. Initial case reports were clustered in several major foci (the Northeast, Wisconsin and Minnesota, California, and Oregon), but this infection is distributed broadly throughout North America and Western Europe. Three days to 3 weeks after the tick bite, of which most individuals are unaware, patients develop a febrile illness, usually associated with headache, stiff neck, myalgias, arthralgias, and erythema chronicum migrans (ECM). ECM begins as a red macule or papule at the site of the tick bite; the surrounding bright red patch expands to a diameter of up to 15 cm. Partial central clearing is often seen. The centers of lesions may become indurated, vesicular, or necrotic. Several red rings may be found within the outer border. Smaller secondary lesions may appear within several days. Lesions are warm but nontender. Enlargement of regional lymph nodes is common. The rash usually fades in about 1 month.

Several weeks after the onset of symptoms, important neurologic manifestations occur in more than 15% of patients. Most characteristic is meningoencephalitis with cranial nerve involvement and peripheral radiculoneuropathy. Bell's palsy may occur as an isolated phenomenon; when associated with fever, this finding is strongly suggestive of Lyme disease. The cerebrospinal fluid (CSF) at this time shows about 100 lymphocytes per milliliter. Heart involvement may also be manifested as atrioventricular block, myopericarditis, or cardiomegaly.

Joint involvement eventually occurs in 60% of patients. Early in the course, arthralgias and myalgias may be quite severe. Months later, arthritis often develops, with marked swelling and little pain in one or two large joints, typically the knee. Episodes of arthritis may recur for months or years; in about 10% of patients, the arthritis becomes chronic, and erosion of cartilage and bone occurs. Diagnosis is suspected on clinical grounds and confirmed by demonstration of IgM antibody, which peaks by the third to sixth week. Total serum IgM is increased, as are IgM-containing immune complexes and cryoglobulins. The level of IgM is reflective of disease activity and predictive of neurologic, cardiac, and joint involvement. However, serologic studies are not precise. Antibody titers may be negative in early disease, and early antibiotic therapy may blunt the antibody response. Synovial fluid contains an average of 25,000 cells/mL, most of them neutrophils. An emerging and sensitive means of diagnosis is blood, synovial fluid, or cerebrospinal fluid polymerase chain reaction.

Treatment of the early manifestations of Lyme disease with doxycycline, 100 mg twice daily for 14 to 21 days, usually prevents late complications. Meningitis, cardiac involvement, or arthritis should be treated with aqueous penicillin G, 20 million U; intravenous ceftriaxone, 4 g/day for 14 to 21 days; or prolonged doxycycline therapy. Repeated courses may be necessary if relapses occur.

A vaccine that offers some protection against Lyme disease is now available, but the precise indications for its use have not been fully defined.

FEVER AND LYMPHADENOPATHY

Many infectious diseases are associated with some degree of lymphadenopathy. However, in some, lymphadenopathy is a major manifestation of the disease. These can be further divided according to whether lymphadenopathy is generalized or regional.

Generalized Lymphadenopathy

The mononucleosis syndromes are important causes of fever and generalized lymphadenopathy.

Mononucleosis Syndromes

Primary HIV Infection (Acute Retroviral Syndrome). Typical presenting features of primary HIV infection overlap those of the mononucleosis syndrome (see Chapter 108). Although most patients with the acute retroviral syndrome seek medical attention, the correct diagnosis is missed in a large proportion of cases because of physician failure to consider HIV infection. Because it is of critical importance to both the patient and his or her sexual partners to establish this diagnosis

(see Chapter 108), primary HIV infection must be considered in all patients with mononucleosis syndromes.

Epstein-Barr Virus Infection. Approximately 90% of American adults have serologic evidence of EBV infection; most infections are subclinical and occur before the age of 5 years or midway through adolescence.

Clinically manifest infectious mononucleosis usually develops late in adolescence after intimate contact with asymptomatic oropharyngeal shedders of EBV. Patients develop sore throat, fever, and generalized lymphadenopathy and sometimes experience headache and myalgias. Five to 10 percent of patients have a transient rash that may be macular, petechial, or urticarial. Palatal petechiae are often present, as is pharyngitis, which may be exudative. Cervical lymphadenopathy, particularly involving the posterior lymphatic chains, is prominent, although some involvement elsewhere is common. The spleen is enlarged in about 50% of patients. Autoimmune hemolytic anemia, thrombocytopenia, encephalitis or aseptic meningitis, Guillain-Barré syndrome, hepatitis, or splenic rupture, although rare, may dominate the clinical presentation. Three fourths of patients present with an absolute lymphocytosis. At least one third of their lymphocytes are atypical in appearance: large, with vacuolated basophilic cytoplasm; rolled edges often deformed by contact with other cells; and lobulated, eccentric nuclei. Immunologic studies indicate that some circulating B cells are infected with EBV and that the cells involved in the lymphocytosis are mainly cytotoxic T cells capable of damaging EBV-containing lymphocytes. Atypical lymphocytes may also be seen in other viral illnesses (Table 95–4).

B-cell infection with EBV is a stimulus to production of polyclonal antibodies. The Monospot rapid diagnostic test is sensitive and specific; false-positive results occur in rare cases in patients with lymphoma or hepatitis. The presence of IgM antibody to viral capsid antigen is diagnostic of acute infectious mononucleosis. The appearance of antibody to EBV nuclear antigen is also indicative of EBV infection.

Infectious mononucleosis usually pursues a benign course even in patients with neurologic involvement. The fever resolves after 1 to 2 weeks, although residual

TABLE 95–4 Most Common Infectious Causes of Heterophile-Negative Atypical Lymphocytosis

Babesiosis
Chickenpox
Cytomegalovirus
Epstein-Barr virus (particularly in children)
Human herpesvirus 6
Human immunodeficiency virus (especially during acute seroconversion)
Infectious mononucleosis
Malaria
Measles
Toxoplasmosis
Varicella
Infectious hepatitis

fatigue may be protracted. Occasional patients have a persistent or recurrent syndrome with fever, headaches, pharyngitis, lymphadenopathy, arthralgias, and serologic evidence of chronic active EBV infection. Patients should be managed symptomatically. Acetaminophen may be useful for sore throat. Antibiotics, particularly ampicillin, should be avoided. The use of ampicillin causes a rash in almost all patients with EBV infection, and this phenomenon can also be a diagnostic clue to the occurrence of EBV infection. Corticosteroids are indicated in the rare individual with serious hematologic involvement (i.e., thrombocytopenia, hemolytic anemia) or impending airway obstruction as a result of massive tonsillar swelling.

Acute bacterial superinfections of the pharynx and peritonsillar tissues should be considered when the course is unusually septic.

The differential diagnosis of Monospot-negative mononucleosis is shown in Table 95–5.

Cytomegalovirus. Serologic surveys indicate that most adults have been infected with cytomegalovirus (CMV). The ages of peak incidence of CMV infection are in the perinatal period (transmission by breast milk) and during the second to fourth decades. CMV shares with the other herpesviridae the propensity to reactivate, particularly in immunosuppressed patients.

Two modes of transmission of CMV are particularly important in the development of lymphadenopathy in otherwise healthy adults. CMV can be transmitted sexually. Semen is an excellent source for viral isolation. The frequency of antibody to CMV and active viral excretion is particularly high in male homosexuals. Blood transfusions carry a risk of approximately 3% per unit of blood for transmitting CMV infection. This risk becomes substantial in the setting of open-heart surgery or multiple transfusions for other indications.

Primary infection with CMV causes a major proportion of cases of Monospot-negative mononucleosis (see Table 95–5). The distinction between CMV and EBV may be impossible on clinical grounds alone. However, CMV tends to involve older patients (mean age, 29) and produce milder disease, and it may be typhoidal in its presentation; that is, it causes fever with little or no adenopathy. The infrequent but serious forms of neurologic and hematologic involvement that occur in EBV infection can also occur with CMV. In addition, pneumonitis and hepatitis (which may be granulomatous) may be found. Isolation of CMV from urine or semen and demonstration of conversion of serologic studies (in-

direct fluorescent antibody test or complement fixation) from negative to positive are useful in establishing etiology. However, in groups such as male homosexuals, in whom asymptomatic excretion of CMV is found frequently, viral isolation alone is inadequate for determining the etiology of lymphadenopathy. CMV mononucleosis is a self-limited disease that does not require or respond to specific therapy. CMV infection in the immunocompromised host may be life threatening; in this setting it often responds to long-term therapy with ganciclovir or foscarnet (see Chapter 108).

Acute Acquired Toxoplasmosis. *T. gondii* is acquired by ingesting oocysts contaminating meat and other foods or by exposure to cat feces. In certain geographic areas, such as France, 90% of individuals have serologic evidence of *Toxoplasma* infection. In the United States, the figure is close to 50% by age 50. Ten percent to 20% of infections in normal adults are symptomatic. Presentation may take the form of a mononucleosis-like syndrome, although maculopapular rash, abdominal pain caused by mesenteric and retroperitoneal lymphadenopathy, and chorioretinitis may also occur. Striking lymph node enlargement and involvement of unusual chains (occipital, lumbar) may necessitate lymph node biopsy to exclude lymphoma. More commonly, cervical adenopathy is observed in symptomatic cases. Overall, however, toxoplasmosis accounts for less than 1% of mononucleosis-like illnesses. Histologically, focal distention of sinuses with mononuclear phagocytes, histiocytes blurring the margins of germinal centers, and reactive follicular hyperplasia indicates *Toxoplasma* infection. Acute acquired toxoplasmosis is suggested by conversion of the indirect fluorescent antibody test from negative to positive or a fourfold increase in titer. Usually the titer is greater than 1:1000 and is associated with increased specific IgM antibody. Acute acquired toxoplasmosis is generally self-limited in the immunologically intact host and does not require specific therapy. Significant involvement of the eye is an indication for treatment with pyrimethamine plus sulfadiazine.

Granulomatous Disease. Disseminated tuberculosis, histoplasmosis, and sarcoidosis may be associated with generalized lymphadenopathy, although involvement of certain lymph node chains can predominate. Lymph node biopsy shows granulomas or nonspecific hyperplasia.

Regional Lymphadenopathy

Pyogenic Infection. *S. aureus* and group A streptococcal infections produce acute suppurative lymphadenitis. The most frequently affected lymph nodes are submandibular, cervical, inguinal, and axillary, in that order. Involved nodes are large (>3 cm), tender, and firm or fluctuant. Pyoderma, pharyngitis, or periodontal infection may be present at the presumed primary site of infection. Patients are febrile and have a leukocytosis. Fluctuant nodes should be aspirated. Otherwise, antibiotic therapy should be directed toward the most common pathogens. Penicillin G therapy is appropriate if pharyngeal or periodontal origin implicates a streptococcal or mixed anaerobic infection. Skin involvement sug-

---

TABLE 95–5 Differential Diagnosis of Monospot-Negative Mononucleosis

Acute HIV infection
EBV mononucleosis (particularly in children)
Cytomegalovirus
Acute toxoplasmosis
Streptococcal pharyngitis
Acute hepatitis B infection

EBV = Epstein-Barr virus; HIV = human immunodeficiency virus.

gests possible staphylococcal infection and is an indication for nafcillin (or dicloxacillin) therapy. The dosage and route of administration of the drug should be determined by the severity of the infection.

Tuberculosis. Scrofula, or tuberculous cervical adenitis, presents in a subacute to chronic fashion. Fever, if present, is low grade. A large mass of matted lymph nodes is palpable in the neck. If *Mycobacterium tuberculosis* is the causative organism, other sites of active infection are usually present. The most common causative agent in children in the United States is *Mycobacterium scrofulaceum*. Infection with this and other drug-resistant nontuberculous mycobacteria usually requires surgical excision.

Cat-Scratch Disease. Chronic regional lymphadenopathy after exposure to cats or cat scratches should suggest the diagnosis. About 1 week after contact with the cat, a local papule or pustule may develop. One week later, regional adenopathy appears. Lymph nodes may be tender (sometimes exquisitely so) or just enlarged (1 to 7 cm). Fever is low grade if present at all. Lymph node enlargement usually persists for several months. The diagnosis can usually be established on clinical grounds. Lymph node biopsy shows necrotic granulomas with giant cells and stellate abscesses surrounded by epithelial cells. Pleomorphic gram-negative bacilli (*Bartonella henselae*) can be identified in the lymph node biopsy specimens during the first 4 weeks of illness. Serologic testing can confirm the diagnosis. The course is usually self-limited and benign in immunocompetent individuals but may be life threatening in persons with severe immunodeficiency. The best approach to treatment of cat-scratch disease in the immunocompromised patient is not known. Erythromycin or doxycycline may be helpful.

Ulceroglandular Fever. Tularemia is the classic cause of ulceroglandular fever. The syndrome is acquired by contact with tissues or fluids from an infected rabbit or the bite of an infected tick. Patients have chills, fever, an ulcerated skin lesion at the site of inoculation, and painful regional adenopathy. When infection is acquired by contact with rabbits, the skin lesion is usually on the fingers or hand and lymph node involvement is epitrochlear or axillary. In tick-borne transmission, the ulcer is on the lower extremities, perianal region, or trunk and the adenopathy is inguinal or femoral. Most cases are diagnosed serologically, because Gram-stained preparations are usually negative and culture of the causative organism, *Francisella tularensis*, is hazardous. A fourfold rise in agglutination titer is diagnostic. Patients should be treated presumptively with streptomycin, 15 to 20 mg/kg/day for 7 to 10 days.

Oculoglandular Fever. Conjunctivitis with preauricular lymphadenopathy can occur in tularemia, cat-scratch disease, sporotrichosis, lymphogranuloma venereum infection, listeriosis, and epidemic keratoconjunctivitis caused by adenovirus.

Inguinal Lymphadenopathy. Inguinal lymphadenopathy associated with sexually transmitted diseases (see Chapter 107) may be bilateral or unilateral. In primary syphilis, enlarged nodes are discrete, firm, and nontender. Early lymphogranuloma venereum causes tender lymphadenopathy with later matting of involved nodes and sometimes fixation to overlying skin, which assumes a purplish hue. The lymphadenopathy of chancroid is most often unilateral, is very painful, and is composed of fused lymph nodes. Tender inguinal lymphadenopathy also occurs in primary genital herpes simplex virus infection.

Plague. Bubonic plague usually presents as fever, headache, and a large mat of inguinal or axillary lymph nodes, which go on to suppurate and drain spontaneously. Plague is an important consideration in the acutely ill patient in the southwestern United States with possible exposure to fleas and rodents. If plague is suspected, blood cultures and aspirates of the buboes should be obtained, and tetracycline, 30 to 50 mg/kg/day, plus streptomycin, 20 to 30 mg/kg/day, instituted. Gram-stained preparations of the aspirate reveal gram-negative rods in two thirds of cases. A fluorescent antibody test allows rapid specific diagnosis and is available through the Centers for Disease Control and Prevention.

Fever of Unknown Origin

Fever of undetermined origin (FUO) is the term applied to febrile illnesses with temperatures exceeding 38.3°C (101°F) that are of at least 3 weeks' duration and remain undiagnosed after 3 days in the hospital or after three outpatient visits. Improvements in noninvasive diagnostic testing have resulted in newly proposed categories of FUO (Table 95–6). They include (1) classic FUO, for which the common causes are infections, malignancy, inflammatory diseases, and drug fever; (2) nosocomial FUO; (3) neutropenic (≤500 neutrophils/mm³) FUO; and (4) HIV-associated FUO (see later discussion). The evaluation of FUO remains among the most challenging problems facing the physician. The majority of illnesses that cause FUO are treatable, making pursuit of the diagnosis particularly rewarding. There is no substitute for a meticulous history and physical examination. These should be repeated frequently during the patient's hospital course, because recurrent questioning of the patient may jar an important historical clue from the patient and important physical findings may develop while the patient is in the hospital. These clues may direct the next series of diagnostic studies. Patients with unexplained fevers should always be offered HIV testing. Directed biopsy specimens of lesions should be stained and cultured for pathogenic microbes. In many instances, however, localizing clues are not present or fail to yield rewarding information. In these cases, bone marrow biopsy can reveal granulomatous or neoplastic disease, even in the absence of clinical evidence of bone marrow involvement. Similarly, liver biopsy may also reveal the etiology of an FUO but seldom in the absence of any clinical or laboratory evidence of liver disease. Exploratory laparotomy is generally not helpful unless signs, symptoms, or laboratory data point

TABLE 95-6 Fever of Unknown Origin (FUO)—Definitions

Classic FUO

Fever ≥ 38.3°C (101°F) on multiple occasions
Duration ≥ 3 wk
Uncertain diagnosis after investigations (3 hospital days or 3 outpatient visits)

Nosocomial FUO

Fever ≥ 38.3°C (101°F) on multiple occasions in hospitalized patient
Infection not incubating on admission
Uncertain diagnosis after 3-day evaluation, including 2-day microbiologic culture incubation

Neutropenic FUO

Fever ≥ 38.3°C (101°F) on multiple occasions
Absolute neutrophil count <500/μL
Uncertain diagnosis after 3-day evaluation, including 2-day microbiologic culture incubation

HIV-Associated FUO

Fever ≥ 38.3°C (101°F) on multiple occasions
Confirmed diagnosis of HIV infection
Fever > 1 mo (outpatients) or >3 days (inpatients)
Uncertain diagnosis after 3-day evaluation, including 2-day microbiologic culture incubation

HIV = human immunodeficiency virus.

to abdominal pathology. Computed tomography (CT) may assist in determining the need for laparotomy in cases of FUO. If tuberculosis remains a reasonable possibility after careful workup fails to establish a diagnosis, an empirical trial of antituberculous therapy may be initiated while awaiting results of bone marrow, liver, and urine cultures.

Table 95–7 indicates the final diagnoses in a study of over 100 cases of FUO observed in the decade from 1970 to 1980. More recent series of FUO cases have emphasized an increasing occurrence of malignancy-associated FUO, decreases in intra-abdominal abscesses because of the increasing sensitivity of CT, and more frequent identification of prolonged viral illnesses, especially CMV, in adolescents and young adults. Table 95–7 simply emphasizes the range of diagnostic possibilities to be considered. Numbers in each category are not presented, because regional and temporal variations in the frequency of specific diagnoses are great. Infectious diseases continue to cause about one third of these cases; another third are caused by neoplasms; and the remainder are caused by connective tissue disorders, granulomatous diseases, and other illnesses.

CAUSES OF FUO

Infections

Abscesses account for approximately one third of infectious causes of FUO. Most of these abscesses are intra-abdominal or pelvic, because abscesses elsewhere (e.g., lung, brain, or superficial abscesses) are readily identifi-

able radiographically or as a result of the signs or symptoms they produce.

Intra-abdominal abscesses generally occur as a complication of surgery or leakage of visceral contents, as might be seen with perforation of a colonic diverticulum. Surprisingly, large abdominal abscesses may be present with few localizing symptoms. This is especially so in the elderly or immunocompromised host. Abscesses of the liver (see Chapter 102) occur as a consequence of inflammatory disease of the biliary tract or of the bowel; in the latter instance, bacteria reach the liver through portal blood flow. Occasionally, blunt trauma predisposes to abscesses of the liver or spleen. Hepatic, splenic, or subdiaphragmatic abscesses are generally readily detected by ultrasonography or CT scan. However, diagnosis of intra-abdominal abscess may be challenging, because even large abscesses in the pericolonic spaces may be difficult to distinguish from fluid-filled loops of bowel on CT. Gallium or tagged white blood cell scanning, ultrasonography, or barium enemas may assist if the diagnosis is suspected and CT is not definitive.

Endovascular infections (infective endocarditis, mycotic aneurysms, infected atherosclerotic plaques) are uncommon causes of FUO, because blood cultures are

TABLE 95-7 Fever of Undetermined Origin

Infections
  Intra-abdominal abscesses
    Subphrenic
    Splenic
    Diverticular
    Liver and biliary tract
    Pelvic
  Mycobacterial
  Cytomegalovirus
  Infection of the urinary tract
  Sinusitis
  Osteomyelitis
  Catheter infections
  Other infections

Neoplastic Diseases
  Hematologic neoplasms
    Non-Hodgkin's lymphoma
    Leukemia
    Hodgkin's disease
    Other
  Solid tumors

Collagen Diseases

Granulomatous Diseases

Miscellaneous

Factitious Fever

Undiagnosed

Adapted from Larson EB, Featherstone HJ, Petersdorf RG: Fever of undetermined origin: Diagnosis and follow-up of 105 cases, 1970–1980. Medicine 1982; 61:269–292. ©1982, The Williams & Wilkins Company, Baltimore.

generally positive unless the patient has received antibiotics within the preceding 2 weeks. Infections of intravascular catheter sites are generally also associated with bacteremia unless the infection is limited to the insertion site. Diagnosis of endovascular infection is more difficult to make when blood cultures are negative and infection is with slow-growing or fastidious organisms, such as *Brucella* species, *C. burnetii* (Q fever), or *Haemophilus* species. It is especially difficult among patients who have been treated with antimicrobial agents. If endocarditis is suspected, blood cultures should be repeated for at least 1 week after antimicrobial agents are discontinued, the bacteriology laboratory should be alerted to the possibility of infection with a fastidious organism, and evidence of valvular vegetations should be sought by transesophageal echocardiography. Occasionally, the suspicion of valvular infection is strong enough to warrant empirical antibiotic treatment of a presumed culture-negative endocarditis.

Although most patients with osteomyelitis have pain at the site of infection, localizing symptoms are occasionally absent and patients present only with fever. Technetium pyrophosphate bone scans and gallium scans demonstrate uptake at sites of osteomyelitis, but positive scans are not always specific for infection. Magnetic resonance imaging can be especially useful in differentiating between bone and soft tissue infection.

Mycobacterial infections, generally with *M. tuberculosis*, are important causes of FUO. Patients with impaired cell-mediated immunity are at particular risk for disseminated tuberculosis, and occult infection with this organism is seen with particular frequency among elderly patients or those who are undergoing hemodialysis. Fever may be the only sign of this infection. Among both immunocompromised patients and previously well persons with disseminated tuberculosis, purified protein derivative (PPD) skin tests are often negative. In some patients, careful review of chest radiographs reveals apical calcifications or upper lobe scars suggestive of remote tuberculous infection. A diffuse, often subtle radiographic pattern of "millet seed" densities, which is best appreciated on the lateral chest views, is highly suggestive of disseminated tuberculosis. In this setting, transbronchial or open lung biopsy will establish the diagnosis. Similar radiographic patterns may be seen in sarcoidosis, disseminated fungal infection (e.g., histoplasmosis), and some malignancies. Bone marrow or liver biopsy often reveals granulomas, and cultures of these sites are positive in 50% to 90% of cases of disseminated tuberculosis.

Viral infections such as those caused by CMV or EBV can produce prolonged fevers. Both infections may be seen in young, healthy adults. Recipients of blood are at risk for acute post-transfusion CMV infection. Recipients of organ transplantation and other immunosuppressed patients may experience reactivation of latent CMV infection producing fever, leukopenia, and pulmonary and hepatic disease. Lymph nodes are often enlarged in EBV infection, and a peripheral blood smear usually reveals a lymphocytosis with increased numbers of atypical lymphocytes. Occasionally, the atypical lymphocytosis is delayed several weeks after the onset of fever. A positive Monospot test result may clarify the diagnosis. Unexplained fever may be a complication of infection with HIV; most such fevers are attributable to complicating opportunistic pathogens (see Chapter 108).

Simple lower urinary tract infections are readily diagnosed by symptoms and urinalysis. Complicated infections such as perirenal or prostatic abscess may be occult and present as FUO. In general, there is a history of antecedent urinary tract infection or disorder of the urinary tract. In prostatic abscess the prostate is usually tender on rectal examination. In suspected cases of perirenal and prostatic abscesses, the urinalysis should be repeated if it is initially normal, because abnormalities of the sediment may be intermittent. Ultrasonography or CT detects most of these lesions.

Although most patients with sinusitis have localizing symptoms, infections of the paranasal sinuses may occasionally present as fever only, particularly among hospitalized patients who have had nasotracheal and/or nasogastric intubation. Sinus films reveal fluid in the sinuses. Infection of the sphenoidal sinus may be difficult to detect unless special views or CT scans are obtained.

Neoplastic Diseases

Neoplasms account for approximately one third of cases of FUO. Some tumors, particularly those of hematologic origin and hypernephromas, release endogenous pyrogens. In others, the mechanism of fever is less clear but may result from pyrogen release by infiltrating or surrounding inflammatory cells. Lymphomas can present as FUO; there is usually enlargement of lymph nodes or the spleen. Some lymphomas present with intra-abdominal disease only. CT may be helpful in detecting these tumors. Leukemia may also present as FUO, sometimes with a normal peripheral blood smear. Bone marrow examination reveals an increased number of blast forms. Renal cell carcinoma, atrial myxoma, primary hepatocellular carcinoma, and tumor metastatic to the liver may also present as FUO. Liver function abnormalities (predominantly alkaline phosphatase) are common in all these tumors except atrial myxoma. Myxoma can be suspected in the presence of heart murmur and multisystem embolization (mimicking endocarditis) and is readily diagnosed by echocardiogram. Radiographic studies of the abdomen and retroperitoneum (CT or ultrasonography) generally detect the other tumors. Colon carcinoma must also be considered in the differential diagnosis, because one third or more of patients with this diagnosis may present with low-grade fever, and in some this is the only sign of disease.

Other Causes

Collagen vascular diseases account for approximately 10% of cases of FUO. Systemic lupus erythematosus is readily diagnosed serologically and thus accounts for a small proportion of cases of FUO. Vasculitis remains an important cause of FUO and should be suspected in febrile patients with "embolization/infarctions" or with "multisystem disease." Giant cell arteritis should be considered in older patients with FUO, particularly in the presence of polymyalgia rheumatica symptoms (see Chapter 86). Juvenile rheumatoid arthritis, or Still's disease, can present as FUO with joint symptoms. An evanescent rash, sore throat, adenopathy, and leukocytosis may occur in this disorder, which is diagnosed on the basis of clinical criteria in the absence of other potential causes of fever.

Granulomatous diseases without a defined etiology have been associated with FUO. Sarcoidosis often involves the lungs, skin, and lymph nodes. The majority of patients are anergic to skin test antigens. Diagnosis is based on the demonstration of discrete, noncaseating granulomas on biopsy of bone marrow, liver, lung, or other tissues. Granulomatous hepatitis can present as prolonged fevers, occasionally lasting for years. Serum alkaline phosphatase levels are generally elevated; liver biopsy reveals granulomas, and no underlying etiology can be demonstrated.

A number of miscellaneous disorders, including Crohn's disease, familial Mediterranean fever, and hypertriglyceridemia, make up the remainder of FUO cases. Drug-related fevers and recurrent pulmonary emboli always demand consideration in the differential diagnosis. A significant minority of FUO (approximately 10%) remain undiagnosed after careful evaluation. The majority of these patients have experienced an undefinable but self-limited illness, with fewer than 10% of these patients developing an underlying serious disorder after several years' follow-up.

FUO IN SPECIAL GROUPS

Besides patients with "classic" FUO, several other groups of patients with fever in whom the diagnosis is not readily apparent deserve special attention. These special groups are encountered more frequently in clinical practice and include patients with nosocomial FUO (see Table 95–6).

Nosocomial FUO

Most patients in this group have significant underlying comorbidities that led to hospitalization and complex treatment. The hospital environment (especially intensive care units), invasive procedures, foreign devices, antibiotic resistance, and alteration of host defenses by diseases or therapy set the stage for potentially unique infectious complications. Bacterial and fungal infections of the urinary tract, surgical wounds, respiratory tract, blood stream, the sinuses, and vascular catheter sites are significant concerns. A frequent cause of nosocomial FUO is *Clostridium difficile*–associated colitis, especially if diarrhea is minimal or absent. Other noninfectious causes of nosocomial FUO include tissue injury or infarction, drug reactions, or thromboembolic disease.

Neutropenic FUO

Neutropenic FUO refers to patients with undiagnosed fever in the context of persistent and severe neutropenia. In general, most patients in this category will have received cytotoxic/immunosuppressive therapy for their underlying disease. Regardless of the cause, complicating infections are frequently encountered when the absolute neutrophil count (mature neutrophils and bands) falls below $1000/\mu L$ (and especially below $500/\mu L$). Occult bacterial infections are the most frequent causes of fever, and deterioration may be rapid; empirical broad-spectrum antibiotics are mandated in febrile neutropenic patients after appropriate cultures are obtained. If the cultures are negative and the patient remains febrile, the patient is considered to have neutropenic FUO. Etiologic considerations include perirectal or periodontal disease, occult fungal infections, reactivation of viral or mycobacterial disease, drug-induced fever, relapse of underlying disease (especially lymphoreticular malignancy), and thromboembolic conditions.

HIV-Associated FUO

Fever is one of the most common symptoms seen in HIV-infected patients. HIV-associated FUO is considered when the HIV-infected person has fever for more than 1 month as an outpatient or more than 3 days when hospitalized. With advanced HIV disease, more frequent causes of FUO include mycobacterial disease (especially disseminated *Mycobacterium avium* complex), cytomegalovirus (retinitis or colitis) infection, drug reactions, and bacterial line infections (see Chapter 108).

Factitious or Self-Induced Fever

Patients with factitious or self-induced illness present unique ethical and therapeutic problems. Once the possibility of factitious or self-induced illness is considered, the doctor-patient relationship is changed. Typically, the physician can rely on the good faith of the patient's history. In the case of factitious or self-induced illness, the physician must assume a more detached role to establish the diagnosis. Patients with factitious fever are typically young and often female. Many have been or are employed in health-related professions. Usually articulate and well educated, these patients are adept at manipulating their family, friends, and physicians. In these instances, a consultant new to the patient may provide a detached and helpful perspective on the problem.

Clues to factitious fever include the absence of a toxic appearance despite high temperature readings, lack of an appropriate rise in pulse rate with fever, and absence of the physiologic diurnal variation in temperature. Suspected factitious readings can be evaluated by immediately repeating the reading with the nurse or physician in attendance. The use of electronic thermometers allows rapid and accurate recording of a patient's temperature (see also Chapter 112).

Self-injection of pyrogen-containing substances, usually bacteria-laden culture medium, urine, or feces, can produce bacteremia and high fever; usually these bacteremic episodes are polymicrobial and intermittent, often suggesting a diagnosis of intra-abdominal abscess. However, patients with self-induced bacteremia may appear remarkably well between episodes of fever. The occurrence of polymicrobial bacteremia in an otherwise healthy person should suggest the possibility of self-induced infection. Illicit ingestion of medications known by the patient to produce fever can also present a difficult diagnostic problem. Clues to the presence of self-induced illness are subtle. The patients are often emotionally immature; some exaggerate their importance and fabricate unrelated aspects of their history. Some are surprisingly stoic about the apparent seriousness of their illness and the procedures employed to diagnose or treat them. In some instances, interviewing family members can elicit clues to the possibility of factitious or self-induced illness. Confirming the diagnosis is crucial and, in many instances, requires a search of the patient's hospital room. Although most will deny their role in inducing or feigning illness, the diagnosis must be explained, and psychiatric care is essential. These complicated patients are at risk for inducing life-threatening disease; some respond to psychiatric counseling.

REFERENCES

Armstrong WS, Katz JT, Kazanjian PH: Human immunodeficiency virus–associated fever of unknown origin: A study of 70 patients in the United States and review. Clin Infect Dis 1999; 28:341–345.

Arnow PM, Flaherty JP: Fever of unknown origin. Lancet 1997; 350: 575–580.

Dinarello CA, Cannon JG, Wolff S: New concepts of the pathogenesis of fever. Rev Infect Dis 1988; 10:168–169.

Durack D, Street A: Fever of unknown origin—reexamined and redefined. *In* Remington J, Swartz M (eds): Current Clinical Topics in Infectious Diseases. St. Louis: Mosby–Year Book, 1991, pp 35–51.

Engels E, Marks PW, Kazanjian P: Usefulness of bone marrow examination in the evaluation of unexplained fevers in patients infected with the human immunodeficiency virus. Clin Infect Dis 1995; 21: 427–428.

Knockaert D, Vanneste LJ, Vanneste SB, Bobbaers HJ: Fever of unknown origin in the 1980s: An update of the diagnostic spectrum. Arch Intern Med 1992; 152:51–55.

Mackowiak PA, LeMaistre DF: Drug fever: A critical appraisal of conventional concepts: An analysis of 51 episodes in two Dallas hospitals and 97 episodes reported in the English literature. Ann Intern Med 1987;106:728–733.

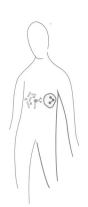

96

BACTEREMIA

Robert A. Salata

Sepsis syndrome, the systemic response to an infectious process, is a leading cause of morbidity and mortality in hospitalized patients. A major advance since 1990 has been the growing understanding of the pathophysiology of sepsis. Novel therapeutic approaches now being tested in the sepsis syndrome are a direct result of the elucidation of the molecular mechanisms of sepsis and the practical application of modern techniques of biochemistry and molecular biology to rational drug design.

The bases for current definitions of sepsis syndrome and related disorders are presented in Table 96–1 and Figure 96–1. Infection, defined by the presence of microbial pathogens in normally sterile sites, can be symptomatic or inapparent. Bacteremia implies the presence of organisms that can be cultured from blood. Septicemia implies bacteremia with greater severity. Sepsis indicates clinical settings in which there is evidence of infection as well as a systemic response to infection (fever/hypothermia, tachycardia, tachypnea, or leukocytosis/leukopenia). Sepsis syndrome emphasizes an increased degree of severity with evidence of altered organ perfusion with one of the following: hypoxemia, oliguria, altered mentation, or elevated serum lactate level. Severe sepsis represents a more advanced degree of organ compromise. Septic shock indicates sepsis plus hypotension despite adequate intravenous fluid challenge. Refractory septic shock is defined as shock lasting more than 1 hour unresponsive to fluids and/or vasopressors. Noninfectious insults (e.g., thermal burns, severe trauma, severe pancreatitis, certain toxins, therapy with monoclonal antibodies for solid organ transplant rejection) can also be associated with a severe systemic reaction simulating the sepsis syndrome. The term *systemic inflammatory response syndrome* encompasses both infectious and noninfectious causes of a profound host inflammatory response with systemic symptoms and signs; sepsis syndrome is the predominant cause of the systemic inflammatory response syndrome.

Epidemiology

The incidence of sepsis and associated deaths has increased dramatically in the United States, and evidence suggests that this rise will continue. Septic shock is the most common cause of death in intensive care units, and the thirteenth most common cause of death in the United States. The incidence is approximately 400,000 cases per year.

The National Nosocomial Infection System indicates marked increases in the frequency of septicemia caused by gram-positive infections since 1985. Highest rates for hospital-acquired septicemias occur in oncology patients and burn/trauma victims and in high-risk nurseries. Hospital-acquired blood stream infections are associated with 7.4 extra days of hospitalization and $4000 of extra hospital charges per occurrence. The most commonly identified blood stream pathogens include staphylococci, streptococci, *Escherichia coli*, *Enterobacter* species, and *Pseudomonas aeruginosa*. Fungal blood stream isolates are less frequent. Major epidemiologic factors that have contributed to the increased occurrence of sepsis include the growing number of immunocompromised hosts resulting from more intense chemotherapy regimens, an aging population, and the aggressive employment of more invasive procedures and complex surgery.

Table 96–2 lists organisms important in the sepsis syndrome as they relate to host factors. Factors that have negatively influenced survival in the setting of bacteremia have included severity of underlying disease, delayed initiation of appropriate antimicrobial therapy, virulence of the pathogen (e.g., *P. aeruginosa*), extremes of age, site of infection (respiratory being more common than abdominal, which is more common than urinary), nosocomial acquisition, polymicrobial infection, and development of end-organ complications (adult respiratory distress syndrome, anuria, disseminated intravascular co-

TABLE 96–1 **Definitions of Sepsis and Related Disorders**

Disorder	Definition
Infection	Microorganisms in a normally sterile site; subclinical or symptomatic
Bacteremia	Bacteria present in blood stream; may be transient
Septicemia	Same as bacteremia but greater severity
Sepsis	Clinical evidence of infection plus systemic response to infection (fever/hypothermia, tachycardia, tachypnea, leukocytosis/leukopenia)
Sepsis syndrome	Sepsis plus altered organ perfusion (hypoxemia, oliguria, altered mentation)
Severe sepsis	Sepsis syndrome plus hypotension/hypoperfusion
Septic shock	Sepsis with hypotension despite adequate fluid resuscitation; patients on vasopressors may not be hypotensive at the time hypoperfusion abnormalities are evident
Refractory septic shock	Shock lasting more than 1 hr unresponsive to fluid administration and/or vasopressors
Systemic inflammatory response syndrome (SIRS)	Wide variety of insults (infectious and noninfectious) that initiate profound systematic responses; sepsis syndrome is a subset of SIRS

agulation [DIC], coma). When there is evidence of dysfunction in two or more systems, the diagnosis of multiorgan system failure can be made. Mortality rises in proportion to the number of organ systems involved and is near 100% when four or more systems are dysfunctional.

Pathogenesis

The pathogenesis of sepsis is shaped largely by the infected host's complex response to the invading pathogen (Fig. 96–2). Gram-negative bacterial lipopolysaccharide

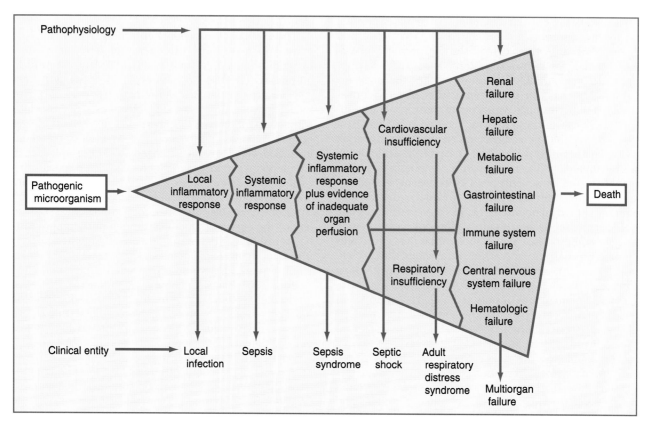

FIGURE 96–1 Natural history of the sepsis process.

TABLE 96–2 **Microorganisms Involved in Sepsis Syndrome in Relation to Host Factors**

Host Factors	Organisms of Particular Importance
Asplenia	Encapsulated organisms: *Streptococcus pneumoniae, Haemophilus influenzae, Neisseria meningitidis,* bacillus (DF-2)
Cirrhosis	*Vibrio, Yersinia,* and *Salmonella* species, other gram-negative rods encapsulated organisms
Alcoholism	*Klebsiella* species, *Streptococcus pneumoniae*
Diabetes	Mucormycosis and *Pseudomonas* species, *Escherichia coli*
Steroids	Tuberculosis, fungi, herpesviruses
Neutropenia	Enteric gram-negative rods, *Pseudomonas, Aspergillus, Candida,* and *Mucor* species, *Staphylococcus aureus*
T cell dysfunction	*Listeria, Salmonella,* and *Mycobacterium* species, herpesvirus group (herpes simplex virus, cytomegalovirus, varicella-zoster virus)

(LPS), or endotoxin, is representative of a larger class of bacterial products causally linked to the septic shock syndrome. Cell wall products of gram-positive bacteria, such as teichoic acid and peptidoglycan, induce inflammatory responses similar to those produced by LPS. Indeed, the sepsis syndrome may complicate infections with bacteria, viruses, fungi, rickettsiae, mycobacteria, and parasites. The pathogenesis of shock involves a series of events initiated by the invading pathogen or its products and is effected through a causally related sequence of host responses. Endotoxin, for example, activates the clotting, fibrinolytic, and complement pathways both directly and indirectly through its effects on platelets, macrophages, polymorphonuclear leukocytes, and hepatocytes.

Endotoxin induces macrophages to produce a number of proinflammatory cytokines including tumor necrosis factor-α, interleukin (IL)-1, IL-6, IL-8, interferon-γ, and granulocyte colony-stimulating factor. Each of these cytokines exerts multiple effects related directly or indirectly to the development of septic shock, and each cytokine modulates its own production and that of other mediators and, in some cases, acts synergistically with one or more of the cytokines. These macrophage-associated cytokines can also stimulate B and T lymphocytes, natural killer cells, and bone marrow cells. Mediators released from macrophages can stimulate T lymphocytes to generate IL-2, IL-4, and IL-10 and granulocyte-macrophage colony-stimulating factor (Table 96–3).

Endotoxin stimulates membrane phospholipid metabolism, leading to the generation of platelet-activating factor and other bioactive metabolites of arachidonic acid, including prostaglandins and leukotrienes. These compounds, in turn, exert a variety of synergistic and antagonistic effects on vascular endothelium, smooth muscle, platelets, and leukocytes and thus contribute to or modulate pathophysiologic events associated with septic shock. Endotoxin may also serve as a cofactor to prime granulocytes to produce toxic oxidative radicals. Lastly, endotoxin induces the production of β-endorphins (which have been implicated in the pathogenesis of sepsis) as well as counterregulatory hormones such as cortisol, glucagon, and catecholamines, which may oppose certain of the shock-producing actions of endorphins and other mediators.

Clinical Manifestations

The clinical manifestations of the sepsis syndrome are multiple and often do not point to the specific cause (Table 96–4). The clinician is faced with the challenge of early recognition and sorting through the various possible causes of the systemic inflammatory response syndrome so that appropriate therapy can be initiated. Patients presenting with the clinical picture of sepsis of uncertain etiology should be presumed to have bacteremic infection and treated accordingly. Prompt careful cultures of blood and suspicious local sites should be followed immediately by initiation of antibiotics appropriate for the most likely pathogens.

Fever and chills are usually present, but elderly or debilitated patients (especially with renal or liver failure)

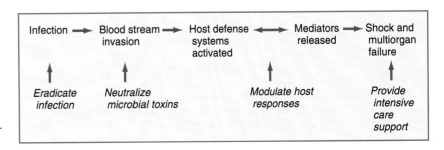

FIGURE 96–2 The pathogenesis and treatment of sepsis syndrome.

TABLE 96-3 Cytokines with a Potential Role in Systemic Inflammatory Response Syndrome

Cytokine	Source	Target Cell	Function
Granulocyte-macrophage colony-stimulating factor (GM-CSF)	T cells, macrophages, endothelial cells, fibroblasts	Myeloid precursor cells, neutrophils, eosinopils, macrophages	Proliferation of progenitor cells Differentation and maturation of neutrophils and macrophages
Granulocyte colony-stimulating factor (G-CSF)	Monocytes, endothelial cells, fibroblasts, neutrophils	Neutrophils, promyelocytes	Proliferation of myeloid progenitor cells Enhanced neutrophil survival and function
Interleukin-1 (IL-1) (α and β)	Macrophages, fibroblasts, T cells, endothelial cells, hepatocytes	Fibroblasts, T cells, monocytes, neutrophils	Induces cytokines (IL-2, IL-3, IL-6, TNF). Induces B- and T-cell activation, growth, and differentiation Synthesis of acute phase reaction, induces fever, catabolism
Interleukin-2 (IL-2)	Activated T cells	Activated lymphoid cells	Enhances T- and B-cell immune responses Promotes cytotoxic T cells Induces INF-γ and TNF
Interleukin-4 (IL-4)	TH2 T cells	B and T cells, macrophages, mast cells	Induces B-cell activation, proliferation and differentiation and IgGl and IgE production Enhances MHC Cl and II receptors
Interleukin-6 (IL-6)	Macrophages, fibroblasts, TH2 T cells	Lymphocytes, monocytes	Stimulates B-cell growth, differentiation, and activation Induces synthesis of acute phase reactivants
Interleukin-8 (IL-8)	Monocytes, fibroblasts, endothelial cells	Neutrophils, monocytes	Enhanced neutrophil activity and histamine release
Interleukin-12 (IL-12)	Macrophages, B cells	T cells	Induces differentiation of TH1 cells Initiates production of IFN-α
Interferon gamma (INF-γ)	T cells	Macrophages, monocytes, T and B cells	Pronounced monocyte/macrophage activation Increased MHC class II expression
Tumor necrosis factor: TNF-α (cachectin) TNF-β (lymphotoxin)	Monocytes, macrophages, lymphocytes, mast cells	Monocytes, macrophages, lymphocytes, neutrophils, fibroblasts	Induces cascade of inflammatory reactions (fever, catabolism, acute phase reactants) Induces multiple cytokines (IL-1, GM-CSF) Increases MHC class I expression Enhances B-cell proliferation and immunoglobulin production

MHC, major histocompatibility complex.

may not develop fever. Hypothermia may occur and is associated with a poor prognosis. One of the early clues to a systemic infectious process is hyperventilation and respiratory alkalosis.

Skin manifestations in sepsis can occur with any infectious agent and at times may represent the earliest sign of the sepsis syndrome. Staphylococci and strepto-cocci can be associated with cellulitis or diffuse erythroderma in association with toxin-producing strains. Blood stream infection with gram-negative bacteria can be associated with a skin lesion called ecthyma gangrenosum (round/oval 1- to 15-cm lesions with a halo of erythema and usually a vesicular or necrotic central area). Although ecthyma gangrenosum is most com-

TABLE 96-4   Signs and Symptoms Indicative of the Sepsis Syndrome

Fever, chills
Hyperventilation
Hypothermia
Mental status changes
Hypotension
Leukopenia, thrombocytopenia
End-organ failure: lung, kidney, liver, heart, disseminated intravascular coagulation

monly associated with *P. aeruginosa, Aeromonas* organisms, *Klebsiella* organisms, *E. coli,* and *Serratia* organisms may also cause ecthyma gangrenosum (see also Chapter 101). *Neisseria meningitidis* bacteremia is often heralded by petechial and hemorrhagic skin lesions and followed by rapidly progressive shock.

The sepsis syndrome is characteristically associated with hypotension and oliguria. In many patients, hypotension will initially respond to intravenous fluids. Other patients progress from an initial stage of hypotension, tachycardia, and vasodilatation (warm shock) to deep pallor, vasoconstriction, and anuria (cold shock). Of all infectious causes of the sepsis syndrome, gram-negative bacilli most often cause shock; up to 35% of patients with gram-negative sepsis develop shock, often with mortality rates between 40% and 70%.

As the sepsis syndrome progresses, myocardial function becomes profoundly depressed. This greatly complicates fluid management and necessitates continuous cardiopulmonary monitoring in an intensive care setting.

Pulmonary complications of the sepsis syndrome are frequent. The adult respiratory distress syndrome, characterized by PaO_2 less than 50 mm Hg despite FIO_2 greater than 50%, diffuse alveolar infiltrates, and pulmonary capillary wedge pressure less than 18 mm Hg, occurs in 10% to 40% of sepsis syndrome patients and is most frequent in conjunction with gram-negative organisms. Increased pulmonary capillary permeability, resulting from inflammatory cytokines released during sepsis, is a major causative factor in adult respiratory distress syndrome and makes administration of intravenous fluids, often given in an attempt to improve cardiac output, extremely hazardous. Failure of respiratory muscles can also complicate sepsis and contribute significantly to morbidity and mortality.

Most patients with sepsis have a neutrophilic leukocytosis. Leukopenia may occur, most often with overwhelming bacteremias, but also with severe systemic viral infections. Alcoholics and the elderly are at greater risk for sepsis-associated neutropenia. A low platelet count and evidence of coagulopathy occur in up to 75% of patients with gram-negative bacillary bacteremia. Disseminated intravascular coagulation occurs in roughly 10% of septic patients.

Renal insufficiency in the sepsis syndrome is multifactorial and depends to varying degrees on the host, the microbe, and the therapy administered. Most often in sepsis, acute tubular necrosis is the basis for renal

dysfunction and may be secondary to hypotension, volume depletion, or cytokines elaborated in the sepsis syndrome. Tubulointerstitial disease caused by specific pathogens and/or antimicrobial therapy may also occur.

Upper gastrointestinal tract bleeding may be a life-threatening complication in septic patients with coagulopathy and thrombocytopenia. Liver dysfunction may occur, with evidence of cholestatic jaundice or of hepatocellular injury. With bacteremia related to gram-negative bacilli, "hyperbilirubinemia of sepsis" often occurs, with little change in other liver enzymes. Large increases in transaminase values usually indicate ischemia in the liver; these abnormalities usually resolve rapidly with restoration of blood pressure.

Hypoglycemia may complicate sepsis syndrome and can be a correctable cause of mental status change or seizures. Hypoglycemia occurs more frequently in individuals with underlying liver disease.

Diagnosis

The initial evaluation of the patient with possible sepsis syndrome ideally begins with a careful history. However, in patients with the fully developed sepsis syndrome, the working diagnosis is made on the basis of physical findings, and the detailed history must necessarily follow correction of hemodynamic problems, obtaining appropriate microbial cultures, and empirical initiation of antimicrobial therapy. Attention should be focused on underlying diseases or predispositions to sepsis, previous infections and antimicrobial therapy, available microbiologic information, and symptoms suggesting localization of infection. A history of travel, environmental exposure, and any contact with infectious agents should be carefully obtained. Information on the complications of previous treatment (e.g., toxic effects of drugs or drug allergies) can be critical in the selection of therapy.

Physical examination should focus on discovering clues to infection and localizing sites thereof. Appropriate specimens for microbiologic evaluation must be obtained. Two or three sets of blood cultures from bacteremic patients yield the organism in 89% and 99% of patients, respectively.

The selection of additional laboratory studies should be based on the clinical manifestations. Obtaining appropriate diagnostic studies expeditiously is critical. These studies are usually aimed at delineating the focus of infection (e.g., cerebrospinal fluid examination, computed tomography scans) and determining whether adjunctive surgical therapy (e.g., abscess drainage, foreign body removal) is indicated.

Therapy

Time does not allow holding antimicrobial therapy until bacteremia or an infectious source is proven in patients with the sepsis syndrome. The key to management of sepsis is the early recognition of the systemic response and initiation of therapy before hypotension and complications ensue.

Patients with sepsis syndrome, especially if hypotensive, are best managed in the intensive care unit. The essential therapies of the sepsis syndrome and septic shock include antibiotics, judicious fluid administration, oxygen, and vasopressors. Antibiotic choices should reflect epidemiologic concerns (see Table 96–2), antibiotic resistance patterns, and potential sites of infection. Until culture results and other diagnostic studies are completed, empirical broad-spectrum antimicrobial therapy, covering both gram-positive and gram-negative pathogens, is necessary in sepsis patients. Initiation of appropriate empirical antimicrobial therapy has a major impact on survival of these patients. As soon as a specific microbial etiology has been established by culture, antibiotics should be changed, if necessary, to target the etiologic agent.

The limitations of currently available therapy for sepsis and septic shock are evidenced by the continued high mortality rates associated with this disease, despite improvement in antibiotic therapy and critical care techniques. Standard approaches to therapy for sepsis and septic shock are crucial. If various steps in the pathogenesis of septic shock are recognized, beginning with tissue invasion by the offending organism and culminating in pathophysiologic phenomena associated with the septic shock syndrome, current therapy addresses only the initial and final stages of this process (see Figs. 96–1 and 96–2). Few currently employed therapies target intermediate steps in the pathogenesis of septic shock, even though these steps dominate the disease process in the fully developed sepsis syndrome. Newer strategies entail attempts to amplify selectively or modulate the host responses to the invading pathogen or its pathogenic products. Targets include the bacterium, endotoxin (or other bacterial products), host cells that respond to endotoxin, mediators produced by these cells in response to endotoxin, and cells injured by endotoxin-induced mediators (see Fig. 96–2).

A multicenter evaluation of monoclonal antibodies against endotoxin and tumor necrosis factor showed no significant benefit. These studies have emphasized that targeting a specific molecule as adjunctive therapy for sepsis may be inadequate given the complex cascade and temporal relationships of factors involved in the pathophysiology of the systemic inflammatory response syndrome.

REFERENCES

Bone RG: The pathogenesis of sepsis. Ann Intern Med 1991; 115: 457–469.

DeSocio GV, Marroni M, Menichetti F: Sepsis with multiple organ dysfunction. Lancet 1998; 351:1552.

Hoffman WD: Anti-endotoxin therapies in septic shock. Ann Intern Med 1994; 120:771–783.

Members of the ACCP/SCCM Consensus Conference Committee: American College of Chest Physicians/Society of Critical Care Medicine Consensus Conference: Definitions for sepsis and organ failure and guidelines for the use of innovative therapies in sepsis. Crit Care Med 1992; 20:864–874.

Parrillo JE: Pathogenetic mechanisms of septic shock. N Engl J Med 1993; 328:1471–1477.

Wenzel RP, Pinsky MR, Ulevitch RJ, Young LG: Current understanding of sepsis. Clin Infect Dis 1996; 22:407–413.

Young L: Sepsis syndrome. In Mandell GM, Bennett JE, Dolin R (eds): Principles and Practice of Infectious Diseases, 5th ed. New York: Churchill Livingstone, 2000, pp 806–819.

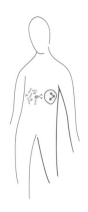

97

INFECTIONS OF THE NERVOUS SYSTEM

Robert A. Salata

Infections of the central nervous system (CNS) range from fulminant, readily diagnosed septic processes to indolent illnesses requiring exhaustive investigation to identify their presence and define their cause. Neurologic outcome and survival depend largely on the extent of CNS damage present before effective treatment begins. Accordingly, it is essential that the physician move quickly to achieve a specific diagnosis and institute appropriate therapy. The initial evaluation must, however, take into account both the urgency of beginning antibiotic treatment in bacterial meningitis and the potential hazard of performing a lumbar puncture in the presence of focal neurologic infection or mass lesions.

Patients with CNS infection usually present with some combination of fever, headache, altered mental status, depressed sensorium, seizures, focal neurologic signs, and stiff neck. The history and physical examination, results of lumbar puncture (Table 97–1), and neuroradiographic procedures provide the mainstays of diagnosis. The order in which the last two procedures are performed is critical. A subacute history, evolving over 7 days to 2 months, of unilateral headache with focal neurologic signs and/or seizures implies a mass lesion that may or may not be infectious. A brain-imaging procedure should be performed first; lumbar puncture is potentially dangerous because it may precipitate cerebral herniation, even in the absence of overt papilledema. However, patients admitted with fulminating symptoms of fever, headache, lethargy, confusion, and stiff neck should have an immediate lumbar puncture and, if this test proves abnormal, antibiotics should be instituted for presumed bacterial meningitis. If the distinction between focal and diffuse CNS infection is unclear or not adequately evaluable, as in the comatose patient, cultures of blood, throat, and nasopharynx should be obtained, antibiotic therapy started, and an emergency scanning procedure performed. If the last is unavailable, lumbar puncture should be delayed pending evidence that no danger of herniation exists. Inevitably, this approach means that some patients will receive parenteral antibiotics several hours before a lumbar puncture is performed. In acute bacterial meningitis, 50% of cerebrospinal fluid (CSF) cultures will be negative by 4 to 12 hours after institution of antibiotics; negative CSF cultures are even more likely if the causative organism is a sensitive pneumococcus. Should the CNS infection actually represent acute bacterial meningitis, however, the characteristics of the CSF still would suggest the diagnosis, because neutrophilic pleocytosis and hypoglycorrhachia (low CSF glucose) usually persist for at least 12 to 24 hours after antibiotics are instituted. Furthermore, Gram-stained preparation (or assay for microbial antigen in the CSF by latex agglutination) should indicate the causative organism even after antibiotics have rendered the CSF culture negative. Blood and nasopharyngeal cultures obtained before therapy also are likely to be positive in view of the high frequency of isolation of causative organisms from these sites. The approach of treating suspected CNS infections promptly ("shoot first, tap later") is often lifesaving and does not significantly compromise management. This approach to the use of scanning procedures is germane only for adults with community-acquired CNS infection. In children, technically adequate computed tomography (CT) requires heavy sedation; therefore, scanning procedures must be reserved for more stringent indications.

Armed with the clinical presentation and the results of the lumbar puncture and CT scan, the clinician must decide on a probable cause and develop a plan for initial management and definitive evaluation. The task is simplified by addressing the following issues:

1. Is the host normal? The spectrum of CNS diseases and their causes shifts dramatically in the immunocompromised host (Table 97–2). The possibility of human immunodeficiency virus (HIV) infection must be determined expeditiously by serologic testing. Acute HIV infection may cause CNS signs and symptoms before seroconversion, requiring additional testing (e.g., HIV polymerase chain reaction [PCR] assay) if the suspicion is sufficiently high (see Chapter 108).

TABLE 97-1 **Typical Cerebrospinal Fluid Findings in Central Nervous System Infection**

Infection	Cells	Neutrophils	Glucose	Protein
Bacterial meningitis	500–10,000/μL	>90%	<40 mg/dL	>150 mg/dL
Aseptic meningitis	10–500/μL	Early >50%; late <20%	Normal	<100 mg/dL
Herpes simplex virus encephalitis	0–1000/μL	<50%	Normal	<100 mg/dL
Tuberculous meningitis	50–500/μL	Early >50%; late <50%	<30 mg/dL	>150 mg/dL
Syphilitic meningitis	50–500/μL	<10%	<40 mg/dL	<100 mg/dL

2. Are there relevant exposures? Exposure to persons with syphilis, tuberculosis, or HIV infection may be associated with acquisition of these diseases. Ticks may transmit Lyme disease or spotted fever, and mosquitoes may transmit arboviral encephalitis. Exposure to livestock or unpasteurized dairy products suggests brucellosis. Residence in the Ohio and Mississippi River valleys increases the risk of histoplasmosis and blastomycosis; coccidioidomycosis is endemic to semiarid regions of the Southwest. Travel and particularly residence in developing countries may suggest cysticercosis, echinococcal cyst disease, and cerebral malaria.

3. Does the patient have meningitis, encephalitis, or meningoencephalitis? Is the disease acute, subacute, or chronic? These distinctions narrow the differential diagnosis considerably and form the basis for organization of the sections that follow. The meningitis syndrome consists of fever, headache, and stiff neck. Confusion and a depressed level of consciousness may occur as part of the metabolic encephalopathy in patients with acute bacterial meningitis. Seizures are rare and may indicate complicating processes such as cortical

vein thrombosis. In contrast, encephalitis characteristically causes confusion, bizarre behavior, depressed levels of consciousness, focal signs, and seizures (grand mal or focal). A presentation suggestive of encephalitis raises a variety of issues quite different from those surrounding a patient with bacterial meningitis.

Meningitis

Meningitis is an inflammation of the leptomeninges caused by infectious or noninfectious processes. The most common types of infectious meningitis are bacterial, viral, tuberculous, and fungal. The most common noninfectious causes are subarachnoid hemorrhage, cancer, and sarcoidosis. Infectious meningitis is considered in three categories: acute bacterial meningitis, aseptic meningitis, and subacute to chronic meningitis.

ACUTE BACTERIAL MENINGITIS

Epidemiology

Three fourths of cases of acute bacterial meningitis occur before the age of 15 years. *Neisseria meningitidis* causes sporadic disease or epidemics in closed populations. Most cases occur in winter and spring and involve children younger than 5 years of age. *Haemophilus influenzae* meningitis is even more selectively a disease of childhood, with most cases developing by the age of 10 years. Infections are sporadic, although secondary cases may occur in close contacts. The incidence of *H. influenzae* meningitis has significantly declined with the widespread use of effective conjugated vaccines. In contrast, pneumococcal meningitis is a disease seen in all age groups and increasing generally in pediatric groups. In addition, pneumococcus is becoming increasingly resistant to penicillin, making therapy much more challenging (see later discussion). Extensive clinical series of adults hospitalized in 1980 showed a relative frequency of 68% pneumococcal, 18% meningococcal, and 10% *H. influenzae* meningitis.

Close contact with a patient with meningococcal or *H. influenzae* disease is particularly important in the development of secondary cases of meningitis and other severe disease manifestations (sepsis, epiglottitis) as well.

TABLE 97-2 **Meningitis and Meningoencephalitis in the Immunocompromised Host**

Abnormality	Infectious Agent
Complement deficiencies (C6–C8)	*Neisseria meningitidis*
Splenectomy and/or antibody defect	*Streptococcus pneumoniae* *Haemophilus influenzae* Enterovirus *Neisseria meningitidis*
Sickle cell disease	*Streptococcus pneumoniae* *Haemophilus influenzae*
Impaired cellular immunity	*Listeria monocytogenes* *Cryptococcus neoformans* *Toxoplasma gondii* *Histoplasma capsulatum* *Coccidioides immitis* *Mycobacterium tuberculosis* *Treponema pallidum* JC virus Cytomegalovirus

For example, the risk of meningococcal disease is 500 to 800 times greater in a close contact of a patient with meningococcal meningitis than in a noncontact. Asymptomatic pharyngeal carriers of *H. influenzae* also can spread infection to their contacts.

Pathogenesis and Pathophysiology

The bacteria that cause most community-acquired meningitis transiently colonize the oropharynx and nasopharynx of healthy individuals. Meningitis may occur in nonimmune hosts after bacteremia from an upper respiratory site (meningococcus or *H. influenzae*) or pneumonia and by direct spread from contiguous foci of infection (nasal sinuses, mastoids).

The pathogenesis of acute bacterial meningitis is best understood for meningococcal disease. The carrier state occurs when meningococci adhere to pharyngeal epithelial cells by means of specialized filamentous structures termed *pili*. The production of IgA protease by pathogenic *Neisseria* species favors adherence by inactivating IgA, a major host barrier to colonization. Organisms enter and pass through epithelial cells to subepithelial tissues, where they multiply in the nonimmune individual and produce bacteremia. The localization of organisms to the CSF is not well understood but presumably depends on invasive properties of the capsular polysaccharide, which permit penetration of the blood-brain barrier. Immunity is conferred by bactericidal antibody and presumably is acquired by earlier colonization of the pharynx with nonpathogenic meningococci and cross-reacting bacteria. The presence of blocking IgA antibody may increase susceptibility transiently in some individuals.

Table 97–2 summarizes host factors conferring a particular risk of meningitis. Bacterial meningitis remains confined to the leptomeninges and does not spread to adjacent parenchymal tissue. Focal and global neurologic deficits develop because of involvement of blood vessels coursing in the meninges and through the subarachnoid space; in addition, cranial nerves and cerebral tissue can be affected by the attendant inflammation, edema, and scarring as well as by the development of obstructive hydrocephalus.

Gram-negative enteric meningitis occurs mainly in severely debilitated persons or individuals whose meninges have been breached or damaged by head trauma, a neurosurgical procedure, or a parameningeal infection.

Clinical Presentation

Patients with bacterial meningitis may present with fever, headache, lethargy, confusion, irritability, and stiff neck. There are three principal modes of onset. About 25% of cases begin abruptly with fulminant illness; mortality is high in this setting. More often, meningeal symptoms progress over 1 to 7 days. Finally, meningitis may superimpose itself on 1 to 3 weeks of an upper respiratory–type illness; diagnosis is most difficult in this group. Occasionally, no more than a single additional neurologic symptom or sign hints at disease more seri-

ous than a routine upper respiratory tract infection. Stiff neck is absent in about one fifth of all patients with meningitis, notably in the very young, the old, and the comatose. A petechial or purpuric rash is found in one half of patients with meningococcemia; although not pathognomonic, palpable purpura is very suggestive of *N. meningitidis* infection. About 20% of patients with acute bacterial meningitis have seizures, and a similar fraction have focal neurologic findings.

Laboratory Diagnosis

The CSF in acute bacterial meningitis usually contains 1,000 to 10,000 cells/μL, mostly neutrophils (see Table 97–1). Glucose concentration falls below 40 mg/dL, and the protein level rises above 150 mg/dL in most patients. The Gram-stained preparation of CSF is positive in 80% to 88% of cases. However, certain cautionary notes are appropriate. Cell counts can be lower (occasionally zero) early in the course of meningococcal and pneumococcal meningitis. Also, predominantly mononuclear cell pleocytosis may occur in patients who have received antibiotics before the lumbar puncture (Table 97–3). A similar mononuclear pleocytosis may be seen in *Listeria monocytogenes* meningitis, tuberculous meningitis, and acute syphilitic meningitis. Gram-stained preparations of CSF may be negative or misinterpreted when meningitis is caused by *H. influenzae*, *N. meningitidis*, or *L. monocytogenes*; the presence of gram-negative diplococci and coccobacilli may be difficult to appreciate, particularly when the background consists of amorphous pink material. In addition, bacteria tend to be pleomorphic in CSF and may assume atypical forms. Compared with patients with acute meningitis due to other bacterial pathogens, patients with *Listeria* infection have a significantly lower incidence of meningeal signs, and the CSF profile is significantly less likely to have a high white blood cell count or a high protein concentration. Gram's stain is negative in two thirds of cases of listerial meningitis and meningoencephalitis and may be misleading in many of the remaining cases. Gram's stain of CSF is negative in two thirds of cases of CNS listeriosis. If interpretation of the Gram-stained CSF is not clear-cut, broad-spectrum antibiotics should be instituted while the results of cultures are being awaited. If the initial Gram-stained preparation does not contain organisms, examining the stained sediment prepared by concentrating up to 5 mL of CSF with a cytocentrifuge may reveal the causative organism.

Cultures of CSF, blood, fluid expressed from purpu-

TABLE 97–3 Presentations of Bacterial Meningitis Without Polymorphonuclear Neutrophil Predominance

Antecedent antimicrobial therapy
Listeria monocytogenes meningitis
Tuberculous meningitis
Syphilitic meningitis

ric lesions, and nasopharyngeal swabs have a high yield. The last mentioned is particularly valuable in patients who have received antibiotic therapy before hospitalization, because most such drugs do not achieve substantial levels in nasopharyngeal secretions.

Recognition of meningitis may be difficult after head trauma or neurosurgery, because the symptoms, signs, and laboratory findings of infection can be difficult to separate from those of trauma. A low CSF glucose level usually indicates infection but can also be seen after subarachnoid hemorrhage. The causative organism, characteristically an enteric gram-negative rod, may already have been cultured from an extraneural site, such as a wound or urine. The known antibiotic sensitivities of such isolates, therefore, may provide a valuable guide to the initial treatment of meningitis.

All patients with meningitis caused by unusual agents or mixed infections and certain patients with meningitis caused by *Streptococcus pneumoniae* and *H. influenzae* should undergo radiography of nasal sinuses and mastoids to exclude a parameningeal focus of infection.

Differential Diagnosis

Classic acute bacterial meningitis resembles few other diseases. Ruptured brain abscess should be considered, particularly if the CSF white blood cell count is unusually high and focal neurologic signs are present. Parameningeal foci of infection usually cause fever, headache, and local signs. CSF characteristically shows modest neutrophilic pleocytosis and moderately increased protein, but the CSF glucose level is usually normal. In patients with bacterial meningitis who have already been given antibiotic treatment, the CSF may be sterile, but neutrophils commonly are present in CSF and the glucose level is depressed. Early in the evolution of viral or tuberculous meningitis, the pleocytosis may be predominantly neutrophilic. Serial examinations, however, will show a progressive shift to a mononuclear cell predominance. Acute viral meningoencephalitis may be difficult to distinguish clinically from bacterial meningitis; the evolution of CSF findings and the clinical course usually decide the matter.

Treatment and Outcome

Bacterial meningitis requires the prompt institution of appropriate antibiotics. If the Gram-stained smear of CSF indicates pneumococcal or meningococcal disease, penicillin G or a third-generation cephalosporin (e.g., ceftriaxone 2 g every 12 hours) should be administered intravenously based on the occurrence of penicillin-resistant *S. pneumoniae* in the locale. The alternative drug for patients with severe penicillin allergy is chloramphenicol, 25 mg/kg, given intravenously every 6 hours. Given the increasing occurrence of highly penicillin-resistant *S. pneumoniae*, additional therapy with vancomycin (pending cultures and sensitivity testing) is indicated. Clinical failure has been observed in some cases of drug-resistant pneumococcal meningitis treated with third-generation cephalosporins in children. Suspected cases of *H. influenzae* meningitis should be treated with cefotaxime, 2 g, given intravenously every 4 hours, or ceftriaxone, 2 g, given intravenously every 12 hours. In a case of suspected community-acquired meningitis, if the Gram-stained preparation of CSF is negative but clinical and laboratory findings suggest bacterial meningitis, penicillin and cefotaxime therapy should be started. Third-generation cephalosporins are the indicated choice for treating sensitive gram-negative enteric organisms causing meningitis. Agents such as ceftazidime, 2 g, given intravenously every 6 to 8 hours, may be effective against *Pseudomonas aeruginosa*. If the organism is resistant to cephalosporins, the patient should be treated with a combination of intraventricular plus parenteral aminoglycoside and a β-lactam antibiotic selected on the basis of the sensitivity of the isolate (e.g., mezlocillin or piperacillin). The placement of an intraventricular reservoir facilitates treatment of such patients. Regardless of the results of sensitivity testing, chloramphenicol is not an adequate drug for treatment of gram-negative bacillary meningitis; its use has been associated with unacceptably high mortality rates.

The management of bacterial meningitis extends beyond the patient. Contacts must be protected, because they are at substantial risk of developing meningococcal meningitis or serious *H. influenzae* disease. At the time one first suspects bacterial meningitis, respiratory isolation procedures should be initiated. One should begin antibiotic prophylaxis of contacts when the clinical course or Gram-stained preparation of CSF suggests meningococcal or *H. influenzae* meningitis. The recommended drug for household and other intimate contacts of patients with meningococcal meningitis is rifampin, 10 mg/kg (up to 600 mg), twice daily for 2 days. The goal of prophylaxis of contacts of *H. influenzae* type B meningitis is to protect children younger than 4 years of age. Because the organism may be passed from patient to asymptomatic adults to an at-risk child, rifampin, 20 mg/kg (up to 600 mg) daily for 4 days, should be given to all members of the household and day care center of the index case who have contact with children younger than 4 years old. Despite parenteral antibiotic therapy, patients with *N. meningitidis* or *H. influenzae* meningitis may have persistent nasopharyngeal carriage and should also receive rifampin treatment before discharge from the hospital. *L. monocytogenes* is resistant to cephalosporins. Ampicillin for a minimum of 15 to 21 days (with an aminoglycoside for the first 7 days) is the treatment of choice.

Although hospital contacts of patients with meningococcal meningitis are at low risk of acquiring the carrier state and disease, occasional secondary cases do occur. Thus, personnel in close contact with the patient's respiratory secretions should receive prophylactic antibiotics. All persons receiving rifampin prophylaxis should be warned that their urine and tears will turn orange and that oral contraceptives will be inactivated temporarily by the antiestrogen effects of the drug.

About 30% of adults with bacterial meningitis die of the infection. In the survivors, deafness (6% to 10%) and other serious neurologic sequelae (1% to 18%) are common. The prognosis in individual cases depends largely on the level of consciousness and extent of CNS damage at the time of the first treatment. Misdiagnosis (>50% of patients) and attendant delays in starting antibiotics are factors in morbidity that the physician must try to offset. Patients with fulminant meningitis should be treated with antibiotics within 30 minutes of reaching medical care. Even after antibiotic therapy and presumed cure, bacterial meningitis may recur. The pattern of recurrence usually suggests a parameningeal infective focus or dural defect (Table 97–4).

The most common types of bacterial meningitis can be prevented by vaccinating susceptible individuals. Effective polysaccharide vaccines are available for some strains of *N. meningitidis, S. pneumoniae,* and *H. influenzae* type B.

ASEPTIC MENINGITIS

Leptomeningitis associated with negative Gram's stains of CSF and negative cultures for bacteria has been designated aseptic meningitis, a somewhat unfortunate designation that implies a benign illness that resolves spontaneously. It is important, however, to assume a high level of vigilance in this group of patients, because they may have a potentially treatable but progressive illness.

Epidemiology

Viral infections are the most frequent cause of aseptic meningitis. Of those cases in which a specific causal agent can be established, 97% are due to enteroviruses (particularly coxsackievirus B, echovirus, mumps virus, and lymphocytic choriomeningitis virus), herpes simplex virus (HSV), and *Leptospira.* Viral meningitis is a disease mainly of children and young adults (70% of patients are younger than 20 years of age). Seasonal variation reflects the predominance of enteroviral infection, so that most cases occur in summer or early fall. Mumps usually occurs in winter, and lymphocytic choriomeningitis usually occurs in fall or winter.

Pathogenesis and Pathophysiology

Localization to the meninges occurs during systemic viremia. The basis for the meningotropism of those viruses that cause aseptic meningitis is not understood.

TABLE 97–4   "Three Rs" of Central Nervous System Infection

"R"	Deterioration	Possibilities
Recrudescence	During therapy, same bacteria	Wrong therapy
Relapse	3–14 days after stopping treatment, same bacteria	Parameningeal focus
Recurrence	Delayed, same, or other bacteria	Congenital or acquired dural defects

HSV type 2 may cause meningitis during the course of primary genital herpes.

Clinical Presentation

The syndrome of aseptic meningitis of viral origin begins with the acute onset of headache, fever, and meningismus associated with CSF pleocytosis. The headache often is described as the worst ever experienced and is exacerbated by sitting, standing, or coughing. In typical cases, the course is benign. The development of changes in sensorium, seizures, or focal neurologic signs shifts the diagnosis to encephalitis or meningoencephalitis. Additional clinical features may suggest a particular infectious agent. Patients with mumps may have or may develop parotitis or orchitis and usually give a history of appropriate contact. Lymphocytic choriomeningitis often follows exposure to mice, guinea pigs, or hamsters and causes severe myalgias; an infectious mononucleosis–like illness can ensue, with rash and orchitis. Leptospirosis often follows exposure to rats or mice or swimming in water contaminated by their urine; aseptic meningitis occurs in the second phase of the illness. Aseptic meningitis also can be seen in persons with HIV infection, either as a manifestation of primary infection by the virus or as a later complication. The pleocytosis generally is modest, the protein level is only slightly elevated, and the glucose concentration is normal or slightly depressed. HIV serology may be negative during acute HIV infection, but the diagnosis is readily established by detectable plasma HIV RNA (see Chapter 108).

Laboratory Diagnosis

In viral meningitis, the CSF shows a pleocytosis of 10 to 2000 white blood cells/μL (see Table 97–1). Two thirds of patients have mainly neutrophils in the initial CSF specimen. However, serial lumbar punctures reveal a rapid shift (within 6 to 8 hours) in the CSF differential count toward a mononuclear cell predominance. CSF protein is normal in one third of cases and almost always less than 100 mg/dL. The CSF glucose level characteristically is normal, although minimal depression occurs in mumps (30% of cases), in lymphocytic choriomeningitis (60%), and, less frequently, in echovirus and HSV meningitis. Serial lumbar punctures show a 95% reduction in cell count by 2 weeks. Stool cultures have the highest yield for enterovirus isolation (40% to 50%); CSF and throat cultures are positive in about 15% of cases. Serologic studies also may indicate a specific causative agent; a fourfold rise in antibody titer is helpful in confirming the significance of a virus isolated from the throat or stool. Serologic studies are seldom useful in acute diagnosis, but PCR-based diagnosis is becoming available for enterovirus infections.

Differential Diagnosis

Partially treated bacterial meningitis and a parameningeal focus of infection may be particularly difficult to distinguish from aseptic meningitis. Serial lumbar punctures may be helpful in establishing the former, and radiographs of paranasal sinuses and mastoids may help confirm the latter. Also in the differential diagnosis are infectious agents that are not cultured on routine bacterial media and are considered to be causes of subacute meningitis (see later). Infective endocarditis may cause aseptic meningitis and is an important diagnostic consideration in the appropriate setting (see Chapter 100).

Treatment and Course

Viral meningitis is generally benign and self-limited. HSV meningitis associated with primary genital herpes occasionally causes sufficient symptoms to warrant treatment with acyclovir.

SUBACUTE AND CHRONIC MENINGITIS

Certain infectious and noninfectious diseases can present as a subacute or chronic meningitis. Chronic meningitis refers to a clinical syndrome of at least 4 weeks' duration and is discussed in Chapter 120. More germane to the differential diagnosis of aseptic meningitis is a neurologic disease that develops over a course of several days to weeks, clinically takes the form of meningitis or meningoencephalitis, and is associated with a predominantly mononuclear pleocytosis in the CSF. The infectious causes of this syndrome may present as a subacute to chronic meningitis (Table 97–5).

At the outset, it is important to consider the possible role of HIV as directly causing this syndrome or predisposing to specific opportunistic infections, such as cryptococcosis or toxoplasmosis, which frequently present as subacute meningitis. The patient in a high-risk category for the acquired immunodeficiency syndrome requires special consideration in this regard (see Chapter 108).

Tuberculous meningitis results from the rupture of a parameningeal focus into the subarachnoid space. The presentation is generally one of semiacute or subacute meningitis, with a neurologic syndrome being present for less than 2 weeks in over half of patients. Headache, fever, meningismus, and altered mental status are characteristic, with papilledema, cranial nerve palsies (II, III,

TABLE 97–5 Subacute to Chronic Meningitis

Causative Agent	Association
Human immunodeficiency virus	Direct involvement or opportunistic infection
Mycobacterium tuberculosis	May have extraneural tuberculosis
Cryptococcus neoformans	Compromised host
Coccidioides immitis	Southwestern United States
Histoplasma capsulatum	Ohio and Mississippi River valleys
Treponema pallidum	Acute syphilitic meningitis, secondary meningovascular syphilis
Lyme disease	Tick bite, rash, seasonal occurrence

IV, VI, or VII), and extensor plantar reflexes each occurring in about one fourth of cases. The initial CSF sample may show predominance of neutrophils, but the differential shifts to mononuclear cells within the next 7 to 10 days. Acid-fast bacilli are identified in the CSF of 10% to 20% of patients; the intermediate-strength tuberculin skin test is positive in 65%. Because delay in institution of treatment is associated with increased mortality, therapy is initiated before confirmation of the diagnosis in most cases. The clinical suspicion of tuberculosis is heightened by a history of remote tuberculosis in one half of patients; concurrent pulmonary disease occurs in about one third, so that the diagnosis may be supported by smears or culture of pulmonary secretions. Appropriate therapy consists of isoniazid, rifampin, ethambutol, and pyrazinamide. "Vasculitis" related to entrapment of cerebral vessels in inflammatory exudate may lead to stroke syndromes. This has been offered as a rationale for the use of corticosteroids as adjunctive therapy. Although evidence of their advantage remains unproved, some authorities believe that corticosteroids should be given, in tapering doses, for 4 weeks when the diagnosis of tuberculosis is established, particularly if cranial palsies appear or stupor or coma supervenes.

Cryptococcal meningitis is the most common fungal meningitis and can occur in apparently normal as well as immunocompromised hosts. The presentation is of insidious onset, followed by weeks to months of progressive meningoencephalitis, sometimes clinically indistinguishable from the course of tuberculosis. Certain associations are useful in this differential diagnosis. The presence of immunosuppression suggests cryptococcosis, whereas chronic debilitating disease, miliary infiltrates on chest radiograph, or the syndrome of inappropriate secretion of antidiuretic hormone suggests tuberculosis. An India ink preparation of CSF reveals encapsulated yeast in 50% of cases. More than 90% of patients have cryptococcal polysaccharide antigen in CSF or serum. Fungal cultures of urine, stool, sputum, and blood should be obtained; they may be positive in the absence of clinically apparent extraneural disease. Treatment of cryptococcal meningitis requires amphotericin B. Addition of flucytosine allows use of less amphotericin B. Fluconazole is also effective but causes less rapid sterilization of the CSF. Daily fluconazole is effective for lifelong maintenance therapy to prevent relapses in persons with the acquired immunodeficiency syndrome.

Coccidioides immitis is a major cause of granulomatous meningitis in semiarid areas of the southwestern United States; Histoplasma capsulatum may cause a similar syndrome in endemic areas (Ohio and Mississippi River valleys).

Neurosyphilis reflects the fact that the spirochete causing syphilis invades the CNS in most instances of systemic infection. The organism then may be either cleared by host defenses or persist to produce a more chronic infection expressed symptomatically only years later. The most common form of neurosyphilis is asymptomatic; patients harbor a few white cells in the CSF and have a positive serologic test for syphilis. Symptomatic neurosyphilis can appear as acute or subacute meningitis (meningitic form), resembling that of other bacterial infections and usually occurring during the stage of secondary syphilis when there are cutaneous changes as well. Hydrocephalus and cranial nerve (VII and VIII) abnormalities may develop. CSF and serum serologic studies usually are strongly positive, and the disease is responsive to penicillin.

Vascular syphilis begins 2 to 10 years after the primary lesion. The disorder is characterized by both meningeal inflammation and a vasculitis of small arterial vessels, the latter leading to arterial occlusion. Clinically, the disorder produces few signs of meningitis but results in monofocal or multifocal cerebral or spinal infarction. The disorder may be mistaken for an autoimmune vasculitis or even arteriosclerotic cerebrovascular disease. The early and prominent spinal cord signs should lead one to expect syphilis, whereas the findings in the CSF of pleocytosis, elevated gamma globulin, and a positive serologic test for syphilis establish the diagnosis. Patients respond to antibiotic therapy, although recovery from focal abnormalities may be incomplete. Syphilis is more difficult to diagnose and may have an accelerated course in the HIV-infected individual. Meningovascular syphilis may develop within months of primary infection, despite treatment with intramuscular benzathine penicillin (see Chapter 107).

General paresis, once a common cause of admission to mental institutions, is now rare. The disorder results from syphilitic invasion of the parenchyma of the brain and begins clinically 10 to 20 years after the primary infection. Paresis is characterized by progressive dementia, sometimes with manic symptoms and megalomania and often with coarse tremors affecting facial muscles and tongue. The diagnostic clue is the presence of Argyll Robertson pupils. The CSF is always abnormal. The diagnosis is made by serologic tests. Early treatment with antibiotics usually leads to improvement but not complete recovery.

Tabes dorsalis is a chronic infective process of the dorsal roots that appears 10 to 20 years after primary syphilitic infection. The disorder is characterized by lightning-like pains and a progressive sensory neuropathy affecting predominantly large fibers supplying the lower extremities. There is profound loss of vibration and position sense as well as areflexia. Autonomic fibers are also affected, causing postural hypotension, trophic ulcers of the feet, and traumatic arthropathy of joints. Argyll Robertson pupils are usually present. CSF serologic tests are usually positive. The disorder responds only partially to treatment with antibiotics.

Rare complications of syphilis include progressive optic atrophy, gumma (a mass lesion in the brain), congenital neurosyphilis, and syphilitic infection of the auditory and vestibular system. Descriptions can be found in appropriate texts.

Lyme disease, a tick-borne spirochetosis (see Chapter 95), is associated in 15% of clinically affected individuals with meningitis, encephalitis, or cranial or radicular neuropathies. Characteristically, the neurologic disease begins several weeks after the typical rash of erythema chronicum migrans. Furthermore, the rash may have been so mild as to go unnoticed and usually has faded by the time neurologic manifestations appear. The diagnosis should be suspected when a patient develops subacute or chronic meningitis during late summer or early fall, with CSF changes consisting of a modest mononuclear pleocytosis, protein values below 100 mg/dL, and normal glucose levels. The diagnosis is established serologically. PCR analysis of CSF provides a sensitive diagnostic approach to the diagnosis of CNS Lyme disease. Patients with early Lyme disease usually respond to oral doxycycline. Patients with later, or disseminated, Lyme disease respond less predictably to prolonged (14 to 21 days) courses of intravenous ceftriaxone.

Several noninfectious diseases may manifest as a subacute or chronic meningitis. Typical of this group is a CSF containing 10 to 100 lymphocytes, elevated protein levels, and a mild to severely lowered glucose level. Meningeal carcinomatosis represents diffuse involvement of the leptomeninges by metastatic adenocarcinoma, lymphoma, or melanoma. Cytologic analysis often identifies malignant cells. Sarcoidosis may cause a basilar meningitis and asymmetric cranial nerve involvement, as well as a low-grade pleocytosis, sometimes associated with borderline low CSF glucose levels. Granulomatous angiitis and Behçet's disease also belong in this category.

Approach to Diagnosis

Diagnosing the specific cause of subacute or chronic meningitis may be quite difficult. In patients with tuberculous or fungal meningitis, cultures may not become positive for 4 to 6 weeks or longer; moreover, meningitis caused by some fungi (e.g., *H. capsulatum*) is often associated with negative cultures of the CSF.

Because of the uncertainties involved in establishing the diagnosis of infectious cases, and even the question of whether a particular patient has an infectious or noninfectious disease, an organized approach must be taken. In addition to routine laboratory tests (on multiple samples of CSF), including India ink and cultures for bacteria, mycobacteria, and fungi, the patient with chronic meningitis of unknown cause should have the following: Venereal Disease Research Laboratories (VDRL) testing and cryptococcal antigens (and, when appropriate, antibody to *Borrelia burgdorferi*) determined on blood and CSF; fluorescent treponemal antibody (FTA)–absorbed and antinuclear antibody on blood, *Histoplasma* antigen in urine and CSF, antibody to HIV and *H. capsulatum* (and, where appropriate, *C. immitis*) on serum; and cytologic studies (×3) on CSF. A tuberculin skin test (intermediate strength, 5 TU) should be done, along with anergy skin testing (mumps, *Candida*, tetanus). Diagnosis by PCR of specific pathogens in CSF should greatly expedite evaluation of patients with chronic meningitis in the future.

The appropriate management is decided by the patient's clinical status and the results of these tests. If the CSF pleocytosis consists of more than 50 to 100 cells/μL, then an infectious disease is likely. Empirical therapy for tuberculous meningitis is appropriate. If the tuberculin skin test is negative, however, fungal meningitis becomes more likely. Repeated cytologic and microbiologic studies of the CSF may reveal the diagnosis. If the pleocytosis is low grade (fewer than 50 to 100 cells/μL), a noninfectious cause becomes more likely; the condition even may be self-limited, the so-called chronic benign lymphocytic meningitis. The approach to treating such patients must be individualized. Only rarely is brain or meningeal biopsy necessary or helpful. If all CSF studies are nondiagnostic and the patient's clinical condition is stable, a period of careful observation is almost always preferable to an invasive diagnostic procedure.

Encephalitis

Acute viral and other infectious causes of encephalitis usually produce fever, headache, stiff neck, confusion, alterations in consciousness, focal neurologic signs, and seizures.

Epidemiology

A large number of viral and nonviral agents can cause encephalitis (Table 97–6). Seasonal occurrence may help to limit the differential diagnosis. Arthropod-borne viruses peak in the summer (California encephalitis [La Crosse virus] and western equine encephalitis in August, St. Louis encephalitis slightly later). The tick-borne infections (Rocky Mountain spotted fever) occur in early summer, enterovirus infections in later summer and fall, and mumps in the winter and spring. Geographic distribution is also helpful. Eastern equine encephalitis is confined to the coastal states. Serologic surveys indicate that infections by encephalitis viruses are most often subclinical. It is not clear why so few among the many infected subjects develop encephalitis.

HSV is the most frequent, treatable, and devastating cause of sporadic, severe focal encephalitis; overall it is implicated in 10% of all cases of encephalitis in North America. There is no age, sex, seasonal, or geographic preference.

TABLE 97–6   Viral Etiology of Encephalitis and Meningoencephalitis

Herpes simplex
Epstein-Barr
Varicella-zoster
Cytomegalovirus
Mumps
Measles
La Crosse virus
St. Louis encephalitis
Eastern equine encephalitis
Western equine encephalitis
Coxsackievirus
Echovirus
Rabies
Human immunodeficiency virus

Pathogenesis

Viruses reach the CNS by the blood stream or peripheral nerves. HSV presumably reaches the brain by cell-to-cell spread along recurrent branches of the trigeminal nerve, which innervate the meninges of the anterior and middle fossae. Although this would explain the characteristic localization of necrotic lesions to the inferomedial portions of the temporal and frontal lobes, it is not clear why such spread is so rare, with one case of HSV encephalitis occurring per million in the population per annum.

Clinical Features

The course of HSV encephalitis is considered here in detail because of the importance of establishing the diagnosis of this treatable entity. Patients affected by HSV commonly describe a prodrome of 1 to 7 days of upper respiratory tract symptoms followed by the sudden onset of headache and fever. The headache and fever may be associated with acute loss of recent memory, behavioral abnormalities, delirium, difficulty with speech, and seizures (often focal). Disorders of the sensorium are not, however, always apparent at the time of presentation and are not essential for the working diagnosis of this eminently treatable, but potentially lethal, infection of the CNS.

Laboratory Diagnosis

In HSV encephalitis, the CSF can contain 0 to 1000 white blood cells/μL, predominantly lymphocytes. Protein is moderately high (median, 80 mg/dL). CSF glucose is reduced in only 5% of individuals within 3 days of onset but becomes abnormal in additional patients later in the course. In about 5% the CSF is normal. Other laboratory findings at onset are of little help, although focal abnormalities may be present in the electroencephalogram and develop in computed tomographic or magnetic resonance imaging brain scan by the third day in most patients. Acyclovir offers such high likelihood of therapeutic benefit in HSV encephalitis, with so little risk in this highly fatal and neurologically damaging disease, that brain biopsy should not be performed unless an alternative, treatable diagnosis seems very likely. A low CSF glucose level should increase suspicion that a granulomatous infection (e.g., tuberculosis, cryptococcosis) is present. If the initial CSF shows a low glucose level, roughly one third of individuals will have an alternative treatable infection. If CSF studies and brain imaging remain inconclusive in such circumstances, biopsy may be appropriate.

Viral cultures of stool, throat, buffy coat, CSF, and brain biopsy specimens and indirect immunofluorescence or immunoperoxidase staining of tissues may provide a specific diagnosis, but both viral isolation and serologic evidence of a rise in antibody titer usually come too late to guide initial treatment. In the case of HSV encephalitis, serologic studies are particularly helpful in the 30% of individuals with a primary infection.

Also, CSF titers of antibody to HSV, which reflect intrathecal production of antibody, may show a diagnostic fourfold rise. Cerebrospinal fluid HSV DNA detection by PCR is highly sensitive and specific in HSV encephalitis.

Differential Diagnosis

Acute (demyelinating) encephalomyelitis, infective endocarditis producing brain embolization, meningoencephalitis caused by *Cryptococcus neoformans, Mycobacterium tuberculosis,* or the La Crosse virus, acute bacterial abscess, acute thrombotic thrombocytopenic purpura, cerebral venous thrombosis, vascular disease, and primary and metastatic tumors may all simulate HSV encephalitis.

Treatment and Outcome

The course of viral encephalitis depends on the etiologic agent. Untreated HSV encephalitis has a high mortality (70%), and survival is associated with severe neurologic residua. Acyclovir therapy improves survival and greatly lessens morbidity in patients if initiated early, before deterioration to coma. Prognosis is particularly favorable in patients younger than 30 years old with a preserved mental status at the time of presentation.

Rabies

Rabies encephalitis is always fatal, requiring major attention on prevention. Currently, zero to six cases of rabies occur each year in the United States, and approximately 20,000 people receive postexposure prophylaxis.

The incubation period for rabies is generally 20 to 90 days, during which the rabies virus replicates locally and then migrates along nerves to the spinal cord and brain. Rabies begins with fever, headache, fatigue, and pain or paresthesias at the site of inoculation; confusion, seizures, paralysis, and stiff neck follow. Periods of violent agitation are characteristic of rabies encephalitis. Attempts at drinking produce laryngospasm, gagging, and apprehension. Paralysis, coma, and death supervene. When rabies is suspected, protective isolation procedures should be instituted to avoid additional exposure of the hospital staff to saliva and other infected secretions. Confirmation of the diagnosis is possible by assaying rabies-neutralizing antibody or isolating virus from saliva, CSF, and urine sediment. Immunofluorescent rabies antibody staining of a skin biopsy specimen taken from the posterior neck is a rapid means of establishing the diagnosis.

Indications for prophylaxis are based on the following principles. (1) The patient must have been exposed. Nonbite exposure is possible if mucous membranes or open wounds are contaminated with animal saliva; exposure to bat urine in heavily contaminated caves has been followed by rabies. (2) Small rodents (rats, mice, chipmunks, squirrels) and rabbits rarely are infected and have not been associated with human disease. Consultation with local or state health authorities is essential, because certain areas of the United States are considered rabies free. In other areas, if rabies is present in wild animals, dogs and cats have the potential to transmit rabies. Domestic dogs and cats should be quarantined for 10 days after biting someone; if they develop no signs of illness, there is no risk of transmission by their earlier bite. Nondomestic animals should be destroyed and their brains examined for rabies virus by direct fluorescent antibody testing. Bites by bats, skunks, and raccoons always require treatment if the animal is not caught. Unusual behavior of animals and truly unprovoked attacks can be signs of rabies.

Currently, postexposure management consists of (1) thorough wound cleansing; (2) human rabies immune globulin, 20 IU/kg, one half infiltrated locally in the area of the bite and one half intramuscularly; and (3) human diploid cell rabies vaccine, 1.0 mL given intramuscularly five times during a 1-month period. Individuals at high risk of exposure (e.g., veterinarians, spelunkers) should be vaccinated.

Spectrum of Tuberculous, Fungal, and Parasitic Infections

The spectrum of tuberculous, fungal, and parasitic infections of the CNS is briefly considered. Many, but not all, of these infections are increasing in incidence as the direct result of the increasing prevalence of HIV infection in the population (see Chapter 108).

TUBERCULOSIS

CNS tuberculosis can occur in several forms, sometimes without evidence of active infection elsewhere in the body. The most common form is *tuberculous meningitis.* This disorder is characterized by the subacute onset of headache, stiff neck, and fever. After a few days, affected patients become confused and disoriented. They often develop abnormalities of cranial nerve function, particularly hearing loss due to marked inflammation at the base of the brain. Most patients, if untreated, lapse into coma and die within 3 to 4 weeks of onset. An accompanying arteritis may produce focal signs, including hemiplegia, during the course of the disorder. Tuberculous meningitis must be distinguished from other causes of acute and subacute meningeal infection, a process that often is not easy even after examination of the CSF. The pressure and cell count are elevated with up to a few hundred cells, a mixture of leukocytes and lymphocytes. The protein level is elevated, usually above 100 mg/dL and often to very high levels, and the glucose concentration is depressed. Smears for acid-fast bacilli are positive in only 10% to 20% of samples. Tuberculosis organisms grow on culture but only after several weeks. Pending complete availability and accuracy of such measures, patients with subacutely developing meningitis suspected of having tuberculosis should

TABLE 97–7   Some Fungal and Parasitic Causes of Central Nervous System Infections

Fungal Infection

Cryptococcosis
Coccidioidomycosis
Aspergillosis
Mucormycosis
Actinomycosis
Histoplasmosis
Blastomycosis
Candidiasis

Helminthic Infection

Trichinosis
Cysticercosis
Echinococcosis
Schistosomiasis
Angiostrongyliasis
Ascariasis

Protozoan Infection

Toxoplasmosis
Amebiasis
Malaria
Chagas' disease
Trypanosomiasis (African)

be treated with antituberculous agents before definitive diagnosis. Large samples of CSF should be sent for culture, and a careful search should be made for tuberculosis elsewhere in the body. Seventy-five percent of such patients have a positive tuberculin skin test, and a careful search may yield evidence of systemic tuberculosis.

Tuberculomas of the brain produce symptoms and signs either of the mass lesion or of meningitis, with the tuberculomas being found incidentally. One or multiple lesions are identified on CT scan, but the scan itself does not distinguish tuberculomas from brain tumor or other brain abscesses. In the absence of evidence of meningeal or systemic tuberculosis, biopsy is necessary for diagnosis. Patients with tuberculomas, like those with tuberculous meningitis, respond to antituberculous therapy, but brain lesions may remain visible in the CT scan long after the patient has improved clinically; the clinical course, not the scan, predicts the outcome.

Less common manifestations of CNS tuberculosis include chronic arachnoiditis characterized by a low-grade inflammatory response in the CSF and progressive pain with signs of either cauda equina or spinal cord dysfunction. The diagnosis of arachnoiditis is suggested by a myelogram showing evidence of fibrosis and compartmentalization instead of the usually smooth subarachnoid lining. The disorder responds poorly to treatment. Tuberculous myelopathy probably results from direct invasion of the organism from the subarachnoid space. Patients present with a subacutely developing myelopathy characterized by sensory loss either in the legs or in all four extremities, depending on the site of the spinal cord invasion. Many patients have additional signs of meningitis, including fever, headache, and stiff neck.

The CSF usually contains cells and tuberculous organisms. The myelogram may show evidence of arachnoiditis and frequently demonstrates an enlarged spinal cord or complete block to the passage of contrast material in the thoracic or cervical region.

FUNGAL AND PARASITIC INFECTIONS

Fungal and parasitic infections of the CNS are less common than viral and bacterial infections and often affect immunosuppressed patients. Table 97–7 lists the more common of these infections. Like bacterial infections, fungal and parasitic infections may cause either meningitis or parenchymal abscesses. The meningitides, when they occur, manifest with clinical symptoms that, while similar, are usually less severe and abrupt than those of acute bacterial meningitis. The common fungal causes of meningitis include cryptococcosis, coccidioidomycosis, and histoplasmosis. *Cryptococcal meningitis* is a sporadic infection that affects both immunosuppressed patients (50%) and nonimmunosuppressed patients. The disorder is characterized by headache and sometimes fever and stiff neck. The clinical symptoms may evolve for periods as long as weeks or months; diagnosis can be made only by identifying the organism or its antigen in the CSF. *Histoplasma* and coccidioidomycosis meningitides occur in endemic areas and often affect nonimmunosuppressed individuals. The diagnosis is suggested by a history of residence in the appropriate geographic area and is confirmed by CSF and serologic evaluation. Antifungal treatment, particularly in the nonimmunosuppressed patient, is usually effective.

Parasitic infections of the nervous system usually produce focal abscesses rather than diffuse meningitis. The most common infection to affect the nonimmunosuppressed host is cysticercosis, a disorder caused by the larval form of the *Taenia solium* tapeworm and contracted by ingesting food or water contaminated with parasite eggs. The disorder is common in the underdeveloped world and parts of the United States having a large Hispanic population. The brain may be invaded in as many as 60% of infected persons. Invasion of the brain leads to formation of either single or multiple cysts, which often lie in the parenchyma but sometimes reside in the ventricles or subarachnoid space. Seizures and increased intracranial pressure are the most common clinical symptoms. Computed tomography identifies

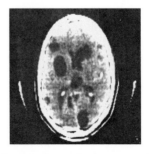

FIGURE 97–1   Neurocysticercosis. A computed tomographic scan shows multiple confluent cysts.

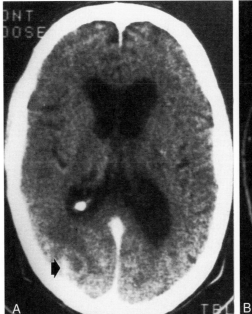 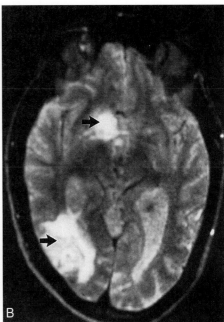

FIGURE 97–2 *Toxoplasma* abscesses in a patient with acquired immunodeficiency syndrome. *A,* Computed tomography shows a contrast medium–enhanced mass *(arrow).* *B,* Magnetic resonance image reveals multiple masses *(arrows)* not seen by computed tomography, leading physicians to suspect abscesses rather than tumor.

small intracranial calcifications and hypodense cysts (Fig. 97–1). Serum indirect hemagglutination tests are usually positive and confirm the diagnosis. Where cysts obstruct the ventricular system to cause symptoms, shunting procedures may be necessary. The anthelmintic praziquantel is effective therapy.

Toxoplasmosis of the brain, when it occurs in the adult, is a manifestation of immunosuppression. Patients with abnormal cellular immunity may develop single or multiple abscesses, which appear usually as ring-enhancing lesions on CT scan (Fig. 97–2). The management of CNS toxoplasmosis is discussed in Chapter 108.

REFERENCES

Bacterial Meningitis

Gripshover BM, Ellner JJ: Chronic meningitis syndrome and meningitis of noninfective or uncertain etiology. *In* Scheld WM, Whitley RJ, Durack DT (eds): Infections of the Central Nervous System, 2nd ed. Philadelphia: Lippincott-Raven, 1997, pp 881–896.

Quagliarello VJ, Scheld WM: New perspectives on bacterial meningitis. Clin Infect Dis 1993; 17:603–610.

Swartz MN, Apicella MA, Simberhaff MS: Bacterial meningitis. *In* Goldman L, Bennett JC (eds): Cecil Textbook of Medicine, 21st ed. Philadelphia: WB Saunders, 2000, pp 1645–1662.

Aseptic Meningitis

Lepow ML, Carver DH, Wright HT, et al: A clinical, laboratory and epidemiologic investigation of aseptic meningitis during the 4-year period 1955–1958. N Engl J Med 1962; 266:1181.

Encephalitis

Johnson RT: Acute encephalitis. Clin Infect Dis 1996; 23:219–226.

Nahmias AJ, Whitley RJ, Visintine AN, et al: HSV encephalitis: Laboratory evaluations and their diagnostic significance. J Infect Dis 1982; 145:829.

Whitley RJ: Viral encephalitis. N Engl J Med 1990; 323:242–250.

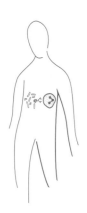

98

INFECTIONS OF THE HEAD AND NECK

Michael M. Lederman

Infections of the Ear

Otitis externa is an infection of the external auditory canal. The process may begin as a folliculitis or pustule within the canal. Staphylococci, streptococci, and other skin flora are the most common pathogens. Some cases of otitis externa have been associated with the use of hot tubs. This infection (swimmer's ear) is usually caused by *Pseudomonas aeruginosa*.

Patients with otitis externa complain of ear pain that is often quite severe, and they may also complain of itching. Examination shows an inflamed external canal; the tympanic membrane may be uninvolved. (Patients with otitis media, in contrast, do not have involvement of the external canal unless the tympanic membrane is perforated.) Otitis externa with cellulitis can be treated with systemic antibiotics such as dicloxacillin or erythromycin and local heat. In the absence of cellulitis, irrigation and administration of topical antibiotics such as neomycin and polymyxin are sufficient. Patients with diabetes mellitus are at risk for an invasive external otitis (malignant otitis) caused by *P. aeruginosa*. In malignant otitis externa, pain is a presenting complaint, and infection rapidly invades the bones of the skull and may result in cranial nerve palsies, invasion of the brain, and death. Computed tomography or magnetic resonance imaging of the cranial bones can establish the extent of disease. Treatment must include debridement of as much necrotic tissue as is feasible and at least 4 to 6 weeks of treatment with an aminoglycoside plus a penicillin derivative active against *Pseudomonas* (e.g., ticarcillin). Ceftazidime, imipenem, or ciprofloxacin may also be effective for this infection.

Otitis media is an infection of the middle ear seen primarily among preschool children but occasionally in adults as well. Infection caused by upper respiratory tract pathogens is promoted by obstruction to drainage through edematous, congested eustachian tubes. *Streptococcus pneumoniae*, *Haemophilus influenzae*, and *Moraxella catarrhalis* are the most common pathogens, and viral infection with serous otitis may predispose to acute otitis media. Fever, ear pain, diminished hearing, vertigo, or tinnitus may occur. In young children, however, localizing symptoms may not be present. The tympanic membrane may appear inflamed, but to diagnose otitis media with certainty, either fluid must be seen behind the membrane or diminished mobility of the membrane must be demonstrated by tympanometry or after air insufflation into the external canal.

Treatment with amoxicillin-clavulanic acid, trimethoprim-sulfamethoxazole, or cefaclor is generally effective; addition of decongestants is of no proven value. Complications of otitis media are uncommon but include infection of the mastoid air cells (mastoiditis), bacterial meningitis, brain abscess, and subdural empyema.

Infections of the Nose and Sinuses

Rhinitis is a common manifestation of numerous respiratory viral infections. It is characterized by a mucopurulent or watery nasal discharge that may be profuse. When rhinitis is caused by respiratory virus infection, pharyngitis, conjunctival suffusion, and fever may be present. Rhinitis can also be caused by hypersensitivity responses to airborne allergens. Patients with allergic rhinitis often have a transverse skin crease on the bridge of the nose a few millimeters from the tip. The demonstration of eosinophils in a wet preparation of nasal secretions readily distinguishes allergic rhinitis from rhinitis of infectious origin. (Eosinophils can be identified in wet preparations by the presence of large refractile cytoplasmic granules.) Occasionally, after head trauma

782

or neurosurgery, cerebrospinal fluid (CSF) may leak through the nose. "CSF rhinorrhea" places patients at risk for bacterial meningitis. CSF is readily distinguished from nasal secretions by its low protein and relatively high glucose concentrations.

Sinusitis is an infection of the air-filled paranasal sinuses that may complicate viral upper respiratory tract infections. Allergic rhinitis and structural abnormalities of the nose that interfere with sinus drainage also predispose to sinusitis. Acute sinusitis is primarily caused by upper respiratory tract bacterial pathogens *S. pneumoniae* and *H. influenzae*, perhaps by *Chlamydia pneumoniae*, and less often by anaerobes and staphylococci. Nosocomial sinusitis may be caused by *S. aureus* or gram-negative bacteria. With chronic sinusitis, anaerobic bacteria play a more important role.

Sinusitis may be difficult to distinguish from a viral upper respiratory tract illness, which in many instances precedes sinus infection. Patients may complain of persistent cough, headache, "stuffiness," a "toothache," or purulent nasal discharge. Headache may be exacerbated by bending over. Sinusitis should be suspected in a person with a febrile upper respiratory tract illness that lasts more than 7 to 10 days. There may be tenderness over the involved sinus, and pus may be seen in the turbinates of the nose. Failure of a sinus to light up on transillumination may suggest the diagnosis; computed tomography is more sensitive than sinus radiographs in establishing the diagnosis of sinusitis. Most patients with sinusitis can be treated with a 10- to 14-day course of amoxicillin-clavulanate, clarithromycin, or trimethoprim-sulfamethoxazole, along with nasal decongestants. Patients who appear toxic or otherwise are severely ill or those with nosocomial sinusitis should undergo sinus puncture for drainage, Gram's stain, and culture. Sinusitis may be complicated by bacterial meningitis, brain abscess, or subdural empyema. Therefore, patients with sinusitis and neurologic abnormalities must be evaluated carefully for these complications by computed tomography if a space-occupying lesion is suspected or by CSF examination if meningitis is suspected (see Chapter 97).

Rhinocerebral mucormycosis is an invasive infection arising from the nose or sinuses and is caused by fungi of the order *Mucorales*. This infection can result in progressive bony destruction and invasion of the brain. Rhinocerebral mucormycosis is seen primarily among poorly controlled diabetics with ketoacidosis, recipients of organ transplants, and patients with hematologic malignancy. Black necrotic lesions of the palate or nasal mucosa are characteristic. Most patients have a depressed sensorium at presentation. Vascular thrombosis and cranial nerve palsies are common. Diagnosis is made by demonstration of the broad, ribbon-shaped, nonseptate hyphae on histologic examination of a scraping or biopsy specimen. Differential diagnosis includes infection caused by *P. aeruginosa* or to fungi such as *Aspergillus* species, and cavernous sinus thrombosis. Rhinocerebral mucormycosis is a surgical emergency. Treatment involves correction of the underlying process if possible, broad surgical debridement, and administration of amphotericin B.

Infections of the Mouth and Pharynx

STOMATITIS

Stomatitis, or inflammation of the mouth, can be caused by a wide variety of processes. Patients with stomatitis may complain of diffuse or localized pain in the mouth, difficulty in swallowing, and difficulty in managing oral secretions. Various nutritional deficiencies (vitamins B_{12} and C, folic acid, and niacin) and cytotoxic chemotherapies can produce stomatitis.

Thrush is an infection of the oral mucosa by *Candida* species. Thrush may be seen among infants and also in patients receiving broad-spectrum antibiotics or corticosteroids (systemic or inhaled), among patients with leukopenia (e.g., acute leukemia), and among patients with impairments in cell-mediated immunity (e.g., acquired immunodeficiency syndrome). In its milder form, thrush is manifested by an asymptomatic white, "cheesy" exudate on the buccal mucosa and pharynx, which, when scraped, leaves a raw surface. In more severe cases, there may be pain and also erythema surrounding the exudate. The diagnosis is suggested by the characteristic appearance of the lesions and is confirmed by microscopic examination of a potassium hydroxide preparation of the exudate, which reveals yeast and the pseudohyphae characteristic of *Candida*. Thrush related to administration of antibiotics and corticosteroids should resolve after the drugs are withdrawn. Otherwise, thrush can be managed with clotrimazole troches. Refractory thrush or candidal infection involving the esophagus should be treated with fluconazole or itraconazole.

ORAL ULCERS AND VESICLES (Table 98–1)

Aphthous Stomatitis

Aphthae are discrete, shallow, painful ulcers on erythematous bases; they may be single or multiple and are usually present on the labial or buccal mucosa. Attacks of aphthous stomatitis may be recurrent and quite debilitating. Symptoms may last for several days to 2 weeks. The cause of these ulcerations is unknown, and treatment is symptomatic with saline mouthwash or topical anesthetics. Giant aphthous ulcers may occur in persons with the acquired immunodeficiency syndrome and may respond to topical or systemic corticosteroids or to thalidomide.

Herpes Simplex Virus Infection

Although most recurrences of oral herpes simplex infections occur on or near the vermillion border of the lips, the primary attack usually involves the mouth and pharynx. Generalized symptoms of fever, headache, and malaise often precede the appearance of oral lesions by as much as 24 to 48 hours. The involved regions are swollen and erythematous. Small vesicles soon appear; these rupture, leaving shallow, discrete ulcers that may coalesce. Autoinoculation may spread the infection; her-

TABLE 98-1 **Oral Vesicles and Ulcers**

Aphthous stomatitis
Primary herpes simplex infection
Vincent's stomatitis
Syphilis
Coxsackievirus A (herpangina)
Fungi (histoplasmosis)
Behçet's syndrome
Systemic lupus erythematosus
Reiter's syndrome
Crohn's disease
Erythema multiforme
Pemphigus
Pemphigoid

petic keratitis is one of the major infectious causes of blindness in the industrialized world. The diagnosis can be made by scraping the base of an ulcer. Wright's or Giemsa's stain of this material may reveal the intranuclear inclusions and multinucleated giant cells characteristic of herpes simplex infection. Viral cultures are more sensitive but more expensive. Diagnosis may also be established by immunoassay for viral antigen in the scraping. Treatment of primary infection with acyclovir or valacyclovir will decrease the duration of symptoms but has no effect on the frequency of recurrence.

Vincent's Stomatitis

Vincent's stomatitis is an ulcerative infection of the gingival mucosa caused by anaerobic fusobacteria and spirochetes. The patient's breath is often foul, and the ulcerations are covered with a purulent, dirty-appearing, gray exudate. Gram's stain of the exudate reveals the characteristic gram-negative fusobacteria and spirochetes. Treatment with penicillin is curative. If not treated, the infection may extend to the peritonsillar space (quinsy) and even involve vascular structures in the lateral neck (see later).

Syphilis

Syphilis may produce a painless primary chancre in the mouth or a painful mucous patch that is a manifestation of secondary disease. The diagnosis should be considered in the sexually active patient with a large (>1 cm) oral ulceration and should be confirmed serologically, because darkfield examination may be confounded by the presence of nonsyphilitic oral spirochetes.

Herpangina

Herpangina is a childhood disease that causes tiny, discrete ulcerations of the soft palate and is caused by infection with coxsackievirus A.

Fungal Disease

Occasionally, an oral ulcer or nodule may be a manifestation of disseminated infection resulting from histoplas-

mosis. These ulcers are generally mildly or minimally symptomatic and are overshadowed by the constitutional symptoms of disseminated fungal illness.

Systemic Illnesses Causing Ulcerative or Vesicular Lesions of the Mouth

Recurrent aphthous oral ulcerations may be part of Behçet's syndrome. Oral ulcerations have been associated with connective tissue diseases, such as systemic lupus erythematosus and Reiter's syndrome, and with Crohn's disease. Although isolated oral bullae and ulcerations may be seen in patients with erythema multiforme, pemphigus, and pemphigoid, almost all patients have an associated rash. The "iris" or "target" lesion of erythema multiforme is diagnostic. Otherwise, biopsy will establish the diagnosis. Corticosteroids may be life-saving for patients with pemphigus. Corticosteroids are also used in the treatment of erythema multiforme majorum (Stevens-Johnson syndrome), although proof of their efficacy is not available.

APPROACH TO THE PATIENT WITH "SORE THROAT"

When evaluating a patient with a sore throat, it is first important to distinguish between the relatively common and benign sore throat syndromes (viral or streptococcal pharyngitis) and the less common but more dangerous causes of sore throat. Patients with viral or streptococcal pharyngitis often give a history of exposure to individuals with upper respiratory tract infections. Symptoms of cough, rhinitis, and hoarseness (indicating involvement of the larynx) suggest a viral upper respiratory tract infection, although it is important to remember that hoarseness may also be seen with more serious infections, such as epiglottitis.

Examination of the Throat

Two points regarding examination of the throat need emphasis. The first is that complete examination of the oral cavity is important. Not only will a thorough examination give clues to the cause of the complaint, but it may also provide early diagnosis of an asymptomatic malignancy at a time when cure is feasible. The second point is that the normal tonsils and mucosal rim of the anterior fauces are generally a deeper red than the rest of the pharynx in healthy subjects. This should not be mistaken for inflammation. Patients with pharyngitis often have a red, inflamed posterior pharynx. The tonsils are often enlarged and red and may be covered with a punctate or diffuse white exudate. Lymph nodes of the anterior neck are often enlarged.

If any of the seven *danger signs* listed in Table 98-2 is present, the clinician must suspect an illness other than viral or streptococcal pharyngitis. Symptoms persisting longer than 1 week are rarely caused by streptococci or viruses and should prompt consideration of other processes (see later section Persistent or Penicillin-Unresponsive Pharyngitis). Respiratory difficulty, particularly stridor, difficulty in handling oral secretions, or

TABLE 98–2   Seven Danger Signs in Patients with "Sore Throat"

1. Persistence of symptoms longer than 1 week without improvement
2. Respiratory difficulty, particularly stridor
3. Difficulty in handling secretions
4. Difficulty in swallowing
5. Severe pain in the absence of erythema
6. A palpable mass
7. Blood, even in small amounts, in the pharynx or ear

difficulty in swallowing should suggest the possibility of epiglottitis or soft tissue space infection. Severe pain in the absence of erythema of the pharynx may be seen with some of the "extrarespiratory" causes of sore throat, as well as in some cases of epiglottitis or retropharyngeal abscess. A palpable mass in the pharynx or neck suggests a soft tissue space infection, and blood in the ear or pharynx may be an early indication of a lateral pharyngeal space abscess eroding into the carotid artery.

A good history and careful examination will distinguish between the common and benign causes of a sore throat and the unusual but often more serious causes.

Pharyngitis

Agents that have been associated with pharyngitis are presented in Table 98–3. More than half of all cases are caused by respiratory viruses or group A streptococci. Most of the remainder are without defined etiology. Most cases occur during the winter months. In practice, once a diagnosis of pharyngitis is established clinically, it is most important to distinguish between group A streptococcal infections, which should be treated with penicillin, and viral infections, which should be treated symptomatically (e.g., salicylates, saline gar-

TABLE 98–3   Causes of Pharyngitis

Viral
Respiratory viruses*
Adenovirus
Herpes simplex
Epstein-Barr virus
Coxsackievirus A (herpangina)
Human immunodeficiency virus
Mycoplasma pneumoniae
Bacterial
Group A *Streptococcus**
Group C *Streptococcus*
Vincent's fusospirochetes
Corynebacterium diphtheriae
Arcanobacterium hemolyticum
Neisseria gonorrhoeae
Fungal
Candida (thrush)

* Most frequent identifiable causes of pharyngitis.

gles). Because clinical criteria do not reliably distinguish streptococcal from nonstreptococcal pharyngitis, all patients with presumed bacterial pharyngitis should have a throat swab specimen obtained for a rapid streptococcal antigen test. This test is highly specific, so that a positive test result establishes the diagnosis of streptococcal pharyngitis. The test is less sensitive, so that a negative test result does not exclude this diagnosis.

Pharyngitis and Respiratory Virus Infections. Many patients with common colds caused by rhinovirus, coronavirus, adenovirus, or influenza virus have an associated pharyngitis. Other signs of rhinorrhea, conjunctival suffusion, and cough suggest a cold virus; fever and myalgias suggest influenza. Symptoms generally resolve in a few days without treatment.

Infectious mononucleosis caused by Epstein-Barr virus is often associated with pharyngitis. Patients often also complain of malaise and fever. On examination, the pharynx may be inflamed and the tonsils hypertrophied and covered by a white exudate. Cervical lymph node enlargement is often prominent, and generalized lymph node enlargement and splenomegaly are common. Examination of a peripheral blood smear shows atypical lymphocytes, and the presence of heterophil antibodies (e.g., monospot test) or a rise in antibodies to Epstein-Barr virus viral capsid antigen will confirm the diagnosis. Patients with acute Epstein-Barr virus infection should be advised to abstain from contact sports, because traumatic rupture of the enlarged spleen may be fatal.

Primary human immunodeficiency virus seroconversion illness is often manifested by fever, pharyngitis, and lymph node enlargement and is sometimes associated with a generalized maculopapular rash. A high index of suspicion is essential, because this diagnosis is often missed in clinical practice. Diagnosis is established by demonstration of human immunodeficiency virus RNA in plasma (see Chapter 108).

Streptococcal Pharyngitis. Streptococcal pharyngitis may produce mild or severe symptoms. The pharynx is generally inflamed, and exudative tonsillitis is common but not universal. Fever may be present, and cervical lymph nodes may be enlarged and tender. Clinical distinction between streptococcal and nonstreptococcal pharyngitis is inaccurate, and patients with pharyngitis should therefore have a swab of the posterior pharynx tested for streptococcal infection. The growth of group A β-hemolytic streptococci or detection of group A streptococcal antigen is an indication for treatment with penicillin (or erythromycin if the patient is penicillin-allergic). Antibiotics may shorten the duration of symptoms caused by this infection but are given primarily to decrease the frequency of rheumatic fever, which may follow untreated streptococcal pharyngitis.

Pharyngitis Caused by Other Bacteria. Diphtheria, caused by *Corynebacterium diphtheriae*, is a rare disease in the United States, with five or fewer cases recognized annually since 1980. The gray pseudomembrane bleeds when removed and in rare cases may cause death by means of airway obstruction. Most morbidity and mortality in diphtheria are related to the elaboration of a toxin with neurologic and cardiac effects. Treatment consists of antitoxin plus erythromycin. A self-limited pharyngitis, often associated with a diffuse scarlatiniform rash, may be caused by *Arcanobacterium* (formerly *Corynebacterium*) *haemolyticum*. This infection can be treated with penicillin or erythromycin.

Epiglottitis

Epiglottitis, usually an aggressive disease of young children, occurs in adults as well. Early recognition of this entity is critical, because delay in diagnosis or treatment frequently results in death, which may occur abruptly, within hours after the onset of symptoms. This diagnosis must be considered in any patient with a sore throat and any of the following key symptoms or signs: (1) difficulty in swallowing; (2) copious oral secretions; (3) severe pain in the absence of pharyngeal erythema (the pharynx of patients with epiglottitis may be normal or inflamed); and (4) respiratory difficulty, particularly stridor.

Patients with epiglottitis often display a characteristic posture; they lean forward to prevent the swollen epiglottis from completely obstructing the airway and resist any attempt at placement in the supine position. The diagnosis can be confirmed by lateral radiographs of the neck or by indirect laryngoscopy with visualization of the swollen erythematous epiglottis. This examination should be performed with the patient in the sitting position to minimize the risk of laryngeal spasm. Furthermore, the physician must be prepared to perform emergency tracheostomy should spasm occur. Therapy has two major objectives: protecting the airway and providing appropriate antimicrobial coverage. Prophylactic endotracheal intubation or tracheotomy is often indicated if respiratory distress increases under observation. Because the most likely pathogen is *H. influenzae,* which may produce β-lactamase, good antibiotic choices are a second- or third-generation cephalosporin or ampicillin-sulbactam. Corticosteroids may relieve some inflammatory edema; however, their role in this disease remains unproven. Patients with respiratory difficulty should have their airway protected by endotracheal intubation or tracheostomy. Patients without respiratory complaints may be monitored continuously in an intensive care setting and intubated at the first sign of respiratory difficulty. Young children who are close contacts of patients with invasive disease caused by *H. influenzae* are themselves at particular risk of serious infection. Children younger than 4 years of age who are close contacts of the index patient and all family members in a household with children younger than 4 years of age should receive prophylaxis with rifampin (20 mg/kg given orally, up to 600 mg twice daily for four doses).

Soft Tissue Space Infections

Quinsy. Quinsy is a unilateral peritonsillar abscess or phlegmon that is an unusual complication of tonsillitis. The patient has pain and difficulty in swallowing and often trouble in handling oral secretions. Trismus (inability to open the mouth because of muscle spasm)

may be present. Examination shows swelling of the peritonsillar tissues and lateral displacement of the uvula. A mass may be felt on digital examination. In the phlegmon stage, penicillin therapy may be adequate; abscess can be identified by computed tomography and requires surgical drainage (Table 98–4). If untreated, quinsy may result in glottic edema and respiratory compromise or lateral pharyngeal space abscess.

Septic Jugular Vein Thrombophlebitis. An uncommon complication of bacterial pharyngitis or quinsy is septic jugular vein thrombophlebitis (syndrome of postanginal sepsis). Several days after a "sore throat," the patient (in general, a teenager or young adult) will note increasing pain and tenderness in the neck. Often there is swelling at the angle of the jaw. The patient will have a high fever; bacteremia, usually with *Fusobacterium* species; and often septic pulmonary emboli. Treatment is intravenous penicillin, 10 million U/day, plus metronidazole, 500 mg every 6 hours. Patients with persistent fevers may require surgical excision of the jugular vein.

Lateral Pharyngeal Space Abscess. This rare infection is associated with serious morbidity because of its proximity to vascular structures. Extension to the jugular vein may result in thrombophlebitis with septic pulmonary emboli and bacteremia (syndrome of "postanginal sepsis"), discussed earlier. Erosion of the carotid artery may also complicate this infection, with resultant exsanguination. This may be preceded by small amounts of blood in the ear or pharynx. This infection is generally associated with tenderness and a mass at the angle of the jaw. Prompt surgical intervention may be lifesaving.

Retropharyngeal Space Abscess. This complication of tonsillitis is rare in adults, because by adulthood the lymph nodes that give rise to this infection are generally atrophied. Most cases in adults are secondary to trauma (e.g., endoscopic) or to extension of a cervical osteomyelitis. The patient often has difficulty in swallowing and may complain of dyspnea, particularly when sitting upright. Diagnosis may be suspected by the presence of a posterior pharyngeal mass and confirmed by lateral neck films.

TABLE 98–4   **Indications for Surgical Drainage: Parapharyngeal Soft Tissue Space Infections**

Infection	Indications for Surgery
Quinsy	Abscess or respiratory compromise
Lateral pharyngeal space abscess	Abscess
Jugular vein septic thrombophlebitis	Febrile after 5 to 6 days of medical therapy
Retropharyngeal abscess	Abscess or respiratory compromise
Ludwig's angina	Abscess or respiratory compromise

Ludwig's Angina. This cellulitis/phlegmon of the floor of the mouth is generally secondary to an odontogenic infection. The tongue is pushed upward, and there is often firm induration of the submandibular space and neck. Laryngeal edema and respiratory compromise may also occur and necessitate protection of the airway. Penicillin is the antibiotic of choice; protection of the airway is crucial in this setting, and endotracheal intubation should be provided if there is any suggestion of airway compromise.

Extrarespiratory Causes of Sore Throat

Several extrarespiratory causes of sore throat should be kept in mind. The older patient who complains of soreness in the throat when climbing stairs or when upset may be suffering from angina pectoris with an unusual radiation. The hypertensive patient who presents with an abrupt onset of a "tearing pain" in the throat may have a dissecting aortic aneurysm. In these patients, swallowing is generally unaffected. Patients with de Quervain's subacute thyroiditis may present as fever and pain in the neck radiating to the ears. In patients with thyroiditis, the thyroid is generally tender and the sedimentation rate is increased. Patients with vitamin deficiencies may complain of soreness in the mouth and throat (see Table 98–1). Examination may reveal a red "beefy" tongue with flattened papillae, resulting in a smooth appearance.

Persistent or Penicillin-Unresponsive Pharyngitis

Most cases of viral or streptococcal pharyngitis are self-limited, and symptoms generally resolve within 3 to 4 days. In addition to acute human immunodeficiency virus infection, infectious mononucleosis, and soft tissue abscess, as discussed earlier, persistent sore throat should prompt consideration of the following possibilities.

Soft Tissue Abscess or Phlegmon. In rare cases, tonsillitis extends to the soft tissues of the pharynx, producing a potentially life-threatening infection (see earlier discussion).

Pharyngeal Gonorrhea. Although most cases of pharyngeal gonorrhea are asymptomatic, mild pharyngitis may be seen occasionally. This infection will not respond to doses of penicillin used for pharyngitis; moreover, the gonococcus is relatively resistant to phenoxymethylpenicillin (Pen-V). The gonococcus will not likely be identified on routine culture medium; isolation generally requires culture of a fresh throat swab on a selective medium such as Thayer-Martin (see Chapter 107).

Acute Lymphoblastic Leukemia. Persistent exudative tonsillitis may be a presentation of acute lymphoblastic leukemia (ALL). Diagnosis can be suspected by examination of the peripheral blood smear; however, some experience may be required to distinguish between the blasts of ALL and the atypical lymphocytes of infectious mononucleosis.

Other Leukopenic States. Stomatitis or pharyngitis may be the presenting complaint of patients with *aplastic anemia* or *agranulocytosis*. Because some of these cases are drug-induced (e.g., propylthiouracil, phenytoin), a complete medication history on initial presentation may suggest this possibility. Prompt discontinuation of the offending drug may be lifesaving.

Although sore throat is a common complaint of patients with relatively benign illness, it is sometimes the presenting complaint of a patient with a serious or life-threatening disease. Any of the key signs or symptoms shown in Table 98–2 should alert the clinician to the possibility of an extraordinary process.

REFERENCES

Gwaltney JM: Pharyngitis. *In* Mandell GL, Bennett JC, Dolin R (eds): Principles and Practice of Infectious Diseases, 4th ed. New York: Churchill Livingstone, 1995, pp 566–572.

Mayo-Smith MF, Spinale JW, Donsky CJ, et al: Acute epiglottitis: An 18-year experience in Rhode Island. Chest 1995; 108:1640–1647.

Mufson MA: Viral pharyngitis, laryngitis, croup, and bronchitis. *In* Goldman L, Bennett JC (eds): Cecil Textbook of Medicine, 21st ed. Philadelphia: WB Saunders, 2000, pp 1793–1794.

Stevens DL: Streptococcal infections. *In* Goldman L, Bennett JC (eds): Cecil Textbook of Medicine, 21st ed. Philadelphia, WB Saunders, 2000, pp 1619–1624.

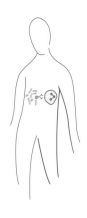

99

INFECTIONS OF THE LOWER RESPIRATORY TRACT

Michael M. Lederman

Pneumonia accounts for about 10% of admissions to adult medical services in North America and is one of the leading causes of death during the productive years of life. This potentially lethal illness is readily reversible. Every physician must therefore be adept at the rapid diagnosis and management of pneumonia. Viruses, chlamydiae, rickettsiae, mycoplasmas, bacteria, protozoans, and parasites can all produce serious infection of the lower respiratory tract. A careful history and physical examination can provide clues to the likely cause of infection. The clinical spectra of pneumonias caused by different pathogens overlap considerably, however. Microscopic examination of respiratory secretions provides a rapid and important step in the differential diagnosis of pneumonia.

Pathogenesis

Microbes can enter the lung to produce infection by hematogenous spread, by spread from a contiguous focus of infection, by inhalation of aerosolized particles, or, most commonly, by aspiration of oropharyngeal secretions. In the last instance, the organisms colonizing the oropharynx will determine the flora of the aspirated secretions and presumably the nature of the resultant pneumonia. Some organisms such as *Streptococcus pneumoniae* may transiently colonize the oropharynx in healthy individuals. Colonization often results in the development of protective antibodies to that strain. Others, such as gram-negative bacilli, are more prevalent in the upper respiratory tract of debilitated and hospitalized patients. Aspiration of normal oropharyngeal flora may lead to necrotizing pneumonia caused by mixtures of oral anaerobic bacteria.

Inoculum size (the number of bacteria aspirated) is an important factor in the development of pneumonia.

Studies using radioisotopes have shown that up to 45% of healthy men aspirate some oropharyngeal contents during sleep. In most instances, the bacteria aspirated are relatively avirulent and back-up defenses, including cough and mucociliary clearance, are adequate to prevent the development of pneumonia. Individuals with structural disease of the oropharynx or patients with cough reflexes impaired as a result of drugs, alcohol, or neuromuscular disease are at particular risk for the development of pneumonia as a result of aspiration. The specialized ciliated cells of the bronchial mucosa are covered by a layer of mucus that traps foreign particles, which are propelled upward by rhythmic beating of the cilia to a point where a cough can expel the particles. Impaired mucociliary transport, as seen in persons with chronic obstructive pulmonary disease, predisposes to bacterial infection. Denuding of the respiratory epithelium by infection with the influenza virus is one mechanism by which influenza predisposes to bacterial pneumonia. Within the alveoli and smaller airways, alveolar macrophages and humoral opsonins, including antibody and complement, serve as host defenses against infection.

Infection by *Mycobacterium tuberculosis* is usually acquired through inhalation of aerosolized contaminated droplet nuclei. A primary infection is established in the parenchyma of the lungs and in the draining lymph nodes, which may result in a progressive primary infection, but in most instances it resolves after producing a mild respiratory illness. The organism remains alive, sequestered within host macrophages, and is contained by host cell-mediated defenses. Reactivation of infection may never occur, may occur without apparent precipitating events, or may become active at times when host cell-mediated immune responses are impaired. Examples of these impairments include starvation, intercurrent viral infections, administration of corticosteroids or cytotoxic drugs, and illnesses associated with immuno-

TABLE 99–1 Important Pathogens Causing Pneumonia

Population (see also Chapters 108 and 109)	Pathogens
Young, healthy adult	*Streptococcus pneumoniae, Mycoplasma pneumoniae, Chlamydia pneumoniae*, respiratory viruses
Elderly	*S. pneumoniae*, influenza virus, *Mycobacterium tuberculosis*
Debilitated	*S. pneumoniae*, influenza virus, oral flora, *M. tuberculosis*, gram-negative bacilli
Hospitalized	Oral flora, *Staphylococcus aureus*, gram-negative bacilli, *Legionella* spp.

TABLE 99–2 Specific Disorders and Associated Pneumonias

Disorder	Pneumonia
Seizures	Aspiration (mixed anaerobes)
Alcoholism	Aspiration, *Streptococcus pneumoniae*, gram-negative bacilli
Diabetes mellitus	Gram-negative bacilli, *Mycobacterium tuberculosis*
Sickle cell disease	*S. pneumoniae, Mycoplasma pneumoniae*
Chronic lung disease	*S. pneumoniae, Haemophilus influenzae, Moraxella catarrhalis*, gram-negative bacilli, *Legionella pneumophila*
Chronic renal failure	*S. pneumoniae, M. tuberculosis, L. pneumophila*

suppression, such as Hodgkin's disease and human immunodeficiency virus (HIV) infection.

Epidemiology

Common pathogens of community-acquired and nosocomial pneumonia are shown in Table 99–1. As a general rule, the pneumococcus is an important pathogen in all age groups, and influenza and tuberculosis become more frequent with increasing age. Although *Mycoplasma* occasionally produces pneumonia in the elderly, it is primarily a pathogen of the young. Certain systemic disorders appear to be associated with pneumonias caused by particular organisms (Table 99–2). The exposure history may be helpful in suggesting specific causative agents (Table 99–3). Pneumonias associated with bone marrow suppression and malignant disorders are discussed in Chapter 109.

Differential Diagnosis

A critical historical point in the differential diagnosis of pneumonia is the duration of symptoms. Pneumonia caused by pneumococci, *Mycoplasma*, or virus is usually an acute illness. Symptoms are measured in hours to a few days, although there may occasionally be a longer viral prodrome before bacterial superinfection. In contrast, symptoms of pneumonia lasting 10 days or more are rarely caused by the common bacterial pathogens and should raise suspicion of mycobacterial, fungal, or anaerobic pneumonia (anaerobes can produce acute or chronic infection), or the presence of an anatomic defect such as an endobronchial mass.

Occupational exposure and travel history often provide clues to the etiology of some less common pneumonias (see Table 99–3). Although these pneumonias are uncommon, they should be considered in the appropriate setting because, if improperly treated, some may be fatal.

A history of rhinitis or pharyngitis suggests respiratory virus or *Mycoplasma* or *Chlamydia* pneumonia. Diarrhea has been associated with *Legionella* pneumonia in some outbreaks. A persistent hacking, nonproductive cough characterizes some *Mycoplasma* infections; symptoms of grippe (malaise and myalgias) are common in influenza and may also be seen with *Mycoplasma* pneumonia. A true rigor is very suggestive of a bacterial (often pneumococcal) pneumonia. Whereas small pleural effusions may be seen in nonbacterial pneumonias, severe pleuritic pain in a patient with pneumonia is highly suggestive of bacterial infection. Night sweats in the absence of rigors are seen in chronic pneumonias and suggest tuberculous or fungal disease.

Most patients with pneumonia have cough, fever, tachypnea, and tachycardia. Fever without a concomitant rise in pulse rate may be seen in legionellosis, *Mycoplasma* infections, and other "nonbacterial" pneumonias. Patients with pulmonary tuberculosis often have high fever that is relatively asymptomatic when compared with patients with acute bacterial pneumonia. Respirations may be shallow in the presence of pleurisy. Increasing tachypnea, cyanosis, and the use of accessory muscles for respiration indicate serious illness. Foul breath suggests anaerobic infection. Mental confusion in

TABLE 99–3 Exposures Associated with Pneumonia

Source/Location	Pneumonia
Cattle, goats, sheep	Q fever, brucellosis
Rabbits	Tularemia
Birds	Psittacosis, histoplasmosis*
Rodents	Hantavirus
Dog ticks	Ehrlichiosis
Southwestern United States	Coccidioidomycosis
Mississippi and Ohio River valleys	Histoplasmosis, blastomycosis
Developing countries	Tuberculosis

* Exposure to bird and bat droppings.

a patient with pneumonia should immediately raise the suspicion of meningeal involvement, which occurs most commonly in patients with pneumococcal pneumonia. Confusion may, however, be the most prominent clinical feature of pneumonia in elderly patients in the absence of associated meningitis. Nonetheless, patients with pneumonia who are confused must be evaluated by examination of cerebrospinal fluid.

Physical evidence of consolidation, dullness to percussion, bronchial breath sounds, crackles, increased fremitus, and whispered pectoriloquy suggest bacterial pneumonia. Early in the course of pneumonia, however, the physical examination may be normal.

RADIOGRAPHIC PATTERNS

Clinical-radiographic dissociation is seen often in patients with *M. pneumoniae* or viral pneumonia. Chest radiographs of patients with *Mycoplasma* infection often suggest a more serious infection than does the appearance of the patient or the physical examination. The converse is true in patients with *Pneumocystis carinii* infection, who may appear quite ill despite normal or nearly normal chest radiographs. This may also be true early in the course of acute bacterial pneumonias, when pleuritic chest pain, cough, purulent sputum, and inspiratory crackles may precede specific radiographic findings by many hours. A "negative" radiograph can never rule out the possibility of acute bacterial pneumonia when the patient's symptoms and signs point to this diagnosis. A lobar consolidation suggests a bacterial pneumonia; however, patients with chronic lung disease often fail to manifest clinical or radiographic evidence of consolidation during the course of bacterial pneumonia. Interstitial infiltrates suggest a nonbacterial process but may also be seen in early staphylococcal pneumonia. Enlarged hilar lymph nodes suggest a concomitant lung tumor but may also be seen in primary tuberculous, viral, or fungal pneumonias. Large pleural effusions should suggest streptococcal pneumonia or tuberculosis. Pneumatoceles are seen in patients after ventilator-mediated barotrauma but occur frequently in the evolution of staphylococcal pneumonia, particularly among children and also in patients with *P. carinii* pneumonia. The presence of cavitation identifies the pneumonia as necrotizing. This finding virtually excludes viruses and *Mycoplasma* and makes pneumococcal infection unlikely (Table 99–4). Lateral radiographs are especially important in showing infiltrates, which may be obscured by the heart on posteroanterior projections.

OTHER LABORATORY FINDINGS

In patients with bacterial pneumonia, the white blood cell count is often (but not invariably) elevated. Among patients with pneumococcal infection, white blood cell counts of 20,000 to 30,000/μL or more may be seen. A left shift with immature forms is common. Patients with nonbacterial pneumonias tend to have lower white blood cell counts. Modest elevations of serum bilirubin (conjugated) level may be noted in many bacterial infec-

TABLE 99–4 **Necrotizing Pneumonias**

Common
Tuberculosis
Staphylococcus
Gram-negative bacilli
Anaerobes
Fungi
Pneumocystis carinii

Rare
Streptococcus pneumoniae
Legionella
Viruses

Unknown
Mycoplasma pneumoniae

tions but are particularly common in patients with pneumococcal pneumonia.

Diagnosis

When the patient presents with abrupt onset of shaking chills, followed by cough, pleuritic chest pain, fever, rusty or yellow sputum, and shortness of breath, and the physical examination shows tachypnea and even minimal signs of alveolar inflammation (e.g., harsh breath sounds at one lung base), the presumptive diagnosis of bacterial pneumonia should be made, sputum should be examined, and appropriate therapy should be begun regardless of radiographic findings. The radiographic abnormalities may lag for several hours after the clinical onset of pneumonia.

Empirical treatment of community-acquired pneumonia without laboratory examination of sputum may be successful in the management of many patients. However, this practice promotes indiscriminate use of broad-spectrum antibiotics with attendant increases in antibiotic resistance. This approach also will result in occasional misdiagnoses and may place nonresponding patients at risk for increased morbidity and death.

Examination of respiratory secretions is essential for accurate diagnosis and proper treatment of pneumonia. When the history and physical examination suggest pneumonia, a specimen of sputum must be Gram-stained and examined immediately. The adequacy of the specimen can be ascertained by (1) the absence of squamous epithelial cells and (2) the presence of polymorphonuclear leukocytes (10 to 15 per high-power field). The presence of alveolar macrophages and bronchial epithelial cells confirms the lower respiratory tract origin of the specimen. A specimen with many (>5 per high-power field) squamous epithelial cells is of no value for either culture or Gram's stain, because it is contaminated with upper respiratory tract secretions.

In some cases, the patient cannot produce an adequate sputum sample, despite vigorous attempts at sputum induction using an aerosolized solution of 3% hy-

TABLE 99–5 Sputum Gram's Stain Showing Inflammatory Cells and No Organisms

Possibilities	Clinical Setting	Confirmation of Diagnosis	Treatment
Prior antibiotic treatment			
Viral pneumonia	Winter months influenza, may be mild or life-threatening	Serologic studies, virus culture, antigen detection	Rimantadine for influenza A, ribavirin for respiratory syncytial virus, oseltamavir or zanamivir for influenza A or B
Mycoplasma pneumoniae infection	Hacking, nonproductive cough	Cold agglutinins, serologic studies	Erythromycin or tetracycline
Legionella pneumophila infection	Chronic lung disease, hospital acquired, summer predominance	DFA of sputum, bronchial brush biopsy, or pleural fluid, culture, serologic studies	Erythromycin, with or without rifampin, or fluoroquinolone
Chlamydia psittaci infection	Exposure to birds (e.g., parrots, turkeys)	Serologic studies	Tetracycline
Chlamydia pneumoniae infection	Hacking cough, sinusitis	Serologic studies, antigen detection	Tetracycline or erythromycin
Q fever	Exposure to cattle, South Africa	Serologic studies	Tetracycline or chloramphenicol

DFA = direct immunofluorescence assay.

pertonic saline. The sicker the patient and the greater the likelihood of a penicillin-resistant pathogen, the more important it is to get an adequate sample of sputum for examination and culture. This can often be achieved by nasotracheal aspiration, which is done by placing the patient supine, hyperextending the neck, and passing a well-lubricated, clear, flexible plastic catheter from the nose to the posterior pharynx. During inspiration, the tube is then passed swiftly past the glottis into the trachea, suction is applied, and secretions are collected in a Lugen trap. The vigorous coughing stimulated by this procedure often produces an additional excellent expectorated specimen. (*Note:* Expectorated sputum and sputum obtained through nasotracheal aspiration cannot be cultured anaerobically because of universal contamination with oral flora.)

The Gram-stained specimen should be examined using an oil immersion lens. The presence of a predominant organism, particularly if found within white blood cells, suggests that this is the likely pathogen. In cases of aspiration of mouth flora, a mixture of oral streptococci, gram-positive rods, and gram-negative organisms is found. In some cases, there may be inflammatory cells and no organisms seen on Gram's stain. This finding suggests a number of possibilities, many of which are "nonbacterial" pneumonias (Table 99–5). The importance of obtaining a good-quality sputum specimen for examination and culture for patients with community-acquired pneumonia has been debated. A good-quality baseline sputum specimen is of value primarily in those patients who do not show an expected clinical response to therapy (see later discussion). Because these persons are not readily identifiable at presentation, a good baseline sample is routinely recommended.

Unless the diagnosis of acute bacterial pneumonia is clear, an acid-fast stain or fluorescent auramine-rhodamine stain of sputum for mycobacteria should be per-

formed. If legionellosis is suspected, immunofluorescence stains for *Legionella* can be used, although the yield on expectorated sputum is low. The demonstration of elastin fibers in a potassium hydroxide preparation of sputum establishes a diagnosis of necrotizing pneumonia (see Table 99–4). Of importance is that this test may be positive in the absence of radiographic evidence of cavitation. Blood cultures should be obtained and may be positive in 20% to 30% of patients with bacterial pneumonia.

Results of sputum cultures must be interpreted with caution, because pathogens causing pneumonia may fail to grow and sputum isolates may not be the pathogens responsible for infection. Careful screening of sputum specimens with Gram's stain increases the accuracy of culture results. A tuberculin skin test and at least two control skin tests (e.g., mumps, *Candida*, or *Trichophyton*) should be applied in all cases of pneumonia of uncertain etiology. If the tuberculin test is negative but tuberculosis remains a diagnostic possibility, the test should be repeated in 2 weeks. In severely ill patients, a negative tuberculin test may occur despite active pulmonary and/or disseminated tuberculosis.

Specific Pathogenic Organisms

VIRAL AGENTS

Viral infection is usually limited to the upper respiratory tract, and only a small proportion of infected adults develop pneumonia. In children, viruses are the most common cause of pneumonia and respiratory syncytial virus is the most frequent organism. In adults, viruses are estimated to account for fewer than 10% of pneumonias, and the influenza virus is the most common organism. Patients at increased risk of influenzal pneumonia include the aged; patients with chronic disease of the heart, lung, or kidney; and women in the last trimester of pregnancy. Cytomegalovirus may cause severe pneumonia in immunosuppressed patients, especially in organ transplant recipients. When varicella occurs in adults, some 10% to 20% develop pneumonia, which commonly leaves a pattern of diffuse punctate calcification on chest radiograph. Measles is occasionally complicated by pneumonia. Cases of pneumonia and adult respiratory distress syndrome caused by hantavirus have been reported, primarily among persons residing in the southwestern United States. This severe, rapidly progressive, and often fatal infection occurs largely among otherwise healthy young adults who have been exposed to rodent droppings. Hemoconcentration caused by a generalized increase in capillary permeability appears to be the most critical pathophysiologic defect. Treatment is supportive. Although ribavirin has been used in the treatment of this infection, its value is unproven.

Other viral pneumonias, of which influenza is the prototype in adults, typically occur in community epidemics and usually develop 1 to 2 days after the onset of flulike symptoms. Major features include a dry cough, dyspnea, generalized discomfort, unremarkable physical examination, and an interstitial pattern on the chest radiograph. Influenza-induced necrosis of respiratory epithelial cells predisposes to bacterial colonization. This may result in superimposed bacterial pneumonia, most often caused by *Streptococcus pneumoniae* or *Staphylococcus aureus*. A presumptive diagnosis may be made on the basis of the clinical presentation and the epidemiologic setting. Gram's stain of sputum reveals inflammatory cells and rare bacteria. Detection of viral antigens in sputum can confirm the diagnosis rapidly. Viral isolation or serology also can establish the diagnosis but not in time to guide management decisions.

BACTERIAL AGENTS

Streptococcus pneumoniae

The pneumococcus is still the most common bacterial cause of pneumonia in the community. The organism colonizes the oropharynx in up to 25% of healthy adults. An increased predisposition to pneumococcal pneumonia is seen in persons with sickle cell disease, prior splenectomy, chronic lung disease, hematologic malignancy, alcoholism, HIV infection, and renal failure. Clinical features include fever, rigors, chills, cough, respiratory distress, signs of pulmonary consolidation, confusion, and herpes labialis. By the second or third day of illness, the chest radiograph typically shows lobar consolidation with air bronchograms, but a patchy bronchopneumonic pattern may also be found. Abscess or cavitation rarely occurs. Sterile pleural effusions occur in up to 25% of cases, and empyema occurs in 1%. Typically, a leukocytosis of 15,000 to 30,000 cells/μL with neutrophilia is found, but leukopenia may be observed with fulminant infection among alcoholics and persons with HIV infection. Demonstration of gram-positive diplococci on Gram's stain of sputum is helpful in the rapid diagnosis of pneumonia but may fail to show organisms in some cases of pneumococcal pneumonia. Positive blood cultures are found in 20% to 25% of patients. In most regions of the world, penicillin G remains the treatment of choice. In regions with higher frequency of penicillin-resistant pneumococci, cephalosporins or vancomycin may be indicated, depending on regional antibiotic sensitivity patterns.

Staphylococcus aureus

Staphylococcus aureus infection accounts for 2% to 5% of community-acquired pneumonias, 11% of hospital-acquired pneumonias, and up to 26% of pneumonias after a viral infection. Persistent nasal colonization is observed in 15% to 30% of adults, and 90% of adults display intermittent colonization. Presentation is similar to that of pneumococcal pneumonia, but contrasting features include the development of parenchymal necrosis and abscess formation in up to 25% of patients and empyema in 10%. A hematogenous source of infection, such as septic thrombophlebitis, infective endocarditis, or an infected intravascular device should be suspected in cases of staphylococcal pneumonia, particularly if the chest radiograph shows multiple or expanding nodular or wedge-shaped infiltrates. Early in staphylococcal pneumonia of hematogenous origin, sputum is rarely available. Blood cultures are usually positive, and associated skin lesions occur in 20% to 40%. When sputum is available, Gram's stain shows grapelike clusters of gram-positive cocci. *S. aureus* is recovered very easily from mixed culture samples, so that its absence in a purulent specimen usually excludes it as a cause of the pneumonia. Treatment requires a penicillinase-resistant agent, such as nafcillin or vancomycin. In hospital-acquired infections or in communities with endemic methicillin-resistant *S. aureus*, vancomycin should be used until sensitivity studies indicate that the isolate is sensitive to semisynthetic penicillins.

Streptococcus pyogenes

Streptococcus pyogenes is now an uncommon cause of pneumonia, probably accounting for less than 1% of all cases. Carriage rate in the pharynx (about 3% in adults) is less than with the other gram-positive cocci. Presentation is similar to that observed with *S. pneumoniae* and *S. aureus*, except that empyema, often massive, is found in 30% to 40% of cases, and the illness may show very rapid progression. Gram's stain shows gram-positive cocci in pairs or chains. Penicillin G is the treatment of choice. Some authorities recommend coadministration of clindamycin. Early decortication is indicated if empyema is present.

Haemophilus influenzae

Haemophilus influenzae is a gram-negative coccobacillus often present in the upper respiratory tract, particularly among patients with chronic obstructive pulmonary disease. Its isolation from sputum in these patients is to be expected. Confirmation of its role in the pathogenesis of pneumonia depends on isolating the organism in the blood, pleural fluid, or lung tissue. Nevertheless, many cases of pneumonia caused by this organism will not be confirmed using these rigid criteria, and in a patient with pneumonia the demonstration of gram-negative coccobacilli on Gram's stain of sputum should prompt institution of treatment with ampicillin plus a β-lactamase inhibitor or a second- or third-generation cephalosporin.

Gram-Negative Bacilli

Gram-negative bacilli have emerged as pathogens of major importance with the introduction of potent antibiotics and the proliferation of intensive care units. They are frequently encountered in patients with debilitating diseases such as chronic alcoholism, cystic fibrosis, neutropenia, diabetes mellitus, malignancy, and chronic diseases of the lungs, heart, or kidney. They are ubiquitous throughout the hospital, contaminating equipment and instruments, and are the major source of nosocomial pneumonia.

Specific organisms are associated with certain situations; for example, *Klebsiella pneumoniae* is particularly common in chronic alcoholics, *Escherichia coli* pneumonia is associated with bacteremias arising from the intestinal or urinary tract, and *Pseudomonas* species commonly infect the lungs of patients with cystic fibrosis. Precise etiologic diagnosis is confounded by the frequency with which these organisms colonize the upper airways in predisposed patients. Treatment in this situation generally includes the use of a penicillinase-resistant penicillin or a cephalosporin plus a fluoroquinolone or aminoglycoside.

OTHER CAUSES OF ACUTE PNEUMONIA

Mycoplasma pneumoniae

Not only is this a common cause of pneumonia in young adults, but it also produces a wide range of extrapulmonary features that may be the only findings. Fewer than 10% of infected patients develop symptoms of lower respiratory tract infection. Respiratory findings resemble those of viral pneumonia. Hacking, nonproductive cough is characteristic. Nonpulmonary features include myalgias, arthralgias, skin lesions (rashes, erythema nodosum and multiforme, Stevens-Johnson syndrome), and neurologic complications (meningitis, encephalitis, transverse myelitis, cranial nerve, or peripheral neuritis). The occurrence of acute, multifocal neurologic abnormalities may be helpful in distinguishing *Mycoplasma* pneumonia from that caused by *Chlamydia* or *Legionella*. The neurologic abnormalities characteristically resolve completely as the acute illness subsides.

In some patients, cold agglutinins may be seen at the bedside by observing red blood cell clumping on the walls of a glass tube containing anticoagulated blood incubated on ice for at least 10 minutes; they are also occasionally positive in other respiratory infections. Complement fixation antibody testing can suggest the diagnosis. Treatment for 2 to 3 weeks with tetracycline or erythromycin decreases the duration of symptoms and hastens radiographic resolution but does not eradicate the organism from the respiratory tract.

Chlamydia pneumoniae

Five percent to 15% of cases of community-acquired pneumonia may be caused by *Chlamydia pneumoniae* (formerly called the TWAR agent). Infection is spread, presumably through the respiratory route, from person to person; and onset of disease is generally subacute, often manifested by pharyngitis, sinusitis, bronchitis, and pneumonia. The radiographic appearance of pneumonia caused by *C. pneumoniae* resembles that of *Mycoplasma* infection. Illness is relatively mild and often prolonged. Diagnosis of this infection is difficult and requires cultivation of the organism in special cell lines or testing of acute and convalescent sera for antibody levels. Although the organism is sensitive to erythromycin and tetracyclines, treatment may have little effect on the course of disease.

Legionella Species

Legionella species are fastidious gram-negative bacilli that were responsible for respiratory infections long before the well-publicized outbreak of legionnaires' disease in 1976, which led to the recognition of this distinct disease entity and to the identification of the responsible bacillus. (The high mortality rate from this outbreak of a hitherto unrecognized disease among participants at an American Legion Convention destroyed the reputation of one of Philadelphia's finest hotels.) These organisms are distributed widely in water, and outbreaks have been related to their presence in water towers, air conditioners, condensers, potable water, and even hospital showerheads. Infection may occur sporadically or in outbreaks. Although healthy subjects can be affected, there is an increased risk in patients with chronic diseases of the heart, lungs, or kidneys; malignancy; and impairment of cell-mediated immunity. After an incubation period of 2 to 10 days, the illness usually begins gradually with a dry cough, respiratory distress, fever, rigors, malaise, weakness, headache, confusion, and gastrointestinal disturbance. The chest radiograph shows alveolar shadowing that may have a lobar or patchy distribution, with or without pleural effusions. The diagnosis is suggested clinically by the combination of a rapidly progressive pneumonia, dry cough, and multiorgan involvement. Gram's stain of sputum shows neutrophils and no organisms.

Diagnosis can be made by four methods:

1. Indirect fluorescent antibody testing of serum is positive in 75% of patients, but up to 8 weeks is required for seroconversion.
2. Direct fluorescence antibody testing of respiratory secretions is technically demanding and has a

specificity of 95%. Sensitivity of this method is low when using expectorated sputum but greater in specimens obtained from bronchoscopy or transtracheal aspirate.

3. *Legionella* antigen can be detected in urine in up to 70% of cases but only for certain types.

4. The organism can be cultured on charcoal yeast extract medium, but up to 10 days is required for growth.

Macrolides, tetracyclines, or fluoroquinolones are effective therapy. Prompt treatment results in fourfold to fivefold reduction in mortality. Patients usually respond within 12 to 48 hours, and it is very unusual for fever, leukocytosis, and confusion to persist beyond 4 days of therapy. In severe cases, rifampin may be added to the treatment regimen.

COMMUNITY-ACQUIRED PNEUMONIA OF UNCERTAIN ETIOLOGY

There are instances in which, because of difficulty in obtaining adequate sputum specimens or lack of laboratory facilities, empirical treatment of acute community-acquired pneumonia may be necessary. In such instances, initial therapy with cefuroxime and erythromycin is reasonable.

TUBERCULOSIS

Approximately 25,000 new cases of tuberculosis occur in the United States each year, with a worldwide incidence of 7 to 10 million. The worldwide figures are now increasing dramatically because tuberculosis is the major communicable complication of the acquired immunodeficiency syndrome. In North America, a disproportionately high number of cases occur among the foreign born, racial and ethnic minorities, and the poor. *Mycobacterium tuberculosis* is transmitted by the respiratory route from an infected patient with cavitary pulmonary tuberculosis to a susceptible host not previously infected with the organism. Primary infection usually is manifested only by development of a positive tuberculin skin test. Occasionally, the patient develops sufficient symptoms of fever and nonproductive cough to visit a physician, and a chest radiograph is taken; patchy or lobular infiltrates are noted in the anterior segment of the upper lobes or in the middle or lower lobes, often with associated hilar adenopathy. Pleurisy with effusion is a less common manifestation of primary tuberculosis. Primary infection usually is self-limited, but hematogenous dissemination seeds multiple organs, and latent foci are established and become niduses for delayed reactivation. Overall, 5% to 15% of infected individuals develop disease. Factors associated with progression to clinical disease are age (the periods of greatest biologic vulnerability to tuberculosis being infancy, childhood, adolescence, and old age); underlying diseases that depress the cellular immune response (see Chapter 109); diabetes mellitus, gastrectomy, silicosis, and sarcoidosis; and the interval since primary infection, with disease progression most likely in the first few years after infection.

Early progression of infection to disease is known as progressive primary tuberculosis and may manifest as miliary tuberculosis, sometimes with meningitis, or as pulmonary disease of the apical and posterior segments of the upper lobes or lower lobe disease.

Most commonly, tuberculosis represents delayed reactivation. Symptoms begin insidiously with night sweats or chills and fatigue; fever is noted by fewer than 50% of patients, and hemoptysis by fewer than 25%. Physical examination may be unremarkable or may show dullness and crackles in the upper lung fields, occasionally with amphoric breath sounds. The chest radiograph may show cavitary disease with infiltrates in the posterior segment of the upper lobes or apical segments of the lower lobes.

Extrapulmonary tuberculosis also reflects reactivation of latent foci and accounts for approximately 15% of cases. Miliary tuberculosis is discussed in Chapter 95, meningeal tuberculosis in Chapter 97, and tuberculosis of bones and joints in Chapter 104.

Because of the growing proportion of elderly individuals in our society and the growing prevalence of HIV infection, "atypical" presentations of tuberculosis are increasingly common. The elderly and patients with diabetes mellitus are more likely to have lower lobe tuberculosis. In HIV-infected patients, involvement of the lower lobes is frequent, extrapulmonary tuberculosis is almost as common as pulmonary involvement, and tuberculin skin tests are likely to be negative. The index of suspicion must be high in these settings.

Before starting antituberculosis drug treatment, two or three sputum samples should be obtained for cultures; bronchoscopy and bronchial washing are indicated only if sputum smears are negative for acid-fast bacilli. It is important to obtain baseline evaluation of liver function for individuals who are to receive potentially hepatotoxic drugs (isoniazid, rifampin, pyrazinamide); color vision, visual fields, and acuity when ethambutol will be used; and audiometry for patients who are to receive streptomycin.

The main principle of chemotherapy for tuberculosis is to avoid resistance by treating with at least two drugs to which the organism is likely to be sensitive. Pulmonary tuberculosis should be treated with daily isoniazid (5 mg/kg, up to 300 mg), rifampin (10 mg/kg, up to 600 mg), ethambutol (15 to 25 mg/kg, up to 2.5 g), and pyrazinamide (15 to 30 mg/kg, up to 2.0 g) for 2 months, followed by isoniazid and rifampin for 4 more months. A longer treatment duration (6 more months) is suggested for persons infected with HIV who have a slow response to treatment. Additional or alternative drugs are necessary if there is reason to believe that the patient is infected with multidrug-resistant isolates until drug sensitivities are known. At that point, the regimen can be tailored to include at least two drugs to which the organism is sensitive. One of these drugs must be bactericidal. Close monitoring during treatment is mandatory to maximize compliance and minimize side effects. Directly observed therapy using twice- or thrice-weekly treatment regimens is indicated for HIV-infected persons or persons who are not adherent to therapy.

Contact tracing is critical, because recent infection or additional cases of tuberculosis are likely in some household contacts. Preventive therapy with isoniazid is discussed later.

Treatment and Outcome

BACTERIAL PNEUMONIA

As soon as the causative organism is identified on Gram's stain, antibiotics must be administered without delay. If the pathogen is readily identified, the antibiotic choices are straightforward (Table 99–6). Patients with *Mycoplasma* and viral pneumonia can generally be treated on an ambulatory basis. An occasional young patient with no underlying disease can also be managed at home, provided that the patient is reliably attended by friends or family and has ready access to a physician or hospital. Otherwise, patients with bacterial pneumonia should be hospitalized.

Supplemental oxygen should be provided if the patient is tachypneic or hypoxemic. Patients at risk for the development of respiratory failure should be monitored in a critical care setting. Patients who are not capable of adequately coughing up respiratory secretions should have frequent clapping and drainage; meticulous attention must be paid to suctioning of oral secretions. Patients with suspected pulmonary tuberculosis should be placed in isolation rooms with negative pressure, frequent air exchange, and germicidal lamps to prevent nosocomial transmission of infection.

Patients treated for pneumococcal pneumonia should begin to improve within 48 hours after institution of antibiotics; patients with pneumonia caused by gram-negative bacilli, staphylococci, *Pneumocystis carinii*, and oral anaerobes may remain ill for longer periods after initiation of treatment. Several possibilities should be considered among patients who fail to improve or whose condition deteriorates during treatment.

ENDOBRONCHIAL OBSTRUCTION

Physical examination may fail to show sounds of consolidation, and radiographs may show evidence of lobar collapse. Bronchoscopy can establish the diagnosis.

UNDRAINED EMPYEMA

Radiographs may not always distinguish between fluid and consolidation; ultrasonography and computed tomography can identify the fluid and provide direction for its drainage.

PURULENT PERICARDITIS

Purulent pericarditis should be suspected in a very ill patient with pneumonia involving a lobe adjacent to the pericardium. Chest pain, pulsus paradoxus, and electrocardiographic evidence of pericarditis are helpful when present but do not occur in all cases. Likewise, distended neck veins and pericardial friction rubs are present in only a minority of cases. Echocardiography or chest ultrasonography shows fluid in the pericardium. If purulent pericarditis is suggested, emergency pericardiocentesis can be lifesaving (see Chapter 11).

INCORRECT DIAGNOSIS OR TREATMENT

In cases in which clinical response is poor, the patient's hospital course and admission sputum stains should be reviewed by a clinician with expertise in the diagnosis and treatment of pneumonia. Pulmonary embolism with infarction, a treatable disease, can prove fatal if misdiagnosed as bacterial pneumonia. Misinterpretation of sputum Gram-stained preparations with either failure to recognize an important pathogen or a treatment decision based on examination of an inadequate specimen is an avoidable pitfall of medical practice. Bronchoscopy should be considered, both to obtain better specimens

TABLE 99–6 Initial Antibiotics for Treatment of Pneumonia

Pathogen	Treatment
Streptococcus pneumoniae	Ceftriaxone, 2 g IV*
Mycoplasma pneumoniae	Erythromycin, 500 mg PO qid
Chlamydia pneumoniae	Erythromycin, 500 mg PO qid
Haemophilus influenzae	Ampicillin/sulbactam, 500 mg q8h IV, or cefuroxime, 1 g q8h IV
Staphylococcus aureus	Nafcillin, 3 g IV q6h, or vancomycin, 1 g IV q12h
Legionella pneumophila	Erythromycin, 750 mg q6h, or fluoroquinolone (e.g., levofloxacin, 500 mg/day) or doxycycline, 100 mg bid
Ehrlichia chaffeensis	Doxycycline, 100 mg bid
Mixed oral flora (anaerobes)	Ampicillin/sulbactam, 500 mg q8h, or clindamycin, 600 mg IV q8h
Gram-negative rods	Fluoroquinolone (e.g., ciprofloxacin, 500 mg/day) or aminoglycoside (e.g., gentamicin, 7 mg/kg IV q24h) plus third-generation cephalosporin (e.g., ceftazidime, 6 g/day)†
Tuberculosis	Isoniazid, 300 mg/day, plus rifampin, 600 mg/day, ethambutol, 15–25 mg/kg/day, and pyrazinamide, 1500 mg/day

* Levofloxacin, 500 mg q24h for penicillin-allergic patients. Vancomycin, 1 g IV q12h for penicillin-resistant isolates.
† Antibiotics can be adjusted when sensitivity data are available.
IV = Intravenously; PO = orally.

TABLE 99-7 Prevention of Pneumonia: Candidates for Pneumococcal and Influenza Vaccines

Factor	Pneumococcal Vaccine (may be repeated after 5–7 yr)	Influenza Vaccine (Yearly)
Patient ≥ 65 years	Yes	Yes
Chronic lung or heart disease	Yes	Yes
Sickle cell disease	Yes	Consider
Asplenic patients	Yes	No
Hodgkin's disease	Yes	Consider
Multiple myeloma	Yes	Consider
Cirrhosis	Yes	Consider
Chronic alcoholism	Yes	Consider
Chronic renal failure	Yes	Consider
Cerebrospinal fluid leaks	Yes	No
Residents of chronic care facilities	Consider	Yes
Diabetes mellitus	Yes	Yes
Human immunodeficiency virus infection	Yes	Consider
Children receiving long-term aspirin therapy	No	Yes
Pregnant women in the second or third trimester during influenza season	No	Yes
Health care workers	No	Yes

for diagnosis and to exclude underlying endobronchial obstruction.

THE PATIENT WITH PLEURAL EFFUSION AND FEVER

The approach to such patients is quite straightforward: the fluid must be examined. If a bacterium other than *S. pneumoniae* is seen on Gram's stain of pleural fluid or grown in culture, chest tube drainage is required. A pleural effusion infected with pneumococcus can often be treated with simple needle aspiration and antibiotics. Among patients with pneumonia, fluids that do not show organisms on Gram's stain but are grossly purulent or have a pH of less than 7 and/or a glucose concentration below 40 mg/dL may require chest tube drainage for satisfactory resolution. Patients with empyema complicating an aggressive bacterial pneumonia such as that caused by group A streptococci may benefit from early surgical debridement of the pleural space (decortication).

Pleurisy caused by *M. tuberculosis* is often an acute illness. In most cases, pneumonia is not present or readily appreciated. Inflammatory cells—polymorphonuclear leukocytes, mononuclear leukocytes, or both—are present in the pleural fluid. Mesothelial cells are usually sparse (<0.5% of the total cell count). Pleural fluid glucose levels are often low but may be normal. Mycobacteria are rarely seen on stains of pleural fluid. As many as one third of patients do not have positive tuberculin skin tests. Other causes of pleural effusion in this setting may be pulmonary infarction (fewer than half of patients produce a hemorrhagic exudate), malignancy (most do not have fever), and connective tissue diseases such as systemic lupus erythematosus and rheumatoid arthritis. If the cause of the effusion is not evident, a biopsy of the pleura is needed.

Prevention

Pneumococcal pneumonia may be preventable by immunizing patients at high risk with polyvalent pneumococcal polysaccharide vaccine. The current polyvalent

TABLE 99-8 Indications for Prophylaxis with Isoniazid

Documented new skin test conversion to tuberculin over past 2 yr
Tuberculin-positive contacts of patients with active TB
Tuberculin-negative contacts of patients with active TB*
Tuberculin-positive persons with HIV infection
Anergic HIV-infected patients at high risk for TB
Positive tuberculin skin test of unknown duration in patients younger than 35 years of age
Patients with radiographic evidence of inactive TB who have never received an adequate course of antituberculosis drugs
Consider isoniazid prophylaxis for patients with positive tuberculin skin tests and gastrectomy, diabetes mellitus, organ transplantation, silicosis, and prolonged (>1 mo) administration of corticosteroids or immunosuppressive drugs

* These individuals should have repeat skin tests 3 mo after isoniazid is begun. If the repeat test is negative, isoniazid may be discontinued.
HIV = human immunodeficiency virus; TB = tuberculosis.

vaccine is 60% to 80% effective in individuals with normal immune responses. Yearly immunization with influenza vaccine is also advised for many of these patients; by decreasing the attack rate of influenza, immunization also decreases morbidity and mortality resulting from secondary bacterial pneumonia (Table 99–7).

Patients without active tuberculosis but with skin test reactivity to purified protein derivative are at risk for reactivating their infection. The development of active tuberculosis can be prevented in most instances by treatment for 6 to 12 months with isoniazid, 300 mg/day. Indications for prophylaxis are shown in Table 99–8.

REFERENCES

Bartlett JG, Breiman RF, Mandell LA, File TM: Community acquired pneumonia in adults: Guidelines for management. Clin Infect Dis 1998; 26:811–838.

Duma RJ: Pneumococcal pneumonia. *In* Goldman L, Bennett JC (eds): Cecil Textbook of Medicine, 21st ed. Philadelphia: WB Saunders, 2000, pp 1603–1609.

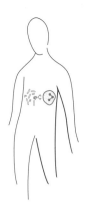

100

INFECTIONS OF THE HEART AND VESSELS

Michael M. Lederman

Infective Endocarditis

Infective endocarditis (IE) ranges from an indolent illness with few systemic manifestations, readily responsive to antibiotic therapy, to a fulminant septicemic disease with malignant destruction of heart valves and life-threatening systemic embolization. The varied features of endocarditis relate in large measure to the different infecting organisms. *Streptococcus viridans* is the prototype of bacteria that originate in the oral flora, infect previously abnormal heart valves, and may cause minimal symptoms despite progressive valvular damage. *Staphylococcus aureus*, in contrast, can invade previously normal valves and destroy them rapidly.

EPIDEMIOLOGY

The average age of patients with endocarditis has increased in the antibiotic era to the current median of 54 years. This change can be attributed to the decreasing prevalence of rheumatic heart disease, the increasing prevalence of underlying degenerative heart disease, and the increasing frequency of procedures and practices predisposing older patients to bacteremia (genitourinary instrumentation, intravenous catheters, hemodialysis shunts). Rheumatic heart disease is now a predisposing factor in fewer than 25% of patients with IE. About 15% of patients have congenital heart disease (exclusive of mitral valve prolapse). The propensity to develop endocarditis varies with the congenital lesion. For example, infection of a bicuspid aortic valve accounts for one fifth of cases of IE occurring in persons over the age of 60; a secundum atrial septal defect, however, rarely becomes infected. Mitral valve prolapse is associated with more than one third of cases of endocarditis of the mitral valve. Intravenous drug users have a unique propensity to develop IE of the tricuspid valve; infection of the mitral or aortic valve is less common. Patients with prosthetic heart valves have a 5% to 10% lifetime risk of IE.

PATHOGENESIS

Endocarditis ensues when bacteria entering the blood stream from an oral or other source lodge on heart valves that may already bear platelet-fibrin thrombi as a consequence of prior valvular damage or turbulent blood flow. The frequency of bacteremia is quite high after dental extraction (18% to 85%) or periodontal surgery (32% to 88%) but also is significant after everyday activities such as tooth brushing (0% to 26%) and chewing candy (17% to 51%). The ability of certain organisms to adhere to platelet-fibrin thrombi, such as for example through production of extracellular dextran by some streptococcal strains, promotes occurrence of endocarditis after bacteremia caused by these organisms. The localization of infection is partly determined by the production of turbulent flow, with left-sided infection more common than right-sided infection, except among intravenous drug users. Vegetations usually are found on the valve surface facing the lower pressure chamber (i.e., atrial surface of the mitral valve), a relative haven for deposition of bacteria from the swift blood stream. Occasionally, "jet lesions" develop in foci in which the regurgitant stream strikes the heart wall or the chordae tendineae. Once infection begins, bacteria proliferate freely within the interstices of the enlarging vegetation; in this relatively avascular site, they are protected from serum bactericidal factors and leukocytes.

The infection may cause rupture of the valve tissue itself or of its chordal structures, leading to either gradual or acute valvular regurgitation, with resultant congestive heart failure. Some virulent bacterial (e.g., *S. aureus*, *Haemophilus* species) or fungal vegetations may become large enough to obstruct the valve orifice or create a large embolus. Aneurysms of the sinus of Valsalva may occur and can rupture into the pericardial space. The conducting system may be affected by valve ring or myocardial abscesses. The infection may invade the interventricular septum, causing intramyocardial abscesses or septal rupture that can also damage the conduction system of the heart. Systemic septic emboli may occur with left-sided endocarditis, and septic pulmonary emboli may occur with right-sided endocarditis.

CLINICAL FEATURES

Some cases of endocarditis caused by oral streptococci become clinically manifest within 2 weeks of initiating events, such as dental extraction. However, diagnosis usually is delayed an additional 4 to 5 weeks or more because of the paucity of symptoms. If the causative organism is slow growing and produces an indolent syndrome, symptoms may be extremely protracted (6 months or longer) before definitive diagnosis. The symptoms and signs of IE relate to systemic infection, emboli (bland or septic), metastatic infective foci, congestive heart failure, or immune complex–associated lesions. The most common complaints in patients with IE are fever, chills, weakness, shortness of breath, night sweats, loss of appetite, and weight loss. Musculoskeletal symptoms develop in nearly one half of patients and may dominate the presentation. Fever is present in 90% of patients. Fever is more often absent in elderly or debilitated patients or in the setting of underlying congestive heart failure, liver or renal dysfunction, or previous antibiotic treatment. Heart murmurs are frequent (85%); changing murmurs (5% to 10%) and new cardiac murmurs, when observed, suggest the diagnosis of IE. With endocarditis involving the aortic or the mitral valve, congestive heart failure occurs in up to two thirds of patients; it may occur precipitously with perforation of a valve or rupture of chordae tendineae. At least one of the peripheral manifestations of endocarditis occurs in one half of patients (Table 100–1). Splenomegaly (25% to 60%) and clubbing (10% to 15%) are more likely when symptoms have been prolonged.

The clinical syndrome of IE differs in users of intravenous drugs. Tricuspid valve infection is most common; this may be related to scarring of the tricuspid valve by injected particulate matter. Patients most often present with fever and chills but may present with pleuritic chest pain caused by septic pulmonary emboli. Round, cavitating infiltrates may be found on the chest radiograph. The infective foci are initially centered in blood vessels; only after they erode into the bronchial system does cough develop, productive of bloody or purulent sputum.

Serious systemic emboli, associated with infection of the aortic or mitral valve, may cause dramatic findings, at times masking the systemic nature of IE. Embolism to the splenic artery may lead to left upper quadrant pain, sometimes radiating to the left shoulder, a friction rub, and/or left pleural effusion. Renal, coronary, and mesenteric arteries are frequent sites of clinically important emboli.

Central nervous system (CNS) embolization is one of the most serious complications of IE, because it often produces irreversible and disabling neurologic deficits. Infective endocarditis must always be considered in the differential diagnosis of stroke in young adults, as well as in all patients with valvular heart disease.

Overall, neurologic manifestations occur in one third of patients with IE. The diagnosis is easily missed when CNS signs and symptoms are the presenting features of IE, as occurs in approximately 10% of cases. Patients with IE may complain of headache or may develop seizures. The pathophysiologic explanation for these symptoms is not always apparent. In addition, stroke caused by vascular occlusion by an infected embolus, toxic encephalopathy, which may mimic psychosis, and meningoencephalitis also occur. The aseptic meningitis or meningoencephalitis seen in patients with IE is not readily distinguished from viral and other causes of a similar syndrome.

Clinical syndromes caused by CNS emboli may be more distinctive. The consequences of embolization depend on the site of lodging and the bacterial pathogen. Organisms such as S. viridans initially produce a syndrome entirely attributable to the vascular occlusion; however, damage to the blood vessel can result in formation of a mycotic aneurysm that may leak or burst at a later date. Resolution of aneurysms may occur after antimicrobial therapy. In many patients, however, surgical clipping is necessary to prevent recurrent hemorrhage. Single aneurysms in accessible areas should be considered for prompt surgical clipping. S. aureus, in contrast, produces progressive infection extending from the site of embolization; brain abscess and purulent meningitis are common sequelae.

The kidney can be the site of abscess formation, multiple infarcts, or immune complex glomerulonephritis. When renal dysfunction develops during antibiotic therapy, drug toxicity is an additional consideration.

TABLE 100–1   Peripheral Manifestations of Infective Endocarditis (IE)

Physical Finding (Frequency)	Pathogenesis	Most Common Organisms
Petechiae (20–40%) (red, nonblanching lesions in crops on conjunctivae, buccal mucosa, palate, extremities)	Vasculitis or emboli	*Streptococcus, Staphylococcus*
Splinter hemorrhages (15%) (linear, red-brown streaks most suggestive of IE when proximal in nail beds)	Vasculitis or emboli	*Staphylococcus, Streptococcus*
Osler's nodes (10–25%) (2- to 5-mm painful nodules on pads of fingers or toes)	Vasculitis	*Streptococcus*
Janeway's lesions (<10%) (macular, red or hemorrhagic, painless patches on palms or soles)	Emboli	*Staphylococcus*
Roth's spots (<5%) (oval, pale retinal lesions surrounded by hemorrhage)	Vasculitis	*Streptococcus*

TABLE 100-2 **Frequency of Infecting Microorganisms in Endocarditis**

Native Valve (%)		Prosthetic Valve Endocarditis			Endocarditis in IVDU (%)	
			Early	Late		
Streptococci	50	Coagulase-negative staphylococci	33	29	*S. aureus*	60
Enterococci	10	*S. aureus*	15	11	Streptococci	13
Staphylococcus aureus	20	Gram-negative bacilli	17	11	Gram-negative bacilli	8
HACEK	5	Fungi	13	5	Enterococci	7
Culture negative	5	Streptococci	9	36	Fungi	5
		Diphtheroids	9	3	Polymicrobial	5
					Culture negative	5

HACEK = *Haemophilus, Actinobacillus, Cardiobacterium, Eikenella, Kingella;* IVDU = intravenous drug user.
From Levison ME: Infective endocarditis. *In* Bennett JC, Plum F (eds): Cecil Textbook of Medicine, 20th ed. Philadelphia, WB Saunders, 1996, pp 1596–1605.

LABORATORY FINDINGS

Nonspecific laboratory abnormalities occur in IE and reflect chronic infection. These include anemia, reticulocytopenia, increased erythrocyte sedimentation rate, hypergammaglobulinemia, circulating immune complexes, false-positive serologic tests for syphilis, and rheumatoid factor. The presence of rheumatoid factor may be a helpful clue to diagnosis in patients with culture-negative endocarditis. Urinalysis frequently shows proteinuria (50% to 60%) and microscopic hematuria (30% to 50%). The presence of red blood cell casts is indicative of immune complex–mediated glomerulonephritis. The finding of gram-positive cocci in the urine of a febrile patient with microscopic hematuria should always prompt consideration of the possibility of infective endocarditis.

The bacteremia of IE is continuous and low grade (often 1 to 100 bacteria per milliliter in subacute cases). Thus, in most instances, all blood cultures are positive. With subacute IE, three sets of blood cultures should be obtained in the first 24 hours of hospitalization. However, with acute IE, blood cultures should be obtained more rapidly (over 60 to 90 minutes) and the patient should be placed on appropriate antibiotics as soon as possible. Two or three additional blood cultures are important if the patient has received antibiotic therapy in the preceding 1 to 2 weeks and if initial blood cultures are negative at 48 to 72 hours. Five percent to 10% of patients with the clinical diagnosis of IE may have negative blood cultures, usually because of previous antibiotic therapy.

Transesophageal echocardiography is a very useful technique for identifying vegetations in endocarditis. The great majority of patients with infective endocarditis have valvular vegetations demonstrable by transesophageal echocardiography. With such a high sensitivity, this study must be interpreted with care, particularly in persons with prosthetic heart valves, because nonspecific echoes may be incorrectly read as vegetations. Transesophageal echocardiography also provides improved visualization of valve ring abscesses and may be helpful in difficult determinations concerning the need for surgery. Magnetic resonance imaging of the heart similarly may demonstrate myocardial, septal, or valve ring abscesses.

DIFFERENTIAL DIAGNOSIS

The diagnosis of IE usually is firmly established on the basis of the clinical findings and the results of blood cultures. In some instances, the distinction between IE and nonendocarditis bacteremia may be difficult. Because the bacteremia is usually continuous in IE and intermittent in other bacteremias, the fraction of blood cultures that are positive may be helpful in distinguishing between these entities. The more frequent causative agents of infective endocarditis are shown in Table 100–2. In streptococcal infection, the speciation of the blood culture isolate may provide circumstantial evidence for or against infection of the heart valves (Table 100–3). The identity of the causative organism may be helpful for other bacteria as well; the ratio of IE to non-IE bacteremias is approximately 1:1 for *S. aureus,* 1:7 for group B streptococci, and 1:200 for *Escherichia coli.* *Streptococcus bovis* bacteremia and endocarditis are often (>50%) associated with colonic carcinomas or polyps. Isolation of this organism warrants thorough evaluation of the lower gastrointestinal tract.

The initial presentation of IE can be misleading: the young adult may present with a stroke, pneumonia, or meningitis; the elderly patient may present with confusion or simply with fatigue or malaise without fever. The index of suspicion for IE, therefore, must be high, and blood cultures should be obtained in these varied settings, particularly if antibiotic use is contemplated.

Major problems in diagnosis arise if antibiotics have

TABLE 100-3 **Relative Frequency of Infective Endocarditis (IE) and Non-IE Bacteremias for Various Streptococci**

Species	IE: Non-IE
Streptococcus mutans	14:1
Streptococcus bovis	6:1
Streptococcus faecalis	1:1
Group B streptococci	1:7
Group A streptococci	1:32

Modified from Parker MT, Ball LC: Streptococci and aerococci associated with systemic infection in man. J Med Microbiol 9:275, 1976.

been administered before blood is cultured or if blood cultures are negative. Attempts to culture slow-growing organisms, including those with particular nutritional requirements, should be done in consultation with a clinical microbiologist. The differential diagnosis of culture-negative endocarditis includes acute rheumatic fever, multiple pulmonary emboli, atrial myxoma, and nonbacterial thrombotic endocarditis. Nonbacterial thrombotic endocarditis (sometimes called marantic endocarditis) occurs in patients with severe wasting, whether caused by malignancy or other conditions. Also, patients with systemic lupus erythematosus may develop sterile valvular vegetations, termed *Libman-Sacks lesions*, on the undersurfaces of the valve leaflets. These diagnoses should be considered and excluded, if possible, before beginning a prolonged course of therapy for presumed culture-negative IE. As noted earlier, the absence of vegetations on transesophageal echocardiography makes a diagnosis of endocarditis unlikely.

MANAGEMENT AND OUTCOME

The outcome of endocarditis is determined by the extent of valvular destruction, the size and friability of vegetations, the presence and location of emboli, and the choice of antibiotics. These factors, in turn, are influenced by the nature of the causative organism and delays in diagnosis. The goal of antibiotic therapy is to halt further valvular damage and to cure the infection. Surgery may be necessary for hemodynamic stabilization, prevention of embolization, or control of drug-resistant infection.

Antibiotics should be selected on the basis of the clinical setting (Tables 100–4 and 100–5) and started as soon as blood cultures are obtained if the diagnosis of IE appears highly likely and the course is suggestive of active valvular destruction or systemic embolization. The antibiotics can be adjusted later on the basis of culture and sensitivity data.

Antibiotics

A number of different regimens have been advocated for the treatment of IE resulting from each of the causative organisms. Because few have been subjected to valid comparative trials, the selection of drugs, dosages, and duration is somewhat empirical. Similarly, although sophisticated laboratory tests such as serum bactericidal activity are used to monitor and adjust drug regimens, they have not been standardized or validated adequately. Nonetheless, each regimen must be capable of bactericidal activity against the offending pathogen and must be of sufficient duration, usually 4 to 6 weeks in left-sided endocarditis, to sterilize the affected heart valves.

Most strains of *S. viridans* and nonenterococcal group D streptococci, such as *S. bovis,* are exquisitely sensitive to penicillin. The penicillin concentration inhibiting growth of such organisms is less than 0.1 μg/mL, and they are killed by similar concentrations of penicillin. A variety of antibiotic regimens have been advocated to treat this form of IE, and several appear to

TABLE 100–4   Syndromes Suggesting Specific Bacteria Causing Infective Endocarditis

Indolent Course (Subacute)

Streptococcus viridans
Streptococcus bovis
Streptococcus faecalis
Fastidious gram-negative rods

Aggressive Course (Acute)

Staphylococcus aureus
Streptococcus pneumoniae
Streptococcus pyogenes
Neisseria gonorrhoeae

Drug Users

S. aureus
Pseudomonas aeruginosa
S. faecalis
Candida species
Bacillus species

Frequent Major Emboli

Haemophilus species
Bacteroides species
Candida species

be equally effective. Aqueous penicillin G, 12 million U/day given intravenously for 4 weeks, is curative in almost all patients, as is a 2-week course of penicillin G plus gentamicin in younger patients with uncomplicated disease. In the stable patient at low risk of complications, some of the antibiotic course can be administered on an outpatient basis.

Treatment of enterococcal endocarditis and IE caused by other penicillin-resistant streptococci is much less satisfactory because of frequent relapses and high mortality. The recommended regimen is intravenous aqueous penicillin G, 20 million U/day, plus intravenous gentamicin, 3 mg/kg/day. This relatively low dose of aminoglycoside is associated with a lower incidence of nephrotoxicity. The aminoglycoside dose should be adjusted according to measured serum levels and the bactericidal activity of serum. Streptomycin, 0.5 g administered intramuscularly every 12 hours, can be substituted as the aminoglycoside if the organism is sensitive; however, streptomycin may be associated with irreversible vestibular and auditory toxicity in some patients, particularly the elderly.

Although the value of serum bactericidal determinations has not been firmly established, most experts rely on them as a general guide to the adequacy of antibiotic regimens for enterococcal endocarditis. A drug regimen is considered adequate for treatment of IE if trough serum bactericidal activity is present at dilutions of 1:8 or greater. In view of the high frequency of relapses, regimens to treat enterococcal infection should be continued for 4 to 6 weeks. Culture-negative endocarditis should be treated similarly.

S. aureus endocarditis should be treated with intravenous nafcillin, 12 g/day, unless the isolate is penicillin-

TABLE 100-5   Treatment of Endocarditis*

Staphylococcus aureus	Nafcillin or cefazolin or vancomycin ± gentamicin
Streptococcus pneumoniae	PCN G/ampicillin + gentamicin
Streptococcus viridans, Streptococcus bovis	PCN G/ampicillin ± gentamicin
Enterococcus	PCN G/ampicillin + gentamicin
HACEK organisms	Ampicillin + gentamicin or ceftriaxone
Fungal	Amphotericin B + surgery
Pseudomonas	Antipseudomonal penicillin (e.g., ticarcillin) + tobramycin

* See text for details. Always individualize treatment based on sensitivity results.
PCN G = penicillin G; HACEK = *Haemophilus, Actinobaccilus, Cardiobacterium, Eikenella, Kingella.*

sensitive, in which case penicillin, 12 million U/day, is the treatment of choice. Infection with a methicillin-resistant species of *Staphylococcus* necessitates the use of vancomycin. The addition of an aminoglycoside hastens clearance of bacteremia and is indicated. Once sepsis is controlled, the aminoglycoside should be discontinued. The duration of antibiotic therapy for staphylococcal endocarditis of the mitral or aortic valve is a minimum of 6 weeks.

In the patient with streptococcal or staphylococcal IE and a history of serious penicillin allergy, vancomycin can be substituted for penicillin. Among patients at risk for complicated disease, consideration should be given to penicillin desensitization.

Pseudomonas endocarditis is a particular problem in intravenous drug users. Therapy should be initiated with tobramycin, 8 mg/kg/day given intravenously, plus either an extended-spectrum penicillin such as ticarcillin, 3 g, given intravenously every 4 hours. The unusually high doses of aminoglycosides have improved the outcome of medical therapy of *Pseudomonas* infection of the tricuspid valve with surprisingly little nephrotoxicity. Left-sided *Pseudomonas aeruginosa* infections, however, most often requires surgery for cure. It is particularly critical to measure serum drug levels and adjust dosages as appropriate when aminoglycosides are used. Quinolones may be of value in combined antibiotic treatment of *Pseudomonas* endocarditis, but experience with these agents is largely anecdotal.

Fungal endocarditis is refractory to antibiotics and requires surgery for management. Amphotericin B generally is administered to such patients but is not in itself curative.

Surgery

The indications for early surgery in IE need to be individualized and forged by discussions with the cardiac surgeon. Refractory infection is a clear indication for surgery; as noted, the requirement for surgery is predictable in IE caused by certain organisms. Persistence of bacteremia for longer than 7 to 10 days, despite the administration of appropriate antibiotics, frequently reflects paravalvular extension of infection with development of valve ring abscess or myocardial abscesses. Medical cure is not likely in this setting. Intravenous drug users are more likely to have IE caused by organisms refractory to medical therapy (e.g., *Pseudomonas*

species, fungi). Refractory tricuspid endocarditis may be amenable to valve debridement or excision without immediate placement of a prosthetic valve. Valvulectomy may, however, be associated with the eventual onset of right-sided congestive heart failure.

Protracted fever is not unusual in patients undergoing treatment of endocarditis and should not automatically be equated with refractory infection. In fact, 10% of patients remain febrile for more than 2 weeks, and persistent fever is not an independent indication for surgery, particularly when tricuspid endocarditis is complicated by multiple septic pulmonary emboli with necrotizing pneumonia. Delayed defervescence also is common, despite appropriate antimicrobial therapy, with endocarditis caused by *S. aureus* and enteric bacteria.

Congestive heart failure refractory to medical therapy is the most frequent indication for early cardiac surgery. The extent of valvular dysfunction may be difficult to gauge clinically, particularly in patients with acute aortic regurgitation; in the absence of compensatory ventricular dilatation, classic physical signs associated with aortic regurgitation, such as wide pulse pressure, may not be present. Echocardiography, fluoroscopy, and cardiac catheterization may be necessary to evaluate the extent of aortic regurgitation in some instances. However, when congestive heart failure develops in the patient with *S. aureus* IE, aortic valvular destruction usually is extensive, necessitating early surgery. Delaying surgery to prolong the course of antibiotic therapy is never appropriate if the patient is hemodynamically unstable or fulfills other criteria for surgical intervention. Prosthetic valve endocarditis (PVE) seldom occurs after cardiac valve replacement for IE, and its incidence is not influenced by duration of preoperative antibiotics.

Recurrent major systemic embolization is another indication for surgery. If valvular function is preserved, vegetations sometimes can be removed without valve replacement. Septal abscess, although often difficult to recognize clinically, and aneurysms of the sinus of Valsalva are absolute indications for surgery.

Prosthetic Valve Endocarditis

Prosthetic valve endocarditis complicates approximately 3% of cardiac valve replacements. Two separate clinical syndromes have been identified. Early PVE occurs within 60 days of surgery and most often is caused by *Staphylococcus epidermidis*, gram-negative enteric bacilli, *S. aureus,* or diphtheroids. The prosthesis may be contaminated at the time of surgery or seeded by bacteremia from extracardiac sites (intravenous cannula, indwelling urinary bladder catheter, wound infection, pneumonia). In addition to forming vegetations, which may be quite bulky and cause obstruction, particularly of mitral valve prostheses, circumferential spread of infection often causes dehiscence and paravalvular leak at the site of an aortic prosthesis. The combination of intravenous vancomycin, 2 g/day, and intravenous tobramycin, 3 to 5 mg/kg/day, plus oral rifampin, 600 mg/day, is indicated to treat *S. epidermidis* infection. Other infections should be treated with synergistic bactericidal combinations of antibiotics based on in vitro sensitivity testing. Surgery is mandatory in the presence of moderate to severe congestive heart failure. The rate of mortality from early PVE remains high.

Late PVE is most frequently caused by *S. viridans* bacteremia from an oral site that seeds a re-endothelialized valve surface. Treatment with intravenous aqueous penicillin G, 12 to 20 million U/day, plus intravenous tobramycin, 3 to 5 mg/kg/day, is appropriate. The prognosis for cure with antibiotic therapy alone is better in patients infected with penicillin-sensitive streptococci. Moderate to severe congestive heart failure is the main indication for surgery. The rate of mortality from late PVE is approximately 40%.

Prophylaxis of Infective Endocarditis

Patients with prosthetic heart valves or mitral or aortic valvular heart disease are at relatively high risk of developing IE. Mitral valve prolapse associated with a systolic murmur is another risk factor. Neither the value of antibiotic prophylaxis nor the optimal regimens have been definitively established. Patients who are at risk for endocarditis are presented in Table 100–6. Procedures for which prophylaxis is given are listed in Table 100–7, and appropriate prophylactic antibiotic regimens are presented in Tables 100–8 and 100–9.

Administration of antibiotics has become an accepted practice for patients undergoing open heart surgery, including valve replacement. Intravenous cefazolin, 2.0 g at induction of anesthesia, repeated 8 and 16 hours later, or intravenous vancomycin, 1.0 g at induction and 0.5 g 8 and 16 hours later, is an appropriate regimen. Cardiac diagnostic procedures (catheterization), pacemaker placement, and coronary artery bypass do not pose sufficient risk to warrant the use of prophylactic antibiotics for IE or PVE.

Devices that are associated with high rates of infection and bacteremia (intravenous cannulas, indwelling urinary bladder catheters) should be avoided in hospitalized patients at risk for IE if at all possible; established local infections should be treated promptly and vigorously.

TABLE 100–6   Prophylaxis of Infective Endocarditis

Prophylaxis for Specific Procedures Recommended
High-Risk Category
Prosthetic heart valves
Prior endocarditis
Complex cyanotic congenital heart disease
Surgical systemic pulmonary shunts
Moderate-Risk Category
Most other congenital cardiac malformations
Acquired valvular dysfunction (e.g., rheumatic heart disease)
Hypertrophic cardiomyopathy
Mitral valve prolapse with regurgitation or thickened leaflets
Prophylaxis *Not* Recommended
Mitral valve prolapse without murmur and without regurgitant or myxomatous leaflets on echocardiogram
Physiologic murmurs
Isolated secundum atrial septal defect
Surgically repaired atrial septal defect, ventricular septal defect, patent ductus arteriosus (after 6 months)
Cardiac pacemakers and defibrillators
History of rheumatic fever or Kawasaki's disease without valvular dysfunction
Previous coronary artery bypass surgery

TABLE 100–7   Procedures That Require Antimicrobial Prophylaxis Against Infective Endocarditis

Dental Procedures Involving Significant Bleeding from Hard or Soft Tissues
Extractions
Periodontal procedures
Implant placement
Endodontic (root canal) procedures
Subgingival placement of orthodontic bands but not brackets
Intraligamentary local anesthetic injections
Prophylactic cleaning of teeth or implants where bleeding is expected
Respiratory Tract Procedures
Tonsillectomy/adenoidectomy
Surgical procedures that involve respiratory mucosa
Rigid bronchoscopy
Gastrointestinal Tract Procedures
Sclerotherapy for varices
Dilatation of esophageal stricture
Endoscopic retrograde cholangiopancreatography with biliary obstruction
Biliary tract surgery
Surgery involving gastrointestinal mucosa
Genitourinary Tract Procedures
Prostatic surgery
Cytoscopy
Urethral dilatation

TABLE 100–8 Prophylactic Regimens Recommended for Dental, Oral, Respiratory Tract, or Esophageal Procedures in Susceptible Patients

Amoxicillin, 2.0 g 1 hour before the procedure
Allergic to penicillin: clindamycin, 600 mg 1 hour before the procedure, or cephalexin, 2.0 g 1 hour before the procedure

Bacterial Endarteritis and Suppurative Phlebitis

Bacterial endarteritis usually develops by one of three mechanisms. (1) Arteries, particularly those with intimal abnormalities, may become infected as a consequence of transient bacteremia. (2) During the course of IE, septic emboli to vasa vasorum may lead to mycotic aneurysms. (3) Blood vessels also may be infected by direct extension from contiguous foci and trauma.

A septic presentation is characteristic of endarteritis caused by organisms such as *S. aureus*. Besides sepsis, the major problem caused by endarteritis is hemorrhage. Three to 4 percent of patients with IE develop intracranial mycotic aneurysms. Mycotic aneurysms in

TABLE 100–9 Prophylactic Regimens for Genitourinary or Gastrointestinal (Excluding Esophageal) Procedures

High-risk patients: ampicillin, 2.0 g IM/IV, plus gentamicin, 1.5 mg/kg (not to exceed 120 mg) IM/IV within 30 minutes of starting the procedure; 6 hours later: ampicillin, 1 g IM/IV, or amoxicillin, 1 g PO
High-risk patients allergic to penicillin: vancomycin, 1.0 g IV over 1 to 2 hours, plus gentamicin, 1.5 mg/kg (not to exceed 120 mg) IM/IV within 30 minutes of starting the procedure
Moderate-risk patients: amoxicillin, 2 g orally 1 hour before the procedure, or ampicillin, 2 g IM/IV within 30 minutes of starting the procedure
Moderate-risk patients allergic to penicillin: vancomycin, 1 g IV over 1 to 2 hours within 30 minutes of starting the procedure

IE typically are situated peripherally and in the distribution of the middle cerebral artery. Focal seizures, focal neurologic signs, or aseptic meningitis may herald catastrophic rupture of such aneurysms. These premonitory findings, therefore, indicate the need for evaluation with arteriography; neurosurgical intervention should be contemplated if accessible lesions are demonstrated. Infection of an atherosclerotic plaque can occur as a complication of bacteremia, particularly in elderly patients with bacteremia caused by *Salmonella* species. Traumatic endarteritis with pseudoaneurysm often complicates arterial injection of illicit drugs and rarely complicates arterial catheterizations. Treatment often requires combined medical and surgical management; antibiotic selection should be based on the results of in vitro sensitivity testing.

Suppurative thrombophlebitis usually is a complication of the use of intravenous plastic cannulas. Burn patients, especially those with lower extremity catheterization, are at particular risk. Typically, intravenous cannulas have been left in place 5 days or more. Often, the vein is sclerosed and tender, and the surrounding skin is erythematous. The vein should be milked to identify pus. If pus is present or if bacteremia and fever persist despite antibiotic therapy, involved segments of vein must be excised. Antibiotics should be selected to ensure coverage of the most common pathogens, *Staphylococcus* species (vancomycin, 2 g/day IV) and Enterobacteriaceae (gentamicin, 5 mg/kg/day IV). When infection of an intravenous cannula is suggested, the catheter should be removed and 2-inch segments rolled across a blood agar plate. The growth of more than 15 colonies suggests infection (see also Chapter 106).

Suppurative phlebitis is preventable. Peripheral intravenous cannulas should be inserted aseptically and replaced at least every 72 hours by well-trained personnel.

REFERENCES

Bayer AS, Bolger AF, Taubert KA, et al: Diagnosis and management of infective endocarditis and its complications. Circulation 1998; 98: 2936–2948.

Dajani AS, Taubert KA, Wilson W, et al: Prevention of bacterial endocarditis: Recommendations by the American Heart Association. JAMA 1997; 277:1794–1801.

Lederman MM, Sprague L, Wallis RS, Ellner JJ: Duration of fever during infective endocarditis. Medicine 1992; 71:52.

Levison ME: Infective endocarditis. *In* Goldman L, Bennett JC (eds): Cecil Textbook of Medicine, 21st ed. Philadelphia: WB Saunders, 2000, pp 1631–1640.

101

SKIN AND SOFT TISSUE INFECTIONS

Michael M. Lederman

Normal skin is remarkably resistant to infection. Most common infections of the skin are initiated by breaks in the epithelium. Hematogenous seeding of the skin by pathogens is less frequent.

Some superficial infections, such as folliculitis and furuncles, may be treated with local measures. Other superficial infections (e.g., impetigo and cellulitis) necessitate systemic antibiotics. Deeper soft tissue infections, such as fasciitis and myonecrosis, necessitate surgical debridement. As a general rule, infections of the face and hands should be treated particularly aggressively because of the risks of intracranial spread in the former and the potential loss of function as a result of closed-space infection in the latter.

Superficial Infections of the Skin

CIRCUMSCRIBED INFECTIONS OF THE SKIN

Vesicles, pustules, nodules, and ulcerations are the lesions in this category (Table 101–1).

Folliculitis is a superficial infection of hair follicles. The lesions are crops of red papules or pustules that are often pruritic; careful examination using a hand lens shows hair in the center of most papules. Staphylococci, yeast, and, occasionally, *Pseudomonas* species are the responsible pathogens. Local treatment with cleansing and hot compresses is usually sufficient. Topical antibacterial or antifungal agents also may be useful. The skin lesions of disseminated candidiasis seen in neutropenic patients may resemble folliculitis. In this setting, skin biopsy readily distinguishes these two processes; in disseminated disease, yeast is found within blood vessels and not simply surrounding the hair follicle.

Furuncles and carbuncles are subcutaneous abscesses caused by *Staphylococcus aureus*. The lesions are red, tender nodules that may have a surrounding cellulitis and occur most prominently on the face and back of the neck. They often drain spontaneously. Furuncles may be treated with local compresses. If fluctuant, the larger carbuncles necessitate incision and drainage. Antistaphylococcal antibiotics should be given if the patient has systemic symptoms, such as fever or malaise, if there is accompanying cellulitis, or if the lesions are on the head.

Impetigo is a superficial infection of the skin caused by group A streptococci, although *S. aureus* may also be found in the lesions. Impetigo is seen primarily among children, who initially develop a vesicle on the skin surface; this rapidly becomes pustular and breaks down, leaving the characteristic dry, golden crust. This pruritic lesion is highly contagious and spreads by the child's hands to other sites on the body or to other children. Gram's stain shows gram-positive cocci in chains (streptococci); occasionally, clusters of staphylococci are also seen. Certain strains of streptococci causing impetigo have been associated with the later development of poststreptococcal glomerulonephritis. The differential diagnosis of impetigo includes herpes simplex infection and varicella. These viral lesions may become pustular; Gram's stain of an unruptured viral vesicle or pustule should not, however, contain bacteria. A Tzanck preparation (see Chapter 93) (or assay for viral antigens for optimal sensitivity) can establish the diagnosis of herpes simplex or varicella if the differential diagnosis is uncertain. Penicillin is the treatment of choice for impetigo, because staphylococci represent secondary infection and will disappear when the streptococci are eradicated. Antibiotics do not appear to affect the development of poststreptococcal glomerulonephritis but will prevent the spread of infection to others. Large bullous lesions, particularly in children, suggest bullous impetigo caused by *S. aureus*. This should be treated with penicillinase-resistant penicillins such as dicloxacillin or erythromycin for the penicillin-allergic patient.

Ecthyma gangrenosum is a cutaneous manifestation of disseminated gram-negative rod infection, usually caused by *Pseudomonas aeruginosa* in neutropenic patients. The initial lesion is a vesicle or papule with an erythematous halo. Although generally small (<2 cm),

TABLE 101–1 Circumscribed Cutaneous Infections (Predominant Organism)

Folliculitis (*Staphylococcus aureus*, *Candida* species)
Furuncles, carbuncles (*Staphylococcus aureus*)
Impetigo (group A streptococci, *Staphylococcus aureus*)
Ecthyma gangrenosum (gram-negative bacilli [systemic infection])
Vesicular or vesiculopustular lesions of the skin
  Impetigo
  Folliculitis
  Herpes simplex virus infection
  Varicella-zoster virus infection
  Rickettsialpox
Ulcerative lesions of the skin
  Pressure sores
  Stasis ulcerations
  Diabetic ulcerations
  Sickle cell ulcers
  Mycobacterial infection
  Fungal infection
  Ecthyma gangrenosum
  Syphilis
  Chancroid

the initial lesion may exceed 20 cm in diameter. In a short time, the vesicle ulcerates, leaving a necrotic ulcer with surrounding erythema or a violaceous rim. Gram's stain of an aspirate may show gram-negative rods; cultures of the aspirate are generally positive. Biopsy of the lesion shows venous thrombosis, often with bacteria demonstrable within the blood vessel walls. Because these lesions are manifestations of gram-negative rod bacteremia, treatment should be instituted immediately with an aminoglycoside plus a third-generation cephalosporin with good activity against *P. aeruginosa* (e.g., ceftazidime) until the results of culture and sensitivity studies are known (see also Chapter 96).

Herpes Simplex Virus

Oral infections caused by this virus are discussed in Chapter 98, and genital infections are discussed in Chapter 107. On occasion, infection with this virus occurs on extraoral or extragenital sites, usually on the hands. This is most often the case in health care workers but also may result from sexual contact or from autoinoculation. The virus may produce a painful erythema, usually at the junction of the nail bed and skin (whitlow). This progresses to a vesiculopustular lesion. At both stages of infection, herpetic whitlow can resemble a bacterial infection (paronychia). When more than one digit is involved, herpes is much more likely. It is important to distinguish between herpetic and bacterial infections, because incision and drainage of a herpetic whitlow are contraindicated. Puncture of the purulent center of a paronychia and Gram's stain of the exudate allow prompt and accurate diagnosis. In the case of herpetic whitlow, bacteria are not present unless the lesion has already drained and become superinfected. In the case of a bacterial paronychia, bacteria are readily

seen. Recurrences of herpetic whitlow may be seen but are generally less severe than the primary infection. Treatment with oral acyclovir may shorten the duration of symptoms.

Varicella-Zoster Virus

Primary infection with varicella-zoster virus (chickenpox) is thought to occur through the respiratory route but may also occur through contact with infected skin lesions. Viremia results in crops of papules that progress to vesicles and then to pustules, followed by crusting. The lesions are most prominent on the trunk. This is almost always a disease of childhood. Systemic symptoms may precede development of the characteristic rash by 1 or 2 days but are mild except in the case of an immunocompromised patient or primary infection in the adult. In the immunocompromised patient, chickenpox can produce a fatal systemic illness. In otherwise healthy adults, chickenpox can be a serious illness with life-threatening pneumonia. Clinical diagnosis is based on the characteristic appearance of the rash. Impetigo and folliculitis are readily distinguished clinically by Gram's stain or Tzanck's preparation of the pustule contents. Disseminated herpes simplex virus infection is seen only in the immunocompromised host or in patients with eczema. Viral culture or viral antigen detection will distinguish herpes simplex from herpes zoster in these settings. Most patients with rickettsialpox, which in rare cases is confused with chickenpox, also have an ulcer or eschar that precedes the generalized rash by 3 to 7 days and represents the bite of the infected mouse mite, which transmits the disease.

Immunocompromised children exposed to varicella should receive prophylaxis with zoster immune globulin. Immunocompromised persons and seriously ill patients with varicella should be treated with acyclovir.

After primary infection, the varicella-zoster virus persists in a latent state within sensory neurons of the dorsal root ganglia. The infection may reactivate, producing the syndrome of zoster (shingles). Pain in the distribution of the affected nerve root precedes the rash by a few days. Depending on the dermatome, the pain may mimic pleurisy, myocardial infarction, or gallbladder disease. A clue to the presence of early zoster infection is the finding of dysesthesia, an unpleasant sensation when the involved dermatome is gently stroked by the examiner's hand. The appearance of papules and vesicles in a dermatomal distribution confirms the diagnosis. Herpes zoster infections of certain dermatomes merit special attention. The Ramsay Hunt syndrome can be caused by infection involving the geniculate ganglia and presents with painful eruption of the ear canal and tympanic membrane, often associated with an ipsilateral seventh cranial nerve (facial nerve) palsy. Infection involving the second branch of the fifth cranial nerve (trigeminal nerve) often produces lesions of the cornea. This infection should be treated promptly with systemic acyclovir to prevent loss of visual acuity. A clue to possible ophthalmic involvement is the presence of vesicles on the tip of the nose (see Chapter 114).

In most instances, dermatomal zoster is a disease of the otherwise healthy adult. However, immunocompromised patients (e.g., persons with human immunodeficiency virus infection) are at greater risk for reactivation of this virus. Patients with zoster should receive a careful history and physical evaluation; in the absence of specific suggestive findings or recurrent episodes of zoster, these patients do not require an exhaustive evaluation for a malignancy or immunodeficiency.

In older, nonimmunocompromised patients, postherpetic neuralgia (severe, prolonged burning pain, with occasional lightning-like stabs in the involved dermatomes) may persist for 1 to 2 years and become disabling. A brief course of corticosteroids (40–60 mg of prednisone, tapered over 3 to 4 weeks) during the acute episode of zoster shortens the duration of acute neuritic pain but does not prevent postherpetic neuralgia. Initiation of treatment during the first 72 hours with antiviral drugs such as famciclovir or acyclovir accelerates the healing of lesions and also may decrease the occurrence of postherpetic neuralgia. The constant burning pain may be diminished by tricyclic antidepressants. When this fails, an anesthetic approach, with either subcutaneous local injection or sympathetic blockage, is sometimes helpful.

Cutaneous Mycobacterial and Fungal Diseases

Mycobacteria and fungi can produce cutaneous infection, manifesting generally as papules, nodules, ulcers, crusting lesions, or lesions with a combination of these features. *Mycobacterium marinum,* for example, can produce inflammatory nodules that ascend through lymphatic channels of the arm among individuals who keep or are exposed to fish; similar lesions caused by *Sporothrix schenckii* may be seen among gardeners. *Blastomyces dermatitidis* and *Coccidioides immitis* are other fungi that produce skin nodules or ulcerations.

As a general rule, a biopsy should be done on a chronic inflammatory nodule, crusted lesion, or nonhealing ulceration that is not readily attributable to pressure, vascular insufficiency, or venous stasis. Mycobacteria and fungi should be carefully sought, using acid-fast and silver stains and appropriate cultures.

Ulcerative Lesions of the Skin

A common factor in the pathogenesis of many skin ulcers is the presence of vascular insufficiency. Microbial infection of these lesions is secondary but often extends into soft tissue and bone.

Pressure sores occur at weight-bearing sites among individuals incapable of moving. Patients with strokes, quadriplegia, or paraplegia or patients in a coma who remain supine rapidly develop skin necrosis at the sacrum, spine, and heels, because pressures at these weight-bearing sites can exceed local perfusion pressure. Patients kept immobile on their sides will ulcerate over the greater trochanter of the femur. As the skin sloughs, bacteria colonize the necrotic tissues; abetted by further pressure-induced necrosis, the infection extends to deeper structures. Infected pressure sores are common causes of fever and occasional causes of bacteremia in debilitated patients. Not infrequently, a necrotic membrane hides a deep infection. The physician should probe the extent of a pressure sore with a sterile glove; potential sites of deeper infection should be probed with a sterile needle. Necrotic material must be debrided, and the ulceration may be treated with topical antiseptics and relief of pressure. Systemic antibiotics are indicated when bacteremia, osteomyelitis, or significant cellulitis is present. Anaerobes and gram-negative rods are the most frequent isolates. Skin grafting can be used to repair extensive ulceration in patients who can eventually be mobilized. Prevention of pressure sores by frequent turning and by inspection of pressure sites among immobilized patients is far more effective than treatment. The use of specialized beds that distribute pressure more evenly may be of particular value among these patients.

Stasis Ulceration

Patients with lower extremity edema are at risk for skin breakdown and formation of stasis ulcers. These may become secondarily infected but, unless cellulitis is present, systemic antibiotics are not necessary and treatment is aimed at reducing the edema.

Diabetic Ulcers

Patients with diabetes mellitus often develop foot ulcers. Peripheral neuropathy may result in the distribution of stress to sites on the foot not suited to weight bearing and may also result in failure to sense foreign objects stepped on or caught within the shoe. The resulting ulceration heals poorly. This may be related to vascular disease, poor metabolic control, or both. Secondary infection with anaerobes and gram-negative bacilli progresses rapidly to involve bone and soft tissue. Prevention of these events requires meticulous foot care, avoidance of walking barefoot, the use of properly fitting shoes, and checking the inside of the shoe before use. Once an ulcer develops, the physician should evaluate the patient promptly. Bed rest and topical antiseptics are always indicated. Systemic antibiotics active against anaerobes and gram-negative bacilli should be employed for all but the most superficial and clean wounds. In most instances, this treatment requires admission to the hospital. Aggressive management is indicated because, if the ulcer is left untreated or improperly treated, the proximate bones and soft tissues of the entire foot may become involved. Once this involvement occurs, eradication of infection without amputation may be difficult.

Other Ulcerative Lesions of the Skin

Ulcerative lesions of the skin, particularly in the genital region, may be caused by *Treponema pallidum,* the agent of syphilis, or by *Haemophilus ducreyi,* the agent of chancroid (see Chapter 107).

DIFFUSE LESIONS OF SKIN

Erysipelas

Erysipelas is an infection of the superficial layers of the skin (Table 101–2); it is almost always caused by group A streptococci. This infection, seen primarily among children and the elderly, most commonly occurs on the face. Erysipelas is a bright red to violaceous raised lesion with sharply demarcated edges. This sharp demarcation distinguishes erysipelas from the deeper tissue infection cellulitis, the margins of which are not raised and merge more smoothly with uninvolved areas of skin. Fever is generally present, but bacteremia is uncommon; in rare cases, the pathogen can be isolated by aspiration or biopsy of the leading edge of the erythema (clysis culture). Penicillin, 2 to 6 million U/day, is curative, but defervescence is gradual.

Cellulitis

Cellulitis is an infection of the deeper layers of the skin. Cellulitis has a particular predilection for the lower extremities, where venous stasis predisposes to infection. It predisposes to recurrent infection, perhaps by impairing lymphatic drainage. A breakdown in normal skin barriers almost always precedes this infection. Lacerations, small abscesses, or even tiny fissures between the toes caused by minor fungal infection antedate the onset of pain, swelling, and fever. Although shaking chills often occur, bacteremia is infrequently documented. Linear streaks of erythema and tenderness indicate lymphatic spread. Regional lymph node enlargement and tenderness are common. Patches of erythema and tenderness may occur a few centimeters proximal to the edge of infection; this is probably caused by spread through subcutaneous lymphatics. Cellulitis of the calf is often difficult to distinguish from thrombophlebitis. Rupture of a Baker cyst or inflammatory arthritis may also mimic cellulitis (Table 101–3). Pain within the joint on passive motion suggests arthritis, but after a Baker cyst rupture, examination of the joint may be relatively benign. Lymph node enlargement and lymphatic streaking virtually confirm the diagnosis of cellulitis. Most cases of lower extremity cellulitis are caused by group A

TABLE 101–2 Diffuse Cutaneous and Subcutaneous Bacterial Infections

Description	Predominant Organisms
Erysipelas	Group A streptococci
Cellulitis	Group A streptococci, *Staphylococcus aureus*, *Haemophilus influenzae*, *Clostridium perfringens*, other anaerobic organisms, gram-negative bacilli
Fasciitis	Group A streptococci, *Clostridium perfringens*, other anaerobic organisms, gram-negative bacilli
Myonecrosis	*Clostridium perfringens*, streptococci, mixed anaerobes, gram-negative bacilli

TABLE 101–3 Processes That May Resemble Cellulitis

Process	Diagnosis
Thrombophlebitis	Tender cord, no lymphangitis, ultrasound
Arthritis	Pain on passive joint movement, joint effusion, joint aspiration
Ruptured Baker's cyst	History of arthritis, joint effusion, arthrogram, MRI
Brown recluse spider bite	Exposure history
Fasciitis	MRI, surgical exploration
Myositis	Muscle tenderness, less prominent skin involvement, MRI, surgical exploration

MRI = magnetic resonance imaging.

β-hemolytic streptococci, but on occasion *S. aureus* is responsible. Gram-negative bacilli often cause cellulitis in neutropenic and other immunosuppressed patients. Cellulitis of the face or upper extremities, particularly among children, may be caused by *Haemophilus influenzae*. Among patients with diabetes mellitus, streptococci and staphylococci are the predominant pathogens of cellulitis. However, if the cellulitis is associated with an infected ulceration of the skin, there is a good chance that anaerobic bacteria and gram-negative rods are also involved.

Occupational exposures are often associated with painful cellulitis of the hands. Erysipeloid cellulitis (caused by *Erysipelothrix rhusiopathiae*) most often occurs in fish or meat handlers and responds to high doses of penicillin (12 to 20 million U/day). Freshwater exposures are associated with cellulitis caused by *Aeromonas* species, and saltwater exposures may result in aggressive cellulitis caused by *Vibrio* species; third-generation cephalosporins are usually effective in the treatment of these potentially lethal infections.

As in the case of erysipelas, cultures of blood and clysis cultures of the leading edge of infection rarely yield the pathogen. Patients with cellulitis who appear toxic or who have underlying diseases causing impaired immune response should be hospitalized. Cellulitis should be treated with a semisynthetic penicillin active against *S. aureus* such as nafcillin (or in regions where methicillin resistance among *S. aureus* is high, with vancomycin). If *Haemophilus* infection is suspected, ampicillin/sulbactam is usually effective. Diabetics with foot ulcers complicated by cellulitis should be treated with agents active against anaerobes and enteric gram-negative rods (e.g., ampicillin/sulbactam). Radiologic studies should be performed on patients with ulcers to determine if osteomyelitis is present (see Chapter 104). Prevention of cellulitis can be achieved by institution of measures aimed at reducing venous stasis and edema. Patients with recurrent cellulitis may benefit from eradication of fungal infection of toes or interdigital regions, if present. Repeated attacks of cellulitis may be prevented by monthly 1-week courses of an oral antibiotic such as erythromycin.

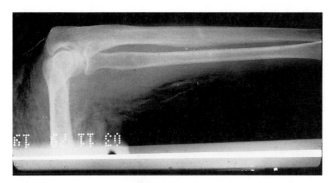

FIGURE 101–1 Radiograph of patient with clostridial myonecrosis shows gas within tissues. (Courtesy of Dr. J. W. Tomford.)

Soft Tissue Gas

Crepitus on palpation of the skin indicates the presence of gas in the soft tissues. Although this often reflects anaerobic bacterial metabolism, subcutaneous gas can also be found after ventilator-induced barotrauma or after application of hydrogen peroxide to open wounds.

In the setting of soft tissue infection, crepitus suggests the presence of gas-forming anaerobes that may include clostridia or facultative bacteria such as streptococci or gram-negative rods. Roentgenograms will occasionally demonstrate gas before crepitus is detected (Fig. 101–1). Magnetic resonance imaging is more sensitive than other techniques in detecting soft tissue gas. The presence of gas necessitates emergency surgery to determine the extent of necrosis and requirements for debridement. Involvement of the muscle establishes the diagnosis of myonecrosis (see later discussion) and mandates extensive debridement. Despite the often extensive crepitus seen in clostridial cellulitis, exploration shows the muscles to be uninvolved, and proper treatment is limited to debridement of necrotic tissue, open drainage, and antibiotics, usually penicillin G, 10 to 20 million U/day, and metronidazole, 500 mg every 6 hours. Thus, the principles of treatment for necrotizing soft tissue infections are (1) removal of necrotic tissue, (2) drainage, and (3) appropriate antibiotics. These apply to superficial necrotizing infections (clostridial cellulitis), deeper anaerobic infections (necrotizing fasciitis [see later discussion]), and deepest infections (necrotizing myonecrosis [see later discussion]).

Deeper Infections of the Skin and Soft Tissue

NECROTIZING FASCIITIS

Necrotizing fasciitis is a deep infection of the subcutaneous tissues that generally occurs after trauma (sometimes minor) or surgery. Most cases are caused by β-hemolytic streptococci with or without staphylococci; some, especially among diabetics, are caused by mixtures of anaerobic organisms and gram-negative ba-

cilli. Because fasciitis involves subcutaneous tissues, the skin may appear normal or may have a red or dusky hue. The clue to this diagnosis is pain and the presence of subcutaneous swelling, particularly in the absence of cellulitis. In some instances, crepitus is present. In time, skin necrosis and dark bullae may develop. The patient appears more toxic than one would expect from the superficial appearance of the skin. Radiographs may show gas within tissues; its absence does not exclude the diagnosis. Men with diabetes mellitus, urethral trauma, or obstruction may develop an aggressive fasciitis of the perineum called Fournier's gangrene. Perineal pain and swelling may antedate the characteristic discoloration of the scrotum and perineum. Prompt debridement of all necrotic tissue is critical to the cure of these infections. Once the diagnosis is suspected, the patient must be taken immediately to the operating room, where incision and exploration will determine if fasciitis is present. Gram's stain of necrotic material will guide antibiotic choice.

INFECTIONS OF MUSCLE

Pyomyositis

Pyomyositis is a deep infection of muscle usually caused by S. aureus and occasionally by group A β-hemolytic streptococci or enteric bacilli. Most cases occur in warm or tropical regions, and most occur among children. Nonpenetrating trauma may antedate the onset of symptoms, suggesting that infection of a minor hematoma during incidental bacteremia may be causative. Patients present with fever and tender swelling of the muscle; the skin is uninvolved or minimally involved. In older patients, myositis may mimic phlebitis. Diagnosis can be readily made, if suspected, by needle aspiration, ultrasonography, or computed tomography. Early aggressive debridement and appropriate antibiotics are usually curative.

Myonecrosis

Myonecrosis generally occurs after a contaminated injury to muscle. Within 1 or 2 days of injury, the involved extremity becomes painful and begins to swell. The patient appears toxic and is often delirious. The skin may appear uninvolved at first but eventually may develop a bronzed-blue discoloration. Crepitus may be present but is not as prominent as in patients with necrotizing cellulitis (a more benign lesion). Most of these infections are caused by clostridial species (gas gangrene); some are caused by streptococci, mixtures of anaerobes, or gram-negative rods. In rare cases, clostridial myonecrosis occurs spontaneously in the absence of trauma; most of these patients have an underlying malignancy, usually involving the bowel. Regardless of etiology, this illness progresses rapidly, producing extensive necrosis of muscle. Hypotension, hemolytic anemia caused by clostridial lecithinase, and renal failure can complicate this illness. Gram's stain of the thin and watery wound exudate reveals large gram-positive rods and very few inflammatory cells. Emergency surgery with wide debridement is essential if the patient is to survive. Large doses of penicillin (10 to 20 million U/day) plus clindamycin, 600 mg every 6 hours, may prevent further spread of the bacilli. Chloramphenicol may be used in patients with hypersensitivity to penicillin. If gram-negative rods are seen in the exudate, treatment with an extended-spectrum penicillin that also has excellent anaerobic activity such as piperacillin-tazobactam is indicated. Hyperbaric oxygen therapy is of uncertain value.

REFERENCES

Stevens DL: Clostridial myonecrosis and other clostridial diseases. *In* Goldman L, Bennett JC (eds): Cecil Textbook of Medicine, 21st ed. Philadelphia: WB Saunders, 2000, pp 1668–1670.

Swartz MN: Skin and soft tissue infections. *In* Mandell GL, Douglas RG, Bennett JE (eds): Principles and Practice of Infections Diseases, 4th ed. New York: Churchill Livingstone, 1995, pp 909–929.

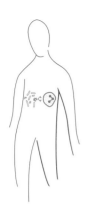

102

INTRA-ABDOMINAL ABSCESS AND PERITONITIS

Michael M. Lederman

Intra-Abdominal Abscess

There are two general categories of intra-abdominal abscess. The first is an infection of a solid intra-abdominal viscus, generally arising as a consequence of hematogenous or enteral spread. The second includes extravisceral abscesses, which are localized collections of pus within the peritoneal or retroperitoneal space. These abscesses usually follow peritonitis or contamination by rupture or leakage from the bowel. Most patients with an intra-abdominal abscess are febrile. The fever may be recurrent and may be associated with rigors, suggesting intermittent bacteremia. Nausea, vomiting, and paralytic ileus are common with extravisceral abscesses. Clues to the presence of intra-abdominal abscess may be subtle and may include extravisceral gas or air-fluid levels on plain radiographs. The availability of computed tomography (CT) has simplified both the diagnosis and the management of these potentially life-threatening infections.

With the exception of amebic abscess or multiple microabscesses of the liver, antibiotic therapy alone is rarely curative. Failure of the antibiotic to penetrate the abscess cavities, inactivation of antibiotics within the abscess by bacterial enzymes, low pH, and low redox potential all contribute to the failure of medical management. Drainage is essential; antibiotics are important primarily to prevent bacteremia and seeding of other organs.

Abscesses of Solid Organs

HEPATIC ABSCESS

Pyogenic liver abscess is a disease that occurs predominantly among individuals with other underlying disorders, most commonly biliary tract disease. Obstruction to biliary drainage allows infected bile to produce ascending infection of the liver. Inflammatory diseases of the bowel, such as appendicitis and diverticulitis, may also lead to hepatic abscess through spread of infection through portal veins (Table 102–1). Hepatic abscesses are also recognized complications of liver transplantation. Penetrating or nonpenetrating trauma may also result in pyogenic liver abscess.

Clinical findings in patients with pyogenic hepatic abscess are often nonspecific. Most patients are febrile, but only about half have abdominal pain and tenderness. Two thirds have palpable hepatomegaly, but fewer than one in four is clinically jaundiced.

The chest roentgenogram may show an elevated right hemidiaphragm and atelectasis or effusion at the right lung base. The diagnosis is best achieved by contrast medium–enhanced CT of the abdomen or ultrasonography of the right upper quadrant. Pyogenic abscesses may be single or multiple; multiple abscesses often arise from a biliary source of infection.

Anaerobic bacilli, microaerophilic streptococci, and gram-negative bacilli are the predominant microorganisms in pyogenic liver abscess. Occasionally, *Staphylococcus aureus* causes hepatic abscesses during the course of bacteremic seeding of multiple organs. Positive blood cultures are obtained from about half the patients with pyogenic liver abscess.

Clinical laboratory studies generally show a moderate elevation of the alkaline phosphatase level, which is disproportionate to the modest elevation in bilirubin level that occurs in roughly half of patients. In contrast, patients with the nonspecific jaundice that occasionally accompanies bacterial infection at other sites generally have elevated bilirubin levels of as much as 5 to 10 mg/dL or more and only slightly elevated alkaline phosphatase levels. In patients with leukemia, multiple hepatic abscesses caused by *Candida* species may present as fever and poorly localized abdominal pain, and an ele-

TABLE 102-1   Intra-Abdominal Abscesses

Site	Predisposing Factors	Likely Pathogens	Diagnosis	Empirical Treatment*
Solid Organs				
Hepatic	Gastrointestinal or biliary sepsis, trauma	Gram-negative bacilli, anaerobes, streptococci, amebae	CT, MRI, ultrasonography	Ampicillin/sulbactam, drainage; metronidazole for amebic abscess
Splenic	Trauma, hemoglobinopathy, endocarditis, injection drug use	Staphylococci, streptococci, gram-negative bacilli	CT	Ampicillin/sulbactam or vancomycin/tobramycin, splenectomy
Pancreatic	Pancreatitis, pseudocyst	Gram-negative bacilli, streptococci	CT	Ampicillin/sulbactam or clindamycin/tobramycin, drainage
Extravisceral				
Subphrenic	Abdominal surgery, peritonitis	Gram-negative bacilli, streptococci, anaerobes	CT	Ampicillin/sulbactam or clindamycin/tobramycin, drainage
Pelvic	Abdominal surgery, peritonitis, pelvic or gastrointestinal inflammatory disease	Gram-negative bacilli, streptococci, anaerobes	CT	Ampicillin/sulbactam or clindamycin/tobramycin, drainage
Perinephric	Renal infection/obstruction, hematogenous	Gram-negative bacilli, staphylococci	CT	Ampicillin/sulbactam or vancomycin/tobramycin, drainage
Psoas	Vertebral osteomyelitis, hematogenous	Staphylococci, gram-negative bacilli, mycobacteria	CT	Ampicillin/sulbactam or vancomycin/tobramycin, drainage

* Ampicillin/sulbactam, 2 g/1 g given intravenously (IV) q8h; vancomycin, 1 g IV q12h; tobramycin, 7 mg/kg q24h; clindamycin, 600 mg IV q8h.
CT = computed tomography; MRI = magnetic resonance imaging.

vated serum alkaline phosphatase level may be the only abnormality pointing to the hepatic origin. Magnetic resonance imaging (MRI) provides the most sensitive radiologic technique for diagnosis.

Hepatic abscess caused by *Entamoeba histolytica* is rare in North America, although it should be suspected in a patient with fever and right upper quadrant pain who has traveled to or emigrated from the developing world. Amebic abscesses are generally single and are usually located in the right lobe of the liver. Only a minority of patients with amebic liver abscess have concurrent intestinal amebiasis. Antibody titers against *E. histolytica* are nearly always positive.

The Fitz-Hugh–Curtis syndrome, or gonococcal perihepatitis, may share some clinical manifestations suggestive of hepatic abscess and should be suspected in young, sexually active women with fever and right upper quadrant tenderness. Tumors involving the liver may produce fever and a clinical and radiologic picture that may mimic hepatic abscess. This is complicated by the occasional concurrence of malignancy and abscess. Patients with hepatic abscesses generally present with a less acute illness than patients with cholecystitis or cholangitis. Ultrasonography, CT, and MRI are all useful in defining liver abscesses; MRI is most effective when the abscesses are less than 1 cm in diameter.

If pyogenic abscess is suggested, needle aspiration is indicated. With the guidance of ultrasonography or CT, a percutaneous catheter can be inserted into the abscess cavity for both diagnostic and therapeutic purposes. The pus should be Gram-stained and cultured aerobically and anaerobically. Unless the Gram stain indicates otherwise, initial therapy for pyogenic liver abscess should include drugs active against enteric aerobic and anaerobic bacteria (see Table 102–1). Antibiotics should

be continued for at least 4 to 6 weeks. Patients with multiple hepatic abscess caused by *Candida* or *Candida*-like species (e.g., *Torulopsis glabrata*) require long-term therapy with either amphotericin B or fluconazole, as determined by the microbiology of the fungus. Surgery is required to relieve biliary tract obstruction and to drain abscesses that do not respond to percutaneous drainage and antibiotics. Patients with pyogenic liver abscess should be evaluated for a primary intra-abdominal source of infection.

If epidemiologic features strongly suggest an amebic abscess, metronidazole is the drug of choice. Needle aspiration is necessary only to exclude pyogenic infection or, if the abscess is large or close to other viscera, to prevent rupture. In the case of amebic abscess, the "anchovy paste" material obtained by needle drainage is not pus but necrotic liver tissue. Large numbers of white cells suggest pyogenic abscess or bacterial superinfection. Trophozoites of *E. histolytica* are infrequently seen on aspiration of abscesses but are often seen on biopsy of the abscess capsule.

SPLENIC ABSCESS

Splenic abscesses are generally the result of hematogenous seeding of the spleen. In the preantibiotic era, splenic infarction and abscess were common complications of infective endocarditis. Now the most common predisposing factors are trauma and (in children) sickle cell disease. Patients with splenic abscess most often present with left upper quadrant abdominal pain, which may be pleuritic. The left hemidiaphragm may be elevated, and there may be an associated pleural rub or effusion. The diagnostic approach, most likely etiologic agents, and initial antimicrobial therapy are outlined in

Table 102–1. Splenectomy is usually the definitive treatment, but CT-guided percutaneous drainage of large, solitary abscesses may also be successful in selected cases.

PANCREATIC ABSCESS

Pancreatic abscess is an uncommon complication of pancreatitis. The symptoms of pancreatic abscess (fever, nausea, vomiting, and abdominal pain radiating to the back) resemble those of pancreatitis. Thus, abscess should be suspected in cases of persistent recurrent fever after pancreatitis. The inflamed organ becomes colonized and infected with microbes inhabiting the upper gastrointestinal tract. Enterobacteriaceae, anaerobes, and streptococci (including the pneumococci) are likely pathogens. The diagnosis may be made by CT; however, radiographic definition of the pancreatic bed is often difficult. Initial antibiotic therapy (see Table 102–1) should be followed by surgical drainage of the abscess as soon as the patient's condition is stable. The mortality rate exceeds 30% even with optimal management.

Extravisceral Abscesses

Extravisceral abscesses most often arise after peritonitis, after intra-abdominal surgery, as a consequence of rupture of the bowel, or after extension of infection of a viscus, such as diverticulitis or appendicitis. Abscesses may occur in the subphrenic, pelvic, or retroperitoneal spaces. Fever, nausea, vomiting, and paralytic ileus are common. Although fever is almost always present, localizing symptoms may be very subtle, making the diagnosis difficult. Predisposing factors, most likely etiologic pathogens, and appropriate initial antimicrobial therapy are outlined in Table 102–1.

When an abscess is suspected, CT or ultrasound scans should be obtained. CT can identify abscesses in the retroperitoneal and abdominal spaces and guide percutaneous drainage. Ultrasonography may be more helpful in the identification of pelvic fluid collections. Fluid-filled abscesses may be difficult to distinguish from loops of viscera on CT or ultrasonography; review of such studies by an experienced radiologist is essential before they are considered negative. Radionuclide imaging using indium-111–labeled leukocytes may be useful in localizing collections of pus when other studies are not diagnostic. Drainage of an abscess either by radiologic guidance or by surgery in conjunction with antibiotics is the mainstay of treatment.

Peritonitis

Peritonitis may occur spontaneously (primary peritonitis) or as a consequence of trauma, surgery, or peritoneal soilage by bowel contents (secondary peritonitis). Peritonitis also may be caused by chemical irritation. Patients with peritonitis generally complain of diffuse abdominal pain. They may have nausea and vomiting; some have diarrhea, and others have paralytic ileus. Patients are usually febrile and uncomfortable and prefer to lie quietly in the supine position. Physical examination may reveal diffuse tenderness, diminished bowel sounds, and evidence of peritoneal inflammation, including rebound tenderness and involuntary guarding. In patients with underlying ascites, the signs and symptoms of peritonitis may be more subtle, with fever as the only manifestation of infection.

PRIMARY PERITONITIS

Primary or spontaneous peritonitis occurs principally among persons with ascites associated with chronic liver disease or the nephrotic syndrome. Bacteria may infect ascitic fluid by means of bacteremic spread, transmural migration through the bowel, or through the fallopian tubes. In cirrhotic patients, clearance of portal bacteremia by hepatic reticuloendothelial cells may be impaired by intrahepatic portosystemic shunting. Not surprisingly, therefore, gram-negative rods, especially *Escherichia coli*, are the predominant pathogens in spontaneous bacterial peritonitis; enteric streptococci are isolated in approximately one third of cases. Staphylococci, *Streptococcus pneumoniae*, or anaerobic bacilli are isolated in a smaller proportion of cases (Table 102–2).

In patients with ascites, the presenting symptoms may be nonspecific abdominal pain, nausea, vomiting, diarrhea, or altered mental status. Thus, febrile patients with ascites should undergo paracentesis unless there is another certain explanation for fever; inoculation of the culture media should be performed at the bedside; and a white blood cell count in the fluid that exceeds 250/μL is suggestive of infection. Gram's stain may reveal the responsible pathogen. Antibiotic penetration into the peritoneum is excellent, and medical therapy is the treatment of choice (see Table 102–2). If Gram's stain or culture reveals a mixed flora with anaerobes, secondary peritonitis caused by leakage of bowel contents should be suspected. Bacteria may be cultured from ascitic fluid in the absence of clinical findings of peritonitis (bacterascites), and as many as one third of patients with clinical and laboratory findings consistent with peritonitis have sterile ascitic fluid cultures. Treatment is indicated in these settings. Among patients with cirrhosis and ascites, prophylactic administration of norfloxacin or trimethoprim-sulfamethoxazole decreases the risk of spontaneous peritonitis.

SECONDARY PERITONITIS

Secondary peritonitis may follow penetrating abdominal trauma or surgery or may result from contamination of the peritoneum with bowel contents. This syndrome may be heralded by the sudden presentation of visceral rupture (e.g., perforated duodenal ulcer or appendix) or visceral infarction. In the postoperative setting, secondary peritonitis should be suspected in the patient whose abdominal discomfort and fever do not resolve, or even worsen, after the first few postoperative days. If peritonitis is secondary to the leakage of bowel contents, im-

TABLE 102–2 Causes, Diagnosis, and Treatment of Peritonitis

Site	Predisposing Factors	Causative Agent	Clues to Diagnosis	Empirical Treatment*
Primary				
Spontaneous	Cirrhosis, nephrotic syndrome	Gram-negative bacilli, streptococci	>250 neutrophils/μL of ascites	Ampicillin/sulbactam or clindamycin/tobramycin
Secondary				
Postoperative	Hemorrhage, visceral rupture	Gram-negative bacilli, streptococci, staphylococci, anaerobes	Postoperative fever, pain, prolonged ileus	Ampicillin/sulbactam or metronidazole/tobramycin
Chemical	Abdominal surgery	Bile, starch, talc	Postoperative fever, pain	Biliary drainage when indicated
Visceral rupture	Perforating ulcer, ruptured appendix, bowel infarction	Gram-negative bacilli, anaerobes, streptococci	Polymicrobial Gram's stain or culture	Ampicillin/sulbactam or metronidazole/tobramycin; surgery
Peritoneal dialysis		Staphylococci, gram-negative bacilli	Pain, fever, neutrophilic pleocytosis	Vancomycin/tobramycin;† consider catheter removal
Periodic peritonitis	Familial		Recurrent, familial	Colchicine prophylaxis, 0.6 mg two to three times daily
Tuberculosis	Infection of fallopian tubes or ileum	*Mycobacterium tuberculosis*	Lymphocytic pleocytosis, high protein level (<3 g/dL) in ascitic fluid	Isoniazid, rifampin, pyrazinamide, ethambutol

* Ampicillin/sulbactam, 2 g/1 g intravenously (IV) q8h; vancomycin, 1 g IV q12h; tobramycin, 1.7 mg/kg q24h; clindamycin, 600 mg IV q8h; isoniazid, 300 mg/d; rifampin, 600 mg/d; ethambutol 15–25 mg/kg/d; pyrazinamide, 25 mg/kg/d (maximum, 2.5 gm/d), metronidazole, 500 mg IV q8h.
† Intraperitoneal vancomycin, initially 1 g/L dialysate, followed by 25 mg/L dialysate; intraperitoneal tobramycin, initially 8 mg/L dialysate, followed by 4–8 mg/L dialysate.

mediate surgical intervention is mandatory. Despite the use of appropriate antibiotics (see Table 102–2) and intensive support systems, the rate of mortality from generalized peritonitis approaches 50%. Peritonitis is also a common complication of peritoneal dialysis. Most infections are caused by staphylococci, followed by gram-negative bacilli and yeast. Intraperitoneal antibiotics are generally effective. Refractory or recurrent peritonitis may necessitate dialysis catheter removal.

TUBERCULOUS PERITONITIS

Tuberculous peritonitis may occur as a result of hematogenous or local extension of tuberculous infection into the peritoneal cavity. Fever, abdominal pain, and weight loss are common. In patients with underlying ascites, a lymphocytic pleocytosis in the peritoneal fluid should suggest the diagnosis. Laparoscopy, with biopsy of the granulomatous peritoneal nodules, is the most effective approach to diagnosis. Antituberculous therapy is generally curative (see Table 102–2).

REFERENCES

Bhuva M, Ganger D, Jensen D: Spontaneous bacterial peritonitis: An update on evaluation, management, and prevention. Am J Med 1994; 97:169–175.

Levison ME, Bush LM: Peritonitis and other intra-abdominal infections. In Mandell GL, Bennett JE, Dolin R (eds): Principles and Practice of Infectious Diseases, 5th ed. New York: Churchill Livingstone, 2000, pp 821–856.

Maddrey WC: Parasitic, bacterial, fungal and granulomatous liver diseases. In Goldman L, Bennett JC (eds): Cecil Textbook of Medicine, 21st ed. Philadelphia: WB Saunders, 2000, pp 797–801.

Singh N, Gayowski T, Yu VL, Wagene MM: Trimethoprim-sulfamethoxazole for the prevention of spontaneous bacterial peritonitis in cirrhosis: A randomized trial. Ann Intern Med 1995; 122:595–598.

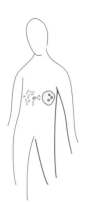

103

INFECTIOUS DIARRHEA

Michael M. Lederman

Acute diarrheal illnesses caused by bacterial, viral, or protozoal pathogens vary from mild bowel dysfunction to fulminant, life-threatening diseases. Worldwide, acute diarrheal illnesses are the most common cause of death in childhood. With the best techniques available, a specific causative agent can be identified in 70% to 80% of cases (Table 103–1).

Pathogenesis and Pathophysiology: General Concepts

In general, pathogens or microbial toxins that produce acute diarrhea must be ingested. Therefore, socioeconomic conditions that result in crowding, poor sanitation, and contaminated water sources lead to increased risk of diarrheal illnesses. Normally, the low pH of the stomach, the rapid transit time of the small bowel, and antibody produced by cells in the lamina propria of the small bowel are adequate to keep the jejunum and proximal ileum free of pathogenic microorganisms (although not sterile). Furthermore, the ileocecal valve inhibits retrograde migration of the huge numbers of bacteria that reside in the large bowel.

Pathogenic microorganisms can pass through the hostile environment of the stomach if (1) they are acid resistant (e.g., *Shigella*) or (2) they are ingested with food and are therefore partially protected in the neutralized environment. People with decreased gastric acidity are at increased risk of acute diarrheal disease.

In the small bowel, the organisms either colonize (*Vibrio cholerae, Escherichia coli*) or invade (rotavirus, Norwalk agent) the local mucosa or must pass through to colonize and invade the mucosa of the terminal ileum (*Salmonella*) or colon (*Shigella*). Small bowel peristalsis deters colonization of most organisms. Special colonization factors such as fimbria (hairlike projections from the cell wall) or lectins (proteins that attach to mucosal cell surface carbohydrates) facilitate adherence of successful colonists to mucosal cell surfaces.

Organisms that do not have special colonization properties pass into the terminal ileum and colon, where they may compete with the established flora. The normal fecal flora produce substances that prevent intraluminal proliferation of most newly introduced bacterial species (*Bacteroides* produces inhibitory fatty acids; other enteric bacteria produce inhibitory colicins). The ability of the colonic enteropathogens (e.g., *Shigella dysenteriae*) to invade intestinal mucosa allows these microorganisms to multiply preferentially.

Types of Microbial Diarrheal Diseases

Microbes can cause diarrhea either directly by invasion of the gut mucosa or indirectly through elaboration of one of three classes of microbial toxins: secretory enterotoxins, cytotoxins, or neurotoxins.

SECRETORY TOXIN-INDUCED DIARRHEAS

Patients infected with secretory toxin-producing pathogens seldom have fever or other major systemic symptoms, and there is little or no inflammatory response. Characteristically, large numbers of bacteria (10^5 to 10^8) must be ingested with grossly contaminated food or water (although a small inoculum may produce disease in individuals with achlorhydria). The enterotoxin-producing bacteria then colonize, but do not invade, the small bowel. After multiplying to large numbers (10^8 to 10^9 organisms per milliliter of fluid), the bacteria produce enterotoxins that bind to mucosal cells, causing hypersecretion of isotonic fluid at a rate that overwhelms the reabsorptive capacity of the colon. The diarrhea is watery with a low protein concentration and an electrolyte content that reflects its source. Rapid loss of this diarrheal fluid results in predictable saline depletion, base-deficit acidosis, and potassium deficiency. The amount and rate of fluid loss determine the severity of the illness. Certain of the secretory diarrheas, such as those caused by *V. cholerae* or *E. coli* enterotoxins, can result

815

TABLE 103–1   Major Etiologic Agents in Acute Diarrheal Illnesses

Invasive/Destructive Pathogens
*Shigella**
Salmonella
Campylobacter jejuni
*Vibrio parahaemolyticus**
Yersinia enterocolitica
Enterohemorrhagic *Escherichia coli* (EHEC)*
Clostridium difficile†
Rotavirus
Other viruses
Entamoeba histolytica
Noninvasive Pathogens
Enterotoxigenic *E. coli*† (ETEC)
Vibrio cholerae†
Giardia lamblia
Isospora belli
Cryptosporidium parvum
Bacterial Causes of Toxin-Induced Food Poisoning
Staphylococcus aureus (short incubation, 2–6 hr)
Clostridium perfringens (longer incubation, 8–14 hr)
Bacillus cereus (short and longer incubation)

* Mucosal destruction mediated by a toxin.
† Diarrhea mediated by a secretory enterotoxin.

in massive intestinal fluid losses, exceeding 1 L/hr in adults. The *V. cholerae* enterotoxin rapidly binds to monosialogangliosides of the gut mucosa and causes sustained stimulation of cell-bound adenylate cyclase. This results, through both increased secretion and decreased absorption of electrolytes, in net movement of large quantities of isotonic fluid into the gut lumen. The disease runs its course in 2 to 7 days, during which time continued fluid and electrolyte repletion is of critical importance.

Enterotoxigenic *E. coli*, probably the major cause of traveler's diarrhea worldwide, produces two major types of plasmid-encoded bacterial enterotoxins. The labile toxin (LT) of *E. coli* is nearly identical in mode of action to cholera enterotoxin. The *E. coli* stable toxins (ST) include STa, which causes gut fluid secretion through activation of guanylate cyclase, and STb, which causes gut fluid secretion by an as yet unknown mechanism. Both STa and STb have a more rapid onset and shorter duration of action than *E. coli* LT. Secretory enterotoxins may also be produced by other enteropathogenic bacteria that cause diarrhea primarily through direct invasion (e.g., *Salmonella typhimurium*, *Shigella dysenteriae*).

CYTOTOXIN-INDUCED DIARRHEAS

Cytotoxins are soluble factors that directly destroy mucosal epithelial cells. *Shigella dysenteriae* elaborates a toxin (Shiga toxin) that causes the destructive colitis seen in patients with shigellosis. A closely related cytotoxin is produced by enterohemorrhagic *E. coli* strains that are associated with hemorrhagic colitis and hemolytic-uremic syndrome. Other bacteria that can produce cytotoxins include *Clostridium perfringens* and *Vibrio parahaemolyticus*. *C. perfringens*, often ingested in contaminated meat or poultry, replicates within the small bowel and produces a secretory enterotoxin that also has cytotoxin activity. Toxin-induced diarrhea caused by *C. perfringens*, like that caused by *Staphylococcus aureus* and *Bacillus cereus*, has a short incubation period and brief (<36 hours) duration. *Clostridium difficile* can colonize the large bowel and, in the presence of antibiotic therapy that limits the growth of normal microbial flora, can produce cytotoxins that can cause severe mucosal damage, producing a colitis that may have a pseudomembranous appearance or may resemble the diffuse colitis seen in shigellosis.

FOOD POISONING (CAUSED BY CYTOTOXINS, SECRETORY ENTEROTOXINS, AND/OR NEUROTOXINS)

Some toxins are ingested directly in food, as with staphylococcal and *Bacillus cereus* food poisoning. These organisms grow to a high concentration in the food, and the toxins they produce cause the symptoms of food poisoning. Distinctive features of acute food poisoning include a short incubation period (2 to 6 hours), high attack rates (up to 75% of the population at risk), and prominent vomiting (probably caused by the effect of absorbed neurotoxins on the central nervous system).

Food poisoning syndromes of somewhat longer incubation (8 to 16 hours) can be caused by organisms ingested in food that produce toxins during replication in the bowel. In this setting, *Bacillus cereus* produces a cytotoxin similar to *E. coli* LT. Thus the longer incubation food poisoning syndrome caused by *B. cereus* (often associated with ingestion of contaminated rice) may resemble the diarrhea caused by enterotoxigenic *E. coli* (ETEC). *Clostridium perfringens* can produce both secretory and cytotoxic enterotoxins after ingestion and replication in the bowel, also producing a longer incubation food poisoning. Nausea and vomiting are less prominent than diarrhea in these food poisoning syndromes with longer incubation times.

DIARRHEAS CAUSED BY INVASIVE PATHOGENS

Diarrheas caused by invasive pathogens are usually accompanied by fever and other systemic symptoms, including headache and myalgia. Cramping abdominal pain may be prominent, and small amounts of stool are passed at frequent intervals, often associated with tenesmus. The invasive microorganisms often induce a marked inflammatory response, so that the stool contains pus cells, large amounts of protein, and often gross blood. Significant dehydration rarely results from this kind of diarrhea, because the diarrheal fluid volume is small, seldom exceeding 750 mL/day in adults. Although certain clinical features are statistically more frequent in invasive diarrheas caused by specific enteropathogens (e.g., more severe myalgias with shigellosis, higher temperature spikes with salmonellosis), epidemiologic characteristics are more helpful than signs or symptoms in determining the etiologic agent in invasive diarrheal illnesses (Table 103–2).

Acute Shigellosis

Acute shigellosis occurs when susceptible individuals ingest fecally contaminated water or food. Shigellosis can occur after ingestion of only 10 to 100 microorganisms. Largely for this reason, direct person-to-person transmission (e.g., in day care centers) is more common with shigellosis than with other bacterial enteric infections. The organism initially multiplies in the small intestine, producing watery, noninflammatory diarrhea. Later, the organisms invade the colonic epithelium, causing the characteristic bloody stool. Unlike *Salmonella*, *Shigella* rarely causes bacteremia. The disease usually resolves spontaneously after 3 to 6 days, but the clinical course can be shortened by antimicrobial agents (see Table 103–2).

Acute Salmonellosis

Acute salmonellosis usually results from ingestion of contaminated meat, dairy, or poultry products. In the industrialized world, *Salmonella* is often transmitted by means of commercially prepared dried, processed foodstuffs. Unlike *Shigella*, *Salmonella* is remarkably resistant to desiccation. The nontyphoidal salmonellae invade primarily the distal ileum. The organism typically causes a short-lived (2 to 3 days) illness characterized by fever, nausea, vomiting, and diarrhea. (This is in marked contrast to the 3- to 4-week febrile illness, usually not associated with diarrhea, that is caused by *Salmonella typhi*.)

Campylobacter jejuni Infection

Campylobacter jejuni may be responsible for up to 10% of acute diarrheal illnesses worldwide. This organism may invade both the small intestine and the colon. Thus the range of symptoms is broad, ranging from an acute *Shigella*-type syndrome to a milder, but more protracted, diarrheal illness.

Other Invasive Enteropathogens

Three other organisms—*Yersinia enterocolitica*, *V. parahaemolyticus*, and enteroinvasive *E. coli* (EIEC)—also cause tissue invasion and acute diarrheal illnesses that may be clinically indistinguishable from those caused by the more commonly recognized invasive bacterial enteropathogens (see Table 103–2). Another distinct *E. coli* strain, enterohemorrhagic *E. coli*, produces bloody diarrhea without evidence of mucosal inflammation (grossly bloody stool with few or no leukocytes).

Although most diarrhea-causing pathogens produce either invasive or enterotoxic diarrhea, both processes contribute to the illness in some situations. Certain strains of *Shigella*, nontyphoidal *Salmonella*, *Y. enterocolitica*, and *C. jejuni* both invade and produce secretory enterotoxins in vitro. Such enterotoxins may play a contributory role in the acute disease process. The invasive capacity of these organisms is, however, of paramount importance in their ability to produce disease.

Viral Causes of Diarrhea

Both the rotavirus and the Norwalk agent invade and damage villous epithelial cells, with the degree of injury ranging from modest distortion of epithelial cells to sloughing of villi. Presumably, both the rotavirus and the Norwalk agent cause diarrhea by interfering with the

TABLE 103–2   Epidemiologic Characteristics of Common Invasive Enteric Pathogens

Microorganisms	Epidemiologic Features	Antibiotics
Shigella species	Outbreaks in child care centers or custodial institutions; person-to-person transmission	Yes
Nontyphoidal *Salmonella* species	Zoonosis; survives desiccation in processed dairy, poultry, and meat products	Rarely
Campylobacter jejuni	Zoonosis; worldwide distribution; transmitted in dairy products	Early treatment for severely ill patients
Yersinia enterocolitica	Zoonosis; occasionally transmitted in dairy products	Maybe
Vibrio parahaemolyticus	Coastal salt waters; transmitted by inadequately cooked shrimp and shellfish	No
Clostridium difficile	Almost always follows antimicrobial therapy	Yes
Rotavirus	Outbreaks among children; worldwide distribution; unusual and mild in adults	No
Norwalk virus	Microepidemic pattern; no specific age predilection	No
Entamoeba histolytica	Person-to-person transmission; very rare in United States, Canada, and Western Europe	Yes

absorption of normal intestinal secretions. This may occur through selective destruction of absorptive villous tip cells with sparing of secretory crypt cells. Affected patients may have low-grade fever and mild to moderate cramping abdominal pain. The stool is usually watery, and its contents resemble those of a noninvasive process, with few inflammatory cells, probably because of lack of damage to the colon.

Protozoan Causes of Diarrhea

In North America, Rocky Mountain water sources are frequent origins of *Giardia lamblia* microepidemics. As is the case in shigellosis, ingestion of only a few organisms is required to establish infection. The organisms multiply in the small bowel, attach to and occasionally invade the mucosa, but do not cause gross damage to the mucosal cells. Clinical manifestations span the spectrum from an acute, febrile diarrheal illness to chronic diarrhea with associated malabsorption and weight loss. Diagnosis may be made by identification of the organism in either the stool or the duodenal mucus or by small bowel biopsy. *Entamoeba histolytica* may cause intestinal syndromes ranging from mild diarrhea to fulminant amebic colitis with multiple bloody stools, fever, and severe abdominal pain. Although *E. histolytica* has a worldwide distribution, it is an uncommon cause of diarrhea in the United States. Two other protozoa, *Cryptosporidium parvum* and *Isospora belli,* occasionally cause self-limited acute diarrheal illness in otherwise healthy individuals and may cause voluminous, life-threatening diarrheal disease in patients with acquired immunodeficiency syndrome. Stool examination will distinguish *Giardia, Entamoeba, Isospora,* and *Cryptosporidium.*

General Epidemiologic Considerations

In developing countries where sanitation is inadequate, young children (up to 2 years of age) contract multiple episodes of diarrhea, a process that engenders intestinal immunity to the majority of enteropathogens in their environment. Most of these diarrheal episodes are mild, but some are life-threatening. In these areas, ETEC and rotavirus together cause the large majority of diarrheal illnesses. *Shigella* infections are far less common during this period.

Infants and small children in industrialized countries have fewer episodes of diarrhea than do those in developing countries, and the most common etiologic agent is the rotavirus. Most episodes are mild. ETEC and *Shigella* infections are infrequent except in a few defined population groups (e.g., individuals in custodial institutions).

Throughout the world, clinically significant diarrhea is relatively unusual in adults except in specific defined epidemics or common-source outbreaks caused by contaminated food or water. However, when immunologically inexperienced adults from the developed world visit developing countries and have an extremely high incidence of diarrheal disease (traveler's diarrhea), the organisms responsible are the same ones as those causing most childhood diarrhea in the country visited.

In addition to the pathogens listed earlier, certain sexually transmissible pathogens that may cause acute diarrheal illnesses among sexually active homosexual men (see Chapter 107) may differ from those that most commonly occur in the general population.

Diagnosis

In managing life-threatening diarrheal illnesses, determining the specific etiologic agent is not as important as promptly repleting lost electrolytes. Fluid losses represent the chief cause of serious morbidity and mortality in diarrheal illness. Moreover, antimicrobial therapy has proven of value in only a minority of cases (see Table 103–2). Discerning the epidemiology of the illness is often more helpful than are laboratory techniques in identifying cases in which antimicrobial therapy is likely to be helpful! Figure 103–1 provides a schematic approach to diagnosis and management.

The examination of a methylene blue–stained stool preparation for erythrocytes and pus cells may be helpful in distinguishing between acute diarrheal illnesses caused by invasive pathogens and those caused by noninvasive pathogens. This is easily accomplished by adding one drop of methylene blue dye to one drop of liquid stool or mucus, allowing the preparation to air dry, and examining the specimen under the high dry microscope lens. Few, if any, leukocytes or erythrocytes are seen in the stools of patients with diarrhea caused by noninvasive organisms (e.g., ETEC). Variable numbers of leukocytes and erythrocytes are present in diarrheas secondary to invasive bacteria (e.g., *Shigella*) or cytopathic toxins (*C. difficile* toxin).

The precise diagnosis of any diarrheal illness lasting longer than 4 to 5 days is important because these illnesses (e.g., giardiasis) may be responsive to specific antimicrobial therapy. Furthermore, among patients with negative stool examinations and cultures, endoscopy may yield a diagnosis of a noninfectious disease (e.g., ulcerative colitis or Crohn's disease).

Management: General Principles of Electrolyte Repletion Therapy

INTRAVENOUS FLUIDS

All acute diarrheal diseases respond to a similar fluid repletion regimen because voluminous infectious diarrhea in adults consistently produces the same pattern of electrolyte loss. The fluid losses of massive diarrhea can rapidly be corrected by infusing fluids intravenously that approximate those that have been lost. Lactated Ringer's

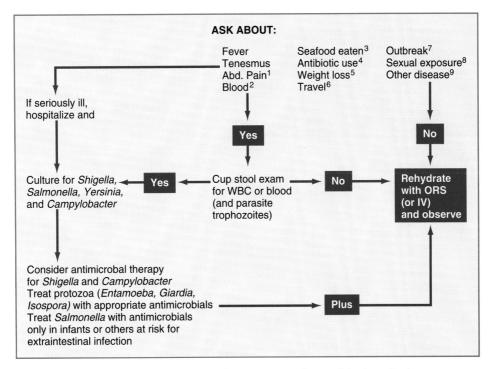

FIGURE 103–1 Approach to the diagnosis and management of acute infectious diarrhea.

1. If unexplained abdominal pain and fever suggest an appendicitis-like syndrome, culture for *Yersinia enterocolitica.*
2. Bloody diarrhea, in the absence of fecal leukocytes, suggests enterohemorrhagic *Escherichia coli* or amebiasis (where leukocytes are destroyed by the parasite).
3. Ingestion of inadequately cooked seafood prompts consideration of *Vibrio* infections or Norwalk-like viruses.
4. Associated antibiotics should be stopped and *Clostridium difficile* considered.
5. Persistence of diarrhea (>10 days) with weight loss prompts consideration of giardiasis, cryptosporidiosis, or inflammatory bowel disease.
6. Travel to tropical areas increases the chance of enterotoxic *E. coli* (ETEC) as well as viral, protozoal *(Giardia, Entamoeba, Cryptosporidium),* and, if fecal leukocytes are present, invasive bacterial pathogens.
7. Outbreaks should prompt consideration of *Staphylococcus aureus, Bacillus cereus, Clostridium perfringens,* ETEC, *Vibrio, Salmonella, Campylobacter,* or *Shigella* infection.
8. Sigmoidoscopy in symptomatic homosexual males should distinguish proctitis in the distal 15 cm (caused by herpesvirus, gonococcal, chlamydial, or syphilitic infection) from colitis (*Campylobacter, Shigella,* or *C. difficile* infections).
9. Immunocompromised hosts should have a wide range of viral (e.g., cytomegalovirus [CMV], herpes simplex virus [HSV], rotavirus), bacterial (e.g., *Salmonella, Mycobacterium avium* complex, *C. difficile*), and protozoal (e.g., *Cryptosporidium, Isospora, Microsporidia, Entamoeba,* and *Giardia*) agents considered.

IV = intravenous; ORS = oral rehydration solution; WBC = white blood cell. (Adapted from Guerrant RL, Shields DS, Thorson SM, et al: Evaluation and diagnosis of acute infectious diarrhea. Am J Med 1985; 78:91–98.)

solution is readily available and provides uniformly good results. With patients who are hypotensive, the intravenous fluids should initially be infused rapidly. Subsequent maintenance fluid administration can be guided by the patient's clinical appearance, including the vital signs, the appearance of neck veins, and skin turgor. Clinical evaluation alone provides an adequate guide to fluid replacement in most acute diarrheal illnesses. If intravenous fluids are administered in adequate quantities throughout the diarrheal illness, virtually every patient with diarrhea caused by toxigenic bacteria should be restored to health. Complications (e.g., acute renal failure secondary to hypotension) are exceedingly rare if these principles are followed.

ORAL FLUIDS

In most patients with acute diarrheal illness, fluid repletion can also be achieved through the oral route, using isotonic glucose–containing electrolyte solutions. A uniformly effective solution can be prepared by the addition of 20 g of glucose, 3.5 g of sodium chloride, 2.5 g of sodium bicarbonate, and 1.5 g of potassium chloride to a liter of drinking water (Table 103–3). These fluids should be administered initially in large quantities, 250 mL every 15 minutes in adults, until clinical observations indicate that fluid balance has been restored. Thereafter, one administers fluids in quantities sufficient to maintain normal balance; if stool output is measured, approximately 1.5 L of glucose-electrolyte solution should be given orally for each liter of stool. The oral glucose-electrolyte fluid does not decrease the volume of fluid lost through the intestinal tract but rather facilitates absorption of adequate fluid to counterbalance the toxin-induced fluid secretion.

Patients with fluid depletion caused by invasive microbial agents (e.g., rotavirus, *Salmonella*) also respond well to oral glucose-electrolyte therapy, although the

TABLE 103-3   Oral Rehydration Fluid

Constituents (g/L)	Electrolyte Content (mmol/L)
NaCl—3.5 g	Na—90
NaHCO₃—2.5 g	Cl—80
KCl—1.5 g	K—20
Glucose—20 g	HCO₃—30
	Glucose—110

pathogenesis of diarrheal disease caused by invasive microbes is quite different from that caused by enterotoxigenic bacteria.

ANTIMICROBIAL THERAPY

Most acute infectious diarrheas do not require antibiotic therapy (see Table 103–2). Of the noninvasive bacterial diarrheas, antibiotics dramatically decrease the volume of diarrhea only in cholera. Doxycycline, 300 mg in a single dose, is the drug of choice.

Of the invasive bacterial diarrheas, short-term antimicrobial treatment significantly decreases the duration and severity of shigellosis. In North America, both ciprofloxacin, 500 mg, and trimethoprim-sulfamethoxazole, one double-strength tablet, given twice daily for 5 days are generally active. Because of the increasing frequency of plasmid-mediated antimicrobial resistance, sensitivity testing is necessary to determine the appropriate antibiotic in many other areas of the world.

Antimicrobial therapy may also be helpful in decreasing the duration and severity of enteritis caused by *Yersinia* and *Campylobacter*. Ciprofloxacin, 500 mg twice daily for 5 days, is useful against these pathogens as well. Antimicrobial agents are of no known value in *V. parahaemolyticus* infections. In uncomplicated nontyphoidal *Salmonella* enteritis, antibiotics may prolong the fecal shedding of salmonellae. Treatment of nontyphoidal salmonella gastroenteritis may, however, be indicated in certain settings to prevent bacteremia and its complications (e.g., meningitis, endovascular infection, or infections of joint or vascular prostheses). Treatment until defervescence with a third-generation cephalosporin or a quinolone is therefore indicated for immunocompromised patients, patients with advanced atherosclerotic disease, patients with sickle cell disease, and patients with bone or vascular prostheses.

Antimicrobial therapy is indicated, paradoxically, for treatment of antibiotic-associated diarrhea. Antibiotic-associated diarrhea develops in 1% to 15% of patients who receive broad-spectrum antimicrobial agents and is caused by cytotoxins produced by *C. difficile,* which proliferate in the colonic mucosa when the normal flora is disturbed. Although generally characterized by mild diarrhea, antibiotic-associated diarrhea may result in a potentially lethal pseudomembranous colitis. In all cases, the responsible antibiotic should be stopped. In moderately ill patients (fever, mucosal ulceration, and/or pseudomembranes), metronidazole (500 mg q8h for 7 days) should be started on the basis of strong clinical suspicion, before the diagnosis is confirmed by stool assay for *C. difficile* toxins. Oral vancomycin should be used only in severe cases. Empirical treatment with these agents should be avoided in patients with mild diarrhea because this may result in the emergence of antibiotic-resistant bacteria, such as vancomycin-resistant enterococci.

Antimicrobial agents decrease the duration and severity of giardiasis. In adults, metronidazole, 250 mg every 8 hours for 3 days, and quinacrine, 300 mg/day for 7 days, appear to be equally effective in adults. Acute intestinal amebiasis demands antimicrobial therapy. Metronidazole, 750 mg every 8 hours for 5 days, is the drug of choice in adults. The duration of diarrhea caused by *Isospora belli* is significantly shortened by administration of trimethoprim-sulfamethoxazole twice daily for 5 days.

ANTIMICROBIAL PROPHYLAXIS

Prophylactic antimicrobial agents are effective in preventing traveler's diarrhea, which is caused most often by ETEC. Doxycycline, trimethoprim-sulfamethoxazole, and a quinolone such as norfloxacin are each effective when taken once daily for up to 3 weeks. However, because of the rapid response of most patients to early treatment with any of these three agents, the advantages of prophylactic drugs are, in most instances, outweighed by their potential risks (adverse reactions).

SYMPTOMATIC THERAPY

Adjuvant symptomatic therapy is not essential but may provide modest symptomatic relief in acute infectious diarrheas associated with cramping abdominal pain. Bismuth subsalicylate, 0.6 g every 6 hours, may ameliorate symptoms of traveler's diarrhea. Agents that decrease intestinal motility (e.g., codeine, diphenoxylate, loperamide) also relieve the cramping abdominal pain associated with many acute diarrheal illnesses but are potentially hazardous because they may enhance the severity of illness in shigellosis, the prototype of invasive bacterial diarrheas.

REFERENCES

Guerrant RL: Enteric *Escherichia coli* infections. *In* Goldman L, Bennett JC (eds): Cecil Textbook of Medicine, 21st ed. Philadelphia: WB Saunders, 2000, pp 1693–1696.

Guerrant RL, Steiner TS: Principles and syndromes of enteric infections. *In* Mandell GL, Bennett JE, Dolin R: Principles and Practice of Infectious Diseases, 5th ed. New York: Churchill Livingstone, 2000, pp 1076–1093.

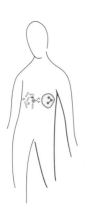

104

INFECTIONS INVOLVING BONES AND JOINTS

Michael M. Lederman

Arthritis

In adults, almost all cases of infective arthritis of natural joints occur through hematogenous seeding. In rare cases, intra-articular trauma can result in septic arthritis. Causative agents for infective arthritis include bacteria, viruses, mycobacteria, and fungi. In addition, certain viruses such as hepatitis B virus can produce a polyarthritis by means of immune complex deposition. Immune mechanisms also underlie arthritis syndromes seen after diarrhea caused by *Salmonella, Shigella, Yersinia,* and *Clostridium difficile* infections; the majority of individuals with postdysentery arthritis syndrome share the human leukocyte antigen HLA-B27 (see Chapter 80).

ACUTE ARTHRITIS

Underlying joint disease, particularly rheumatoid arthritis, predisposes to septic arthritis. Many patients with septic arthritis give a history of joint trauma antedating symptoms of infection. Conceivably, disruption of capillaries during an unrecognized and transient bacteremia allows bacteria to spill into hemorrhagic and traumatized synovium or joint fluid, resulting in the initiation of infection.

Microbiology

Staphylococcus aureus is the most common cause of septic arthritis (Table 104–1). Patients with underlying joint disease and intravenous drug users are at particular risk for infection with this organism. *Pseudomonas aeruginosa* is another important cause of septic arthritis among intravenous drug users.

Other gram-negative bacilli are infrequent causes of septic arthritis and are found primarily among elderly debilitated patients with chronic arthritis. In adults younger than age 30, *Neisseria gonorrhoeae* is the most likely pathogen. Isolates causing disseminated gonococ-cal infection with arthritis are generally resistant to killing by normal serum.

Clinical Presentation

Symptoms of septic arthritis are generally present for only a few days before the patient seeks medical attention. Fever is usual; shaking chills may occur. The knee is the most commonly affected joint and is generally painful and swollen. Fluid can be found in most infected joints, and limitation of motion is marked. In some cases, however, particularly among patients with underlying rheumatoid arthritis who are receiving corticosteroids, physical findings indicating infection may be subtle. In these individuals, who are at particular risk for septic arthritis, superimposed infection may be difficult to distinguish from a flare-up of underlying disease. Symmetric symptoms in multiple joints are more indicative of a rheumatoid flare-up. Approximately 10% of cases of septic arthritis, however, involve more than one joint.

Differential Diagnosis of Acute Monoarticular or Oligoarticular Arthritis

Crystal deposition (uric acid gout; calcium pyrophosphate pseudogout), rheumatoid arthritis, systemic lupus erythematosus, and degenerative joint disease can also produce an acute monoarticular arthritis. Radiographs may show evidence of osteoarthritis, gouty tophi, or the linear densities of chondrocalcinosis, which are characteristic of pseudogout. All red, warm, tender joints must be aspirated. The synovial fluid should be cultured anaerobically and aerobically. A Gram-stained preparation should be examined, and a wet mount of fluid should be examined using a polarized microscope to look for crystals. Synovial fluid leukocyte counts and chemistries are of limited value in the differential diagnosis of a suspected septic joint. As a general rule, however, synovial fluid white blood cell (WBC) counts in excess of

TABLE 104-1   Infective Arthritis—Acute

	Etiologic Agent	Characteristics
Bacterial	*Staphylococcus aureus*	Most common overall; usually monarticular, large joint involvement
	Neisseria gonorrhoeae	Most common in young, sexually active adults; commonly polyarticular in onset; often associated with skin lesions
	Pseudomonas aeruginosa	Largely restricted to intravenous drug users; often involves sternoclavicular joint
Viral	Hepatitis B, rubella, mumps, parvovirus	Usually polyarticular, with minimal joint effusions, normal peripheral white blood cell count

$100,000/\mu L$ suggest either infection or crystal-induced disease (see Table 78–3). Blood cultures should be obtained in all cases of suspected septic arthritis.

Treatment

The two major modalities for treatment of acute septic arthritis are drainage and antibiotics. The first needle aspiration of a septic joint should remove as much fluid as possible. Initial antibiotic choice should be based on the clinical presentation and the results of the Gram stain. Staphylococcal infection can be treated with penicillinase-resistant penicillin or vancomycin. Gonococcal infections should be treated with ceftriaxone, 1 g every 24 hours for 10 days. Arthritis caused by gram-negative rods should be treated with an aminoglycoside or a quinolone such as ciprofloxacin plus another drug active against gram-negative bacilli, such as a cephalosporin. In intravenous drug users, the second drug should be active against *Pseudomonas;* therefore, an extended-spectrum penicillin, such as piperacillin, or a third-generation cephalosporin, such as ceftazidime, is indicated. Arthritis caused by *S. aureus* or gram-negative bacilli should be treated with antibiotics for 4 to 6 weeks. Otherwise, 2 to 3 weeks of antibiotic treatment is sufficient to eradicate infection.

Septic joints (with the notable exception of joints infected with the gonococcus) generally reaccumulate fluid after treatment is initiated. These reaccumulations must be removed by repeated needle aspirations as often as necessary. Indications for open surgical drainage of the joint include failure of the synovial fluid white blood cell count to fall after 5 days of antibiotic treatment and repeated needle aspirations, and the presence of loculated fluid within the joint. Septic arthritis of the hip is generally drained surgically because of the difficulty and potential hazard of repeated needle aspirations of this joint. Early surgical drainage also should be considered for joint infections with gram-negative rods and with *S. aureus*. Osteomyelitis is an uncommon complication of untreated or inadequately treated septic arthritis. In instances in which the diagnosis and treatment have been delayed, radiographs of the involved joint should be obtained at the beginning and termination of treatment.

POLYARTICULAR ARTHRITIS

Arthritis involving multiple joints is infrequently attributable to direct microbial invasion. In many instances, a polyarticular arthritis represents an immunologically mediated process. Acute rheumatic fever, a delayed immune-mediated response to group A streptococcal infection, may manifest as a migratory, asymmetric arthritis of the knees, ankles, elbows, and wrists. Heart involvement, subcutaneous nodules, or erythema marginatum is present in a minority of cases. Most patients have serologic evidence of recent streptococcal infection. Antistreptolysin-O, anti-DNAse, and antihyaluronidase antibodies are usually present. The importance of making this diagnosis lies primarily in the requirement for long-term prophylaxis against streptococcal infection and the clinical response of this process to salicylates.

Viral infections including hepatitis B, rubella, parvovirus, and mumps may be associated with polyarthritis. In mumps and rubella, the arthritis results from direct infection of articular tissue; with hepatitis B, the joint inflammation is a secondary result of the host immune response to the virus. These processes are self-limited. Serum sickness, polyarticular gout, sarcoidosis, rheumatoid arthritis, and other connective tissue disorders must be considered in the differential diagnosis. Because 10% of cases of septic arthritis involve more than one joint, all acutely inflamed joints containing fluid should be tapped to exclude bacterial infection.

Disseminated gonococcal infection (see Chapter 107) may manifest with fever, tenosynovitis, or arthritis involving several joints and a characteristic rash. The rash may be petechial but usually consists of a few to a few dozen pustules on an erythematous base. Cultures of the joint fluid are usually negative at this stage, but blood cultures are often positive; Gram's stain of a pustule may reveal the pathogen. Ceftriaxone, 1 g/day for 10 days, is curative.

CHRONIC ARTHRITIS

Mycobacteria and fungi may produce an indolent, slowly progressive arthritis, usually involving only one joint or contiguous joints, such as those of the wrist and hand (Table 104–2). Fever may be low grade or absent. Cultures of joint fluid may be negative. Some patients with

TABLE 104-2 Causes of Infective
Arthritis—Chronic

Tuberculosis
Nontuberculous mycobacteria
Fungi
Lyme disease (oligoarticular)

tuberculous arthritis have no evidence of active disease in the lungs. As a general rule, patients with inflammatory chronic monoarticular arthritis should have a synovial biopsy for culture and histology. Granulomas indicate the likelihood of fungal or mycobacterial infection. Cultures should confirm the diagnosis.

Fungal arthritis is treated with amphotericin B. Mycobacterial arthritis must be treated for 18 months with at least two drugs active against the isolate. Because some mycobacterial isolates causing joint disease are nontuberculous, extensive susceptibility testing may be needed to guide antimicrobial therapy.

A spirochete, *Borrelia burgdorferi,* is the pathogen responsible for Lyme disease. Several months to 2 years after the bite of the ixodid tick and the characteristic rash of erythema chronicum migrans, some patients develop an intermittent arthritis involving one or more joints, usually including the knees. This chronic arthritis may result in joint destruction, but fever is unusual. Treatment with intravenous ceftriaxone, 2 g/day for 14 to 21 days, will halt the progression of disease in the majority of cases (see Chapter 95).

Septic Bursitis

Septic bursitis is almost always caused by *Staphylococcus aureus* and involves either the olecranon or the prepatellar bursa. In most instances, there is a history of antecedent infection or irritation of the skin overlying the bursa. On examination, the skin over the bursa is red and often peeling. The bursa has a doughy consistency and fluid may be present on careful examination. Needle aspiration or surgical drainage and antistaphylococcal antibiotics are generally curative. Occasionally, long courses of antibiotics (>4 weeks) may be required for cure.

Osteomyelitis

Infections of the bone occur either as a result of hematogenous spread or through extension of local infection.

HEMATOGENOUS OSTEOMYELITIS

This infection occurs most commonly in the long bones or vertebral bodies (Table 104–3). The peak age distributions are in childhood and old age. Individuals predisposed to hematogenous osteomyelitis include intrave-

nous drug users, who are at risk for infections with *S. aureus* and *P. aeruginosa,* and patients with hemoglobinopathy, in whom nontyphoidal salmonellae often infect infarcted regions of bone. *Staphylococcus epidermidis* has emerged as an important nosocomial pathogen among patients with infected intravenous catheters. Like patients with septic arthritis, patients with hematogenous osteomyelitis often give a history of trauma antedating symptoms of infection, suggesting that transient, unrecognized bacteremia might result in infection of traumatized tissue.

Patients with acute hematogenous osteomyelitis generally present with acute onset of pain, tenderness, and fever; there may also be soft tissue swelling over the affected bone. In most instances, physical examination distinguishes acute osteomyelitis from septic arthritis, because range of joint motion is preserved in osteomyelitis. In the first 2 weeks of illness, roentgenograms may be negative or show only soft tissue swelling; technetium scans or gallium scans are almost always positive, but technetium scans may also be positive in the setting of increased vascularity or increased bone formation of any etiology. Magnetic resonance imaging demonstrates bone erosion with a decreased signal intensity on T1-weighted images and generally an increased signal intensity on T2-weighted images before it is apparent on plain films. After 2 weeks of infection, plain radiographs generally show some abnormality, and untreated osteomyelitis may produce areas of periosteal elevation or erosion followed by increased bone formation (sclerosis). The erythrocyte sedimentation rate is generally elevated, as is the white blood cell count.

A patient with back pain and fever must be considered to have a serious infection until proven otherwise. Spasm of the paravertebral muscles is common in patients with vertebral osteomyelitis but nonspecific. Point tenderness over bone suggests the presence of local infection. A good history should be obtained and a careful neurologic examination performed. Abnormalities of bowel or bladder or of strength or sensation in the lower extremities suggest the possibility of spinal cord involvement by means of spinal epidural abscess with or without osteomyelitis. Acute spinal epidural abscess is a surgical emergency. The challenge is to make the diagnosis before neurologic signs appear (see Chapter 127). Magnetic resonance imaging provides excellent definition of epidural or paravertebral abscess and is the diagnostic procedure of choice. Demonstration of an epidural abscess mandates prompt intervention, either by

TABLE 104-3 Factors Predisposing to
Hematogenous Osteomyelitis

Setting	Likely Pathogens
Intravenous drug use	*Staphylococcus aureus*
	Pseudomonas aeruginosa
Intravenous catheters	*Staphylococcus aureus*
	Staphylococcus epidermidis
	Candida species
Urinary tract infection	Enterobacteriaceae

surgical intervention or, in selected cases, by computed tomographic–guided drainage. As an alternative, emergency myelography can confirm the diagnosis.

Although most cases of hematogenous osteomyelitis have an acute presentation, some cases, particularly those involving the vertebral bodies among intravenous drug users, may have an indolent course. These patients may have an illness of more than 1 year's duration characterized by pain and low-grade fever. Radiographs are abnormal but may show only collapse of a vertebral body. This most often occurs in infections with *P. aeruginosa,* but *Candida* species and *S. aureus* may also occasionally present in this manner.

Blood cultures are positive in about half of acute cases of osteomyelitis. Patients with acute osteomyelitis should have a needle biopsy and culture of the involved bone unless blood culture results are known beforehand. Antibiotic treatment should be continued for 4 to 6 weeks, using agents active against the pathogen.

OSTEOMYELITIS SECONDARY TO EXTENSION OF LOCAL INFECTION

Local infection predisposes to osteomyelitis in several major settings (Table 104–4). The first is after penetrating trauma or surgery where local infection gains access to traumatized bone. In postsurgical infections, staphylococci and gram-negative bacilli predominate. Generally, there is evidence of wound infection with erythema, swelling, increased postoperative tenderness, and drainage. A traumatic incident often associated with osteomyelitis is either a human or an animal bite. Human bites, if deep enough, may result in osteomyelitis caused by anaerobic mouth flora. Cat bites notoriously result in the development of osteomyelitis because the thin, sharp, long cat's teeth often penetrate the periosteum. *Pasteurella multocida* is a frequent pathogen in this setting. A 4- to 6-week course of penicillin G, 10 million U/day, is indicated.

The intimate relationship of the teeth and periodontal tissues to the bones of the maxilla and mandible may predispose to osteomyelitis after local infection. Debridement of necrotic tissue and penicillin constitute the treatment of choice, because penicillin-sensitive anaerobes are the usual agents of these infections.

TABLE 104–4   Osteomyelitis Secondary to Contiguous Spread

Setting	Likely Microorganisms
Surgery, trauma	*Staphylococcus aureus* Aerobic gram-negative bacilli
Cat or dog bites	*Pasteurella multocida*
Human bites	Penicillin-sensitive anaerobes
Periodontal infections	Penicillin-sensitive anaerobes
Cutaneous ulcers	Mixed aerobic and anaerobic organisms

The third setting in which local infection predisposes to osteomyelitis is that of an infected sore or ulcer. Pressure sores of the sacrum or femoral region may erode into contiguous bone and produce an osteomyelitis (see Chapter 101) because of a mixed flora containing anaerobic organisms. Patients with diabetes mellitus often develop ulcerations of their toes and feet, with eventual development of osteomyelitis. Anaerobes, streptococci, staphylococci, and gram-negative bacilli are often involved in these infections (see Chapter 101). Treatment involves debridement (often amputation in the case of diabetics) and antibiotics active against the pathogens involved.

CHRONIC OSTEOMYELITIS

Untreated or inadequately treated osteomyelitis results in avascular necrosis of bone and the formation of islands of nonvascularized and infected bone called sequestra. Patients with chronic osteomyelitis may tolerate their infection reasonably well, with intermittent episodes of disease activity manifested by increased local pain and the development of drainage of infected material through a sinus tract. Some patients have tolerated chronic osteomyelitis for decades. A normochromic normocytic anemia of chronic disease is common in this setting, and occasionally amyloidosis and, in rare cases, osteogenic sarcoma complicate this disorder.

S. aureus is responsible for the great majority of cases of chronic osteomyelitis; the major exception is among patients with sickle cell anemia, in whom nontyphoidal salmonellae may cause chronic infection of the long bones.

Cultures of sinus tract drainage do not reliably reflect the pathogens involved in the infection. Diagnosis and cure are best effected by surgical debridement of necrotic material followed by long-term administration of antibiotics active against the organism found in the surgical specimens.

Mycobacteria, especially *Mycobacterium tuberculosis,* can produce a chronic osteomyelitis. The anterior portions of vertebral bodies are the most common sites of infection. Hematogenous dissemination and lymphatic spread are the most likely routes of infection. Paravertebral abscess (often termed *cold abscess* because of lack of signs of acute inflammation) may complicate this infection. Diagnosis is usually confirmed by histologic examination and culture of biopsy material. Treatment with antituberculous drugs is usually curative.

REFERENCES

Baker DG, Shumacher HR: Acute monoarthritis. N Engl J Med 1995; 329:1013–1020.
Brause BD: Osteomyelitis. *In* Goldman L, Bennett JC (eds): Cecil Textbook of Medicine, 21st ed. Philadelphia: WB Saunders, 2000, pp 1662–1664.
Goldenberg DL, Reed JI: Bacterial arthritis. N Engl J Med 1985; 312: 764–770.

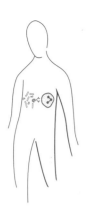

105

INFECTIONS OF THE URINARY TRACT

Michael M. Lederman

The urethra, bladder, kidneys, and prostate are all susceptible to infection. Most urinary tract infections (UTIs) cause local symptoms, yet clinical manifestations do not always pinpoint the site of infection. In addition, the criteria used by different clinical laboratories to confirm infection of the urinary tract are variable. The purpose of this chapter is to simplify the clinical and laboratory approach to diagnosis and treatment of UTIs. Infections associated with indwelling urinary catheters are discussed in Chapter 106.

Urethritis

Urethritis is predominantly an infection of sexually active individuals, usually men. The symptoms are pain and burning of the urethra during urination, and there is generally some discharge at the urethral meatus. Urethritis may be gonococcal in origin. However, nongonococcal urethritis is now more frequent in North America. Nongonococcal urethritis may be caused by *Chlamydia trachomatis* or *Ureaplasma urealyticum* and less commonly by *Trichomonas vaginalis* or herpesviruses. Diagnosis and management of urethritis are considered in Chapter 107.

Cystitis and Pyelonephritis

EPIDEMIOLOGY

Bacterial infection of the bladder (cystitis) and kidney (pyelonephritis) is more frequent in women, and the incidence of infection increases with age. Factors that predispose to UTI include instrumentation (e.g., catheterization, cystoscopy), pregnancy, anatomic abnormalities of the genitourinary tract, and diabetes mellitus.

PATHOGENESIS

Although some infections of the kidney may arise as the result of hematogenous dissemination, most UTIs ascend through a portal of entry in the urethra. Most pathogens responsible for community-acquired UTIs are part of the patient's normal bowel flora. *Escherichia coli* is the most common isolate; and, in women, colonization of the vaginal and periurethral mucosa may antedate infection of the urinary tract. Bacteria capable of adherence to epithelial cells are more likely to cause UTIs. The longer and protected male urethra may account for the lower incidence of UTI in men. Motile bacteria may swim upstream, and reflux of urine from the bladder into the ureters may predispose to the development of kidney infection.

CLINICAL FEATURES

Suprapubic pain, discomfort, or burning sensation on urination and frequency of urination are common symptoms of infection of the urinary tract. Back or flank pain or the occurrence of fever suggests that infection is not limited to the bladder (cystitis) but involves the kidney (pyelonephritis) or prostate as well. However, clinical presentation often fails to distinguish between simple cystitis and pyelonephritis. Approximately one half of infections that appear clinically to involve the bladder can be shown by instrumentation and other specialized techniques to affect the kidneys. Elderly or debilitated patients with infection of the urinary tract may have no symptoms referable to the urinary tract and may present only with fever, altered mental status, or hypotension.

LABORATORY DIAGNOSIS

Analysis of a midstream urine sample obtained from patients with infection of the bladder or kidney shows white blood cells (WBCs) and may also reveal red blood cells and slightly increased amounts of protein. The presence of an increased number of WBCs (pyuria) in a midstream urine sample indicates the likelihood of a UTI. However, because most laboratories count WBCs by examining the sediment of a centrifuged urine sample, and since the urinary WBC count may vary according to the degree of urine concentration, quantitation of pyuria is imprecise. As a general rule, more than 5 to 10 WBCs per high-power field on a centrifuged specimen of urine is abnormal. Resuspending a sedimented urine should be done gently with a Pasteur pipette so that casts are not disrupted. The presence of WBC casts in an infected urine sample indicates the presence of pyelonephritis. Bacteria may be seen in sedimented urine and can be readily identified by means of Gram's stain.

At present, most clinical laboratories consider bacterial growth of greater than 10^5 colony-forming units/mL to be indicative of infection. Studies have indicated that smaller numbers of bacteria also can produce UTIs. A hazard in interpreting results of urine culture is that if the sample is allowed to stand at room temperature for a few hours before being cultured, bacteria can multiply. This results in spuriously high bacterial counts. For this reason, urine for culture should not be obtained from a catheter bag. Specimens that are not plated immediately should be refrigerated. Biochemical tests to detect bacteriuria are not reliable.

TREATMENT AND OUTCOME

Most patients with cystitis are cured by a single high dose of antibiotic (e.g., one double-strength trimethoprim-sulfamethoxazole tablet or norfloxacin, 800 mg). Culture and sensitivity confirm the diagnosis and ascertain if the antibiotic is active against the pathogen. Because of the difficulty in clinical distinction between cystitis and upper urinary tract disease, some patients treated for cystitis with a single dose of an antibiotic may experience relapse because of unrecognized upper urinary tract disease.

Occasionally, urine cultures obtained from a patient with symptoms of UTI and pyuria are reported as exhibiting "no growth" or "insignificant growth." This situation has been labeled the "urethral syndrome." Low numbers of bacteria (as few as 100/mL of urine) may produce such infections of the urinary tract. In other instances, the urethral syndrome may be caused by *Chlamydia* or *Ureaplasma*, which will not grow on routine culture media. Thus, if a patient with the urethral syndrome has responded to antibiotics, the course should be completed; otherwise, if symptoms and pyuria persist, the patient should receive a 7- to 10-day course of tetracycline, which is active against *Chlamydia* and *Ureaplasma*. Other considerations for patients with lower urinary tract symptoms and no or "insignificant" growth on cultures of urine include vaginitis, herpes simplex infection, and gonococcal infection. (*Neisseria gonorrhoeae* will not grow on routine media used for urine culture.) Thus, a pelvic examination and culture for gonococci may be indicated in this setting if the patient is sexually active. Men with urethral discomfort and discharge should be evaluated for urethritis (see Chapter 107). Men with suprapubic pain, frequency,

and urgency should be evaluated for cystitis, as discussed earlier.

The presence of fever suggests that infection involves more than just the bladder. Young, otherwise healthy, febrile patients with UTI may be treated on an ambulatory basis with trimethoprim-sulfamethoxazole or a fluoroquinolone for 2 weeks, provided that (1) they do not appear toxic, (2) they are able to take oral fluids and medications, (3) they have friends or family at home, (4) they have good provisions for follow-up, and (5) they have no potentially complicating features, such as diabetes mellitus, history of renal stones, history of obstructive disease of the urinary tract, or sickle cell disease. Gram's stain of urine in patients hospitalized for pyelonephritis will guide initial therapy. Gram-negative rod infection may be treated initially with an aminoglycoside plus ampicillin/sulbactam or a cephalosporin. The aminoglycoside should be promptly discontinued if antibiotic sensitivity studies indicate that it is not essential. The finding of gram-positive cocci in chains suggests that enterococci are the pathogens. This infection should be treated, at least initially, with ampicillin plus an aminoglycoside. Gram-positive cocci in clusters may indicate staphylococci. *Staphylococcus saprophyticus* is a likely agent in otherwise healthy women and is sensitive to most antibiotics used in the treatment of UTI. In the older patient, *Staphylococcus aureus* should be considered, and this infection may be treated with a penicillinase-resistant penicillin, such as nafcillin. Gram-positive cocci in the urine may represent endocarditis with septic embolization to the kidney.

Therapy should be simplified when reports of antimicrobial susceptibility are available. A repeat urine culture after 2 days of effective treatment should show sterilization, or a marked decrease in the urinary bacterial count. If the patient fails to demonstrate some clinical improvement after 2 to 3 days of treatment, or presents with the clinical picture of sepsis and has been febrile for more than 1 week, a complicating feature should be suspected. Intranephric or perinephric abscess or obstruction caused by a stone or an enlarged prostate may underlie this presentation. Plain films of the abdomen may occasionally show a radiopaque stone, but ultrasonography is a good first diagnostic procedure in this setting. This will generally detect obstruction and collections of pus and will also detect stones greater than 3 mm in diameter. If ultrasonography is negative in this setting, computed tomography is indicated. Obstruction must be relieved and abscesses drained to result in cure. Computed tomographic–guided percutaneous drainage is the procedure of choice whenever possible.

All patients with complicated UTI should have repeat urine cultures 1 to 2 weeks after treatment is completed to check for relapse. If relapse occurs, the patient may have pyelonephritis, prostatitis, or neuropathic or structural disease of the urinary tract. If a 6-week course of antibiotics active against the bacterial isolate is not effective in eradicating infection, the possibility of structural abnormalities or prostatic infection should be investigated. Urologic evaluation should be performed for all men with UTI (except urethritis) because of the high frequency of correctable anatomic lesions in this population.

Some women have frequent episodes of UTI that are caused by different bacterial isolates. In some instances, these reinfections are related to sexual activity. Prompt voiding and a single dose of an active antibiotic such as cephalexin just after sexual contact can decrease the reinfection rate in these women. In other women, in whom no precipitating factor can be found and infections are frequent, prophylaxis with one half of a tablet of trimethoprim-sulfamethoxazole nightly has been effective.

On occasion, urine cultures show bacterial growth in the absence of symptoms. If the sample has been obtained properly and repeat culture reveals the same organism, this is termed *asymptomatic bacteriuria*. This condition is generally observed in elderly or middle-aged individuals and, in the absence of structural disease of the urinary tract or diabetes mellitus, does not require treatment. Asymptomatic bacteriuria occurring during pregnancy or in immunocompromised patients should be treated because of the high risk of pyelonephritis in these settings.

The occurrence of pyuria in the absence of bacterial growth on culture of urine ($< 10^2$ colonies/mL) may be termed *sterile pyuria*. If this occurs in the patient with lower urinary tract symptoms, chlamydial or gonococcal infection, vaginitis, or herpes simplex infection should be considered. In the absence of lower urinary tract symptoms, sterile pyuria may be seen among patients with interstitial nephritis of numerous causes or with tuberculosis of the urinary tract. Patients with renal tuberculosis often have nocturia and polyuria. More than half of male patients also have involvement of the genital tract, most commonly the epididymis. Diagnosis can be made by biopsy of genital masses, when present, and by three morning cultures of urine for mycobacteria.

Prostatitis

Although prostatic fluid has antibacterial properties, the prostate can become infected, usually by direct invasion through the urethra. Symptoms of back or perineal pain and fever are common. Some patients have pain with ejaculation. Rectal examination usually shows a tender prostate. Patients with acute prostatitis generally have an abnormal urinary sediment and pathogenic bacteria (usually gram-negative enteric rods) in cultures of urine.

Acute prostatitis may be caused by the gonococcus but is most often caused by gram-negative bacilli. Treatment is directed against the pathogen observed on Gram's stain of urine and is generally effective. Chronic prostatitis may be asymptomatic and should be suspected in men with recurrent UTI. The urine sediment may be relatively benign in patients with chronic prostatitis. In this instance, comparison of the first part of the urine sample, midstream urine, excretions expressed by massage of the prostate, and postmassage urine should reveal bacterial counts more than 10-fold greater in the prostatic secretions and postmassage urine samples than in first-void and midstream samples. Treatment of chronic prostatitis is hampered by poor penetration of the prostate by most antimicrobial agents. Long-term (4 to 12 weeks) treatment with a fluoroquinolone or trimethoprim-sulfamethoxazole is indicated and is effective in a minority of cases.

REFERENCES

Komaroff AL: Acute dysuria in women. N Engl J Med 1984; 310:368–374.

Kunin CM: Urinary tract infections and pyelonephritis. *In* Goldman L, Bennett JC (eds): Cecil Textbook of Medicine, 21st ed. Philadelphia: WB Saunders, 2000, pp 613–617.

Stam WE, Horton TM: Management of urinary tract infection in adults. N Engl J Med 1993; 329:1328–1334.

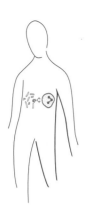

106

NOSOCOMIAL INFECTIONS

Michael M. Lederman

A nosocomial or hospital-acquired infection is an infection not present on admission to the hospital that first appears 72 hours or more after hospitalization. A patient admitted to a hospital in the United States has a 5% to 10% chance of developing a nosocomial infection. These infections result in significant morbidity and mortality (approximately 1% of these infections are fatal, and an additional 4% contribute to death) and greatly increased medical costs (approximately $10 billion per year).

Numerous factors are associated with a greater risk of acquiring a nosocomial infection. These include factors that are not avoidable by optimal medical practice, such as age and severity of underlying illness. Contributing factors that can be minimized by thoughtful management of the patient include prolonged duration of hospitalization, the inappropriate use of broad-spectrum antibiotics, the prolonged use of indwelling catheters, and the failure of health care personnel to wash their hands.

Infection Control

Hospitals now have teams charged with surveillance of nosocomial infections and the implementation of practices to limit these occurrences. These practices include isolation of patients with specific infectious diseases or impairments of host defenses and the education of hospital staff to ensure appropriate compliance with infection control practices, such as the simple rule that hands must be washed before and after examining every patient. In addition, all hospitals now must employ "universal precautions" that consider all blood and certain body fluids (e.g., cerebrospinal, amniotic, perivisceral, seminal, vaginal, and blood-contaminated) as potentially infectious. Gloves must be worn when exposure to these fluids, nonintact skin, or mucosal surfaces is expected, and masks and gowns are worn when splashes are expected.

Approach to the Hospitalized Patient with Possible Nosocomial Infection

The first clue to the presence of a nosocomial infection is often a rise in temperature. The only sign of infection, particularly in the elderly or demented patient, may be a change in mental status (Table 106–1). Some patients with serious infection do not initially develop fever but instead become tachypneic or confused for no apparent reason. Analysis of arterial blood gases may show at first a respiratory alkalosis, followed by a metabolic acidosis caused by increased levels of lactate. Arterial oxygen content may be normal or depressed.

When evaluating a hospitalized patient for a new fever (Table 106–2) or suspected nosocomial infection, the physician should first assess the stability of the patient. Hypotension, tachypnea, or new obtundation mandates rapid evaluation and treatment. The patient's problem list must be reviewed; the physician must ascertain if the patient was recently subjected to a potentially hazardous intervention (e.g., genitourinary tract instrumentation or administration of blood products). If the patient can cooperate, the physician should elicit a history directed at possible causes of the fever. Often the patient has a specific complaint that helps identify the source of the fever. The skin must be examined carefully. Maculopapular rashes often accompany drug fevers; ecthyma gangrenosum can be a sign of gram-negative sepsis (see Chapter 96). Surgical wounds should be examined for the presence of infection. Among debilitated patients, pressure sores located near the sacrum or over the greater trochanters may become infected and produce fever. Abscesses at these sites may be covered by a necrotic membrane, so that exploration with a gloved finger or sterile needle may be required to demonstrate a focus of pus. Patients receiving multiple intramuscular injections may develop fever as a result of the development of sterile abscesses at the injection sites. Headache or sinus tenderness may be present in patients with sinusitis; this can be a problem among patients after nasogastric or nasotracheal intubation. Nuchal rigidity may be a sign of nosocomial meningitis, although it is absent in some cases, particularly after neurosurgery or head trauma. Furthermore, generalized rigidity is often seen in elderly demented patients without central nervous system infection. The physician should examine the nose and oropharynx and look for symptoms of viral upper respiratory tract infections, because these do occur in hospitals. A pleural friction rub may indicate a recent pulmonary thromboembolism as a cause of fever. Crackles or other evidence of consolidation may indicate a nosocomial pneumonia, and basilar crackles, egophony, and bronchial breath sounds can be caused by atelectasis in debilitated patients. A new S_4 gallop or pericardial friction rub may be the only clinical manifestation of a myocardial infarction.

The abdomen is also a source of fever in the hospitalized patient. The patient with antibiotic-induced colitis generally has fever, diarrhea, and abdominal pain. Leukocytosis is common. Patients with indwelling urinary catheters are at particular risk of infection. The urine should be examined, looking for white blood cells and bacteria. Catheterized men should undergo careful examination of the prostate in a search for tenderness or a mass suggestive of prostatic infection or abscess.

The extremities must be examined carefully, particularly the sites of current and old intravenous catheter placements, for evidence of phlebitis. If no other source of fever is found and an intravenous catheter has been in place, it should be replaced and a segment of the catheter should be rolled on an agar plate for culture.

Deep vein thrombophlebitis and pulmonary thromboemboli are life-threatening complications of hospitalization whose only clinical manifestations may be fever. The lower extremities should be examined and measured carefully. An asymmetry in leg or calf circumference, which may not be obvious without a measurement, may be an important clue to an underlying thrombosis. Crystal-induced arthritis is another potential source of fever in a hospitalized patient. Gout and pseudogout may be precipitated by acute infections.

The patient's medication list should be reviewed for drugs likely to produce fever. In this regard, antimicrobial agents (particularly penicillins, sulfa drugs, and cephalosporins) are among the most common causes of drug-induced fevers. A drug fever can occur at any time but usually occurs during the second week of drug administration. A review of the peripheral blood smear can give important clues to the cause of the fever. Eosinophilia may suggest a drug reaction, and lymphocytosis may suggest a viral process. A left shift and vacuolization within neutrophils suggest a bacterial infection. Unless the cause of the fever is apparent, cultures of blood and urine and a chest radiograph should be obtained.

Nosocomial Pneumonia

Although some hospital-acquired pneumonias occur as a result of bacteremic spread, the vast majority occur by means of aspiration of oropharyngeal contents. The oropharynx of the patient admitted to the hospital rapidly becomes colonized with aerobic gram-negative bacilli and often staphylococci. The administration of broad-spectrum antibiotics, severe underlying illness (e.g., chronic lung disease), respiratory intubation, advanced age, and prolonged duration of hospitalization predispose to colonization.

Sedation, loss of consciousness, and other factors that depress the gag and cough reflexes place the colonized patient at greater risk for aspiration and the development of nosocomial pneumonia. The development of a new pulmonary infiltrate in a hospitalized patient may represent pneumonia, atelectasis, aspiration of gastric contents, drug reaction, or pulmonary infarction. If pneumonia is suspected, prompt definition of the pathogen and appropriate treatment are critical, because nosocomial pneumonia carries a 20% to 50% mortality. If the patient cannot produce a sputum specimen adequate for interpretation, nasotracheal aspiration should be performed (see Chapter 99). Antibiotic therapy is guided by the results of Gram's stain of the sputum or of the aspirate. Gram-negative rods are the predominant pathogens in this setting; these infections should be treated with a fluoroquinolone or aminoglycoside plus an extended-spectrum penicillin or cephalosporin until results of culture and sensitivity testing are known. If gram-positive cocci in clusters are seen, vancomycin should be administered; a mixed flora suggestive of aspiration of oral anaerobes should prompt treatment with clindamycin or a penicillin/β-lactamase inhibitor combination such as piperacillin-tazobactam. In certain hospitals, nosocomial pneumonia caused by *Legionella* species is frequent, and erythromycin should be included in the initial treatment regimen. (*Legionella* species are rarely

TABLE 106–2   Common Causes of Fever in the Hospitalized Patient

Pneumonia
Catheter-related infection
Surgical wound infection
Urinary tract infection
Drugs
Pulmonary emboli
Infected pressure sores

TABLE 106–1   Signs of Infection in the Hospitalized Patient

Fever
Change in mental status
Tachypnea
Hypotension
Oliguria
Leukocytosis

detectable on Gram's stain.) Patients with nosocomial pneumonia should also receive respiratory therapy consisting of clapping, postural drainage, and promotion of coughing to assist in bringing up secretions.

The patient in the intensive care unit with an endotracheal tube in place is at particular risk for nosocomial pneumonia. This patient has an ineffective gag reflex and often a depressed cough as well. Many are paralyzed to facilitate ventilator-dependent respiration. The patient is therefore entirely dependent on suctioning by the staff to clear secretions from the airways. The airways of these patients become rapidly colonized with bacteria. Epidemics of nosocomial pneumonia have sometimes been associated with contamination of tubing and machinery used for ventilation or respiratory therapy, but infection is often caused by transmission of pathogens on the hands of medical personnel. Large-volume nebulizers, when contaminated, are also capable of delivering droplets containing bacteria to the lower respiratory tract. Patients whose airways are simply colonized but whose lower respiratory tracts are not infected should not be treated with antibiotics, despite positive sputum cultures. Premature treatment of colonization results in replacement of the initial colonists by more resistant organisms, whereas delay in treatment of nosocomial pneumonia can result in death from overwhelming infection. The physician must therefore be able to distinguish accurately between colonization and infection. The development of new fever, leukocytosis, pulmonary infiltrate, or deterioration of respiratory status as ascertained by blood gas determinations suggests pneumonia rather than colonization. A Gram stain of sputum should be performed to identify the predominant organism or organisms. A potassium hydroxide (KOH) preparation of sputum may identify elastin fibers indicative of necrotizing pneumonia. The appearance of these fibers may actually precede the development of infiltrates on chest radiograph. This test, however, detects fewer than one half of nosocomial pneumonias in the intensive care unit.

Nosocomial pneumonias are best prevented by (1) avoiding excessive sedation, (2) providing frequent suctioning and respiratory therapy—drainage and clapping—to patients who have difficulty managing secretions, (3) avoiding the use of large-volume reservoir nebulizers, (4) avoiding the injudicious use of broad-spectrum or high-dose antibiotic therapy, (5) frequent hand washing by medical and nursing personnel, and (6) weaning the patient from mechanical respiratory support as soon as possible.

Intravascular Catheter–Related Infections

Infections related to intravascular catheters may occur by means of bacteremic seeding or through infusion of contaminated material, but the vast majority of these infections occur through bacterial invasion at the site of catheter insertion.

Intravenous catheters may produce a sterile phlebitis. Certain drugs such as tetracycline or erythromycin, when administered intravenously, are particularly likely to produce phlebitis. Bacteria migrating through the catheter insertion site may colonize the catheter and then produce a septic phlebitis or bacteremia without evidence of local infection. Factors associated with a greater risk of intravenous catheter–related infection are shown in Table 106–3. *Staphylococcus epidermidis* and *Staphylococcus aureus* are the predominant pathogens in this setting, followed by the enteric gram-negative rods. A peripheral catheter (and all readily removable foreign bodies) should be replaced if bacteremia occurs and no other primary site of infection is found. The catheter should also be removed if fever without an obvious source occurs or if local phlebitis develops. The value of culturing a peripheral catheter tip is uncertain unless semiquantitative techniques are used (i.e., rolling the catheter across an agar plate). During the evaluation of a hospital-acquired fever, an inflamed vein should be examined carefully, and after the catheter is removed, the inflamed portion of the vein should be compressed in an attempt to express pus through the catheter entry site. If pus can be expressed or the patient remains febrile or bacteremic while on appropriate antibiotics, the vein should be surgically explored and excised if septic phlebitis is found. Routine replacement of peripheral indwelling intravascular catheters every 72 hours decreases the risk of catheter-related infections.

Central venous catheters remain in place longer than peripheral catheters and are therefore associated with a greater overall infection rate. This is particularly true if total parenteral nutrition is provided by this route. Patients receiving parenteral nutrition are at particular risk for systemic infection with *Candida* species and gram-negative bacilli as well as with staphylococci. Pus at the catheter insertion site or positive blood cultures without another source are indications for catheter removal. In an attempt to decrease percutaneous spread of bacteria to intravascular sites, most centers are now placing long Silastic catheters into the subclavian vein after subcutaneous tunneling. These catheters may be kept in place for prolonged periods with a lower infection risk. As a general rule, persistent bacteremia while the patient is taking appropriate antibiotics, recurrent bacteremia, and fungemia with *Candida* or related yeasts are indications for removal of these catheters.

TABLE 106–3 **Factors Associated with Greater Risks of Intravenous Catheter-Related Infection**

Failure of staff to wash hands
Duration of catheterization > 72 hr
Plastic catheter > steel needle
Lower extremities and groin > upper extremity
Cutdown > percutaneous insertion
Emergency > elective insertion
Breakdown in skin integrity (e.g., burns)
Inserted by physician > intravenous therapy teams

> = greater risk.

Pressure Sores

The reader is referred to Chapter 101.

Nosocomial Urinary Tract Infection

Urinary tract infections are the most common nosocomial infections, and infection of the urinary tract accounts for 15% of nosocomial bacteremias. Placement of an indwelling catheter into the urethra of a hospitalized patient facilitates access of pathogens to an ordinarily sterile site. Factors that predispose to infection are shown in Table 106–4. The most common pathogens are enteric gram-negative rods; however, among immunocompromised patients and patients receiving broad-spectrum antibiotics, *Candida* species are also important causes of infection. Prophylactic antibiotics, irrigation, urinary acidification, and use of antiseptics are of no value in prevention of infection in this setting. Nosocomial urinary tract infections can be best prevented by adherence to the following guidelines:

1. Catheterize only when necessary. (Monitoring of intake and output and urinary incontinence are generally not appropriate indications for catheterization.)
2. Remember that repeated straight ("in-and-out") catheterizations are less likely to produce infection than indwelling catheters. Many patients with dysfunctional bladders (e.g., those with multiple sclerosis) have used this technique for years without developing significant urinary tract infections. Thrice-daily straight catheterization, with the use of aseptic technique, is preferable to a chronic indwelling catheter.
3. If the use of an indwelling catheter is unavoidable, observe the following guidelines:
   a. Remove the catheter as soon as possible.
   b. Emphasize hand washing.
   c. Maintain a closed and unobstructed drainage system. (Urine specimens for culture and analysis may be obtained by inserting a 22-gauge needle aseptically through the distal end of the catheter wall.) Do not disconnect the catheter from the drainage bag.
   d. Secure the catheter in place.
   e. Keep the catheter bag below the level of the bladder.
   f. Irrigate the catheter only if it is obstructed.

Asymptomatic bacterial colonization of the catheterized bladder need not be treated. If the patient has fever or local symptoms, antibiotic treatment is indicated. *Candida* infection of the bladder often resolves once broad-spectrum antibiotics are discontinued. If *Candida* infection persists, the catheter may be changed; if infection persists, twice-daily irrigation of the bladder with amphotericin B or oral fluconazole will often eradicate the organism.

The best way to prevent catheter-related infections of the urinary tract is to avoid catheterization unless absolutely necessary.

TABLE 106–4 Factors Predisposing to Nosocomial Urinary Tract Infection

Indwelling catheters
Duration of catheterization
Open drainage (vs. closed-bag drainage)
Interruption of closed drainage system
Use of broad-spectrum antibiotics *(Candida)*

REFERENCES

Jernigan JA: Nosocomial infections. *In* Goldman L, Bennett JC (eds): Cecil Textbook of Medicine, 21st ed. Philadelphia: WB Saunders, 2000, pp 1581–1586.

Salata RA, Lederman MM, Shlaes DM, et al: Diagnosis of nosocomial pneumonia in intubated, intensive-care unit patients. Am Rev Respir Dis 1987; 135:426–432.

Warren JW: Nosocomial urinary tract infections. *In* Mandell GL, Bennett JE, Dolin R (eds): Principles and Practice of Infectious Diseases, 5th ed. New York: Churchill Livingstone, 2000, pp 3028–3038.

107

SEXUALLY TRANSMITTED DISEASES

Robert A. Salata

Sexually transmitted diseases (STDs) are a diverse group of infections caused by multiple microbial pathogens. These infections are grouped because of common epidemiologic and clinical features. Since the mid-1980s, the field of STDs has evolved from one emphasizing the traditional venereal diseases of gonorrhea and syphilis to one concerned also with infections associated with *Chlamydia trachomatis*, herpes simplex virus, and human papillomavirus. More recently, the field has become focused on the human immunodeficiency virus (HIV).

Changes in sexual attitudes and practices have contributed to a resurgence of all venereal infections. Gonorrhea, for example, has increased in incidence in the United States since 1963; approximately 2 million cases now occur each year. The number of new cases of syphilis has increased each year since 1986. The incidence of syphilis began to decrease in homosexual males in the same period, in association with safer sex practices. The increase in cases is predominantly a result of heterosexual spread and results in part from the widespread exchange of sex for drugs.

At the outset, two common errors in approaching the patient with STD should be avoided. The first is to fail to consider that an individual is at risk for STD. All sexually active persons are at risk, not just because of their own sexual behavior but because of that of their sexual partners as well. Failure to consider risk factors often results in mistakes in diagnosis, inappropriate treatment, poor follow-up of infected sexual contacts, and, ultimately, recurrent or persistent infection. A second problem with STDs is the failure to recognize and diagnose co-infection. The most serious co-infection is with HIV. The worldwide epidemic of STDs fuels the global spread of HIV. STDs, many of which can be readily diagnosed and treated, may greatly enhance the transmission of HIV infection. HIV, in turn, may alter the natural history of other STDs.

STDs can be considered in broad groups according to whether major initial manifestations are (1) genital ulcers; (2) urethritis, cervicitis, and pelvic inflammatory disease; or (3) vaginitis. All patients with any STD should be strongly encouraged to undergo screening for HIV infection (see Chapter 108).

Genital Sores

Six infectious agents cause most genital lesions (Table 107–1). The appearance of the lesions, natural history, and laboratory findings allow a clear-cut distinction among the possible causes in most instances. The two most common and significant infections in North America are herpes simplex virus infection and syphilis.

HERPES SIMPLEX VIRUS INFECTION

Genital herpes infection has reached epidemic proportions, causing a corresponding increase in public awareness and concern. Genital herpes differs from other STDs in its tendency for spontaneous recurrence. Its importance stems from the morbidity, both physical and psychological, of the recurrent genital lesions and the danger of transmission of a fulminant, often fatal, disease to newborns.

Epidemiology

Herpes simplex virus (HSV) has a worldwide distribution. Humans are the only known reservoir of infection, which is spread by direct contact with infected secretions. Of the two types of HSV, HSV-2 is the more frequent cause of genital infection. The major risk of infection is in the 14- to 29-year-old cohort and varies with sexual activity. Prevalence rates for HSV-2 infection are as high as 40% to 50% in some North American populations.

After exposure, HSV replicates within epithelial cells and lyses them, producing a thin-walled vesicle. Multinucleated cells are formed with characteristic intranuclear inclusions. Regional lymph nodes become enlarged

TABLE 107-1   Differentiation of Diseases Causing Genital Sores

Disease	Primary Lesion	Adenopathy	Systemic Features	Diagnosis/Treatment
Herpes genitalis (primary 20% sexually active adults, due to HSV-2)	Incubation 2–7 days; multiple painful vesicles on erythematous base; persist 7–14 days	Tender, soft adenopathy, often bilateral	Fever	Tzanck smear positive; tissue culture isolation, HSV-2 antigen, fourfold rise in antibodies to HSV-2; Rx: acyclovir
Recurrent	Grouped vesicles on erythematous base, painful; last 3–10 days	None	None	Tzanck, HSV-2 antigen, tissue culture positive; titers not helpful; Rx: acyclovir
Syphilis (90,000 cases in U.S. per year, caused by *Treponema pallidum*)	Incubation 10–90 days (mean, 21); chancre: papule that ulcerates; painless, border raised, firm, ulcer indurated, base smooth; usually single; may be genital or almost anywhere; persists 3–6 wk, leaving thin, atrophic scar	One week after chancre appears; bilateral or unilateral; firm, discrete, movable, no overlying skin changes, painless, nonsuppurative; may persist for months	Later stages	Cannot be cultured; positive darkfield; VDRL positive; 77%; FTA-ABS positive, 86% (see Table 107–2)
Chancroid (2000 cases in U.S. per year, caused by *Haemophilus ducreyi*)	Incubation 3–5 days; vesicle or papule to pustule to ulcer; soft, not indurated; very painful	One week after primary in 50%; painful, unilateral (two thirds), suppurative	None	Organism in Gram's stain of pus; can be cultured (75%) but direct yields highest from lymph node; Rx: ceftriaxone, 250 mg once intramuscularly, or ciprofloxacin, 500 mg twice daily for 3 days
Lymphogranuloma venereum (600–1000 cases per year in U.S., due to *Chlamydia trachomatis*)	Incubation 5–21 days; painless papule, vesicle, ulcer, evanescent (2–3 days), noted in only 10%–40%	5–21 days post primary, one third bilateral, tender, matted iliac/femoral "groove sign"; multiple abscesses; coalescent, caseating, suppurative, sinus tracts; thick yellow pus; fistulas; strictures; genital ulcerations	Fever, arthritis, pericarditis, proctitis, meningoencephalitis, keratoconjunctivitis, preauricular adenopathy, edema of eyelids, erythema nodosum	LGV CF positive 85%–90% (1–3 wk); must have high titer (>1:16), cross reacts with other *Chlamydia;* also positive STS, rheumatoid factor, cryoglobulins; Rx: doxycycline, 100 mg twice daily for 7 days
Granuloma inguinale (50 cases in U.S. per year, caused by *Calymmatobacterium granulomatis*	Incubation 9–50 days; at least one painless papule that gradually ulcerates; ulcers are large (1–4 cm), irregular, nontender, with thickened, rolled margins and beefy red tissue at base; older portions of ulcer show depigmented scarring, while advancing edge contains new papules	No true adenopathy; in one fifth, subcutaneous spread through lymphatics leads to indurated swelling or abscesses of groin "pseudobuboes"	Metastatic infection of bones, joints, liver	Scraping or deep curetting at actively extending border; Wright's or Giemsa's stain reveals short, plump, bipolar staining; "Donovan's bodies" in macrophage vacuoles; Rx: tetracycline, 2 g/day for 21 days
Condyloma acuminatum (genital warts, frequent, due to human papillomavirus)	Characteristic large, soft, fleshy, cauliflower-like excrescences around vulva, glans, urethral orifice, anus, perineum	None	None per se; association with cervical dysplasia/neoplasia	Chief importance is distinction from syphilis and chancroid; Rx: topical podophyllin ± cryosurgery, laser resection

CF = complement fixation; FTA-ABS = fluorescent treponemal antibody absorption; HSV = herpes simplex virus; LGV = lymphogranuloma venereum; Rx = prescription; STS = serologic test for syphilis; VDRL = Venereal Disease Research Laboratory.

and tender. HSV also migrates along sensory neurons to sensory ganglia, where it assumes a latent state. Inside the sacral ganglia, HSV DNA can be demonstrated, but the virus does not replicate and is inactive metabolically. Just how viral reactivation occurs is uncertain. During reactivation, the virus appears to migrate back to skin along sensory nerves.

Clinical Presentation

Primary genital lesions develop 2 to 7 days after contact with infected secretions. In males, painful vesicles appear on the glans or penile shaft; in females, they occur on the vulva, perineum, buttocks, cervix, or vagina. A vaginal discharge frequently is present, usually accompanied by inguinal adenopathy, fever, and malaise. Sacroradiculomyelitis or aseptic meningitis can complicate primary infection. Perianal and anal HSV infections are common, particularly in male homosexuals; tenesmus and rectal discharge often are the main complaints.

The precipitating events associated with genital relapse of HSV infection are poorly understood. In individual cases, stress or menstruation may be implicated. Overall, genital recurrences develop in about 60% of HSV-infected patients. Clinically apparent recurrences are more frequent in males with HSV-2 infection. The frequency of asymptomatic cervical recurrence in women is not known. Many patients describe a characteristic prodrome of tingling or burning for 18 to 36 hours before the appearance of lesions. Recurring HSV genital lesions are fewer in number, are usually stereotyped in location, are often restricted to the genital region, heal more quickly, and are associated with few systemic complaints.

Laboratory Diagnosis

The appearance of the characteristic vesicles is strongly suggestive of HSV infection. However, diagnosis should be confirmed by a Tzanck smear (66% sensitive) (see Chapter 93), Papanicolaou smear, immunofluorescent assay for viral antigen, or viral isolation. Serologic studies for HSV can be useful in the diagnosis of primary infection. Culture remains the gold standard for diagnosis. Direct antigen detection, by means of an enzyme immunoassay test, shows greater sensitivity than culture for later-stage HSV lesions and is equivalent to culture for early-stage infection.

Treatment

Topical or oral administration of acyclovir shortens the course of primary genital HSV infection. Intravenous or oral administration is recommended for severe cases with fever, systemic symptoms, and extensive local disease. Antiviral agents do not, however, prevent the latent stage of virus and cannot prevent recurrent infections. Prophylactic oral acyclovir decreases the frequency of symptomatic recurrences by 60% to 80% when used over a 4- to 6-year period, but asymptomatic viral shedding may occur despite prophylaxis. Oral acyclovir also hastens recovery from severe recurrent epi-

sodes. New antiviral agents with excellent activity against HSV have been introduced, including valacyclovir and famciclovir. Cervical shedding of HSV from active lesions late in pregnancy, near the time of parturition, is an indication for cesarean section. This is especially true in primary HSV infection, which carries the greatest risk of neonatal infection. The risk to neonates exposed to asymptomatic shedding of HSV during parturition is uncertain.

SYPHILIS

Syphilis is of unique importance among the venereal diseases because early lesions heal without specific therapy; however, serious systemic sequelae pose a major risk to the patient, and transplacental infections can occur.

Epidemiology

Primary syphilis occurs mostly in sexually active 15- to 30-year olds, and the incidence of primary syphilis increased sharply in North America during the 1990s. Approximately 50% of the sexual contacts of a patient with primary syphilis become infected. The long incubation period of syphilis becomes a key factor in designing strategies for contact tracing and management. Unless successful follow-up seems certain, contacts of proven cases must be treated with penicillin. The most rapid increase in syphilis has occurred in groups of individuals at increased risk of HIV infection. This poses a serious problem, because the mucosal lesions of primary syphilis facilitate transmission of HIV infection (see Chapter 108). In turn, HIV appears to accelerate the course of syphilis with more rapid and frequent involvement of the neurologic system.

Pathogenesis

Treponema pallidum penetrates intact mucous membranes or abraded skin, reaches the blood stream by means of the lymphatics, and disseminates. The incubation period for the primary lesion depends on inoculum size, with a range of 3 to 90 days.

Natural History and Clinical Presentation

Primary syphilis is considered in Table 107–1. Secondary syphilis develops 6 to 8 weeks after the chancre, if it has not been treated. This time period can be accelerated in HIV-infected persons. Skin, mucous membranes, and lymph nodes are involved. Skin lesions may be macular, papular, papulosquamous, pustular, follicular, or nodular. Most commonly, they are generalized, symmetric, and of like size and appear as discrete, erythematous, macular lesions of the thorax or as red-brown hyperpigmented macules on the palms and soles. In moist intertriginous areas, large, pale, flat-topped papules coalesce to form highly infectious plaques or condylomata lata; darkfield microscopy reveals that they are teeming with spirochetes. Mucous patches are painless, dull erythematous patches or grayish-white erosions. They, too, are infectious and darkfield positive. Systemic manifestations of secondary syphilis include malaise, anorexia, weight loss, fever, sore throat, arthralgias, and generalized, nontender, discrete adenopathy. Specific organ involvement also may develop: gastritis (superficial, erosive); hepatitis; nephritis or nephrosis (immune complex–mediated); and symptomatic or asymptomatic meningitis. One fourth of patients have relapses of the mucocutaneous syndrome within 2 years of onset. Thereafter, infected patients become asymptomatic and noninfectious except through blood transfusions or transplacental spread.

Late syphilis develops after 1 to 10 years in 15% of untreated patients. The skin gumma is a superficial nodule or deep granulomatous lesion that may develop punched-out ulcers. Superficial gummas respond dramatically to therapy. Gummas also may involve bone, liver, and the cardiovascular or central nervous system. Deep-seated gummas may have serious pathophysiologic consequences; treatment of the infection often does not reverse organ dysfunction.

Gradually progressive cardiovascular syphilis begins within 10 years in more than 10% of untreated patients, most frequently men. Patients develop aortitis with medial necrosis secondary to an obliterative endarteritis of the vasa vasorum. There may be asymptomatic linear calcifications of the ascending aorta or (in decreasing frequency) aortic regurgitation, aortic aneurysms (saccular or fusiform, most commonly thoracic), or obstruction of coronary ostia.

Central nervous system syphilis develops in 8% of untreated patients 5 to 35 years after primary infection and includes meningovascular syphilis, tabes dorsalis, and general paresis (see Chapter 120). Although general paresis and tabes are classified as separate neurologic syndromes, many patients show elements of both. Late central nervous system syphilis also may be asymptomatic despite cerebrospinal fluid (CSF) abnormalities indicating active inflammation. The natural history of syphilis may be altered by co-infection with HIV. Patients with dual infections may develop signs and symptoms of secondary syphilis more rapidly, sometimes even before healing of the primary chancre (see Chapter 108).

Diagnosis and Treatment

The clinical diagnosis of syphilis must be confirmed by darkfield examination and/or serologic studies. Spirochetes are seen in darkfield preparations of chancres or moist lesions of secondary syphilis. Saprophytic treponemes confuse darkfield diagnosis of oral lesions. Serologic diagnosis is considered in Table 107–2. The differential diagnosis of primary syphilis consists of herpes simplex and three conditions that are relatively rare in the United States: chancroid, lymphogranuloma venereum, and granuloma inguinale. The characteristics of these diseases are presented in Table 107–1.

The presence of neurosyphilis requires modifying the standard antibiotic treatment of syphilis. For this reason, a lumbar puncture should be considered in all patients with latent syphilis (positive Venereal Disease Research Laboratory [VDRL] test at least 1 year after primary syphilis) or syphilis of unknown duration. An elevated CSF white blood cell count, elevated protein, and positive VDRL test on diluted samples of CSF establish the

TABLE 107–2   Serologies in Syphilis

	VDRL	FTA-ABS
Technique	Standard nontreponemal test; antibody to cardiolipin-lecithin	Standard treponemal test; antibody to Nichol's strain of *Treponema pallidum* after absorption on nontreponemal spirochetes
Indications	Screening and assessing response to therapy; should be quantified by diluting serum	Confirmation of specificity of positive VDRL; remains reactive longer than VDRL; useful or late syphilis, particularly neurosyphilis
Percent positive in syphilis		
Primary	77%	86%
Secondary	98%	100%
Early latent	95%	99%
Late latent and late	73%	96%
False positives	Weakly reactive VDRL is common (~30% of normals); positive VDRL should be repeated and, if confirmed, FTA-ABS performed; relative frequency of false positives determined by prevalence of syphilis in the population	Borderline positive is frequent (80%) in pregnancy; should be repeated

FTA-ABS = fluorescent treponemal antibody absorption; VDRL = Venereal Disease Research Laboratory.

diagnosis of neurosyphilis. A patient with persistent positive blood VDRL and a positive CSF VDRL should be considered to have neurosyphilis and treated accordingly. However, the sensitivity of CSF VDRL in proven cases of neurosyphilis is only 40% to 50%. Treatment of neurosyphilis is therefore indicated in patients with a consistent neurologic syndrome, characteristic CSF changes, and a positive serum VDRL. Because the VDRL may be negative in late syphilis, the presence of a positive serum fluorescent treponemal antibody absorption (FTA-ABS) test in a patient with a neurologic syndrome consistent with syphilis is a sufficient indication for treatment. A small proportion (2% to 3%) of patients with neurosyphilis may undergo abrupt deterioration after treatment with penicillin; this Jarisch-Herxheimer reaction, thought to represent a systemic response to penicillin-induced lysis of spirochetes, may be ameliorated by concomitant treatment with corticosteroids. This is especially important in secondary syphilis with meningeal involvement. After treatment of neurosyphilis, lumbar puncture should be repeated at 6-month intervals for 3 years to ensure adequacy of treatment, as reflected by normalization of CSF and progressive decline in CSF VDRL titer. Re-treatment may be necessary if CSF abnormalities persist or recur. Treatment protocols are shown in Table 107–3.

Serologic studies for syphilis must be followed after treatment. With the recommended treatment schedules, 1% to 5% of patients with primary syphilis will develop relapse or be reinfected. In adequately treated primary syphilis, the VDRL should become negative by 2 years after therapy (usually by 6 to 12 months). The FTA-ABS, however, often remains positive for life. Seventy-five percent of adequately treated patients with secondary syphilis will have a negative serum VDRL by 2 years. If the VDRL does not become negative or achieve a low fixed titer, lumbar puncture should be performed to evaluate the possibility of asymptomatic neurosyphilis, and the patient should be re-treated with penicillin. Two percent to 10% of patients with central nervous system syphilis will experience relapse after treatment. However, it is rare for asymptomatic patients to develop symptomatic disease after penicillin therapy;

the only major exception is the HIV-infected patient, in whom meningovascular syphilis can develop within months of the standard treatment for primary syphilis. Every patient who is treated for syphilis should be seronegative or *serofast* with a low fixed titer before termination of follow-up. If not, therapy should be repeated.

Because of the documented progression to neurosyphilis in some HIV-infected individuals who have received treatment for primary syphilis, the following approach is suggested. All patients with syphilis should be tested for HIV infection. All HIV-infected individuals should be tested for syphilis. If dual infection is likely or documented, a lumbar puncture is indicated regardless of the stage or activity of the syphilis. Any CSF abnormality warrants a 10- to 14-day course of intravenous penicillin to treat neurosyphilis. If the CSF is unremarkable, three weekly doses of benzathine penicillin plus a 10-day course of amoxicillin may be appropriate. In any event, careful clinical and laboratory follow-up is essential.

Urethritis, Cervicitis, and Pelvic Inflammatory Disease

These syndromes can be considered broadly as gonococcal and nongonococcal in etiology.

GONORRHEA

Neisseria gonorrhoeae is second only to *C. trachomatis* as a cause of sexually transmitted diseases in the United States, and the incidence of gonorrhea rose sharply during the 1990s. An estimated 3 million cases now occur annually in the United States.

Epidemiology

The incidence of gonorrhea reached a plateau in the United States between 1975 and 1980, possibly reflective of a decrease in the size of the at-risk cohort.

TABLE 107–3   Treatment for Syphilis in the Normal Host

Clinical Category	Regimen of Choice	History of Penicillin Allergy
Primary	Benzathine penicillin, 2.4 MU IM	Tetracycline or erythromycin, 2 g/day for 15 days
Secondary		
Early latent		
Healthy contact*		
Late latent or late	Benzathine penicillin, 2.4 MU IM per week for 3 weeks	No regimen adequately evaluated; ? tetracycline or erythromycin, 2 g/day for 30 days
Neurosyphilis	Aqueous penicillin G, 20 MU IV per day for 10 days	Same as for late latent or late

* Contact of patient with active skin or mucous membrane lesions.
IM = intramuscularly; IV = intravenously; MU = million units.

Reinfection is common, and it is not unusual for one sexually active patient to have 20 or more discrete infections. Particular risk factors are urban habitat, low socioeconomic status, unmarried status, and large numbers of unprotected sexual contacts. Fifty percent of females having intercourse with a male with gonococcal urethritis will develop symptomatic infection. The risk for males is 20% after a single sexual contact with an infected female. Orogenital contact and anal intercourse also transmit infection. Asymptomatic infection of males is an important factor in transmission. Forty percent of male contacts of symptomatic women have asymptomatic urethritis. If untreated, about one fourth develop symptomatic infection within 7 days; a like number spontaneously become culture negative within this period. The rest remain culture positive and asymptomatic but capable of transmitting infection for periods of up to 6 months. Co-infection with *C. trachomatis* is observed in up to 30% to 40% of patients with gonorrhea.

Pathogenesis

Neisseria gonorrhoeae is a gram-negative, kidney bean–shaped diplococcus. Specialized projections from the organism, pili, aid in attachment to mucosal surfaces, contribute to resistance to killing by neutrophils, and constitute an important virulence factor. Production of an IgA protease by the organism contributes to pathogenicity. In females, several factors alter susceptibility to infection. Group B blood type increases susceptibility, whereas vaginal colonization with normal flora, IgA content of vaginal secretions, and high progesterone levels may be protective. Spread from the cervix to the upper genital tract is associated with menstruation because changes in the pH and biochemical constituents of cervical mucus lead to increased shedding of gonococci; cervical dilation, reflux of menses, and binding of the gonococcus to spermatozoa may be additional factors in ascending genital infection and dissemination. Intrauterine contraceptive devices increase the risk of endometrial spread of infection twofold to ninefold (oral contraceptives are associated with a twofold decrease).

Clinical Presentation

In males who develop symptomatic urethritis, symptoms of purulent discharge and severe dysuria usually occur 2 to 7 days after sexual contact. Prompt treatment usually follows, so that more extensive genital involvement is uncommon.

In females, cervicitis is the most frequent manifestation and results in copious yellow vaginal discharge. Overall, 20% of females with gonococcal cervicitis develop pelvic inflammatory disease (PID), usually beginning at a time close to the onset of menstruation. PID is manifest as endometritis (abnormal menses, midline abdominal pain), salpingitis (bilateral lower abdominal pain and tenderness), or pelvic peritonitis. Salpingitis can cause tubal occlusion and sterility. Gonococcal perihepatitis (Fitz-Hugh–Curtis syndrome) also may complicate PID and present as right upper quadrant pain.

Females also may develop urethritis with dysuria and frequency. In certain populations of sexually active women, one fourth of women complaining of urinary tract symptoms and 60% of those with symptoms but no bacteriuria have urethral cultures positive for *N. gonorrhoeae*.

Anorectal gonorrhea occurs in both homosexual males and heterosexual females. In males, the resultant rectal pain, tenesmus, mucopurulent discharge, and bleeding may represent the only site of infection. Anorectal infection may be recognized only by cultures of asymptomatic contacts of patients with gonorrhea. In females, asymptomatic anorectal involvement is a frequent complication of symptomatic genitourinary disease even in the absence of anal intercourse (44%); isolated anorectal infection (4%) as well as acute or chronic proctitis (2% to 5%) is rare. Treatment failures are frequent in anorectal gonorrhea (7% to 35%).

Because of the frequency of asymptomatic infection in each of the potential sites, patients with symptoms suggestive of gonococcal infection should have cultures from the urethra, anus, pharynx, and (when applicable) cervix.

Pharyngeal gonorrhea occurs in homosexual males or heterosexual females after oral sex and less frequently in heterosexual males. The pharynx is rarely the sole site of gonococcal infection (5% to 8%).

Extragenital dissemination occurs in approximately 1% of males and 3% of females with gonorrhea. Strains of *N. gonorrhoeae* causing dissemination differ from other gonococci in several respects. They are generally more penicillin-sensitive and resist the normal bactericidal activity of antibody and complement. The latter finding may result from their binding of a naturally occurring blocking antibody. Complement deficiency states can predispose patients to disseminated gonorrhea. Dissemination of gonococcal infection may take the form of the arthritis-dermatitis syndrome, with 3 to 20 papular, petechial, pustular, necrotic, or hemorrhagic skin lesions usually found on the extensor surfaces of the distal extremities. An associated finding is an asymmetric polytenosynovitis, with or without arthritis, which predominantly involves wrists, fingers, knees, and ankles. Joint fluid cultures usually are negative in the arthritis-dermatitis syndrome, leading to speculation that circulating immune complexes, demonstrable in most patients, are important in its pathogenesis. Synovial biopsies may yield positive cultures. Biopsy of skin lesions reveals gonococcal antigens (by immunofluorescent antibody staining) in two thirds of cases. Blood cultures are positive in 50%. Septic arthritis is another manifestation of dissemination; *N. gonorrhoeae* is the most frequent cause of septic arthritis in 16- to 50-year olds. The joint fluid cultures usually are positive (particularly when the leukocyte count in joint fluid exceeds $80,000/\mu L$), and blood cultures are usually negative. Gonococcemia may in rare cases lead to endocarditis, meningitis, myopericarditis, or toxic hepatitis.

Laboratory Diagnosis and Management

Gram's stain of the urethral discharge will determine the cause of urethritis in most males with gonorrhea,

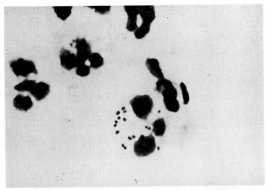

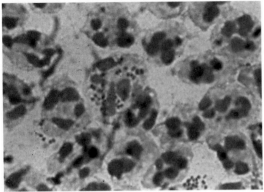

FIGURE 107–1   Gram's stain of urethral discharge, showing typical intracellular diplococci associated with neutrophils.

because typical intracellular diplococci are diagnostic (Fig. 107–1). The finding of only extracellular gram-negative diplococci is equivocal. The absence of gonococci on a smear of urethral discharge from a male virtually excludes the diagnosis. Diagnosis by Gram's staining of cervical exudates is relatively specific but insensitive (<60%). Modified Thayer-Martin medium contains antibiotics that inhibit the growth of other organisms and increase the yield of gonococci from samples likely to be contaminated; it is not necessary for culture of normally sterile fluids, such as joint fluid, blood, and CSF. Specimens from these sites should be cultured on chocolate agar. Other important considerations for the isolation of gonococci include the use of synthetic swabs (unsaturated fatty acids in cotton may be inhibitory), the introduction of a very thin calcium alginate swab or a loop 2 cm into the male urethra, and the avoidance of vaginal douching (12 hours), urination (2 hours), and vaginal speculum lubricants before culture. In all suspected cases of gonorrhea, the urethra, anus, and pharynx should be cultured. In females, 20% of cases in which initial cervical cultures were negative yield *N. gonorrhoeae* when cultures are repeated. Gene probes are less sensitive than culture in diagnosis.

Gonococcal resistance to penicillin is increasing worldwide. The current recommendation for the treatment of uncomplicated gonorrhea is ceftriaxone, 250 mg given intramuscularly once. This should be followed by a course of doxycycline (100 mg orally twice daily for 7 days) or azithromycin (1 g orally as single dose) to treat concurrent chlamydial infection. Alternative therapies include cefixime, 400 mg once orally; ciprofloxacin, 500 mg once orally; or levofloxacin, 500 mg once. Quinolones are contraindicated in pregnancy. In patients with severe β-lactam allergies, spectinomycin, 2 g intramuscularly, can be used; this is inadequate therapy for pharyngeal infection. PID should be treated with cefoxitin, 2 g given intramuscularly, followed by doxycycline, 100 mg twice daily administered orally for 10 days. Seriously ill females with PID should be hospitalized. Evaluation by ultrasonography for the presence of a pelvic abscess or peritonitis usually is warranted in this setting. Surgery may be indicated to drain a tubo-ovarian or pelvic abscess.

Disseminated gonococcal infection should be treated with ceftriaxone, 1 g every 24 hours for 10 days. Cephalosporins should not be used, however, if the history suggests an IgE-mediated allergy to penicillin (anaphylactoid reaction, angioedema, urticaria). In such a case, ciprofloxacin, 500 mg twice daily for 7 days, is an effective alternative.

A VDRL test should be performed in all patients with gonorrhea. If negative, no further follow-up is necessary, because ceftriaxone in the dosage used is probably effective in treating incubating syphilis. If alternative drugs are used, the VDRL test should be repeated after 4 weeks. Anal cultures should be part of the routine follow-up of females, because persistent anorectal carriage may be the source of relapse. Postgonococcal urethritis occurs in 30% to 50% of males 2 to 3 weeks after penicillin therapy if this treatment is not followed by tetracycline. It usually is caused by *C. trachomatis* or *Ureaplasma urealyticum*.

NONGONOCOCCAL URETHRITIS, CERVICITIS, AND PID

The diagnosis of nongonococcal urethritis (NGU) requires the exclusion of gonorrhea, because considerable overlap exists in the clinical syndromes.

Epidemiology

At least as many cases of urethritis are nongonococcal as gonococcal. Typically, NGU predominates in higher socioeconomic groups. *C. trachomatis* causes 30% to 50% of NGU and can be isolated from 0% to 11% of asymptomatic, sexually active males. *C. trachomatis* also can be isolated from 30% of males with gonorrhea and presumably represents a concurrent infection. Some cases of *Chlamydia*-negative NGU are caused by *U. urealyticum* or *Trichomonas vaginalis*.

Clinical Syndromes

Nongonococcal urethritis is less contagious than gonococcal infection. The incubation period is 7 to 14 days. Characteristically, patients complain of urethral discharge, itching, and dysuria. Importantly, the discharge is not spontaneous but becomes apparent after milking

TABLE 107–4 Organisms Causing Proctocolitis in Homosexual Men

Neisseria gonorrhoeae
Chlamydia trachomatis
Herpesvirus hominis
Treponema pallidum
Shigella species
Salmonella species
Campylobacter species
Entamoeba histolytica
Giardia lamblia
Strongyloides stercoralis

the urethra in the morning. The mucopurulent discharge consists of thin, cloudy fluid with purulent specks; these characteristics do not always allow clear distinction from gonococcal disease. *T. vaginalis* causes a typically scanty discharge.

C. trachomatis also is a common cause of epididymitis in males younger than 35 years of age and can produce proctitis in men and women who practice receptive anal intercourse.

Chlamydial infections are also more common than gonococcal infections in females but frequently escape

detection. Two thirds of women with mucopurulent cervicitis have chlamydial infection. Similarly, many females with the acute onset of dysuria, frequency, and pyuria, but sterile bladder urine, have *C. trachomatis* infection. *C. trachomatis* is at least as common a cause of salpingitis as is the gonococcus.

Laboratory Diagnosis

Ordinarily, the distinction between gonococcal and nongonococcal infections relies mainly on Gram-stained preparations of exudate and cultures. In a male with urethritis and typical gram-negative diplococci associated with neutrophils, the diagnosis of gonococcal urethritis is clear-cut and the culture is unnecessary. Coincident NGU cannot be excluded, however. Whenever interpretation of the Gram stain is not straightforward in males, and in all females, culture on Thayer-Martin medium is appropriate. Techniques for isolation and detection (DNA probes) of chlamydiae are widely available and should be used routinely in evaluating genital infections.

Treatment

The patient and all sexual contacts should be treated with azithromycin, 1 g orally as a single dose, or doxycy-

TABLE 107–5 Vaginitis

Disease	Epidemiology/ Pathogenesis	Clinical Findings	Laboratory Diagnosis	Treatment
Candidiasis	Yeast are part of normal flora; overgrowth favored by broad-spectrum antibiotics, high estrogen levels (pregnancy, before menses, oral contraceptives), diabetes mellitus, may be early clue to HIV infection	Itching, little or no urethral discharge, occasional dysuria; labia pale or erythematous with satellite lesions; vaginal discharge thick, adherent, with white curds, balanitis in 10% of male contacts	Vaginal pH = 4.5 (normal), negative whiff test, yeast seen on wet mount in 50%, culture positive	Miconazole, butoconazole, terconazole, or clotrimazole cream or suppositories for 3–7 days; fluconazole, 150 mg orally as a single dose
Trichomonas vaginalis infection	STD; incubation 5–28 days; symptoms begin or exacerbate with menses	Discharge, soreness, irritation, mild dysuria, dyspareunia; copious loose discharge, one fifth yellow/green, one third bubbly	Elevated pH; wet mount shows large numbers of WBCs, trichomonads; positive whiff test (10% KOH causes fishy odor)	Metronidazole, 2 g as single dose; treat sexual contacts
Bacterial vaginosis	Synergistic infection, *Gardnerella vaginalis* and anaerobes (*Mobiluncus* sp.)	Vaginal odor, mild discharge, little inflammation; grayish, thin, homogeneous discharge with small bubbles	Elevated pH; positive whiff test; wet prep contains clue cells (vaginal epithelial cells with intracellular coccobacilli), few WBCs	Metronidazole, 500 mg bid for 7 days; alternatives include metronidazole gel (0.75%) 5 g intravaginally twice daily for 7 days, or clindamycin cream (2%) 5 g intravaginally daily at night for 7 days; do not treat contacts unless recurrent vaginitis

HIV = human immunodeficiency virus; KOH = potassium hydroxide; STD = sexually transmitted disease; WBCs = white blood cells.

cline, 100 mg orally twice daily for 7 days. Recurrence may occur and requires longer periods (2 to 3 weeks) of treatment. In pregnancy, erythromycin base, 500 mg orally four times daily for 7 days, is an acceptable regimen.

Proctocolitis in Homosexual Men

Men who practice receptive anal intercourse may present with proctitis/proctocolitis, causing anorectal pain, mucoid or bloody discharge, tenesmus, diarrhea, or abdominal pain. Sigmoidoscopy should be performed with culture and Gram's stain of the discharge. Potential causative organisms are shown in Table 107–4. The diarrheal syndromes are considered in Chapter 103. Ten percent of patients harbor two or more pathogens. Proctitis also may occur without a definable pathogen (42%).

Diarrhea in the patient infected with HIV has an entirely different set of implications (see Chapter 108).

Vaginitis

Table 107–5 considers salient features in the diagnosis and management of patients with vaginitis.

REFERENCES

Centers for Disease Control and Prevention: 1998 Sexually transmitted diseases treatment guidelines. MMWR Morbid Mortal Wkly Rep 1998; 47:(RR-1):1–116.

Cohen MS, Hook EW III, Hitchcock PJ: Sexually transmitted diseases in the AIDS era. Infect Dis Clin North Am 1993; 7:739–914 and 1994; 8:751–925.

Sparling PF, Hook EW: Sexually transmitted diseases. *In* Goldman L, Bennett JC (eds): Cecil Textbook of Medicine, 21st ed. Philadelphia, WB Saunders Co, 2000, pp 1738–1742.

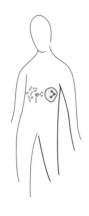

108

HIV INFECTION AND THE ACQUIRED IMMUNODEFICIENCY SYNDROME

Charles C. J. Carpenter • *Timothy P. Flanigan*
Michael M. Lederman

The acquired immunodeficiency syndrome (AIDS) is the expression of a spectrum of disorders caused by cellular and humoral immune dysfunction resulting from infection by the human immunodeficiency virus (HIV-1). Since AIDS was recognized as a distinct, new disease entity in 1981, over 50 million individuals worldwide have been infected by HIV-1. Of these, more than 90% are in the developing world and approximately 90% have acquired the infection through heterosexual intercourse.

A second human immunodeficiency virus (HIV-2) was identified in West Africa in the mid 1980s. HIV-2 infection also results in AIDS, but HIV-2 infection has a considerably longer clinically latent period than HIV-1.

Although HIV-2 shares many biologic and genetic characteristics with HIV-1, each of the two viruses has regulatory and structural genes that are unique. Whereas HIV-1 is closely related to the simian immunodeficiency virus (SIV) isolated from a subspecies of chimpanzee (SIV_{cpz}), HIV-2 is more closely related to an SIV that is commonly found in the sooty mangaby (SIV_{sm}). The rare HIV-2 infections in the United States to date have been of West African origin. Throughout the remainder of this chapter, the abbreviation *HIV* refers to the HIV-1 virus.

Epidemiology

AIDS was first recognized as a clinical entity in previously healthy men who had serious infections with unusual opportunistic pathogens, most frequently *Pneumocystis carinii* pneumonia (PCP), an illness previously found only among patients with severe cellular immunodeficiency. Studies confirmed profound immunodeficiency in these individuals, leading to the name *acquired immunodeficiency syndrome*.

When similar opportunistic infections (OIs) were subsequently observed in injecting drug users and men with hemophilia and their female sexual partners, it became clear that this syndrome was caused by an agent transmitted through sexual contact or through infusion of contaminated blood or blood products. The HIV virus was identified in 1984 as the causative agent of AIDS. Subsequently, recognition of a wide spectrum of HIV disease has emerged, ranging from asymptomatic infection to severe immunodeficiency associated with life-threatening OIs and/or neoplasms.

The Centers for Disease Control and Prevention (CDC) surveillance criteria for the diagnosis of AIDS, as modified in 1987, included a large number of OIs (Table 108–1) indicative of defects in cellular and/or humoral immunity, as well as certain neoplasms and other conditions associated with severe immunodeficiency (Table 108–2). The occurrence of any one of these conditions in an individual with no other cause of immunosuppression constituted the diagnosis of AIDS. In 1992, the CDC broadened the surveillance definition of AIDS to include all HIV-infected persons with severely depressed levels of cell-mediated immunity as indicated by $CD4^+$ T lymphocyte counts (CD4 counts) less than 200 cells/mm³. In 1993, AIDS had become the leading cause of death of American adults aged 25 to 44 (Fig. 108–1). By the year 2000, over 700,000 HIV-infected persons in the United States had been diagnosed with AIDS; at least 400,000 additional persons were living with asymptomatic HIV infection.

TABLE 108-1 Opportunistic Infections Indicative of a Defect in Cellular Immune Function Associated with Acquired Immunodeficiency Syndrome (AIDS)

Protozoan Infection

Pneumocystis carinii pneumonia
Toxoplasma gondii encephalitis
Cryptosporidium parvum enteritis (>1 mo)
Isospora belli enteritis (>1 mo)

Fungal Infection

Candida esophagitis
Cryptococcus neoformans meningitis
Disseminated histoplasmosis*
Disseminated coccidioidomycosis*

Bacterial Infection

Disseminated *Mycobacterium avium* complex
Active *Mycobacterium tuberculosis* infection*
Recurrent *Salmonella* septicemia*
Recurrent bacterial pneumonia*

Viral Infection

Chronic (>1 mo) mucocutaneous or esophageal herpes simplex virus infection
Cytomegalovirus retinitis, esophagitis, or colitis
Progressive multifocal leukoencephalopathy (JC virus)

Helminthic Infection

Strongyloidiasis (disseminated beyond the gastrointestinal tract)

* Requires laboratory evidence of human immunodeficiency virus (HIV) infection.

TABLE 108-2 Other Conditions Fulfilling Clinical Criteria for AIDS

Neoplasms

Kaposi's sarcoma (in a person <60 years old)
High-grade, B-cell non-Hodgkin's lymphoma*
Undifferentiated non-Hodgkin's lymphoma*
Immunoblastic sarcoma*
Primary brain lymphoma*
Invasive carcinoma of the cervix*†

Systemic Illness

HIV wasting syndrome*
(Unintentional loss of >10% of body weight)

* Requires laboratory evidence of HIV infection.
† Recognized as AIDS-defining condition in 1992.

ence of other sexually transmissible diseases (STDs), especially those associated with genital ulcerations, strongly facilitates sexual transmission of HIV-1 (see Chapter 107). Women are now the group in which HIV infection is increasing most rapidly in the United States. In several rural areas in the Southeast, women accounted for over half of new cases in 1999.

Sharing of needles used for drug injection transmits the virus efficiently. Because of the concentration of injecting drug users in impoverished inner-city areas, a disproportionate number of North American men and women infected by HIV are African-American or Hispanic. Differences in regional patterns of intravenous drug use largely explain the greater than 100-fold re-

Retrospective analysis of stored serum specimens has revealed that HIV infection had been present in parts of Central Africa for at least two decades before recognition of the clinical syndrome of AIDS. Since the early 1980s, HIV infection has spread widely to become a major worldwide pandemic. HIV infection continues to spread, albeit at strikingly different rates, throughout all continents. During the 1990s exceptionally rapid transmission occurred throughout India, Southeast Asia, and Southern Africa.

Because of latency between HIV infection and the development of AIDS-associated illnesses, the clinically recognized epidemic of AIDS has lagged 6 to 8 years behind the spread of the virus into new populations. Although initially recognized among homosexual men and intravenous drug users in the United States, heterosexual intercourse has been the dominant mode of HIV transmission throughout most of the world. In the United States through 1985, fewer than 1% of the recognized cases of AIDS in the United States had been acquired through heterosexual contact; by 2000, heterosexual transmission accounted for more than 25% of the cases of AIDS and a considerably higher proportion of persons with asymptomatic HIV infection. The virus is present in both semen and cervicovaginal secretions of infected individuals and can be transmitted by either partner during vaginal intercourse. The concurrent pres-

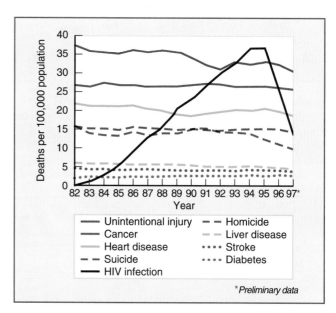

FIGURE 108-1 Death rates in persons aged 25 to 44, United States, 1982–1997. In 1993, AIDS became the leading cause of death of Americans in this age group. Since the widespread adoption of effective combination antiretroviral therapy in 1996, AIDS-related death rates have fallen sharply. By 1998, AIDS ranked fourth among the causes of death in this age group. (Data from Centers for Disease Control and Prevention.)

gional variation in prevalence of AIDS cases in the United States (Fig. 108–2).

Vertical transmission of HIV from infected mother to child may occur in utero, during labor, or through breast-feeding. Twenty-five to 30 percent of infants born to HIV-seropositive mothers who are not receiving antiretroviral therapy are infected by HIV. The rate of vertical transmission can be reduced to 5% or less by prenatal and perinatal treatment of the mother and postnatal treatment of the infant with antiretroviral drugs.

The HIV virus is almost universally present in the blood of infected patients in the absence of effective antiretroviral therapy. Thus, before the nationwide implementation of a blood screening test in late 1985, infection by means of transfused blood or blood products (e.g., factors VIII and IX for hemophiliacs) accounted for nearly 3% of AIDS cases in the United States. Since 1985, all blood products in North America have been screened for antibodies to HIV, and factor VIII and factor IX concentrates are now heat-treated to inactivate HIV. The risk of transfusion-acquired HIV infection in North America and Western Europe is now extremely small, but not absent. It is possible that persons recently infected with HIV donate blood during the weeks before they develop detectable HIV antibodies (window period). However, most such cases should be identified by p24 antigen screening, which has been mandated by the U.S. Food and Drug Administration since 1996.

HIV infection also has occurred after accidental parenteral exposures of health care workers. After injury by an HIV-contaminated hollow needle, the risk of infection is approximately 0.3%. The possibility that HIV-infected health care workers who perform invasive procedures may transmit HIV to patients has been carefully investigated; this risk is extremely small.

Pathophysiology

HIV is a member of the lentivirus family of retroviruses, which includes the agents of visna, equine infectious anemia virus, and the simian immunodeficiency viruses (SIV). The core of HIV contains two single-stranded copies of the viral RNA genome, together with the vi-

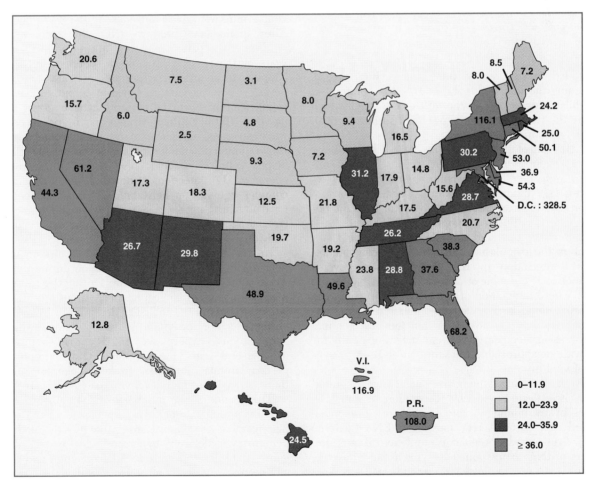

FIGURE 108–2 The rates of male adult/adolescent acquired immunodeficiency syndrome (AIDS) cases per 100,000 population in the United States, July 1997 through June 1998. The rates show tremendous regional variation, from 329 in the District of Columbia to 3 in North Dakota. Rates for women show generally similar regional variation, with an overall rate roughly 20% that of men. (From Centers for Disease Control and Prevention: HIV/AIDS Surveillance Report 1998; 10[No. 1]:10.)

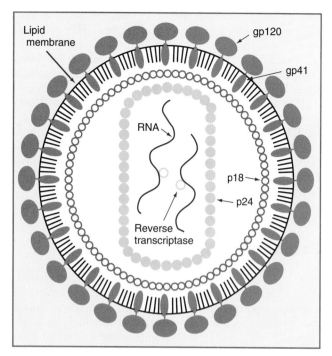

FIGURE 108–3 Structure of human immunodeficiency virus (HIV). (Adapted from "The AIDS virus," copyright © 1987 by Scientific American, Inc., George V. Kelvin, all rights reserved.)

rus-encoded enzyme reverse transcriptase (Fig. 108–3). Surrounding the core (p24) and matrix (p18) proteins is a lipid bilayer derived from the host cell, through which protrude the transmembrane (gp41) and surface (gp120) envelope glycoproteins.

The HIV envelope glycoproteins have a high affinity for the CD4 molecule on the surface of T helper lymphocytes and other cells of monocyte/macrophage lineage. After HIV binds to CD4 and a specific cellular co-receptor (CCR5 is an essential co-receptor on T helper lymphocytes, CXCR4 on macrophages) the viral and cellular membranes fuse and the HIV nucleoprotein complex enters the cytoplasm. The RNA viral genome undergoes transcription by the virally encoded reverse transcriptase. The double-stranded viral DNA enters the nucleus, where integration of the DNA provirus into the host chromosome is catalyzed by another retroviral enzyme, integrase (Fig. 108–4). Within the host genome the provirus may remain in a latent state, apparently for years, without appreciable transcription of RNA or synthesis of viral protein.

When a T helper lymphocyte-containing integrated provirus is activated (e.g., by recognition of antigenic peptides or by binding of proinflammatory cytokines), increased expression of HIV messenger RNA (mRNA) occurs. Virus-encoded regulatory proteins *tat* and *rev* facilitate mRNA expression and cytoplasmic transport, respectively. Core proteins, viral enzymes, and envelope proteins are encoded by the *gag, pol,* and *env* genes of HIV, respectively. Viral polyproteins are cleaved by viral-encoded proteases (see Fig. 108–4), and the envelope protein is glycosylated by host glycosylases. Viral particles are assembled, each containing two copies of

unspliced mRNA within the core as the viral genome, and virions then are released from the cell by budding. Productive viral replication is lytic to infected T cells. A number of other host cells, including macrophages, dendritic cells, and Langerhans cells, also are infected by HIV, but these cells do not appear to be lysed by the virus.

IMMUNE DEFICIENCY IN HIV INFECTION

Shortly after HIV infection, rapid viral multiplication occurs in blood and lymphatic tissue (and presumably other organs), and plasma HIV-RNA levels (plasma viral load [PVL]) may exceed 1 million copies/mL during the second to fourth weeks after infection. During the subsequent weeks, the PVL decreases, often very rapidly. Presumably, the decrease in viremia results from a partially effective, but incomplete, immune response by the patient. After 8 to 12 months, the PVL generally stabilizes, at a level often called the viral "set point," and remains roughly at this level for several years (Fig. 108–5). The PVL at 8 to 12 months after infection is a powerful predictor of the subsequent rate of progression of HIV disease.

During the burst of viral replication shortly after infection, the majority of patients develop an acute retroviral syndrome, which subsides as the PVL decreases. After spontaneous recovery from the acute retroviral syndrome, the patient may feel entirely well for several years and may have little or no decrease in CD4+ T lymphocyte count in the peripheral blood. During this period of clinical latency, however, rapid viral multiplication continues. In the asymptomatic infected individual, over 100 billion new virions may be produced daily, while an equal number are removed from circulation. Rapid production and turnover of circulating CD4+ T helper cells (CD4 cells) also occurs throughout the course of HIV infection. Although a highly dynamic and complex equilibrium between HIV and CD4 cells may be maintained for several years, eventually a decline in circulating CD4 cells occurs in the great majority of individuals; this is preceded by an increase in PVL.

An HIV-specific immune response contributes to the decrease in the rate of viral replication during the initial weeks after acute HIV infection. During the subsequent months to years of clinical latency, virions are present in large numbers in the follicular dendritic processes of the germinal centers of lymph nodes and spleen, which undergo intense hyperplasia. As HIV disease progresses over several years, the lymphatic tissue atrophies and plasma viremia intensifies. In later-stage HIV disease, there is persistent high-level viremia (see Fig. 108–5).

The decline in the number of CD4 cells is accompanied by profound functional impairment of the remaining lymphocyte populations. Anergy—the failure to demonstrate delayed hypersensitivity to recall antigens—may develop early in HIV infection and eventually occurs in virtually all persons with AIDS. With development of anergy, T helper lymphocyte proliferation in response to antigenic stimuli is dramatically impaired. T cell cytotoxic responses are diminished, and natural killer cell activity against virus-infected cells is greatly impaired, despite normal or increased numbers of these

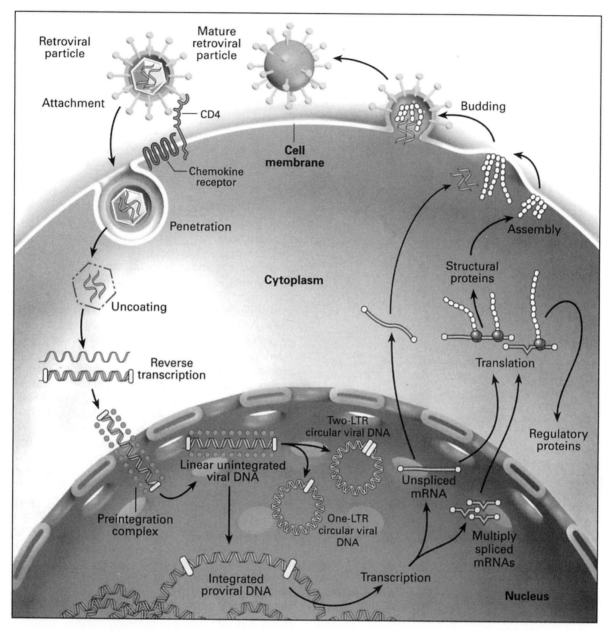

FIGURE 108-4 Essential steps in the life cycle of human immunodeficiency virus-1 (HIV-1). The first step is the attachment of the virus particle to receptors on the cell surface. The HIV-1 RNA genome then enters the cytoplasm as part of a nucleoprotein complex. The viral RNA genome is reverse-transcribed into a collinear DNA duplex (site of action of reverse transcriptase inhibitors, see text). Once the viral DNA has been synthesized, the linear viral DNA molecule is incorporated into a preintegration complex that enters the nucleus. In the nucleus, unintegrated viral DNA is found in both linear and circular forms. The linear unintegrated viral DNA is the precursor of integrated proviral DNA, which remains indefinitely in the host-cell genome and serves as a template of viral transcription. Transcription of the proviral DNA template and alternative messenger RNA (mRNA) splicing creates spliced viral mRNA species encoding the viral accessory proteins, including Tat, Rev, and Nef, and the unspliced viral mRNA encoding the viral structural proteins, including the gag-pol precursor protein. (Cleaving of the precursor proteins is prevented by protease inhibitors; see text.) A shift in the transcriptional pattern from the expression of predominantly multiply spliced viral mRNA to predominantly unspliced viral mRNA is indicative of active viral replication. All the viral transcripts are exported into the cytoplasm, where translation, assembly, and processing of the retroviral particle take place. The cycle is completed by the release of infectious retroviral particles from the cell. (Modified from Wolinsky SM, et al: Persistence of HIV-1 transcription in patients receiving potent antiretroviral therapy. N Engl J Med 1999; 340:1614–1622, with permission.)

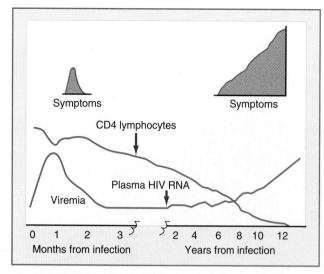

FIGURE 108–5 Natural history of HIV-1 infection in the untreated adult. Note the long period of clinical latency between the acute retroviral syndrome and AIDS-related disease. Note also the relative stability of the plasma HIV RNA level for several years after recovery from the initial burst of viremia, followed by an increase before the onset of AIDS-related symptoms. (Modified from Goldman L, Bennett JC [eds]: Cecil Textbook of Medicine, 21st ed. Philadelphia: WB Saunders, 2000, p 1896.)

cells. Decrease in function as well as number of CD4+ T helper lymphocytes is central to the immune dysfunction. Despite a polyclonal or oligoclonal hypergammaglobulinemia, B lymphocyte function is also diminished, as measured by impaired capacity to synthesize antibody in response to new antigens. The profound impairment of multiple arms of the immune system underlies the enhanced risk of acquiring the OIs that are characteristic of AIDS.

INADEQUACY OF HOST DEFENSE MECHANISMS

A characteristic feature of HIV infection is the ability of the virus to continue to replicate despite brisk host immune responses to the virus. Humoral responses to viral proteins are readily demonstrable in all infected persons. Neutralizing antibodies develop rapidly but generally in relatively low titer, in comparison with neutralizing antibodies generated in response to other viral infections. Cell-mediated immune responses to several HIV-derived proteins are also readily seen and are temporally associated with the decrease in plasma viremia after acute HIV infection.

There are several possible explanations for the inability of host responses to control HIV infection. The viral replication cycle allows integrated provirus to persist in the host genome in a transcriptionally latent state, in which it is not recognized by either humoral or cellular immune mechanisms (see Fig. 108–4). The CD4 binding domain of the HIV envelope, a potential conserved target for neutralizing antibody, is relatively inaccessible to antibody. Other envelope regions vary among different isolates. Errors in retroviral reverse transcription underlie this high degree of genetic variability. Selective

pressure (e.g., the development of antibodies against a nonconserved region of the envelope) results in the emergence of viral mutants resistant to neutralizing activity of a specific antibody species. The frequency of transcription errors may prove to be a major obstacle to the development of an effective vaccine.

Diagnosis and Testing for HIV Infection

Because HIV transmission is preventable, antiretroviral therapy is increasingly effective, and prophylaxis against the major OIs can be achieved, it is important that persons at risk for HIV infection undergo serologic testing. Testing should not be confined to individuals at highest risk (e.g., injecting drug users) but should be strongly recommended for all sexually active persons with any risk, including all individuals with current or past partners whose HIV status is unknown. Testing must be provided in a confidential environment consistent with relevant state laws. Pretest discussion is essential to ensure that persons appreciate the importance and consequences of the test results. All individuals should be counseled regarding safer sexual practices. Injecting drug users should strongly be advised not to share needles. Positive test results should be given in a face-to-face meeting, during which the patient is given assurance that, with currently available therapy, he or she may live asymptomatically with HIV infection for many years. Appropriate arrangements for continuing medical care should be made at this time. All patients should be encouraged to notify their sexual partners and persons with whom they have shared needles. This is often difficult; regional health authorities may be of great assistance in confidential notification of persons at risk.

Diagnosis of HIV infection is established by detection of serum or salivary antibody to HIV by enzyme-linked immunosorbent assay (ELISA) and confirmed by Western blot. These techniques are very sensitive in detecting HIV antibody, but individuals who have been infected recently may be antibody negative. During this "window period," infected individuals have detectable HIV RNA in plasma. For recently exposed individuals whose initial ELISA test is negative, a repeat ELISA test at 6 weeks and 3 months is indicated. False-positive ELISA tests are rare. Western blot reactivity with at least two different HIV proteins confirms infection. In a person at high risk for HIV exposure, an indeterminate Western blot reaction pattern often represents early seroconversion; in such cases, detectable plasma HIV RNA is indicative of acute HIV infection.

Although 25% to 30% of infants born to HIV-infected mothers who are not receiving antiretroviral therapy acquire HIV infection, all such infants have positive ELISA tests because of circulating maternal anti-HIV antibodies. Maternal antibodies generally disappear by 9 to 12 months. Early diagnosis of HIV infection in this setting may be achieved by sensitive plasma HIV RNA or DNA assays.

Rapid and more accessible testing methods play an

increasingly important role in the diagnosis and confirmation of HIV infection. Oral mucosal transudate and urine testing offer noninvasive ways of testing; home testing offers easier access.

Sequential Clinical Manifestations of HIV-1 Infection

ACUTE HIV INFECTION AND THE ACUTE RETROVIRAL SYNDROME

Forty to 70 percent of HIV-infected persons experience a mononucleosis-like syndrome (acute retroviral syndrome) from 2 to 8 weeks after initial infection (see Fig. 108–5). Acute symptoms may include fever, sore throat, lymph node enlargement, rash, arthralgias, and headache and usually persist for several days to 3 weeks (Table 108–3). A maculopapular rash is common, is short-lived, and usually affects the trunk or face. Acute, self-limited aseptic meningitis, documented by cerebrospinal fluid (CSF) pleocytosis and isolation of HIV from CSF, is the most common clinical neurologic presentation and occurs in 10% to 20% of patients.

The acute retroviral syndrome varies greatly in both severity and duration, but a large proportion of patients seek medical attention. In the absence of a high index of suspicion, these symptoms are often mislabeled as an "acute viral syndrome." This is especially unfortunate, because a very high plasma HIV-RNA level during or shortly after infection indicates a high likelihood of HIV transmission to sexual or needle-sharing partners, or from mother to infant.

During the acute retroviral syndrome, HIV antibody is generally not detectable, but HIV infection can be demonstrated by plasma HIV RNA or p24 antigen assays. Within 4 to 12 weeks after HIV infection, specific antibodies develop that are directed against the three main gene products of HIV: gag (p55, p24, p15), pol (p34, p68), and env (gp160, gp120, gp41).

ASYMPTOMATIC PHASE

HIV infection usually results in a slow, nonlinear progression to severe immunodeficiency marked by progressive depletion of CD4 cells. Approximately 50% of untreated individuals develop AIDS within 10 years after HIV infection (see Fig. 108–5); an additional 30%

TABLE 108–3 Acute HIV Retroviral Syndrome: Common Signs and Symptoms

Sign/Symptom	Frequency (%)
Fever	98
Lymph node enlargement	75
Sore throat	70
Myalgia or arthralgia	60
Rash	50
Headache	35

have milder symptoms related to immunodeficiency, and less than 20% are entirely asymptomatic 10 years after infection. Progression of disease varies greatly among individuals. Adolescents with HIV progress to AIDS at a slower rate than older persons, with fewer than 30% developing AIDS within 10 years after HIV infection. The rate of progression of immunodeficiency is not influenced by the route of HIV transmission. The PVL obtained 8 to 12 months after primary infection is a highly significant predictor of the subsequent rate of disease progression (Fig. 108–6).

The majority of HIV-infected individuals are not diagnosed during the acute retroviral syndrome, are unaware of their infection, and are asymptomatic, with CD4 counts greater than 200 cells/mm^3. Major life-threatening OIs seldom occur until the CD4 count is less than 200 cells/mm^3. Despite abundance of antibody manifested by elevated gamma globulin levels, patients show diminished antibody response to protein and polysaccharide antigens. This is manifest clinically by a threefold to fourfold increase in incidence of bacterial pneumonias caused by common pulmonary pathogens such as *Streptococcus pneumoniae* and *Haemophilus influenzae*. Acute bacterial pneumonias are even more frequent in HIV-infected individuals who continue injection drug use.

Clinically recognized lymph node enlargement occurs in 35% to 60% of asymptomatic HIV-infected persons and is not significantly associated with either the rate of progression of immunodeficiency or with subsequent development of lymphoma. During early HIV infection, thrombocytopenia, probably caused by autoimmune platelet destruction, is common. Mucocutaneous lesions may be the first manifestations of immune dysfunction, especially recurrent genital herpes simplex virus (HSV) infections, polydermatomal varicella-zoster infection (shingles), and oral hairy leukoplakia. Mucocutaneous manifestations become more frequent and severe as immune function deteriorates (see later discussion). Clinical manifestations of infection by *Mycobacterium tuberculosis* often occur with CD4 counts over 200 cells/mm^3.

SYMPTOMATIC PHASE: OPPORTUNISTIC INFECTIONS

With more advanced immunodeficiency, indicated by CD4 counts below 200, patients are at high risk of developing OIs (Table 108–4). For example, in the absence of specific prophylaxis, 60% of HIV-infected North American men develop *Pneumocystis carinii* pneumonia. Local and/or disseminated fungal infections with *Cryptococcus neoformans*, *Histoplasma capsulatum*, or *Coccidioides immitis* may occur. (The incidence of each infection varies, depending on geographic locale.) Protozoal infections with *Toxoplasma gondii* (encephalitis) or with *Cryptosporidium parvum* or *Isospora belli* (enteritis) may prove lethal.

SEVERE IMMUNODEFICIENCY

CD4 counts less than 50 cells/mm^3 indicate profound immunosuppression and, in the absence of effective antiretroviral therapy, are associated with a high mortal-

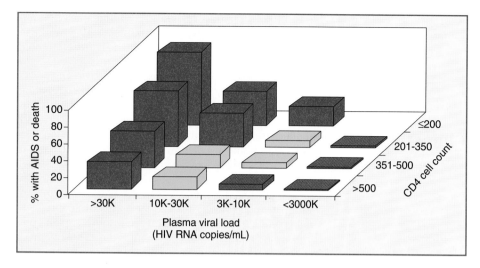

FIGURE 108–6 Likelihood of developing symptomatic AIDS-related illness or death within 3 years. Values in the red zone indicate more than 25% likelihood of disease progression within 3 years and are considered a strong indication for initiation of antiretroviral therapy. Values in the yellow zone indicate a 6 to 24% likelihood of progression in 3 years and suggest initiation of patient-physician discussion of antiretroviral therapy (see text). Values in the green zone indicate small (<5%) likelihood of 3-year progression.

ity within the subsequent 24 to 36 months. Cytomegalovirus (CMV) retinitis and disseminated *Mycobacterium avium* complex (MAC) infection occur frequently. They respond adequately to specific therapy only when it is accompanied by effective control of viral replication.

SEX-SPECIFIC MANIFESTATIONS

Several sex-specific-manifestations are relevant to the management of HIV infection in women. Recognition of

these manifestations is especially important because they are responsive to specific therapy; each manifestation may serve as the signal for HIV testing in a person with no prior clinical manifestations of immunodeficiency.

1. The earliest clinical manifestation of HIV infection in women may be the frequent recurrence of *Candida* vaginitis in the absence of predisposing factors. Because recurrent *Candida* vaginitis may develop at a time of only moderate immunodefi-

TABLE 108–4   Relation of CD4 Lymphocyte Counts to the Onset of Certain HIV-Associated Infections and Neoplasms in North America

CD4 Count Cells/mm³ *	Opportunistic Infection or Neoplasm	Frequency (%)†
>500	Herpes zoster, polydermatomal	5–10
200–500	*Mycobacterium tuberculosis* infection, pulmonary and extrapulmonary	2–20
	Oral hairy leukoplakia	40–70
	Candida pharyngitis (thrush)	40–70
	Kaposi's sarcoma, mucocutaneous	15–30 (M)
	Bacterial pneumonia, recurrent	15–20
	Cervical neoplasia	1–2 (F)
100–200	*Pneumocystis carinii* pneumonia	20–60
	Histoplasmosis capsulatum infection, disseminated	0–20
	Kaposi's sarcoma, visceral	3–8 (M)
	Progressive multifocal leukoencephalopathy	2–3
	Lymphoma, non-Hodgkin's	2–5
<100	*Candida* esophagitis	15–20
	Cytomegalovirus retinitis	20–35
	Mycobacterium avium complex, disseminated	20–35
	Toxoplasma gondii encephalitis	5–25
	Cryptosporidium parvum enteritis	2–10
	Cryptococcus neoformans encephalitis	3–5
	Herpes simplex virus, chronic, ulcerative	4–8
	Cytomegalovirus esophagitis or colitis	4–8
	Lymphoma, central nervous system	4–8

* Table indicates CD4 count at which specific infections or neoplasms generally begin to appear. Each infection may recur or progress during the subsequent course of HIV disease.

† Even within the United States, great regional differences in the incidence of specific opportunistic infections are apparent. For example, disseminated histoplasmosis is common in the Mississippi River drainage area but rare in individuals who have lived exclusively on the east or west coast.

F = exclusively in women; M = usually in men.

ciency (CD4 count above 200 cells/mm³), it may serve as a trigger to discuss HIV testing and lead to earlier diagnosis in otherwise asymptomatic women.

2. Recurrent large painful genital, perianal, or perineal ulcers, caused by HSV-2, are significantly more frequent in women than in men. Occurring at a time of more advanced immunodeficiency, such lesions should always prompt HIV testing, as well as specific antiviral therapy (see Chapter 107).

3. A rare but potentially life-threatening consequence of HIV infection in women may be development of cervical dysplasia/neoplasia, which appears to result from impaired host defenses against the human papillomavirus (HPV). HIV-infected women show an increased prevalence of high-grade squamous intraepithelial lesions on Papanicolaou (Pap) smear. HIV-infected women should therefore obtain two Pap smears at a 6-month interval; if the initial two Pap smears are both normal, smears should be repeated once a year. Conversely, all women with high-grade squamous intraepithelial lesions on a Pap smear should be encouraged to undergo testing for HIV infection, in addition to specific management of the cervical lesions.

Management of HIV Infection

Because patients are asymptomatic during most of the course of HIV-1 infection (see Fig. 108–5), and even seriously immunocompromised individuals often function productively between bouts of OIs, the ambulatory management of persons with HIV infection deserves major emphasis.

INITIAL AMBULATORY EVALUATION

Once HIV infection is recognized, the physician should discuss, in an unhurried manner, the clinical course and treatment of HIV infection and the use of immunologic and virologic studies (e.g., CD4 counts, PVL assays) to guide therapy. The physician should emphasize that most patients, even without antiviral therapy, survive for 10 to 12 years after acquiring HIV infection and are asymptomatic during most of that time. The physician should then stress the fact that, with effective currently available antiretroviral therapy, HIV disease progression can be prevented for a long period of time, and gradual immunologic recovery will take place in the majority of patients. Such recovery can be maintained for up to 5 years in many patients, and there is a sound basis to believe that, with judicious management, many patients may remain asymptomatic, on maintenance antiretroviral therapy, for much longer periods of time.

Prevention of further transmission through unprotected sex and sharing of needles must be discussed not only at the first visit but also periodically thereafter.

Initial evaluation should include both an HIV-oriented review of systems and a complete physical examination (Table 108–5). In particular, the skin must be examined for HIV-associated rashes and Kaposi's sarcoma. Examination of the oral cavity may reveal thrush, gingivitis, hairy leukoplakia, superficial ulcers caused by HSV, aphthous ulcers, or lesions characteristic of Kaposi's sarcoma. The optic fundi may have hemorrhagic lesions characteristic of CMV retinitis. Lymph node enlargement, hepatomegaly, splenomegaly, and any genital lesions should all be carefully noted. Neurologic examination for both peripheral neuropathy and decreased global cognition deserves close attention. Pelvic examination with Pap smear should be routine for women.

Purified protein derivative (PPD) testing, in conjunction with baseline chest radiograph, is mandatory. PPD skin testing should be performed as early in the course of HIV infection as possible. Induration of 5 mm or more should be considered positive. Any patient with a positive PPD should be evaluated for the presence of active tuberculosis; if no active disease is present, the patient should receive 1 year of prophylaxis with isoniazid or combination drug therapy for a shorter time period (see Chapter 99). If active tuberculosis is identified, multidrug therapy should be initiated.

Serologic testing for *T. gondii* infection is important in the event that a person subsequently develops an intracerebral lesion (see later discussion). Serologic testing for syphilis should be done at the first visit and followed by prompt treatment if positive (see Chapter 107). Antibody responses to pneumococcal polysaccharides are better among patients with higher CD4 counts; therefore, the pneumococcal vaccine should be administered as soon as the diagnosis of HIV infection is established.

Because the most helpful laboratory guides to the degree of immunodeficiency and to appropriate therapy are the CD4 count and the PVL assay, these determinations should be obtained at the first visit and repeated at intervals of 2 to 3 months. The patient should understand that the CD4 count and the PVL are rough

TABLE 108–5 Management of Early HIV Disease

Monitoring

Confirm positive HIV test
Complete baseline history and physical examination: directed-interval interview and examination every 6 months

Laboratory Evaluation

Baseline plasma HIV-RNA level and CD4 cell count with repeat every 2 to 3 months
Baseline purified protein derivative (PPD) and anergy panel
Baseline *Toxoplasma* antibody, syphilis serology, hepatitis B and C antibodies, cytomegalovirus antibody, liver function tests, and chest radiograph

Health Care Maintenance

Assessment for ongoing counseling needs and referral for significant psychiatric or social problems
Pneumococcal vaccine, hepatitis B vaccine (if HBV seronegative)
Yearly influenza vaccine

guides to the degree of immunodeficiency and the rate of viral replication, respectively, and that modest fluctuations in these measurements may not be indicative of a change in clinical course. It is helpful for the physician to utilize graphic illustrations of the interaction between PVL and CD4 count as predictors of the course of illness in the absence of treatment, as well as a guide to the initiation of antiretroviral therapy (see Fig. 108–6).

ANTIRETROVIRAL THERAPY

Clarification of the mechanisms of HIV replication has identified several potential sites at which retroviral replication might be limited or blocked (see Fig. 108–4). The drugs approved by the U.S. Food and Drug Administration for treatment of HIV infection include six nucleoside analogues that inhibit HIV reverse transcriptase (nRTIs): zidovudine (ZDV, formerly azidothymidine [AZT]), didanosine (ddI), zalcitabine (ddc), stavudine (d4T), lamivudine (3TC), and abacavir (ABC); three non-nucleoside reverse transcriptase inhibitors (NNRTIs): nevirapine, efavirenz, and delavirdine; and five drugs that are HIV protease inhibitors (PIs): indinavir, nelfinavir, ritonavir, saquinavir, and amprenavir.

Currently recommended combination therapy can cause marked and sustained decreases in PVL to levels below current limits of detection in the majority of patients for at least 48 months. The ensuing discussion provides guidelines based on controlled clinical trials. Additional clinical trials are in progress, and therapeutic recommendations will change periodically over the next few years.

The laboratory objective of antiretroviral therapy should be to maintain the lowest PVL for as long as possible. Treatment with a single antiretroviral agent has only a transient effect on PVL and HIV progression and predictably results in development of HIV resistance against the single drug. Monotherapy with any available antiretroviral drug should therefore not be used to treat established HIV infection. Therapy with two nucleoside RTIs (e.g., zidovudine/lamivudine), although more effective in decreasing PVL and delaying HIV progression than monotherapy, usually results in viral resistance to both agents, usually within 18 to 24 months, and is

therefore not recommended. Three-drug combinations are currently recommended for the initiation of treatment in all patients.

The three-drug regimens that currently provide the most profound, durable suppression of viral replication include either a potent PI or the NNRTI efavirenz, in combination with two NRTIs (Table 108–6). Such regimens can maintain PVL below currently detectable limits (50 RNA copies/mL) for 2 or more years in over half of patients who adhere closely to the regimen. However, interruptions in the regimen (e.g., by missing midday doses) can lead to development of HIV resistance to the antiviral agents, first reflected by increasing PVL. It is important for the patient to understand the rationale for, and be fully committed to, an effective treatment plan before initiation of antiretroviral therapy. Drug resistance may eventually occur with even the most effective antiviral regimens.

Although a number of factors (e.g., adverse drug reactions, development of viral resistance to multiple drugs, suboptimal compliance with complicated regimens) will make it impossible to achieve maximal suppression of PVL in every patient, every effort should be made to achieve this objective.

WHEN TO INITIATE THERAPY

Symptomatic Patients

All patients with symptomatic AIDS (with active or past OIs listed in Table 108–1) should receive antiretroviral therapy as outlined later. Without effective antiretroviral therapy, patients with symptomatic AIDS have a high risk of death within 3 to 18 months.

Some experts recommend treatment of patients in whom the acute retroviral syndrome is documented. There is suggestive evidence that initiation of effective antiretroviral therapy at this early stage may lead to full restoration of immune function and may lower the PVL "set point" to a level consistent with long-term nonprogression of HIV disease.

Asymptomatic Patients

In most patients, treatment should be initiated when HIV infection is asymptomatic. PVL assays in conjunc-

TABLE 108–6 Guidelines for the Initiation of Antiretroviral Therapy in the Chronically HIV-Infected Patient*

Clinical Category	CD4⁺ T Cell Count and HIV RNA	Recommendation
Symptomatic (AIDS, thrush, unexplained fever)	Any value	Treat.
Asymptomatic	CD4⁺ T cells < 350 mm³ or HIV RNA > 30,000 copies/mL	Treatment generally recommended.
Asymptomatic	CD4⁺ T cells between 350 and 500 and HIV RNA between 10,000 and 30,000	Treatment should be considered based on prognosis for disease-free survival (see Fig. 108–6).
Asymptomatic	CD4⁺ T cells > 500 mm³ and HIV RNA < 10,000 copies/mL	Most clinicians would delay therapy and observe; however, some would treat under certain circumstances.

* These general guidelines should be used only in conjunction with the text. There are no absolute laboratory thresholds on which the initiation of therapy can be based. This decision must always be made jointly by the informed patient and the physician.

tion with CD4 counts provide the tools essential to guide the initiation and change of antiviral treatment regimens. The PVL reflects the magnitude of viral replication in the patient; the rate of HIV disease progression is directly related to PVL. Although the optimal time to initiate therapy in a given asymptomatic patient is uncertain, there is general agreement that patients with CD4 counts below 350 cells/mm^3, and patients with PVLs greater than 30,000 copies/mL, will benefit from effective antiretroviral therapy (see Table 108–6). For patients with CD4 counts greater than 500 cells/mm^3 and PVLs less than 10,000 copies/mL, the disadvantages of antiretroviral therapy (short- and long-term toxicities, development of antiretroviral resistance because of lapses in adherence) generally outweigh the potential advantage (prevention of progressive immunologic damage). For patients with CD4 counts between 350 and 500 cells/mL associated with PVLs between 10,000 and 30,000 copies/mL, the risk of clinical HIV progression over a 3-year period is less than 20%, and it is not clear whether the potential long-term advantages of treatment outweigh the known disadvantages.

In all cases, it is critical that initiation of therapy be based on a joint decision by the informed patient and his or her physician. Initiation of antiretroviral therapy in an asymptomatic patient is never an urgent issue, and the physician should spend whatever time is necessary (e.g., three patient visits over an 8-week period) for the patient to understand both the potential benefits and risks of the specific regimen that is to be undertaken. Graphs such as shown in Figure 108–6 can be very effective in helping the patient to understand the importance of the CD4 count and PVL in providing the prognostic information essential to determining when to initiate therapy. Therapy should be individualized to the extent possible (e.g., a patient with chronic colitis should not initiate therapy with a PI with major gastrointestinal side effects, a patient with recurrent nephrolithiasis should avoid a PI with renal toxicity). Because, with currently available antiretroviral agents, the patient may anticipate lifelong antiretroviral therapy, and because inadequate adherence to any antiretroviral regimen will result, over time, in resistance to the antiretroviral drugs, it is essential that the patient has as full an understanding of the regimen as possible before initiating antiretroviral therapy.

DRUGS TO INITIATE THERAPY

The goal of antiretroviral therapy is to ensure that the patient has the highest possible quality of life for as long as possible. In general, this requires therapy that durably suppresses the PVL below levels that are detectable by the most sensitive available assays (<50 copies/HIV-RNA mL). Achievement of this objective demands that the patient take combination antiretroviral therapy with a minimum of three antiretroviral drugs. Current consensus guidelines recommend antiretroviral drug combinations outlined in Table 108–7.

Although each of the recommended regimens can result in durable suppression of PVL, associated with gradual recovery of immunologic function, each regimen has specific advantages and potential toxicities of which the patient must be aware. For example, an efavirenz-based regimen has the advantage of simplicity of administration (once a day for efavirenz, twice a day for the associated nucleoside reverse transcriptase inhibitors) but the disadvantage of more rapid development of resistance if adherence is poor. A triple nucleoside regimen appears less likely than a PI-containing one to result in long-term toxicities (lipodystrophy, insulin resistance), but it may be less effective in patients with very high initial viral loads. The choice of the regimen should always be made jointly by the physician and the informed patient.

WHEN TO CHANGE THERAPY

When an effective antiretroviral regimen is initiated in an asymptomatic patient, with no previous antiretroviral therapy, the PVL should decrease sharply, generally by 100-fold in 8 weeks and to an undetectable level (<50 copies/mL) within 16 weeks. If a reduction of this magnitude is not achieved, the physician should, with the patient, assess whether adherence has been adequate. If adherence has been nearly complete (>90%), the physician and patient should consider changing to another effective regimen. If a given regimen achieves a reduction of PVL below detectable limits and continuing adherence is achieved, the patient can anticipate effective viral suppression for at least 2 to 3 years. The PVL should be monitored at 2- or 3-month intervals throughout the course of therapy. If, after months or years of adequate viral suppression, the viral load again becomes detectable on two consecutive determinations, consideration of a change in therapy is indicated.

There are currently no data that critically define the threshold at which a change in therapy should occur. Some experts recommend change as soon as the viral load is above detectable limits on two determinations. Other experts would not change until the viral load again exceeded an arbitrary figure of 10,000 to 20,000 copies/mL. Once the decision for the first change is made, all three antiretroviral agents should be changed if possible (e.g., efavirenz/zidovudine/lamivudine might be changed to nelfinavir/stavudine/didanosine).

After failure of a second combination antiretroviral regimen, change is more difficult, because the remaining options are fewer. Although antiretroviral resistance testing, both phenotypic and genotypic, has the potential for determining antiretroviral resistance patterns in a given patient, such testing is not now sufficiently precise to be of general clinical utility. This situation may change rapidly.

There is now evidence that many treated patients continue to do well clinically, with stable CD4 counts, for months to years after viral "escape" (increasing PVL). In such patients, stopping antiretroviral therapy does generally result in clinical deterioration. The basis for continued clinical well-being, despite increasing PVL, during long-term antiretroviral therapy is uncertain. However, these observations make it clear that many patients continue to receive clinical and immunologic benefit from antiretroviral therapy despite loss of viral control. How long the clinical benefit will be sustained in such patients is unknown.

TABLE 108–7   Recommended Antiretroviral Agents for Treatment of Established HIV Infection

Preferred	Strong evidence of clinical benefit and/or sustained suppression of plasma viral load. One choice each from column A and column B. Drugs are listed in random, not priority, order.
	Column A *Column B* Indinavir ZDV + ddI Nelfinavir d4T + ddI Efavirenz ddI + 3TC Saquinavir − SGC* ZDV + 3TC Ritonavir ZDV + ddC Ritonavir + saquinavir d4T + 3TC Amprenavir
Alternative	Less likely to provide sustained virus suppression, or data inadequate. Nevirapine or delavirdine + 2 NRTIs (column B, above).† Abacavir + ZDV + 3TC‡
Not Generally Recommended	Strong evidence of clinical benefit but initial virus suppression is not sustained in most patients. Two NRTIs (column B, above)
Not Recommended	Evidence against use, virologically undesirable, or overlapping toxicities. All monotherapies§

* *Only* the soft-gel capsule (SGC) preparation of saquinavir (Fortovase) is recommended.

† The combination of any of the three available NNRTIs + two NRTIs can suppress viremia to undetectable levels in the majority of patients remaining on treatment for > 28 weeks. An efavirenz-containing regimen has been shown to compare favorably to a PI-containing regimen with regard to suppression of viremia through 72 weeks; such head-to-head comparative trials have not been performed with nevirapine or delavirdine. Of note, use of efavirenz, nevirapine, or delavirdine may result in resistance that precludes efficacy of any other member of this drug class.

‡ Virologic and immunologic responses obtained with abacavir + ZDV + 3TC are similar to those obtained with indinavir + ZDV + 3TC at 48 weeks. The durability of viral load suppression with this regimen is uncertain; in addition, abacavir is associated with a potentially life-threatening hypersensitivity reaction. For these reasons, a PI-containing or efavirenz-containing regimen is preferred until longer-term data are available for an abacavir-containing three-drug regimen.

§ Zidovudine (ZDV) monotherapy may be considered for prophylactic use in pregnant women with low viral load and high CD4+ T-cell counts to prevent perinatal transmission.

3TC = lamivudine; d4T = stavudine; ddI = didanosine; NRTIs = nucleoside reverse transcriptase inhibitors; NNRTIs = non-nucleoside reverse transcriptase inhibitors; PI = protease inhibitor; ZDV = zidovudine; ddc = zalcitabine.

Modified from DHHS guidelines for the use of antiretroviral agents in HIV-infected adults and adolescents. (www.hivatis.org/guidelines).

PROPHYLAXIS AGAINST OPPORTUNISTIC INFECTIONS

During the first 15 years of the HIV pandemic, the most effective medical interventions for persons with HIV infection were prophylactic measures against OIs. The greatest success was the prevention of PCP for individuals with CD4 counts less than 200 cells/mm³; routine use of prophylaxis has resulted in a greater than fourfold (from 60% to <15%) decrease in the frequency of PCP as the initial OI in North American men with HIV infection. Specific antimicrobial prophylaxis (Table 108–8) is also effective for prevention of *T. gondii* encephalitis in patients with anti-*Toxoplasma* antibodies with CD4 counts less than 100 cells/mm³ and for prevention of active tuberculosis in patients with positive tuberculin skin tests at any CD4 level (see Table 108–8). Prophylaxis is moderately effective against CMV retinitis and disseminated MAC infections in patients with CD4 counts less than 50 cells/mm³; in both instances, the value of prophylaxis must be carefully weighed against potential toxicities of the prophylactic agents. Prophylaxis is very effective against recurrent HSV-2 infection (acyclovir, famcyclovir, or valacyclovir) and against recurrent *Candida* esophagitis (fluconazole) but should generally be reserved for those patients with recurrent symptomatic disease.

Management of Specific Clinical Manifestations of Immunodeficiency: A Problem-Oriented Approach

In persons with HIV infection OIs vary considerably in time of onset (see Table 108–4). For example, some patients may develop multidermatomal herpes zoster with CD4 counts greater than 500 cells/mm³ and then have no other OIs until they develop PCP with CD4 counts less than 200 cells/mm³. On the other hand, occasional patients may remain entirely asymptomatic until their CD4 counts are below 50 cells/mm³, at which time they may develop major life-threatening OIs, such

TABLE 108-8 **Prophylaxis Against Certain Opportunistic Infections (OIs) in HIV-Infected Adults***

Pathogen	Indication	First Choice	Alternatives
Pneumocystis carinii†	CD4 count < 200, or history of thrush	Trimethoprim-sulfamethoxazole (TMP-SMZ), 1 double-strength tablet qd	Dapsone, 100 g qd Pentamidine, aerosolized, 300 mg q mo Atovaquone, 1500 mg qd
Mycobacterium tuberculosis† Isoniazid-sensitive	TST (t) reaction > 5 mm, or prior positive TST without treatment, or contact with case of active tuberculosis	Isoniazid, 300 mg, PO plus pyridoxine, 50 mg, qd × 9 mo	Rifampin, 600 mg, and pyrizinamide, 800 mg, qd × 2 mo
Isoniazid-resistant	Same as above	Rifampin, 600 mg qd plus pyrizinamide, 20 mg/kg qd × 2 mo	Rifabutin, 300 mg qd × 4 mo
Toxoplasma gondii†	IgG antibody to *Toxoplasma* and CD4 count < 100	TMP-SMZ, 1 double-strength tablet qd	Dapsone, 50 mg PO qd plus pyrimethimine, 50 mg, PO q wk plus leucovorin, 25 mg, PO q wk
Mycobacterium avium complex‡	CD4 count < 50	Azithromycin, 1200 mg q wk	Clarithromycin, 500 mg PO bid
Cytomegalovirus	CD4 count < 50	Gancyclovir, 1 g, qid§	

* DHHS recommendations for prophylaxis against OIs are updated regularly and are available at www.hivatis.org.
† Strongly recommended as standard of care in all patients.
‡ Recommended for consideration in all patients.
§ The benefit: risk ratio of prophylaxis versus early recognition and treatment of cytomegalovirus retinitis is uncertain.
TST (t) = tuberculosis skin test.

as *T. gondii* encephalitis. In general, life-threatening OIs do not occur with CD4 counts greater than 200 cells/mm³ (see Table 108–4).

In general, OIs that occur with higher CD4 counts respond to routine therapy for the specific infection (e.g., appropriate β-lactam antibiotic for pneumococcal pneumonia, standard multidrug therapy for pulmonary tuberculosis) whereas OIs occurring with CD4 counts less than 200 cells/mm³ require chronic suppressive therapy after treatment of acute infection (e.g., PCP, CMV retinitis, or *Cryptococcus neoformans* meningitis).

An important principle in the management of OIs is that the great majority respond well to appropriate antimicrobial therapy. A history of a life-threatening OI does not appear to influence the subsequent response to effective combination antiretroviral therapy.

The development of durable and effective antiretroviral therapy has had a dramatic impact on the incidence of OIs in all areas in which treatment is available. Although the impact on specific OIs has varied, with decreases greater than 80% in CMV retinitis and over 70% in PCP, all recognized OIs have significantly decreased in frequency in the United States since 1995. Furthermore, after partial restoration of immunologic function in response to effective therapy, withdrawal of prophylaxis against specific OIs is reasonable. Current data support withdrawal of prophylaxis against PCP after two consecutive CD4 counts greater than 200 cells/mm³ in patients with effective reduction in PVL. Specific recommendations are not yet available as to when suppressive therapy may be withdrawn after successful treatment of other specific OIs (e.g., CMV retinitis, MAC infection).

Because of the highly significant reduction in OIs

associated with effective antiretroviral therapy, rates of hospitalization and mortality for AIDS-related illnesses have dropped sharply from 1995 to 1999, with decreases of as much as 80% in several major North American and Western European cities.

CONSTITUTIONAL SYMPTOMS

Nonspecific symptoms may be the initial clinical manifestations of severe immunodeficiency. Patients may develop unexplained fever, night sweats, anorexia, weight loss, or diarrhea. These symptoms may last for weeks or months before the development of identifiable OIs in patients who do not receive effective antiretroviral therapy. These constitutional symptoms may represent manifestations of specific, but unidentified, OIs.

Mucocutaneous Diseases

Disorders of the skin and mucosa are among the most common clinical manifestations of HIV disease (Table 108–9).

CUTANEOUS DISEASE

HIV-infected patients may have a variety of dermatologic ailments; many of these are readily treatable (see Table 108–9). Rashes occur in response to a variety of medications, particularly sulfa-containing drugs. Staphylococcal folliculitis occurs frequently. Severe seborrheic dermatitis, often manifested as a scaly eruption between the eyebrows and the nasolabial fold, is common. Psori-

TABLE 108-9   Dermatologic Conditions Common in HIV Infection

Condition	Description	Treatment
Herpes simplex	Clear or crusted vesicles with an erythematous base; ulceration common when chronic; location: oral or genital mucous membranes, face, and hands	Acyclovir, 200 mg, five times/day
Herpes zoster (shingles)	Cluster of vesicles in a dermatomal distribution; may involve adjacent dermatomes or may disseminate	Acyclovir, 800 mg, five times/day; if disseminated or involvement of ophthalamic branch of trigeminal nerve, IV acyclovir, 10 mg/kg, q8h
Staphylococcal folliculitis	Erythematous pustules on face, trunk, and groin, often pruritic	Dicloxacillin, 500 mg qid, or erythromycin, 500 mg qid
Bacilliary angiomatosis	Friable vascular papules or subcutaneous nodules on skin; may involve liver, spleen, and lymph nodes	Clarithromycin, 500 mg bid, or doxycycline, 200 mg qd
Molluscum contagiosum	Chronic, flesh-colored papules, often umbilicated, on face or anogenital area	Cryotherapy and curettage
Seborrheic dermatitis	White scaling or erythematous patches on scalp, eyebrows, face, trunk, axilla, and groin	Hydrocortisone cream 2.5% and ketoconazole cream
Psoriasis	Scaling, marginated patches on elbows, knees, and lumbosacral areas	Triamcinolone acetonide cream 0.1%
Candidal dermatitis	Urticarial scaling or erythematous patches on face, trunk, axilla, and groin	Hydrocortisone cream 1% and ketokonazole cream

asis, a scaling eruption usually most prominent on the elbows, also occurs frequently.

Herpes zoster, manifested by crops of vesicular lesions on erythematous bases in a dermatomal or polydermatomal distribution, is often preceded for several days by unexplained pain in the involved dermatome(s). Molluscum contagiosum, umbilicated pearly papules caused by poxvirus infection, may occur in crops on the face, neck, abdomen, and genitalia of HIV-infected persons. Facial and genital warts caused by HPV infection also occur with increased frequency.

Cutaneous lesions of Kaposi's sarcoma may be flat or raised; may be red, brown, or blue; and may resemble insect bites, nevi, or cutaneous ecchymoses. On examination, Kaposi's sarcoma lesions often have a firm texture when rolled between the fingers, whereas many benign lesions are not distinguishable from normal skin by this maneuver. Definitive diagnosis is established by biopsy.

Treatment

Many of the minor mucocutaneous problems can be readily treated, but recurrence is frequent (see Table 108–9). Thrush and *Candida* vaginitis usually respond to topical therapy. Fungal skin infections usually respond to antifungal creams. Esophageal candidiasis necessitates systemic therapy (fluconazole, 200 mg daily for 10 days).

Recurrent or chronic ulcerative perioral, perianal, or genital herpes simplex lesions usually respond rapidly to specific therapy (e.g., oral acyclovir, 400 mg five times per day for 10 days), but chronic suppressive therapy may be required to prevent frequent relapses. Although the effectiveness of therapy for uncomplicated multidermatomal herpes zoster is uncertain, most clinicians pre-

scribe specific therapy (e.g., acyclovir, 800 mg orally five times per day for 7 days).

Seborrheic dermatitis often responds to hydrocortisone cream. Warts caused by HPV, as well as lesions of molluscum contagiosum, may be treated with ablative procedures (e.g., cryotherapy, laser).

ORAL DISEASE

Candida stomatitis, or thrush, is often the earliest recognized OI. Early thrush may be entirely asymptomatic; as infection becomes more extensive, it causes pain and discomfort on eating. The characteristic cheesy white exudate on the mucous membranes can easily be scraped off. The underlying mucosa may be normal or inflamed.

Oral hairy leukoplakia (OHL) is a white lichenified, plaquelike lesion, most commonly seen on the lateral surfaces of the tongue. Unlike thrush, the lesions of OHL cannot be scraped off with a tongue depressor. OHL may also be an early manifestation of moderately severe immunodeficiency. OHL is painless and may remit and relapse spontaneously.

Patients may develop painful ulcers in the mouth. These may be caused by HSV but often represent aphthous lesions of uncertain etiology. Aphthous mucosal ulcers are difficult to treat. Small oral ulcers may respond to topical corticosteroids, whereas giant oral or esophageal ulcers require oral administration of thalidomide or corticosteroids. It is important to obtain cultures for HSV and CMV to be sure that the ulcers are not viral in origin before initiating corticosteroid or thalidomide therapy. Thalidomide should be used, if at all, only when birth control can be ensured in women with childbearing potential because of its well-documented adverse effects on fetal development.

Kaposi's sarcoma has a predilection for the oral cavity and skin. Oral lesions may be purple, red, or blue and may be raised or flat. Usually painless, these lesions cause symptoms when they enlarge, bleed, or ulcerate.

ESOPHAGEAL DISEASE

Symptomatic esophageal disease seldom occurs with CD4 counts greater than 50 cells/mm³. Pain on swallowing and substernal burning are common and may indicate *Candida* esophagitis, particularly when oral thrush is present. Esophagoscopy with biopsy, cytology, and culture should only be performed if symptoms do not rapidly respond (within 3 to 5 days) to antifungal therapy. If esophagoscopy shows ulcerative lesions, they are usually caused by CMV (50%), aphthae (45%), or HSV (5%). Because each of these lesions is responsive to appropriate therapy, definitive etiologic diagnosis is strongly recommended (Table 108–10). CMV esophageal ulcers respond well to intravenous gancyclovir or foscarnet therapy for 2 to 3 weeks, or until resolution is confirmed endoscopically. Esophageal ulcerations caused by HSV usually respond well to intravenous acyclovir (see Table 108–10).

GENITAL DISEASE

Recurrent genital ulcers are most often caused by HSV. Tzanck preparation reveals multinucleated giant cells, and culture or specific immunofluorescence of ulcer scrapings confirms the diagnosis; biopsy is rarely indicated. Primary syphilis also occurs with increased frequency (see Chapter 107). Chancroid is unusual in North America.

VAGINAL AND CERVICAL DISEASE

Candida species, most often *Candida albicans*, can cause an irritating vulvovaginitis in women with HIV infection as well as among healthy HIV-seronegative women. A potassium hydroxide preparation of the cheesy white exudate will reveal budding yeast or pseudohyphae.

Bacterial vaginosis and trichomoniasis are common and both respond well to specific treatment.

Infection with HPV is associated not only with proliferation of genital warts but also with a greater frequency of cervical dysplasia in HIV-infected women. Pap smears indicative of cervical dysplasia should be followed by prompt colposcopy, biopsy when indicted, and appropriate treatment of any dysplastic lesions. With this approach, progression of cervical dysplasia to invasive cervical cancer is exceedingly rare.

Nervous System Diseases

Nervous system complications ultimately occur in the majority of untreated HIV-infected persons and range from mild cognitive disturbances or peripheral neuropathy to severe dementia or life-threatening central nervous system (CNS) infections. The physician must be alert to the development of early signs of treatable neurologic complications of HIV disease. As with other lentiviruses, HIV enters microglial cells of the CNS early in the course of HIV infection. This process may be associated with neuronal cell loss, vacuolization, and occasional lymphocytic infiltration. Both direct neuronal destruction and effects of viral proteins on neuronal cell function contribute to nervous system disease in AIDS.

COGNITIVE DYSFUNCTION

Intellectual impairment rarely occurs early in the course of HIV infection, but it is common among persons with advanced immunodeficiency. AIDS dementia complex (ADC) often begins insidiously and usually progresses over months to years (Table 108–11). ADC is charac-

TABLE 108–11 Major Clinical Manifestations of AIDS Dementia Complex

Cognition	Inattention, reduced concentration, forgetfulness, impaired memory	Global dementia
Motor performance	Slowed movements, clumsiness, ataxia	Paraplegia
Behavior	Apathy, altered personality, agitation	Mutism

TABLE 108–10 HIV-Associated Esophagitis

Condition	Characteristics	Treatment
Candida infection	Thrush usual, esophageal plaques	Fluconazole, 200 mg/day
CMV infection	Large shallow esophageal ulcers on endoscopy	Ganciclovir, 5 mg/kg bid
Herpes simplex	Deep ulceration on endoscopy	Acyclovir, 200–800 mg five times/day
Aphthae	Giant ulcers on endoscopy; no virus on biopsy	Prednisone, 40–60 mg/day or thalidomide, 200 mg/day*

* Thalidomide must *never* be given during pregnancy.
CMV = cytomegalovirus.

terized by poor concentration, diminished memory, slowing of thought processes, motor dysfunction, and occasionally behavioral abnormalities characterized by social withdrawal and apathy. Symptoms of clinical depression overlap with many of the characteristics of early ADC and must be considered carefully in differential diagnosis and therapy. Computed tomography (CT) of the head in ADC reveals only atrophy, with enlarged sulci and ventricles. Examination of CSF is most often normal.

Motor abnormalities may include a progressive gait ataxia. As the disease progresses, patients may develop focal neurologic complications characterized by spastic weakness of the lower extremities and incontinence secondary to vacuolar myelopathy.

A large variety of neurologic problems may complicate the later stages of HIV infection. A neuroanatomic classification of these manifestations is presented in Table 108–12, and several of the more frequent or treatable problems are discussed next.

FOCAL LESIONS OF THE CNS

Several opportunistic complications of HIV infection produce focal CNS lesions. Patients with focal neuro-

TABLE 108–12 Neuroanatomic Classification of the Common Complications of HIV-1 Infection

Meningitis and Headache
Aseptic meningitis
Cryptococcal meningitis
Tuberculous meningitis

Diffuse Brain Diseases
With preservation of consciousness
  AIDS dementia complex
With concomitant depression of arousal
  Toxoplasma encephalitis
  Cytomegalovirus encephalitis

Focal Brain Diseases
Cerebral toxoplasmosis
Primary CNS lymphoma
Progressive multifocal leukoencephalopathy
Tuberculous brain abscess (*M. tuberculosis*)

Myelopathies
Subacute/chronic, progressive
  vacuolar myelopathy
Subacute with polyradiculopathy
  Cytomegalovirus myelopathy

Peripheral Neuropathies
Predominantly sensory polyneuropathy
Toxic neuropathies (zalcitabine, didanosine, stavudine)
Autonomic neuropathy
Cytomegalovirus polyradiculopathy

Myopathies
Polymyositis
Noninflammatory myopathy
Zidovudine myopathy

logic signs, seizures of new onset, or recent onset of rapidly progressive cognitive impairment should undergo magnetic resonance imaging (MRI) and/or CT of the brain.

Toxoplasmosis, CNS lymphoma, and progressive multifocal leukoencephalopathy (PML) are the most common causes of CNS focal lesions in this setting (Table 108–13).

In the absence of antiretroviral therapy, *Toxoplasma gondii* encephalitis occurs in up to one third of HIV-1–infected patients who have serologic evidence of *T. gondii* infection, but it is rare in individuals who have no such antibodies. Thus, the importance of toxoplasmosis as an OI varies according to region. Patients with CNS toxoplasmosis often present with progressive headache and focal neurologic abnormalities, usually associated with fever. CT with contrast dye usually shows multiple ring-enhancing lesions, but it may show only focal edema. MRI is a more sensitive technique and often shows multiple small lesions that are not apparent on CT. Management of symptomatic, ring-enhancing brain lesions in persons with AIDS includes initiation of empirical therapy with pyrimethamine, sulfadiazine, and folinic acid. Brain biopsy should be reserved for patients with atypical presentations, those with no serum antibodies to *T. gondii*, or those whose lesions do not respond after 10 to 14 days of antiprotozoal treatment. Because cyst forms of toxoplasmosis are not eradicated with current therapy, patients must remain on chronic suppressive therapy; although many experts believe that suppressive therapy may be withdrawn if a sustained rise in CD4 count above 200 cells/mm^3 is achieved with effective antiretroviral therapy, conclusive data supporting this approach are not available.

Primary CNS lymphoma complicates HIV infection in 3% to 6% of cases. On CT or MRI, lesions are characteristically located in the periventricular space, are often single but may be oligofocal, and usually enhance weakly with contrast medium (see Table 108–13). Irradiation often provides transient remission.

PML is a demyelinating disease caused by a papovavirus (JC virus). Presenting symptoms may include progressive dementia, visual impairment, seizures, and/or hemiparesis. MRI usually shows multiple lesions predominantly involving the white matter. These lesions are usually not visible on CT, which helps to distinguish PML from other mass lesions of the CNS in AIDS patients. There is no effective specific treatment for PML, but the disease often regresses in response to effective antiretroviral therapy.

CNS DISEASES WITHOUT PROMINENT FOCAL SIGNS

Evaluation of the HIV-infected patient who presents with fever and headache is complicated by the often subtle manifestations of serious CNS lesions in immunocompromised patients. Patients with bacterial meningitis (see Chapter 97) are managed the same as noncompromised patients. Meningeal diseases in HIV-infected patients often, however, fall into the broad categories of

TABLE 108–13 Comparative Clinical and Radiologic Features of Cerebral Toxoplasmosis, Primary CNS Lymphoma, and Progressive Multifocal Leukoencephalopathy

Condition	Clinical Onset			Neuroradiologic Features		
	Temporal Profile	Level of Alertness	Fever	Number of Lesions	Characteristics of Lesions	Location of Lesions
Cerebral toxoplasmosis	Days	Reduced	Common	Usually multiple	Spherical, ring-enhancing on CT	Basal ganglia, cortex
Primary CNS lymphoma	Days to weeks	Variable	Absent	One or few	Irregular, weakly enhancing on CT	Periventricular
Progressive multifocal leukoencephalopathy	Days to weeks	Variable	Absent	Multiple	Multiple lesions, seen on MRI only	White matter

CT = computed tomography; MRI = magnetic resonance imaging.

aseptic meningitis, chronic meningitis, and meningoencephalitis.

Aseptic Meningitis

Patients with aseptic meningitis complain most often of headache; the sensorium is generally intact, and the neurologic examination is normal (see Chapter 97). Aseptic meningitis may occur as a manifestation of the acute retroviral syndrome. In the person with established HIV infection, aseptic meningitis may result from several potentially treatable causes (see Chapters 97 and 107).

Chronic Meningitis

Patients with chronic meningitis characteristically present with a history of headache, fever, difficulty in concentrating, and/or changes in sensorium. CSF examination shows a low glucose concentration, an elevated protein level, and a mild to modest lymphocytic pleocytosis. Cryptococcal meningitis is the most common cause. The presence of cryptococcal antigen in CSF or a positive India ink preparation establishes the diagnosis of cryptococcal infection (see Chapter 97). Treatment with amphotericin B for at least 2 weeks followed by lifelong suppression with fluconazole is indicated.

Mycobacterium tuberculosis is an eminently treatable cause of subacute to chronic meningitis in the HIV-infected patient, although it is rare in North America. Antituberculosis therapy should be considered in the setting of chronic meningitis if the cryptococcal antigen test is negative (see Chapter 97).

Coccidioidomycosis and histoplasmosis are possible causes of chronic meningitis in patients residing in, or with a travel history to, endemic regions (desert Southwest, and Ohio and Mississippi River drainage areas, respectively) (see Chapter 97).

Meningoencephalitis

Patients with meningoencephalitis present with alterations in sensorium varying from mild lethargy to coma. Patients are usually febrile, and neurologic examination often shows evidence of diffuse CNS involvement. CT or MRI may show only nonspecific abnormalities, whereas electroencephalography often is consistent with diffuse disease of the brain.

CMV encephalitis is difficult to diagnose. Patients may present with confusion, cranial nerve abnormalities, or long tract signs. CSF findings may resemble bacterial meningitis, with a predominantly polymorphonuclear leukocyte pleocytosis. Many patients have CMV disease elsewhere, most often retinitis. Polymerase chain reaction detection of CMV antigens in CSF appears to be a sensitive and specific method for diagnosis of CMV encephalitis and polyradiculopathy.

Meningoencephalitis caused by HSV is unusual in HIV infection (see Chapter 97).

Pulmonary Diseases

Pulmonary manifestations are common in persons living with HIV and range from nonspecific interstitial pneumonitis to life-threatening pneumonias (Table 108–14). Pneumonia is the most frequent serious infectious complication of HIV disease.

HIV-infected patients have a threefold to fourfold increased risk of bacterial pneumonia, which is generally caused by encapsulated bacteria, including *S. pneumoniae* and *H. influenzae*. The intracellular bacterium *Legionella pneumophila* also causes pneumonia with increased frequency. The increased risk begins with modest degrees of immunodeficiency (CD4 counts of 200 to 500 cells/mm^3). The onset of bacterial pneumonia is often abrupt; patients may have rigors and cough productive of purulent sputum. Physical examination and chest radiographs often show evidence of consolidation. The response to prompt initiation of therapy is usually good, but delay in appropriate antimicrobial therapy may result in a fulminant downhill course. Initial therapy is guided by the results of Gram stain of sputum (see Chapter 99).

PCP was the most common life-threatening infection in North American persons with AIDS until prophylaxis against it became routine. Patients with PCP frequently complain of gradual onset of nonproductive cough, fever, and shortness of breath with exertion; a productive cough suggests another process. In contrast to the acute onset of PCP in other immunocompromised patients, AIDS patients with PCP may have pulmonary symptoms for weeks before presentation to a physician. Arterial hypoxemia is usual and rapidly worsens with slight exertion; the chest radiograph generally shows a subtle interstitial pattern but may be entirely normal. The patient usually appears more sick than the radiograph would suggest. The presence of pleural effusions is suggestive of a cause other than PCP.

If PCP is suspected clinically, therapy should be started immediately; treatment for several days does not interfere with the ability to make a specific diagnosis. Confirmation of PCP is essential; treatment is often complicated by drug reactions, and delay in establishing a correct diagnosis of another treatable condition may be lethal. The diagnosis may often be made by examination of induced sputum. If this fails, bronchoalveolar lavage, with silver staining or immunofluorescence of specimens, is adequate to diagnose PCP in more than 95% of patients.

Treatment with high-dose intravenous trimethoprim-sulfamethoxazole for 3 weeks is effective therapy; this drug combination, however, frequently produces side effects (rash, fever, and/or granulocytopenia). Alternative therapies include atovaquone, trimethoprim plus dapsone, or primaquine plus clindamycin. Patients with advanced PCP and arterial hypoxemia (PO$_2$ ≤ 75 mm on breathing room air) benefit from administration of corticosteroids (40 mg of prednisone twice daily), with tapering of the drug over a 3-week period.

Some AIDS patients (most often children) with inter-

TABLE 108-14 Pulmonary Disease Associated with HIV Infection

Condition	Characteristic	Chest Radiograph	Diagnosis	Treatment
Pneumocystis carinii pneumonia	Subacute onset, dry cough, dyspnea	Interstitial infiltrate most common	Sputum or bronchoalveolar lavage for organism by stain	Trimethoprim-sulfamethoxazole, pentamidine, or atovaquone
Bacterial (pneumococcus, *Haemophilus* most common)	Acute productive cough, fever, chest pain	Lobar or localized infiltrate	Sputum Gram's stain and culture, blood culture	Cefuroxime or alternative antibiotics
Mycobacterial (*Mycobacterium tuberculosis* or *M. kansasii*)	Chronic cough, weight loss, fever	Localized infiltrate, lymphadenopathy	Sputum acid-fast stain and mycobacterial culture	Isoniazid, rifampin, pyrazinamide, ethambutol
Kaposi's sarcoma	Asymptomatic or mild cough	Pulmonary nodules, pleural effusion	Open lung biopsy	Chemotherapy

stitial pneumonitis may have no pathogen identified on transbronchial biopsy.

M. tuberculosis infection occurs with greater frequency in regions having a high prevalence of tuberculosis. Active pulmonary tuberculosis may develop at a time when the CD4 count remains well above 200 cells/mm³ (see Table 108–4). Chest radiographs in HIV-infected patients may show features of primary tuberculosis, including hilar adenopathy, lower or middle lobe infiltrates, miliary pattern, or pleural effusions, as well as classic patterns of reactivation. Extrapulmonary *M. tuberculosis* infection also occurs with increased frequency. Specific blood cultures may yield *M. tuberculosis* in the severely immunocompromised patient.

Both pulmonary and extrapulmonary tuberculosis generally respond promptly to standard antituberculosis therapy, although several outbreaks of multidrug-resistant *M. tuberculosis* have occurred in people with HIV infection. Treatment therefore should begin with four antituberculosis drugs (see Chapter 99). Once initial therapy is completed, long-term monitoring for reactivation is critical. Because nosocomial transmission of multidrug resistant *M. tuberculosis* may occur both in hospitals and in ambulatory care centers, physicians must take adequate precautions to prevent spread of *M. tuberculosis* in the health care setting.

Disseminated histoplasmosis and coccidioidomycosis occur with much greater frequency in persons with HIV infection. Either fungal infection may present with nodular infiltrates or with a miliary pattern on chest radiograph. Histoplasmosis usually involves bone marrow as well as skin; bone marrow examination often shows the organism. Standard treatment of disseminated mycoses in AIDS patients is high-dose amphotericin. Because relapse is common, oral azole therapy (fluconazole for coccidioidomycosis, itraconazole for histoplasmosis) must be continued after resolution of signs and symptoms.

Gastrointestinal Diseases

With advanced immunodeficiency (CD4 count <50 cells/mm³) gastrointestinal disease presenting as dysphagia, diarrhea, or colitis is common. Each of these processes may contribute to inadequate nutrition, compounding the weight loss associated with advanced HIV disease. Dysphagia was discussed earlier.

NAUSEA AND VOMITING

Nausea and vomiting are frequent in advanced HIV disease. Symptoms are often related to medications; these must be reviewed and the likely offending drug (or drugs) withheld as a therapeutic trial. If symptoms of nausea and vomiting remain undefined and do not respond to empirical therapy with histamine (H_2) antagonists or an antiemetic, more extensive gastrointestinal evaluation with endoscopy should be performed.

Abnormalities of liver function tests are common in HIV disease and often are nonspecific. Elevations of serum alanine aminotransferase and aspartate amino-

transferase often represent chronic active hepatitis B or C but may reflect hepatic inflammation caused by medications, including trimethoprim-sulfamethoxazole and/or antiretroviral agents. Marked elevations in serum alkaline phosphatase levels may reflect infiltrative disease of the liver (e.g., MAC or CMV) but also may occur in patients with acalculous cholecystitis, cryptosporidiosis, or AIDS-associated sclerosing cholangitis.

DIARRHEA

Diarrhea occurs, at least intermittently, in more than half of persons with advanced immunodeficiency and may be caused by a variety of microorganisms (Table 108–15). In many cases no clear etiology is found, and the diarrhea is attributed to HIV-associated enteropathy. Stool specimens should be cultured for the common bacterial pathogens. *Salmonella, Campylobacter,* and *Yersinia* species frequently cause diarrhea in HIV-infected persons; patients usually respond to standard antimicrobial therapy (see Chapter 103). Patients may also have recurrent episodes of diarrhea associated with *Clostridium difficile* toxin; this may reflect the frequent use of broad-spectrum antibiotics in this population.

In cases of persistent diarrhea, a fresh stool specimen should be examined for parasites, using a modified acid-fast stain for *C. parvum* and *I. belli,* the most common enteric protozoal infections in AIDS patients throughout the world. Although cryptosporidiosis may be self-limited, massive diarrhea (up to 10 L/day) may occur. Isosporiasis frequently responds to oral trimethoprim-sulfamethoxazole. All symptoms of both cryptosporidiosis and isosporiasis resolve in response to effective antiretroviral therapy.

If stool diagnostic studies are negative and diarrhea persists, patients should undergo endoscopy (see Chapter 33). Biopsy of the duodenum or small bowel may show histologic evidence of cryptosporidial, microsporidial, MAC or CMV infection, or villous atrophy characteristic of HIV enteropathy. Biopsy of the colon may show histologic abnormalities indicative of HSV proctitis, CMV colitis, or MAC infection.

For patients with refractory diarrhea, symptomatic treatment may improve the quality of life.

Unexplained Fever

Most persistent fevers late in the course of HIV infection reflect a definable OI.

The most common cause of unexplained fever in patients with CD4 counts less than 50 cells/mm³ is disseminated MAC infection. This is most rapidly diagnosed by bone marrow biopsy, but blood cultures are usually positive within 5 days. Treatment (see Table 108–8) usually results in resolution of fever and weight gain.

Aggressive non-Hodgkin's lymphoma may cause unexplained fever and weight loss. A rapidly enlarging spleen or asymmetric lymph node enlargement may suggest the diagnosis. The lymphomas often have an intra-abdomi-

TABLE 108–15   Diarrhea in Advanced HIV Infection

Etiology	Characteristic	Diagnosis	Treatment
Frequent			
Cryptosporidium parvum	Varies from increased frequency to large-volume diarrhea	Acid-fast stain of stool	Antiretroviral therapy
Clostridium difficile	Abdominal pain, fever common	*Clostridium difficile* toxin in stool or endoscopy	Metronidazole or vancomycin
Cytomegalovirus	Small bowel movements with blood or mucus (colitis)	Colonoscopy and biopsy	Ganciclovir
Mycobacterium avium complex	Abdominal pain, fever, retroperitoneal lymphadenopathy	Blood culture or endoscopy with biopsy	Multidrug regimen, including clarithromycin; ethambutol
Less Frequent			
Salmonella or *Campylobacter*	Sometimes with blood or mucus in bowel movements (colitis)	Stool culture	Norfloxacin (check sensitivities)
Isospora belli	Watery diarrhea	Acid-fast stain of stool	Trimethoprim-sulfamethoxazole

nal presentation. CT-guided biopsy of enlarged intra-abdominal nodes may provide the diagnosis.

Weight Loss and Anorexia

Cachexia may be a prominent feature of advanced HIV disease. In some instances, the wasting is caused by an intercurrent infectious process. In many instances, however, no opportunistic process is identified. Heightened production of tumor necrosis factor/cachectin may contribute to fever, cachexia, and hypertriglyceridemia in advanced HIV disease.

If orthostatic hypotension occurs, especially if associated with hyperkalemia, an adrenocorticotropin (ACTH) stimulation test should investigate the possibility of adrenal insufficiency, which can rarely result from CMV infection.

Most patients with AIDS-associated cachexia gain weight and achieve a sense of well-being after initiation of effective antiretroviral therapy. Some also gain weight after administration of recombinant growth hormone, non-methylated androgens, or megestrol, but definitive indications for hormone therapy have not been established.

AIDS-Associated Malignancies

In the United States, Kaposi's sarcoma occurs primarily among homosexual and bisexual men. Among HIV-infected homosexual men, the frequency of Kaposi's sarcoma has fallen from 40% at the outset of the epidemic to less than 15% in 1999. Current data suggest that this Kaposi's sarcoma results from an OI by a newly recognized herpesvirus, human herpesvirus-8. In many instances, lesions resolve after institution of effective antiretroviral therapy. Systemic chemotherapy can provide remissions in many patients with disseminated disease or symptomatic visceral disease.

Non-Hodgkin's B-cell lymphomas may also complicate advanced HIV-1 infection. Most AIDS-associated lymphomas are of small noncleaved or immunoblastic histology. Extranodal presentation of these tumors is the rule, with a high frequency of gastrointestinal or intracranial presentation. Chemotherapy for systemic disease or radiation therapy for CNS disease generally provides only brief clinical responses.

Other Complications of HIV Infection

RENAL DISORDERS

Renal insufficiency in AIDS patients may be a consequence of nephrotoxic drug administration, heroin injection, or HIV-associated nephropathy. Certain histologic features such as focal and segmental glomerulosclerosis may distinguish HIV-associated nephropathy from renal failure associated with intravenous heroin use. The disease usually presents as heavy proteinuria and progressive renal insufficiency. Without treatment, most patients develop end-stage renal disease within several months. Short-term, high-dose corticosteroid therapy often arrests the progression of renal disease in persons with HIV-associated nephropathy. Renal biopsy may be helpful in excluding other potentially treatable causes of renal failure.

RHEUMATOLOGIC DISORDERS

Musculoskeletal complaints are common; the relationship of circulating autoantibodies to these manifestations is unknown. Muscle weakness, if localized, may be indicative of myelopathy-neuropathy (see Table 108–11). When weakness is proximal or is associated with myalgia and tenderness, myopathy should be suspected. The myopathy may be HIV-associated or may, rarely, represent zidovudine toxicity. Muscle biopsy may distinguish between these two processes, with inflammation most prominent in AIDS-associated myopathy and mitochondrial abnormalities in zidovudine-related myopathy. Arthralgias are common, and both a Reiter-like syndrome and a Sjögren-like syndrome occur with increased frequency.

Prevention of HIV Infection

Three approaches—behavioral modification, community-wide treatment of STDs, and antiretroviral therapy of seropositive pregnant women—have been shown to have major impact on HIV transmission.

In several communities at increased risk for HIV (e.g., homosexually active men in the United States and Western Europe), adaptation of safer sexual practices has resulted in a decrease in incidence of HIV infection. Sustaining these behavioral changes over long periods is difficult, and thus behavioral reinforcement is important.

Studies in Central Africa have clearly demonstrated that periodic community-wide STD-treatment programs may result in a nearly 50% reduction in HIV transmission in communities with an overall HIV infection prevalence less than 10%. Such programs are less effective in communities with higher (>20%) rates of HIV infection.

Treatment of HIV-infected women with zidovudine during the third trimester of pregnancy and during delivery, followed by zidovudine treatment of the infant for 6 weeks, decreases maternal-fetal transmission by 67% (from 25% to 8%), without harm to the newborn child. More recent experience indicates that administration of combination antiretroviral therapy can further decrease perinatal HIV transmission to less than 5%.

The use of universal blood and body fluid precautions is routinely recommended to protect health care workers. Meticulous attention to utilization and disposal of sharp instruments is most important, because most nosocomial acquisition of HIV infection has occurred through accidental needlestick. Prompt administration of zidovudine significantly decreases the likelihood of HIV infection in health care workers after needlestick injuries. Current provisional recommendations by the United States Public Health Service for prophylaxis after high-risk occupational exposure include a combination regimen of a potent protease inhibitor and two nucleoside reverse transcriptase inhibitors, initiated as soon as possible after exposure and continuing for 4 weeks.

The development of an effective vaccine is the target of active research. Early clinical trials of vaccine candidates are ongoing.

REFERENCES

Carpenter CCJ, Cooper DA, Fischl MA, et al: Antiretroviral therapy in adults: Updated recommendations of the International AIDS Society—USA panel. JAMA 2000; 283, 381–391.

DHHS Guidelines for the use of antiretroviral agents in HIV-infected adults and adolescents. Ann Intern Med 1998; 128:1079–1100.

HIV and the acquired immunodeficiency syndrome. *In* Goldman L, Bennett JC (eds): Cecil Textbook of Medicine, 21st ed. Philadelphia: WB Saunders, 2000, pp 1889–1946.

Ho DD, Newman AU, Perelson AS, et al: Rapid turnover of plasma virions and CD4 lymphocytes in HIV-1 infection. Nature 1995; 362: 355–358.

Mellors J, Munoz AM, Giorgi VJ, et al: Plasma viral load and CD4 lymphocytes as prognostic markers of HIV-1 infection. Ann Intern Med 1997; 126:946–954.

Palella FJ, Delaney KM, Moorman AC, et al. Declining morbidity and mortality among patients with advanced human immunideficiency virus infection. N Engl J Med 1998; 338:853–860.

Saag M, Holodniy M, Kuritzkes DR, et al: HIV viral load markers in clinical practice: Recommendations of an International AIDS Society—USA expert panel. Nat Med 1996; 2:625–629.

1999 USPHS/IDSA Guidelines for prevention of opportunistic infections in persons infected with human immunodeficiency virus. Clin Infect Dis 2000; 30:529–565.

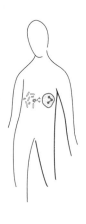

109

INFECTIONS IN THE IMMUNOCOMPROMISED HOST

Robert A. Salata

Immunosuppression is an increasingly common by-product of diseases and modern approaches to their treatment. The immunocompromised host suffers from increased susceptibility to *opportunistic infection,* defined as infection caused by organisms of low virulence that constitute normal mucosal and skin flora or by pathogenic microbial agents that are usually maintained in a latent state. Until the 1980s, compromised hosts mainly included patients with congenital immunodeficiencies or those who became immunocompromised as a consequence of cancer and its treatment, bone marrow failure, or treatment with steroids and cytotoxic therapy. The advent of the human immunodeficiency virus (HIV) brought new meaning and relevance to the term *immunocompromised host.*

Immunocompromise is not an all-or-none phenomenon. The extent of immunosuppression varies with the underlying cause and must exceed a threshold to predispose to opportunistic infections. The type of immunosuppression predicts the spectrum of agents likely to cause infections. Accordingly, opportunistic infections can best be considered in categories that reflect the nature of the immune deficiency.

Disorders of Cell-Mediated Immunity

Cell-mediated immunity is the major host defense against facultative and some obligate intracellular parasites, as discussed in Chapter 92. A partial list of diseases and situations that produce impaired cell-mediated immunity is presented in Table 109–1. However, only certain of these conditions result in increased susceptibility to infection with intracellular parasites. Foremost

among acquired immunodeficiencies are HIV infection (see Chapter 108), Hodgkin's disease and other lymphomas, hairy cell leukemia, and disseminated solid tumors. Severe malnutrition, as well as treatment with high-dose corticosteroids, cytotoxic drugs, or radiation therapy, can produce a similar predilection to infections. Congenital immunodeficiencies are associated with severe infections early in childhood and are not considered here. Patients with impaired cell-mediated immunity are especially susceptible to the organisms shown in Table 109–2. The relative frequency of occurrence varies with the underlying disease (e.g., *Mycobacterium avium* complex is frequent in HIV infection, whereas *Listeria* is not), the geographic area (*Mycobacterium tuberculosis* is more frequent in developing countries), and the extent of immunosuppression (*M. tuberculosis* is an early, and *M. avium* complex a late, complication of HIV infection).

Thus, with depression of cell-mediated immunity, organisms ordinarily constituting the normal flora, such as *Candida* species, act as virulent opportunistic pathogens capable of causing aggressive infections. Latent viruses, fungi, mycobacteria, and parasites reactivate to cause locally progressive or disseminated disease. Often, the signs, symptoms, and laboratory abnormalities suggesting the diagnosis are subtle and nonspecific.

The association between defective cell-mediated immunity and disease produced by the infectious agents listed in Table 109–2 is clear-cut. Sometimes, treatment of the underlying disease causing immunodeficiency or progression of this disease produces a more severe and generalized compromised state, which predisposes to infection by additional microorganisms. For example, during chemotherapy for lymphoma, bacterial infections initially predominate. Disease progression also results in local factors that favor bacterial infections such as mucosal breakdown and obstruction by tumor masses of the

TABLE 109–1 Conditions Causing Impaired Cell-Mediated Immunity

Infectious Diseases
Measles, chickenpox, typhoid fever, tuberculosis, leprosy, histoplasmosis, human immunodeficiency virus infection

Vaccinations
Measles, mumps, rubella

Malignant Diseases
Hodgkin's disease, lymphomas, advanced solid tumors

Drugs
Corticosteroids, cytotoxic drugs

Miscellaneous
Congenital immunodeficiency states, sarcoidosis, uremia, diabetes mellitus, malnutrition, old age

bronchi, the ureters, or the biliary tract. The result is a marked increase in severe bacterial infection and septicemia late in the course of many diseases associated with impaired cell-mediated immunity.

Disorders of Humoral Immunity

The *acquired disorders of antibody production* associated with increased frequency of infection in adults are common variable immunodeficiency, chronic lymphocytic leukemia, lymphosarcoma, multiple myeloma, nephrotic syndrome, major burns, and protein-losing enteropathy. The paraproteinemic states belong in this category because of secondary decreases in levels of functioning antibody. Therapy with cytotoxic drugs may produce similar immunocompromise.

TABLE 109–2 Infections in Patients with Impaired Cell-Mediated Immunity

Viruses
Varicella-zoster, herpes simplex, cytomegalovirus, Epstein-Barr virus, JC virus, human herpesvirus 6, human herpesvirus 8

Fungi
Pathogenic: *Histoplasma, Coccidioides*
Saprophytic: *Cryptococcus, Candida;* less commonly, *Aspergillus, Zygomycetes*

Bacteria
Listeria monocytogenes, Nocardia, Mycobacterium tuberculosis, Legionella pneumophila, nontuberculous mycobacteria, *Salmonella* species

Protozoa
Pneumocystis carinii, Toxoplasma gondii, Cryptosporidium parvum, Leishmania donovani

Helminths
Strongyloides stercoralis

Infections with pneumococci, *Haemophilus influenzae*, streptococci, and staphylococci predominate early in the course of the humoral immunodeficiency. As the underlying disease itself progresses, infections with gram-negative bacilli become more frequent. Treatment of the underlying condition with corticosteroids and cytotoxic drugs causes additional defects in cell-mediated immunity and provides susceptibility to infections with the group of pathogens presented in Table 109–2.

In *sickle cell anemia*, heat-labile opsonic activity is abnormal. Complement depletion by erythrocyte stroma impairs opsonization of pneumococci and *Salmonella* species and leads to frequent infections with these organisms. Impaired reticuloendothelial system function resulting from erythrophagocytosis and functional asplenia also may predispose patients with sickle cell disease to serious bacterial infections. The predisposition to infection is related to age; once children with sickle cell disease develop antibodies to pneumococcal capsular polysaccharide, they lose their thousandfold increased susceptibility to severe pneumococcal infection.

Splenectomy results in a loss of mechanisms for the clearing of opsonized organisms. Over a period of years, the liver may partially compensate for this filtration function. The splenic tissue also represents a major source of production of antibody as well as other opsonic factors such as tuftsin, which opsonizes staphylococci. Splenectomy therefore predisposes to fulminant infections caused by encapsulated bacteria.

Impaired Neutrophil Function

Many inherited and acquired diseases impair neutrophil function. The defect may be extrinsic or intrinsic to the neutrophil. *Impaired chemotaxis* is a significant factor predisposing patients with inherited C3 and C5 deficiencies to frequent bacterial infections (see Chapter 92). *Corticosteroid therapy* also interferes with chemotaxis. Whereas circulating neutrophil counts may be normal or increased in patients treated with corticosteroids, these cells are dysfunctional because they do not localize normally to the site of infection. Defective cell-mediated immunity also contributes to the spectrum of infections associated with corticosteroid therapy. Other conditions and situations associated with impaired neutrophil function include myelodysplasia, paroxysmal nocturnal hemoglobinuria, radiation therapy, and cytotoxic drug therapy.

Intrinsic defects in neutrophils are rare but provide insights into the microbicidal mechanisms of these cells. Neutrophils from patients with *chronic granulomatous disease* cannot develop an oxidative burst. Catalase-negative organisms produce sufficient hydrogen peroxide to faciliate their own killing by neutrophils in chronic granulomatous disease through the myeloperoxidase pathway. Catalase-producing organisms such as staphylococci, *Serratia, Nocardia,* and *Aspergillus* scavenge the hydrogen peroxide that they produce; these infectious agents therefore cannot be killed by neutrophils of chronic granulomatous disease and thus produce serious recurrent, deep-seated infections.

The most severe intrinsic neutrophil defects occur in the *Chédiak-Higashi syndrome.* Patients have giant granules in their leukocytes and defective microtubule assembly. The results are impaired chemotaxis, abnormal phagolysosomal fusion, delayed bacterial killing, and recurrent infections. Diagnosis of this rare syndrome is aided by phenotypic abnormalities: partial albinism, depigmentation of the iris, peripheral neuropathies, and nystagmus are characteristic.

Neutropenia

Neutropenia is among the most important risk factors for serious infection in the compromised host. Frequently, other alterations in host defense mechanisms coexist with granulocytopenia; these alterations further increase the risk of infection and determine the types of infectious complications. As the neutrophil count falls to less than 500/μL, an exponential increase occurs in the frequency and severity of infections. Most reliable data derive from patients with acute leukemia. For example, in one study, neutrophil counts of 100 to 500/μL were associated with infections during 35% of hospitalized days, whereas at counts below 100/μL, infections increased to 55% of days. However, granulocytopenia of other causes, when sustained, may result in a comparable risk of infection. In patients with chronic and cyclic neutropenias, the susceptibility to infection varies inversely with the monocyte count; the mononuclear phagocytes provide some of the antibacterial capacity of the missing neutrophils. After chemotherapy of acute leukemia, neutropenia usually is profound and sustained and is associated with damage to mucosal barriers to infection. Patients become susceptible to organisms that are ubiquitous in the environment and ordinarily make up the normal flora (Table 109–3).

Diagnostic Problems in the Compromised Host

PULMONARY INFILTRATES

The immunocompromised patient with *pulmonary infiltrates* presents a particularly vexing diagnostic problem. The pulmonary infiltrates can represent infection, extension of underlying tumor, complication of chemotherapy, fluid overload, pulmonary infarction, hemorrhage, or some combination of these conditions. Specific diagnosis is necessary. Unfortunately, noninvasive serodiagnostic tests rarely are helpful in this setting, yet concomitant thrombocytopenia too often increases the risk of lung biopsy.

The clinical setting and radiographic appearance of the pulmonary infiltrate influence the probable yield of lung biopsy and the decision about whether to proceed. For example, in patients with leukemia, parenchymal infiltrates occurring before or within 3 days of initiating chemotherapy usually are bacterial, as are focal infil-

TABLE 109–3 Infectious Agents that Frequently Cause Infections in Neutropenic Patients

Bacteria
Pseudomonas, Klebsiella, Serratia, Escherichia coli, Staphylococcus aureus, coagulase-negative staphylococci, *Corynebacterium* group JK, streptococci (α-hemolytic)
Fungi
Candida, Aspergillus, Zygomycetes
Viruses
Cytomegalovirus, herpesviruses
Protozoa
Pneumocystis carinii

trates developing later in the course of treatment. Major efforts should be directed at obtaining adequate sputum samples for Gram's stain and culture (see Chapter 99); the evolution of pneumonitis during antibiotic therapy becomes a useful factor in deciding whether to proceed with lung biopsy.

In contrast, diffuse infiltrates occurring *after* treatment of leukemia are more suggestive of opportunistic infection. *Pneumocystis carinii* is an important preventable, treatable cause of diffuse infiltrates and occurs most often after treatment of acute lymphocytic leukemia or in patients with an acquired deficiency of cell-mediated immunity (see Chapter 108). In these settings, the diagnosis should be established by examination of induced sputum, by bronchoalveolar lavage, or, less commonly, by transbronchial biopsy. If these diagnostic approaches are not helpful, empirical therapy with trimethoprim-sulfamethoxazole may be initiated.

The indications and timing of *lung biopsy,* when needed, must be individualized. Delay in proceeding with biopsy, to a point at which the patient is severely hypoxic, reduces the chances of affecting the outcome with therapy, even if the biopsy shows a potentially treatable disease.

Once the decision has been made to perform a biopsy, the next question is which procedure to use. *Fiberoptic transbronchial biopsy* has provided a good diagnostic yield, particularly in the evaluation of diffuse pulmonary lesions. This technique should not be performed in the patient with thrombocytopenia. The tissue obtained must be processed and examined quickly. *Open-lung biopsy* has an additional yield of 50% to 75% in the patient with a nondiagnostic transbronchial biopsy and should be performed without delay if the tempo of progression of the patient's illness mandates immediate diagnosis. Open-lung biopsy can generally be performed in patients with thrombocytopenia if prophylactic transfusions can achieve an increment in the platelet count and can diminish the bleeding time.

Early treatment of most pulmonary infections in immunocompromised hosts, even *aspergillosis* (Fig. 109–1), is associated with an initially favorable outcome. The long-term result, however, depends on the natural history of the underlying disease process.

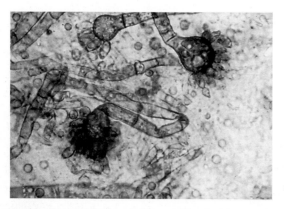

FIGURE 109-1 Fruiting head of *Aspergillus fumigatus* on a lung biopsy. Aspergillosis usually causes an expanding perihilar pulmonary infiltrate. Prompt institution of amphotericin B therapy may lead to a good clinical response.

DISSEMINATED MYCOSES

Disseminated mycoses represent another major diagnostic problem in the immunocompromised host. Fungal infections are found post mortem in more than one half of patients with leukemia and lymphoma; usually, the nature of the infection is not established ante mortem. Culture of a saprophytic organism such as *Candida* from superficial sites does not establish pathogenicity. Even in patients with widespread infection, however, detectable fungemia is generally a late event.

How, then, can the diagnosis of fungal infection be established early, at a time when the infection is potentially curable? The physician should search for superficial lesions accessible to scraping, aspiration, or biopsy (Fig. 109–2). Dissemination of *Candida tropicalis* frequently causes hyperpigmented macular or pustular skin lesions that show the organisms within blood vessel walls on biopsy. *Hepatosplenic candidiasis* is most frequently encountered in patients with fever after recovery from neutropenia. The presence of "bull's-eye" lesions on computed tomographic scans of the liver and spleen suggests hepatosplenic candidiasis. Cryptococcal polysaccharide antigen may be present in the serum or cerebrospinal fluid of the patient with *disseminated cryptococcosis*. Serodiagnosis for other fungi has, in general, been disappointing. Acute invasive *pulmonary aspergillosis* occurs most often in patients with prolonged, profound neutropenia who present with fever and pleuritic chest pain during or after broad-spectrum antibacterial therapy.

In the absence of adequate diagnostic procedures, empirical use of antifungal drugs is often indicated in the immunocompromised host when clinical suspicion of disseminated mycoses is appropriate (e.g., in the patient with neutropenia and fever for more than 5 to 7 days despite broad-spectrum antibiotic therapy).

Prevention and Treatment of Infections in the Patient with Neutropenia

PREVENTION

Acute bacterial infections and septicemia arising from organisms comprising the gut flora occur frequently in patients with granulocytopenia and may have fever as their sole manifestation. *Prophylactic nonabsorbable antibiotics* and protective isolation have generally failed to prevent such infection. Trimethoprim-sulfamethoxazole, given prophylactically, may decrease the number of infections and bacteremic episodes in some patients with neutropenia, in addition to preventing the development of *P. carinii* pneumonia. However, the bone marrow toxicity of this drug and selection of resistant organisms make it less suitable for widespread use as a prophylactic agent in patients with neutropenia. Quinolones, such as ciprofloxacin, may be at least as effective in preventing bacterial infections and are less toxic; quinolones lack activity, however, against *P. carinii* and have been associated with severe α-hemolytic streptococcal infection in some patients. Prophylactic administration of imidazoles to prevent systemic fungal infections is of uncertain value in this setting.

Prophylactic granulocyte transfusions decrease the occurrence of bacterial sepsis in patients with acute myelogenous leukemia, but they are costly and do not affect the overall remission rate and duration of survival. These transfusions should be reversed for selected patients with profound and persistent neutropenia and gram-negative bacillary or fungal infection that is refractory to appropriate antimicrobial agents.

TREATMENT

Empirical antibiotic therapy is indicated in febrile granulocytopenic patients, because up to two thirds have an underlying infection. Selection of two drugs with activity against gram-negative enteric bacilli, such as tobramycin

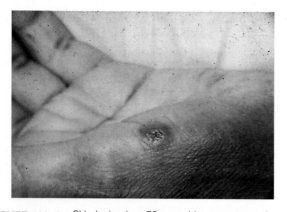

FIGURE 109-2 Skin lesion in a 76-year-old woman treated with corticosteroids and cytotoxic drugs for chronic lymphocytic leukemia and presenting with nodular pulmonary infiltrates and lymphocytic meningitis. Fluid expressed from the lesion contained encapsulated yeast seen on India ink preparation and yielded *Cryptococcus neoformans* on culture.

and piperacillin, is usually necessary. Initial empirical therapy for staphylococci is necessary only when clinical concern exists about infections of vascular catheters or of skin or soft tissue. Despite the early empirical use of antibiotics, the outcome of patients with bacterial infections is poor unless the initial neutrophil count exceeds $500/\mu L$, the count rises during treatment, or the pathogen is a gram-positive organism. Treatment with granulocyte colony-stimulating factors may result in shorter duration of neutropenia and fewer infectious complications.

The appropriate duration of antimicrobial therapy of febrile patients with neutropenia is uncertain. Many physicians continue to administer antibiotics until the neutropenia resolves. The empirical addition of antifungal therapy is indicated in the patient with neutropenia who remains febrile for at least 5 days despite broad-spectrum antibiotics. In this setting, the best approach is often to continue broad-spectrum antibiotics for the duration of the neutropenia unless the cause of the patient's fever can be clearly defined.

REFERENCES

Hughes WT, Armstrong D, Bodey GP, et al: 1997 guidelines for the use of antimicrobial agents in neutropenic patients with unexplained fever: Infectious Diseases Society of America. Clin Infect Dis 1997; 25:551–573.

Pizzo PA: The compromised host. In Goldman L, Bennett JC (eds): Cecil Textbook of Medicine, 21st ed. Philadelphia: WB Saunders, 2000, pp 1569–1581.

Rubin RH, Young LS (eds): Clinical Approach to Infection in the Compromised Host, 3rd ed. New York: Plenum Medical Book Company, 1994.

110

INFECTIOUS DISEASES OF TRAVELERS; PROTOZOAL AND HELMINTHIC INFECTIONS

Robert A. Salata

The medical preparation of patients for overseas travel, some common clinical symptoms that may develop on their return, and the diagnosis and treatment of common parasitic diseases endemic in the United States and abroad are reviewed in this chapter.

Preparation of Travelers

More than 10 million Americans travel to developing countries each year. Major increases in international travel, the resurgence of malaria and other infectious diseases worldwide, and the widespread concern for new and emerging infections such as "mad cow" disease in the United Kingdom bring the issues of prevention and management of health problems in travelers into the office of every physician.

Risks associated with international travel are dependent on the destination, duration of the trip, underlying health and age of the traveler, and activities while abroad. In general, destinations within the industrialized world require no specific health precautions. In contrast, travelers to developing areas, especially the tropics, can be exposed to life-threatening infections. Major issues to be addressed in the pretravel period include immunizations, malaria prophylaxis, traveler's diarrhea, and other problems that can be avoided or prevented. Information about health risks in specific geographic areas, updated weekly, can be obtained from the Centers for Disease Control and Prevention (CDC) through its publications or by calling the International Traveler's Hotline (1-888-232-3299; website: www.cdc.gov/travel).

IMMUNIZATIONS

In general, only yellow fever vaccination may be required by law for international travel. Both polio and meningococcal meningitis vaccinations may be required during outbreak situations. Although some immunizations are not generally considered "travel" immunizations, many Americans have allowed routine diphtheria-tetanus immunizations to lapse or may not have been fully immunized against measles and polio. Finally, other immunizations are often strongly recommended, depending on the type and duration of travel. With a few exceptions, vaccines can be given simultaneously. Before immunization, a careful history should be obtained to determine allergies to eggs or chicken embryo cells. Pregnant women and individuals immunocompromised by human immunodeficiency virus (HIV), malignancy, or chemotherapy pose specific and important challenges; most live virus vaccines are contraindicated in these patients.

Yellow Fever

This live attenuated virus vaccine is highly effective and recommended if traveling to areas in South America and Africa where yellow fever is endemic. Vaccination is highly effective and lasts for 10 years but must be given at designated vaccination centers.

Cholera

Cholera has returned to South and Central America, where it is a major concern to travelers. The currently available vaccine is not recommended for travel into endemic areas. Health education on likely sources of transmission is far more effective in preventing disease than vaccine. Cholera vaccination is, however, still a legal requirement for travel between some developing countries.

Measles

Up to 20% of first-year college students have no serologic evidence of prior measles infection or immunization and must be presumed to be susceptible. Individuals with no physician-documented record of immunization born after 1956 are at greatest risk for measles. In addition, a single immunization with measles vaccine at 15 months of age may permit breakthrough infection as a young adult. As a result, a second measles vaccination is now recommended for international travel for individuals who have never experienced the clinical illness. All live virus vaccines should be given at least 2 weeks before gamma globulin administration.

Diphtheria-Tetanus

Tetanus is a ubiquitous problem and is most prevalent in tropical countries. A booster within the past 5 years is recommended. This eliminates the need for a tetanus booster if the traveler sustains a tetanus-prone injury overseas. This recommendation is made primarily because of the uncertainty of obtaining sterile, disposable needles in many overseas locations. Given the resurgence of diphtheria in countries of the former Soviet Union and the occurrence of disease in travelers to these areas, diphtheria toxoid should be co-administered with tetanus toxoid.

Polio

Polio remains endemic in some regions of Asia and Africa. Most young adults have been immunized with at least four doses of trivalent oral polio vaccine (OPV); an additional booster dose is recommended for international travel. Many adults (>18 years of age) cannot remember, however, whether they received OPV; such individuals should be given inactivated polio vaccine (IPV).

Hepatitis A

Hepatitis A is a major risk for travelers to areas of poor sanitation, affecting an estimated 1 in 1000 travelers per 2- to 3-week trip in some areas. As such, hepatitis A is the most important vaccine-preventable infection for travelers. Hepatitis A vaccine should be given at least 2 weeks before departure. This vaccine is safe and immunogenic.

Meningococcal Meningitis

Meningococcal meningitis is a worldwide disease, but cases in international travelers are infrequent except with prolonged contact with the local population. Vacci-

nation with the quadrivalent polysaccharide vaccine (A, C, Y, +W135) is recommended for travel to northern India, Nepal, Saudi Arabia during the Moslem haj, certain parts of sub-Saharan Africa, and other locations where travel advisories have been issued.

Typhoid

American international travelers are at greatest risk of contracting typhoid in the Indian subcontinent, Mexico, western South America, and sub-Saharan Africa. Vaccination is recommended for travel to endemic areas where exposure to contaminated food and water is likely. Vaccination is also strongly indicated for travelers with achlorhydria, immunosuppression, or sickle cell anemia and for those taking broad-spectrum antibiotics. Adequate vaccination with the injectable vaccine takes time (2 injections 1 month apart) and is associated with significant side effects (frequently a sore arm and a flulike reaction). An oral vaccine (4 enteric-coated capsules given over 7 days) is equally efficacious and has fewer side effects.

Other Vaccines

Some travelers, including missionaries, physicians, and anthropologists, need special consideration. These individuals live for prolonged periods in developing countries or are at special risk for contracting certain highly contagious diseases. Consideration should be given to immunization with hepatitis B, Japanese B encephalitis, plague, and rabies vaccines. In general, such consultations should be referred to a qualified travelers' clinic.

MALARIA PROPHYLAXIS

Malaria prophylaxis is a major problem for international travelers because of the high and increasing prevalence of drug resistance by the parasite. The need for, as well as the type of, prophylaxis is dependent on the exact itinerary within a given country, since transmission risk is quite regional. Recommended chemoprophylactic regimens have changed frequently within the past few years. In general, travelers to areas where chloroquine-sensitive *Plasmodium falciparum* strains are exclusively found (Central America, the Caribbean, North Africa, and the Middle East) should take chloroquine phosphate (300 mg base or 500 mg salt) weekly starting 2 weeks before, during, and for 6 weeks after leaving areas in which malaria is endemic. Travelers to areas where chloroquine-resistant *P. falciparum* is common should take mefloquine (Lariam), 250 mg a week starting a week before travel, during travel, and for 4 weeks after. These areas currently include Southeast Asia, sub-Saharan Africa, South America, and South Asia. No antimalarial regimen is completely effective in Myanmar, rural Thailand, or some parts of East Africa, where mefloquine resistance is a growing problem. Because of these facts, emphasis must be given to the use of netting, screens, and insect repellents as well as to the prompt diagnosis and treatment of any febrile episodes (temperature >102°F [39°C]) overseas.

TRAVELER'S DIARRHEA

Between 20% and 50% of individuals traveling to developing countries will develop diarrhea during or shortly after their trip. The risk is highest when traveling to India, Latin America, Africa, the Middle East, and South Asia. The average duration of an episode of traveler's diarrhea is 3 to 6 days. About 10% of episodes last longer than 1 week. The diarrhea may be accompanied by abdominal cramping, nausea, headache, low-grade fever, vomiting, or bloating. Fewer than 5% of persons have fever greater than 101°F (38°C), bloody stools, or both. Travelers with these symptoms may not have simple traveler's diarrhea and should see a physician at once (see Chapter 103).

Diarrheal illness (including cholera) can be avoided through precautions with food and beverage. All water should be presumed to be unsafe. Salads are often contaminated by protozoal cysts and, along with street vendor foods, are the most dangerous foods encountered by most travelers. Food should be well cooked, including meat, seafood, and vegetables. Dairy products should be avoided.

Bismuth subsalicylate (Pepto-Bismol) can be used as a prophylactic measure (2 tablets four times a day) or used to treat acute bouts of diarrhea (1 oz every 30 minutes for eight doses). Diphenoxylate (Lomotil) and loperamide (Imodium) may give some symptomatic relief of diarrhea but should be avoided if the diarrhea is severe, fever exists, or blood is present in the stool. Trimethoprim-sulfamethoxazole (Bactrim), doxycycline (Vibramycin), or one of the newer quinolones can be taken orally for 3 to 5 days to reduce the duration of symptoms and are effective against a wide variety of bacterial pathogens, including most *Shigella* and *Salmonella* species. Prophylactic antibiotics are not generally recommended except for very short trips.

GENERAL HEALTH INFORMATION

Other potentially dangerous activities overseas include exposure to dogs and cats (rabies), swimming in fresh water (schistosomiasis or leptospirosis), walking barefoot (hookworm or strongyloidiasis), and insect bites. In addition to malaria, many diseases, including dengue, sleeping sickness, and yellow fever, are transmitted by biting insects.

SPECIAL PROBLEMS

Pregnant Women

Live virus vaccines are contraindicated in pregnant women and greatly complicate pretravel preparations. Chloroquine probably can be used safely. Travel to areas of chloroquine-resistant malaria should be strongly discouraged. No drug regimen to prevent or treat chloroquine-resistant malaria is safe in pregnant women, and malaria during pregnancy is a medical emergency for both the mother and her fetus.

Acquired Immunodeficiency Syndrome

Many countries, including the United States, now bar entry to patients with the acquired immunodeficiency syndrome (AIDS). Several countries require HIV serologic testing for all travelers applying for more than a 3-month visa, which requires official documentation well in advance of travel. Patients with HIV infection need special preparation before travel to developing countries because of their increased susceptibility to certain illnesses (e.g., pneumococcal infection and tuberculosis).

Most international travelers are concerned about the risk of acquiring AIDS while abroad. Most concerns center on untested blood or nonsterile needles, which might be used in an emergency. In general, a few hospitals in almost all countries frequented by tourists now have sterile needles and screen their blood supply.

The Returning Traveler

With the exception of skin testing for tuberculosis, asymptomatic returning travelers generally do not need screening tests. The clinical problems that most often arise in travelers soon after return are fever and diarrhea, whereas eosinophilia is the most common cause for later referral. Fever is most important, since delay in the diagnosis of *P. falciparum* malaria is often fatal. Fever should always prompt consideration of malaria until proved otherwise in travelers returning from countries where malaria is endemic, even if they are still taking prophylactic drugs. It is important to speciate the malaria with a blood film, because this affects therapy. Chloroquine-sensitive *P. falciparum* is treated with 1 g of chloroquine given orally, followed by 500 mg at 6, 24, and 48 hours. For *P. vivax* and *P. ovale* (also generally chloroquine-sensitive), this regimen is followed by primaquine daily for 14 days to eradicate hepatic forms. Resistant *P. falciparum* is treated with quinine sulfate, 650 mg given orally every 8 hours for 3 days, and doxycycline, 100 mg orally twice daily for 7 days. All patients with suspected resistant infection should be hospitalized. In smear-negative cases in which clinical suspicion remains high, repeated smears every 8 to 12 hours should be obtained. If fever is not caused by malaria, then tuberculosis, typhoid fever, and amebic liver abscess should be considered.

Traveler's diarrhea unresponsive to empirical antibiotics and persistent until the traveler returns home often represents giardiasis. Three stool specimens for ova and parasites and a stool culture are warranted. Unfortunately, *Giardia lamblia* may be missed in up to one third of cases even after this work-up. If clinical suspicion is high, an empirical course of metronidazole (500 mg orally three times a day for 7 days) is usually justified. Antibiotic-resistant bacteria, amebiasis, temporary lactose intolerance, bacterial overgrowth, and tropical sprue should also be considered.

Eosinophilia in a returning traveler usually manifests weeks or months after travel. It is usually caused by any one of a variety of helminth infections. A stool specimen for ova and parasites is indicated but may be negative during the tissue-migrating phase of many intestinal worms or in tissue nematode infections, such as filariasis or onchocerciasis. Management of the more common parasitic infections encountered in travelers is included in the next section.

Protozoal and Helminthic Infections

PROTOZOAL INFECTIONS IN THE UNITED STATES

Worldwide, the incidence of parasitic infections is increasing. This is due in part to the emergence of antimicrobial resistance (e.g., malaria) and an increasing number of susceptible hosts, especially those with HIV infection. Protozoal infections in the United States occur more frequently in immunocompromised hosts (Table 110–1) (see Chapter 108). Babesiosis is very severe in asplenic individuals, and *Toxoplasma* encephalitis primarily affects patients with AIDS.

Giardiasis and Amebiasis

Giardiasis is a common cause of persistent, nonbloody diarrhea in returning travelers. *G. lamblia* is prevalent throughout much of the developing world. Homosexual men also have a high prevalence of infection because of specific sexual practices. The diagnosis is generally made by identification of ova or trophozoites on stool examination (at least three stool specimens should be examined). The drug of choice for adults is metronidazole, 500 to 750 mg three times a day for 7 days.

Like *Giardia*, *Entamoeba histolytica* is transmitted by the fecal-oral route; the vast majority of infected individuals are asymptomatic. When *E. histolytica* causes acute illness, it is generally manifested by bloody diarrhea. In the United States, amebic dysentery is occasionally misdiagnosed as ulcerative colitis or Crohn's disease and the administration of corticosteroids may cause significant worsening and toxic megacolon. Stool examination for ova and parasites is generally diagnostic, but sigmoidoscopy may be required. Serology is useful to rule out this diagnosis. This is especially important in individuals from industrialized countries, because the background serologic positivity is quite low in this population. Extraintestinal amebiasis generally presents as hepatic liver abscess (see Chapter 102).

PROTOZOAL INFECTIONS COMMON IN TRAVELERS AND IMMIGRANTS

Leishmaniasis

Cutaneous and mucocutaneous leishmaniasis (see Table 110–1) should be considered in any traveler returning from the Middle East or endemic areas of Latin America who has a persistent skin or mucous membrane lesion. Diagnosis is made by tissue biopsy. Visceral leishmaniasis should be suspected in immigrants with fever and splenomegaly. Diagnosis is made by bone marrow biopsy and culture. Cutaneous leishmaniasis is generally self-limited. Other types are treated with sodium stibogluconate (Pentostam), 20 mg/kg/day for up to 20 days.

African Trypanosomiasis

This protozoal infection, endemic in Africa, causes sleeping sickness. Rarely imported into developed countries, it should be suspected in systemically ill patients from Africa presenting with fever, headache, and confusion (see Table 110–1). Many patients will remember a painful chancre at the site of an insect bite. Diagnosis is made by direct examination of the blood, lymph aspirate, or cerebrospinal fluid. Treatment should be supervised by an expert in the field.

Chagas' Disease (American Trypanosomiasis)

Trypanosoma cruzi is the most common cause of heart failure in Brazil. Transmission is through contact with feces from infected reduviid bugs (kissing bugs), and cases of transfusion-associated *T. cruzi* infection have been recognized in the United States (see Table 110–1). Most cases are asymptomatic for decades and then manifest as cardiomegaly, megaesophagus, or megacolon. Diagnosis of acute disease is made by direct examination of the blood. Early diagnosis is critical, because patients may respond to nitrofuran or nitroimidazole derivatives. Treatment of chronic Chagas' disease is largely supportive.

HELMINTHIC INFECTIONS COMMON IN THE UNITED STATES

Pinworm

Enterobiasis is common in the United States (Table 110–2), particularly among children. Perianal pruritus is the major clinical presentation. Infection is maintained by fecal-oral contamination. Diagnosis is made by the application of cellophane tape to the anus and subsequent direct examination for ova. Treatment is with mebendazole, 100 mg given once. It is advisable to treat all family members.

Other Intestinal Nematodes

Ascaris (giant roundworm), *Ancylostoma duodenale* and *Necator americanus* (hookworm), and *Trichuris* (whipworms), still endemic in the United States, are extremely common in immigrants and are ubiquitous in the developing world (see Table 110–2). Most individuals are asymptomatic. Ascariasis and hookworm may cause transient pulmonary infiltrates with eosinophilia during the tissue migratory phase of infection. Heavy

TABLE 110–1　Protozoal Infections

Protozoan	Setting	Vectors	Diagnosis	Special Considerations	Treatment
Endemic in the United States					
Babesia microti	New England	Ixodid ticks, transfusions	Thick or thin blood smear	Severe disease in asplenic persons	Quinine and clindamycin
Giardia lamblia	Mountain states	Humans, ? small mammals	Microscopic examination of stool or duodenal fluid	Common in homosexual men, travelers, children in day care centers	Quinacrine or metronidazole
Toxoplasma gondii	Ubiquitous	Domestic cats, raw meat	Clinical; serologic confirmation	Pregnant women, immunosuppressed host (AIDS)	Pyrimethamine and sulfadiazine
Entamoeba histolytica	Southeast	Human	Microscopic examination of stool or "touch prep" from ulcer	Common in homosexual men, travelers, institutionalized persons	Metronidazole
Cryptosporidium sp.	Ubiquitous	Human	Acid-fast stain of stool	Severe in immunosuppressed hosts (AIDS)	None
Trichomonas vaginalis	Ubiquitous	Human	"Wet prep" of genital secretions	Common cause of vaginitis	Metronidazole
Primarily Seen in Travelers and Immigrants					
Plasmodium sp.	Africa, Asia, South America	*Anopheles* mosquito	Thick and thin blood smear	Consider in returning travelers with fever	Dependent on regional resistance pattern (see text)
Leishmania donovani	Middle East	Sandfly	Tissue biopsy	Consider in immigrants with fever and splenomegaly	Pentostam
Trypanosoma sp.	Africa, South America	Reduviid bugs, transfusion	Direct examination of blood or CSF	Very rare in travelers, transfusion-associated	Supportive

AIDS = Acquired immunodeficiency syndrome; CSF = cerebrospinal fluid.

TABLE 110–2　Helminthic Infections

Helminth	Setting	Vectors	Diagnosis	Treatment
Endemic in the United States				
Pinworm (enterobiasis)	Ubiquitous	Human	Direct examination for ova	Mebendazole, albendazole
Ascaris lumbricoides	Southeast	Human	Stool examination for ova	Mebendazole, albendazole
Trichuris trichiura	Southeast	Human	Stool examination for ova	Mebendazole, albendazole
Hookworm	Southeast	Human	Stool examination for ova	Mebendazole, albendazole
Common in Travelers and Immigrants				
Strongyloides stercoralis	Developing world	Human	Stool examination for larvae	Thiabendazole, ivermectin
Schistosoma sp.	Developing world	Snails	Stool examination for ova	Praziquantel
Wuchereria sp.	Asia	Mosquitoes	Nocturnal blood examination	Ivermectin
Onchocerca volvulus	Africa, South and Central America	Blackfly	Biopsy	Ivermectin
Loa loa	Africa	Mosquitoes	Blood examination, clinical setting	Ivermectin

Ascaris infection may cause intestinal, biliary, or pancreatic obstruction. Hookworm infection can be associated with iron deficiency. Diagnosis is made on the basis of stool examination for ova and parasites. Each of these worms can be eradicated with appropriate anthelmintic therapy such as mebendazole, 100 mg orally twice daily for 3 days.

HELMINTH INFECTIONS COMMON IN TRAVELERS AND IMMIGRANTS

Strongyloidosis

Strongyloides stercoralis is a common cause of eosinophilia in returning long-term travelers and immigrants, particularly those from Southeast Asia (see Table 110–2). Infection can persist for years; many men who served in the Pacific theater during World War II or in Vietnam still harbor infections. Although usually asymptomatic, infection can cause diarrhea, abdominal pain, and malabsorption. This helminth can cause life-threatening disseminated infection in individuals immunosuppressed by cancer chemotherapy, corticosteroids, or HIV infection. Diagnosis may be made by stool examination, but this is not a very sensitive technique. Treatment with thiabendazole, 25 mg/kg (maximum, 3 g/day) orally twice daily for 2 days is curative in more than 90% of immunocompetent hosts.

Schistosomiasis

Schistosoma mansoni (Africa, South America, and the Caribbean), *S. japonicum* (Philippines, China, and Indonesia), and *S. mekongi* (Cambodia, Laos, and Vietnam) are the most common causes of hepatosplenic enlargement in the world (see Table 110–2). Chronic infection can lead to periportal hepatic fibrosis, obstruction of portal blood flow, and bleeding esophageal varices. Cases in the United States are often misdiagnosed as hepatitis B or alcohol-induced liver disease. A clue to the correct diagnosis is that the liver is enlarged, in contrast to the small, shrunken liver of alcoholic cirrhosis. *S. haematobium* (Africa) commonly causes hematuria and leads to urinary obstruction. Diagnosis is made by examination of stool or urine for ova and parasites.

Lymphatic Filariasis

Wuchereria bancrofti and *Brugia malayi* cause elephantiasis throughout the tropics (see Table 110–2). Patients may present with acute lymphadenitis or asymptomatic eosinophilia. Occasional patients have pulmonary symptoms, infiltrates, and marked eosinophilia (tropical pulmonary eosinophilia). The diagnosis is made by finding microfilariae in blood specimens obtained at midnight. Treatment currently consists of a single oral dose of ivermectin, 100–400 μg/kg.

Loa Loa

Eyeworm is endemic in West and Central Africa (see Table 110–2). Patients present with transient pruritic subcutaneous swellings. Eosinophilia is universal. In the United States, cases are often misdiagnosed for years as chronic urticaria. In rare patients, the adult worm can be visualized as it crosses the anterior chamber of the eye, giving this worm its common name. Diagnosis is generally suspected on clinical grounds and is confirmed by biopsy. Diethylcarbamazine can be given over 21 days for effective therapy: days 1 and 2, 50 mg tid; day 3, 100 mg tid; days 4–21, 2 mg/kg tid.

River Blindness

Infection with *Onchocerca volvulus* occurs in West and Central Africa as well as in South and Central America (see Table 110–2). Although the most severe manifestations occur in the eye, the most common clinical presentation in the United States is recurrent pruritic dermatitis. The diagnosis can be made by direct examination of skin snips for microfilariae; a specific serologic test is also available. Ivermectin, 150 μg/kg orally for one dose, is the treatment of choice. Ivermectin should be repeated after 6 months to suppress cutaneous and ocular microfilariae.

Clonorchiasis

The Chinese liver fluke, *Clonorchis sinensis*, is important to diagnose in Asian immigrants. Symptoms may be confused with those of biliary tract disease. If untreated, infection can lead to cholangiocarcinoma. Praziquantel is curative.

Cysticercosis

The invasive larval form of pork tapeworm is the most common cause of seizures throughout the world, as well as in young adults in Los Angeles, chiefly immigrants from Mexico. Typically, patients present with new onset of seizures or severe headache. A single ring-enhancing lesion is the characteristic finding on computed tomography. The diagnosis may be confirmed by an immunoblot assay using peripheral blood. Praziquantel (50 mg/kg/day in three divided doses for 15 days) or albendazole (for 30 days, dosed by weight: >60 kg, 400 mg orally twice daily; <60 kg, 15 mg/kg/day in divided doses twice daily) is curative but may precipitate focal cerebral edema and seizures by killing other cysticercariae within the cerebrospinal fluid. An expert should be consulted before treatment.

Intestinal Tapeworms

Three intestinal tapeworms commonly infect humans: *Taenia saginata* from raw beef, *Taenia solium* from raw pork, and *Diphyllobothrium latum* from raw fish. Most individuals are asymptomatic, but *T. solium* can cause invasive disease (cysticercosis) if ova of the adult worm are ingested by humans. *D. latum* is associated with vitamin B$_{12}$ deficiency. All three are treated with praziquantel.

Hydatid Disease

Hydatid disease commonly manifests as a cystic liver mass in emigrants from sheep-raising parts of the world. Early diagnosis is important, because rupture of the cyst can lead to dissemination. Diagnosis is often suspected from the appearance of the cyst (calcified wall and dependent hydatid "sand") on abdominal computed tomography. Serology can be helpful but is occasionally negative if the cyst has not leaked. Currently, primary therapy is the surgical removal of the cyst without spillage of its contents.

REFERENCES

Freedman DO (ed): Travel medicine. Infect Dis Clin North Am 1998; 12(2):249–549.

Mahmoud AAF: Tropical medicine: Current problems and possible solutions. Infect Dis Clin North Am 1995; 9:265–274.

US Public Health Service, Department of Health and Human Services, Centers for Disease Control and Prevention: Health Information for International Travel. Washington, DC: US Government Printing Office, 2000 [updated on a weekly basis with the blue summary sheet].

SECTION XVI

Neurologic Disease

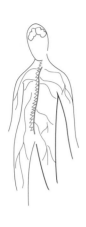

111

NEUROLOGIC EVALUATION OF THE PATIENT

Frederick J. Marshall

To arrive at an accurate neurologic diagnosis, the clinician must generate and test hypotheses about both the location and the mechanism of injury to the nervous system. Hypotheses are refined as one progresses from the interview to the physical examination to the laboratory assessment of the patient. The focus is first placed on those entities that are common, serious, and treatable. Typical presentations of common diseases account for 80% of all cases, unusual presentations of common diseases account for 15%, typical presentations of rare diseases account for 5%, and unusual presentations of rare diseases account for less than 1%.

Taking a Neurologic History

The clinician must determine the location, quality, and timing of symptoms. He or she must avoid hearsay and ask the patient to report the progression of actual symptoms rather than a litany of diagnostic procedures and specialty evaluations. It is important to establish when the patient last felt perfectly normal. Ambiguous descriptors such as "dizzy" should be rejected in favor of evocative descriptors such as "light-headed" (which might implicate cardiovascular insufficiency) or "off balance" (which might implicate cerebellar or posterior column dysfunction).

Historical information must be corroborated by family members and other witnesses when appropriate. This should include the past medical and surgical history; current medications; allergies; family history; review of systems; and social history, including the patient's level of education, work history, possible toxin exposures, substance use, sexual history, and current life circumstance.

Clues are sought to localization during the interview. For example, pain is generally due to a lesion of the peripheral nervous system, whereas aphasia (disordered language processing) indicates an abnormality of the central nervous system. Because sensory and motor functions are anatomically relatively distant in the cerebral cortex but progressively closer together as fibers converge in the brain stem, spinal cord, roots, and peripheral nerves, the coexistence of sensory loss and motor dysfunction in a limb implies either a large lesion at the level of the cortex or a smaller lesion lower down in the neuraxis. Small lesions in areas of "high traffic" such as the spinal cord or brain stem can result in widespread neurologic dysfunction, whereas small lesions elsewhere may be asymptomatic.

Table 111–1 lists common neurologic symptoms with regard to how much potential they have to help settle the issue of lesion localization. Tables 111–2 and 111–3 list symptoms commonly associated with lesions at specific locations in the nervous system. Some symptoms can result from a lesion at any of several levels of the nervous system. For example, double vision can result from a focal lesion in the brain stem, peripheral nerves (cranial nerve III, IV, or VI), neuromuscular junction, or extraocular muscles or can be nonfocal from an increase in intracranial pressure. Associated symptoms (or lack thereof) may lead the interviewer to reject certain hypotheses that at first seemed most likely.

Table 111–4 lists the most important types of neurologic pathology and provides examples of diseases in each category.

Some locations of neurologic pathology point to a specific diagnosis or a limited number of diagnoses. For example, disease of the neuromuscular junction is usually caused by an autoimmune process: myasthenia gravis (common) or Eaton-Lambert myasthenic syndrome (uncommon). The exceptions are rare: botulism and congenital myasthenic disorders. Alternatively, some areas of the nervous system (e.g., the cerebral hemispheres) are vulnerable to practically any of the categories of disease outlined in Table 111–4.

TABLE 111–1 Potential Localizing Value of Common Neurologic Symptoms

Potential Localizing Value	Symptom
High	Focal weakness, sensory loss, or pain
	Focal visual loss
	Language disturbance
	Neglect or anosognosia
Medium	Vertigo
	Dysarthria
	Clumsiness
Low	Fatigue
	Headache
	Insomnia
	Dizziness
	Anxiety, confusion, or psychosis

The pace and temporal order of symptoms is important. Degenerative diseases generally progress gradually, whereas vascular diseases (e.g., stroke, aneurysmal subarachnoid hemorrhage) present rapidly. Certain symptoms, such as double vision, almost invariably present abruptly, even if the underlying disorder has been developing gradually over days to weeks.

The Neurologic Examination

Although it is imperative to perform the main elements of a general screening neurologic examination (Table 111–5), the examination should be tailored to confirm or disprove the clinical hypotheses generated from the history. Unexpected signs must be explained (often by a return to the history for further clarification).

The examination is approached as if only one of two possible injuries had occurred: either the "final common pathway" to a structure is disrupted or the input to that pathway is disrupted (Fig. 111–1). In the case of the motor system, the "final common pathway" includes the anterior horn cells giving rise to axons in a nerve, the nerve itself, neuromuscular junctions, and the muscle. Injury to any of these structures will result in dysfunction of the muscle. On the other hand, if these structures are intact, it may be possible to observe the muscle function under the right circumstances. If all modes of engaging the final common pathway fail to elicit a

TABLE 111–2 Clues to Symptom Localization in the Central Nervous System

Symptom	Location
Cerebral Hemispheres	
Unilateral weakness or sensory complaints	Contralateral cerebral hemisphere
Language dysfunction	Left hemisphere (frontal/temporal)
Spatial disorientation	Right hemisphere (parietal/occipital)
Anosognosia (lack of insight into deficit)	Right hemisphere (parietal)
Hemivisual loss	Contralateral hemisphere (occipital/temporal/parietal)
Flattening of affect or social dysinhibition	Bihemispheric (frontal/limbic)
Alteration of consciousness	Bihemispheric (diffuse)
Alteration of memory	Bihemispheric (hippocampus/fornix/amygdala/mammillary bodies)
Cerebellum	
Limb clumsiness	Ipsilateral cerebellar hemisphere
Unsteadiness of gait or posture	Midline cerebellar structures
Basal Ganglia	
Slowness of voluntary movement	Substantia nigra and striatum
Involuntary movement	Striatum/thalamus/subthalamus
Brain Stem	
Contralateral weakness or sensory complaints in the body, with ipsilateral weakness or sensory complaints in the face	Midbrain/pons/medulla
Double vision	Midbrain/pons
Vertigo	Pons/medulla
Alteration of consciousness	Midbrain/pons/medulla (reticular formation)
Spinal Cord	
Weakness and spasticity (ipsilateral) and anesthesia (contralateral) below a specified level	Corticospinal and spinothalamic tracts
Unsteadiness of gait	Posterior columns
Bilateral (can be asymmetric) weakness and sensory complaints in multiple contiguous radicular distributions	Central cord

TABLE 111-3 Clues to Symptom Localization in the Anterior Horn Cell and the Peripheral Nervous System

Symptom	Location
Anterior Horn Cell	
Weakness and wasting with muscle "twitching" (fasciculation) but no sensory complaints	Anterior horn of spinal cord (diffuse or segmental)
Spinal Root	
Weakness and sensory loss confined to a known radicular distribution (pain, a common feature, may spread)	Cervical/thoracic/lumbar/sacral
Plexus	
Pain, weakness, and sensory loss in a limb, not limited to a single radicular or peripheral nerve distribution	Brachial/lumbosacral (may also be due to polyradiculopathy)
Nerve	
Pain, distal weakness, and/or sensory changes confined to a single peripheral nerve distribution	Peripheral nerve (mononeuropathy)
Pain, distal weakness, and/or sensory changes affecting both sides symmetrically (generally starting in feet)	Peripheral nerves (polyneuropathy)
Pain, distal weakness, and/or sensory changes affecting scattered single peripheral nerve distributions	Peripheral nerves (mononeuropathy multiplex)
Unilateral special sensory loss	Cranial nerve I/II/V/VII/VIII/IX
Unilateral facial weakness involving entire half of face	Cranial nerve VII (ipsilateral)
Neuromuscular Junction	
Progressive weakness with repeated use of a muscle; no sensory complaints	Ocular/pharyngeal/skeletal
Muscle	
Proximal weakness; no sensory complaints	Diffuse/various patterns

response, the clinician can conclude that the lesion is located somewhere within the final common pathway.

For example, a man with paralysis of facial movement on one side that is caused by a lesion of cranial nerve VII cannot voluntarily smile, close his eye, or wrinkle his forehead on the affected side. Spontaneous laughter or smiling as an automatic response to a joke also fails to be evident on the paretic side. If the problem is central, however, facial movement with involuntary (spontaneous) smiling may be preserved or even increased. This is commonly observed in patients with facial weakness caused by a stroke.

Central input to a final common pathway in the nervous system is usually tonically inhibitory. Damage to this input typically results in overactivity of the involved muscle group. Signs of damage to central inhibitory systems include (1) spasticity and hyperreflexia (motor cortex, subcortical white matter, corticospinal pathways in the brain stem and spinal cord); (2) dystonia, rigidity, tremor, and tic (basal ganglia, extrapyramidal systems); and (3) ataxia and dysmetria (cerebellum). An exception is hypotonia caused by cerebellar disease.

Technologic Assessment

Laboratory investigations and special testing should be used to confirm clinical suspicions and finalize the diag-

nosis. Testing should be done selectively, because of expense, risk, and discomfort to the patient. Frequently helpful tests are discussed here. Diagnostic tests should never be ordered without a specific differential diagnosis firmly in mind. Many neurodiagnostic tests disclose "diagnoses" unrelated to a patient's symptomatic disease process.

LUMBAR PUNCTURE

Investigation of the cerebrospinal fluid (CSF) is indicated in a small number of specific circumstances (usually suspected meningitis and encephalitis) (Table 111–6). A CSF specimen should routinely be sent for cell count and differential, determination of protein and glucose levels, and bacterial cultures. The CSF should be looked at for its color and clarity. Cloudy or discolored CSF should be centrifuged and examined for xanthochromia in comparison with water. Special studies may be supplemented as appropriate, including Gram's stain; fungal, viral, and tuberculous cultures; cryptococcal and other antigens; tests for syphilis; Lyme titers; malignant cytology; or oligoclonal bands. Polymerase chain reaction for specific viruses holds promise for many conditions. It is important to record the opening and closing pressure. Tissue infection in the region of the puncture site is an absolute contraindication to lumbar puncture. Relative contraindications include known or probable intracranial or spinal mass lesion, increased intracranial pressure as

TABLE 111-4 Categories of Neurologic Disease

Disease Category	Example
Genetic	
Autosomal dominant	Huntington's disease
Autosomal recessive	Friedreich's ataxia
Sex-linked recessive	Duchenne's dystrophy
Sporadic	Down's syndrome
Neoplastic	
Intrinsic	Glioblastoma
Extrinsic	Metastatic melanoma
Paraneoplastic	Cerebellar degeneration
Vascular	
Stroke	Thrombotic, embolic, lacunar, hemorrhagic
Structural	Arteriovenous malformation
Inflammatory	Cranial arteritis
Infectious	
Bacterial	Meningococcal meningitis
Viral	Herpes encephalitis
Protozoal	Toxoplasmosis
Fungal	Cryptococcal meningitis
Helminthic	Cysticercosis
Prion	Creutzfeldt-Jakob disease
Degenerative	
Central	Parkinson's disease
Central and peripheral	Amyotrophic lateral sclerosis
Autoimmune	
Central demyelinating	Multiple sclerosis
Peripheral demyelinating	Guillain-Barré syndrome
Neuromuscular junction	Myasthenia gravis
Toxic/metabolic	
Endogenous	Uremic encephalopathy
Exogenous	Alcoholic neuropathy
Other structural	
Trauma	Spinal cord injury
Hydrodynamic	Normal pressure hydrocephalus
Psychogenic	Hysterical paraparesis

a result of mass lesions, coagulopathy caused by thrombocytopenia (usually correctable), anticoagulant therapy, or bleeding disorders. Rare but severe complications include transtentorial or foramen magnum herniation, spinal epidural hematoma, spinal abscess, herniated or infected disc, meningitis, and adverse reaction to local anesthetic agent. More common and relatively benign complications include headache and backache.

TISSUE BIOPSIES

In selected specialty centers, diagnostic biopsy is performed on various tissues, including brain, peripheral nerve (see Chapter 129), muscle (see Chapter 130), and skin. On occasion, biopsy provides the only means of arriving at a definitive diagnosis.

ELECTROPHYSIOLOGIC STUDIES

Electrophysiologic studies include electroencephalography, electromyography, nerve conduction studies, and

evoked potentials. They are helpful in situations in which the patient cannot be adequately examined or interviewed.

Electroencephalography is most often used to investigate seizures (see Chapter 125). It can document encephalopathy, in which case the background electrical activity of the brain is slowed, and it is also used in the evaluation of brain death.

Electromyography is useful in the differential diagnosis of muscle disease, neuromuscular junction disease, peripheral nerve disease, and anterior horn cell disease (see Chapters 129 and 130). Nerve conduction studies (see Chapters 129 and 130) may show decreased amplitude (characteristic of axonal neuropathy) or decreased velocity (characteristic of demyelinating neuropathy).

Visual evoked potential studies are commonly used in the evaluation of suspected multiple sclerosis (see Chapter 128). Asymmetric slowing of the cortical response to visual pattern stimulation suggests demyelination in the optic nerve or central optic pathways. Brain stem auditory evoked potential studies are useful in the diagnosis of diseases affecting cranial nerve VIII or its central projections. Lesions at the cerebellopontine angle and the brain stem cause abnormal delay in conduction.

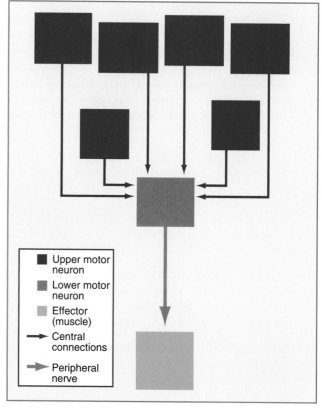

■ Upper motor neuron
■ Lower motor neuron
■ Effector (muscle)
→ Central connections
→ Peripheral nerve

FIGURE 111-1 The nervous system can be conceptually reduced to a series of higher order inputs converging on final common pathways. For example, upper motor neurons converge on lower motor neurons, whose axons form the final common pathway to an effector muscle.

TABLE 111–5 Elements of a General Screening Neurologic Examination

General Systemic Physical Examination

Head (trauma, dysmorphism, bruits)
Neck (tone, bruits, thyromegaly)
Cardiovascular (heart rate, rhythm, murmurs; peripheral pulses, jugular venous distention)
Pulmonary (breathing pattern, cyanosis)
Abdomen (hepatosplenomegaly)
Back/extremities (skeletal abnormalities, peripheral edema, straight-leg raising)
Skin (neurocutaneous stigmata, hepatic stigmata)

Mental Status

Level of consciousness (awake, drowsy, comatose)
Attention (coherent stream of thought, serial 7s)
Orientation (temporal and spatial)
Memory (short-term and long-term)
Language (naming, repetition, comprehension, fluency, reading, writing)
Visuospatial skills (clock drawing, figure copying)
Judgment/insight/thought content (psychotic)
Mood (depressed, manic, anxious)

Cranial Nerves

Olfactory (smell in each nostril)
Optic (afferent pupillary function, funduscopic examination, visual acuity, visual fields, structural eye findings)
Oculomotor, trochlear, abducens (smooth pursuit and saccadic eye movements, nystagmus, efferent pupillary function, eyelid opening)
Trigeminal (jaw jerk, facial sensation, afferent corneal reflex, muscles of mastication)
Facial (efferent corneal reflex, facial expression, eyelid closure, nasolabial folds, power and bulk)
Vestibulocochlear (nystagmus, speech discrimination, Weber, Rinne)
Glossopharyngeal, vagus (afferent and efferent gag reflex, uvula position)
Spinal accessory (power and bulk of sternocleidomastoids and trapezii)
Hypoglossal (position, bulk, and fasciculations of tongue)

Motor Examination

Pronator drift (subtle corticospinal lesion)
Tone and bulk of muscles (basal ganglia lesion yields rigidity, cerebellar lesion yields hypotonia, corticospinal lesion yields spasticity, nonspecific bihemispheric disease yields paratonia, hypertrophy indicates dystonia, pseudohypertrophy indicates muscle disease, atrophy indicates lower motor neuron disease)
Adventitious movements (tremor, tic, dystonia, and chorea indicate disease of the basal ganglia; asterixis and myoclonus may indicate toxic metabolic process)
Power of major muscle groups (scale 0–5)
    Upper extremities: deltoid, biceps, triceps, wrist extension and flexion, finger extension and flexion, interossei

Lower extremities: hip flexion, extension, abduction, and adduction; knee extension and flexion; ankle dorsiflexion, plantarflexion, inversion, and eversion; toe extension and flexion)

Sensory Examination

Light touch (posterior columns)
Pinprick (spinothalamic tract)
Temperature (spinothalamic tract)
Joint position sense (posterior columns)
Vibration (posterior columns)
Graphesthesia (cortical sensory)
Double simultaneous stimulation (cortical sensory)
Two-point discrimination (posterior columns, cortical sensory)

Reflex Examination

Standard reflexes (grade 0–3)
  Biceps
  Triceps
  Brachioradialis
  Knee jerk
  Ankle jerk
Pathologic reflexes
  Babinski sign (if present)
  Myerson sign (if present)
  Snout (if present)
  Jaw jerk (if brisk)
  Palmomental (if present)
  Hoffmann sign (if brisk)

Coordination and Gait

Finger-nose-finger (intention tremor suggesting cerebellar disease)
Rapid alternating movements (dysdiadokokinesia suggesting cerebellar disease)
Fine motor movements (slowness and small amplitude suggesting basal ganglia or corticospinal tract abnormalities)
Heel-to-shin (ataxia suggesting cerebellar disease)
Arising from chair with arms folded across chest (inability in advanced basal ganglia, cerebellar, corticospinal, or muscle disease)
Walking naturally (look for decreased arm swing, spasticity, broad base, festination, waddle, footdrop, start hesitation, dystonia)
Tandem gait (look for ataxia)
Walking with feet everted or inverted (look for latent dystonia)
Hopping on each foot separately (look for latent dystonia)
Stand with feet together and eyes open, eyes closed (sensory ataxia, cerebellar disease)
Response to retropulsive stress (loss of postural righting mechanisms)

Brain stem auditory evoked potentials are helpful in the diagnosis of deafness in infants. Somatosensory evoked potentials are used to identify slowing of central sensory conduction that results from demyelinating disease, compression, or metabolic derangements. They are also used to evaluate spinal cord–mediated sensory abnormalities.

IMAGING STUDIES

Magnetic resonance imaging (MRI) and computed tomography (CT) are high-resolution imaging techniques that provide extraordinary diagnostic precision for central nervous system (CNS) lesions. Most neurologic diseases, however, can have normal CT and MRI findings. More-

TABLE 111–6   Indications for Lumbar Puncture

Urgent (do not wait for brain imaging):
   Acute central nervous system infection in the absence of focal neurologic signs
Less urgent (wait for brain imaging):
   Vasculitis, subarachnoid hemorrhage, or cryptic process
   Increased intracranial pressure in the absence of mass lesion on magnetic resonance imaging or computed tomography
   Intrathecal therapy for fungal or carcinomatous meningitis
   Symptomatic treatment for headache from idiopathic intracranial hypertension or subarachnoid hemorrhage

TABLE 111–8   Some Neurologic Conditions for Which Genetic Tests Are Available

Peripheral neuropathies (Charcot-Marie-Tooth 1A, Kennedy)
Neuromuscular diseases (myotonic dystrophy, Duchenne, Becker, spinal muscular atrophy, MELAS, MERRF, familial amyotrophic lateral sclerosis)
Movement disorders (spinocerebellar ataxia types 1, 2, 3, 6, and 7; Friedreich; dystonia DYT1; Huntington)
Mental retardation (fragile X)

MELAS = mitochondrial encephalomyelopathy—lactic acidosis—and stroke-like symptoms (syndrome); MERRF = myoclonus epilepsy with ragged red fibers (syndrome).

over, many abnormal findings on CT and MRI bear no relationship to the diagnosis responsible for the patient's symptoms. Table 111–7 compares CT and MRI. MRI is used for most purposes, although CT has the advantage of wider accessibility, greater speed of acquisition, and better tolerability by the patient. CT detects acute hemorrhage and is preferred for emergencies. MRI provides more detail and obtains images in horizontal, vertical, and coronal planes simultaneously. Contrast media for CT or MRI are useful in the diagnosis of tumors, abscesses, and other processes that derange the blood-brain barrier. MRI can now be used for functional imaging and spectroscopy; both techniques have great promise for the evaluation of cognitive and metabolic disorders, epilepsy, multiple sclerosis, and many other conditions.

Magnetic resonance angiography allows noninvasive visualization of the major vessels of the head and neck. Conventional angiography with an intra-arterial injection of contrast agent is used for evaluation of many intracranial vascular abnormalities: small aneurysms and arteriovenous malformations and inflammation of small blood vessels.

Noninvasive ultrasonography of the carotid and vertebral arteries can define stenotic vessels and has been supplemented by transcranial Doppler technology, which allows characterization of blood flow in intracranial arteries.

TABLE 111–7   Magnetic Resonance Imaging (MRI) vs. Computed Tomography (CT)

MRI
Resolution 1–2 mm
Gadolinium contrast relatively safe
Unaffected by bone
Multiple planes of imaging available
Functional (physiologic) imaging capacity

CT
Resolution >5 mm
Iodine contrast associated with anaphylaxis, rash
Faster acquisition than MRI
Metallic objects such as pacemaker or aneurysm clip preclude MRI
Acute hemorrhage well visualized
Better tolerated by severely ill or claustrophobic patients

Single photon emission CT is useful for the evaluation of intracranial blood flow. Moreover, the development of new radioligands may make it possible to visualize the dopamine transporter on nigral-striatal dopaminergic projection neurons by using a ligand (β-CIT) to follow cell loss in Parkinson's disease. As the techniques of neural transplantation for Parkinson's disease improve, it may be possible to image restoration of function.

Positron emission tomography is an extremely useful functional imaging technology that can demonstrate specific metabolic derangements. It remains a largely investigational method but is particularly useful for evaluating local abnormalities of glucose and oxygen metabolism. The high cost of the cyclotron technology needed to generate the radioactive ligands limits its clinical use to specialized centers. Positron emission tomography is of particular value in defining the site of origin of focal seizures.

GENETIC AND MOLECULAR TESTING

There are many more neurologic diseases than diseases of all other systems combined. Continuing scientific discoveries have yielded a revolution in the diagnostic approach to many of these diseases, and each passing year new genetic tests are added to our armamentarium. Table 111–8 outlines a number of tests that are now commercially available. The use of a genetic test for a given disorder requires that the clinician perform a thoughtful and caring evaluation of the patient, usually with input from and evaluation of the patient's family. There are many important ethical issues surrounding the use of genetic tests, including the ability to ensure privacy, to ensure adequate psychological and social support for patients who may be given devastating news, and to adequately address the appropriateness of prenatal screening or presymptomatic testing when no treatment is available.

REFERENCES

Patten J: Nuerological Differential Diagnosis, 2nd ed. London: Springer, 1996.
Samuels MA, Feske S (eds): Office Practice of Neurology. New York: Churchill Livingstone, 1996.

112

DISORDERS OF CONSCIOUSNESS

Roger P. Simon

Coma is a sleeplike state in that the eyes are closed even when the person is vigorously stimulated. A poorly responsive state in which the eyes are open, or an agitated confused state or delirium, is not coma but it may represent early stages of the same disease processes and should be investigated in the same manner.

Consciousness requires an intact and functioning brain stem reticular activating system and its cortical projections. The reticular formation begins in the mid-pons and ascends through the dorsal midbrain to synapse in the thalamus; it then innervates higher centers through thalamocortical connections. Knowledge of this anatomic substrate provides the short list of regions to be investigated in the search for a structural cause of coma; brain stem or bihemispheric dysfunction must satisfy these anatomic requirements or it is not the cause of the patient's unconsciousness. In addition to structural lesions, meningeal inflammation, metabolic encephalopathy, and seizures diffusely affect the brain and complete the differential diagnosis of the patient in coma.

Pathophysiology

Meningeal irritation caused by infection or blood in the subarachnoid space is an essential early consideration in coma evaluation because its cause requires immediate attention (especially with purulent meningitis) and may not be diagnosed by computed tomography (CT).

Hemispheric mass lesions result in coma either by expanding across the midline laterally to compromise both cerebral hemispheres or by impinging on the brain stem to compress the rostral reticular formation. These processes—*lateral herniation* (lateral movement of the brain) and *transtentorial herniation* (vertical movement of hemispheric content)—most commonly occur to-

gether. At the bedside, clinical signs of an expanding hemispheric mass evolve in a level-by-level, rostral-caudal manner (Fig. 112–1). Hemispheric lesions of adequate size to produce coma are readily seen on CT.

Brain stem mass lesions produce coma by directly affecting the reticular formation. As the pathways for lateral eye movements (the pontine gaze center, medial longitudinal fasciculus, and oculomotor—third nerve—nucleus) traverse the reticular activating system, impairment of reflex eye movements is often the critical element of diagnosis. A comatose patient without impaired reflex lateral eye movements does not have a mass lesion compromising brain stem structures in the posterior fossa. CT is not able to show some lesions in this region. Posterior fossa lesions may block the flow of cerebrospinal fluid from the lateral ventricles, and the result may be the dangerous situation of *noncommunicating hydrocephalus*.

Metabolic abnormalities are caused by deficiency states (e.g., thiamin, glucose), by derangements of metabolism (e.g., hyponatremia), or by the presence of *exogenous toxins* (drugs) or *endogenous toxins* (organ system failure). Metabolic abnormalities result in diffuse dysfunction of the nervous system without localized signs such as hemiparesis or unilateral pupillary dilatation. The diagnosis of *metabolic encephalopathy* means that the examiner has found no focal anatomic features on examination or neuroimaging studies to explain coma, but it does not state that a specific metabolic cause has been established. Drugs have a predilection for affecting the reticular formation in the brain stem and producing paralysis of reflex eye movement on examination. *Multifocal structural disorders* may simulate metabolic coma (Table 112–1).

In the late stages of status epilepticus, motor movements may be subtle even though *seizure activity* is continuing throughout the brain. Once seizures stop, the so-called *postictal state* can also cause unexplained coma.

883

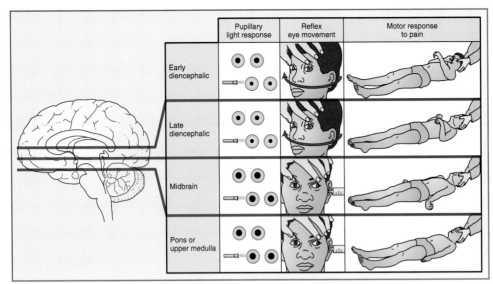

	Pupillary light response	Reflex eye movement	Motor response to pain
Early diencephalic			
Late diencephalic			
Midbrain			
Pons or upper medulla			

FIGURE 112–1   The evolution of neurologic signs in coma from a hemispheric mass lesion as the brain becomes functionally impaired in a rostral caudal manner. Early and late diencephalic refer to levels of dysfunction just above (early) and just below (late) the thalamus. (From Aminoff MJ, Greenberg DA, Simon RP: Clinical Neurology. Stamford, CT: Appleton and Lange, 1996.)

Diagnostic Approach

The history and examination are essential in the diagnosis and are not replaced by CT (Table 112–2). History of a premonitory headache supports a diagnosis of meningitis, encephalitis, or intracerebral or subarachnoid hemorrhage. A preceding period of intoxication, confusion, or delirium points to a diffuse process such as meningitis or endogenous or exogenous toxins. The sudden apoplectic onset of coma is particularly suggestive of ischemic or hemorrhagic stroke affecting the brain stem or of subarachnoid hemorrhage or intracerebral hemorrhage with intraventricular rupture. Lateralized symptoms of hemiparesis or aphasia before coma occur in patients with hemispheric masses or infarctions.

The physical examination is critical, quickly accomplished, and diagnostic. The issues are three: (1) Does the patient have meningitis? (2) Are signs of a mass lesion present? (3) Is this a diffuse syndrome of exogenous or endogenous metabolic cause? Emergency management should then be instituted (Table 112–3).

IDENTIFICATION OF MENINGITIS

Although signs of meningeal irritation are not invariably present and have differing sensitivity in regard to cause

TABLE 112–1   Multifocal Disorders Presenting as Metabolic Coma

Disseminated intravascular coagulopathy
Sepsis
Pancreatitis
Vasculitis
Thrombotic thrombocytopenic purpura
Fat emboli
Hypertensive encephalopathy
Diffuse micrometastases

(extremely common with acute pyogenic meningitis and subarachnoid hemorrhage, less common with indolent, fungal meningitis), the presence of these signs on examination is the central clue to the diagnosis. Missing these signs results in time-consuming additional tests such as CT and the potential loss of a narrow therapeutic window of opportunity. Passive neck flexion should be carried out (Fig. 112–2) in all comatose patients unless there is a history of head trauma. When the neck is passively flexed, by attempting to bring the chin within a few fingerbreadths of the chest, patients with irritated meninges reflexively flex one or both knees. This sign (*Brudzinski's reflex*) is usually asymmetric and not dramatic, but any evidence of knee flexion during passive neck flexion requires that the cerebrospinal fluid be examined. Is CT required before lumbar puncture in this setting? In the absence of lateralized signs (such as hemiparesis) supporting a superimposed mass lesion, a spinal puncture should be performed immediately. Although rare cases of herniation after lumbar puncture have been reported in children with bacterial meningitis, the urgency of diagnosis and treatment at the point of coma is paramount. The time needed for CT may result in a fatal therapeutic delay. An alternative approach involves obtaining blood cultures and immediately initiating antibiotic therapy with subsequent lumbar puncture; cerebrospinal fluid cell count, glucose determination, and protein content are unchanged and Gram's stain and culture often remain positive despite a short period of antibiotic treatment.

SEPARATION OF STRUCTURAL FROM METABOLIC CAUSES OF COMA

This goal is achieved by neurologic examination. Because the evaluation and potential treatments for structural and metabolic coma are widely divergent and the disease processes in both categories are often rapidly progressive, initiating the evaluation medically or surgi-

TABLE 112–2 Causes of Coma with Normal Computed Tomography Scan

Meningeal Disorders
Subarachnoid hemorrhage (uncommon)
Bacterial meningitis
Encephalitis
Subdural empyema

Exogenous Toxins
Sedative drugs and barbiturates
Anesthetics and γ-hydroxybutyrate*
Alcohols
Stimulants
    Phencyclidine†
    Cocaine and amphetamine‡
Psychotropic Drugs
    Cyclic antidepressants
    Phenothiazines
    Lithium
Anticonvulsants
Opioids
Clonidine§
Penicillins
Salicylates
Anticholinergics
Carbon monoxide, cyanide, and methemoglobinemia

Endogenous Toxins/Deficiencies/Derangements
Hypoxia and ischemia
Hypoglycemia
Hypercalcemia
Osmolar
    Hyperglycemia
    Hyponatremia
    Hypernatremia
Organ system failure
    Hepatic encephalopathy
    Uremic encephalopathy
    Pulmonary insufficiency (carbon dioxide narcosis)

Seizures
Prolonged postictal state
Spike-wave stupor

Hypothermia or Hyperthermia

Brain Stem Ischemia

Basilar Artery Stroke

Brain Stem or Cerebellar Hemorrhage

Conversion or Malingering

* General anesthetic, similar to γ-aminobutyric acid; recreational drug and body building aid. Rapid onset, rapid recovery often with myoclonic jerking and confusion. Deep coma (2–3 hr; Glasgow Coma Scale = 3) with maintenance of vital signs.
† Coma associated with cholinergic signs: lacrimation, salivation, bronchorrhea, and hyperthermia.
‡ Coma after seizures or status (i.e., a prolonged postictal state).
§ An antihypertensive agent active through the opiate receptor system; frequent overdose when used to treat narcotic withdrawal.

cally may be life-saving. This task is accomplished by focusing on three features of neurologic examination: the *motor response* to a painful stimulus, *pupillary function*, and *reflex eye movements*.

Motor Response

Asymmetric or reflex function of the motor system provides the clearest indication of a mass lesion. Elicitation of a *motor response* requires that a painful stimulus be applied to which the patient will react. The patient's arms should be placed in a semiflexed posture, and a painful stimulus should be applied to the head or trunk. Strong pressure on the supraorbital ridge or pinching of the skin on the anterior chest or inner arm is the most useful method; finger nail bed pressure is also used, but it makes the interpretation of upper limb movement difficult.

The neurologic examination of a patient with an expanding hemispheric mass lesion is shown in Figure 112–1. Hemispheric masses at their early stage (*early diencephalic,* i.e., compromising the brain above the thalamus) produce appropriate movement of one upper extremity toward the painful stimulus. The attenuated contralateral arm movement reflects a hemiparesis. This lateralized motor movement in a comatose patient establishes the working diagnosis of a hemispheric mass. As the mass expands to involve the thalamus (*late diencephalic*), the response to pain becomes reflex arm flexion associated with extension and internal rotation of the legs (*decorticate posturing*); asymmetry of the response in the upper extremities is seen. With further brain compromise at the midbrain level, the reflex posturing changes in the arms, so both arms and legs respond by extension (*decerebrate posturing*); at this level, the asymmetry tends to be lost. At this point, the pupils become midposition in size, and the light reflex is lost, first unilaterally and then bilaterally. With further progression to the level of the pons, no response to painful stimulation is the most frequent finding, although spinal movements of leg flexion may occur. The classic postures illustrated in Figure 112–1, and particularly their asymmetry, strongly support the presence of a mass le-

TABLE 112–3 Emergency Management

Ensure airway adequacy
Support ventilation and circulation
Obtain blood for glucose, electrolytes, hepatic and renal function, prothrombin and partial thromboplastin time, complete blood count, and drug screen
Administer 25 g of dextrose IV (typically 50 mL of 50% dextrose) to treat possible hypoglycemic coma*
Administer 100 mg of thiamine IV
Treat opiate overdose with naloxone (0.4–1.2 mg IV)
The specific benzodiazepine antagonist flumazenil (0.2 mg IV repeated once and followed by 0.1 mg IV to 1–3 mg total) can be given for the reversal of benzodiazepine-induced coma or conscious sedation†

* The glucose level is poorly correlated with the level of consciousness in hypoglycemia; stupor, coma, and confusion are reported with blood glucose concentrations ranging from 2 to 60 mg/dL.
† Not recommended in coma of unknown origin because seizures may be precipitated in patients with polydrug overdoses containing benzodiazepines with tricyclic antidepressants or cocaine.

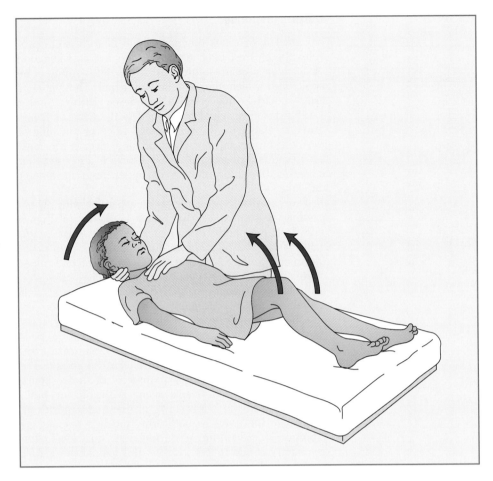

FIGURE 112–2 Elicitation of Brudzinski's sign of meningeal irritation as seen in infectious meningitis or subarachnoid hemorrhage. (From Aminoff MJ, Greenberg DA, Simon RP: Clinical Neurology. Stamford, CT: Appleton and Lange, 1996.)

sion. However, these motor movements, especially early in coma, are most frequently fragments of abnormal, asymmetric flexion or extension in the arms, rather than the complete decorticate and decerebrate postures illustrated in Figure 112–1. A small amount of asymmetric flexion or extension of the arms to painful stimulus carries the same implications as the full-blown postures.

Metabolic lesions do not compromise the brain in a progressive, level-by-level manner as do hemispheric masses, and they rarely produce the asymmetric motor signs typical of masses. Reflex posturing may be seen, but it lacks the asymmetry of decortication from a hemispheric mass and is not associated with the loss of pupillary reactivity at the stage of decerebration.

Pupillary Reactivity

In metabolic coma, one feature is central to the examination: pupillary reactivity is present. This reactivity is seen both early in coma, when an appropriate motor response to pain may be retained, and late, when no motor responses can be elicited. The pupillary reaction is lost only when coma is so deep that the patient requires ventilatory and blood pressure support.

Reflex Eye Movements

The presence of inducible lateral eye movements reflects the integrity of the pons and midbrain. These reflex eye movements (see Fig. 112–1) are brought about by passive head rotation to stimulate the semicircular canal input to the vestibular system (so-called doll's eyes maneuver) or by inhibiting the function of one semicircular canal by infusion of ice water against the tympanic membrane (caloric testing).

In metabolic coma, reflex eye movements may be lost or retained. Lack of inducible eye movements with the doll's eyes maneuver, in the setting of preserved pupillary reactivity, is virtually diagnostic of drug toxicity. With metabolic coma of non–drug-induced origin such as organ system failure, electrolyte disorders, or osmolar disorders, reflex eye movements are preserved.

Brain stem mass lesions are most commonly caused by hemorrhage or infarction. Reflex lateral eye movements, the pathways for which traverse the pons and midbrain, are particularly affected, and the reflex postures of decortication and decerebration typical of brain stem injury are common. Lesions restricted to the midbrain (e.g., embolization from the heart to the top of the basilar artery) are manifested by sluggish pupillary reflexes or their absence, with or without impaired medial eye movements (both are controlled by the third cranial nerve). With lesions restricted to the pons (e.g., intrapontine hypertensive hemorrhage), pupils are reactive but very small (pinpoint or pontine pupils), which reflects focal impairment of descending sympathetic fibers; these are rare. Ocular bobbing (spontaneous symmetric or asymmetric rhythmic vertical ocular oscillations) may be seen.

Seizures occurring in a patient with acute brain injury (e.g., that resulting from encephalitis, hypertensive encephalopathy, hyponatremia or hypernatremia, hypoglycemia or hyperglycemia) or chronic brain injury (e.g., dementia, mental retardation) often result in a prolonged postictal coma. The examination shows reactive pupils and inducible eye movements (in the absence of overtreatment with anticonvulsants) and often upgoing toes or focal signs (Todd's paresis). Nonconvulsive seizures, particularly spike-wave stupor, may occur in a patient without a history of epilepsy. The diagnosis is made by electroencephalogram (see Chapter 125).

Prognosis in Coma

In coma after cardiac arrest, the prognosis for meaningful recovery can be assessed from clinical signs. Return of pupillary reactivity within 24 hours and purposeful motor movements within the first 72 hours after cardiac arrest are highly correlated with a favorable outcome (Table 112–4). Rare late recoveries, however, have been reported.

Coma-like States

Locked-in patients are those in which a lesion (usually a hemorrhage or an infarct) transects the brain stem at a point below the reticular formation (therefore sparing consciousness) but above the ventilatory nuclei of the medulla (therefore maintaining cardiopulmonary function). Such patients are awake, with eye opening and sleep-wake cycles, but the descending pathways through the brain stem necessary for volitional vocalization or limb movement have been transected. Voluntary eye movement, especially vertical, is preserved, and patients open and close their eyes or produce appropriate num-

TABLE 112–4   Probability (%) of Recovering Independent Function from Coma After Cardiac Arrest

Sign	Days After Cardiac Arrest			
	0	1	3	7
No verbal response	13	8	5	6
No eye opening	11	6	4	0
Unreactive pupils	0	0	0	0
No spontaneous eye movements	6	5	2	0
No caloric response	5	6	6	0
Extensor posturing	18	0	0	0
Flexor posturing	14	3	0	0
No motor response	4	3	0	0
From Levey et al (*N* = 210)				
No eye opening to pain	31	8	0	0
Absent or reflex motor response	25	9	0	0
Unreactive pupils	17	7	0	0
From Edgren et al (*N* = 131)				

Data from Levey DE, Caronna JJ, Singer BH: Predicting the outcome from hypoxic coma. JAMA 1985; 523:1420–1426; and from Edgren E, Hedstrand U, Kelsey S: Assessment of neurological prognosis in comatose survivors of cardiac arrest. Lancet 1994; 343:1055–1059.

bers of blinking movements in answer to questions. The electroencephalogram is usually normal, reflecting normal cortical function.

Psychogenic unresponsiveness is a diagnosis of exclusion. The neurologic examination shows reactive pupils and no reflex posturing to pain. Eye movements during the doll's eyes maneuver show volitional override rather than the smooth uninhibited reflex lateral eye movements of coma. Ice water caloric testing either arouses the patient because of the discomfort produced or induces cortically mediated nystagmus rather than the tonic deviation typical of coma. The slow conjugate roving eye movements of metabolic coma cannot be imitated and, therefore, rule out psychogenic unresponsiveness. In addition, the slow, often asymmetric and incomplete eye closure seen after passive eye opening of a comatose patient cannot be feigned. These signs, therefore, rule out psychogenic coma. In contrast, conscious patients usually exhibit some voluntary muscle tone in the eyelids during passive eye opening. The electroencephalogram in psychogenic unresponsiveness is that of normal wakefulness with reactive posterior rhythms on eye opening and eye closing. In patients with catatonic stupor, lorazepam administration may produce awakening.

In *persistent vegetative states (PVSs)*, patients have awakened from coma but have not regained awareness. Wakefulness is manifested by eye opening and sleep-wake cycles. The reticular activating system of the brain stem is intact to produce wakefulness, but the connections to the cortical mantle are interrupted, precluding awareness.

Clinical features do not differ by etiology (Table

TABLE 112-5   Persistent Vegetative State: Common Causes*

Trauma (diffuse axonal injury)
Cardiac arrest and hypoperfusion (laminar necrosis of cortical mantle and/or thalamic necrosis)
Bihemispheric infarctions
Purulent meningitis or encephalitis (cortical injury)
Carbon monoxide
Prolonged hypoglycemic coma

* A vegetative state may not necessarily begin with coma but can also develop as the end stage of neurodegenerative diseases (e.g., Alzheimer's disease) of adults or children or also accompany severe congenital developmental abnormalities of the brain such as anencephaly.

112–5). PVS patients open their eyes diurnally and in response to loud sounds; blinking occurs with bright lights. Pupils react and eye movements occur both spontaneously and with the doll's eyes maneuver. Yawning, chewing, swallowing, and, uncommonly, guttural vocalizations and lacrimation may be preserved. Spontaneous roving eye movements (very slow, constant velocity) are particularly characteristic and distressing to the patient's visitors because the patient appears to be looking about the room. The brain stem origin of the eye movements is documented by their being readily redirected by the oculocephalic (doll's eyes) reflex. The limbs may move, but motor responses are only primitive; pain usually produces decorticate or decerebrate postures or fragments of these movements.

A vegetative state is termed *persistent* after 3 months if the brain injury was medical and after 12 months if

TABLE 112-6   Criteria for Cessation of Brain Function*

Anatomic Region Tested	Confirmatory Sign
Hemispheres	Unresponsive and unreceptive to sensory stimuli including pain†
Midbrain	Unreactive pupils‡
Pons	Absent reflex eye movements§
Medulla	Apnea ‖

* Sequential testing is necessary for a clinical diagnosis of brain death; at least 6 hr for all cases and at least 24 hr in the setting of anoxic-ischemic brain injury.
† The patient does not rouse, groan, grimace, or withdraw limbs; purely spinal reflexes (deep tendon reflexes, plantar flexion reflex, plantar withdrawal, and tonic neck reflexes) may be maintained.
‡ Most easily assessed by the bright light of an ophthalmoscope viewed through its magnifying lens when focused on the iris; unreactive pupils may be either midposition (as they will be in death) or dilated, as they often are in the setting of a dopamine infusion.
§ No eye movement toward the side of irrigation of the tympanic membrane with 50 mL of ice water; the oculocephalic response (doll's eyes) will always be absent in the setting of absent oculovestibular testing.
‖ No ventilatory movements in the setting of maximum CO_2 stimulation (≥60 mm Hg; with apnea, PCO_2 will passively rise 2–3 mm Hg/min); disconnect the ventilator from the endotracheal tube and insert cannula with 6 L/min O_2.

TABLE 112-7   Exclusionary Criteria for Brain Death

Seizures
Decorticate or decerebrate posturing
Sedative drugs
Hypothermia (<32.2°C)
Neuromuscular blockade
Shock

the brain injury was traumatic. The determination as to when *persistent* equals *permanent* cannot be stated absolutely; to predict which patients early in the vegetative state will remain persistently vegetative is particularly difficult in trauma. Lesions of the corpus callosum and dorsolateral brain stem seen on magnetic resonance images between 6 and 8 weeks after trauma correlated with persistence of the vegetative state at a year. In rare cases, patients show late improvement, but none return to normal.

Brain imaging studies depict the sequelae of the causative injury but are not diagnostic of PVS. Magnetic resonance spectroscopy has shown a decrease in the neuronal marker of *N*-acetylaspartate. Positron emission tomographic studies have shown decreased glucose usage and cerebral blood flow, but such studies in and of themselves are rarely diagnostic. Evoked responses are not useful.

Brain death characterizes the *irreversible cessation* of brain function. Therefore, death of the organism can be determined on the basis of death of the brain. Although some details may be dictated by local law, the standard definition permits a diagnosis of brain death upon documentation of irreversible cessation of all brain function, including function of the brain stem (Table 112–6).

Documentation of *irreversibility* requires that the cause of the coma be known, that the cause be adequate to explain the clinical findings of brain death, and that exclusionary criteria are absent (Table 112–7). Confirmatory tests are sometimes used but are not required for diagnosis (Table 112–8).

Brain death results in asystole, usually within days (mean = 4) even if ventilatory support is continued.

TABLE 112-8   Confirmatory Tests for Brain Death

EEG Isoelectricity

Deep coma from sedative drugs or hypothermia below 20°C can produce EEG flattening; patients clinically brain dead may have residual EEG activity for a number of days following a brain death diagnosis

No Cerebral Blood Flow at Angiography

The most definitive confirmatory test (the role of transcranial Doppler is still unclear)

EEG = electroencephalogram.

Recovery after appropriate documentation of brain death has never been reported. Removal of the ventilator results in terminal rhythms, most often complete heart block without ventricular response; in junctional rhythms; or in ventricular tachycardia. Purely spinal motor movements may occur in the moments of terminal apnea (or during apnea testing in the absence of passive administration of oxygen): arching of the back, neck turning, stiffening of the legs, and upper extremity flexion.

REFERENCES

Halevy A, Brody B: Brain death: Reconciling definitions, criteria, and tests. Ann Intern Med 1993; 119:519–525.

Medical aspects of the persistent vegetative state. N Engl J Med 1994; 330:1499–1508, 1572–1579.

Plum F, Posner JB: The diagnosis of stupor and coma. *In* Contemporary Neurology Series, 3rd ed, vol 19. Philadelphia: FA Davis, 1980.

Young GB, Ropper AH, Bolton CF: Coma and Impaired Consciousness: A Clinical Perspective. New York: McGraw-Hill, 1998.

Zeman A: Persistent vegetative state. Lancet 1997; 350:795–799.

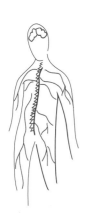

113

DISORDERS OF SLEEP

Roger P. Simon

Neurobiology of Sleep

The precise function of *sleep* is not completely understood. Rest periods are known throughout all biologic systems. Sleep occurs in reptiles and birds, and nearly all mammals sleep and dream. Sleep is necessary for life; deprivation in the rat results in death in about 1 month. Endogenous sleep-inducing factors have been isolated but not fully characterized. Wakefulness is under the control of the reticular activating system of the rostral brain stem, which projects to the thalamus and cortex. The pons contains the rapid eye movement (REM) sleep generator, which may play a role in the random imagery of dreaming.

Sleep stages (Table 113–1), defined by electroencephalogram (EEG) and by behavior, are associated with specific sleep disorders. In *REM sleep*, the EEG is similar to that seen in waking and is characterized by low-voltage mixed frequencies, abrupt rapid eye movements, penile erections, and an absence of electromyographic activity (muscular atonia). REM sleep occupies 20% to 25% of sleep time. Patients awakening during REM sleep report vivid dream imagery. *Non-REM (NREM) sleep* lacks these special features and is associated with EEG slowing.

Insomnia

Insomnia is the perception of inadequate sleep, either in amount or quality, and is usually not associated with daytime sleepiness. The normal duration of sleep in a given person can vary from as little as 4 hours to as many as 11 hours a day.

Diagnosis and treatment of insomnia are based on the patient's history. Is the problem of recent onset or is it chronic? Does the patient have associated psychological, medical, or medication changes (Tables 113–2 and 113–3)? Is the symptom impairment of sleep onset, multiple awakenings during sleep (arousal), early awakenings, or normal but nonrefreshing sleep? Does the patient have partial arousal (history often elicited from the bed partner), breathing abnormalities, or involuntary movements? Each of these forms of insomnia has different differential diagnoses. *Situational insomnia* may be associated with exogenous events: life stresses, death of a family member, stress at work, a new sleeping location or partner, shift work, jet lag, or endogenous depression. *Depression* suppresses REM and stage 4 sleep, which is restored after nonpharmacologic treatment and, to a lesser extent, after pharmacologic treatment of depression. *Chronic behavioral insomnia* occurs in persons with a characteristic personality inducing rumination, emotional arousal, and increased autonomic activity. The focus on the inability to fall asleep becomes self-perpetuating.

The treatment of insomnia (Table 113–4) includes an optimal sleep environment supplemented, as needed, with brief use of sedatives. For patients with persistent insomnia, specific causes should be sought such as sleep apnea or abnormal arousal including periodic limb movements.

Abnormal Arousal

Abnormal arousal results in the perception of inadequate sleep. *Restless leg syndrome*, a need to move the legs or a deep sensory complaint in the lower extremities, occurs at sleep onset and is briefly relieved by walking about or by rubbing or moving the limbs. Sinemet (carbidopa and levodopa) (beginning with 25/100, 30 minutes before bedtime) or bromocriptine (2.5 to 7.5 mg a few hours before sleep) are effective; clonazepam (1 mg at bedtime) or gabapentin may be helpful. Restless leg syndrome is occasionally symptomatic of an underlying neuropathy, but most cases are idiopathic. A family history of restless leg syndrome is common.

Periodic limb movements often accompany restless leg syndrome. The movements are brief and consist of repetitive dorsiflexion of the great toe or plantar flexion of the foot during sleep stages 1 to 2. Clonazepam may

TABLE 113–1   Sleep Stages, Their Characteristics, and Disorders Associated with Them

Sleep Stage	Electroencephalogram*	Eye Movements	Electromyographic Activity	Imagery	Sleep Disorder
Wakefulness	Alpha and beta activity (low voltage fast)	Random, rapid	Active, spontaneous	Vivid, external	Insomnia
Presleep	Reduction of alpha rhythms	Reduced	Reduced	External	Restless leg syndrome; sleep onset myoclonus
Non-REM Sleep (NREM):					
Stage 1 (drowsiness)	Theta activity	Slow, rolling	Attenuated, episodic	Dulled	Periodic limb movements of sleep; sleep myoclonus
Stage 2 (light sleep)	Sleep spindles, K complexes	Slow or absent	Attenuated	Nonvivid	
Stage 3 and 4 (Slow-wave sleep)	Delta activity	Absent	Attenuated		Sleepwalking; sleep terrors
REM Sleep	Low-amplitude, irregular	Abrupt, rapid eye movements	Absent (REM atonia)	Vivid, bizarre	Nightmares; REM behavioral disorder
Sleep-wake transition	Disappearance of slowing	Random	Active	Sleep paralysis; hypnopompic hallucinations	

* Alpha activity: 8–13 Hz (cycles/sec); beta: <13 Hz; theta: 4–7 Hz; delta: <4 Hz.
REM = rapid eye movement.

be useful. *Myoclonus* involving body or limb jerking at the onset of sleep has been reported in nearly 80% of healthy persons. The prolongation of these fragments of myoclonus during NREM sleep constitutes *sleep myoclonus*, which does not usually require treatment.

Sleep Apnea

Obstructive sleep apnea occurs in 2% to 5% of the adult population of the United States and affects primarily middle-aged or elderly men. The classic presentation is the obese patient with loud snoring who has multiple arousals or awakenings during the night, with gasping for breath. One hundred or more events lasting between less than 10 and 30 seconds per night may occur. The resultant sleep fragmentation produces daytime sleepiness and impaired occupational performance. Epi-

TABLE 113–2   Drug-Related Insomnia

Caffeine or caffeine-containing over-the-counter drugs (in susceptible patients)
Alcohol (hastens sleep onset but increases sleep-related breathing abnormalities, sleep fragmentation, and early awakening)
Corticosteroids
Antidepressants
Bronchodilators
Central nervous system stimulants
Short-acting sedatives (on withdrawal)

sodes are exacerbated by alcohol use at bedtime as well as by sedative-hypnotic drugs. The supine position for sleeping is the worst. The diagnosis should be confirmed in a sleep laboratory; the presence or absence of respiratory effort separates obstructive from central causes. Preventive treatments include weight loss and alcohol avoidance. Continuous positive airway pressure during sleep results in symptomatic improvement in most patients.

Parasomnias

Parasomnias are sleep-related motor disorders, with or without autonomic features, that induce brief partial arousals not associated with daytime sleepiness. They are most common in childhood but may occur in adults. *Sleepwalking* occurs in more than 10% of children, many of whom have a family history of the condition. The behavior occurs during sleep stages 3 and 4 and may be fragmentary, such as merely sitting up in bed. Patients are difficult to arouse during the event and do not recollect it. Events usually occur in the first few hours of sleep and are brief (<10 minutes), but they may be recurrent. *Sleep terrors* are often associated; they also occur in NREM sleep and include intense autonomic arousal, marked vocalization and movements, difficulty in arousing the patient, and minimal recall of the episode. The spells may be attenuated by benzodiazepines. *Nightmares* are distinct from sleep terrors because they occur in REM sleep; thus, motor movements are limited, vocalization is much less intense, the patient is relatively easily aroused, and vivid dream recall is evident. *REM behavioral disorder* is an uncommon parasomnia affecting middle-aged or older men or patients with degenerative disease of the central nervous system. The absence of the usual muscle paralysis characteristic of REM (resulting from the absence of electromyographic activity during this sleep stage known as *REM atonia*) allows for REM motor behaviors that are often violent and may injure the patient or the bed partner. Vivid imagery is reported on awakening. Clonazepam is an effective treatment.

Narcolepsy

Narcolepsy, a disorder of excessive daytime sleepiness, is associated with abnormalities in REM sleep. It may be associated with cataplexy or with hypnagogic hallucinations and sleep paralysis. The onset of narcolepsy is between the second and fourth decades. *Narcoleptic hypersomnia* occurs in settings of sedentary activity and boredom but also during conversation, during meals, and while driving. The induced sleep episodes are brief, and their frequency is little changed in patients after the first months of the disorder. The diagnosis is made on the history of excessive daytime sleepiness, the absence of underlying nocturnal sleep disorders, and sleep-onset

TABLE 113-3 Medical or Neurologic Conditions Associated with Insomnia

Pain (especially skeletal pain and arthritis)
Shortness of breath and congestive heart failure (paroxysmal nocturnal dyspnea)
Bowel hypermotility disorders and nocturnal diarrhea
Eating disorders and hunger
Neurologic disorders that impair normal movement during sleep (stroke, multiple sclerosis, or Parkinson's disease)
Nocturnal headaches (cluster and hypnic headache)
Aging (increased awakenings between non-REM and REM sleep; daytime napping shortens nocturnal sleep; sundowning)
Arrival at high altitude (hypoxia, altered ventilatory drive, periodic breathing, and multiple awakenings)

REM = rapid eye movement.

TABLE 113-4 Treatment of Insomnia

Treat depression
Eliminate stimulant drugs
Provide an optimal sleep environment (optimal temperature, light, and ambient noise; a regular sleep time; increased daytime exercise; "winding down" before sleep, i.e., quiet, reading)
Avoid drugs and alcohol
Medications (prescribe only briefly because tolerance develops within weeks)
    Triazolam (Halcion) or zolpidem (Ambien) (rapid acting, short half-life for sleep onset)
    Flurazepam (Dalmane) or quazepam (Doral) (longer acting for sleep maintenance)
    For sundowning: trazodone or zolpidem

REM with an abnormal multiple sleep latency test performed in a sleep laboratory. False-positive results occur in patients with depression, drug withdrawal, and sleep deprivation.

Treatment of narcolepsy should begin with one to three planned, 15- to 20-minute naps throughout the day. Pharmacologic therapy with stimulants (methylphenidate, 10 to 60 mg, or dextroamphetamine, 5 to 50 mg/day) rarely achieves complete relief of daytime sleepiness. Modafinil (an α-adrenergic agonist), 200 or 400 mg/day, was effective in one controlled trial. The imidazole derivative mazindol, the monoamine oxidase inhibitor selegiline, and pemoline (Cylert) are alternatives.

Cataplexy is eventually associated with narcolepsy in 70% of patients. The cataplectic phenomenon is that of emotion-induced, brief, reflex muscular atonia (partial or generalized), which spares respiratory muscles. Laughter is the most common inducer. Cataplectic attacks can be attenuated by tricyclic antidepressants such as clomipramine (10 to 150 mg/day).

REFERENCES

Hauri PJ: Insomnia. Clin Chest Med 1998; 19:157–168.
Nishino S, Mignot E: Pharmacological aspects of human and canine narcolepsy. Prog Neurobiol 1997; 52:27–28.
US Modafinil in Narcolepsy Multicenter Study Group: Randomized trial of modafinil for the treatment of pathological somnolence in narcolepsy. Ann Neurol 1998; 43:88–97.

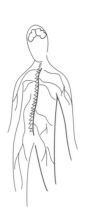

114

FOCAL BRAIN DISEASE

Timothy J. Counihan

Anatomy

The paired cerebral hemispheres are connected by a large band of white matter fibers, the *corpus callosum.* Each hemisphere comprises four anatomically and functionally distinct regions: frontal, temporal, parietal, and occipital lobes. The two cerebral hemispheres supplement each other functionally in a variety of behavioral and sensorimotor tasks; however, certain functions, particularly language, manual dexterity, and visuospatial perception, are strongly lateralized to one hemisphere. Language function, for instance, is lateralized to the left hemisphere in 95% of the population; although 15% of the population are left-handed, only a minority possess a right hemisphere that is dominant for language. Visuospatial functions are largely subserved by the right (nondominant) hemisphere.

The Rolandic fissure separates the motor cortex (precentral gyrus) from the sensory cortex (postcentral gyrus). In these regions, cortical representation of the different parts of the body are arranged as the motor (in the frontal lobe) and sensory (in the parietal lobe) homunculi.

Regional Syndromes

Because many neurologic disorders affect the cerebral hemispheres in a regionally specific or focal manner, a careful history and clinical examination that includes the Mini-Mental Status Examination (see Table 115–3) is helpful not only in localizing brain lesions but also in establishing the etiology. Tables 114–1 to 114–4 summarize some of the core clinical features involved with damage to individual hemispheres. The rate of onset of symptoms and the tempo of progression influence the extent of the clinical deficit. The homuncular arrangement of cortical motor and sensory representation may allow for more precise localization of a lesion (Fig. 114–1). For instance, motor or sensory signs confined to the

lower extremities may suggest a parasagittal lesion, whereas signs involving the face and upper limb may be found in laterally placed cortical lesions.

APHASIA

Aphasia or *dysphasia* refers to a loss or impairment of language function as a result of damage to the specific language centers of the dominant hemisphere. It is distinct from dysarthria, which is a disturbance in the articulation of speech. The principal types of aphasia are summarized in Table 114–5. A good bedside screening test for aphasia is to have the patient read and write a sentence; writing is almost invariably affected in patients with disturbances of language. An exception to this occurs in the syndrome of *alexia without agraphia;* this syndrome results from a vascular lesion of the dominant hemisphere's posterior cerebral artery, in which the patient's language center is "disconnected" from the contralateral (unaffected) visual cortex. Such patients can write a sentence but are unable to read what they have written. Clinical assessment for aphasia requires testing fluency, comprehension, repetition, naming, reading, calculation, and writing. *Anomia* (difficulty in recalling the names of objects) in isolation has little localizing value.

Broca's aphasia is characterized by a severe disruption in the fluency of speech, with profound impairments in expression both in speech and writing. Comprehension may be mildly affected. The language disturbance is almost invariably accompanied by contralateral face and arm weakness as a result of the proximity of the motor homunculus to Broca's speech area.

Wernicke's aphasia is characterized by an inability to comprehend spoken or written language. Affected patients speak fluently but the content is meaningless; they may use words that are close in meaning to the intended word (semantic paraphasias) or words that sound like the intended word (literal paraphasias). Some patients with Wernicke's aphasia have an associated contralateral homonymous hemianopia.

Conduction aphasia is characterized by an inability to repeat a spoken phase such as "no ifs, ands, or buts,"

TABLE 114-1 Frontal Lobe Syndromes

Symptoms	Site of Lesion
Contralateral spastic weakness	Primary motor/premotor cortex
Broca's aphasia	Dominant inferior frontal lobe
Forced eye deviation	Frontal eye fields
Executive dysfunction/poor sequencing	Dorsolateral prefrontal lobe
Akinetic mutism/urinary incontinence	Medial frontal cortex
Disinhibition/emotional lability	Orbitofrontal cortex

TABLE 114-2 Parietal Lobe Syndromes

Symptoms	Site of Lesion
Contralateral sensory loss	Postcentral gyrus
Contralateral sensory neglect	Postcentral gyrus (nondominant)
Wernicke's aphasia, apraxia	Inferior parietal/superior temporal cortex
Acalculia, finger agnosia, right-left confusion, agraphia (Gerstmann's syndrome)	Angular gyrus

TABLE 114-3 Syndromes of Temporal Lobe Lesions

Symptom	Lesion Site
Anomic/sensory aphasia	Lateral temporal lobe (dominant)
Contralateral superior quadratic anopsia	Superior lateral temporal lobe
Amnesia	Hippocampus
Oral-exploratory behavior, passivity, hypersexuality (Klüver-Bucy syndrome)	Amygdala (bilateral)
Visual delusions (déjà vu, jamais vu), olfactory hallucinations	Inferomedial temporal lobe

TABLE 114-4 Occipital Lobe Syndromes

Symptom	Lesion Site
Contralateral homonymous hemianopia	Striate cortex
Alexia without agraphia	Primary visual cortex (dominant) and splenium of corpus callosum
Visual agnosia, denial of blindness (Anton's syndrome), visual hallucinations	Medial occipital lobe
Optic apraxia, absent optokinetic nystagmus	Lateral (visual association) cortex

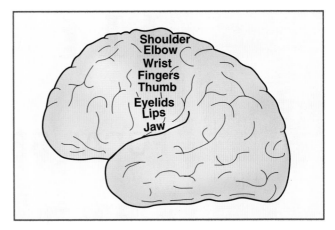

FIGURE 114-1   Diagrammatic representation of parts of the body in the primary motor area (MI) on the lateral aspect of the hemisphere in the human. Parts of the lower extremity are represented in sequential fashion in the anterior portion of the paracentral lobule on the medial aspect of the hemisphere. (From Carpenter MB: Core Text of Neuroanatomy, 4th ed. Baltimore: Williams & Wilkins, 1991, p 421.)

although they have normal comprehension. The responsible lesion lies in the arcuate fasciculus connecting Broca's and Wernicke's areas. *Global aphasia* results from large lesions of the frontal lobe, in which all aspects of language are affected.

In *dysarthria,* language function is intact (which can be confirmed by having the patient write a sentence), but patients are unable to articulate speech. Dysarthria results from either supranuclear, nuclear, or peripheral lesions of the lower cranial nerves or from lesions of the bulbar musculature or neuromuscular junction.

AGNOSIA AND APRAXIA

Agnosia is the inability to recognize a specific sensory stimulus despite preserved sensory function. For instance, visual agnosia is the inability to recognize a visual stimulus despite normal visual acuity. Similar syndromes include the inability to recognize sounds (auditory agnosia), color (color agnosia), and familiar faces (prosopagnosia). Usually the responsible lesions are located in the occipitotemporal region.

Apraxia refers to an inability to perform learned motor tasks despite sufficient memory and sensorimotor function to understand the command. The responsible lesions are usually in the dominant inferior parietal lobe. Lesions of the right parietal lobe often result in hemispatial neglect: the patient does not attend to stimuli in the left visual field or on the left side of the body. In a milder form of neglect, called *extinction,* patients can attend to stimuli contralateral to the side of the brain with the lesion (and the lesion is usually on the right side), but when presented with bilateral stimuli simultaneously, they respond only on the ipsilateral (right) side. Anosognosia, or the lack of awareness of one's deficit, frequently accompanies hemispatial neglect.

TABLE 114-5 Principal Types of Aphasia

Type	Lesion site	Fluency	Comprehension	Repetition	Naming	Other signs
Broca's	Inferior frontal lobe	↓	Good	↓	↓	Contralateral weakness
Wernicke's	Posterior superior temporal lobe	Good	↓	↓	↓	Homonymous hemi-anopia
Conduction	Supramarginal gyrus	Good	Good	↓	↓	None
Global	Frontal lobe (large)	↓	↓	↓	↓	Hemiplegia

AMNESIA

Memory and mechanisms for recall are located in the hippocampus of the temporal lobe. The common memory disorders are summarized in Table 114–6. Degeneration of the hippocampus or its connections results in the inability to form new memories and is a central accompaniment of Alzheimer's disease. Concussion injuries typically induce severe retrograde amnesia (the inability to recall events that occurred before the injury) and mild anterograde amnesia (the inability to recall events that occur after the injury).

Transient global amnesia typically affects persons older than 65 years and consists of abrupt onset of amnesia for time, place, and recent memory and lasts less than 12 hours. Patients are distressed and repeatedly require reorientation to their environment. They are, however, able to carry out complex, previously learned tasks such as driving. A number of precipitants have been identified, including extreme emotion, physical activity, sexual intercourse, and immersion in cold water. Recurrent episodes are rare. The condition is thought to be caused by transient focal hippocampal ischemia.

Korsakoff's syndrome is the end result of untreated or partially treated Wernicke's encephalopathy caused by thiamine deficiency. Affected patients (many of whom are alcoholic or malnourished) present with confusion, gait ataxia, nystagmus, and ophthalmoparesis. The condition may be precipitated by the administration of glucose unless thiamine is given in advance. If it is untreated, a profound inability to form new memories results, with devastating consequences for the patient. In the chronic phase, patients confabulate freely in an attempt to fill the memory void.

Psychogenic amnesia often affects long-term memory as well as recent memory, and patients are occasionally unable to recall their own names. This is in contrast to most organic amnestic states, in which only short-term memory is affected and disorientation is greatest for time and place, but never for self.

TABLE 114-6 Common Disorders of Memory

Benign forgetfulness of aging
Alzheimer's disease and other dementias
Head trauma
Transient global amnesia
Korsakoff's syndrome (thiamine deficiency)
Encephalitis (herpes simplex)
Stroke (posterior cerebral artery)
Temporal lobe seizures
Psychogenic disorders

REFERENCES

Brazis PW, Masdeu JC, Biller J: Localization in Clinical Neurology, 3rd ed. Boston: Little, Brown, 1996.
Cummings JL: Disorders of cognition. In Goldman L, Bennett JC (eds): Cecil Textbook of Medicine, 21st ed. Philadelphia, WB Saunders, 2000, pp 2033–2047.

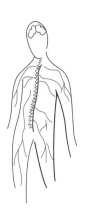

115

DEMENTIA AND MEMORY DISTURBANCES

Frederick J. Marshall

Major Dementia Syndromes

Dementia is defined as the progressive loss of intellectual function. Memory loss is the central feature, and specific dementia syndromes characteristically show particular forms of memory impairment. Dementia syndromes also produce specific abnormalities of cognition: language, spatial processing, *praxis* (learned motor behavior), and *executive function* (the ability to plan and sequence events). *Cortical dementia* and *subcortical dementia* subdivide the dementias (Table 115–1). Table 115–2 provides the differential diagnosis of dementia by underlying origin. Alzheimer's disease (AD), vascular dementia, frontotemporal dementia, and diffuse Lewy body disease are the most common. Most other causes of dementia are rare and untreatable. Treatable structural processes or infections must be considered. Correctable metabolic and nutritional diseases should be sought. Every patient with dementia should have tests of serum electrolytes, liver, renal, and thyroid function, vitamin B_{12} level, and serologic studies for syphilis. Chronic infections (see Chapter 127) and normal pressure hydrocephalus should be considered. Magnetic resonance imaging (MRI) of the brain should be performed in patients with focal signs noted on the neurologic examination and in patients less than 65 years old at the onset of dementia.

Neuropsychological testing characterizes the pattern of cognitive and memory impairments and is helpful in the differential diagnosis. The Mini-Mental Status Exam (Table 115–3) is a standard test that should be used as a bedside or office screening tool for identifying patients with dementia. This examination emphasizes memory and language and is better for detecting cortical rather than subcortical dementia. In addition to the Mini-Mental Status Exam, patients with dementia should have tests of visuospatial processing (clock drawing), praxis ("show how you would comb your hair," "show how you would blow out a match"), and planning and sequencing (draw a set of letters and numbers randomly on a page and have the patient connect them in alternating alphabetic and numeric order, i.e., 1-A, 2-B, 3-C, etc.).

ALZHEIMER'S DISEASE

AD accounts for about 70% of all cases of dementia in the elderly. Nearly 4 million persons in the United States are affected, and this number is likely to double by 2020 as the population ages. AD places enormous burdens on the patient, on the family, and on society; annual direct and indirect expenditures are estimated to exceed $100 billion. The incidence of AD increases with age, and the disease occurs in up to 30% of persons more than 85 years old.

AD has many causes, none fully defined. All causes, however, produce similar clinical and pathologic findings. Pathologically, the disease is characterized by the progressive loss of cortical neurons and the formation of amyloid plaques and intraneuronal neurofibrillary tangles. β-Amyloid ($A\beta$) is the major component of the plaques, whereas hyperphosphorylated tau protein is the major constituent of the neurofibrillary tangles. The process starts in the hippocampus and entorhinal cortex and spreads to involve diffuse areas of association cortex in the temporal, parietal, and frontal lobes. The relative deficiency of cortical acetylcholine (resulting from the loss of neurons in the nucleus basalis) provides the rationale for symptomatic treatment of the disease with centrally acting acetylcholinesterase inhibitors (see later discussion).

Pathogenesis

AD is often categorized into two forms: (1) a young-onset hereditary or familial form, which is extremely uncommon and for which three specific genetic abnormalities have been determined; and (2) a more common, sporadic form that typically occurs in persons more than 65 years old (Table 115–4).

TABLE 115-1 Distinguishing Characteristics of Cortical and Subcortical Dementia

Cortical Dementia

Symptoms: major changes in memory, language deficits, perceptual deficits, praxis disturbances

Affected brain regions: temporal cortex (medial), parietal cortex, and frontal lobe cortex

Examples: Alzheimer's disease, diffuse Lewy body disease, vascular dementia, frontotemporal dementias

Subcortical Dementia

Symptoms: behavioral changes, impaired affect and mood, motor slowing, executive dysfunction, less severe changes in memory

Affected brain regions: thalamus, striatum, midbrain, striatofrontal projections

Examples: Parkinson's disease, progressive supranuclear palsy, normal pressure hydrocephalus, Huntington's disease, Creutzfeldt-Jakob disease, chronic meningitis

The autosomal dominant early-onset forms of AD have provided clues to the molecular pathogenesis of sporadic AD. Progressive dementia and pathologic changes characteristic of AD are almost universal in patients with Down's syndrome (trisomy 21) who are more than 30 years old. This observation suggested that chromosome 21 harbors a gene responsible for AD. $A\beta$ is a cleavage product of the amyloid precursor protein, the gene for which is on chromosome 21. Abnormal processing of amyloid precursor protein into the amyloidogenic fragment, $A\beta_{42}$, may be important in the pathogenesis of AD. The *apolipoprotein E* (ApoE) gene was found to be a susceptibility locus for sporadic AD in late-onset familial AD pedigrees. The gene is polymorphic (ϵ2/3/4), and persons who inherit one or both ϵ4 alleles are at increased risk of developing AD. ApoE-ϵ4 interacts selectively with $A\beta$ and with τ, but how ApoE-ϵ4 increases the risk of AD is still unknown.

Clinical Features

AD begins gradually and affects multiple cognitive functions: memory, orientation, language, visuospatial processing, praxis, judgment, and insight. Depression is frequent early in AD; frank psychosis with agitation and behavioral disinhibition often occur in advanced stages. Patients become dependent on others for all activities of daily living. The rate of progression of AD is variable, usually taking 5 to 15 years to progress from presentation to advanced illness. Diagnostic criteria are outlined in Table 115-5. Although a definitive diagnosis of AD requires biopsy (rarely done) or autopsy confirmation, these diagnostic criteria establish the diagnosis with more than 85% specificity in moderately demented patients.

Treatment

Treatments for AD have been developed. Although their benefits are modest, the cholinesterase-inhibiting drugs tacrine (Cognex), and donepezil (Aricept), and rivastigmine (Exelon) represent important advances. Tacrine can be hepatotoxic and must be given four times a day; donepezil is given once a day and has fewer side effects. In clinical trials, cholinesterase inhibitors benefit fewer than 50% of patients.

Nursing services provide oversight of hygiene, nutri-

TABLE 115-2 Etiologic Diagnosis of Progressive Dementia in Adults

Neurodegenerative Diseases

Alzheimer's disease*
Parkinson's disease*
Diffuse Lewy body disease*
Progressive supranuclear palsy
Corticobasal-ganglionic degeneration
Multisystem atrophy
   Striatonigral degeneration
   Olivopontocerebellar degeneration
   Shy-Drager syndrome
Huntington's disease
Frontotemporal dementias
   Pick's disease
   Frontotemporal dementia without characteristic neuropathology
   Frontotemporal dementia with motor neuron disease
Hallervorden-Spatz disease

Structural Disease or Trauma

Normal pressure hydrocephalus†
Neoplasms†
Dementia pugilistica (multiple concussions in boxers)

Vascular Disease

Vascular dementia*
Vasculitis†

Heredometabolic Disease

Wilson's disease†
Neuronal-ceroid lipofucinosis (Kufs' disease)
Other late-onset lysosomal storage diseases

Demyelinating or dysmyelinating Disease

Multiple sclerosis*
Metachromatic leukodystrophy

Infectious Disease

Human immunodeficiency virus, type 1†
Tertiary syphilis†
Creutzfeldt-Jakob disease
Progressive multifocal leukoencephalopathy
Whipple's disease†
Chronic meningitis†
   Cryptococcal meningitis†
   Others

Metabolic or Nutritional Disease

Vitamin B$_{12}$ deficiency†
Thyroid hormone deficiency or excess†
Thiamine deficiency† (Wernicke-Korsakoff syndrome)
Alcoholism*

Psychiatric Disease

Pseudodementia from depression†

* Denotes those for which symptomatic treatment is available.
† Denotes those for which preventive or corrective treatment is available.

TABLE 115-3   Elements of the Mini-Mental Status Examination

Cognitive Domain	Items	Score
Attention/concentration	Spell "World" backward (or perform "serial 7's" subtraction)	5
Memory		
Orientation		
Temporal	Indicate year, season, month, day, date	5
Spatial	Indicate state, county, city, building, floor	5
Learning		
Immediate recall	Register three words ("apple, table, penny")	3
Delayed recall	Recall three words ("apple, table, penny")	3
Language		
Naming	Name two objects ("pen," "watch")	2
Repetition	Repeat phrase ("no ifs, ands, or buts")	1
Comprehension	Follow three-step verbal command	3
	Follow one-step written command	1
Writing	Write original sentence	1
Visuospatial processing	Copy intersecting pentagons	1
	Total Possible Score =	30

Based on Folstein M, Folstein S, McHugh P: "Mini-mental state"—a practical method for grading the cognitive state of patients for the clinician. J Psychiat Res 1975; 12:189–198.

tion, and medication compliance. Antipsychotics, antidepressants, and anxiolytics are useful for patients with behavioral disturbances, which are the most common cause of nursing home placement.

DIFFUSE LEWY BODY DISEASE

Lewy bodies are pathologic inclusions that are the hallmark of Parkinson's disease when they are restricted to the brain stem (see Chapter 121). Patients with *diffuse Lewy body disease* have clinical parkinsonism (slow movement, rigidity, balance problems) combined with early and prominent dementia. Pathologically, Lewy bodies are found in the brain stem, the limbic system, and the cortex. Visual hallucinations and cognitive fluctuations are common, and patients are sensitive to the adverse effects of neuroleptic medication. Diffuse Lewy body disease may represent the second most common cause of dementia after AD. However, the common concurrence of the pathologic features of diffuse Lewy body disease with the classic neuritic plaques and neu-

rofibrillary tangles of AD complicates the identification of the cause of dementia in a given patient.

VASCULAR DEMENTIA

Approximately 10% to 20% of elderly patients with dementia have radiographic evidence of focal stroke on MRI or computed tomography, combined with focal signs on the neurologic examination. When the dementia syndrome begins with the stroke, and the progression of the illness is step-wise (suggesting recurrent vascular events), the diagnosis of *vascular dementia* is likely. Patients typically develop early incontinence, gait disturbances, and flattening of affect. A subcortical dementing process attributed to small vessel disease in the periventricular white matter has been referred to as *Binswanger's disease,* but it may merely be a radiographic finding rather than a true disease. Appropriate treatment of risk factors for vascular disease is clearly mandatory and may be of benefit: blood pressure control, smoking ces-

TABLE 115-4   Familial Versus Sporadic Alzheimer's Disease

Chromosome/Gene	Age at Onset (yr)	% of All FAD*	% of All AD Cases
Familial Alzheimer's Disease: Early Onset, Autosomal Dominant			
1/Presenilin 2	40–80	5–10	<0.5
14/Presenilin 1	30–60	70	<1
21/Amyloid precursor protein	35–65	5	<0.5
Chromosome/Gene	**Age at Onset (yr)**		**% of All AD Cases**
Sporadic Alzheimer's Disease: Late Onset, ? Polygenetic ± ?Environmental			
No single determinant gene†	Usually >60		98

* FAD = familial Alzheimer's disease.
† Apolipoprotein E-ε4 allele on chromosome 19 yields increased risk compared with ε2 or ε3 allele.

TABLE 115-5 Diagnostic Criteria for Probable Alzheimer's Disease

Progressive functional decline and dementia established by clinical exam and mental status testing and confirmed by neuropsychological assessment

Cognitive deficits in two or more domains (including memory impairment)

Normal level of consciousness at presentation

Not developmentally acquired; onset between 40 and 90 yr

Absence of other illnesses capable of causing dementia

sation, diet modification, and anticoagulation (in selected settings such as atrial fibrillation).

FRONTOTEMPORAL DEMENTIAS

Unlike AD, in which the presenting symptom is typically memory loss, *frontotemporal dementia* often begins with marked behavioral disturbances. Patients with *Pick's disease,* the classic form of frontotemporal dementia, are frequently irascible and socially disinhibited. Like AD, the illness progresses for years; no intervention slows the inevitable decline of these patients. About 50% of patients have a family history of the disease; for some families, a mutation in the tau protein gene on chromosome 17 is the cause.

PARKINSON'S DISEASE

Nearly 50% of patients with *Parkinson's disease* (see Chapter 121) become demented by the time they reach the age of 85 years. The dementia of Parkinson's disease affects executive function out of proportion to its impact on language and visuospatial processing. Thought processes appear to slow down *(bradyphrenia),* analogous to the slowing of movement *(bradykinesia).* Because dementia occurs relatively late in the progression of Parkinson's disease, most patients are taking drugs to improve their movement disorder by enhancing dopaminergic neurotransmission. These drugs can induce psychosis. Dosage reductions should be attempted before one diagnoses underlying dementia in these patients.

NORMAL PRESSURE HYDROCEPHALUS

The triad of dementia (typically subcortical), gait instability, and urinary incontinence suggests *normal pressure hydrocephalus.* These patients walk with their "feet stuck to the floor," without lifting up the knees and with a broad base. Symptoms evolve over the course of weeks to months, and computed tomographic imaging reveals ventricular enlargement out of proportion to the amount of cortical atrophy. Numerous diagnostic tests have been described, including radionuclide cisternography and MRI flow studies. The most important test remains a therapeutic lumbar puncture with removal of a large amount of cerebrospinal fluid, followed by examination of the patient's gait and cognitive function. Neu-

rosurgical placement of a ventriculoperitoneal shunt may correct the problem. Patients likely to benefit from shunt placement have a clear response to the removal of 30 to 40 mL of spinal fluid, with improved gait and alertness within minutes to hours of the procedure. The cause of normal pressure hydrocephalus is a derangement of the cerebrospinal fluid hydrodynamics. Shunt placement is most likely to be effective if normal pressure hydrocephalus is secondary to trauma or subarachnoid hemorrhage.

SLOW VIRUS INFECTION/CHRONIC MENINGITIS/DEMENTIA RELATED TO ACQUIRED IMMUNODEFICIENCY SYNDROME

Creutzfeldt-Jakob (or Jakob-Creutzfeldt) disease is a subacute, dementing, transmissible illness with typical onset between 40 and 75 years of age and incidence of 1 in 1,000,000 (see Chapter 127). The disease causes spongiform degeneration and gliosis in widespread areas of the cortex. Clinical variants of the disorder are differentiated by the relative predominance of cerebellar symptoms, extrapyramidal hyperkinesias, or visual agnosia and cortical blindness *(Heidenhain's variant).* Ninety percent of patients with Creutzfeldt-Jakob disease have myoclonus, compared with 10% of patients with AD. Patients with all forms of the disease share a relentlessly progressive dementia and disruption of personality over weeks to months. The electroencephalogram develops characteristic abnormalities including diffuse slowing and periodic sharp waves or spikes. The transmissible agent, a prion protein, is invulnerable to routine modes of antisepsis. A laboratory test for a characteristic amino acid sequence has been developed, and it is now possible to make the diagnosis by testing cerebrospinal fluid in specialty laboratories (see Chapter 127).

Certain *infectious agents* can cause the subacute to chronic development of subcortical dementia. These chronic meningitides are discussed in Chapter 127.

Human immunodeficiency virus (HIV) accesses the central nervous system through monocytes and the microglial system and causes associated neuronal cell loss, vacuolization, and lymphocytic infiltration. The dementia associated with this infection is characterized by bradyphrenia and bradykinesia. Patients have executive dysfunction, impaired memory, poor concentration, and apathy. Treatment of the underlying viral infection with protease inhibitors and reverse transcriptase inhibitors may slow the progression of the dementia (see Chapter 127).

Other Memory Disturbances

STRUCTURE OF MEMORY

Memory function is divided into introspective processes (declarative, explicit, aware memories) and those that are not accessible to introspection (nondeclarative, implicit, procedural memories). Short-term memory (e.g., for words on a list) is a form of *declarative memory.* Other forms include the conscious recall of episodes from our personal experience *(episodic memory)*, factual knowledge *(semantic memory)* that can be consciously recalled and stated (declared), and the ability to remember to remember *(prospective memory)*. Thus, declarative memories involve consciously "knowing that. . . ." Patients with amnesia resulting from lesions of the medial temporal lobes or midline diencephalic structures have deficits of declarative memory.

Nondeclarative memory encompasses several distinct and neuroanatomically less clearly localized functions related to the performance of specific learned motor, cognitive, or perceptual tasks. Nondeclarative (procedural) memories involve unconsciously "knowing how. . . ." Deficits in nondeclarative memory may involve various areas of association neocortex, depending on the nature of the task (e.g., parieto-occipital cortex for visual perceptual tasks, frontal association cortex for motor tasks). Patients with amnesia resulting from lesions of the medial temporal lobes tend to perform normally on tests of nondeclarative memory.

Anterograde amnesia refers to the inability to learn new information. It commonly occurs after brain injury or in association with dementia. The inability to recollect prior information is known as *retrograde amnesia.* Both types of amnesia usually occur together in brain injury syndromes, although the extent of one type or the other may vary.

ISOLATED DISORDERS OF MEMORY FUNCTION

Memory can be impaired in relative isolation as a consequence of head injury, thiamine deficiency (Korsakoff's syndrome), benign forgetfulness of aging, transient global amnesia, or psychogenic disease.

Head injury typically results in retrograde amnesia in excess of anterograde amnesia, with both forms stretching out in time away from the discrete event. As time passes, these disrupted memories generally gradually return, although rarely to the point at which the events immediately surrounding the trauma are recalled.

Korsakoff's syndrome is characterized by the near-total inability to establish new memory. Patients often confabulate responses when they are asked to convey the details of their current circumstance or to relay the content of a recently presented story. Deficiency of thiamine and other nutritional deficiencies in the context of chronic alcoholism are the most common underlying causes. Thiamine is a necessary cofactor in the metabo-

lism of glucose, and for this reason thiamine must be replenished at the same time glucose is administered whenever a comatose patient presents to the emergency room.

Aging is associated with mild loss of memory, manifested by difficulty in recalling names and forgetfulness for dates. Population-based assessments of neuropsychological function have demonstrated that poor performance on delayed-recall tasks is the most sensitive indicator of cognitive change with advancing age. Verbal fluency, on the other hand, remains intact with advancing age, and vocabulary may increase with time, even into old age.

Transient global amnesia is a dramatic memory disturbance that affects older patients (>50 years). Patients usually have only one episode; occasionally, episodes recur over the course of several years. Patients have complete temporal and spatial disorientation; orientation for person is preserved. Near-total retrograde and anterograde amnesia persists for variable periods, typically 6 to 12 hours. Patients are often anxious and may repeat the same question over and over again. Transient global amnesia may be confused with psychogenic amnesia, fugue state, or partial complex status epilepticus. Transient global amnesia is thought to reflect underlying vascular insufficiency to the hippocampus or midline thalamic projections.

Unlike patients with organic memory disturbances, patients with *psychogenic amnesia* typically have inconsistent loss of recent and remote memory, relatively more loss of emotionally charged memory (rather than relatively less loss of such memory in organic disease), and an apparent indifference to their own plight: they ask few questions. Most characteristically, patients with psychogenic amnesia tend to express disorientation to person (asking "Who am I?"), a phenomenon seldom seen in organic memory disturbance.

Patients with *severe depression* may present with *pseudodementia.* Vegetative signs including changes in appetite, weight, and sleep pattern are common, whereas signs of cortical impairment such as aphasia, agnosia, and apraxia are rare. Memory and bradyphrenia improve with antidepressant therapy.

REFERENCES

Growden JH, Rossor MN (eds): The Dementias. Boston: Butterworth Heinemann, 1998.

Mendez MF, Cummings JL: Amnesia and aphasia. *In* Goldman L, Bennett JC (eds): Cecil Textbook of Medicine, 21st ed. Philadelphia: WB Saunders, 2000, pp 2038–2042.

Troster AI (ed): Memory in Neurodegenerative Disease: Biological, Cognitive, and Clinical Perspectives. Cambridge, UK: Cambridge University Press, 1998.

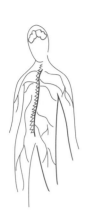

116

DISORDERS OF MOOD AND BEHAVIOR

Frederick J. Marshall

The major disorders of mood and behavior are outlined in Tables 116–1 to 116–3, adapted from the fourth edition of the *Diagnostic and Statistical Manual of Mental Disorders* (DSM-IV). DSM-IV uses a multiaxial classification system for psychiatric illness, medical illness, personality structure, and social and environmental factors. This approach provides an integrated picture of the impediments to an individual's functional adaptation. Table 116–4 outlines the multiaxial diagnostic approach of DSM-IV.

Psychotic Disorders

Psychosis is a disordered pattern of thought, perception, emotion, and behavior. The psychotic person has a bizarre sense of reality, with emotional and cognitive impairment leading to loss of function in the environment. Some primary features of psychosis are outlined in Table 116–5. Psychotic disorders may be *functional* (without known biologic cause) or *organic* (resulting from medical or neurologic illness). Drug intoxication and withdrawal may cause psychosis. Clues to the possible organic basis of psychosis include the following: significant memory loss, clouding of consciousness, absence of a family or personal history of psychiatric illness, presence of a serious underlying medical or neurologic condition, acute onset of symptoms, visual more often than auditory hallucinations, and presence of myoclonus or asterixis.

Schizophrenia, the most common form of psychosis, affects 1% to 2% of people worldwide. The illness places an enormous burden on individuals, families, and society, leads to pervasive dysfunction, and causes downward social mobility. Schizophrenia is more prevalent among those in the lower socioeconomic strata. Between psychotic episodes, patients show social withdrawal, odd manners, flat or inappropriate affect, and eccentric thinking. Patients may be diagnosed with a personality disorder (schizoid, borderline, schizotypal, antisocial) before their first acute psychotic episode, which typically occurs between the ages of 15 and 35 years.

Although schizophrenia has a strong genetic component, the disease has no established origin. The risk of developing schizophrenia is 10% to 15% if one parent is affected and 30% to 40% if both parents are affected. Earlier theories about "schizophrenogenic" parenting styles are poorly supported. Abnormal family dynamics may be the result of (rather than the cause of) a child with schizophrenia.

Schizophrenia is a chronic disorder for which no cure exists. *Positive symptoms* include delusions and hallucinations; *negative symptoms* include emotional withdrawal and apathy. Psychotropic medications are useful to control positive symptoms, but they offer little benefit for negative symptoms.

Evidence for the dopamine hypothesis of schizophrenia (an imbalance of central dopaminergic neurotransmission) includes the following: the antipsychotic activity of dopamine receptor–blocking neuroleptic medications, the propsychotic activity of levodopa in patients with Parkinson's disease, and the propsychotic activity of amphetamines known to cause the central release of dopamine.

Antipsychotic agents are the mainstay of drug treatment during acute psychotic episodes and should usually be continued during periods of relative remission. These medications may cause drug-induced movement disorders and blunting of affect as well as other side effects. Many patients and unwary physicians discontinue medications during times of relative remission. This practice generally hastens the return of active psychosis; long-acting depot formulations may be used to ensure compliance. Newer generations of atypical antipsychotic agents have fewer side effects; they may also prove useful in the management of formerly intractable negative symptoms.

The other psychiatric disorders characterized by psy-

TABLE 116–1   Major Disorders of Mood and Behavior

Psychotic Disorders
Schizophrenia
Schizophreniform disorder
Schizoaffective disorder
Mood disorder with psychotic features
Delusional disorder
Mood Disorders
Major depressive disorder
Dysthymic disorder
Bipolar disorder
Cyclothymic disorder
Anxiety Disorders
Panic disorder
Phobic disorder
Obsessive-compulsive disorder
Post-traumatic stress disorder
Generalized anxiety disorder
Somatoform Disorders
Somatization disorder
Conversion disorder
Pain disorder
Hypochondriasis
Body dysmorphic disorder
Factitious Disorder
Dissociative Disorders
Dissociative amnesia
Dissociative fugue
Dissociative identity disorder
Depersonalization disorder

Adapted with permission from the Diagnostic and Statistical Manual of Mental Disorders, 4th ed. Copyright 1994, American Psychiatric Association.

TABLE 116–2   Personality Disorders

Paranoid
Schizoid
Schizotypal
Antisocial
Borderline
Histrionic
Narcissistic
Avoidant
Dependent
Obsessive-compulsive

Adapted with permission from the Diagnostic and Statistical Manual of Mental Disorders, 4th ed. Copyright 1994, American Psychiatric Association.

Depression and Bipolar Disorder

Disorders of mood include *depression* and *mania*. Classification is based on severity, underlying cause, and whether depression and mania occur together or in isolation. Mood disorders affect up to 30% of the US population. Certain medical conditions are strongly associated with depression: carcinoma of the pancreas, lung cancer, brain tumors (particularly those affecting the frontal lobes), Cushing's disease (and exogenous steroid use), hypothyroidism, aftermath of myocardial infarction, Parkinson's disease, stroke, and Huntington's disease. Table 116–6 outlines important features of depression, and Table 116–7 outlines features of mania.

Depression occurs when sadness or grief lasts longer than usual and causes dysfunction. *Dysthymia* is prolonged but minor depression. *Cyclothymia* is minor depression alternating with hypomania. *Major depression* causes severe and chronic depressive symptoms with vegetative signs (sleep disturbance, change of appetite or weight, loss of libido). Patients vary widely in the duration and pattern of recurrence of these signs and symptoms. Patients may have associated psychotic thought content, generally of self-blame or persecution. Memory may be severely impaired; the distinction between depression and dementia is particularly challenging in elderly patients, in whom both conditions often coexist. Major depression is more common in women. Most young people with one attack of major depression will have another during their lifetime. Approximately 10% develop lifelong dysthymia. An episode of major depression comes on gradually over the course of months and may last up to 3 years or more.

chosis and listed in Table 116–1 differ from schizophrenia in several important respects. *Schizophreniform disorder* is characterized by a more rapid onset and remission of symptoms, by better premorbid adjustment and subsequent functioning, and by a negative family history. *Schizoaffective disorder* is an overlap syndrome of schizophrenia and major affective disorder with depressed mood. Prognosis is worse than in those with pure affective illness. Patients with *delusional disorder* have isolated delusions (generally of persecution, grandeur, or a spouse's infidelity), without other positive or negative symptoms of schizophrenia.

TABLE 116–3   Substance-Related Disorders

Substance	Symptoms
Sedatives: alcohol, barbiturates, benzodiazepines	Acute lethargy, stupor, coma, aware memory loss, apathy
Hallucinogens: cannabis, opioids, mescaline, phencyclidine	Hallucinations
Stimulants: amphetamine, caffeine, cocaine	Agitation, paranoia

TABLE 116-4   Multiaxial Approach to Diagnosis

Axis I	Clinical psychiatric disorders
Axis II	Personality disorders/mental retardation
Axis III	General medical conditions
Axis IV	Psychosocial and environmental problems
Axis V	Global assessment of functioning

Adapted with permission from the Diagnostic and Statistical Manual of Mental Disorders, 4th ed. Copyright 1994, American Psychiatric Association.

Abnormalities of the neurotransmitters norepinephrine and serotonin play a major role in mood disorders: their levels or effects are underactive in depression and are overactive in mania. Treatments that affect these neurotransmitters include tricyclic antidepressants, monoamine oxidase inhibitors, and selective serotonin

TABLE 116-5   Common Features of Psychosis

Disruption of the Form and Flow of Thought and Speech

Flight of ideas (disconnected ideas, incoherent speech, loose associations)
Pressured speech (rapid and unrelenting speech)
Thought blocking (speech halted for variable intervals)
Clanging (rhyming speech without meaningful content)
Echolalia (sing-song repetition of recently heard words or phrases)
Neologisms (idiosyncratic or newly coined words)
Alogia (paucity of speech, mutism)

Disruption of the Content of Thought and Perception

Delusions (false beliefs about reality that are not amenable to revision by fact)
    Persecutory delusions (others intend one harm)
    Delusions of grandeur (one is famous or all powerful)
    Delusions of reference (events or others' actions are directed at one)
    Thought broadcasting (one's thoughts can be sensed by others)
    Thought insertion (others' thoughts are invading one's mind)
    Loss of insight (unawareness of one's illness)
Hallucinations (typically auditory > visual in schizophrenia, visual > auditory in organic psychoses)

Disruption of Emotions

Blunting of affect
Inappropriate affect
Labile affect

Disruption of Behavior

Ritual behavior
Aggressiveness
Sexual inappropriateness
Posturing or grimacing
Mimicking
Withdrawal

Adapted with permission from Tomb DA: Psychiatry, 5th ed. Copyright 1995, Williams & Wilkins.

TABLE 116-6   Clinical Features of Depression

Emotional Content

Interpersonal withdrawal
Anhedonia
Sadness
Irritability
Anxiety

Thought Content

Guilt
Self-criticism, worthlessness
Pessimism, hopelessness
Distractibility
Indecision
Delusions and hallucinations
Memory complaints

Physical Content ("Vegetative Features")

Fatigue
Insomnia
Hypersomnia
Anorexia
Overeating
Weight loss
Weight gain
Poor libido
Somatic complaints
Psychomotor retardation
Psychomotor agitation

Adapted with permission from Tomb DA: Psychiatry, 5th ed. Copyright 1995, Williams & Wilkins.

reuptake inhibitors (SSRIs). All patients with major depression and most patients with chronic minor depressions merit a trial of antidepressant medication (typically starting with an SSRI or tricyclic antidepressant). Adequate trials require increasing doses over the course of

TABLE 116-7   Clinical Features of Mania

Emotional Content

Euphoria
Emotional lability
Irritability

Thought Content

Egocentric
Grandiose
Poor judgment
Pressured speech
Delusions
Hallucinations

Physical Content

Insomnia
Hyperarousal
Loss of appetite
Psychomotor agitation

Adapted with permission from Tomb DA: Psychiatry, 5th ed. Copyright 1995, Williams & Wilkins.

4 to 6 weeks. Therapeutic counseling should also be offered. Electroconvulsive therapy is useful in patients with refractory depression, acute suicidality, or concomitant psychosis unresponsive to antipsychotic drugs.

Bipolar disorder shows 70% concordance in monozygotic twins. Men and women are equally at risk. First-degree relatives have a 5% to 10% lifetime risk (compared with 1% to 2% in the general population). More than 90% of patients have periods of depression. Attacks of mania and depression are usually separated by years, but some patients have *rapid cycling* (four or more episodes per year). Rapid cycling is more common in women. Lithium, carbamazepine, and valproate are used alone or in combination with antidepressants to prevent recurrence of symptoms. Acute mania may require treatment with neuroleptic agents.

Anxiety Disorders

Common clinical features of anxiety disorders are outlined in Table 116–8. *Chronic generalized anxiety* is a familial trait, with depression developing in up to half of all patients at some point in life. Treatment is challenging. Benzodiazepines provide short-term benefit, but they are associated with a risk of long-term addiction. Buspirone (Buspar) and tricyclic antidepressants are useful, especially in patients with concomitant depression.

Panic disorder involves episodic, acute-onset, overwhelming anxiety, accompanied by autonomic symptoms (palpitations, sweating) and a feeling of impending doom. Medical conditions that may present with panic are outlined in Table 116–9.

Phobic disorders involve irrational fear of specific objects or events. The fear may be overwhelming and may result in reclusive, eccentric behavior. *Agoraphobia,* the fear of being in public situations from which escape may be difficult (typically new situations or wide-open

TABLE 116–8 Clinical Features of Anxiety

Emotional Content
Tension
Irritability
Apprehension
Fear
Thought Content
Obsessions
Ruminations
Distractibility
Physical Content
Psychomotor agitation
Insomnia
Loss of appetite
Loss of libido
Palpitations
Diarrhea
Sweating
Urinary frequency

TABLE 116–9 Medical Illnesses That Can Present with Anxiety

Neurologic
Encephalitis
Meniere's disease
Cardiac
Angina
Mitral valve prolapse
Pulmonary
Chronic obstructive pulmonary disease
Asthma
Metabolic or Endocrine
Acute intermittent porphyria
Hyperthyroidism
Hypoglycemia
Pheochromocytoma
Carcinoid tumor
Gastrointestinal
Bleeding ulcer
Ulcerative colitis

Adapted with permission from Tomb DA: Psychiatry, 5th ed. Copyright 1995, Williams & Wilkins.

spaces), is named for the ancient Greek open market-place *(agora).* This is a common phobia in elderly patients or in those with chronic medical illness. It can occur with or without associated panic attacks. *Specific phobias* (formerly known as simple phobias) include discrete, irrational fears of specific objects or situations. Common specific phobias include fear of flying, fear of enclosed spaces, and fear of snakes. Treatment of the phobic disorders often involves desensitization with behavioral therapy.

Obsessive-compulsive disorder has a strong genetic component, but its underlying origin remains unknown. *Obsessions* are recurrent unwanted thoughts (e.g., self-deprecatory preoccupations or fears of contamination); *compulsions* are repetitive unwanted *(ego-dystonic)* behaviors (e.g., hand washing, double-checking whether appliances have been turned off). Treatment with SSRIs may alleviate symptoms in some patients.

Somatoform Disorders

The somatoform disorders involve psychological preoccupation with physical symptoms. Patients with *somatization disorder* have numerous physical symptoms involving several organ systems. Symptoms tend to be migratory (both in time and space) and are presented with dramatic flair. The patient insists on complete medical attention. Symptoms include ill-defined pains, pseudoneurologic symptoms (often poorly described alterations of consciousness), and gastrointestinal, genitourinary, and sexual dysfunction. The disorder is more common in women and is frequently associated with

TABLE 116–10 **Clues to the Nonorganic Basis of Common Conversion Symptoms**

Pseudoseizures

These episodes are often bizarre, without associated loss of bladder continence or self-injury (tongue biting, lacerations). Patients with pseudoseizures commonly also suffer from true epileptic seizures.

Pseudocoma

The coma is light, with responsiveness to noxious stimulation and subtle avoidance of physical threat (e.g., arm suspended above face and dropped does not strike face, patient shifts to avoid falling from table).

Pseudoparalysis

Weakness is variable, with little resistance to passive movement but intact resistance to gravity. Contraction of antagonist muscles is inappropriate when the patient is asked to engage agonist muscles.

Pseudosensory Loss

This may include blindness, deafness, or anesthesia. Blindness may be total, but is commonly tunnel loss. If the examiner defines the perimeter of the tunnel by drawing it on a target paper held close to the patient, the tunnel remains the same size when the examiner subsequently steps back (this does not obey fundamental rules of optics). Sensory loss may not respect the midline, or may deviate from known anatomic distributions of roots and nerves.

Pseudoataxia

The patient may have swooping dives and thrusts, sustained monopedal postures, and clutching to surfaces. The patient rarely falls. This style of gait is also known as *astasia-abasia* or *stasibasiphobia.*

concomitant psychiatric illness, including depression, unsuccessful suicide attempts, anxiety, and irritability.

Conversion disorder involves an obvious loss of neurologic function in the absence of organic neurologic disease. Patients do not consciously realize the nonorganic basis of the illness, yet they frequently demonstrate lack of concern for the deficit *(la belle indifférence).* Clues to the nonorganic nature of common conversion symptoms are outlined in Table 116–10. Patients often have an antecedent psychosocial stressor, as well as unconscious secondary gain (e.g., extra attention from the spouse, relief from onerous work obligations).

Factitious Disorder

Patients with *factitious disorder* intentionally feign physical or psychological symptoms to assume the sick role. Once the condition is diagnosed, patients may disappear, only to present their symptoms to another physician. Patients may change their symptoms once the initial complaints have been thoroughly evaluated. Patients with *Munchausen's syndrome* inflict real physical harm

on themselves (e.g., ingesting anticoagulants to cause hematuria, injecting contaminated fluids to cause abscesses or fever). Rarely, a parent may provoke symptoms in a child; such *Munchausen's syndrome by proxy* can lead to recurrent unexplained pediatric sickness and should raise the physician's suspicion under appropriate circumstances.

In *malingering,* a person consciously feigns disease for concrete personal goals, rather than for psychological goals. The malingerer may intentionally feign disease or may provoke real (although usually not life-threatening) illness to avoid some unwanted outcome (e.g., military service).

Dissociative Disorders

Dissociative disorders disrupt the coherent sense of self, and several variants are recognized. In *dissociative amnesia,* patients are unable to recall traumatic personal events, despite intact cognition and memory in other domains. *Dissociative fugue* involves acting in complex ways, such as traveling away from home, without having personal memory of the events or of details of one's past. *Dissociative identity disorder* (also known as *multiple personality disorder*) involves switching from one internally coherent personality to another; sometimes several distinct personalities are involved. Patients fail to recall important elements of personal history, and transitions among identities are triggered by stress. In *depersonalization disorder,* patients have persistent or recurrent episodes of feeling outside one's body or of dispassionately observing one's mental processes. The differential diagnosis of the dissociative disorders includes complex partial seizures, factitious disorder, malingering, and psychosis.

Personality Disorders and Substance Abuse

The major personality disorders are listed in Table 116–2. These disorders are generalized styles of behavior that persevere over time and interfere with a person's social functioning. Common classes of abused substances are listed in Table 116–3, along with symptoms of intoxication or addiction.

REFERENCES

American Psychiatric Association: Diagnostic and Statistical Manual of Mental Disorders, 4th ed. Washington, DC: American Psychiatric Association, 1994.
Diamond I, Jay CA: Alcoholism and alcohol abuse. *In* Goldman L, Bennett JC (eds): Cecil Textbook of Medicine, 21st ed. Philadelphia: WB Saunders, 2000, pp 49–54.
Samet JH: Drug abuse and dependence. *In* Goldman L, Bennett JC (eds): Cecil Textbook of Medicine, 21st ed. Philadelphia: WB Saunders, 2000, pp 54–59.
Schiffer RB: Psychiatric disorders in medical practice. *In* Goldman L, Bennett JC (eds): Cecil Textbook of Medicine, 21st ed. Philadelphia: WB Saunders, 2000, pp 2047–2056.
Tomb DA: Psychiatry, 5th ed. Baltimore: Williams & Wilkins, 1995.

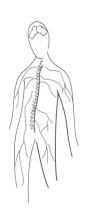

117

DISORDERS OF THERMAL REGULATION

Roger P. Simon

Hypothermia

Hypothermia (core body temperature <35°C [95°F]) may result from disorders that depress the sensorium directly (drug overdose and alcohol abuse), from disorders that affect the anterior hypothalamus directly (Wernicke's encephalopathy and hypoglycemia), or from environmental cold exposure (Table 117–1). Alcohol predisposes to hypothermia by inducing vasodilation and attenuating peripheral vasoconstriction; neuroleptic drugs vasodilate and suppress shivering as well. Because the body's ability to vasoconstrict and shiver diminishes with age, the elderly are at greatest risk.

In mild or early hypothermia, shivering appears and muscle tone increases, coordination is poor, speech becomes slurred, and judgment is impaired; in severe cases, the patient may be presumed dead because of barely detectable pulse or respiration and unmeasurable blood pressure. Patients' bodies are cold to the touch. Mental function remains normal to 34°C (93°F). The neurologic signs and vital sign changes are presented in Table 117–2. Major deviations from the features outlined in Table 117–2 should prompt a search for factors other than hypothermia that are responsible for nervous system dysfunction.

Physiologic responses to hypothermia are noted in Table 117–2. They reflect three responses to progressive temperature reduction:

1. Shivering, which doubles or triples muscle heat output above 30°C to 32°C.
2. Decreasing metabolism (blood pressure, pulse, respiration) at 32°C to 28°C.
3. Poikilothermia below 28°C. The electroencephalogram shows diffuse slowing and is isoelectric below 20°C.

The severity of the underlying disease, not the features of the neurologic examination or the degree of hypothermia, predicts survival. The neurologic abnor-

malities are fully reversible with rewarming. Hypothyroidism causing hypothermia is an exception, because the degree of thyroid dysfunction is related to outcome.

Treatment begins with passive external rewarming, suitable for mild hypothermia. For more severe hypothermia, active external and core rewarming may be required. A number of methods such as heating lamps, hot tubs, warm fluid lavage of body cavities, or cardiopulmonary bypass have been recommended. Warmed (42°C to 45°C), humidified inhaled oxygen should be part of any regimen. All hypothermic patients are hypovolemic and require intravenous fluids.

Hyperthermia

Hyperthermia (core body temperature >41°C [105.8°F]) results from environmental heat exposure with or without exertion (heat stroke, heat exhaustion), from anesthesia (malignant hyperthermia) in those with an inherited defect of calcium transport in skeletal muscle, or as

TABLE 117–1   Causes of Hypothermia*

Alcohol abuse	43%
Wernicke's encephalopathy	18%
Age >70	26%
Sepsis or shock	25%
Exposure without other causes	14%
Hypoglycemia	12%
Sedative overdose	10%
Hepatic encephalopathy, uremia	8%
Structural brain disorder, head trauma, hypothyroidism, diabetic ketoacidosis, renal failure, ethylene glycol poisoning	5% or less

*N = 148; more than one factor occurred in 35 patients.
From Fischbeck KH, Simon RP: Neurological manifestations of accidental hypothermia. Ann Neurol 1981; 10:384–387.

906

TABLE 117-2 Effects of Hypothermia*

	Mild (90°F-95°F; 32°C-35°C)	Moderate (82°F-90°F; 28°C-32°C)	Severe (<82°F; <28°C)
Blood pressure and pulse	Normal	Normal to decreased; atrial fibrillation frequent	Decreased; ventricular fibrillation may occur
Respiration	Normal	Normal	Normal to decreased
Level of consciousness	Alert or lethargic	Lethargic	Nonverbal but purposively responsive
Pupils	Normal	Normal to sluggish	Sluggish to fixed
Tendon reflexes	Normal	Normal	Normal to decreased
Muscle tone	Normal or increased	Increased	Increased
Eye movements, posturing, plantar reflexes	No correlation with temperature		

*N = 97.

Data from Fischbeck KH, Simon RP: Neurological manifestations of accidental hypothermia. Ann Neurol 1981; 10:384–387.

an idiosyncratic reaction to neuroleptics involving blockade of central dopamine receptors (neuroleptic malignant syndrome). The features of these three forms of hyperthermia are compared in Table 117–3.

Heat stroke occurs in young persons who overexert themselves in a hot, humid climate (e.g., military recruits) and the elderly, who cannot dissipate heat generated at rest (sometimes as a result of drugs with anticholinergic properties, such as tricyclic antidepressants and antihistamines; phenothiazine, butyrophenone, and thioxanthene use also predisposes). In its most severe form (heat stroke), core temperature rises very rapidly to 40.4°C (105°F) or greater. Altered consciousness ranges from confusion to coma. Patients may, but more often do not, sweat. Tachycardia is universal. More protracted symptoms of dizziness, fatigue, and weakness developing over a few days constitute heat exhaustion. Rapid reduction in body temperature is mandatory.

Evaporative cooling (water spray plus fans) to reduce temperatures to 38.0°C to 38.8°C is effective; antipyretics and dantrolene are not.

Hyperthermia and diffuse muscle rigidity (*malignant hyperthermia*) occur most often with the use of halothane and succinylcholine. Rigidity of limb, chest, or jaw muscles occurs within 30 minutes of anesthesia. Treatment is drug discontinuation and dantrolene (1 to 10 mg/kg IV until muscular relaxation occurs, followed by 4 to 8 mg/kg every 6 hours for 24 to 48 hours).

The *neuroleptic malignant syndrome* causes hyperthermia, rigidity, and altered mental status; rhabdomyolysis is frequent. Haloperidol is responsible in most cases, but other neuroleptic drugs and withdrawal from levodopa have been implicated. Symptoms begin within 1 to 3 days of drug initiation or dose change. All patients have elevated temperatures (average, 39.9°C). Dysphagia, dysarthria, tremors, and altered mental

TABLE 117-3 Comparative Features of Neuroleptic Malignant Syndrome (NMS), Malignant Hyperthermia, and Heat Stroke

	NMS	Malignant Hyperthermia	Heat Stroke
Hyperthermia	+	+	+
Muscle rigidity	+	+	Rare
Sweating	+	+	Rare
Tachycardia	+	+	+
Acidosis	+	+	+
Coagulopathy	+	+	+
Myoglobinuria	+	+	+
Impaired mental status	+	+	+
Genetic predisposition	−	+	−
Precipitant	Neuroleptics	Halothane, succinylcholine	Heat exposure, exercise
Onset	Hours–days	Minutes–hours	Minutes–hours
Treatment	Dantrolene, dopa agonists	Dantrolene	Rapid external cooling

Modified from Lazarus A, Mann SC, Caroff SN: The Neuroleptic Malignant Syndrome and Related Conditions. Washington, DC: American Psychiatric Press, 1989.

status (agitation to coma) occur early. Treatment is with dantrolene (as discussed earlier) and dopa agonists (bromocriptine, 2.5–10 mg three time daily).

Experimental studies show that elevation of body temperature to 42°C causes a rise in cerebral oxygen consumption, but there is a subsequent fall at higher temperatures. The electroencephalogram slows above 42°C. Neurologic abnormalities resolve with temperature reduction except for a persistent neuropathy in one third of patients. Mortality rises with temperature extremes, but the underlying cause is a better predictor of outcome than the degree of hyperthermia. Temperatures up to 42°C are usually tolerated.

REFERENCES

Danzl DF, Pozos RS: Accidental hypothermia. N Engl J Med 1994; 331:1756–1760.

Simon HB: Hyperthermia. N Engl J Med 1993; 329:483–487.

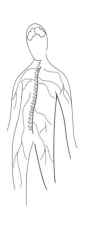

118

HEADACHE, NECK PAIN, AND OTHER PAINFUL DISORDERS

Timothy J. Counihan

Headache

PAIN-SENSITIVE STRUCTURES

Headache is caused by irritation of pain-sensitive intracranial structures; the dural sinuses; the intracranial portions of the trigeminal, glossopharyngeal, vagus, and upper cervical nerves; the large arteries; and the venous sinuses. Many structures are insensitive to pain, including the brain parenchyma, the ependymal lining of the ventricles, and the choroid plexuses. There are also nociceptive nerve endings on many extracranial structures (e.g., muscles, tendons, joints, skin) that when stimulated can produce pain referred to various regions of the head. Nociceptive impulses from these structures probably pass into midbrain serotoninergic centers before being relayed to the cerebral hemispheres where pain is consciously "perceived." Painful stimuli arising from brain tissue above the tentorium are conveyed by means of the trigeminal nerve, whereas the glossopharyngeal, vagus, and first two cervical nerves convey impulses from the posterior fossa.

EVALUATION OF THE PATIENT WITH HEADACHE

It is important to distinguish benign from ominous causes. A detailed history helps decide which patients have a major intracranial lesion. Ask about the quality, location, duration, and time course of the headache. What exacerbates or relieves it? Pain intensity is not of much diagnostic value, except for the patient who complains of the acute onset of the worst headache of his or her life. This headache suggests subarachnoid hemorrhage. The quality of pain ("throbbing," "pressure," "jabbing") and the location may also be helpful, especially if the pain is of extracranial origin such as the temporal

location of temporal arteritis. Posterior fossa lesions cause occipitocervical pain, occasionally associated with unilateral retro-orbital pain. In general, multifocal pain usually implies a benign etiology. Patients should be asked about any known triggers for the headache, such as menses, particular foods, caffeine, alcohol, or stress. Diurnal variation in headache severity may give a clue to etiology; morning headache or headache that awakens a patient from sleep may indicate raised intracranial pressure or sleep apnea as a cause. The presence of associated symptoms such as visual disturbances, nausea, or vomiting should be noted. The history should include inquiries about medications, especially use of analgesics and over-the-counter remedies. Information regarding the patient's past medical history as well as family history should also be taken into consideration. In the majority of patients with headache, the physical and neurologic examination is normal, although special attention may be directed toward examination of the eyes for papilledema.

HEADACHE SYNDROMES

Migraine

Clinical Features. Migraine is an episodic headache disorder characterized by various combinations of neurologic, gastrointestinal, and autonomic changes. The diagnosis is based on the headache's characteristics and associated symptoms. Results of the physical examination as well as the laboratory studies are usually normal.

The prevalence of migraine is about 15% in women and 7% in men. All varieties of migraine may begin at any age from early childhood on, although peak ages at onset are adolescence and early adulthood.

Several varieties of migraine are described (Table 118–1), of which the two most common are migraine without aura (*common migraine*) and migraine with aura

TABLE 118–1   Classification of Migraine

Migraine without aura (common migraine)
Migraine with aura (classic migraine)
Complicated migraine
    Hemiplegic migraine
    Confusional migraine
    Ophthalmoplegic migraine
    Basilar migraine

(classic migraine). Migraine auras are focal neurologic symptoms typified by positive visual phenomena (such as scintillating scotomata) that often precede the headache. The pain of migraine is often pulsating, unilateral, and frontotemporal in distribution and invariably accompanied by anorexia, nausea, and, occasionally, vomiting. In characteristic attacks, patients are markedly intolerant of light (photophobia) and seek rest in a dark site. There may also be intolerance to sound (phonophobia) and occasionally to odors (osmophobia). The diagnosis of migraine requires the presence of at least one of these features, particularly in the absence of aura. In children, migraine is often associated with episodic abdominal pain, motion sickness, and sleep disturbances. Onset of typical migraine late in life (older than age of 50) is rare, although recurrence of migraine that had been in remission is not uncommon. Recurrent migraine headache associated with transient hemiparesis or hemiplegia occurs rarely as a clearly genetically determined disease (familial hemiplegic migraine).

Other rare types of migraine include recurrent ophthalmoplegia and basilar migraine, which occurs primarily in childhood and in which severe episodic headache is preceded, or accompanied by, signs of bilateral occipital lobe, brain stem, or cerebellar dysfunction (e.g., diplopia, bilateral visual field abnormalities, ataxia, dysarthria, bilateral sensory or motor disturbances, other cranial nerve signs, and occasionally coma). The term *complicated migraine* refers to migraine attacks with major neurologic dysfunction (e.g., migraine with hemiplegia or coma) separate from the visual aura; in these cases, neurologic dysfunction outlasts the headache by hours to 1 or 2 days. Acute severe headache can reflect serious central nervous system disease (Table 118–2). Certain symptoms raise suspicion for a structural brain lesion (Table 118–3).

Etiology. A migraine attack is the end result of the interaction of a number of factors of varying importance in different individuals. These include a genetic predisposition, a susceptibility of the central nervous system to certain stimuli, hormonal factors, and a sequence of neurovascular events. A positive family history is reported in up to 65% to 91% of cases. Linkage analysis with DNA polymorphism has mapped some families with hemiplegic migraine to a calcium channel locus on chromosome 19.

The traditional view has been that the neurologic phenomena of migraine were caused by spasm of cerebral vessels and the pain was caused by subsequent dilatation of extracranial arteries. There is good evidence

TABLE 118–2   Differential Diagnosis of Acute Headache—Major Causes

Migraine
Cluster headache
Stroke
    Subarachnoid hemorrhage
    Intracerebral hemorrhage
    Cerebral infarction
    Arterial dissection (carotid or vertebral)
Acute hydrocephalus
Meningitis/encephalitis
Giant cell arteritis (often chronic)
Tumor (usually chronic)

that diminished cerebral blood flow accompanies the aura of the migraine attack. One of the key structures in the mechanism of pain in all migraine is the trigeminal vascular system. Stimulation of the trigeminal nerve or its ganglion can activate serotonin receptors and nerve endings on small dural arteries and result in a state of neurogenic inflammation. It is postulated that in migraine, these processes stimulate, in turn, perivascular nerve endings, with resultant orthodromic stimulation of trigeminal nerve and pain referred to its distribution. The precise role of other factors, such as female sex hormones, environmental triggers, and stress in the pathogenesis of migraine remains unclear.

Treatment. The goals of treatment include (1) the relief of acute attacks and (2) the prevention of pain and associated symptoms of recurrent headaches. The first step is to inform the patient that he or she has migraine. The benign nature of the disorder and the patient's central role in the treatment plan should be emphasized. It is important that the patient keep a headache diary.

Acute Migraine Attack. Acute attacks are alleviated with single agents or varying combinations of drugs (Fig. 118–1) as well as with behavioral modification therapy. Many attacks of migraine respond to simple analgesics, such as acetaminophen, aspirin, or nonsteroidal anti-in-

TABLE 118–3   Clinical Features of Headaches Suggesting a Structural Brain Lesion

Symptoms
Worst of the patient's life
Progressive
Onset > 50 years of age
Worse in early morning—awakens patient
Marked exacerbation with straining
Focal neurologic dysfunction

Signs
Nuchal rigidity
Fever
Papilledema
Pathologic reflexes or reflex asymmetry
Altered state of consciousness

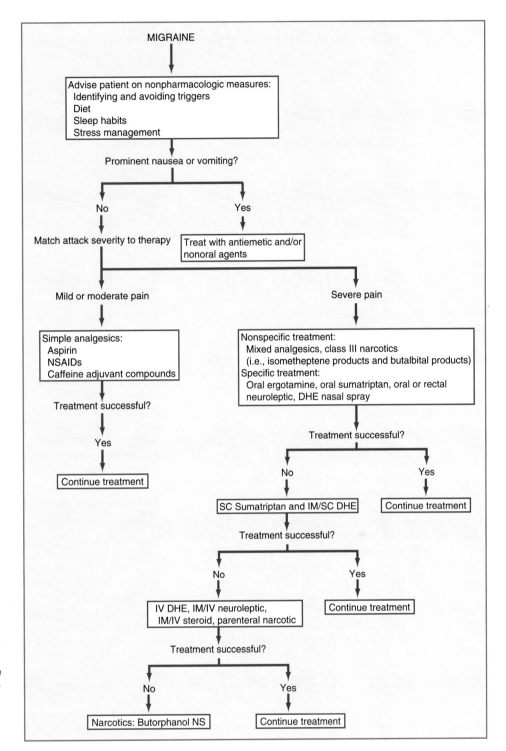

MIGRAINE

Advise patient on nonpharmacologic measures:
Identifying and avoiding triggers
Diet
Sleep habits
Stress management

Prominent nausea or vomiting?

No — Match attack severity to therapy

Yes — Treat with antiemetic and/or nonoral agents

Mild or moderate pain

Simple analgesics:
Aspirin
NSAIDs
Caffeine adjuvant compounds

Treatment successful?

Yes

Continue treatment

Severe pain

Nonspecific treatment:
Mixed analgesics, class III narcotics
(i.e., isometheptene products and butalbital products)
Specific treatment:
Oral ergotamine, oral sumatriptan, oral or rectal
neuroleptic, DHE nasal spray

Treatment successful?

No — SC Sumatriptan and IM/SC DHE

Yes — Continue treatment

Treatment successful?

No — IV DHE, IM/IV neuroleptic,
IM/IV steroid, parenteral narcotic

Yes — Continue treatment

Treatment successful?

No — Narcotics: Butorphanol NS

Yes — Continue treatment

FIGURE 118–1 Algorithm for the treatment of migraine. DHE = dihydroergotamine; IM = intramuscular; IV = intravenous; NS = normal saline; NSAIDs = nonsteroidal anti-inflammatory drugs; SC = subcutaneous. (From Silberstein SD, Young WB, Lipton RB: Migraine and cluster headaches. *In* Johnson RT, Griffin JW (eds): Current Therapy in Neurologic Disease, 5th ed. St. Louis: CV Mosby, 1997, p 88.)

flammatory agents (NSAIDs). Opioid drugs have a limited use in the migraine attack. Overuse of analgesics is particularly frequent in headache patients; and one of the most important aspects of therapy of migraine patients, therefore, is the monitoring of amounts of analgesic used. In patients who are nauseated, it is often helpful to prescribe an antiemetic agent early in an attack. Phenothiazine drugs can produce involuntary movements as an acute adverse effect as well as having a sedative effect (which may be beneficial).

A number of "migraine-specific" serotonin agonist drugs have become available (see Fig. 118–1). Although many are highly effective in alleviating migraine, patients must be carefully instructed in their appropriate use. Moreover, a response to these medications does not confirm a diagnosis of migraine.

Migraine Prevention. Several drugs prevent migraine (Table 118–4). The use of these agents should be restricted to patients who have frequent attacks (usually more than four per month) and who are willing to

TABLE 118-4 Preventive Therapy for Migraine

Drug Class	Agent	Dose	Adverse Effects
β-Adrenergic receptor blockers	Propranolol Nadolol	40–160 mg/day 40–160 mg/day	Contraindicated in asthma; nightmares, fatigue, syncope
Tricyclic antidepressants	Amitriptyline	10–50 mg qhs	Dry mouth, confusion, palpitations
Serotonin reuptake inhibitors	Paroxetine Sertraline	10–50 mg/day 50–200 mg/day	Insomnia, somnolence, sexual dysfunction
Calcium channel blockers	Verapamil	120–900 mg/day	Constipation, edema, hypotension
Serotonin antagonists	Methysergide	2–8 mg/day	Prolonged use associated with fibrotic reactions
Anticonvulsants	Divalproex sodium	500–1000 mg/day	Weight gain, tremor

take daily medication. With any of the medications, an adequate trial period should be given, using adequate doses, before it is declared ineffective. Combination therapy is occasionally required but is not routinely prescribed.

Cluster Headache

Clinical Features. Cluster headache comprises a group of symptoms and has a more or less specific temporal course. It is uncommon, accounting for less than 10% of all headache sufferers. Unlike migraine, it is much more common in men than women and its mean age at onset is later in life than migraine. Also, unlike migraine, cluster headache rarely begins in childhood and there is less often a family history. Cluster headache pain is of extreme intensity and is associated with congestion of the nasal mucosa and injection of the conjunctiva on the side of the pain. Increased sweating of the ipsilateral side of forehead and face may occur. There may be associated ocular signs of Horner's syndrome: miosis, ptosis, and the additional feature of eyelid edema. The pain is usually steady, nonthrobbing, and invariably localized retro-orbitally on one side of the head; it may occasionally spread to the ipsilateral side of the face or neck. Attacks often awaken patients, usually 2 to 3 hours after the onset of sleep. In contrast to migraineurs, the pain is not relieved by resting in a dark, quiet area; on the contrary, patients sometimes seek some activity that can distract them.

As the name implies, cluster attacks frequently recur over a period of several days or weeks. These periods of frequent headaches are separated by headache-free periods of varying duration, often several months or years. Attacks have a striking tendency to be precipitated by even small amounts of alcohol. There are rare variants of cluster headache: a "chronic variety" in which remissions are brief (less than 14 days), "chronic paroxysmal hemicrania" in which attacks are shorter and strikingly more prevalent in women, and "hemicrania continua," in which there is continuous moderately severe unilateral headache. The etiology of all these syndromes is un-

known, although the distribution of the pain suggests dysfunction of the trigeminal nerve.

Treatment. Therapy for cluster headache may be abortive for acute headache or prophylactic to prevent headache. Acute headache may respond to oxygen by mask (7 to 10 L/min for 15 minutes), which is effective within several minutes in 70% of patients. Sumatriptan and dihydroergotamine (DHE) are also effective. Preventive medications include lithium, divalproex sodium, verapamil, methysergide, and corticosteroids. Paroxysmal hemicrania and related syndromes are often strikingly sensitive to indomethacin.

Tension-Type Headache

This headache syndrome is defined by a number of characteristics. The pain is usually not throbbing but rather steady and often described as a "pressure feeling" or a "viselike" sensation. It is usually not unilateral and may be frontal, occipital, or generalized. There is frequently pain in the neck area, unlike in migraine. Pain commonly lasts for long periods of time (e.g., days) and does not rapidly appear and disappear in attacks. Nausea is uncommon and mild when present. There is no "aura." Photophobia and phonophobia are usually absent. Although tension-type headache may be related by the patient to occur or be exacerbated at times of particular emotional stress, the pathophysiology relates to sustained craniocervical muscle contraction; hence, a more appropriate term for this syndrome is *muscle-contraction headache*.

A careful evaluation should be made of the patient's life situations and the presence of anxiety or depression. The tricyclic antidepressant drugs in low doses have proven the most useful for prevention of tension-type headache; although the most well documented is amitriptyline, newer agents with fewer side effects may be equally effective.

Other Defined Headache Syndromes

A variety of acute headache syndromes need to be differentiated from migraine, cluster, or tension headache.

These include "thunderclap" headache, "ice cream" headache, and coital headache. The latter may be indistinguishable from the headache of subarachnoid hemorrhage and usually requires computed tomography (CT) for diagnosis. All three headache syndromes are more common in migraineurs.

Headache Secondary to Structural Brain Disease

Headache may be a manifestation of underlying structural brain disease (Table 118–5). Headache can be seen in all forms of cerebrovascular disease: infarction, transient ischemic attacks, and intracerebral and subarachnoid hemorrhage. The headache in subarachnoid hemorrhage is usually extremely severe and often described by the patient as "the worst headache of my life." Nuchal rigidity, third nerve palsy (usually involving the pupil), and retinal, preretinal, or subconjunctival hemorrhages may be found. CT of the head usually shows subarachnoid, intraventricular, or other intracranial blood.

The patient with headache and fever presents a common diagnostic problem in the emergency department. Neck stiffness is a common symptom. Meningismus is confirmed by eliciting Brudzinski's and Kernig's signs. Vomiting occurs in about 50% of patients. Suspicion for meningitis should prompt further investigation, including a lumbar puncture. If the patient shows focal signs, papilledema, or profound alteration in level of consciousness, CT of the head before lumbar puncture is

required to rule out focal disease such as an abscess or subdural empyema. These lesions, however, are rare.

Acute Sinusitis. Head pain is the most prominent feature of sinusitis. Malaise and low-grade fever are usually present. The pain is dull, aching, and nonpulsatile and exacerbated by movement, coughing, or straining and improved with nasal decongestants. The pain is most pronounced on awakening or after any prolonged recumbency and is diminished with maintenance of an upright posture.

The location of the pain depends on the sinus involved. Maxillary sinusitis provokes ipsilateral malar, ear, and dental pain with significant overlying facial tenderness. Frontal sinusitis produces frontal headache that may radiate behind the eyes and to the vertex of the skull. Tenderness to frontal palpation may be present with point tenderness on the undersurface of the medial aspect of the superior orbital rim. In ethmoidal sinusitis the pain is between or behind the eyes with radiation to the temporal area. The eyes and orbit are often tender to palpation, and, in fact, eye movements themselves may accentuate the pain. Sphenoidal sinusitis causes pain in the orbit and at the vertex of the skull and occasionally in the frontal or occipital regions. Chronic sinusitis is seldom a cause of headache.

Brain Tumors. Posterior fossa tumors (particularly of the cerebellum) frequently produce headache, especially if hydrocephalus occurs because cerebrospinal fluid (CSF) flow is partially obstructed. Supratentorial tumors, however, are less likely to cause headache and are more frequently heralded by altered mental status, focal deficits, or seizures. Although increased intracranial pressure is often associated with headache, it is usually not the primary mechanism, because uniform pressure elevations do not usually produce distortions of pain-sensitive structures.

Idiopathic Intracranial Hypertension (IIH). This syndrome, also called benign intracranial hypertension, is defined as a syndrome of elevated intracranial pressure without evidence of focal lesions, hydrocephalus, or frank brain edema. It occurs usually between the ages of 15 and 45 and is more frequent in obese women. The disorder is characterized by headache. At times, patients have visual disturbances, such as restricted peripheral visual fields, enlarged blind spots, slight visual blurring, or diplopia secondary to abducens nerve palsies. Funduscopic examination shows papilledema, which is often more impressive than the clinical picture. IIH is usually a benign and self-limited disorder, but it may lead to visual loss, including blindness. The headache is usually insidious in onset, is typically generalized, is relatively mild in severity, and is often worse in the morning or after exertion (e.g., straining or coughing).

The condition has been associated with drugs—vitamin A intoxication, nalidixic acid, danazol (Danocrine), and isotretinoin (Accutane)—as well as corticosteroid withdrawal and with systemic disorders such as hypoparathyroidism and lupus.

CT is usually normal but can show small ventricles.

TABLE 118–5   Headache Secondary to Underlying Brain Disease

Cerebrovascular Disease
Ischemic stroke
Intracerebral hemorrhage
Subarachnoid hemorrhage

Inflammatory Disease
Cranial arteritis
Isolated central nervous system vasculitis
Tolosa-Hunt syndrome
Systemic lupus erythematosus

Infectious Disease
Meningitis
Abscess
Encephalitis
Sinusitis

Post-traumatic
Subdural hematoma
Empyema

Neoplastic Disease
Malignant brain tumor
Benign brain tumor
Metastasis

Other
Idiopathic intracranial hypertension

CSF opening pressure is elevated, usually in the range of 250 to 450 mm of water, with the pressure fluctuating markedly when monitored over a prolonged period.

Treatment. After eliminating secondary causes of IIH, the patient should have dietary counseling for weight loss. Carbonic anhydrase inhibitors (acetazolamide) and corticosteroids have proved useful in headache control. As a second-line agent, furosemide also acts to lower CSF production. Serial lumbar punctures are understandably unpopular with patients even though transient headache relief is obtained. CSF shunting procedures (ventriculoperitoneal shunt) are occasionally necessary. For patients with progressive visual loss, optic nerve sheath fenestration has been shown to preserve or restore vision in 80% to 90% of patients and provide headache relief in a majority. Intracranial hypotension (usually secondary to a CSF leak after trauma or lumbar puncture) may also cause headache, exacerbated by standing.

Post-Traumatic Headache. Headache in these individuals has no specific quality and is associated with irritability, concentration impairment, insomnia, memory disturbance, and light-headedness. Anxiety and depression are present to variable degrees. Multiple treatment options are available, and amitriptyline and nonsteroidal anti-inflammatory agents are useful. Occasionally, muscle relaxants and anxiolytics are beneficial.

Giant Cell Arteritis. Headache occurs in 60% of patients with giant cell arteritis, a granulomatous vasculitis of medium and large arteries. More than 95% of patients are 50 years of age or older. Malaise, fever, weight loss, and jaw claudication occur early, in addition to headache. Polymyalgia rheumatica, a syndrome of painful stiffness of the neck, shoulders, and pelvis, is found in half the patients. Visual impairment secondary to ischemic optic neuritis may occur. The headache is usually described as aching and is exacerbated at night and after exposure to cold. The superficial temporal artery is frequently swollen, red, and very tender and may be pulseless. The erythrocyte sedimentation rate is usually elevated; the mean is 100 mm/hr. Anemia is frequently present. Temporal artery biopsy usually confirms the diagnosis, but because the arteritis is segmental, large or multiple sections may be required. Prednisone therapy is often dramatically effective and must be given promptly to preserve vision on the affected side.

HEADACHE IN SYSTEMIC DISEASE

A wide variety of systemic diseases have headache as a prominent symptom; some of the more prevalent disorders are summarized in Table 118–6.

Cranial Neuralgias

Neuralgias are differentiated from other head pains by the brevity of the attacks (usually 1 to 2 seconds or less) and by the distribution of the pain. Neuralgic pain is often responsive to treatment with standard doses of

TABLE 118-6 Headache Secondary to Systemic Disease

Endocrine/Metabolic

Malignant hypertension (e.g., pheochromocytoma)
Acromegaly
Cushing's disease
Carcinoid
Hyperparathyroidism
Paget's disease

Pulmonary

Hypercapnea
Sleep apnea

Pharmacologic

Alcohol
Nitrates
Caffeine withdrawal
Analgesic withdrawal ("rebound") headache
Others: dipyridamole, cyclosporine, tacrolimus, calcium channel antagonists

anticonvulasants such as phenytoin, carbamazepine, or gabapentin and, occasionally, baclofen.

Trigeminal Neuralgia. In trigeminal neuralgia (tic douloureux), stabbing, spasmodic pain occurs unilaterally in one of the divisions of the trigeminal nerve. It lasts seconds, but it may occur many times a day for weeks at a time. It is characteristically induced by even the lightest touch to particular areas of the face, such as the lips or gums. A very small minority of cases are due to multiple sclerosis, cerebellopontine angle tumors, aneurysms, or arteriovenous malformations, although in these cases (unlike "true" trigeminal neuralgia) there are usually objective signs of neurologic deficit such as areas of diminished sensation. In these cases of "symptomatic" neuralgia, the pain is often atypical. Trigeminal neuralgia may be life threatening when it interferes with eating. If medical treatments are unsuccessful, surgical procedures to ablate the sensory portion of the trigeminal nerve are often needed.

Glossopharyngeal Neuralgia. Glossopharyngeal neuralgia is a rare disorder that is much less common than trigeminal neuralgia. Brief paroxysms of severe stabbing unilateral pain radiate from the throat to the ear or vice versa and are frequently initiated by stimulation of specific "trigger zones" (e.g., tonsillar fossa or pharyngeal wall). Swallowing occasionally provokes an attack; yawning, talking, and coughing are other potential triggers.

Postherpetic Neuralgia. Herpes zoster produces head pain by cranial nerve involvement in one third of cases. In some cases a persistent intense burning pain follows the initial acute illness. The discomfort may subside after several weeks or persist (particularly in the elderly) for months or years. The pain is localized over the distribution of the affected nerve and associated with exquisite tenderness to even the lightest touch. The first division of the trigeminal nerve is the most frequent cranial nerve involved (ophthalmic herpes) and is occasionally associated with keratoconjunctivitis. When the seventh nerve is affected ("geniculate herpes"), the pain involves the external auditory meatus and pinna. Occasionally, concomitant facial paralysis may occur (Ramsay Hunt syndrome).

Occipital Neuralgia. This is a syndrome that includes occipital pain starting at the base of the skull and often provoked by neck extension. Physical examination shows tenderness in the region of the occipital nerves and altered sensation in the C2 dermatome. Treatment includes the use of a soft collar, muscle relaxants, physical therapy, and local injections of analgesics and anti-inflammatory agents.

Reflex Sympathetic Dystrophy

Reflex sympathetic dystrophy (RSD) denotes a syndrome that consists of pain and hyperesthesia and autonomic changes. Almost any type of injury can lead to RSD, including blunt trauma, lacerations, and burns.

The symptoms of RSD usually develop gradually over days or weeks and are divided into three stages whose duration may vary considerably. The *acute stage* is characterized by spontaneous aching or burning pain that is restricted to a particular vascular, peripheral nerve, or root territory. Hyperpathia (pain characterized by overreaction and "aftersensation" to a stimulus) may occur with dysesthesia. The *dystrophic stage* usually begins 3 to 6 months after the injury and is characterized by spontaneous burning pain and more marked hyperpathia than in the acute stage. The nails become cracked, grooved, or ridged, and hair growth is decreased. In addition, there is decreased range of joint motion, muscle wasting, osteoporosis, and edema. *Atrophy* usually occurs more than 6 months after the injury. The pain becomes less prominent, and the skin becomes cold, pale, and cyanotic, with increased or decreased sweating. Irreversible trophic changes occur in the skin and subcutaneous tissues and result in smooth, glossy skin, with subcutaneous atrophy, tapering of digits, and fixed joints with contractures. RSD often is associated with marked behavioral changes, which may include emotional instability, anxiety, and social withdrawal. The diagnosis of RSD is primarily clinical, based on the patient's history and physical findings. No diagnostic tests are specific for this condition.

The mechanisms by which the signs and symptoms of RSD develop have not been fully elucidated. Sympathetic blockade by anesthetic block of the sympathetic ganglia innervating the painful part or by systemic α-adrenergic blockade relieves the pain in many patients, suggesting that the pain is sympathetically maintained. Sympathetic blockade is the mainstay of treatment. Systemic intravenous α-adrenergic blockade with phentolamine seems to be a good predictor of response to subsequent sympatholytic treatment. Anti-inflammatory agents, amitriptyline, and other tricyclic antidepressants may be useful in the treatment of chronic burning pain, whereas anticonvulsants (carbamazepine, phenytoin) and antispasmotic drugs (baclofen) may relieve episodic or allodynic pain.

Neck and Back Pain

Most patients with acute neck or back pain have a musculoskeletal disorder that is self-limiting and does not require specific therapy. The pain may originate from a number of sources, including the vertebrae and intervertebral discs, facet joints, or muscles and ligaments of the vertebral column.

Because the thoracic spine is designed for rigidity rather than mobility, thoracic disc rupture is exceedingly rare. Acute onset pain in the thoracic region may be due to dissection of the aorta or anterior spinal artery thrombosis.

CERVICAL SPONDYLOSIS

Cervical spondylosis is a degenerative disorder of the cervical intervertebral discs leading to osteophyte formation and hypertrophy of adjacent facet joints and ligaments. Cervical spondylosis is probably the most common pathology seen in office practice of neurologists and is present radiographically in over 90% of the population older than 60. For unknown reasons, the degree of anatomic abnormality is not directly correlated with the clinical signs and symptoms. Clinical disease may represent a combination of normal, age-related, degenerative changes in the cervical spine and a congenital or developmental stenosis of the cervical canal; the process may be aggravated by trauma. It may present as a painful stiff neck, with or without symptoms or signs of cervical root irritation or spinal cord compression. Patients with root irritation complain of pain and paresthesias radiating down the arm roughly in the dermatomal distribution of the affected nerve root. Discrete sensory loss is uncommon and certainly less prominent than symptoms (Table 118–7). For relief, patients often adopt a position with the arm elevated and flexed behind the head. Objective neurologic findings may be limited to reflex asymmetry because weakness may be obscured by pain. Patients who have some degree of spinal cord compression present with gait and bladder disturbances and evidence of spasticity on examination of the lower extremities. These patients require investigation with an imaging study, ideally magnetic resonance imaging or CT myelography. Plain radiographs of the cervical spine add little information except in patients with rheumatoid arthritis in whom basilar invagination or atlantoaxial subluxation is suspected.

Cervical spondylosis is so common in the general population that it may be present coincidentally in a patient with another disease of the spinal cord. Among other diseases that may mimic cervical spondylosis are multiple sclerosis, amyotrophic lateral sclerosis, and, rarely, subacute combined system disease (vitamin B_{12} deficiency). Conservative treatment includes the use of anti-inflammatory medication, cervical immobilization,

TABLE 118-7   **Common Root Syndromes of Intervertebral Disc Disease**

Disc Space	Root Affected	Muscles Affected	Area of Pain/ Paresthesias	Reflex Affected
C4–5	C5	Deltoid/biceps	Shoulder	Biceps
C5–6	C6	Wrist extensors	Radial forearm	Triceps
C6–7	C7	Triceps	Middle finger	Brachioradialis
C7–T1	C8	Hand intrinsics	Fourth and fifth fingers	Finger flexion
L3–4	L4	Quadriceps	Anterior thigh	Knee jerk
L4–5	L5	Peronei	Great toe/dorsum of foot	
L5–S1	S1	Gastrocnemius/glutei	Lateral foot/sole	Ankle jerk

and physical therapy for isometric strengthening of neck muscles (Fig. 118–2). Surgery should be considered if there is progression of the neurologic deficit.

ACUTE LOW BACK PAIN

The same pathologic changes that affect the cervical spine may also affect the lumbar spine. Since the spinal cord ends at the level of the first lumbar vertebra, lumbar canal stenosis from intervertebral disc disease and degenerative spondylosis will affect the roots of the cauda equina. The most common levels for lumbar degenerative disc disease are at L4–5 and L5–S1, resulting in the common complaint of sciatica due to irritation of the lower lumbar roots. Pain tends to improve with sitting or lying down, in contrast to the pain from spinal or vertebral tumors, which is aggravated by prolonged recumbency. Examination shows loss of the normal lumbar lordosis, paraspinal muscle spasm, and exacerbation of pain with straight leg-raising, owing to stretching of the lower lumbar roots. About 10% of disc herniations occur lateral to the spinal canal, in which case the more rostral root is compressed.

Spinal stenosis of the lumbar region may present as "neurogenic claudication," which is usually described as unilateral or bilateral buttock pain worse on standing or walking and relieved by rest or flexion at the waist. Patients may have pain that is worse when walking downhill in contrast to patients with vascular claudication whose pain is maximal walking up an incline.

Treatment strategies for lumbar pain are similar to

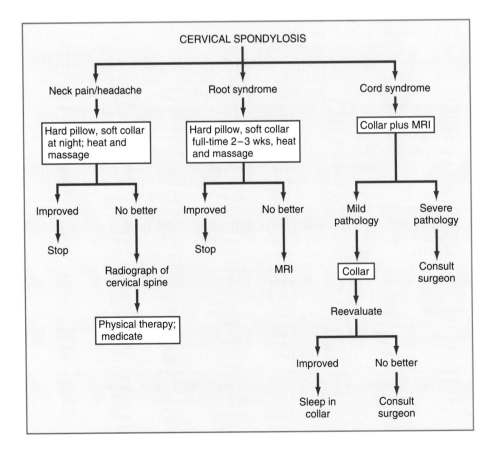

FIGURE 118-2 Algorithm for the treatment of cervical spondylosis. MRI = magnetic resonance imaging. (From Ronthal M, Rachlin JR: Cervical spondylosis. *In* Johnson RT, Griffin JW (eds): Current Therapy in Neurologic Disease, 5th ed. St. Louis: CV Mosby, 1997, p 77.)

those for cervical pain, with surgery reserved for patients with neurologic signs and clear pathologic processes seen on imaging studies. Most cases of acute low back pain, even with rupture of an intervertebral disc, can be treated conservatively with a short period of rest, muscle relaxants, and analgesics. Prolonged bed rest is no longer recommended except for patients in severe pain. Patient education regarding proper posture and appropriate back exercises is helpful, as is a formal physical therapy program. Chiropractic manipulation should be reserved for patients who have no evidence of neurologic injury or spine instability.

REFERENCES

Cutrer FM, Moskowitz MA: Headaches and other head pain. *In* Goldman L, Bennett JC (eds): Cecil Textbook of Medicine, 21st ed. Philadelphia: WB Saunders, 2000.

Johnson RT, Griffin JW (eds): Current Therapy in Neurologic Disease, 5th ed. St. Louis: CV Mosby, 1997.

Malmivaara A, Hakkinen U, Aro T, et al: The treatment of acute low back pain—bed rest, exercises or ordinary activity? N Engl J Med 1995;332:351–355.

Silberstein SD, Lipton RB, Goadsby PJ (eds): Headache in Clinical Practice. Oxford: Isis Medical Media, 1998.

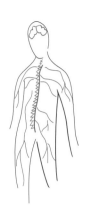

119

DISORDERS OF VISION AND HEARING

Timothy J. Counihan

Disorders of Vision and Eye Movements

EXAMINATION OF THE VISUAL SYSTEM

Acuity

The clinical examination of visual function should begin with the testing of visual acuity. The patient should wear corrective lenses if they are available, and, if possible, testing should be performed with a Snellen chart at a distance of 20 feet to minimize the influence of pupil size and lens accommodation on visual acuity. When errors of refraction are responsible for decreased visual acuity, vision may be improved by having the patient look through a pinhole. Corrected vision in one eye of less than 20/40 suggests damage to the lens (cataract) or retina or a disorder of the anterior visual (prechiasmal) pathway. Color vision in each eye should also be tested; even when visual acuity is normal, patients with lesions of the optic nerve may complain that colors appear "washed out" in the affected eye.

Visual Fields

Careful examination of the visual fields (Fig. 119–1) can often localize lesions interrupting the afferent (sensory) visual system. Visual fields in all four quadrants should be tested by comparing the patient's field with the examiner's (confrontation). Asking the patient to count the number of the examiner's extended fingers is more sensitive than presenting moving objects in detecting visual field deficits. The field should be tested first unilaterally and then bilaterally because uncovering a defect (particularly in the left hemifield) with bilateral testing only (extinction) suggests a lesion in the contralateral parietal lobe.

Partial or complete visual loss in one eye only implies damage to the retina or optic nerve anterior to the optic chiasm, whereas a visual field abnormality involving both eyes implies a defect at or posterior to the optic chiasm. Scotomas are areas of partial or complete visual loss and may be central or peripheral; central scotomas severely disrupt vision as a result of damage to macular fibers. A scotoma impairing half of a visual field is known as a hemianopia. A homonymous hemianopia implies a post-chiasmal lesion. Quadrantanopias are smaller defects in the visual field and may be superior (which suggests a temporal lobe lesion) or inferior (which suggests a parietal lobe lesion). Bitemporal hemianopia implies a lesion at the chiasm such as a pituitary tumor. An altitudinal hemianopia occurs with vascular damage to the retina. Scintillating scotomas refer to hallucinations of flashing lights. If they are monocular, they may be caused by retinal detachment; binocular scintillations suggest occipital oligemia (as in migraine) or seizure. Any suspicious findings on bedside confrontation testing warrant formal visual perimetry testing.

Pupils

Pupil constriction results from stimulation of the parasympathetic division of the oculomotor (third cranial) nerve, whereas dilation is mediated by the sympathetic system. If the balance of these systems is upset, pupillary inequality (anisocoria) results. The pupils should be examined in both dim and bright light; if the anisocoria increases going from dim to bright light, a lesion of the parasympathetic system is likely (Fig. 119–2). *Physiologic anisocoria* is characterized by a difference in pupil size that appears less in bright light and has no associated pathologic findings.

Both the direct and consensual light responses should be noted for each eye, such that when the light is shone in one eye both pupils constrict. This is best tested using the "swinging light test," in which the light is moved quickly from one eye to the other. If there is dilation of one pupil as the light is moved to it from the other side, an abnormality of the optic nerve in that eye

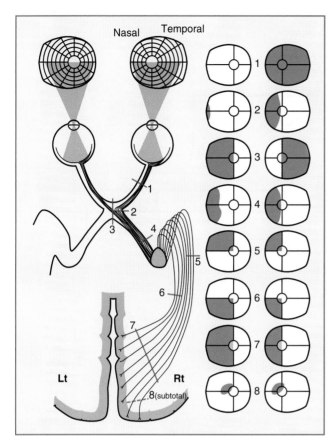

FIGURE 119–1 Visual fields that accompany damage to the visual pathways: 1, Optic nerve: unilateral amaurosis. 2, Lateral optic chiasm: grossly incongruous, incomplete (contralateral) homonymous hemianopia. 3, Central optic chiasm: bitemporal hemianopia. 4, Optic tract: incongruous, incomplete homonymous hemianopia. 5, Temporal (Meyer's) loop of optic radiation: congruous partial or complete (contralateral) homonymous superior quadrantanopia. 6, Parietal (superior) projection of the optic radiation: congruous partial or complete homonymous inferior quandrantanopia. 7, Complete parieto-occipital interruption of optic radiation. Complete congruous homonymous hemianopia with psychophysical shift of foveal point often sparing central vision, giving "macular sparing." 8, Incomplete damage to visual cortex: congruous homonymous scotomas, usually encroaching at least acutely on central vision. (From Baloh RW: Neuro-ophthalmology. *In* Goldman L, Bennett JC [eds]: Cecil Textbook of Medicine, 21st ed. Philadelphia: WB Saunders, 1998, p 2236.)

should be suspected. This abnormality is referred to as an *afferent pupillary defect.* The accommodative pupillary response is tested by asking the patient to look first in the distance and then at the examiner's finger, held 12 inches away. The pupils should constrict symmetrically and rapidly.

The presence of ptosis should be noted. A large unreactive pupil with ptosis indicates a lesion of the oculomotor nerve *(third cranial nerve palsy)* interrupting the parasympathetic nerve supply to the pupil. The associated paralysis of the medial and inferior rectus and inferior oblique muscles (see later discussion) results in distortion of the eye (inferolaterally, "down and out") and a subjective complaint of diplopia by the patient. Com-

mon causes of a third nerve palsy include compression by an aneurysm of the posterior communicating artery, by transtentorial herniation or from ischemia, usually in the setting of diabetes or vasculitis. A third nerve palsy can be assumed to be caused by ischemia only when the pupil is completely spared and there is complete paralysis of the oculomotor and eyelid levator muscles.

A small unreactive pupil with associated ptosis is known as *Horner's syndrome* and results from damage to the sympathetic fibers to the pupil. There may be associated unilateral anhidrosis resulting from damage to sympathetic fibers. Horner's syndrome may result from lesions of the hypothalamus, brain stem, cervical spinal cord, or sympathetic fibers to the pupil. A Horner's syndrome from sympathetic fiber involvement may be the first sign of an apical lung tumor (Pancoast's) or may occur in diseases affecting the carotid artery.

Argyll-Robertson pupils are small, irregular pupils that constrict to near vision but not to light. They are often associated with neurosyphilis and occasionally diabetes. This so-called light-near dissociation may also occur in rostral dorsal midbrain lesions, in which there are abnormalities of vertical gaze, eyelid retraction, and convergence retraction nystagmus.

Tonic (Adie's) pupils constrict slowly and incompletely to light; this is usually an incidental finding on examination but may be associated with areflexia (Adie's syndrome). It has been suggested that the disorder is a result of parasympathetic denervation.

Hippus refers to pupillary unrest with synchronous oscillation of the pupil size; it is considered a normal phenomenon.

Eye Movements

Several elements in the history may help in evaluating the patient with diplopia. Is the diplopia primarily horizontal or vertical, or is it greater looking to the right or to the left? Double vision that varies during the day suggests myasthenia gravis. Is the diplopia maximal with near or distant vision? Greater difficulty with near vision suggests impairment of the medial rectus, oculomotor nerve, or convergence system, whereas abducens nerve weakness results in horizontal diplopia when viewing objects at a distance. Monocular diplopia is usually caused by diseases of the retina or lens and is corrected by having the patient look through a pinhole, unless the cause is psychogenic.

The examination should begin by determining the position of the head and eyes with the eyes in primary gaze. Both smooth pursuit as well as (voluntary) saccadic eye movements in horizontal and vertical directions are checked to determine whether the movements are conjugate or disconjugate. Disconjugate eye movements suggest a disorder of the brain stem (at the level of the ocular motor nuclei or their connections), peripheral nerves (cranial nerves III, IV, or VI), individual eye muscles (ocular myopathy), or neuromuscular junction (myasthenia gravis, botulism). A large deficit in the range of eye movements may provide sufficient diagnostic information. However, in many cases, although the patient complains of diplopia, no clear misalignment is

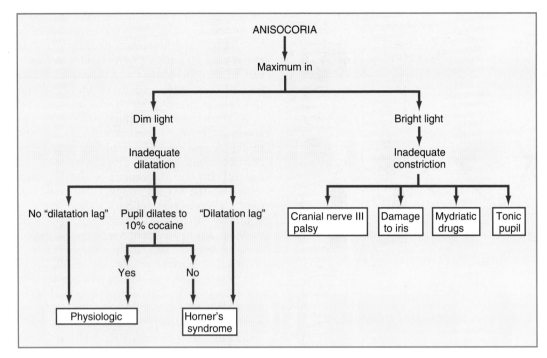

FIGURE 119-2 Algorithm for the approach to unequal pupils (anisocoria).

visible on testing eye movements. The corneal reflection test may help identify misalignment in these cases. The patient is instructed to look at a light shining directly at the eyes. If the eyes are normally aligned, the light reflection will be about 1 mm nasal to the center of the cornea. If one eye is deviated medially, the reflection will be displaced outward and vice versa if the eye is deviated outward.

The abducens (sixth cranial) nerve supplies the lateral rectus muscle. The trochlear (fourth cranial) nerve subserves the superior oblique muscle, which intorts the eye as well as depresses the eye in adduction (such as when a patient tries to look downstairs). All other muscles are supplied by the oculomotor nerve. Abnormalities of the cranial nerves in the brain stem are usually accompanied by other signs, such as weakness, ataxia, or dysarthria. The abducens nerve has a long ascending course through the posterior fossa, where it is prone to compression at multiple sites and as a result of raised intracranial pressure; hence, a sixth nerve palsy may be a false localizing sign. Table 119–1 lists the major causes of acute ophthalmoplegia.

Conjugate eye movement is regulated by supranuclear pathways from the cerebral hemisphere to reach the medial longitudinal fasciculus in the brain stem. A lesion in the cerebral hemisphere resulting from hemorrhage, infarction, or tumor disrupts conjugate gaze to the contralateral side, so that the eyes "look away" from the hemiplegia. Lesions of the brain stem cause conjugate paralysis to the ipsilateral side (eyes looking toward

TABLE 119-1 Major Causes of Acute Ophthalmoplegia

Condition	Diagnostic Features
Bilateral	
Botulism	Contaminated food; high-altitude cooking; pupils involved
Myasthenia gravis	Fluctuating degree of paralysis; responds to edrophonium chloride (Tensilon) IV
Wernicke's encephalopathy	Nutritional deficiency; responds to thiamine IV
Acute cranial polyneuropathy	Antecedent respiratory infection; elevated CSF protein level
Brain stem stroke	Other brain stem signs
Unilateral	
P Comm aneurysm	Third cranial nerve, pupil involved
Diabetic-idiopathic	Third or sixth cranial nerve, pupil spared
Myasthenia gravis	As above
Brain stem stroke	As above

CSF = cerebrospinal fluid; IV = intravenous; P Comm = posterior communicating artery the side of the hemiplegia). Lesions of the medial longitudinal fasciculus, which connects the nuclei of the oculomotor and abducens nerves, leads to *internuclear ophthalmoplegia*. In this case, conjugate gaze toward the side of the lesion results in failure of adduction of the ipsilateral eye and abduction nystagmus in the other eye. The accommodation reflex is normal, indicating that the lesion is supranuclear and not a partial third nerve palsy. Bilateral internuclear ophthalmoplegia in a young person is virtually pathognomonic of multiple sclerosis.

Funduscopy

The retina should be carefully examined in each patient by direct ophthalmoscopy, which provides a magnified view of the fundus without the necessity for dilatation of the pupil.

UNILATERAL VISUAL LOSS

Loss of vision in one eye may be caused by lesions of the cornea, lens, vitreous, retina, or optic nerve. Careful funduscopic examination will usually detect ocular and retinal lesions, but acute lesions of the optic nerve (optic neuritis) may not be associated with abnormalities of the optic nerve head. *Optic neuritis* is a condition characterized by inflammation of the optic nerve accompanied by nonhomonymous defects in vision. The term *papillitis* refers to ophthalmoscopically observable changes in the optic nerve; *retrobulbar neuritis* refers to this condition without observable changes in the funduscopic examination.

The patient with optic neuritis complains of difficulty with vision in the affected eye. Loss of vision may be insidious and recognized only when the unaffected eye is accidentally occluded. The evolution of visual loss is highly variable, progressing over a period ranging from less than a day to several weeks, although most patients will have reached their maximal visual deficit in 3 to 7 days. Patients may describe their vision as blurred or dim, and colors may appear less bright than usual or "gray." At the time the patient is first examined, visual acuity may range from almost 20/20 to the extreme of total blindness. Examination of the visual field shows defects within the central 25 degrees, with central and paracentral scotomas being the most common types. An afferent pupillary defect is frequently present. The funduscopic examination is abnormal in only about one half of the cases. The disc may appear hyperemic with blurred margins, and hemorrhages, when present, are few and found only on the disc or in the area immediately surrounding the disc. By far the most common etiology of optic neuritis is multiple sclerosis.

Ischemic optic neuropathy occurs in two forms. The *atherosclerotic* variety occurs mostly between the ages of 50 and 70, and no evidence of systemic disease is present. The *arteritic* form is usually a manifestation of giant cell arteritis in which there may be systemic manifestations of the disease, including headache, scalp tenderness, and generalized myalgias. Laboratory evaluation shows anemia and elevated erythrocyte sedimentation rate in almost every case. Patients with arteritis should be treated with high doses of corticosteroids to prevent permanent loss of vision.

The optic nerve may be compressed by tumors that originate in the nerve itself or in the region of the optic chiasm. Pathologic processes that appear acutely as optic disc edema frequently result in a secondary optic atrophy, including papilledema, optic neuritis, and ischemic optic neuropathy. Glaucoma is responsible for more cases of optic atrophy in the adult population than any other etiology. In young patients with inherited optic atrophy, Leber's hereditary optic neuropathy should be kept in mind and usually is bilateral.

Acute transient monocular blindness is usually the result of embolization to the central retinal artery from an atheromatous plaque in the carotid artery (*amaurosis fugax*). Any complaint of transient visual loss constitutes an emergency, and steps must be taken to prevent permanent loss of vision by making a prompt diagnosis and initiation of appropriate therapy. Examples of sight-saving procedures include corticosteroid therapy for cranial arteritis, reduction of intraocular pressure for acute glaucoma, and carotid surgery, anticoagulation, or antiplatelet therapy for severe cerebrovascular disease.

BILATERAL VISUAL LOSS

Gradual bilateral visual loss caused by optic nerve lesions is rare but may be from Leber's hereditary optic neuropathy or a toxic-nutritional deficiency state. Acute transient bilateral visual loss (visual obscuration) may be a symptom of raised intracranial pressure caused by a brain tumor or pseudotumor cerebri; papilledema is often severe. Lesions of the optic chiasm or postchiasmal optic pathways lead to specific patterns of partial visual loss summarized in Figure 119–1. Bilateral damage to the optic radiations or visual cortex results in *cortical blindness*. The pupillary light reflex is normal, as is the funduscopic examination, and the patient may occasionally be unaware that he or she is blind (Anton's syndrome). Patients are often misdiagnosed as having a conversion reaction. Transient cortical blindness occurs most often in basilar artery insufficiency but is also seen in hypertensive encephalopathy. Positive visual phenomena (phosphenes, scintillating scotomas) are characteristic of migrainous aura and probably reflect oligemia to the occipital lobes from vasoconstriction. Arteriovenous malformations, tumors, and seizures may produce similar symptoms and should be distinguished from migraine with aura by a careful history and examination as well as by imaging in appropriate cases.

Visual hallucinations are visual sensations independent of external light stimulation; they may be either simple or complex or localized or generalized and occur in patients with a clear or clouded sensorium. Visual illusions are alterations of a perceived external stimulus in which some features are distorted. The simplest visual phenomena consist of flashes of light (photopsias), blue lights (phosphenes), or scintillating zigzag lines, which last a fraction of a second and recur frequently or which appear to be in constant motion. These can arise from dysfunction within the optic pathways at any point from the eye to the cortex. Glaucoma, incipient retinal detachment, retinal ischemia, or macular degeneration can cause simple visual hallucinations based on dysfunction in the eye. Lesions of the occipital lobe are often associated with simple hallucinations; classic migraine is by far the most common condition of this type. Complex visual hallucinations such as seeing objects as people, animals, landscapes, or various indescribable scenes occur most frequently with temporal lobe lesions or parieto-occipital association areas.

Hearing and Its Impairments

SYMPTOMS OF AUDITORY DYSFUNCTION

The main symptoms of lesions within the auditory system are hearing loss and tinnitus. Hearing loss can be classified as conductive, sensorineural, and central based on the anatomic site of pathology (Fig. 119–3). Tinnitus can be either subjective or objective. Conductive hearing loss results from lesions involving the external or middle ear. Patients with a conductive hearing loss can hear speech in a noisy background better than in a quiet background, because they can understand loud speech as well as anyone. The ear often feels full, as if it is blocked. The Weber test localizes to the deaf ear, if the deafness is unilateral.

Sensorineural hearing loss results from lesions of the cochlea or the auditory division of the vestibulocochlear (eighth cranial) nerve. Patients with sensorineural hearing loss often have difficulty hearing speech that is mixed with background noise and may be annoyed by loud speech. They hear low tones better than high-frequency ones. Distortion of sounds is common with sensorineural hearing loss. Central hearing disorders are rare and result from bilateral lesions of the central auditory pathways, including the cochlear and dorsal olivary nuclear complexes, inferior colliculi, medial geniculate bodies, and auditory cortex in the temporal lobes. Damage to both auditory cortices may result in pure word deafness, in which patients are selectively unable to discriminate language but may be able to hear nonverbal sounds.

Tinnitus is a noise or ringing in the ear that is usually audible only to the patient (subjective), although, rarely, an examiner can hear the sound as well. The latter, so-called objective tinnitus, can be heard when the examining physician places a stethoscope against the patient's external auditory canal. Tinnitus that is pulsatory and synchronous with the heart beat suggests a vascular abnormality within the head or neck (Fig. 119–4). Aneurysms, arteriovenous malformations, and vascular tumors can produce this type of tinnitus.

Subjective tinnitus, heard only by the patient, can result from lesions involving the external ear canal, tympanic membrane, ossicles, cochlea, auditory nerve, brain stem, and cortex. The character of the tinnitus does not usually aid in determining the site of the disturbance. For this, one must rely on associated symptoms and signs. When tinnitus results from a lesion of the external or middle ear, it is usually accompanied by a conductive hearing loss. The patient may complain that his or her voice sounds hollow and that other sounds are muffled. Because the masking effect of ambient noise is lost, the patient may be disturbed by normal muscular sounds such as chewing, tight closure of the eyes, or clenching of the jaws. The characteristic tinnitus associated with Meniere's syndrome is low pitched and continuous, although fluctuating in intensity. Often, the tinnitus becomes very loud immediately preceding an acute attack of vertigo and then may disappear after the attack. Tinnitus resulting from lesions within the central nervous system is usually not associated with hearing loss but is nearly always associated with other neurologic symptoms and signs. Salicylate toxicity frequently results in tinnitus.

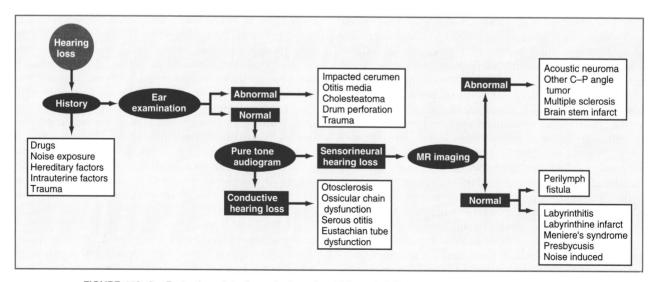

FIGURE 119–3   Evaluation of deafness (unilateral and bilateral). MR = magnetic resonance. (Modified from Baloh RW: Hearing and equilibrium. *In* Goldman L, Bennett JC [eds]: Cecil Textbook of Medicine, 21st ed. Philadelphia, WB Saunders, 1998, p 2250.)

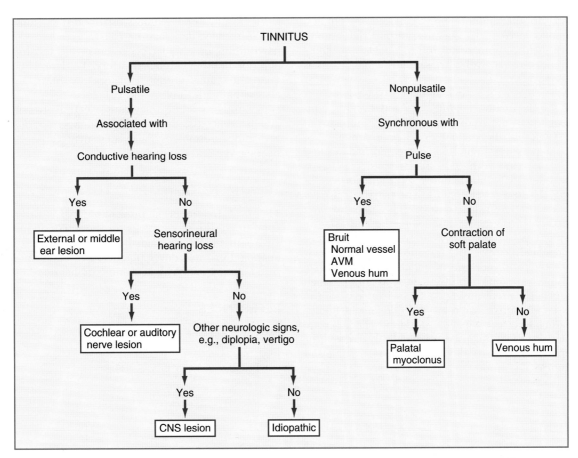

FIGURE 119-4   Algorithm for the approach to the patient with tinnitus. AVM = arteriovenous malformation; CNS = central nervous system.

EXAMINATION OF THE AUDITORY SYSTEM

A quick test for hearing loss in the speech range is to observe the response to spoken commands at different intensities (whisper, conversation, and shouting). The examiner must be careful to prevent the patient from reading his or her lip movement. A high-frequency stimulus such as a watch tick should also be used, because sensorineural disorders often involve only the higher frequencies. Tuning fork tests permit a rough assessment of the hearing level for pure tones of known frequency. The Rinne test compares the patient's hearing by air conduction with that by bone conduction. A 512-cps tuning fork is first held against the mastoid process until the sound fades. It is then placed 1 inch from the ear. Normal subjects can hear the fork about twice as long by air conduction as by bone conduction. If hearing by bone conduction is longer than by air conduction, a conductive hearing loss is suggested. Weber's test compares the patient's hearing by bone conduction in the two ears. The fork is placed at the center of the forehead, and the patient is asked where he or she hears the tone. Normal subjects hear it in the center of the head, patients with unilateral conductive loss hear it on the affected side, and patients with unilateral sensorineural loss hear it on the side opposite the loss. Otoscopic examination may reveal impacted cerumen as a cause of conductive hearing loss.

CAUSES OF HEARING LOSS

The bilateral hearing loss commonly associated with advancing age is called *presbycusis*. Presbycusis is not a distinct disease entity but rather represents multiple effects of aging on the auditory system. Presbycusis may include conductive and central dysfunction, although the most consistent effect of aging is on the sensory cells and neurons of the cochlea; as a result, higher tones are lost early.

Otosclerosis is a disease of the bony labyrinth that usually manifests itself by immobilizing the stapes and thereby producing a conductive hearing loss. Seventy percent of patients with clinical otosclerosis notice hearing loss between the ages of 11 and 30. There is a family history of otosclerosis in approximately 50% of cases.

Unilateral hearing loss that progresses slowly is often caused by a lesion of the cerebellopontine angle, such as an *acoustic neuroma*. Acoustic neuromas (vestibular schwannomas) usually begin on the vestibular nerve in the internal auditory canal; they cause symptoms by compressing the nerves in the narrow confines of the canal. By far the most common symptoms associated with acoustic neuromas are slowly progressive hearing loss and tinnitus from compression of the cochlear nerve. Vertigo occurs in fewer than 20% of patients, but approximately 50% complain of imbalance or disequilibrium. Next to the auditory nerve, the most common cranial nerves involved by compression are the seventh and fifth; such compression produces facial weakness and numbness, respectively. Treatment in most cases is surgical removal.

Meniere's syndrome (endolymphatic hydrops) is characterized by fluctuating hearing loss and tinnitus, episodic vertigo, and a sensation of fullness or pressure in the ear. Typically, the patient develops a sensation of fullness and pressure along with decreased hearing and tinnitus in one ear. Vertigo rapidly follows, reaching a maximum intensity within minutes and then slowly subsiding over the next several hours. The patient is usually left with a sense of unsteadiness and dizziness for days after the acute vertiginous episode. In the early stages, the hearing loss is completely reversible, but in later stages a residual hearing loss remains. Patients with idiopathic Meniere's syndrome frequently have a positive family history (in some reports as high as 50%), which suggests genetic predisposing factors. The key to the diagnosis of Meniere's syndrome is to document fluctuating hearing levels in a patient with the characteristic clinical history. The mainstay of medical therapy for endolymphatic hydrops is dietary sodium restriction and oral diuretics.

Acute unilateral deafness usually results from damage to the cochlea and may be caused by viral or bacterial labyrinthitis or vascular occlusion in the territory of the anterior inferior cerebellar artery. Perilymphatic fistulas may also cause abrupt unilateral deafness, usually in association with tinnitus and vertigo.

A number of drugs may cause acute irreversible bilateral hearing loss: these include aminoglycosides, cisplatin, and furosemide. Salicylates may cause reversible hearing loss and tinnitus.

TREATMENT OF HEARING LOSS

The best treatment is prevention, particularly by the appropriate use of ear plugs for those working in a noisy environment. Hearing aids help patients with conductive hearing loss, and developments with cochlear implants may help patients with sensorineural hearing loss.

REFERENCES

Baloh RW: Dizziness, Hearing Loss, and Tinnitus. Philadelphia: FA Davis, 1998.
Brazis PW, Masdeu JC, Biller J: Localization in Clinical Neurology, 3rd ed. Boston: Little, Brown, 1996.

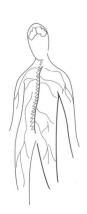

120

DIZZINESS

Roger P. Simon

Dizziness is a nonspecific term that includes *vertigo* (definite rotational sensation), *presyncope* (lightheadedness, impending fainting, dimming of vision), instability, and *disequilibrium* (impaired balance or gait). The symptom can be caused by peripheral or central vestibular disorders (vertigo), systemic or cardiovascular disorders producing impaired cerebral blood flow (presyncope), neurologic disorders producing disordered sensory input into the brain (disequilibrium), or hyperventilation (Table 120–1).

Approach to the Diagnosis

The physician should separate presyncope by history and examination. Its cause may be cardiac arrhythmia, outflow obstruction, or orthostatic hypotension. Its symptoms are wooziness or giddiness, disequilibrium without true vertigo, global weakness, and, finally, dimming of vision. Cardiac causes are suggested by events occurring when the patient is in the recumbent position and/or during exercise. The physician can eliminate a diagnosis of orthostatic hypotension by positional blood pressure examinations. The diagnosis of hyperventilation can be excluded by asking the patient to compare the symptoms of dizziness with those induced by hyperventilation (3 minutes).

VERTIGO

Vertigo is an illusory sense of unidirectional rotational movement. With eyes open, the patient sees the environment move (in a direction opposite the slow component of nystagmus), and with the eyes closed, the patient feels a turning or whirling sensation in space. Both vertigo and nystagmus have characteristics that point to a central or a peripheral cause (Tables 120–2 and 120–3). Peripheral (i.e., vestibular) disorders may be disabling (e.g., severe vertigo with vomiting), but they are rarely life-threatening. Central nervous system disorders may produce only mild symptoms, but those symptoms

may progress to central nervous system dysfunction (e.g., multiple sclerosis) or even death (e.g., basilar artery stroke).

Nystagmus

If the vertigo is peripheral in origin, *nystagmus* is invariably present; the fast phase is directed away from the affected ear. Thus, if the patient has the symptom of vertigo at the moment of the examination and has no nystagmus, then the cause is central. If nystagmus is present and a disassociation of nystagmoid movement exists between the two eyes or if the nystagmus is purely vertical, a central cause is again determined.

Peripheral Vertigo

Acute peripheral vestibular disorders produce acute vertigo, nausea, and vomiting. The patient appears ill, typi-

TABLE 120–1 Common Causes of Dizziness

Cause	Frequency (%)
Peripheral vestibular disorders*	38
Hyperventilation	23
Multiple sensory deficits†	13
Psychiatric disorders	9
Uncertain	9
Brain stem stroke	5
Other neurologic disorders‡	4
Cardiovascular disorders	4
Multiple sclerosis	2
Visual disorders	2
Other	2

N = 104.
* Benign positional vertigo most common.
† Gait apraxia, Parkinson's disease, temporal lobectomy.
‡ Peripheral neuropathy, cervical spondylosis, vestibular abnormalities, visual impairment.
Data from Drachman DA, Hart CW: An approach to the dizzy patient. Neurology 1972; 22:323.

925

TABLE 120–2   Symptoms Suggestive of Central Versus Peripheral Vertigo

Symptom or Sign	Peripheral	Central
Severity	4+	1–4+
Onset	Sudden	Nonparoxysmal
Nausea and vomiting	Common	Uncommon
Nystagmus	*Always* present	Present or absent
Tinnitus and hearing loss	Often present	Vary rare
Visual fixation	Inhibits	No effect

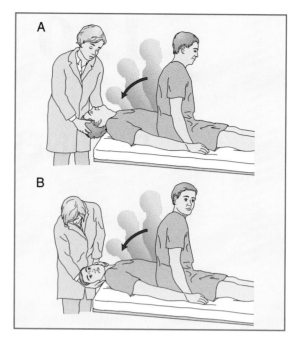

FIGURE 120–1   Nylen Bárány or Dix-Hallpike maneuver to test for position nystagmus. The patient is seated on an examining table with head and eyes directed forward *(A)* and is then quickly lowered to the supine position with the head over the table edge, 45 degrees below the horizontal. The patient is instructed to keep eyes open; nystagmus is observed for, and the patient is asked to report vertigo. When the test is positive, the affected ear is down; the fast phase of nystagmus beats toward the affected ear. The test is repeated with the patient's head turned to the right *(B)* and again to the left. (From Simon RP, et al: Clinical Neurology, 4th ed. Stamford, CT: Appleton & Lange, 1999.)

cally lies on one side with the affected ear upward, and is reluctant to move the head. Horizontal nystagmus with the fast phase directed away from the affected ear is always present.

Vestibular neuronitis refers to repetitive attacks of peripheral vertigo without auditory dysfunction. *Labyrinthitis* is the phenomenon of severe acute vertigo, with autonomic symptoms, in the setting of otitis or viremia. *Peripheral vestibulopathy* refers to recurrent attacks of vertigo in any age group with other neurologic symptoms and with a normal neurologic examination. These various terms are based on unverifiable inferences about the site of disease and the pathogenetic mechanism.

Positional vertigo is extremely common and is most often described as severe vertigo induced by the maneuver of moving from upright to recumbent posture and/or rolling over in bed. The symptom of vertigo and the sign of nystagmus are reproduced by Nylen Bárány or Dix-Hallpike maneuver (Fig. 120–1). The syndrome is caused by freely moving debris within the semicircular canals of the vestibular system. The syndrome can be treated by repositioning maneuvers (see Fig. 120–2). *Positional nystagmus* occurs when the head is placed in the provocative position. This condition must be differentiated from the exacerbation of vertigo by head movement (head movements make all vertigo symptoms worse).

The most common positional nystagmus, termed *benign paroxysmal positional nystagmus*, usually has a 3- to 10-second latency before onset and rarely lasts longer than 15 seconds. The nystagmus is always torsional and is prominent in only one head-hanging position (see Fig. 120–1). Another key feature is fatigability, in which the vertigo and nystagmus disappear with repeated positioning. In most patients, benign paroxysmal positional vertigo occurs as an isolated symptom of unknown cause; it may follow head injury, viral labyrinthitis, or occlusion of the vasculature to the inner ear. The diagnosis is made clinically, with the typical history of abrupt-onset positional vertigo, nausea, and disequilibrium.

Other causes of peripheral vertigo include *Meniere's disease*, an uncommon disorder of vertiginous spells on the background of progressive unilateral hearing loss and tinnitus. *Acoustic neuromas* are extremely rare causes of vertigo; they present most often with hearing loss, tinnitus, and unsteadiness.

TABLE 120–3   Characteristics of Central Versus Peripheral Nystagmus

Characteristic	Peripheral	Central
Direction	Usually horizontal, may have rotary component	Any direction (pure vertical is always central)
Symmetry between eyes	Always symmetric	Dissociation between eyes possible
Lesion side	Fast component away from injured labyrinth	No relation between direction and lesion location
Duration of problem	Minutes to weeks	Days to years
Visual fixation	Decreases	No effect

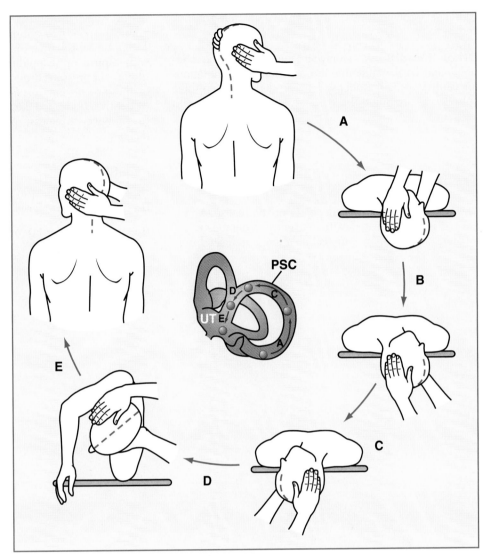

FIGURE 120—2 Repositioning treatment for benign positional vertigo designed to move endolymphatic debris out of the posterior semicircular canal (PSC) of the right ear and into the utricle (UT). The patient is seated, and the head is turned 45 degrees to the right (*A*). The head is lowered rapidly to below the horizontal (*B*). The examiner shifts hand positions (*C*), and the patient's head is rotated rapidly 90 degrees in the opposite direction, so it now points 45 degrees to the left, where it remains for 30 seconds (*D*). The patient then rolls onto the left side without turning the head in relation to the body and maintains this position for another 30 seconds (*E*) before sitting up. The treatment is repeated until nystagmus is abolished. The procedure is reversed for treating the left ear. The patient must avoid the supine position for 2 days. (Adapted from Foster CA, Baloh RW: Episodic vertigo. *In* Rakel RE [ed]: Conn's Current Therapy. Philadelphia: WB Saunders, 1995.)

Central Vertigo

Cerebrovascular Disease. Vertigo can be the presenting sign of *vertebral basilar ischemia,* but vertiginous episodes continuing for more than 6 weeks without other symptoms or signs of a nervous system dysfunction are rarely caused by cerebral ischemia. Cerebral ischemia producing vertigo is in the vertebral basilar distribution. Therefore, carotid Doppler studies are not indicated for this symptom in isolation. Computed tomography of the brain is rarely useful because the brain stem is poorly seen with this technique. Magnetic resonance imaging may show areas of ischemic injury in the brain stem or cerebellum or low flow through the vertebral basilar system.

The sudden onset of dizziness with vomiting, disequilibrium, and truncal ataxia is a common manifestation of *cerebellar hemorrhage or infarction.* Nystagmus is uncommon. Computed tomography enables one to make the diagnosis. *Cerebellar swelling* can produce brain stem compression and death. Surgical decompression is a life-saving procedure.

Vertigo is a common symptom in patients with infarction of the lateral brain stem, which is supplied by the posterior inferior cerebellar artery *(Wallenberg's syndrome).* Characteristic findings include vertigo, ipsilateral facial pain, diplopia, dysphagia, and dysphonia. The diagnosis is confirmed by the neurologic examination, which discloses unilateral Horner's syndrome, ipsi-

TABLE 120-4 **Treatment of Vertigo**

Vestibular Suppressants (Peripheral)*
Meclizine (12.5–25 mg q6h)
Dimenhydrinate (50 mg q6h)
Promethazine (25 mg q6h)

Vestibular Suppressants (Central)*
Low-dose diazepam (2 mg q4–6h) or oxazepam (10–15 mg q6h)
Antiemetics added as needed

* May be more effective in combination.

lateral facial hypesthesia with contralateral sensory loss, and nystagmus.

Other Conditions. Demyelinating disease, mass lesions, and basilar migraine are additional considerations for central vertigo. Epilepsy may produce brief episodic episodes of disequilibrum or a sensation of rotation with "absences."

Treatment

The treatment of vertigo depends on the cause. Meniere's disease is treated with diuretics; spontaneous remissions are common. Surgical ablation is indicated only in severe persistent cases. Vertigo in patients with migraine responds to antimigrainous therapy (see Chapter 118). Vertebrobasilar insufficiency should be treated with aspirin or ticlopidine. For peripheral vertigo, vestibular suppressant drugs may be helpful (Table 120–4), or the patient may respond to desensitization techniques (repetitive body and head rotations and tilts, adequate to produce dizziness, performed two to three times daily).

REFERENCES

Baloh RW: Vertigo. Lancet 1998; 352:1841–1846.
Debery MJ: The diagnosis and treatment of dizziness. Med Clin North Am 1999; 83:13–17.
Halmagyi GM, Cremer PD: Assessment and treatment of dizziness. J Neurol Neurosurg Psychiat 2000; 168:129–134.

121

DISORDERS OF THE MOTOR SYSTEM

Frederick J. Marshall

The human voluntary motor system originates in the motor areas of the frontal lobe cortex, which send their output caudally in the corticospinal tract. The basal ganglia and cerebellum have additional integrating, postural, reinforcing, and coordinating influences (Fig. 121–1). Descending influences from the red nuclei, vestibular nuclei, and brain stem reticular formation converge with descending corticospinal pathways on bulbospinal motor neurons to activate integrated, functionally automatic motor programs. At every level, afferent feedback provides input from muscle, nerve, spinal segment, brain stem, cerebellum, basal ganglia, and cortex to guide the efferent messages from the motor cortex. Figures 121–2 and 121–3 indicate the corticobasal ganglia and corticocerebellar loops that unconsciously precede movement.

Disease can affect selectively every level of the motor system from brain to muscle. Table 121–1 lists the anatomic locations of diseases affecting the motor system.

Symptoms and Signs of Motor System Disease

The patient with motor system disease usually complains of difficulty with accomplishing specific tasks. Patients with a central nervous system (CNS) disorder (see Table 121–1) typically have difficulty with coordination, balance, and rapid movements. Muscle strength is frequently normal, and muscle atrophy (wasting) is usually lacking. Muscle tone is usually increased, characterized by spasticity or rigidity. Patients with a peripheral nervous system (PNS) disorder (see Table 121–1) usually complain of difficulty with tasks: if weakness is proximal, this includes activities such as climbing or descending stairs, rising from a chair, or lifting heavy objects above the head. If weakness is distal, the patient complains of stumbling and tripping or of having problems fastening buttons or opening locks or doors with the hands.

The patient with weakness of gradual onset may not recognize it, emphasizing the useful axiom that "signs of muscle weakness precede symptoms of weakness." Words such as "numbness," "deadness," "tiredness," or "fatigue" may be used by a patient with weakness who is unfamiliar with what is taking place. In contrast, when a patient has complaints of "weakness," it often results from systemic rather than neurologic disease. In such patients, strength is often normal or only mildly reduced, because the complaint is usually loss of stamina and endurance. The patient with a complaint of fatigue should be asked to distinguish between true weakness and the less specific symptoms of lassitude and asthenia. If the patient is unable to perform a specific normal activity, true weakness is suggested. Objective evidence of weakness is established if symptoms exceed the boundaries of normal variation (e.g., double vision, drooping eyelids, difficulty in swallowing, repeated aspiration of food or liquids into the airway) as opposed to the more subjective complaints of inability to lift, carry, or push an object.

CNS motor disorders (see Table 121–1) can result from focal brain or spinal cord disease such as occurs with stroke, tumor, or inflammatory or demyelinating disease, each of which is covered in specific chapters elsewhere in this text. CNS motor disorders can also be the result of a widespread, nonfocal "system" degeneration, which is considered in this chapter. Focal brain disease usually produces abnormalities on neuroimaging procedures. System degeneration, on the other hand, seldom produces detectable abnormalities on neuroimaging and other neurodiagnostic tests until long after patients first report symptoms and have signs of abnormal function on examination.

Corticospinal diseases from system degeneration are uncommon and are characterized by upper motor neuron signs: spasticity and hyperreflexia. The most common is amyotrophic lateral sclerosis, which differs from other CNS motor diseases by the prominent involvement of both CNS and PNS. The hereditary spastic

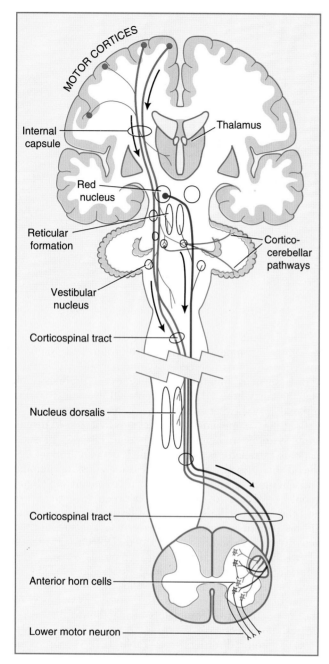

FIGURE 121–1　Normal human voluntary motor system.

paraplegias are rare, usually hereditary diseases with only upper motor neuron signs.

Movement Disorders and Ataxia

Central motor systems are divided into three constituents: pyramidal, extrapyramidal, and cerebellar. The pyramidal system (named for the pyramidal cross-section of fiber tracts in the medulla) is the major outflow from motor cortex to spinal cord. Lesions of the pyramidal system cause motor weakness (paresis), spasticity, and hyperreflexia. Although lesions of this system disturb

motor function, they are not considered "movement disorders." Movement disorders are caused by extrapyramidal or cerebellar dysfunction. The term *extrapyramidal* refers to the basal ganglia and their projections. The main components of the extrapyramidal system are noted in Table 121–2, and their major interconnections are depicted in Figure 121–4.

The basal ganglia receive input from the cortex and give feedback to the cortex through projections from the thalamus. Multiple neurotransmitters are involved in complex feedback loops. The basal ganglia modulate not only motor cortical activity but also the activity of association cortex, particularly in the frontal lobes. Many "movement disorders" therefore involve complex neurobehavioral symptoms (e.g., dementia in Huntington's disease, attentional deficits and obsessive-compulsive behavior in Tourette's disorder, depression in Parkinson's disease). Clinicoanatomic correlations between lesions in a component of the system and development of a characteristic movement disorder or neurobehavioral syndrome remain elusive. An exception is hemiballismus, a dramatic flailing movement of the extremities on one side of the body usually caused by a lesion of the contralateral subthalamic nucleus. Neurosurgical interventions designed to ablate or stimulate specific nuclei and neuropharmacologic treatments designed to modulate selective receptor systems are increasingly widespread.

Movement disorders entail not enough movement (hypokinesia) or too much movement (hyperkinesia). Table 121–3 outlines the hypokinetic disorders in the differential diagnosis of akinetic-rigid syndromes. The disorders listed in Table 121–3 cause progressive immobility. Rigidity refers to increased muscular tone throughout the range of motion. It does not vary with passive acceleration of the limb by the examiner. Lead-pipe rigidity connotes the ductile quality of metal being passively bent. Cogwheel rigidity is the superimposition of tremor on underlying rigidity. Paratonic rigidity or paratonia refers to a velocity-dependent resistance to passive movement. Such resistance increases as one increases the speed of passive limb displacement. Para-

TABLE 121–1　Anatomic Classification of Motor Systems Disease: Principal Disorders of the Motor System from Proximal to Distal

Central Nervous System
Corticospinal diseases (disorders of the upper motor neuron)
Extrapyramidal movement disorders
Cerebellar ataxias
Spinal cord diseases

Peripheral Nervous System
Radiculopathies and lower motor neuron diseases
Peripheral nerve disorders
　Polyneuropathy
　Focal neuropathy
Neuromuscular junction
　Myasthenia, Lambert-Eaton syndrome, botulism
Muscular

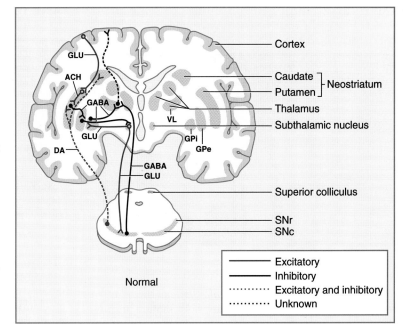

FIGURE 121-2 Anatomy of the basal ganglia and their connections. Note the feedback loop that proceeds from cerebral prefrontal areas to the basal ganglia and eventually back from basal ganglia to thalamus to motor cortex. This ultimately regulates the descending corticospinal motor system. ACH = acetylcholine; DA = dopamine; GABA = γ-aminobutyric acid; GLU = glutamate; GP = globus pallidum (e = external, i = internal); SN = substantia nigra (c = compacta, r = reticulate); VL = ventrolateral. (From Jankovic J: The extrapyramidal disorders: Introduction. *In* Goldman L, Bennett JC [eds]: Cecil Textbook of Medicine, 21st ed. Philadelphia: WB Saunders, 2000, p 2078.)

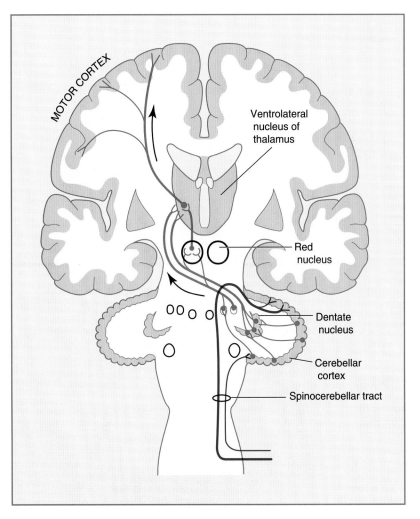

FIGURE 121-3 Corticocerebellar loop.

TABLE 121–2   Major Components of the Basal Ganglia and Extrapyramidal Nervous System

Substantia nigra
  Pars reticulata
  Pars compacta
Striatum
  Caudate
  Putamen
Globus pallidus
  Pars medialis
  Pars lateralis
Subthalamus
Thalamus
  Ventroanterior
  Ventrolateral

TABLE 121–3   Differential Diagnosis of the Akinetic/Rigid Syndrome

Idiopathic Parkinson's disease
Drug-induced parkinsonism
Diffuse Lewy body disease
Progressive supranuclear palsy
Multisystem atrophy
  Olivopontocerebellar atrophy; striatonigral degeneration; Shy-Drager syndrome
Vascular parkinsonism
Other hereditary neurodegenerative disorders: Huntington's disease; Hallervorden-Spatz disease
Toxic parkinsonism: carbon monoxide; manganese; MPTP
Catatonia (psychosis)

tonic patients demonstrate *gegenhalten,* an inability to fully relax a limb for passive range of motion testing. Paratonic patients also demonstrate *mitgehen,* the tendency to "help out" as the examiner attempts to passively move the limb. Paratonia is clinically nonspecific: it is common in patients with diminished cerebral function resulting from a variety of causes. True rigidity always implies basal ganglia dysfunction on the contralateral side.

There are many different hyperkinetic movements (Table 121–4). Accurate identification of these movements is required for proper diagnosis and treatment of

extrapyramidal diseases. For example, chorea occurring in successive generations is most likely caused by Huntington's disease (hereditary chorea). Resting tremor in an elderly patient with rigidity and bradykinesia (slow movement) is most likely caused by Parkinson's disease (paralysis agitans). Action tremor in a patient without rigidity or bradykinesia is most likely caused by essential tremor (a common inherited disorder).

Table 121–5 outlines a number of signs commonly associated with lesions of the cerebellar system. Disorders of proprioceptive function may result in "sensory" ataxia caused by impairment of the spinocerebellar inputs.

The common hypokinetic movement disorders, hyperkinetic movement disorders, and ataxias are discussed as follows.

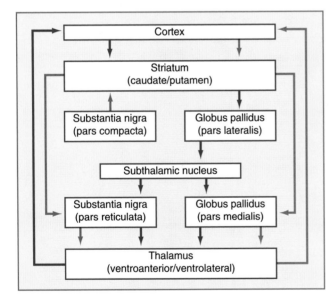

FIGURE 121–4 In this simplified version of the basal ganglia wiring diagram, information flows in one of two ways, either facilitating motor output by means of the "direct" pathway *(red lines)* or inhibiting motor output by means of the "indirect" pathway *(blue lines).* In Parkinson's disease, loss of neurons in the pars compacta of the substantia nigra shifts the balance away from the direct pathway and toward the indirect pathway, resulting in hypokinesia. Conversely, in Huntington's disease, loss of selected neurons in the striatum shifts the balance away from the indirect pathway and toward the direct pathway, resulting in hyperkinesia.

TABLE 121–4   Descriptive Terms of the Hyperkinesias

Asterixis	Transitory loss of motor tone resulting in rapid movement of a joint (the conceptual opposite of myoclonus)
Athetosis	Slow writhing movement
Ballism	Flailing movement (typically unilateral—hemiballism)
Chorea	Irregular flicking, dancelike movement
Choreoathetosis	The combination of chorea and athetosis
Dystonia	Sustained contortion due to excess muscular activity across a joint: generalized, segmental, or focal
Dyskinesia	Nonspecific term for hyperkinesia (generally chorea, athetosis, and dystonia, alone or in combination)
Myoclonus	Rapid jerking muscular movement: multifocal or segmental; rhythmic or irregular
Tic	Semi-suppressible motor or vocal gestural movement (may be simple, such as eye blinking or throat clearing, or complex, such as hopping or swearing)
Tremor	Rhythmic oscillating movement: predominantly at rest or with action

TABLE 121–5 **Signs of Cerebellar System Impairment**

Ataxia	Poorly coordinated, broad-based, lurching gait
Ataxic dysarthria	Abnormal modulation of speech velocity and volume
Dysmetria	Irregular placement of voluntary limb or ocular movement
Hypometria	Movement falling short of the intended target
Hypermetria	Movement overshooting the intended target
Dysdiadochokinesis	Breakdown in precision and completeness of rapid alternating movements (as with a pronation-supination task)
Dysrhythmokinesis	Irregularity of the rhythm of rapid alternating movements or planned movement sequences
Dyssynergia	Inability to perform movement as a coordinated temporal sequence
Hypotonia	Decreased resistance to passive muscular extension (seen immediately after injury to the lateral cerebellum)
Intention tremor	Tremor orthogonal to the direction of intended movement (tends to increase in amplitude as the target is approached)
Titubation	Rhythmic rocking tremor of the trunk and head

Hypokinetic Movement Disorders

IDIOPATHIC PARKINSON'S DISEASE (PARALYSIS AGITANS)

The London physician James Parkinson first described the clinical tetrad of tremor, bradykinesia, rigidity, and postural instability in 1817. These signs remain the diagnostic criteria for Parkinson's disease. Parkinson's disease affects 750,000 to 1 million people in the United States and is a leading cause of neurologic disease in individuals older than 65. Premature death of pigmented dopaminergic neurons in the pars compacta of the substantia nigra is the underlying basis of the disease, but the cause remains unclear. There is neuronal loss in the substantia nigra, with characteristic eosinophilic hyaline intraneuronal inclusions called Lewy bodies. Dopamine containing neurons with cell bodies in the substantia nigra project to the striatum (caudate and putamen), where they synapse on a variety of cell types. Early in the course of the disease, dopamine receptors in the striatum are upregulated in response to decreased dopaminergic input from the substantia nigra. This compensatory ability of the striatum is eventually overwhelmed, and progressive clinical dysfunction ensues.

Symptoms and signs of Parkinson's disease are listed in Table 121–6. The typical patient initially notes unilateral symptoms (characteristically hand tremor, decreased

TABLE 121–6 **Clinical Features of Parkinson's Disease**

Primary Features

Bradykinesia; rest tremor; rigidity; postural instability; therapeutic response to levodopa

Secondary Features

Masked facies (facial hypomimia)
Dysphagia; hypophonia/palilalia; micrographia; stooped posture; festinating gait; start hesitation; dystonic cramps
Autonomic dysfunction: orthostatic hypotension; urinary incontinence; constipation
Behavioral alterations: depression; dementia; sleep disorders including restless legs syndrome
Sensory complaints: aching; numbness; tingling

arm swing, foot dragging, or micrographia). Symptoms and signs subsequently spread to involve both sides. Gradually worsening postural instability ultimately results in wheelchair confinement. Symmetric onset of symptoms and early falls caused by postural instability are atypical of idiopathic Parkinson's disease, whereas they are common in other causes of the akinetic/rigid syndrome outlined in Table 121–3. Tremor may or may not be a prominent feature of idiopathic Parkinson's disease, and it is not usually a prominent feature of other akinetic/rigid disease states.

Treatment of Parkinson's disease is outlined in Table 121–7.

Carbidopa/levodopa (Sinemet) remains the mainstay of treatment for advanced Parkinson's disease. Failure of bradykinesia and rigidity to improve in response to a trial of levodopa treatment raises the possibility of another disease listed in Table 121–3, because these diseases typically involve primary pathology at the level of the striatum rather than the substantia nigra.

Levodopa requires enzymatic conversion to dopamine within substantia nigra neurons. The dopamine agonists

TABLE 121–7 **Medications for Parkinson's Disease**

Anticholinergic agents
　Trihexyphenidyl (Artane)
　Benztropine (Cogentin)
Dopamine precursors (combined with peripheral aromatic-amino-acid-decarboxylase inhibitors)
　Carbidopa/levodopa (Sinemet, Sinemet-CR) (regular and controlled-release forms)
　Benserazide/levodopa (Madopar) (marketed in Europe)
Dopamine agonists
　Bromocriptine (Parlodel)
　Pergolide (Permax)
　Pramipexole (Mirapex)
　Ropinirole (Requip)
Monoamine oxidase type-B (MAO-B) inhibitors
　Selegiline (deprenyl) (Carbex, Eldepryl)
Catechol-*o*-methyltransferase (COMT) inhibitors
　Tolcapone (Tasmar)
　Entacapone (Comtan)

do not compete with other amino acids to cross the blood-brain barrier, require no enzymatic conversion, and act directly at the level of the striatum, bypassing the substantia nigra. There has been concern that treatment with levodopa may eventually provoke motor complications, such as "on-off" fluctuations and dyskinesias. Initiating therapy with dopamine agonists allows the physician to reserve levodopa treatment for later stages of the illness. The amount of levodopa required may be reduced by co-administration with a dopamine agonist in later stages of illness.

Selegiline delays the need for levodopa treatment in patients with early Parkinson's disease. Selegiline inhibits monoamine oxidase type B, an enzyme that breaks down dopamine. Toxic free radicals generated in the normal catabolism of dopamine may damage dopaminergic neurons in the substantia nigra. This may cause Parkinson's disease in patients who are vulnerable as a result of a combination of inherited risk and as yet undetermined environmental exposures. It has been postulated that by inhibiting the formation of free radicals, selegiline may act as a neuroprotective agent. Other monoamine oxidase type B inhibitors are in development.

The newest additions to the list of medications for Parkinson's disease are the catechol-o-methyltransferase (COMT) inhibitors. Like aromatic amino acid decarboxylase, COMT catalyzes the catabolism of levodopa. Co-administration of levodopa with carbidopa and a COMT inhibitor suppresses its peripheral catabolism, maximizing the amount available to cross the blood-brain barrier and prolonging its effective half-life. Tolcapone has been associated with rare but potentially lethal liver toxicity; the hepatic function of patients undergoing treatment with this drug must be regularly monitored.

Because the underlying rationale of drug treatments for Parkinson's disease is to enhance dopaminergic neurotransmission, most antiparkinson drugs have unwanted dopaminergic side effects. These include nausea, orthostatic hypotension, hallucinations, psychosis, and dyskinesia (abnormal involuntary hyperkinetic movements such as chorea and dystonia). Management of progressive Parkinson's disease requires a careful balance between the potential beneficial effects of medication and these potential side effects.

DRUG-INDUCED PARKINSONISM

The most common cause of drug-induced parkinsonism is treatment with neuroleptic medication. A number of other agents may provoke a bradykinetic/rigid syndrome (Table 121-8).

DIFFUSE LEWY BODY DISEASE

Lewy body disease may be classified into three types based on the pathologic distribution of underlying Lewy bodies: brain stem, transitional, and diffuse. When Lewy bodies are restricted to the brain stem, there is no clinical or pathologic difference between Lewy body disease and Parkinson's disease. In the transitional phase,

TABLE 121-8 Drugs Causing Bradykinesia/Rigidity

Established
Neuroleptics (virtually all phenothiazines, butyrophenones, others)
Metoclopramide
Reserpine

Reported
Lithium
Phenytoin
Angiotensin-converting enzyme inhibitors

Lewy bodies spread to involve the limbic system. In diffuse Lewy body disease, there is clinical parkinsonism combined with early and prominent dementia. Visual hallucinations are common, patients may be extremely sensitive to the adverse effects of neuroleptic medication, and cognitive fluctuations occur (see Chapter 115).

PROGRESSIVE SUPRANUCLEAR PALSY

In the early 1960s, Steele, Richardson, and Olszewski described a series of patients who presented with gait disturbance, unheralded falls, bradykinesia, and rigidity. Unlike patients with idiopathic Parkinson's disease, patients with progressive supranuclear palsy typically do not have tremor. There is progressive loss of voluntary eye movements with preservation of oculocephalic reflex eye movements (the hallmark of a supranuclear eye movement abnormality). Patients develop dementia, pseudobulbar affect (affective lability without normal underlying emotional content), and frontal release signs. Progression is faster than in patients with idiopathic Parkinson's disease, and symptomatic response to dopaminergic agents is poor. The cause of progressive supranuclear palsy remains unknown. There are neurofibrillary tangles with neuronal loss and gliosis involving the globus pallidus, subthalamic nucleus, substantia nigra, pons, oculomotor complex, medulla, and dentate nucleus of the cerebellum.

MULTISYSTEM ATROPHY

Three entities are included under the rubric *multisystem atrophy* (see Table 121-3). Each involves progressive loss of neurons in particular brain regions or nuclei, and each may occur sporadically or as a familial condition. Presentation depends on the particular nuclei affected, but all eventually progress to a profoundly akinetic/rigid state. In olivopontocerebellar atrophy the predominant early symptoms are cerebellar dysmetria and ataxia, with abnormalities of vocal modulation, appendicular coordination, and smooth pursuit eye movements. There is dramatic and progressive loss of neurons in the olivary nucleus of the medulla, the pons, and the cerebellum, giving rise to characteristic atrophy of these regions on computed tomography (CT) or magnetic resonance imaging (MRI). In striatonigral degeneration there is predominant bradykinesia, symmetric rigidity, and postural instability relatively early on, typically without prominent resting tremor. These symptoms are relatively refractory to levodopa treatment—a clue to differentiating them from similar symptoms caused by idiopathic Parkinson's disease. In Shy-Drager syndrome, bradykinesia, rigidity, and postural instability are combined with early and prominent loss of autonomic function. Severe orthostatic hypotension results in syncopal events. There may be cardiac arrhythmias, urinary incontinence, constipation, diarrhea, sudomotor instability, and disordered central temperature regulation.

VASCULAR PARKINSONISM

Vascular parkinsonism is a controversial entity because its findings are variable and its pathogenesis is ill defined. Patients have signs of Parkinson's disease and have microangiopathic changes in the basal ganglia that cause periventricular high T2-weighted signals on MRI. However, such changes are commonly seen on MR images from older individuals, regardless of whether they have bradykinesia and rigidity. Vascular parkinsonism is often diagnosed whenever there are known vascular risk factors and clinical evidence of parkinsonism accompanied by periventricular white matter lesions by MRI. The diagnosis is supported by a lack of improvement with levodopa therapy or overt evidence of stroke involving the basal ganglia.

TOXIC PARKINSONISM

Carbon monoxide intoxication may cause bilateral necrosis of the basal ganglia, leading to an akinetic/rigid state. Chronic exposure to manganese has also been associated with the development of parkinsonism. An intriguing clue to a possible toxic basis for idiopathic Parkinson's disease was discovered in the 1970s with the report of a series of formerly asymptomatic individuals who developed bradykinesia, postural instability, tremor, and rigidity after exposure to the designer street drug methylphenyl-tetrahydropyridine (MPTP). Selective uptake of this agent into pigmented cells of the substantia nigra, with conversion by monoamine oxidase type B to the toxic free radical MPP+, accounts for selective cell death of dopaminergic neurons. MPTP has been widely studied in animal models of Parkinson's disease.

Hyperkinetic Movement Disorders

ESSENTIAL TREMOR

The most common cause of tremor is essential tremor. This condition is inherited and ranges in severity from cosmetic to disabling. Unlike the tremor of Parkinson's disease, essential tremor typically affects both sides of the body symmetrically and is more prominent with action than at rest. The frequency of the tremor oscilla-

tion is relatively constant, but the amplitude may vary. As with all forms of tremor, stress, sleep deprivation, and stimulants (e.g., caffeine) make the condition worse. Alcohol relieves essential tremor. When essential tremor occurs in the context of a dominant family history, it is called familial tremor. Essential tremor starts somewhat earlier than Parkinson's disease and may affect the neck and head muscles, the voice, as well as the arms and hands. The most useful medications for essential tremor include propranolol (Inderal) and primidone (Mysoline).

OTHER CAUSES OF TREMOR

Parkinson's tremor is worst at rest, is somewhat slower than essential tremor, and responds best to anticholinergic treatment rather than to medications for essential tremor. Cerebellar tremor has a more irregular rhythm, is coarser than either essential tremor or the tremor of Parkinson's disease, and is more marked as the limb approaches a target (intention tremor). So-called rubral tremor is an extremely coarse tremor with marked intention dysmetria that occurs with lesions in the area of the red nucleus in the mesencephalon. Numerous drugs can provoke tremor, including stimulants (theophylline, methylphenidate), dopamine receptor–blocking drugs, lithium, tricyclic antidepressants, anticonvulsants (valproate, phenytoin, carbamazepine), cardiac agents (amiodarone, calcium channel blockers, procainamide), and immunosuppressive agents (cyclosporin A, corticosteroids).

DYSTONIA

Dystonia consists of sustained muscle contractions that result in abnormal postures and contortions. It may occur as a primary process or as a secondary symptom of an underlying neurologic disease (e.g., Wilson's disease, Huntington's disease, cerebral anoxia). Derangements in the physiology of the dopamine synapse may lead to acute drug-induced dystonic reactions. Such reactions can be life threatening if respiratory function is compromised, but they generally respond to emergent treatment with anticholinergic medication. Metoclopramide (Reglan), commonly prescribed for nausea and vomiting, may induce dystonia.

Although the primary dystonias presumably involve basal ganglia dysfunction, no underlying structural pathology has been convincingly documented. Mutations of the *DYT* gene on chromosome 9 have been defined in some families with generalized dystonia. Five percent to 10% of cases of primary generalized dystonia are responsive to treatment with levodopa (dopa-responsive dystonia), and all patients presenting with symptoms of generalized dystonia should receive a therapeutic trial of levodopa.

There are a large number of common focal dystonias that were once considered emotional disorders: writer's cramp, spasmodic dysphonia, and torticollis (Table 121–9). Intramuscular injection of botulinum toxin is the treatment of choice for symptomatic control of focal dystonia.

TABLE 121–9 **Features of the Primary Dystonias**

Feature	Description
Generalized (usually childhood onset, autosomal dominant with variable penetrance)	
Idiopathic torsion dystonia	Intorsion of a foot, followed by progressive spread of dystonia to involve the muscles of the limbs, trunk, neck, and face.
Dopa-responsive dystonia	As above, with bradykinesia and rigidity common and hyperreflexia in 25%. Dramatic response to low-dose levodopa (50–200 mg).
Focal (usually adult onset, sporadic)	
Spasmodic torticollis	Involuntary contraction of neck musculature resulting in various combinations of twisting, tilting, extension, or flexion.
Meige's syndrome	Lower facial/mandibular dystonia with dyskinetic movements of tongue and lips.
Blepharospasm	Involuntary forced eyelid closure.
Spasmodic dysphonia	Dystonic vocal cord contraction resulting in hoarse or breathy whisper.
Writer's cramp	Task-specific contortion of hand/forearm when attempting to write.

WILSON'S DISEASE

Wilson's disease is a rare (approximately 1 per 40,000 births) but treatable autosomal recessive disorder that is debilitating and eventually fatal if untreated. It should be considered in the differential diagnosis of new-onset hyperkinesia or parkinsonism in a young adult. Wilson's disease almost never presents after the age of 50. Like many movement disorders, Wilson's disease may also present with neuropsychiatric manifestations. Psychosis is common. The disease is a systemic disorder of copper metabolism. In addition to the neurologic signs and symptoms, there are variable degrees of hepatic dysfunction (including death from fulminant hepatic failure). All young adult patients presenting with a movement disorder should be screened for Wilson's disease by means of a ceruloplasmin level. In suspected patients, slit lamp examination for Kayser-Fleischer rings (characteristic depositions of copper pigment in the limbus of the iris), 24-hour urine collection for copper, determination of serum copper level, and hepatic biopsy are indicated. Treatment with copper chelation and zinc can arrest further neurologic decline and occasionally improves neurologic deficits. Mobilization of copper from liver stores can result in neurologic worsening during initial treatment with standard chelation regimens. Patients should be referred to experienced centers for initiation of treatment.

HUNTINGTON'S DISEASE

Huntington's disease is an inexorably progressive autosomal dominant neurodegenerative disorder affecting motor function, cognition, and behavior. The mean age at onset is 40 (10% of cases begin in childhood), and the mean duration of illness is 20 years. In the adult-onset form, chorea affects the limbs and trunk. Other movement abnormalities commonly occur, including dystonia, rigidity, postural instability, and myoclonus. Bradykinesia and rigidity predominate in the juvenile-onset form. Eye movements are often abnormal early in the disease with slowing of saccadic initiation and velocity and eventual breakdown of smooth pursuit movements. The disease involves premature death of selected neurons in the caudate and putamen.

There is an abnormal expansion in the number of trinucleotide CAG repeat sequences in a 350-kd gene on chromosome 4, coding for the protein huntingtin. Excessive CAG sequences encode an overly expanded number of polyglutamine repeats in the protein. There is currently no treatment that slows progression of Huntington's disease. Downregulation of dopaminergic neurotransmission by means of neuroleptics may suppress chorea but often worsens underlying postural instability and rigidity. Treating depression and psychosis may enhance patients' quality of life. Use of antenatal diagnosis and presymptomatic genetic testing of adult patients at risk for the disease raises ethical and personal questions. Presymptomatic testing of at-risk children is not indicated.

OTHER CAUSES OF CHOREA

Sydenham's chorea occurs in childhood as a postinfectious complication of group A β-hemolytic streptococcal pharyngitis. The illness is usually self-limited, but prolonged chorea may occur, as may neuropsychiatric symptoms. The caudate and subthalamic nuclei are affected, presumably on an autoimmune basis. Some patients respond to a short course of corticosteroids.

A number of drugs occasionally cause chorea, including isoniazid, lithium, oral contraceptives, and reserpine. Metabolic causes include thyrotoxicosis, hypoparathyroidism, and hypomagnesemia. Hemichorea may result from stroke or tumor, and autoimmune or vascular mechanisms may underlie the chorea sometimes observed in patients with lupus erythematosus.

MYOCLONUS

Myoclonus occurs in many neurologic disorders, but it may also occur in isolation. *Physiologic* (hypnagogic) *myoclonus* occurs in normal people as they fall asleep. *Essential myoclonus* is a nonprogressive, generalized disorder that can occur as an autosomal dominant trait. Patients suffer from multifocal large-amplitude lightning jerks that are provoked by action and are disabling, or they may have mild, small amplitude jerks that do not disrupt their function. Patients with essential myoclonus almost always also have some degree of underlying dystonia. Myoclonus also occurs in generalized epilepsy syndromes that are not inherently progressive (e.g., benign myoclonus of infancy, juvenile myoclonic epilepsy) or in tonic-clonic epilepsy and progressive encephalopathy (progressive myoclonic encephalopathy). Static myoclonic encephalopathy occurs most commonly as a consequence of severe anoxia (Lance Adams syndrome) or head trauma and may be spontaneous or action-induced, multifocal, or generalized. Secondary causes of focal or multifocal myoclonus include underlying structural lesions of the nervous system (stroke, arteriovenous malformation, demyelinating disease, tumor, abscess, or other infectious process) or toxic-metabolic conditions (hypoxia, uremia, hepatic encephalopathy, sepsis, electrolyte disturbances, and hormonal abnormalities). Treatment should be directed to the underlying cause. Valproate or clonazepam are commonly prescribed for symptomatic treatment of myoclonus.

TOURETTE'S DISORDER

In 1885, Gilles de la Tourette described a series of patients with motor and vocal tics, some of whom had coprolalia (foul language). For most of the ensuing century, Tourette's disorder was considered a rare curiosity, existing on the border zone of neurology and psychiatry. In the past decade there has been an increasing recognition that, while coprolalia is an uncommon manifestation, Tourette's disorder and the related primary tic disorders (chronic motor tics, chronic vocal tics, and transient tic disorder) are common entities. A substantial proportion of children with learning disorders have Tourette's disorder.

Transitory tics are a normal part of child development. Tourette's disorder is defined as the history of both motor and vocal tics (for more than a year) with onset before age 18. The tics are associated with obsessions and compulsive behavior in 50% of cases and are accompanied by attention deficit disorder in 50% of cases. Tourette's disorder is probably an autosomal dominant condition with variable penetrance.

Treatment focuses on the most functionally incapacitating aspect of the disorder (not necessarily the tics), and patients and families should be reassured that the disorder is not progressive or fatal. Approximately two thirds of patients outgrow their tics (but not necessarily the other neuropsychiatric manifestations of the illness)

TABLE 121–10 Medications Used in the Management of Incapacitating Tourette's Disorder

Tics
Neuroleptics (haloperidol, pimozide, others)
Clonidine (oral or transdermal patch)
Calcium channel blockers (diltiazem, verapamil)
Benzodiazepines (clonazepam, others)

Obsessive-Compulsive Behavior
Selective serotonin reuptake inhibitors (fluoxetine, sertraline, others)
Clomipramine

Attention Deficit Disorder
Stimulants (methylphenidate, pemoline)
Clonidine
Selegiline
Tricyclic antidepressants

by adulthood. Useful medications are outlined in Table 121–10. Strategies to reduce stress on the patient, including education of parents, peers, and teachers, are frequently preferable. Treatment of attention deficit with stimulants may exacerbate tics; treatment of tics with neuroleptics may blunt affect, disrupt learning, provoke depression, and lead to unwanted weight gain.

OTHER CAUSES OF TICS

Tics may be drug induced (stimulants, neuroleptics causing tardive tics), or they may be symptomatic of developmental, degenerative, toxic-metabolic, or infectious neurologic disorders. Patients with chromosomal abnormalities (Down's and fragile X syndromes) frequently have tics, as do those with pervasive developmental delay, anoxic encephalopathy, and autism. Tics occasionally occur in patients with Huntington's disease, progressive supranuclear palsy, Creutzfeldt-Jakob disease, and encephalitis, as well as those with sequelae of carbon monoxide poisoning or hypoglycemia.

Cerebellar Ataxias

The cerebellum receives input from the spinal cord (spinocerebellar tracts), from the vestibular nuclei in the brain stem, and from pontine relays carrying information from the motor and premotor cortex. The cerebellar cortex is made up of four main neuronal types. Granule cells input onto Purkinje cells, whose axons form the sole output of the cerebellar cortex, terminating in cerebellar nuclei or select brain stem nuclei. Golgi cells and stellate/basket cells function as inhibitory interneurons within the cerebellar cortex. The cerebellar cortex is organized into three main sagittal zones. The most medial (vermal) zone projects to the fastigial nuclei, which, in turn, project to the vestibulospinal and reticulospinal tracts. Injuries to this zone or its projections lead to

TABLE 121–11   Hereditary Ataxias

Disease	Onset	Associated Signs
Autosomal Recessive Inheritance		
Ataxia-telangiectasia	Childhood	Telangiectasia, recurrent sinus and pulmonary infection, choreoathetosis, mental retardation in 30%, neoplasms (lymphoma, lymphocytic leukemia)
Abetalipoproteinemia (Bassen-Kornzweig syndrome or acanthocytosis)	Childhood	Absent serum apolipoprotein B leads to fat malabsorption with decreased vitamins A, E, and K; retinitis pigmentosa; nystagmus
Friedreich's ataxia	Childhood	Scoliosis, cardiomyopathy, dysarthria, areflexia, Babinski signs, loss of joint position and vibration sense in legs, dysmetria
Autosomal Dominant Inheritance		
Spinocerebellar ataxia Types 1–8	Adulthood	Variable combinations of long-tract signs, parkinsonism, dementia
Dentatorubral-palidoluysian atrophy		Sensory loss, myoclonus, chorea
Other forms of olivopontocerebellar atrophy		Dystonia and seizures

abnormal stance and gait, truncal titubation, and disturbances of extraocular movement. The intermediate (paravermal) zone projects to the interposed nuclei, which in turn project to the red nucleus and the thalamus. Isolated injuries to this zone are rare, and clinical manifestations generally overlap with medial or lateral cerebellar syndromes. The lateral zone projects to the dentate nuclei, which in turn project to the thalamus and cerebral cortex. Injuries to this zone or its projections result in abnormal stance and gait, appendicular dysmetria, eye movement dysmetria, dysdiadochokinesia, dysrhythmokinesia, intention tremor, ataxic dysarthria, and hypotonia.

NONHEREDITARY ATAXIAS

Lesions of the cerebellum, its inflow tracts, or its outflow tracts may all be associated with ataxia. The rapid onset of ataxia suggests an underlying structural condition, an immune-mediated process, drug intoxication, or conversion disorder. Structural lesions of the cerebellum or its connecting tracts include tumors, demyelinating plaques, abscesses, or vascular events such as vertebrobasilar occlusion, cerebellar parenchymal hemorrhage, traumatic hematoma, or arteriovenous malformation. Immune-mediated processes include acute postinfectious cerebellitis or myoclonic encephalopathy with neuroblastoma in children, or paraneoplastic cerebellar degeneration in adults. Migraine headaches, particularly in childhood, may be accompanied by ataxia. Radiographic studies, drug screening, and cerebrospinal fluid analysis will clarify the diagnosis in most cases of acute-onset ataxia.

Chronic or progressive ataxia may result from slow-growing brain tumors (cerebellar astrocytoma, hemangioblastoma, ependymoma, medulloblastoma, supratentorial tumors), congenital malformations (basilar impression, Dandy-Walker malformation, Chiari malformation), drug effects (alcoholic cerebellar vermian degeneration, chronic phenytoin toxicity), or hereditary ataxias.

HEREDITARY ATAXIAS

Progressive ataxia is a feature of numerous hereditary neurologic diseases (Table 121–11). Determining which hereditary disease is responsible depends on careful assessment of the familial pattern of inheritance and knowledge of the typical age at onset and progression of symptoms and signs associated with these conditions.

Molecular tests for a number of specific hereditary ataxias have become available within the past decade, but caution should be used to ensure adequate informed consent, support services, and follow-up before such tests are used to determine a potentially fatal diagnosis, especially in presymptomatic individuals. Genetic test results have immediate implications for the risk status of extended family members. Definitive therapies are generally lacking, genetic testing is expensive, and there are few mechanisms to ensure that genetic testing results are not used by insurers or employers to the disadvantage of the patient or family.

Like Huntington's disease, several of the autosomal dominant spinocerebellar ataxias are caused by abnormal expansions in the number of repeated CAG codons within unique genes. CAG repeat expansion disorders may account for a number of autosomal dominant neurodegenerative diseases. These diseases display the phenomenon of "anticipation": the age at onset is progressively younger in successive generations of a family. This is because the CAG repeat length of the abnormal genes is upwardly unstable during gametogenesis and higher CAG repeat burden results in younger age at onset.

REFERENCES

Jankovic J: The extrapyramidal disorders. *In* Goldman L, Bennett JC (eds): Cecil Textbook of Medicine, 21st ed. Philadelphia: WB Saunders, 2000, pp 2077–2087.
Klockgether T, Evert B: Genes involved in hereditary ataxias. Trends Neurosci 1998; 21:413–418.
Kurlan RM: Treatment of Movement Disorders. Philadelphia: JB Lippincott, 1995.
Watts RL, Koller WC: Movement Disorders: Neurologic Principles and Practice. New York: McGraw-Hill, 1997.

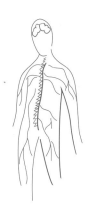

122

DEVELOPMENTAL AND NEUROCUTANEOUS DISORDERS

Robert C. Griggs

Computed tomography and magnetic resonance imaging detect many congenital and developmental diseases that used to go unrecognized. Subarachnoid cysts, ventricular asymmetries, as well as many of the more minor of the malformations and anomalies described here usually have no symptoms and need no treatment.

Spinal Malformations

Developmental anomalies of the vertebral bodies are frequent and may result in pain and neurologic symptoms if they cause scoliosis or lead to accelerated degenerative changes of the spine. Neurologic disability is likely if the anomalies compress neural structures or alter cerebrospinal fluid flow.

Chiari Malformations

A Chiari I malformation is defined as ectopia of the cerebellar tonsils more than 5 mm below the foramen magnum. It is usually asymptomatic but occasionally causes headaches worsened by straining or cough, lower cranial neuropathies, downbeat nystagmus, ataxia, or sensory loss. The malformation is congenital, but symptoms often present in the third decade or later.

Chiari II malformations (also called Arnold-Chiari malformations) are characterized by extension of the cerebellum and lower brain stem through the foramen magnum. A myelomeningocele and hydrocephalus are usually present. Brain stem dysfunction may develop from malformation or compression of neural structures. Treatment is surgical: repair of the myelomeningocele, relief of hydrocephalus, and cervical bony decompression.

Tethered Spinal Cord

Here the filum terminale is anomalous, resulting in either a lack of normal ascent of the conus medullaris to the L1 vertebral level or an ischemic or metabolic disturbance of the caudal spinal cord. Associated spinal anomalies are common: diastematomyelia (split cord), spinal lipomas, dermal sinuses, and fibrolipomas of the filum terminale. Patients present with bladder and sexual dysfunction and lower extremity weakness and spasticity. Symptoms typically develop in childhood or adolescence. Focal hypertrichosis, hemangiomas, and nevi occur in the skin over the lumbar spine.

Syringohydromyelia

In syringohydromyelia the central canal of the spinal cord (hydromyelia), the substance of the spinal cord (syringomyelia), or the brain stem (syringobulbia) is expanded by the presence of fluid under pressure. Symptoms of syringohydromyelia begin in late adolescence or early adulthood and alternate with long periods of stability. The syrinx usually affects the cervical spinal cord. Patients present with asymmetric weakness, atrophy, and decreased reflexes of the hands and arms; dissociated sensory loss (impaired perception of pain and temperature, but preservation of light touch and proprioception) in the neck, arms, and upper trunk; and increased muscle tone and reflexes in the legs. Extension into the medulla may cause nystagmus or lower cranial neuropathies. A syrinx can occur 20 or more years after cord trauma. Diagnosis is made by magnetic resonance imaging, which may show an associated craniocervical junction lesion or tumor. Treatment is directed at the cause of the syrinx. In patients with Chiari II malformations, adequate shunting of the lateral ventricles may result in collapse of the syrinx. Syringohydromyelia in patients with spinal tumors is treated by surgery.

Malformations of Cortical Development

Malformations of cortical development are caused by intrauterine infection, intrauterine ischemia, and gene mutations. When small areas of the brain are involved, patients typically develop epilepsy in the first or second decade and have minor static neurologic dysfunction but normal intellect. Those with involvement of larger areas of the brain often have mental retardation and more severe neurologic dysfunction in addition to epilepsy. Diagnosis is established by magnetic resonance imaging. Table 122–1 lists common malformations.

Developmental and Neurocutaneous Disorders

The neurocutaneous syndromes are congenital, usually hereditary, disorders characterized by lesions involving both the nervous system and skin. Often termed the *phacomatoses* (from the Greek, *phakoma*, meaning "birthmark"), over 40 syndromes have been described. The most important ones are neurofibromatosis (types 1 and 2), tuberous sclerosis, Sturge-Weber syndrome, and von Hippel-Lindau syndrome.

NEUROFIBROMATOSIS TYPE 1

Neurofibromatosis type 1 (NF1) is the classic disorder described by von Recklinghausen, with a prevalence of 1 in 3000 births. Transmission is autosomal dominant, but half of the cases are sporadic. NF1 causes many types of skin and central nervous system (CNS) tumors: in the skin, neurofibromas and plexiform neurofibromas; in the CNS, optic nerve gliomas, meningiomas, and astrocytomas of the brain and spinal cord. The NF1 gene is located on chromosome 17q and expresses a protein designated as neurofibromin (a tumor-suppressor protein). Pathogenic mutations in the NF1 gene are identified in approximately 75% of clinical cases, but there is no correlation between a particular genotype and phenotype. Although NF1 is a congenital disease, most manifestations appear during childhood and adult life. The criteria for the diagnosis include two or more of the following: (1) six or more café-au-lait macules larger than 5 mm in prepubescent patients and more than 15 mm in postpubescent individuals; (2) two or more neurofibromas of any type or one plexiform neurofibroma; (3) axillary or inguinal freckling; (4) sphenoid bone dysplasia; (5) optic glioma (6) Lisch nodules; and (7) a family history of NF1. Diagnosis is based on clinical criteria, supplemented by neuroimaging findings Other manifestations include developmental delay and epilepsy. Important complications include scoliosis, gastrointestinal neurofibromas, pheochromocytomas, and renal artery stenosis. The majority of patients with NF1 do not require treatment. Subcutaneous neurofibromas may be painful and can be excised surgically. Many intraspinal and intracranial tumors are benign and treated surgically. Genetic counseling must be provided in all patients and families in which NF1 is present. Many new mutations occur in the germline of an unaffected parent; siblings of parents with new mutations may therefore be at risk for the disease.

NEUROFIBROMATOSIS TYPE 2

Neurofibromatosis type 2 (NF2) is also called central neurofibromatosis and, like NF1, is transmitted by an autosomal dominant mechanism. It is less frequent than NF1 (approximately 1 in 50,000 individuals). The usual manifestation of NF2 is bilateral eighth nerve schwannomas. However, multiple meningiomas and multiple other schwannomas are also common features. The NF2 gene is located on chromosome 22q. The gene product

TABLE 122–1   Malformations of Central Nervous System Cortical Development Recognized by Magnetic Resonance Imaging

Malformation	Clinical Features	Cause(s)	Treatment
Focal cortical dysplasia	Epilepsy (usual); developmental delay (if extensive)	Multiple	Seizure control*
Lissencephaly (smooth brain)	Epilepsy	Genes: 17q13.3 Xq22	Usually unsatisfactory
Band heterotopia	Females > males; epilepsy; variable developmental delay	Xq22	Seizure control*
Subependymal nodular heterotopia	Males > females; epilepsy; variable developmental delay	Xq28	Seizure control*
Polymicrogyria-schizencephaly	Severe central nervous system dysfunction; epilepsy	Multiple	Seizure control*

*Treatment of seizures with medication is often unsuccessful. Surgical excision of an epileptogenic focus can be curative.

(merlin) is a cytoskeletal protein. Skin lesions are present in up to 30% of patients with NF2, but the diagnosis is based on the following criteria: (1) bilateral eighth nerve tumors detected by magnetic resonance imaging; (2) a family member with either NF2 or unilateral eighth nerve lesions (neurofibroma, meningioma, or schwannoma; and (3) juvenile posterior subcapsular lens opacities. Symptoms of NF2 begin in the second to fourth decades. Surgical treatment of schwannomas and meningiomas is usually indicated, and early recognition is important for successful treatment of eighth nerve tumors. Family members should be screened regularly with hearing tests and magnetic resonance imaging.

TUBEROUS SCLEROSIS

Tuberous sclerosis complex (TSC) causes hamartomatous lesions involving multiple organs at different stages in the course of the disease. Transmission is autosomal dominant, but sporadic cases are frequent because of spontaneous mutations. The incidence of TSC is 1 in 10,000 to 50,000. TSC affects tissues from different embryonic germ layers: cutaneous lesions include adenoma sebaceum, hypomelanotic skin macules (ash leaf spots), shagreen patches, and subungual fibromas. Visceral lesions include cardiac and renal tumors; CNS lesions include hamartomas of cortex and ventricular walls and subependymal giant-cell tumors. There are at least three TSC gene loci. In *TSC-1* the abnormality is localized on chromosome 9q34 but the nature of the gene remains unclear. In *TSC-2* the gene abnormalities are on chromosome 16p. This gene encodes tuberin, a guanosine triphosphatase–activating protein. Hereditary cases not linked to these two loci also occur.

The diagnostic clinical triad is mental subnormality, epilepsy, and skin lesions. CNS imaging reveals multiple calcified subependymal nodules as well as cortical tubers. Retinal hamartomas occur in half of the patients. The diagnosis is usually clinical with confirmation by identification of hamartomas on imaging studies. Treatment is directed at controlling epilepsy and correcting hydrocephalus. Serial cardiac studies and renal ultrasound evaluation may be indicated in some patients.

STURGE-WEBER SYNDROME

Sturge-Weber syndrome is usually sporadic without an established hereditary pattern. The incidence and prevalence are not defined; it occurs in less than 1 in 20,000 births. Usual clinical manifestations include facial vascular nevus (port-wine stain) epilepsy, cognitive deficits, and, less frequently, hemiparesis or hemiplegia, hemianopia, or glaucoma. The facial lesion suggests the presence of venous angiomatosis of the pia mater. Most patients have epilepsy. The diagnosis is usually made by the facial nevus and imaging confirmation of intracranial pathology (ipsilateral cerebral cortical calcifications). The treatment is that of the associated epilepsy. If antiepileptic drugs do not control seizures, surgical excision of epileptogenic areas is often successful.

VON HIPPEL-LINDAU DISEASE (CNS ANGIOMATOSIS)

Von Hippel-Lindau disease is an autosomal dominant disorder caused by a defective tumor suppressor gene at chromosome 3p25-p26. It is characterized by retinal angiomas, brain and spinal cord hemangioblastomas, renal cell carcinomas, pheochromocytomas, angiomas of the liver and kidney, and cysts of the pancreas, kidney, liver, and epididymis. Both sexes are affected equally. The diagnosis is established if patients have more than one CNS hemangioblastoma, one hemangioblastoma with a visceral manifestation of the disease, or one manifestation of the disease and a known family history. Symptoms typically begin during the third or fourth decade. Retinal inflammation with exudates, hemorrhage, and retinal detachment typically antedate cerebellar complaints. Headache, vertigo, and vomiting result from the cerebellar tumor. Cerebellar findings such as incoordination, dysmetria, and ataxia are common.

Retinal detachments and tumors are treated by laser therapy. Brain tumors, renal cell carcinomas, pheochromocytomas, and epididymal tumors are treated surgically. Small CNS tumors may be treated by gamma knife. Early evaluation and repeated imaging studies are indicated once the diagnosis is made, and at-risk subjects should be evaluated.

REFERENCES

Barkovich AJ, Kuzniecky RI: Congenital anomalies of the craniovertebral junction, spine and spinal cord (including syringomyelia). *In* Goldman L, Bennett JC (eds): Cecil Textbook of Medicine, 21st ed. Philadelphia: WB Saunders, 2000, pp 2076–2077.

Barkovich AJ, Kuzniecky RI: Malformations of cortical development. *In* Goldman L, Bennett JC (eds): Cecil Textbook of Medicine, 21st ed. Philadelphia: WB Saunders, 2000, pp 2075–2076.

Barkovich AJ, Kuzniecky RI: Neurocutaneous syndromes. *In* Goldman L, Bennett JC (eds): Cecil Textbook of Medicine, 21st ed. Philadelphia: WB Saunders, 2000, pp 2074–2075.

Milhorat TH, Johnson RW, Milhorat RH, et al: Clinicopathological correlations in syringomyelia using axial magnetic resonance imaging. Neurosurgery 1995; 37:206–213.

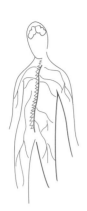

123

CEREBROVASCULAR DISEASE

Timothy J. Counihan

The term *cerebrovascular disease* refers to disorders of the arterial or venous circulatory systems of the central nervous system. The term *stroke* is used when the symptoms begin abruptly, either as a result of inadequate blood flow (ischemic stroke) or hemorrhage into the brain tissue (parenchymal hemorrhage) or surrounding subarachnoid space (subarachnoid hemorrhage). Approximately 80% of strokes are ischemic in origin. *Focal* ischemic stroke is caused by either thrombotic or embolic occlusion of a major artery, whereas *global* ischemia usually results from inadequate cerebral perfusion such as that which occurs after cardiac arrest or ventricular fibrillation. Rarely does isolated hypoxia (from carbon monoxide poisoning or asphyxiation) cause global cerebral ischemia.

Epidemiology

Stroke remains the third leading medical cause of death and the second most frequent cause of morbidity in developed countries. Since 1990, the incidence of stroke in the United States has declined by about 1.5% annually to about 0.5 to 1.0 per thousand population, accounting for about 1 in every 15 deaths. It is believed that this steady decrease is the result of improvements in general public health and is coincident with the decline of cardiovascular deaths and better control of hypertension and other risk factors (Table 123–1). Rates of stroke among men and women are similar, although the incidence and rate of mortality from stroke are higher in blacks than whites.

Although the reasons for the decline in the incidence of stroke remain unclear, a greater understanding of the importance of controlling risk factors in stroke prevention may be in part responsible. The increasingly successful management of hypertension and the reduction in smoking habits have been major factors in reducing the incidence of stroke. In addition, the increasing public awareness of the warning symptoms of stroke as constituting a *brain attack* (analogous to chest pain as a warning of a "heart attack") is beginning to improve primary stroke prevention.

Anatomy

The brain is supplied by two pairs of major arteries, the carotid (anterior circulation) and vertebral (posterior circulation) arteries (Fig. 123–1).

ANTERIOR CIRCULATION

The common carotid artery bifurcates into an internal and external branch at the level of the thyroid cartilage in the neck. The internal carotid artery (ICA) enters the skull through the carotid canal and passes through the cavernous sinus as the carotid siphon. It gives off the ophthalmic, anterior choroidal, and posterior communicating arteries before bifurcating into the anterior cerebral artery (ACA) and middle cerebral artery (MCA). The ACA supplies the medial surfaces of the cerebral hemispheres, and the MCA supplies the lateral surface (convexity), in addition to the basal ganglia and subcortical white matter.

POSTERIOR CIRCULATION

In the neck, the vertebral arteries (VAs) course upward within the transverse processes of the cervical vertebrae. The intracranial VA gives off a branch to form the anterior spinal artery, as well as the posterior inferior cerebellar arteries (PICAs) before the two arteries unite to form the basilar artery (BA) at the pontomedullary junction. The BA supplies the cerebellum via the anterior inferior cerebellar artery (AICA) and superior cerebellar artery (SCA) before bifurcating into the posterior

TABLE 123-1   Risk Factors for Ischemic Stroke

Diabetes
Hypertension
Smoking
Family history of premature vascular disease
Hyperlipidemia
Atrial fibrillation
History of transient ischemic attack (TIA)
History of recent myocardial infarction
History of congestive heart failure (left ventricular [LV] ejection fraction <25%)
Drugs (sympathomimetics, oral contraceptive pill, cocaine)

cerebral arteries (PCAs) at the level of the pontomesencephalic junction.

CIRCLE OF WILLIS

The circle of Willis is formed at the base of the brain by the union of both ACAs via the anterior communicating artery and the union of the MCA with the PCA via the posterior communicating artery (see Fig. 123–1). Hence there is communication between both anterior circulations as well as between the posterior and anterior circulations on each side. Congenital anomalies of the circle are frequent; they include hypoplasia or atresia of a posterior communicating artery or ACA, which may reduce collateral blood supply if an adjacent vessel becomes occluded.

Physiology

Unlike other body tissues, the brain has few energy stores but relies on a sizable and reliable cerebral blood flow (CBF) to meet its energy demands. CBF averages 60 mL per 100 g of brain tissue per minute. A complex system of neural pathways regulates CBF in a process known as *autoregulation,* which serves to maintain CBF at a constant level despite wide fluctuations in cerebral perfusion pressure (Fig. 123–2). CBF remains relatively constant when the mean arterial pressure lies between 50 and 150 mm Hg. In the case of chronic systemic hypertension, however, both the upper and lower levels of autoregulation are raised, which indicates a higher tolerance of hypertension but a greater susceptibility to the effects of hypotension.

Ischemic Stroke

PATHOGENESIS

Cerebral ischemia may result from thrombotic or embolic occlusion of a major vessel that reduces blood flow within the involved vascular territory, or it may be a consequence of diminished systemic perfusion. Pro-

longed brain ischemia results in infarction, characterized histologically by necrosis of neurons, glia, and endothelial cells. Cerebral infarcts are classified as either "pale" (anemic) or "hemorrhagic" (in areas of endothelial necrosis). In transition zones between normally perfused tissue and the infarcted central core is a rim of moderately ischemic tissue known as the *ischemic penumbra,* which is the target area for several emerging neuroprotective agents currently being investigated.

Global cerebral ischemia usually results from cardiac arrest or ventricular fibrillation. Some neuronal populations are selectively vulnerable to transient global ischemia, particularly neurons of the hippocampus, cerebellar Purkinje cells, and the deeper layers of the cerebral cortex (inducing so-called laminar necrosis). Pure hypoxia causes cerebral dysfunction (manifested clinically as lethargy and confusion) but rarely produces irreversible brain injury unless accompanied by other factors such as hypoglycemia. When neurons are rendered ischemic, a number of biochemical changes take place: intracellular membranes are no longer able to control ion fluxes, which leads to increased intracellular concentrations of Ca^{2+} and arrest of mitochondrial function. Activation of membrane lipases further compromises

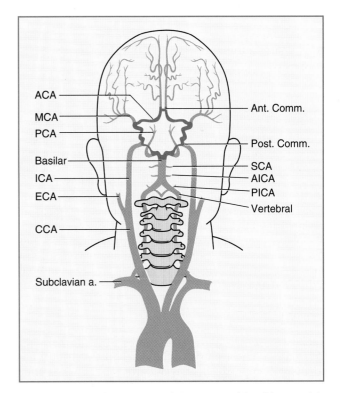

FIGURE 123-1   Coronal view of the extracranial and intracranial arterial supply to brain. Vessels forming the circle of Willis are highlighted. ACA = anterior cerebral artery; AICA = anterior inferior cerebellar artery; Ant. Comm. = anterior communicating artery; CCA = common carotid artery; ECA = external carotid artery; ICA = internal carotid artery; MCA = middle cerebral artery; PCA = posterior cerebral artery; PICA = posterior inferior cerebellar artery; Post. Comm. = posterior communicating artery; SCA = superior cerebellar artery. (Modified from Lord R: Surgery of Occlusive Cerebrovascular Disease. St. Louis: CV Mosby, 1986.)

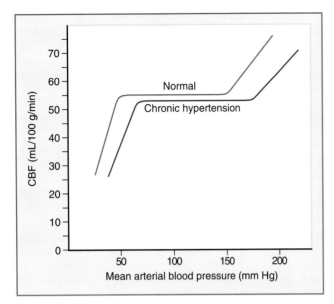

FIGURE 123-2 Autoregulatory cerebral blood flow response to changes in mean arterial pressure in normotensive and chronically hypertensive persons. Note the shift of the curve toward higher mean pressures with chronic hypertension. (From Goldman L, Bennett JC [eds]: Cecil Textbook of Medicine, 21st ed. Philadelphia: WB Saunders, 2000, p 2097.)

cell membrane integrity and leads to release of excitatory neurotransmitters, which in turn may further exacerbate tissue injury. If blood flow is restored within 15 minutes, the effects of these events may be reversible.

CEREBRAL EDEMA

Cerebral edema may be intracellular (cytotoxic) or interstitial (vasogenic). Intracellular edema develops rapidly in ischemic neurons as energy-dependent ion-channel pumps fail, whereas vasogenic edema occurs as a result of damage to endothelial cells, disrupting the blood-brain barrier and allowing macromolecules such as plasma proteins to enter the interstitial space. Fluid accumulates over 3 to 5 days after an ischemic stroke and can increase brain water content by as much as 10%; such large volume increases can lead to transtentorial herniation and death.

ETIOLOGY

Table 123-2 lists the major causes of acute cerebral ischemia. Atherosclerosis of the cerebral vasculature accounts for approximately two thirds of strokes, either through embolization of plaque to distal vessels (artery-to-artery embolus) or by in situ thrombosis. Certain sites of the cerebral vasculature are more prone to the development of atheromatous plaques (Fig. 123-3). Cardiogenic emboli make up the majority of the remaining third of ischemic strokes, arising most commonly as a result of atrial fibrillation. Mural thrombi, valvular vegetations, and atrial myxomas are also potential sources of embolus, as are *paradoxical emboli* (emboli of venous origin passing through a patent foramen ovale).

TABLE 123-2   Causes of Cerebral Ischemia

Focal
Mural Abnormalities
Atherosclerosis
Vasculitis
Vasospasm (migraine, subarachnoid hemorrhage)
Compression (by tumor, aneurysm)
Fibromuscular dysplasia/Moyamoya
Dissection (spontaneous, traumatic)
Embolism
Cardiogenic (atrial fibrillation, mural thrombus, myxoma, valvular vegetations)
Artery-to-artery
Fat
Air
Paradoxical
Hematologic
Hypercoagulable state
Sickle cell disease
Homocystinuria
Antiphospholipid antibodies (lupus anticoagulant, anticardiolipin antibodies)
Protein C or protein S deficiency

Global
Hypoperfusion
Cardiac arrest
Ventricular fibrillation

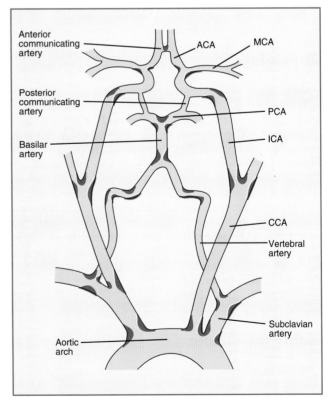

FIGURE 123-3 Site of predilection for atheromatous plaque. (From Caplan LR: Stroke—A Clinical Approach. Boston: Butterworth-Heinemann, 1993.)

TABLE 123-3 Causes of Stroke in Young Adults

Migraine
Arterial dissection
Drugs (cocaine, heroin, oral contraceptive pill)
Premature atherosclerosis (homocystinuria, hyperlipidemia)
Postpartum angiopathy
Cardiac factors
    Atrial septal defect
    Patent foramen ovale
    Mitral valve prolapse
    Endocarditis
Hematologic factors
    Deficiency states (antithrombin III, protein S, protein C)
    Disseminated intravascular coagulation
    Thrombotic thrombocytopenic purpura
Inflammatory factors
    Systemic lupus erythematosus
    Polyarteritis nodosa
    Neurosyphilis
    Cryoglobulinemia
Other factors
    Fibromuscular dysplasia
    Moyamoya syndrome

Certain conditions predispose younger patients to stroke (Table 123–3).

TRANSIENT ISCHEMIC ATTACK VERSUS STROKE

A transient ischemic attack (TIA) is defined arbitrarily as a transient neurologic deficit resulting from reduced blood flow, lasting less than 24 hours, and followed by full functional recovery. Most TIAs resolve within 1 hour, however, and deficits that last longer should prompt a search for an alternative explanation. A *completed stroke* indicates that infarction has taken place. In most instances, the maximal clinical deficit occurs at the onset of symptoms, with variable recovery over time thereafter. Several factors may contribute to symptom progression (often referred to as a *stroke in evolution*) and include propagation of a thrombus or progression of cerebral edema or hemorrhage into an infarcted area. Coexistent medical conditions such as systemic hypotension, fever, hyperglycemia, or hypoxemia may further adversely affect the outcome.

LACUNAR STROKE

A *cerebral lacuna* is a small, deep infarction involving a penetrating branch of a large cerebral artery. Lacunae are usually associated with chronic hypertension, although they are occasionally found in normotensive patients, presumably as a result of microatheroma of penetrating arteries, especially of the basal ganglia, thalamus, and white matter of the internal capsule and pons.

Major Stroke Syndromes
(Fig. 123–4)

The clinical manifestations of ischemic stroke are summarized in Table 123–4.

INTERNAL CAROTID ARTERY

TIAs that occur in the anterior circulation affect either the retinal artery or MCA distribution most frequently.

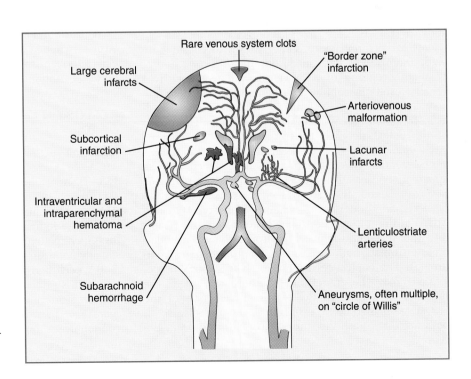

FIGURE 123-4 Major types of stroke. (Modified from Adams RJ: Neurologic complications. *In* Embury S, Hebbel RP, Mohandas N, et al [eds]: Sickle Cell Disease: Basic Principles and Clinical Practice. New York: Raven Press, 1994.)

TABLE 123–4 Clinical Manifestations of Ischemic Stroke

Occluded Vessel	Clinical Signs
ICA	Ipsilateral blindness (variable)
	MCA syndrome
MCA	Contralateral hemiparesis, hemisensory loss (face/arm > leg)
	Aphasia (dominant) or anosognosia (nondominant)
	Homonymous hemianopsia (variable)
ACA	Contralateral hemiparesis, hemisensory loss (leg > arm)
	Abulia (especially if bilateral)
VA/PICA	Ipsilateral facial sensory loss, hemiataxia, nystagmus, Horner's syndrome
	Contralateral loss of temperature/pain sensation
	Dysphagia
SCA	Gait ataxia, nausea, vertigo, dysarthria
BA	Quadriparesis, dysarthria, dysphagia, diplopia, somnolence, amnesia
PCA	Contralateral homonymous hemianopsia, amnesia, sensory loss

ACA = anterior cerebral artery; BA = basilar artery; ICA = internal carotid artery; MCA = middle cerebral artery; PCA = posterior cerebral artery; PICA = posterior inferior cerebellar artery; SCA = superior cerebellar artery; VA = vertebral artery.

Symptoms of retinal artery involvement consist of several seconds of a "graying out" of vision in one eye or monocular blindness (*amaurosis fugax*). An important finding on retinoscopy is the presence of refractile arterial spots, which represent cholesterol crystals (Hollenhorst plaques) that have become detached from an upstream cholesterol plaque. Most anterior circulation TIAs occur in the setting of significant stenosis/ulceration of the ICA (>75%); cardiogenic embolism accounts for the remainder. Other causes to consider include traumatic or spontaneous arterial *dissection*.

Acute occlusion of a previously widely patent ICA usually results in contralateral hemiplegia and hemisensory loss, reflecting ischemia to MCA territory. Headache frequently accompanies ICA occlusion. The extent of the deficit depends on the availability of collateral circulation; in the case of occlusion of a previously severely stenotic ICA, little or no clinical deficit may be apparent, on account of extensive collateral circulation. Severe bilateral ICA stenosis may occasionally cause *border zone* ("watershed") ischemia (between ACA and MCA) in the setting of systemic hypotension; this results in a well-recognized clinical syndrome comprising bilateral proximal limb weakness (*man-in-a-barrel* syndrome). The clinical recognition of ICA stenosis or occlusion may be unreliable, because although the presence of a bruit in the region of the angle of the jaw suggests significant extracranial vascular disease, it does not distinguish the external carotid artery from the ICA.

ANTERIOR CEREBRAL ARTERY

Occlusion of the ACA distal to the anterior communicating artery causes weakness and sensory loss in the contralateral leg. Other clinical manifestations include urinary incontinence and *abulia*, a state of akinetic mutism reflecting bilateral frontal lobe dysfunction.

MIDDLE CEREBRAL ARTERY

Embolism accounts for the majority of MCA occlusion. Emboli may be either cardiogenic or artery-to-artery from the extracranial ICA. Occlusion of the main MCA trunk results in contralateral hemiplegia, hemianesthesia, and homonymous hemianopsia with a gaze preference away from the side of the hemiplegia. A global aphasia occurs with dominant hemisphere lesions, and anosognosia occurs with nondominant hemisphere involvement. Occasionally, selective occlusion of the lenticulostriate branches from the proximal MCA causes capsular infarction without evidence of cortical infarction, as a result of collateral filling of the distal MCA. Occlusion of the superior division of the MCA causes faciobrachial weakness; an expressive (Broca's) aphasia results from dominant hemisphere lesions, or a motor neglect (characterized by motor impersistence and spatial disorientation) results from lesions in the nondominant side. Inferior division occlusion usually produces impairment of sensory perception (astereognosis) and occasionally a visual field disturbance. Dominant hemisphere lesions result in a fluent (Wernicke's) aphasia.

VERTEBROBASILAR ISCHEMIA

Vertebrobasilar ischemia manifests with various combinations of symptoms such as dizziness (vertigo), diplopia, ataxia, bilateral sensory or motor symptoms, and fluctuating episodes of drowsiness. Scintillations or transient visual field deficits may indicate ischemia in the PCA distribution. Distinguishing the vertigo of vertebrobasilar ischemia from labyrinthine vertigo can be difficult, although isolated positional vertigo is more likely to be of labyrinthine origin.

OCCLUSION OF VERTEBRAL ARTERY OR BASILAR ARTERY

Occlusion of these arteries and their branches (PICAs, AICA, SCA) results in discrete syndromes (see Table 123–4). Acute infarction of the cerebellum from occlusion of any of its three supplying vessels may result in significant swelling within the posterior fossa, obstruction of the fourth ventricle, and obstructive hydrocephalus. Such patients require close monitoring and occasionally neurosurgical intervention.

BA occlusion produces massive brain stem dysfunction and is often fatal. If the medulla is spared, a number of syndromes can occur, including the *locked-in syndrome*, in which patients are quadriplegic and can communicate only by means of vertical eye movements.

POSTERIOR CEREBRAL ARTERY OCCLUSION

Proximal PCA occlusions cause contralateral hemiparesis (from damage to the cerebral peduncle), hemisensory loss (thalamus), amnesia (medial temporal lobe), and hemianopsia. Macular (central) vision may be spared because of collateral vessels from the MCA.

CEREBRAL VENOUS THROMBOSIS

Occlusion of the sagittal sinus may occur in several settings, often in the setting of a hyperviscosity or hypercoagulable state. The condition is particularly common in pregnancy. The clinical picture varies; patients may present with headache and papilledema or seizures. The diagnosis frequently rests on imaging findings; bilateral hemorrhagic infarctions in a parasagittal distribution are common; magnetic resonance angiography (MRA) or contrast computed tomography (CT) often shows the sinus filling defect ("delta sign").

Diagnosis

Evaluation of the patient with a suspected stroke should seek to answer two questions: *what* the mechanism is (focal ischemia-thrombotic or embolic; global ischemia/hypoperfusion or hemorrhage) and *where* the lesion is. Some useful bedside pointers that may be elicited from the history and help define the stroke mechanism include the time of symptom onset and the temporal course and progression of symptoms. The type of activity and the presence of accompanying symptoms (such as headache, vomiting, or syncope) are also useful to determine from the history, as is the presence or absence of stroke risk factors.

The physical examination determines lesion localization, as well as identifies clues to pathogenesis. A thorough cardiovascular examination, including measurements of blood pressure and cardiac rhythm, is essential. Palpation of the facial artery occasionally discloses reversal of flow, which indicates ICA occlusion. Ophthalmoscopy can detect platelet and cholesterol emboli, as well as giving information about the chronicity and severity of systemic hypertension. Papilledema may accompany cerebral venous thrombosis.

Ancillary blood tests include a complete blood count, sedimentation rate, glucose, coagulation screen, and a lipid profile. In young patients and those with unexplained venous sinus thrombosis, a search for a hypercoagulable state is necessary (see Table 123–3).

Brain imaging with CT is the most reliable test for differentiating ischemic stroke from hemorrhage, but it has limitations in the acute setting in that only 5% of acute ischemic strokes are readily visible on CT scan in the first 12 hours. MRI may be used to verify infarction if the diagnosis remains in doubt.

The anterior circulation can be assessed with duplex ultrasonography or MRA. Cerebral angiography is reserved for specific indications to exclude vasculitis and carotid dissection or before carotid endarterectomy.

Differential Diagnosis

TIAs need to be distinguished from other paroxysmal events affecting the nervous system. In rare cases, patients with migraine headache have weakness contralateral to the side of the headache *(hemiplegic migraine)*. Some generalized seizures are followed by a transient hemiparesis *(Todd's paralysis)*.

The acute onset of a stroke generally distinguishes it from other brain lesions, although hemorrhage into a primary or metastatic tumor may manifest in a stroke-like fashion. Strokes and seizures may coexist, and 10% of strokes are associated with seizure at the time of onset. As a general rule, stroke rarely manifests with an alteration of consciousness unless there are other signs of brain dysfunction.

Primary Stroke Prevention

The identification and reduction of stroke risk factors (see Table 123–1), including therapy for hypertension, cessation of smoking, and treatment of diabetes and hyperlipidemia, is largely responsible for the decline in the incidence of stroke.

ATRIAL FIBRILLATION

Atrial fibrillation, particularly in the setting of valvular heart disease, increases the yearly risk of stroke 17-fold. For these patients, anticoagulation with warfarin to an international normalized ratio (INR) of 2 to 3 is recommended. Patients with nonvalvular atrial fibrillation in whom there are no other risk factors for stroke may be treated with aspirin, 325 mg/day. Patients with prosthetic heart valves require long-term anticoagulation. Patients with bacterial endocarditis should not receive warfarin because of the risk of cerebral hemorrhage from septic embolization.

TRANSIENT ISCHEMIC ATTACK (Fig. 123–5)

The occurrence of a TIA or stroke is a significant risk factor for recurrent stroke, with an average 5% risk per year, although the annual risk of stroke after an episode of amaurosis fugax is only 1% to 2%. Prophylactic antiplatelet therapy with aspirin, ticlopidine, or clopidogrel has been shown to prevent secondary events. Patients with a significant risk for cardiogenic thromboembolism should be treated with warfarin. Hospital admission is advisable for new-onset and recurrent TIAs unless a confident diagnosis of the etiology of the event can be made. Angiography should be performed and a decision made promptly to treat the patient either medically or surgically.

CAROTID STENOSIS

In patients with an asymptomatic bruit or extracranial carotid stenosis of less than 60%, treatment with antiplatelet therapy has been shown to be effective. For patients with extracranial carotid stenoses of more than 70% (with or without symptoms of ischemia in that vascular distribution) *carotid endarterectomy* reduces the risk of stroke. For patients with moderate (60%–70%) asymptomatic carotid stenosis, the decision to treat with optimal medical therapy versus surgery is made on an individual case-by-case basis.

Management of Acute Stroke

GENERAL MEASURES

Specific medical and nursing measures should be initiated, with particular emphasis on reducing the risk of

complications from immobility, such as pneumonia, deep venous thrombosis, and urinary tract infection. The early introduction of physical, occupational, and speech therapy and a careful evaluation of swallowing ability reduce morbidity. Judicious treatment of hypertension and hyperglycemia and correction of dehydration should be instituted. Prevention and prompt treatment of hyperthermia with antipyretics may reduce the extent of the deficit. Early awareness of poststroke depressive symptoms is especially important in preparing patients for rehabilitation.

USE OF ANTICOAGULANTS (see Fig. 123–5)

Although antiplatelet therapy remains the treatment of choice to prevent recurrent thromboembolism in the majority of patients with stroke, anticoagulation may be appropriate in patients with atrial fibrillation, in patients with recent myocardial infarction, and in cases of suspected propagation of thrombus or of stroke in evolution. Cranial CT is necessary before institution of heparin, to confirm or rule out intracerebral or subarachnoid hemorrhage. Baseline prothrombin time, partial thromboplastin time, and platelet count, as well as tests for hypercoagulable states, should be obtained be-

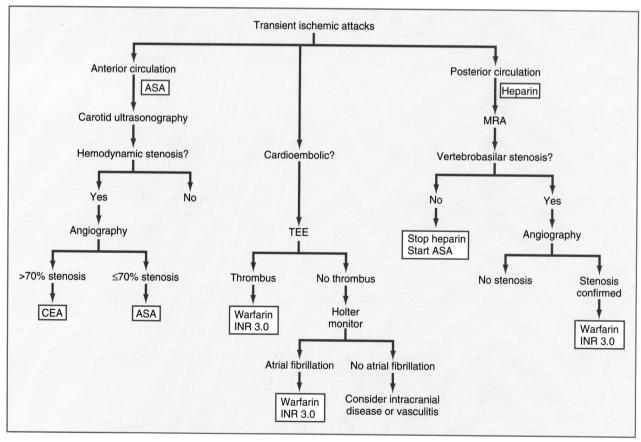

FIGURE 123–5 Algorithm for the treatment of transient ischemic attacks (TIAs). ASA = aspirin; CEA = carotid endarterectomy; INR = International Normalized Ratio; MRA = magnetic resonance angiography; TEE = transesophageal echocardiography. (Modified from Morgenstern LB, Grotta JC: Transient ischemic attacks. *In* Johnson RT, Griffin JW [eds]: Current Therapy in Neurologic Disease, 5th ed. St. Louis: Mosby, 1997, p 188.)

fore initiation of therapy. A history of active peptic ulceration or uncontrolled hypertension (systolic blood pressure consistently >200 mm Hg) precludes the use of anticoagulants, unless the benefits clearly outweigh the risks.

THROMBOLYSIS (Fig. 123–6)

Patients who present within 3 hours of the onset of ischemic stroke should be considered for intravenous recombinant tissue plasminogen activator (rt-PA). A careful clinical evaluation is essential to determine whether the patient is an appropriate candidate for the treatment (see Fig. 123–6). The risks (6% risk of symptomatic intracranial hemorrhage) and benefits (50%

chance of little or no disability at 3 months, compared with 38% chance without rt-PA) must be fully explained to the patient and family so that an informed decision can be made rapidly. Careful monitoring of blood pressure and avoidance of anticoagulants and aspirin are required for 24 hours after rt-PA administration.

Although preliminary results are promising, intra-arterial thrombolysis remains under investigation as an alternative therapy. A potential future development of thrombolytic therapy may be combination therapy with neuroprotective agents (such as glutamate antagonists), which may extend the therapeutic time window beyond 3 hours. Use of antiplatelet agents, such as platelet glycoprotein IIb/IIIa complex antagonists, is also under study.

MANAGEMENT OF CEREBRAL EDEMA

Only in large hemispheric infarction is ischemic cerebral edema sufficient to cause brain shift and transtentorial herniation. If signs of herniation appear, intubation and hyperventilation produce transient cerebral vasoconstriction and may reduce intracranial pressure. Mannitol acts by reducing the volume of the surrounding unaffected brain, but its effects are also transient. Corticosteroids are of no benefit in cytotoxic edema.

HYPERTENSIVE ENCEPHALOPATHY

The term *hypertensive encephalopathy* refers to the diffuse cerebral effects of severe hypertension that are not caused by infarction or hemorrhage and that are potentially reversible with control of the blood pressure. Patients experience headache, visual blurring (obscurations), confusion, and drowsiness. Seizures may develop. The blood pressure is typically very high (250/150), and papilledema and retinal hemorrhages are usually apparent on funduscopy. CT and MRI show diffuse cerebral edema with a predilection for the occipital lobes.

Hypertensive encephalopathy is a medical emergency. Treatment should be directed to the prompt but controlled lowering of blood pressure (e.g., with sodium nitroprusside), with care taken to avoid hypotension. The condition is clinically and pathophysiologically analogous to eclampsia.

REHABILITATION

The majority of stroke-related deaths result from medical complications (pneumonia, myocardial infarction, sepsis) rather than as a consequence of the neurologic deficit. Appropriate rehabilitation optimizes functional recovery and minimizes medical complications.

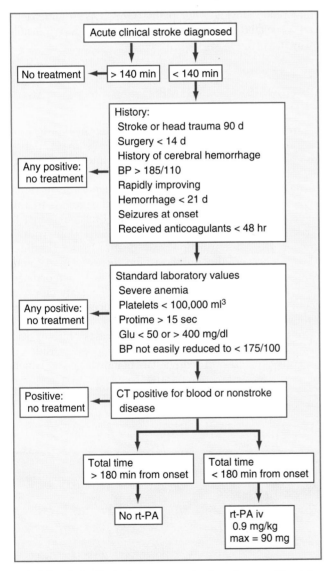

FIGURE 123–6 Evaluating acute stroke for safe recombinant tissue-type plasminogen activator (rt-PA) therapy. (From National Institute of Neurological Disorders and Stroke rt-PA Stroke Study Group: Tissue plasminogen activator for acute ischemic stroke. N Engl J Med 1996; 333:1581–1587.)

Intracerebral Hemorrhage

Intracerebral hemorrhage (ICH) may be diffuse (subarachnoid hemorrhage) or focal (intraparenchymal) and accounts for 20% of all strokes. Table 123–5 lists the causes of spontaneous intracerebral hemorrhage. The

TABLE 123-5 **Causes of Spontaneous Intracerebral Hemorrhage**

> **Intraparenchymal Hemorrhage**
> Trauma
> Hypertension
> Amyloid (congophilic) angiopathy
> Arteriovenous malformation
> Bleeding diathesis (anticoagulants, thrombolytics)
> Drugs (amphetamines, cocaine)
>
> **Subarachnoid Hemorrhage**
> Congenital saccular aneurysm (85%)
> Unknown (15%)

acute rise in intracranial pressure from arterial rupture frequently results in loss of consciousness at the outset; some patients die from herniation.

HYPERTENSIVE INTRACEREBRAL HEMORRHAGE

Hypertensive intracerebral hemorrhage often occurs at the same sites that are affected in lacunar infarction. Pathologically, microaneurysms known as *Charcot-Bouchard aneurysms* have been identified in some cases. The commonest sites for hypertensive hemorrhage are the putamen (40%), thalamus (12%), lobar white matter (15% to 20%), caudate (8%), pons (8%), and cerebellum (8%). Although CT readily identifies the hemorrhage, several clinical findings may help localize the site (Table 123–6). In general, severity of headache correlates with the size of the lesion. Diminished level of alertness is caused by mass effect, increased intracranial pressure, or direct involvement of the brain stem reticular activating system. Seizures are slightly more frequent during the acute phase in ICH than in ischemic stroke. Both basal ganglia and thalamic hemorrhages may rupture into the adjacent ventricle and result in secondary hydrocephalus; cerebellar hemorrhage may cause obstructive hydrocephalus as a result of compression of the fourth ventricle.

With intracerebral hematoma, patients' level of consciousness often deteriorates during the first 24 to 48 hours after the initial symptoms, usually because of the development of edema around the lesion. Edema that is sufficient to cause significant brain shift results in herniation of brain tissue. In addition to causing direct pressure on vital brain stem structures, herniation may cause compression of adjacent blood vessels (particularly the PCAs and ACAs), resulting in infarction.

LOBAR HEMORRHAGE

Lobar hemorrhages occur in a peripheral distribution of the cerebral white matter. They are usually smaller than hypertensive ICHs and have a more benign prognosis. In young persons, they may be secondary to arteriovenous malformations or ingestion of sympathomimetic drugs. In elderly persons, they are usually secondary to congophilic amyloid angiopathy (CAA). As in anticoagulant-associated hemorrhage, signs tend to develop insidiously in CAA.

DIAGNOSIS, MANAGEMENT, AND PROGNOSIS

CT remains the diagnostic test of choice in the diagnosis of ICH, which acutely shows up as a hyperintense area with mass effect and (later) hypointense surrounding edema. MRI is less sensitive for detecting hemorrhage in the early stages. The management of ICH depends on the size and location of the lesion. In the acute phase, the mass effect of a cerebral hematoma is far greater than in a large cerebral infarction, with a greater risk of herniation and death. In the chronic phase, however, the prognosis for recovery in patients who survive is much better for those with hemorrhage than for those with ischemic stroke. Thus therapy for acute hemorrhage is directed at reducing mass effect either by medical decompression with controlled hyperventilation or mannitol or, in rare cases, by surgical decompression. This latter option should be considered urgently in cases of cerebellar hemorrhage in which

TABLE 123-6 **Clinical Manifestations Related to Site of Intracerebral Hemorrhage**

Site	Manifestation				
	Headache	Pupils	Eye Movements	Sensorimotor Signs	Other
Basal ganglia	Severe	Normal	Normal	Hemiparesis	Confusion, aphasia
Thalamus	Moderate	Small, poorly reactive to light	Hyperconvergence Absent vertical gaze	Hemisensory > motor loss	Hypersomnolence
Pons	Severe	Small, reactive	Horizontal gaze paresis	Quadriplegia	Coma
Cerebellum	Severe, occipital	Normal	Normal	Ataxia	Early vomiting

patients are especially at risk of sudden deterioration either through acute obstructive hydrocephalus (because of compression of the fourth ventricle) or as a result of direct pressure on the caudal brain stem.

Intracranial Aneurysms

Intracranial aneurysms occur in three forms: fusiform, mycotic, and saccular (congenital "berry") aneurysms.

Fusiform aneurysms represent ectatic dilatations of large arteries, usually the basilar or intracranial carotid arteries. They rarely rupture but may compress adjacent brain tissue or cranial nerves and cause local neurologic dysfunction. They are rarely accessible to surgical repair.

Mycotic aneurysms occur in the context of bacterial endocarditis when septic emboli lodge in a peripheral vessel. They are often multiple and located distally in the arterial tree, and thus they are accessible to surgical repair should they fail to respond to antibiotic therapy.

Saccular aneurysms form at arterial bifurcations (Fig. 123–7); 80% are located in the anterior circulation. They are thought to arise from a combination of a congenital defect in the arterial media and elastic lamina and gradual deterioration from hemodynamic stress. Higher incidences are found among patients with polycystic kidney disease and Marfan's syndrome.

Approximately 6% of the population harbor saccular aneurysms, which are multiple in 25% of cases. Fortunately, the annual incidence of rupture is only about 10 per 100,000. Of patients with those that do rupture, 33% die before reaching a hospital and another 20% die in the hospital. Overall, only 30% recover without significant disability.

CLINICAL MANIFESTATIONS OF SUBARACHNOID HEMORRHAGE

Aneurysms may rupture at any time, but especially during periods of strenuous activity such as exercise, coitus, or strenuous physical work. The commonest manifestation is sudden severe headache ("the worst headache of my life") often accompanied by neck pain and rigidity. Loss of consciousness and vomiting are common sequelae. Occasionally, with so-called *sentinel hemorrhages,* the onset of symptoms is less cataclysmic and the headache gradually resolves over 24 to 48 hours. Aneurysms may also manifest by compression of adjacent cranial nerves, such as compression of cranial nerve III by an aneurysm of the posterior communicating artery. *Giant aneurysms* (>2.5 cm) may compress cranial nerves III, IV, and VI in the cavernous sinus. In rare instances, aneurysms may manifest as TIAs as a result of embolization from a thrombus within an aneurysm.

DIAGNOSIS

CT of the brain shows subarachnoid hemorrhage in 95% of cases, and its location may suggest a site of rupture. A normal CT scan does not totally rule out subarachnoid hemorrhage and mandates a lumbar puncture in patients with symptoms. Care must be taken to centrifuge cerebrospinal fluid to detect true xanthochromia, the yellow coloration that develops by 6 hours after subarachnoid hemorrhage. Contrast CT or MRI identifies aneurysms larger than 5 mm as well as ateriovenous malformations. Cerebral angiography remains the gold standard for the diagnosis of intracranial aneurysms, and it is usually performed when surgery is being contemplated and deferred in severe cases in which there is significant risk of vasospasm. A small group of patients

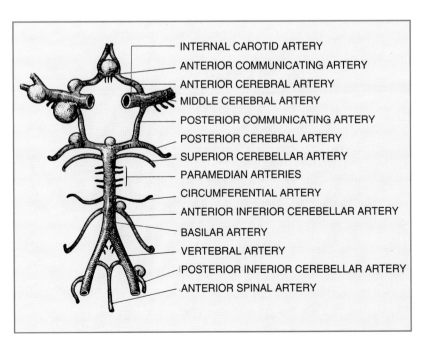

FIGURE 123–7　The more common sites of berry aneurysm. The diagrammatic size of the aneurysm at the various sites is directly proportional to its frequency at that locus.

INTERNAL CAROTID ARTERY
ANTERIOR COMMUNICATING ARTERY
ANTERIOR CEREBRAL ARTERY
MIDDLE CEREBRAL ARTERY
POSTERIOR COMMUNICATING ARTERY
POSTERIOR CEREBRAL ARTERY
SUPERIOR CEREBELLAR ARTERY
PARAMEDIAN ARTERIES
CIRCUMFERENTIAL ARTERY
ANTERIOR INFERIOR CEREBELLAR ARTERY
BASILAR ARTERY
VERTEBRAL ARTERY
POSTERIOR INFERIOR CEREBELLAR ARTERY
ANTERIOR SPINAL ARTERY

TABLE 123-7   Complications of Subarachnoid Hemorrhage

Hypertension (systemic and intracranial)
Vasospasm
Hemorrhage (rebleeding)
Hydrocephalus
Hyponatremia (syndrome of inappropriate antidiuretic hormone; cerebral salt wasting)

with predominantly perimesencephalic hemorrhage on CT have normal cerebral angiograms and a more benign outcome. The electrocardiogram may show deep, symmetric T-wave inversion. Once the diagnosis of subarachnoid hemorrhage has been made (or if clinical suspicion persists, even with inconclusive testing), the patient should be managed under the guidance of a neurosurgical team.

MANAGEMENT AND PROGNOSIS

An essential part of management of patients with subarachnoid hemorrhage is to prevent any one of several complications (Table 123–7). To reduce the risk of rebleeding, patients are placed on bed rest with analgesics for pain relief, mild sedation, and the use of laxatives to reduce straining. Management of hypertension requires balancing the need to maintain a steady cerebral perfusion pressure in the context of raised intracranial pressure and possible vasospasm and, in contrast, the risk of rebleeding. The peak timing for vasospasm is between 5 and 9 days after the hemorrhage, and it may be accompanied by an alteration in the neurologic status.

Vascular Malformations

Vascular malformations of the brain and spinal cord are grouped according to vessel size and composition. *Venous angiomas* are the most common and tend to lie close to the brain surface. Malformations composed of capillaries are called *capillary telangiectases* and are typically located within the brain stem. *Cavernous angiomas* are composed of dilated sinusoidal channels, are readily detectable by CT, and rarely bleed.

Arteriovenous malformations are composed of tangles of arteries connected directly to veins without intervening capillaries. They may produce headache, seizures, or hemorrhage, accounting for 1% of all strokes. The initial hemorrhage typically occurs before the fourth decade, with a 7% risk of rebleeding within the first year afterward. Hemorrhage may occur into the brain parenchyma, subarachnoid space, or intraventricular space.

Treatment of arteriovenous malformations is guided by individual factors, such as the age of the patient, location and composition of the lesion, and manifestation. In general, arteriovenous malformations in older patients (>55 years) are treated conservatively, whereas younger patients are treated either by surgical excision or, less commonly, by irradiation combined with embolization of the arterial feeding vessel.

REFERENCES

Adams RJ: Neurologic complications. *In* Embury S, Hebbel RP, Mohandas N, et al (eds): Sickle Cell Disease: Basic Principles and Clinical Practice. New York: Raven Press, 1994.

Barnett HJ, Mohr JP, Stein BM, et al (eds): Stroke: Pathophysiology, Diagnosis and Management. New York: Churchill Livingstone, 1998.

Caplan LR: Stroke—A Clinical Approach. Boston: Butterworth-Heinemann, 1993.

Pulsinelli WA: Cerebrovascular diseases. *In* Goldman L, Bennett JC (eds): Cecil Textbook of Medicine, 21st ed. Philadelphia: WB Saunders, 2000, pp 2092–2115.

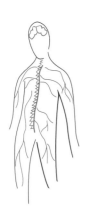

124

TRAUMA TO HEAD AND SPINE

Roger P. Simon

Traumatic injury is the third most common cause of death in the United States; half the deaths result from head injury, and most occur before patients reach the hospital. Men less than 30 years old account for two thirds of these cases; half of these incidents involve alcohol intoxication. Spinal injury is less likely to be fatal and therefore results in long-term residual disability. Injury of the head and spine may coexist; spinal injury should be assumed in unconscious patients or in any patient who has sustained trauma and complains of neck or back pain.

Head Injury

SKULL FRACTURES

Cutaneous signs that suggest *basilar skull fracture* are those resulting from seepage of blood from the fracture site: mastoid *(Battle's sign)*, periocular *(raccoon eye)*, and conjunctival blood extending from the posterior orbit. These signs occur 24 to 72 hours after injury. Clear fluid, leaking from the auditory canal or nose, should be assumed to be cerebrospinal fluid (CSF); it documents a potential portal of entry for infection and mandates close observation, although prophylactic antibiotics are not recommended. Fractures of the base of the skull may also result in cranial nerve injury, particularly olfactory, ocular, oculomotor, or facial nerve injury. Bruits over the orbits occur in patients with traumatic carotid-cavernous fistulas and predict the development of pulsating exophthalmos during the next 24 to 48 hours.

FOCAL BRAIN INJURY

In the extracerebral space, *venous bleeding in the subdural compartment or arterial bleeding in the epidural space* produces expanding masses; these lesions are readily seen on noncontrast computed tomography. The symptoms and signs are variable (Table 124–1), but altered consciousness, with or without a "lucid interval," predominates. Emergency neurosurgical evaluation is mandatory. *Parenchymal hemorrhage* occurs in cortical regions adjacent to the skull base or falx such as the frontal or occipital pole, temporal tip, cerebellar hemispheres, or parasagittal convexity. Bleeding into contused brain may be delayed. Blood is frequently found in the *subarachnoid space*, which may occasionally cause confusion among primary head trauma, an aneurysmal origin of bleeding, or secondary head injury from a fall after loss of consciousness.

DIFFUSE BRAIN INJURY

Diffuse brain injury results from angular (side-to-side) head motion. It causes the immediate phenomenon of *concussion* (brief unconsciousness) and is responsible for prolonged traumatic coma. The pathologic correlate is *diffuse axonal injury*, which is the result of widespread axonal disruption by shearing forces produced as inertia causes the brain to lag behind the skull during head acceleration-deceleration movements.

ACUTE MANAGEMENT

Maintenance of oxygenation and, especially, of blood pressure is essential because cerebral blood flow falls and the protective mechanisms of cerebral blood flow autoregulation are impaired in brain trauma. Systemic hypotension doubles mortality and in adults is not the consequence of the intracranial bleeding itself. Blood pressure needs to be adjusted in proportion to intracranial pressure; the *perfusion pressure* (blood pressure minus intracranial pressure) should be initially maintained at over 60 to 70 mm Hg. Hyperventilation decreases intracranial pressure but worsens outcome because of the induced cerebral vasoconstriction, and possibly also by removing the hydrogen ion block of the postsynaptic glutamate (N-methyl-D-aspartate) receptor. Osmotic agents such as mannitol may be effective briefly in re-

TABLE 124-1 Clinical Features of Subdural Hematoma

	Acute* (82 cases) (%)	Subacute† (91 cases) (%)	Chronic‡ (216 cases) (%)
Symptoms			
Depression of consciousness	100	88	47
Vomiting	24	31	30
Weakness	20	19	22
Confusion	12	41	37
Headache	11	44	81
Speech disturbance	6	8	5
Seizures	6	3	9
Vertigo	0	4	5
Visual disturbance	0	0	12
Signs			
Depression of consciousness	100	88	59
Pupillary inequality	57	27	20
Motor asymmetry	44	37	41
Confusion and memory loss	17	21	27
Aphasia	6	12	11
Papilledema	1	15	22
Hemianopia	0	4	3
Facial weakness	0	3	3

* Within 3 days of trauma.
† 4–20 days after trauma.
‡ >20 days after trauma.
Data from McKissock W, Richardson A, Bloom WH: Subdural hematoma: A review of 389 cases. Lancet 1960; 1:1365–1370.

ducing intracranial pressure. Antiedema agents such as corticosteroids have not been shown to alter outcome. Moderate (whole-body) hypothermia, 32°C to 33°C for the first 24 hours, may increase recovery in patients with severe traumatic brain injury.

QUANTIFYING INJURY

Prognosis

The Glasgow Coma Scale (GCS) (Table 124–2) allows for serial assessment of the head-injured patient and is an excellent guide to the severity of injury. The GCS categorizes injury as mild (13 to 15), moderate (9 to 12),

TABLE 124-2 Glasgow Coma Scale*

Eye Opening	Best Motor Response	Best Verbal Response
4: Spontaneous	6: Obeys commands	5: Oriented
3: To voice	5: Localizes pain	4: Confused
2: To pain	4: Withdraws to pain	3: Inappropriate vocalization
1: None	3: Reflex flexion	2: Incomprehensible
	2: Reflex extension	1: No vocalization
	1: Flaccid	

* Glasgow Coma Scale score is the sum of best scores in eye opening, motor and verbal performance, e.g., normal = 15; flaccid, mute, eyes closed = 3.

or severe (3 to 8), with the motor response being the most sensitive. A patient's GCS score correlates with outcome, as follows:

Death or vegetative state: GCS 3 to 4 (80%), 5 to 7 (54%), 8 to 10 (27%), 11 to 15 (6%).
Residual cognitive disability: CGS 9 to 12 (62%), <8 (80%).

Ninety percent of recovery is determined at 6 months, and 95% is determined at 1 year.

Apolipoprotein E

The putative Alzheimer's susceptibility gene, apolipoprotein E (APOE) ∊4, may also predict the duration of posttraumatic coma and eventual outcome, a concept that suggests a degree of genetic susceptibility to the effects of traumatic brain injury. Patients recovering from traumatic brain injury may be at risk of earlier onset of Alzheimer's disease if they are predisposed to this condition.

CHRONIC SEQUELAE

Postconcussive syndrome often follows relatively minor trauma. The symptom constellation nearly always includes headache of almost any clinical pattern from tension to migraine. Additional symptoms include dizziness, weakness, gait instability, inability to concentrate, memory loss, personality changes, and problems with sleep regulation. Resolution occurs over many months. In patients with more severe injury, cognitive impairment may be permanent.

Focal or generalized seizures may develop immediately (in the first week) or in a delayed fashion after head injury, and they occur in proportion to the severity of injury. Prophylactic anticonvulsants are routinely administered and decrease the incidence of early seizures; the incidence of *posttraumatic epilepsy* is not reduced.

Spinal Cord Injury

Possible spinal cord injuries should be considered in all patients with head injury. Patients who are responsive may complain of neck and back pain suggesting cervical or thoracolumbar fractures. If evidence of injury is noted in an awake patient or if the patient is unconscious, immobilization of the neck must be the first step in treatment. Attention is next focused on maintenance of blood pressure and oxygenation, to preclude secondary injury as blood pressure control will be impaired with injury of descending sympathetic pathways. Bladder catheterization is essential in spinal cord injury, because the patient's awareness of bladder filling is impaired or absent.

On examination of patients with severe spinal cord injury, deep tendon reflexes are usually absent below the level of the lesion (ankle, S1–S2; knee, L3–L4; biceps, C5–C6; triceps, C7–C8). A sensory level to pinprick may be found on the chest. The pattern of motor impairment dictates the focus of imaging studies. High cervical lesions (C3, C4, C5) affect all arm muscles and ventilation; patients with midcervical lesions are able to flex at the elbow but not to extend. Patients with low cervical lesions may preserve elbow flexion and extension but not hand muscle function. Thoracic injury results in paraplegia.

Partial spinal cord injuries may be seen particularly with acute neck extension (e.g., falling and striking the forehead and thereby forcing the neck into hyperextension); typically, a central spinal cord syndrome or anterior spinal artery syndrome results, producing bilateral arm weakness with normal leg strength (Fig. 124–1).

IMAGING

Radiographs of the cervical spine should be obtained with portable equipment, to decrease the need to move the patient. Lateral radiographs must include all seven cervical vertebra and the odontoid. In a patient with neck pain, further assessment for cervical spine stability may be indicated even if plain radiographs are normal. Extension and flexion radiographs should be obtained. *The patient moves his or her own neck*, first in extension (usually reducing subluxations) and, if results are normal, then in flexion. Computed tomography should be used in follow-up of patients with subluxations or fractures and is indicated if plain radiographs are normal

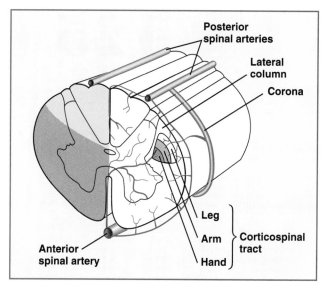

FIGURE 124–1 Blood supply to the cervical spinal cord. *Left*, Major territories supplied by the anterior spinal artery *(dark shading)* and the posterior spinal artery *(light shading)*. *Right*, Pattern of supply by the intramedullary arteries. The descending motor fibers of the corticospinal tract are supplied by both the anterior and the posterior spinal arteries, with the fibers supplying arm movement in a watershed area susceptible to hypoperfusion. (From Simon RP, Aminoff MJ, Greenberg DA: Clinical Neurology. Stamford, CT: Appleton & Lange, 1999.)

but a neurologic abnormality is present. Magnetic resonance images bone poorly but readily demonstrates spinal cord hemorrhage or contusion.

TREATMENT

In controlled trials, only methylprednisolone was effective in improving motor outcome. All patients with spinal cord injury should receive 30 mg/kg within 8 hours of injury, followed by 5.4 mg/kg over the next 23 hours. GM_1 gangliosides appear to increase the rate, but not the ultimate degree, of recovery.

Whiplash

Neck-wrenching injuries such as occur in "rear end" automobile collisions result in neck and head pain in about half these patients. Most symptoms should resolve in a few weeks to 1 month, and all symptoms should resolve by 1 year.

REFERENCES

Chiles BW, Cooper PR: Acute spinal injury. N Engl J Med 1996; 334: 514–520.

White RJ, Likavec MJ: The diagnosis and initial management of head injury. N Engl J Med 1992; 327:1507–1511.

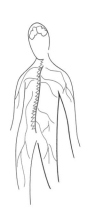

125

EPILEPSY

Robert C. Griggs

Definition

Epilepsy is a chronic condition whose major clinical manifestation is the occurrence of epileptic seizures characterized by sudden and usually unprovoked attacks of subjective experiential phenomena, altered consciousness, or involuntary movements. The diagnosis of epilepsy indicates that a patient has recurrent seizures, but not all seizures imply epilepsy. Seizures result from abnormal brain electrical activity and are a common sign of brain dysfunction. They occur during the course of many medical or neurologic illnesses in which brain function is temporarily deranged (*symptomatic* seizures) (Table 125–1). Such seizures are usually self-limited and do not persist if the underlying disorder can be corrected. Seizures can also occur as a reaction of the brain to physiologic stress, such as sleep deprivation, fever, and alcohol or sedative drug withdrawal. Occurrence of such seizures suggests an increased seizure susceptibility (lowered seizure threshold). Genetic factors or unrecognized previous central nervous system injury may account for such susceptibility. Isolated seizures may also occur for no discoverable reason as unprovoked events in presumably healthy people. None of these kinds of seizures represent epilepsy.

Incidence and Etiology

Seizures can begin at any time of life. In developed countries 2% to 4% of all persons have recurrent seizures at some time during their lives. Developing countries as well as inner-city areas show higher incidence rates. Epilepsy affects about 45 million people worldwide. The incidence is highest among young children and the elderly, and men are affected slightly more often than women (1.5:1). Epilepsy results from many conditions and mechanisms (Fig. 125–1). About 70% of adults and 40% of children with new-onset epilepsy have partial (focal) seizures. In many it is not possible to

identify a specific cause, although focal seizures imply a cerebral injury or lesion. The most common specific lesions are hippocampal sclerosis, gangliogliomas and glial tumors, cavernous malformations, neuronal migrational defects (cortical dysplasia) and hamartomas, encephalitis, cerebral trauma, and hemorrhage. Not all patients with cerebral lesions develop epilepsy; how a particular lesion becomes epileptogenic is poorly understood.

Many specific genetic disorders cause epilepsy, but these disorders are uncommon causes. However, a growing number of epilepsies are recognized to be caused by specific gene lesions. Most others have clear hereditary influences, but the genetic factors have not yet been defined. At least three of the genetic epilepsies are known to be channelopathies. It is likely that channel dysfunction will be the cause of others. Neuronal migration defects (see Chapter 122) are now readily identified by magnetic resonance imaging (MRI) and are a common cause of genetic and acquired epilepsy.

Classification and Clinical Manifestations

The most widely used classification scheme is that of the International League Against Epilepsy (Table 125–2). Seizures are classified by their clinical symptoms and signs. The manifestations of a seizure depend on whether most or only a part of the cerebral cortex is involved at the beginning, the functions of the cortical areas where the seizure originates, and the subsequent pattern of spread within the brain. Seizures are of two types: (1) those with onset limited to part of the cerebral hemisphere (*partial* or *focal* seizures) and (2) those that involve the cerebral cortex diffusely from the beginning (*generalized* seizures). Seizures are dynamic and evolve; a patient's seizure pattern varies depending on the extent and manner of spread of the electrical discharge. Thus, *simple* partial seizures many evolve into *complex* partial seizures, and partial seizures can evolve into *secondarily generalized* tonic-clonic convulsions.

TABLE 125-1 Causes of Symptomatic Seizures

Acute electrolyte disorders
  Acute hyponatremia (<120 mEq/L)—especially acute
  Acute hypernatremia (>155 mEq/L)—especially acute
  Hyperosmolality (>310 mOsm/L)
  Hypocalcemia (<7 mg/dL)
Hypoglycemia (<30 mg/dL)
Drugs
  Isoniazid, pencillins
  Theophylline, aminophylline, ephedrine, phenylpropanol-
    amine, terbutaline
  Lidocaine, meperidine
  Tricyclic antidepressants
  Cyclosporine
  Cocaine (crack), phencyclidine, amphetamines; alcohol
    withdrawal
Central nervous system disease
  Hypertensive encephalopathy, eclampsia
  Hepatic encephalopathy, renal failure
  Sickle cell disease, thrombotic thrombocytopenic
    purpura
  Systemic lupus erythematosus
  Meningitis, encephalitis, brain abscess
  Acute head trauma (impact seizures), stroke, brain
    tumor

TABLE 125-2 International League Against Epilepsy Classification of Epileptic Seizures and Syndromes

Classification of Seizures
Partial (Focal) Seizures
  Simple partial seizures (consciousness not impaired)
    With motor signs
    With sensory signs
    With psychic symptoms
    With autonomic symptoms
  Complex partial seizures (consciousness is impaired)
    Simple partial onset followed by impaired conscious-
      ness
    With impairment of consciousness at onset
    With automatisms
  Partial seizures evolving to secondarily generalized sei-
    zures
Generalized Seizures of Nonfocal Origin
  Absence seizures
  Myoclonic seizures; myoclonic jerks (single or multiple)
  Tonic-clonic seizures
  Tonic seizures
  Atonic seizures
Classification of Epileptic Syndromes
Idiopathic Epilepsy Syndromes (Focal or Generalized)
  Benign neonatal convulsions
  Benign partial epilepsy of childhood
  Childhood absence epilepsy
  Juvenile myoclonic epilepsy
  Idiopathic epilepsy, otherwise unspecified
Symptomatic Epilepsy Syndromes (Focal or Generalized)
  West's syndrome (infantile spasms)
  Lennox-Gastaut syndrome
  Partial continuous epilepsy
  Temporal lobe epilepsy
  Frontal lobe epilepsy
  Post-traumatic epilepsy
Other Epilepsy Syndromes of Uncertain or Mixed Classification
  Neonatal seizures
  Febrile seizures
  Reflex epilepsy
  Adult nonconvulsive status epilepticus

Modified from Pedley TA: The epilepsies. *In* Goldman L, Bennett JC (eds): Cecil Textbook of Medicine, 21st ed. Philadelphia, WB Saunders, 2000, pp 2151–2163.

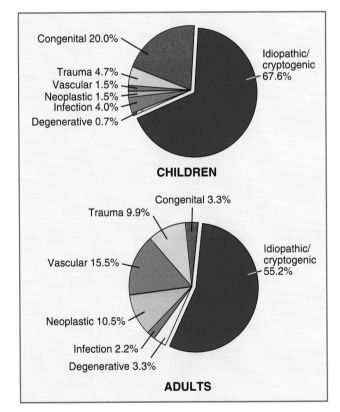

FIGURE 125-1 Etiology of epilepsy, according to age, in all newly diagnosed cases in Rochester, Minnesota, 1935–1984. (Modified from Hauser WA, Annegers JF, Kurland LT: Incidence of epilepsy and unprovoked seizures in Rochester, Minnesota: 1935–1984. Epilepsia 1994; 34:453.)

PARTIAL SEIZURES

The onset of a seizure, as described by the patient and observers, often indicates if a seizure begins focally. Simple partial seizures result when the epileptic electrical discharge remains limited to a focal area of cortex. Patients can interact normally with their environment except for limitations imposed by the seizure on specific localized brain functions. Simple partial seizures include subjective sensory and psychological phenomena. These auras affect about 60% of patients with focal epilepsy. Specific symptoms often localize the epileptogenic focus (Table 125–3). The location of the focus is important for diagnosis: the location often predicts the nature of the pathology and directs diagnostic testing. Moreover,

TABLE 125–3 **Localization of Seizures by Symptoms and Ictal Manifestations**

Locus	Manifestation
Temporal lobe	
Uncus/amygdala	Foul odor
Middle/inferior temporal gyrus	Visual changes: micropsia, macropsia
Parahippocampal-hippocampal area	Déjà vu; jamais vu
Parahippocampal-septal area	Fear, pleasure, anger, dreamy sensation
Auditory association cortex	Voices, music
Insular, anterior temporal cortex	Lip smacking, abdominal symptoms, cardiac arrhythmia
Frontal lobe	
Motor cortex	Clonic movements of face, fingers, hand, foot
Premotor cortex	Arm extension
Language areas	Speech arrest, aphasia
Parietal lobe cortex	Sensory symptoms
Occipital lobe cortex	Visual: teichopsias, metamorphopsias

both medical and surgical treatment are determined by focus location.

Simple partial seizures with motor signs begin with clonic (rhythmic jerking) or tonic (stiffening) movements of a discrete body part. Because of their large cortical representation, muscles of the face and hand are involved often. When the seizure discharge begins in the primary motor cortex and spreads to involve the rest of the precentral gyrus, clonic movements progress in an orderly sequence ("jacksonian march") that reflects the homunculus representation (e.g., thumb to fingers to face to leg). More often, however, ictal discharges involve supplementary or other secondary motor areas of the frontal lobe and produce contralateral flexion and elevation of the arm, contralateral turning of the head and eyes, and tonic extension of the ipsilateral arm (the so-called fencer's posture). Other simple partial motor signs include speech arrest, vocalizations, and eye blinking.

Simple partial seizures may be followed by a transient neurologic abnormality reflecting postictal depression of the epileptogenic cortical area. Thus, focal weakness may follow a simple partial motor seizure, numbness may follow a sensory seizure, and blindness may follow an occipital lobe seizure. These reversible neurologic deficits are referred to as Todd's paralysis and rarely last for more than 48 hours. Prompt examination of a patient after a seizure may show transient focal abnormalities that are useful clues to the site of seizure origin.

Complex partial seizures impair consciousness and produce unresponsiveness. In temporal lobe seizures, loss of consciousness results when the ictal discharge spreads bilaterally to involve both hippocampal and amygdala areas, the parahippocampal gyri, and, to some extent, the entorhinal cortex and subfrontal, especially septal, regions. Seventy percent to 80% of complex partial seizures arise from the temporal lobe, and more than two thirds of these originate in mesial temporal lobe structures, especially the hippocampus, amygdala, and parahippocampal gyrus. Remaining cases of complex partial seizures arise mainly from the frontal lobe, with smaller percentages originating in parietal and occipital lobes. Many complex partial seizures evolve from simple partial seizures; consciousness becomes impaired as the seizure progresses. Complex partial seizures preceded by an olfactory aura are referred to as *uncinate fits* because of their origin in or near the uncus of the medial temporal lobe. Table 125–3 lists other symptoms and signs of limbic and temporal lesions.

Psychomotor, temporal lobe, and *limbic seizures* are all terms that have been used in the past to describe many of the ictal behaviors now classified as complex partial seizures, but they are not synonymous. Not all complex partial seizures arise from the temporal lobe, nor do all involve the limbic system. Some temporal lobe and limbic phenomena reflect unilateral ictal discharges and may not be associated with the significant alteration and awareness that invariably occurs with complex partial seizures.

GENERALIZED SEIZURES

Generalized seizures begin diffusely and involve both cerebral hemispheres simultaneously from the outset. They lack clinical and electroencephalographic (EEG) features that indicate a localized cerebral origin. Generalized seizures are subdivided mainly on the basis of the presence or absence and character of ictal motor manifestations. They must be distinguished from focal seizures that spread to cause *secondary generalized seizures.*

Generalized tonic-clonic seizures (grand mal convulsions) are characterized by abrupt loss of consciousness with bilateral tonic extension of the trunk and limbs (tonic phase), often accompanied by a loud vocalization as air is forcefully expelled across tightly contracted vocal cords (the "epileptic cry"), followed by bilaterally synchronous muscle jerking (clonic phase). In some patients, a few clonic jerks precede the tonic-clonic sequence; in others, only a tonic or a clonic phase is seen. Urinary incontinence is common; fecal incontinence is rare. The actual ictus does not usually last more than 90 seconds. The postictal phase is marked by transient deep stupor, followed in 15 to 30 minutes by a lethargic, confused state with automatic behavior. As recovery progresses, many patients complain of headache, muscle soreness, mental dulling, lack of energy, or mood changes lasting as long as 24 hours.

Generalized tonic-clonic seizures result in a number of striking, but transient, physiologic changes, including blood hypoxia and lactic acidosis, elevated plasma catecholamine levels, and increased concentrations of serum creatine kinase, prolactin, corticotropin, cortisol, β-endorphin, and growth hormone. Complications include oral trauma, vertebral compression fractures, shoulder dislocation, aspiration pneumonia, and sudden death, which may be related to acute pulmonary edema, cardiac arrhythmia, or suffocation.

Absence seizures (petit mal seizures) occur mainly in children and are characterized by sudden, momentary lapses in awareness (the absence attack), staring, rhythmic blinking, and, often, a few small clonic jerks of arms or hands. Behavior and awareness return to normal immediately. There is no postictal period and usually no recollection that a seizure has occurred. Most absence seizures last less than 10 seconds.

Lapses of awareness that have a more gradual onset, do not resolve as abruptly, and are accompanied by autonomic features or loss of muscle tone are referred to as *atypical absence seizures*. These occur most often in children with mental retardation, and they do not respond as well to antiepileptic drug treatment.

Myoclonic seizures manifest as rapid, recurrent, brief muscle jerks that can occur bilaterally, synchronously or asynchronously, or unilaterally without loss of consciousness. The myoclonic jerks range from small movements of the face or hands to massive bilateral spasms that simultaneously affect the head, limbs, and trunk. Repeated myoclonic seizures may seem to crescendo and terminate in a generalized tonic-clonic convulsion. Although they can occur at any time, myoclonic seizures often cluster shortly after waking or while failing asleep.

Atonic seizures ("drop attacks") occur most often in children with diffuse encephalopathies and are characterized by sudden loss of muscle tone that may result in falls with self-injury. *Reflex seizures* are attacks precipitated by a specific stimulus, such as touch, a musical tune, a particular movement, reading, stroboscopic light patterns, or complex visual images.

FEBRILE SEIZURES

This is the most common cause of convulsions in children. They affect between 3% and 5% of all children in the United States and Europe younger than the age of 5 years. Most febrile seizures occur between the ages of 6 months and 4 years, although sometimes they occur in children as old as 6 or 7 years. About 30% of children have more than one attack; the chance of recurrence is greatest if the first seizure occurs before 1 year of age or there is a family history of febrile seizures. Although the great majority of affected children have no long-term consequences, febrile seizures increase the risk of developing epilepsy later. This risk is low for most children, 2% to 3%, but it increases to 10% to 13% in those who have had prolonged or focal seizures, who have a family history of afebrile seizures, or who were neurologically abnormal before the first febrile seizure. Febrile seizures are not associated with, nor do they cause, mental retardation, poor school performance, or behavior problems.

BENIGN PARTIAL EPILEPSY OF CHILDHOOD WITH CENTRAL-MIDTEMPORAL SPIKES (ROLANDIC EPILEPSY)

This is one of the most common epileptic syndromes of childhood, representing about 15% of all pediatric epilepsies. Seizures usually begin between the ages of 4 and 13 years; affected children are otherwise normal. Most have seizures principally or only at night. Because sleep promotes secondary generalization, parents report only tonic-clonic convulsions; the focal signature is usually missed. In contrast, seizures occurring during the day are typically focal: twitching of one side of the face, speech arrest, drooling, and paresthesias of the face, gums, tongue, and inner cheeks. These may be so minor as to escape notice. Seizures may progress to include hemiclonic movements or hemitonic posturing. EEGs show a distinctive pattern of stereotyped epileptiform discharges over the central and midtemporal regions. Prognosis is invariably good, and seizures disappear by mid to late adolescence. Outcome is not affected by treatment, but carbamazepine prevents recurrent attacks.

JUVENILE MYOCLONIC EPILEPSY

This is a frequently encountered type of idiopathic generalized epilepsy. It begins most often between the ages of 8 and 20 years in otherwise healthy individuals. When fully developed, the syndrome is characterized by morning myoclonic jerks, generalized tonic-clonic seizures that occur just after awakening, normal intelligence, and a family history of similar seizures.

LENNOX-GASTAUT SYNDROME

This term is used for a heterogeneous group of early childhood epileptic encephalopathies that have in common physical brain abnormalities, mental retardation, and uncontrolled seizures.

TEMPORAL LOBE EPILEPSY

This is the most common epileptic syndrome of adults, accounting for at least 40% of epilepsy cases. Seizures begin in late childhood or adolescence, and there is often a history of febrile seizures. Virtually all patients have complex partial seizures, some of which secondarily generalize. Temporal lobe epilepsy arises most often from mesial temporal limbic structures, typically in association with a characteristic lesion known as hippocampal sclerosis. In 20% of cases, temporal lobe epilepsy is caused by other structural lesions such as cavernous malformations, hamartomas, cortical dysplasia, glial tumors, and scars related to previous head injuries or encephalitis.

POST-TRAUMATIC EPILEPSY

The chance of developing post-traumatic epilepsy relates directly to the severity of the head injury. After penetrating wounds and other severe head injuries, for example, about one third of patients develop seizures within 1 year. Severe head injuries are defined by the presence of a cerebral contusion, intracerebral or intracranial hematoma, unconsciousness or amnesia lasting more than 24 hours, or persistent abnormalities on neurologic examination, such as hemiparesis or aphasia. Although the majority of patients develop seizures within 1 to 2 years of injury, new-onset seizures may still appear 5 or more years later. Two thirds of patients with post-traumatic epilepsy have partial or secondarily generalized seizures. Mild head injuries (uncomplicated brief loss of consciousness, no skull fracture, absence of focal neurologic signs, no contusion or hematoma) do not increase the risk of seizures.

Diagnosis

Accurate diagnosis is the cornerstone of rational management. The diagnostic evaluation has three objectives: (1) to determine if the patient has epilepsy; (2) to classify the seizures and type of epilepsy accurately and determine if the clinical data fit a particular epilepsy syndrome; and (3) to identify, if possible, a specific underlying cause. The patient's description of the experi-

ence or a witness's accurate observation of an attack usually provides the most rewarding information. The setting of the attack often suggests acute causes such as drug withdrawal, central nervous system infection, trauma, or stroke; a history of recent-onset seizures in an adult suggests an intracranial mass lesion, and a more chronically sustained or remote history of attacks suggests chronic epilepsy. Any focal feature reported either as an aura or during or after the seizure suggests a structural brain lesion demanding appropriate investigation. The pattern of an attack as well as the patient's age immediately suggests the possible types and causes.

The physical examination is normal in most patients with epilepsy. Physical findings that should be sought include for the skin: café-au-lait spots, a facial angioma, hypopigmented macules, axillary freckling, and a shagreen patch; in the retina: pigmentary abnormalities or hamartomas; and focal neurologic signs that indicate localized cerebral pathology. Asymmetry in the size of the hands, feet, or face signifies a long-standing abnormality of the cerebral hemisphere contralateral to the smaller side. Absence seizures can be triggered in untreated patients by having them hyperventilate for 2 or 3 minutes.

LABORATORY TESTS

Electroencephalography (EEG) is the most important diagnostic test for epilepsy. EEG findings are useful and sometimes essential for establishing the diagnosis, classifying seizures correctly, identifying epileptic syndromes, and making therapeutic decisions. In combination with appropriate clinical findings, *epileptiform* EEG patterns termed *spikes or sharp* waves strongly support a diagnosis of epilepsy (Fig. 125–2). In patients with seizures,

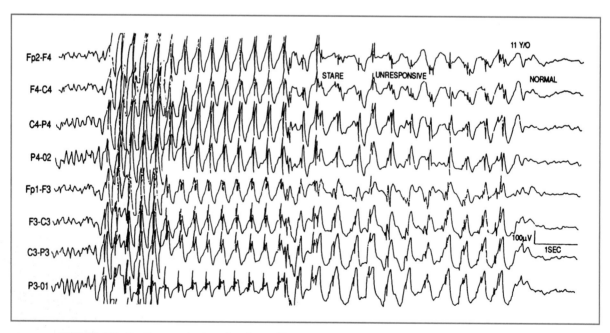

FIGURE 125–2 Absence (petit mal) epilepsy. The electroencephalogram shows the typical pattern of generalized 3-Hz spike-wave complexes associated with a clinical absence seizure. (From Pedley TA: The epilepsies. *In* Goldman L, Bennett JC [eds]: Cecil Textbook of Medicine, 21st ed. Philadelphia: WB Saunders, 2000, p 2155.)

focal epileptiform discharges indicate focal epilepsy, whereas generalized epileptiform activity indicates a generalized form of epilepsy. A note of caution: most EEGs are obtained between seizures, and interictal abnormalities alone can never prove or eliminate a diagnosis of epilepsy. Epilepsy can be definitively established only by recording a characteristic ictal discharge during a representative clinical attack. This is uncommon during routine EEG recordings. A further factor that can confound interpretation of interictal EEGs is the occurrence of similar epileptiform abnormalities in about 2% of normal people; many of these, especially in children, are asymptomatic markers of a genetic trait. Finally, normal epileptiform-like waveforms or artifacts can be misinterpreted and erroneously considered to be evidence of seizure susceptibility.

Forty percent to 50% of patients with epilepsy show epileptiform abnormalities on their initial EEG. The chance of capturing epileptiform activity is enhanced by sleep deprivation for 24 hours before the test and by the patient's sleeping during a portion of the EEG recording. Serial EEGs increase the yield of positive tracings. A small number of persons with epilepsy, however, continue to have normal interictal EEGs despite all efforts to record an abnormality.

NEUROIMAGING STUDIES

Brain MRI complements EEG findings by identifying structural brain pathology that may be causally related to the development of epilepsy. MRI can detect the vast majority of epileptogenic cerebral lesions: hippocampal sclerosis, defects of neuronal migration, and cavernous malformations. It is important to obtain a complete imaging study that includes both T1- and T2-weighted images in coronal and axial planes. Imaging in the coronal plane perpendicular to the long axis of the hippocampus has improved detection of hippocampal atrophy and gliosis, findings that correlate with the pathologic picture of mesial temporal sclerosis and an epileptogenic temporal lobe.

An MRI should be obtained in all patients suspected of having epilepsy over the age of 18 years and in all children with partial seizures (except those with benign focal epilepsy of childhood), abnormal neurologic findings, or focal slow-wave abnormalities on EEG.

In contrast to MRI, positron emission tomography (PET) and single photon emission computed tomography (SPECT) offer functional views of the brain. These techniques use physiologically active, radiolabeled tracers to image the brain's metabolic activity (PET) or blood flow (SPECT). For example, about 70% of patients with temporal lobe epilepsy show focal hypometabolic areas on interictal PET scans that correspond to the epileptogenic focus. Abnormalities using PET or SPECT are often seen even when MRIs are normal.

OTHER TESTS

Routine blood tests rarely offer diagnostic assistance in otherwise healthy patients with epilepsy. Serum electrolytes, liver function tests, and an automated blood cell count are useful as baseline studies before antiepileptic drug therapy is begun. Blood tests are necessary in older patients with acute or chronic systemic disease. Adolescents and young adults with unexplained generalized seizures should be screened for substance abuse (especially cocaine) with blood or urine studies.

Lumbar puncture is indicated only if there is a suspicion of meningitis or encephalitis. It is otherwise unnecessary. Repeated generalized seizures and status epilepticus can increase cerebrospinal fluid protein content slightly and produce a pleocytosis of up to 100 white blood cells/mm³ for 24 to 48 hours, but *cerebrospinal fluid pleocytosis should be attributed to seizures only in retrospect*. An intracranial inflammatory process should always be excluded first.

An electrocardiogram should be obtained in any young person with a first generalized seizure if there is a family history of arrhythmia, sudden unexplained death, or episodic unconsciousness. An electrocardiogram should also be obtained in any patient with a history of cardiac arrhythmia or valvular disease.

Differential Diagnosis

Not every paroxysmal event is a seizure, and misidentification of other conditions as epilepsy leads to ineffective, unnecessary, and potentially harmful treatment. Misdiagnosis accounts for a substantial portion of patients who have not responded to antiepileptic drug treatment. A variety of conditions can be confused with epilepsy, depending on the age of the patient and the nature and circumstances of the attacks (Table 125–4). Nonepileptic paroxysmal disorders have in common the occurrence of sudden, discrete events characterized by abnormal behavior, variable responsiveness, changes in muscle tone, and various postures or movements. These conditions are far more common and variable in their presentation in children than in adults.

Syncope (see Chapter 120) refers to the symptom complex that results when there is a transient, global reduction in cerebral perfusion. Loss of consciousness lasts only a few seconds, uncommonly a minute or more, and recovery is rapid. If the cerebral ischemia is sufficiently severe, the syncopal episode may include brief tonic posturing of the trunk or a few clonic jerks

TABLE 125–4   Nonepileptic Episodic Disorders That May Resemble Seizures

Movement disorders: myoclonus, paroxysmal choreoathetosis, episodic ataxias, hyperexplexia (startle disease)
Migraine: confusional, vertebrobasilar
Syncope
Behavioral and psychiatric: psychogenic seizures, hyperventilation syndrome, panic disorder, dissociative states
Cataplexy (usually associated with narcolepsy)
Transient ischemic attack
Alcoholic blackouts
Hypoglycemia

of the arms and legs (*convulsive syncope*). Similarly, some forms of *migraine* can be mistaken for seizures, especially if headache is atypical or mild. Basilar artery migraine, a variant noted most often in adolescents and young adults, can include lethargy, mood changes, confusion and disorientation, vertigo, bilateral visual disturbances, and alteration or loss of consciousness.

Psychogenic seizures frequently cause intractable "epilepsy" in adults. Many patients with psychogenic seizures have epilepsy as well. Definitive diagnosis requires video-EEG documentation, although a history of atypical and nonstereotyped attacks, emotional or psychological precipitants, psychiatric illness, complete lack of response to antiepileptic drugs, and repeatedly normal interictal EEGs suggests the possibility of psychogenic seizures. *Panic attacks* and anxiety attacks with hyperventilation can superficially resemble partial seizures with affective, autonomic, or special sensory symptoms. Prolonged hyperventilation results in muscle twitching or spasms (tetany); affected patients may faint.

Treatment

If the cause of symptomatic seizures is corrected, antiepileptic drugs are usually unnecessary. Adults with a single, unprovoked seizure and normal clinical and laboratory findings frequently do not have subsequent seizures, so that antiepileptic treatment is not necessarily indicated. However, patients with focal neurologic findings on clinical, radiologic, or EEG examinations are more likely to have repeated seizures. In individual patients, social considerations may dictate treatment after a single seizure. However, in otherwise normal patients who are likely to be poorly compliant with medications, treatment after a single seizure is seldom justified.

If seizures are recurrent, the goal of treatment is to stop attacks completely. Antiepileptic drugs should be used for their indicated conditions (Table 125–5) and according to the following guidelines:

1. The type of seizure should be defined and the preferred medication should be given in usual doses and then increased until seizure control is complete or side effects occur (Table 125–6).
2. Seizures that are infrequent require slow changes in medication doses.
3. If seizures persist at toxic levels, or if major side effects occur, select another agent.

TABLE 125–6   Treatment of Status Epilepticus

Time (min)	Steps
0–5	Give O$_2$; ensure adequate ventilation Monitor: vital signs, electrocardiography, oximetry Establish intravenous access; obtain blood samples for glucose level, complete blood cell count, electrolytes, toxins, and anticonvulsant levels
6–9	Give glucose (preceded by thiamine in adults)
10–20	Intravenously administer either 0.1 mg/kg of lorazepam at 2 mg/min or 0.2 mg/kg of diazepam at 5 mg/min. Diazepam can be repeated if seizures do not stop after 5 min; if diazepam is used to stop the status, phenytoin should be administered promptly to prevent recurrence of status.
21–60	If status persists, administer 15–20 mg/kg of phenytoin intravenously no faster than 50 mg/min in adults and 1 mg/kg/min in children.
>60	If status does not stop after 20 mg/kg of phenytoin, give additional doses of 5 mg/kg to a maximal dose of 30 mg/kg. If status persists, give 20 mg/kg of phenobarbital intravenously at 100 mg/min. When phenobarbital is given after a benzodiazepine, ventilatory assistance is usually required. If status persists, give general anesthesia (e.g., pentobarbital). Vasopressors or fluid volume are usually necessary. Electroencephalogram should be monitored. Neuromuscular blockade may be needed.

4. Do not stop one agent until another has been added. Otherwise, status epilepticus may result.
5. If seizures persist after two agents have been given to toxic levels, consider referral to a specialized center for complex combination therapy and seizure monitoring.
6. Toxic levels of some antiepileptics (particularly phenytoin and carbamazepine) can cause seizures.

EPILEPSY SURGERY

In the majority of patients, epilepsy is controlled with medication. When seizures cannot be controlled by ade-

TABLE 125–5   Drugs Used for Different Types of Seizures

Type of Seizure	Drugs
Simple and complex partial	Carbamazepine, phenytoin, valproate, gabapentin, lamotrigine, topiramate
Secondarily generalized	Carbamazepine, phentoin, valproate, gabapentin, lamotrigine, topiramate
Primary generalized seizures	
Tonic-clonic	Valproate, carbamazepine, phenytoin, lamotrigine
Absence	Ethosuximide, valproate, lamotrigine
Myoclonic and tonic	Valproate, clonazepam

quate trials of two appropriate single agents or by the combination of two agents the epilepsy is termed *medically intractable.* In approximately 20% of patients the epilepsy cannot be fully controlled. Such patients are at considerable risk for the consequences of seizures: inability to drive; stigmatization by schools, employers, and families; and threats to personal educational and occupational goals. In appropriately selected cases, surgery can abolish seizures with restoration of normal neurologic function. The accurate localization of a small, resectable seizure focus requires intensive investigation before surgery. The optimum timing of such monitoring and surgery relative to continued trials of additional medications is under investigation.

SPECIAL TREATMENT CONCERNS

Status Epilepticus

In *major generalized motor status epilepticus,* seizures follow one another so rapidly that new attacks begin before the patient has recovered from the previous one. Status epilepticus can occur with partial or generalized epilepsy and is of great concern because successive or continuous epileptic activity can damage the brain permanently. The most frequent cause is abrupt withdrawal of anticonvulsant medications from a known epileptic. Other precipitants include withdrawal of alcohol or drugs in a habitual user, cerebral infection, trauma, hemorrhage, or neoplasm. However, merely observing that a patient is in the midst of a seizure does not indicate that he or she should be treated for status epilepticus. If status epilepticus is documented, treatment is urgent (Table 125–7). Identification of the cause must be undertaken as soon as possible after seizures stop.

Partial motor status is also known as partial continuous epilepsy. It is uncommon, occurs in several forms, and can last for hours, days, or longer. The seizure frequency can range from one every 3 seconds to several per second. The motor attacks range from highly focal, myoclonic, repetitively localized twitches to jerks that involve most of the limb or half the body. In general, cerebral lesions cause partial motor seizures in the face or distal upper extremity, whereas brain stem or spinal lesions tend to cause proximal myoclonic activity. Causes include stroke, trauma, neoplasms, and encephalitis. Sometimes the cause never becomes clear. Partial continuous epilepsy often resists all efforts at treatment. Severe hyperglycemia can produce partial motor and complex partial status; seizures stop once hyperglycemia is corrected.

Partial complex status produces a sustained state of confusion associated with stereotyped motor and autonomic automatisms. Some attacks produce an abrupt-onset schizophreniform or other bizarre activity, whereas others are marked by a stuporous state. Patients may resist assistance in their abnormal state, which can last for hours or even days. The EEG usually shows continuous slow and spike activity predominating over one or both temporal areas, commonly asymmetrically. Occasionally, surface recordings may be only mildly abnormal, but epileptiform activity can be detected by nasopharyngeal leads or from electrodes placed deep in the brain. Treatment should be initiated promptly, because the effects of prolonged seizures can permanently impair memory and intellect.

Absence status (petit mal status) occurs in two forms. The more common resembles partial complex status and consists of confused automatic behavior accompanied by closely spaced or continuous runs of 3- to 4-Hz spike and wave activity on the EEG. The condition occurs in adolescents or occasionally young adults with known petit mal. Most episodes last less than 30 minutes. Similar attacks of prolonged (days to months) automatisms associated with confusion, EEG abnormality, and sometimes gradual interictal mental deterioration can occur in older persons with no history of epilepsy. Most such attacks can be halted with intravenous diazepam.

Genetic Counseling and Pregnancy

Over 90% of women taking antiepileptic drugs have healthy infants. However, persons with seizure disorders should be advised about the hereditary risks to the fe-

TABLE 125-7 Frequently Prescribed Antiepileptic Drugs

Drug	Dosage	Dose Frequency (hr)	"Therapeutic" Concentrations
Carbamazepine	*Adult:* 800–1600 mg *Child:* 10–40 mg/kg/day	6–8	6–12 μg/mL
Ethosuximide	*Adult:* 750–1500 mg *Child:* 10–75 mg/kg/day	8–12	40–100 μg/mL
Gabapentin	*Adult:* 900–3600 mg	8	Uncertain
Lamotrigine	*Adult:* 75–200 mg *Child:* 1–5 mg/kg	12	4–15 μg/mL
Phenobarbital	*Adult:* 90–180 mg *Child:* 2–6 mg/kg/day	24	15–40 μg/mL
Phenytoin	*Adult:* 300–500 mg *Child:* 4–12 mg/kg/day	24	10–20 μg/mL
Topiramate	200–400 mg	12	2–20 μg/mL
Valproate	*Adult:* 1000–3000 mg *Child:* 10–70 mg/kg/day	8	50–120 μg/mL

tus. Four to 10% of the offspring of patients with generalized primary epilepsy will have one or more seizures. This compares to a risk of about 1.5% in the general population. Women with epilepsy have a 1.5- to 3-fold increased rate of complications of pregnancy, including bleeding, toxemia, abruptio placentae, and premature labor. Anticonvulsant medication dosage often requires adjustment during pregnancy because blood volume increases and drug pharmacokinetics change. Blood level monitoring during the latter half of pregnancy is essential. During pregnancy, it is advisable to give vitamins and supplements, including calcium. Woman of childbearing age should take 1 mg of folic acid daily to protect against developmental defects. Vitamin K, 5 mg twice weekly, should be given orally during the final 6 weeks, with a parenteral supplement administered to the mother and infant at the time of delivery. Breast feeding is not contraindicated in women taking antiepileptic drugs.

Children of both mothers and fathers taking antiepileptic medication have a birth defect risk two to three times that of the general population. Seizures, however pose a greater risk to the mother and fetus than does the generally low rate of birth defects associated with antiepileptic drugs. Two agents, valproate and carbamazepine, have been incriminated in neural tube defects. Phenytoin, phenobarbital, and trimethadione use during pregnancy all have been associated with neurodevelopmental abnormalities. Discontinuation of medication before conception should be considered only if there are clear reasons to believe that seizures will not recur (see later). Medications should not be discontinued during pregnancy.

Psychosocial Problems

The presence of incompletely controlled epilepsy and its frequent association with other neurologic limitations often create major emotional problems for the patient. In addition, disorders that cause partial complex seizures often cause aberrant personality traits that intensify isolation. Outbreaks of frustration, depression, and suicide are more frequent among patients with epilepsy than in the general population. A reduced libido and hyposexuality have been noted in men with partial complex seizures. However, in the absence of associated brain damage, most persons with epilepsy score in the normal range on intelligence tests. Many persons with controlled epilepsy have performed superbly at every level of professional, artistic, and business life.

Patients with seizure disorders are helped most by bringing the attacks under complete control, but reassurance, sensitivity, and optimistic social guidance aid immeasurably. Once seizures are under control, affected persons should be encouraged to live a normal life, using common sense as their guide. Body contact and high-risk sports are best avoided unless seizures have been completely controlled for well over a year; high diving, deep water or underwater swimming, high alpine climbing, boxing, and head-contact football should be avoided. Most states grant automobile driver's licenses to patients with epilepsy provided that no seizures have occurred for at least a year. Life and health insurance policies are available under special circumstances. The Epilepsy Foundation of America can assist patients with these and other social-vocational considerations.

Prognosis

Sixty percent to 70% of people with epilepsy achieve a 5-year remission of seizures within 10 years of diagnosis. About half of these patients eventually become seizure free without anticonvulsant drugs. Factors favoring remission include an idiopathic form of epilepsy, a normal neurologic examination, and an onset in early to middle childhood (excluding neonatal seizures).

Thirty percent of patients, usually those with severe epilepsy starting in early childhood, continue to have seizures and never achieve a remission. In the United States, the prevalence of intractable epilepsy cases approximates 1 to 2 per 1000 population.

Discontinuing Antiepileptic Drugs

Many patients with epilepsy become seizure free on medication for an extended period. Some patients can discontinue antiepileptic drugs without a relapse. Successful drug withdrawal is most likely if initial seizure control was readily achieved using monotherapy, there were relatively few seizures before remission, and the EEG and neurologic examination are normal just before drugs are discontinued. In addition, seizure-free intervals of 4 years reduce the likelihood of relapse. Conversely, risk of relapse is high if seizure control was difficult to establish and required polytherapy, if there were frequent generalized tonic-clonic seizures before control was achieve, and if the EEG demonstrates moderate or severe disturbances of background activity or active epileptiform activity at the time drug withdrawal is considered.

REFERENCES

Engel J Jr, Pedley TA (eds): Epilepsy: A Comprehensive Textbook. Philadelphia: Lippincott-Raven, 1997.
Pedley TA: The Epilepsies. In Goldman L, Bennett JC (eds): Cecil Textbook of Medicine, 21st ed. Philadelphia: WB Saunders, 2000, pp 2151–2163.

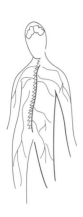

126

CENTRAL NERVOUS SYSTEM TUMORS

Jennifer J. Griggs

Central nervous system (CNS) tumors produce devastating effects and are associated with high mortality rates. Even histologically benign tumors may be unresectable and thus incurable. Malignant tumors are considered malignant because they cannot be removed completely, rather than because they metastasize to other organs.

After childhood, when brain tumors are the second most common cancers, the incidence of CNS tumors increases with advancing age and reaches a plateau between the ages of 65 and 79 years. Some evidence indicates a rise in the incidence of primary brain tumors among elderly patients, but such an increase may be the result of better detection rather than increasing incidence. The incidence of primary CNS lymphoma is clearly increasing, accounted for only in part by the acquired immunodeficiency syndrome (AIDS).

The cause of most CNS tumors is unknown. With the exception of gliomas associated with vinyl chloride and various tumors that occur after CNS irradiation, no environmental agents are known to be causative. Moreover, no evidence supports a viral origin of CNS tumors. Hereditary syndromes associated with an increased risk of CNS tumors, including von Hippel–Lindau disease, tuberous sclerosis, Li-Fraumeni syndrome, and neurofibromatosis, account for fewer than 1% of primary CNS tumors. Although the chromosomal abnormality associated with many of these syndromes is known, the specific mechanisms leading to CNS neoplasia have not been defined.

Classification

The World Health Organization has classified primary CNS tumors on the basis of cell of origin. Most primary CNS tumors are of neuroepithelial origin and result from malignant transformation of astrocytes, ependymocytes, and oligodendrocytes. Gliomas, which arise from astrocytes, are the most common. In a patient with a known systemic malignant disease, metastases to the CNS are more likely than a primary CNS tumor.

Clinical Manifestations

Symptoms caused by intracranial tumors result from either (1) compression of the brain by tumor and the presence of associated edema or (2) infiltration and destruction of brain parenchyma by tumor cells. Because of the uncompromising rigidity of the cranial vault, both histologically benign and malignant tumors may cause symptoms even when these tumors are small. Symptoms caused by primary brain tumors tend to be slowly progressive rather than acute. In contrast, metastatic tumors are more likely to produce acute symptoms because they grow more rapidly and are associated with edema. Moreover, hemorrhage into metastatic tumors, particularly renal cell cancer, melanoma, lung tumors, and choriocarcinomas, causes acute symptoms.

Patients with brain tumors may present with generalized symptoms that arise from increased intracranial pressure or with focal symptoms resulting from specific areas of compromise. Among the generalized symptoms, *headache* is the most common and is the first symptom in half of adults with brain tumors. Headache is only infrequently the result of tumor; tumor-related headache is often worse in the morning and with maneuvers that increase intracranial pressure. The pain may localize to the side of the tumor in patients with supratentorial tumors; patients with infratentorial tumors frequently describe pain in the retro-orbital, retroauricular, or occipital regions. Other generalized symptoms include changes in mood or personality, a decrease in appetite, and nausea. Projectile vomiting, common in children, is rare in adults. Generalized or focal seizures occur in 20% of patients.

Other focal symptoms of brain tumors depend on the location of the tumor. *Tumors of the frontal lobe* may grow to massive proportion before symptoms prompt the patient or the patient's family to seek medical help. Progressive difficulty with concentration and memory, personality changes, and lack of spontaneity may occur with a frontal lobe tumor. Urinary incontinence and gait disorder may appear. Bifrontal disease, most commonly seen with gliomas (the "butterfly glioma") or lymphomas, may cause the appearance of primitive reflexes.

Parietal lobe tumors cause subtle signs or more dramatic findings such as hemianesthesia. Tumors of the right parietal lobe may present with spatial disorientation or left homonymous hemianopia, whereas left parietal lobe tumors cause receptive aphasia or right homonymous hemianopia.

Involvement of the *temporal lobes* by tumor can lead to personality changes, auditory hallucinations, complex partial seizures, and quadrantanopia. If tumors are large enough, they can cause herniation of the uncus through the tentorial notch *(uncal herniation)*.

Metastatic spread of primary CNS tumors to sites outside the CNS is exceedingly rare. Spread along the neuraxis to the meninges and spinal cord, however, can occur with most malignant CNS tumors.

Evaluation of the Patient

RADIOGRAPHIC EVALUATION

A careful neurologic examination helps in localizing the site of a suspected brain tumor. All patients should have either a contrast-enhanced *computed tomography* (CT) scan or a *magnetic resonance imaging* (MRI) scan. MRI is superior to CT scanning in almost all patients because it is more useful in imaging the posterior fossa and is more sensitive in detecting parenchymal invasion by tumor. If MRI is not available, a contrast-enhanced CT scan should be done. CT scans done without contrast enhancement are not adequate for evaluation of either primary tumors or metastatic tumors. CT scans may be superior in the evaluation of oligodendrogliomas, tumors of the pineal region, and calcified meningiomas. *Cerebral angiography* is indicated only when an understanding of tumor blood supply is deemed necessary before surgical resection, such as in patients with highly vascularized meningiomas.

BIOPSY

Biopsy of a suspected brain tumor is essential to make an accurate histologic diagnosis and to detect non-neoplastic disease such as abscess. Exceptions include brain stem tumors with radiographic characteristics of astrocytomas. Tissue may be obtained either by open craniotomy or with MRI-guided or CT-guided stereotactic techniques. Because the histologic features of the tumor may be mixed, small biopsy specimens can be misleading. When the suspicion of a primary brain tumor is high, the tissue diagnosis may be made at the time of surgical resection. This approach yields the greatest amount of tissue for pathologic examination. In 20% of patients with metastatic tumors to the CNS, the primary tumor site is not evident; biopsy can be helpful in identifying the most likely primary sites.

OTHER DIAGNOSTIC TESTS

Lumbar puncture is helpful only if the patient is suspected of having leptomeningeal involvement with tumor; it is contraindicated when an intracranial mass lesion is present. *Electroencephalography* is not routinely performed in patients with brain tumors, even if seizures are part of the clinical presentation.

Treatment

SURGICAL RESECTION

Surgical resection is attempted in most patients with primary brain tumors and in many patients with solitary brain metastases. Even when surgical cure is unlikely, resection of a large portion of the tumor may relieve symptoms for many months. Such "debulking" of primary brain tumors may lead to improvement in survival, but a clear correlation between extent of resection and survival time has not been established. Extensive tumor resection is not possible in most patients with brain stem tumors. Additionally, radical resection is not recommended for tumors that lie in language or sensorimotor areas, the basal ganglia, or the corpus callosum because of the risk of permanent and debilitating neurologic dysfunction. Surgical resection is not recommended for patients with CNS lymphomas because these tumors are often multifocal and respond to the combination of chemotherapy and radiation therapy.

ACUTE TREATMENT OF INCREASED INTRACRANIAL PRESSURE

Most patients with CNS tumors have brain edema. Some patients benefit from the use of glucocorticoids. Dexamethasone is usually given because of its long half-life. Doses used for treatment of tumor-related edema range from 16 to 60 mg/day given in divided doses (two to four times daily). Dexamethasone can be given orally because it is well absorbed from the gastrointestinal tract. Patients with symptoms related to edema often have an improvement in symptoms within 48 hours.

In patients with life-threatening edema with signs of brain herniation, mannitol can be given at a dose of 0.5 to 2 g/kg IV to reduce intracranial pressure. Dexamethasone should be given concurrently.

ANTICONVULSANTS

Patients who develop seizures and many patients who are at risk of developing seizures are given anticonvulsants before they undergo biopsy or surgical procedures. Many of these patients do not need to continue anticonvulsant therapy postoperatively.

RADIATION THERAPY

Radiation therapy can be delivered in three ways: as external beam (conventional) radiation therapy, as brachytherapy, or as "radiosurgery." *External beam radiation therapy* uses x-rays directed either at the whole brain or to the focal area involved by tumor. Whole-brain radiation therapy is associated with long-term toxicity, manifested as dementia and gait disturbance. Although rates of such toxicity are low in people who die within 1 to 2 years of treatment, long-term survivors have increasingly high rates of these complications. *Brachytherapy* involves the implantation of either permanent or temporary radiation "seeds" within the tumor. This approach allows higher doses of radiation therapy to be delivered to the tumor while the surrounding normal tissue is protected. The third approach, *radiosurgery,* involves converging more than 200 beams of radiation onto a small, well-defined tumor. This can be done either with cobalt-60 (the so-called *gamma knife)* or with linear accelerators. Radiosurgery is indicated for the treatment of small tumors that are not surgically accessible.

CHEMOTHERAPY

Chemotherapy is not used as sole therapy for primary CNS neoplasms but rather as part of multimodality therapy. Fewer than 10% of patients with glioblastomas benefit from therapy. The major obstacle to the effective use of chemotherapy is the blood-brain barrier, often disrupted by large tumors but not to the extent that would allow treatment of the entire tumor. Attempts to overcome the blood-brain barrier by giving intra-arterial chemotherapy have not been successful. In addition, CNS tumor cells are often drug resistant.

One development is the use of biodegradable polymer wafers impregnated with the nitrosourea BCNU (*bis*-chloroethyl-nitrosourea; carmustine), an alkylating agent. The wafers are placed into the tumor bed after resection of recurrent glioblastoma multiforme and slowly release the drug into the surrounding tissues. Early studies of this approach have shown improvements in 6-month survival rates. The use of the wafers is being investigated in the treatment of other CNS tumors.

Oligodendrogliomas are unusually sensitive to chemotherapy. The combination of procarbazine, vincristine, and lomustine (CCNU) produces responses in 80% or fewer of patients treated with this regimen. CNS lymphomas are treated with a combination of chemotherapy and radiation therapy (see later discussion).

Specific Tumors

MALIGNANT ASTROCYTOMAS

The term *malignant astrocytoma* refers to a group of heterogenous tumors and includes glioblastoma multiforme, anaplastic astrocytoma, and anaplastic oligoden-droglioma. Some patients with these types of tumors have mixed histologic features with both high-grade and low-grade characteristics.

Of the anaplastic gliomas, *glioblastoma multiforme* is associated with the worst prognosis, with a median survival of less than 12 months. Surgery and radiation therapy are used together to improve symptoms and quality of life. In younger patients and in those with good function, chemotherapy may prolong survival, but studies showing such prolongation may merely reflect the effects of selection bias. When disease relapse occurs in patients with glioblastoma multiforme, surgical resection, brachytherapy, radiosurgery, and chemotherapy are all occasionally helpful, but, in general, benefit is short-lived.

In contrast, *anaplastic astrocytomas* and *anaplastic oligodendrogliomas* are associated with median survival times of 4 to 5 years. Patients with anaplastic oligodendrogliomas or tumors with mixed histologic features benefit most from chemotherapy given after surgical resection. Both BCNU (carmustine) and the combination of procarbazine, CCNU, and vincristine have been used in this setting. Patients with recurrent tumors are treated with the same approach as those with recurrent glioblastoma multiforme.

MENINGIOMAS

Meningiomas arise outside the brain and generally grow slowly; they may be found incidentally during the evaluation of unrelated symptoms. These tumors are histologically benign in 90% of cases and tend to arise along the dorsal surface of the brain, along the falx cerebri, on the sphenoid ridge, within the lateral ventricles, at the base of the skull, or close to the optic nerves.

Complete resection of meningiomas should be attempted; the risk of recurrent disease is proportionate to the extent of resection. For example, in patients who do not have resection or coagulation of dural attachments, the risk of recurrent disease within the subsequent two decades is close to 20%. In these patients and in those who have only partial resection of tumor, postoperative radiation therapy should be given. In the patient with malignant meningioma, radiation therapy should be recommended regardless of the extent of resection. Chemotherapy is not used in the treatment of meningiomas.

CENTRAL NERVOUS SYSTEM LYMPHOMA

Primary CNS lymphomas are increasing in incidence among both immunocompromised and immunocompetent people. These lymphomas may arise from lymphocytes that travel into and out of the CNS. By definition, a patient with primary CNS lymphoma has no evidence of lymphoma outside the CNS. Primary CNS lymphomas most often occur deep within the frontal lobe and are therefore less likely to present with seizures than are other primary and metastatic CNS neoplasms. Headache, personality changes, and focal symptoms corresponding to the location of the tumor are usual presenting complaints. Forty percent of immunocompetent patients and close to 100% of patients with AIDS have multifocal lymphoma at the time of diagnosis. More than 40% of patients have involvement of the leptomeninges, but such involvement is rarely symptomatic. An additional site of involvement is one or both eyes in 20% of patients.

Treatment of primary CNS lymphomas requires first that the correct diagnosis be made. Because the disease is often multifocal, it may be confused with metastatic disease from other solid tumors. Surgical resection is not indicated in the management of CNS lymphoma. Treatment includes corticosteroids, which, because of the cytotoxic effects of steroids on lymphoma cells, can result in dramatic responses. Treatment with steroids is not sufficient, however, and most patients are treated with a combination of systemic chemotherapy given before whole-brain radiation therapy. The chemotherapy combinations used are the same used in the treatment of systemic non-Hodgkin's lymphoma. The 5-year survival rates associated with combined modality therapy are as high as 30%. In some patients who have a complete response to chemotherapy, whole-brain radiation therapy may be deferred in an attempt to decrease the late effects associated with brain radiation.

METASTATIC TUMORS TO THE BRAIN

Most intracranial tumors are metastatic from other sites. The tumors that commonly metastasize to the brain are lung cancer, breast cancer, and melanoma, but nearly any solid tumor can metastasize to the CNS. Patients present with headache, seizures, and focal symptoms reflecting the area of involvement, as well as depression and changes in mental status. Metastases are usually multifocal, although non–small cell lung cancer and renal cell cancer often present with solitary metastases. Rapidly growing tumors may cause massive edema.

Treatment of metastases is usually with corticosteroids and radiation therapy. Symptomatic improvement may be seen within hours of giving dexamethasone in patients with brain edema. Surgical resection is indicated in selected patients with solitary or easily resectable tumors if the systemic malignant disease is well controlled and the patient is otherwise doing well. Because most chemotherapeutic agents do not cross the blood-brain barrier, CNS metastases other than small cell lung cancer do not usually respond to systemic chemotherapy.

SPINAL CORD TUMORS

Much less common than tumors of the brain, spinal cord tumors are described as *extradural* (outside of the dural sac) or *intradural*. Most extradural tumors are metastases from other sites, including lung, breast, and prostate cancers. Intradural tumors are further described as either extramedullary (arising outside the spinal cord) or intramedullary (arising within the spinal cord). Examples of extramedullary tumors are schwannomas (neurilemmomas) and meningiomas. Ependymomas and astrocytomas are the most common intramedullary tumors. The most common location for spinal tumors is the thoracic region.

Patients with spinal cord tumors usually develop symptoms as a result of compression of normal structures by the tumor or impairment of the vascular supply, rather than by invasion of the parenchyma by tumor. Back pain and distal paresthesias are among the earliest symptoms, followed by loss of sensation and weakness below the level of the tumor and loss of bowel and bladder control.

MRI is most useful in the evaluation of the patient with suspected spinal cord tumor and has replaced myelography in most cases. In patients with progressing deficits, urgent evaluation and treatment are indicated.

Treatment of primary spinal tumors is with surgical resection. Resection of high-grade astrocytomas is followed by radiation therapy; the usefulness of radiation therapy for other tumors is not clear. Patients with epidural metastatic tumors are treated with high doses of corticosteroids and surgery or radiation. Although radiation therapy is probably as effective as surgery in many patients, surgical decompression is recommended in patients with an acute onset of symptoms and in those in whom the pathologic features of the tumor have not yet been identified.

REFERENCES

Blumenthal DT, Raizer JJ, Rosenblum MK, et al: Primary intracranial neoplasms in patients with HIV. Neurology 1999, 52:1648–51.

Scott JN, Rewcastle NB, Brasher PM, et al: Which glioblastoma multiforme patient will become a long-term survivor? A population-based study. Ann Neurol 1999; 46:183–185.

Vick NA: Intracranial and spinal tumors. *In* Goldman L, Bennett JC (eds): Cecil Textbook of Medicine, 21st ed. Philadelphia: WB Saunders, 2000, pp 2164–2168.

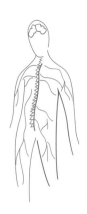

127

INFECTIOUS DISEASES OF THE NERVOUS SYSTEM

Robert C. Griggs • Roger P. Simon

The central nervous system can be infected with the same spectrum of infectious agents as the rest of the body. Specific bacterial, fungal, parasitic, and viral infections are covered in Section XV. In this chapter we focus on brain and spinal cord infections that are localized to the central nervous system, either as abscesses within the parenchyma itself or as parameningeal infections. Also discussed are the central nervous system manifestations of infections elsewhere in the body. Finally, a category of infections with clinical signs confined to the brain and spinal cord—prion diseases—are considered.

Brain Abscess

Brain abscesses produce symptoms and findings similar to those of other space-occupying lesions, such as brain tumors, but often progress more rapidly than tumors and more frequently affect meningeal structures. They originate or extend from extracerebral locations, resulting from (1) bloodborne metastases from unknown sources, lung, or heart, and (2) direct extension from parameningeal sites of infection (otitis, cranial osteomyelitis, sinusitis), sites of recent or remote head trauma or neurosurgical procedures, and sites of infections associated with cyanotic congenital heart disease. The most commonly isolated pathogens are aerobic and microaerobic streptococci and gram-negative anaerobes such as *Bacteroides* and *Prevotella*. Less common are gram-negative aerobes and *Staphylococcus. Actinomyces, Nocardia,* and *Candida* are less frequently found. Infection is often polymicrobial. Culture-negative abscesses from surgical specimens occur in 30% of antibiotic-treated patients and in 5% of patients operated on before antibiotic administration.

DIAGNOSIS

Systemic signs of infection may be minimal or absent. Almost half of patients do not have fever or leukocytosis. Neck stiffness is rare unless there is increased intracranial pressure. The presenting features are, instead, those of an expanding intracranial mass (Table 127–1). A headache of recent onset is the most common symptom. If the process is untreated, headache increases in severity and focal signs appear, such as hemiparesis or aphasia, followed by obtundation and coma. The period of evolution may be as brief as hours or as long as days to weeks with more indolent organisms. Seizures may occur with abscesses involving the cortical gray matter. Cerebrospinal fluid (CSF) examination should not be performed for diagnosis; it is seldom diagnostic and can be normal. Moreover, abscesses often expand rapidly, and lumbar puncture may aggravate impending transtentorial herniation. Contrast-enhanced computed tomography (CT) and magnetic resonance imaging (MRI) are used for diagnosis and for monitoring response to therapy. MRI is superior for detecting multiple and posterior fossa abscesses; and with intravenous gadolinium contrast, MRI is superior in demonstrating cerebritis, the extent of mass effect, associated venous thrombosis, and the response to therapy.

TREATMENT

Pyogenic abscesses are treated with antibiotics alone or with antibiotics combined with surgical aspiration or excision. Surgery is required if there is a major mass effect or if the abscess adjoins the ventricular surface (raising the possibility of catastrophic rupture into the ventricular system). Also, if the lesion is in the posterior fossa (with the potential of brain stem compression), is large (> 3 cm diameter), or is refractory to medical

TABLE 127–1 Brain Abscess: Presenting Features in 43 Patients

Feature	%
Headache	72
Lethargy	71
Fever	60
Nuchal rigidity	49
Nausea, vomiting	35
Seizures	35
Ocular palsy	27
Confusion	26
Visual disturbance	21
Weakness	21
Dysarthria	12
Stupor	12
Papilledema, dysphasia, hemiparesis, dizziness	10 or less

From Chun CH, Johnson JD, Hofstetter M, et al: Brain abscess: A study of 45 consecutive cases. Medicine 1986; 65:415.

therapy, surgery is indicated. Antibiotics alone are appropriate for a surgically inaccessible abscess, multiple abscesses (seen in 10% of patients), or those in the early cerebritis stage. If the causal organism is not identified, antibiotics should cover the most likely organisms (streptococci and anaerobes). A suggested regimen includes penicillin G, 3 to 4 million units given intravenously every 4 hours, and metronidazole, 7.5 mg/kg given intravenously or orally every 6 to 8 hours. If staphylococcal or aerobic gram-negative infection is suggested (e.g., because of a history of trauma or intravenous drug abuse), nafcillin plus cefotaxime or ceftriaxone is recommended. Concomitant corticosteroid therapy may attenuate edema surrounding abscesses and may be warranted if the abscess produces life-threatening mass effect. Antibiotics must be continued until the abscess cavity resolves completely, usually in 4 to 8 weeks. If the abscess does not decrease in size after 4 weeks, this constitutes an antibiotic failure. The outcome correlates inversely with the abscess size and the degree of neurologic dysfunction at presentation but less well with age, cause, number of abscesses, or corticosteroid use.

Subdural Empyema

Subdural empyema refers to infection in the space separating the dura and arachnoid. It is responsible for one fifth of localized intracranial infections and results from direct or indirect extension from infected paranasal sinuses through a retrograde thrombophlebitis or, less frequently, from untreated chronic otitis. Unilateral empyema is most common, because the falx prevents passage across the midline, but bilateral or multiple empyemas can occur. Cortical venous thrombosis or brain abscess develops in approximately one fourth of cases.

Symptoms initially reflect those of chronic otitis or sinusitis, on which lateralized headache (a universal fea-

ture), fever, and obtundation become superimposed. Vomiting, meningeal signs, and focal neurologic abnormalities (hemiparesis or seizures) usually follow. If the disease remains untreated, obtundation progresses and the septic mass and swollen underlying brain soon lead to venous thrombosis or death from herniation. The major differential diagnosis is that of meningitis. Nuchal rigidity and obtundation occur in both, but papilledema and lateralizing deficits are more common in empyema. Contrast-enhanced CT or MRI can be diagnostic of empyema, showing an extra-axial, crescent-shaped mass with an enhancing rim lying just below the inner table of the skull over the cerebral convexities or the interhemispheric fissures. MRI better detects underlying parenchymal edema as well as the infection itself. Treatment requires both prompt surgical drainage of the empyema cavity and high-dose intravenous antibiotics directed toward organisms found at the time of craniotomy.

Malignant External Otitis

Malignant external otitis occurs in elderly patients with diabetes and is caused by *Pseudomonas aeruginosa*. An external otitis progresses rapidly, with ear pain, facial swelling, osteomyelitis of the base of the skull, and purulent meningitis accompanied by multiple cranial nerve palsies. Urgent treatment with an antipseudomonal penicillin or a third-generation cephalosporin combined with an aminoglycoside or ciprofloxacin, as well as surgical debridement and drainage, is essential. The mortality rate is high.

Spinal Epidural Abscess

Infection within the epidural space about the spinal cord can cause paralysis and death but usually responds to treatment. Its incidence is 0.5 to 1.0 per 10,000 hospital admissions in the United States, but the frequency is higher in intravenous drug users. Patients are usually febrile (38°C to 39°C [100.4°F to 102.2°F]) and present with acute or subacute neck or back pain, with focal percussion tenderness being a prominent sign; stiff neck and headache are common. The pain can be mistaken for sciatica, a visceral abdominal process, chest wall pain, or cervical disc disease. If the condition goes unrecognized at this stage, the symptoms can rapidly evolve, over a few hours to a few days, to produce weakness and finally paralysis occurring distal to the spinal level of the infection. In this clinical setting, spinal epidural abscess should be assumed, systemic antibiotics begun, and urgent neuroradiologic confirmatory diagnostic procedures pursued. The differential diagnosis includes compressive and inflammatory processes involving the spinal cord (transverse myelitis, intervertebral disc herniation, epidural hemorrhage, metastatic tumor), which can usually be detected by MRI.

PATHOPHYSIOLOGY

Infections of the epidural space originate from contiguous spread or through hematogenous routes from a distant source. Cutaneous sites of infection are the most common remote sources, especially in intravenous drug users. Abdominal, respiratory tract, and urinary sources are also common. The anatomy of the epidural space dictates the location of the abscess, the frequency of epidural infections being proportional to the volume of the epidural space. Because the size of the intravertebral canal remains relatively constant while the circumference of the spinal cord changes, abscess formation is maximal in the thoracic and lumbar regions and least at the cervical spine enlargement.

BACTERIOLOGY

Causative organisms can be identified by culture or Gram stain from pus obtained at exploration (90% of cases), blood cultures (60 to 90% of cases), or CSF (20% of cases). *Staphylococcus aureus* accounts for most infections, followed by streptococci and gram-negative anaerobes. Tuberculous abscesses remain common, representing as many as 25% of cases in high-risk populations.

TREATMENT

Unless culture and sensitivities dictate otherwise, penicillinase-resistant penicillin (nafcillin, 12 g/day, or oxacillin, 12 g/day) should be started empirically as antistaphylococcal treatment for presumed bacterial infection. Considering the severity of the disease, most authorities would provide additional gram-negative coverage with a third-generation cephalosporin, a quinolone, or an aminoglycoside. Surgical decompression was once thought to be mandatory in all cases; now, early diagnosis by MRI allows for effective medical therapy before the occurrence of neurologic complications.

Septic Cavernous Sinus Thrombosis

Septic cavernous sinus thrombosis presents as headache or lateralized facial pain, followed in a few days to weeks by fever and involvement of the orbit, which produces proptosis and chemosis secondary to obstruction of the ophthalmic vein. Paralysis of oculomotor nerves follows rapidly. At times there is sensory dysfunction in the first and second divisions of the trigeminal nerve and a decrease in the corneal reflex. Further involvement of the contiguous orbital contents follows, with mild papilledema and decreased visual acuity, sometimes progressing to blindness. Extension to the opposite cavernous sinus or to other intracranial sinuses with cerebral infarction or increased intracranial pressure secondary to impaired venous drainage can result in stupor, coma, and death. The CSF is abnormal in almost all cases, sometimes with a profile resembling that of purulent meningitis or parameningeal infection. The most common causative organism is *S. aureus*, with streptococci and pneumococci being less common; anaerobic infection has been reported. Radiologic evaluation includes sinus imaging, with attention to the sphenoidal and ethmoidal sinuses. MRI (with and without intravenous gadolinium) can often show venous thrombosis by illustrating the lack of the normal "flow void" within a vascular structure. Treatment requires early diagnosis and consists of the prompt drainage of infected paranasal sinuses as well as specific antistaphylococcal agents, such as nafcillin or oxacillin, given intravenously.

Lateral Sinus Thrombosis

Septic thrombosis of the lateral sinus results from acute or chronic infections of the middle ear. The symptoms comprise ear pain followed over several weeks by fever, headache, nausea, vomiting, and vertigo. Results of otologic examination are abnormal; mastoid swelling may be seen. Sixth cranial nerve palsies and papilledema can occur, but other focal neurologic signs are rare. Treatment includes intravenous antibiotics to cover staphylococci and anaerobes (nafcillin or oxacillin with penicillin or metronidazole), but surgical drainage (mastoidectomy) may be required.

Septic Sagittal Sinus Thrombosis

Septic sagittal sinus thrombosis is uncommon and occurs as a consequence of purulent meningitis, infections of the ethmoidal or maxillary sinuses spreading through venous channels, infected compound skull fractures, or, rarely, neurosurgical wound infections. Symptoms include manifestations of elevated intracranial pressure (headache, nausea, and vomiting) that evolve rapidly to stupor and coma.

Neurologic Complications of Infectious Endocarditis

Neurologic complications occur in one third of patients with bacterial endocarditis and triple the mortality rate of the disease. Most of these complications derive from valvular vegetations. Cerebral (but not systemic) emboli are more common from mitral valve endocarditis. The time of embolization during the course of endocarditis depends on the virulence of the organism and whether it produces acute or subacute disease. With acute endocarditis (predominantly staphylococci or enterococci), embolization occurs early, often during the first week, whereas in subacute disease (predominantly viridans group streptococci or enterococci) emboli occur over the full course of treatment and occasionally after treatment is completed. Cerebral emboli are distributed in the brain in proportion to cerebral blood flow. Therefore, most emboli lodge in the branches of the middle cerebral artery peripherally, with resultant hemiparesis. Focal seizures may result.

Mycotic aneurysms complicate endocarditis in 2% to 10% of cases and are more common in acute than subacute disease. The middle cerebral artery is most commonly involved, with the aneurysms being located distally in the vessel, differentiating them from congenital berry aneurysms. Small brain abscesses may complicate the course of endocarditis, but macroscopic abscesses are rare, most occurring in the setting of acute, rather than subacute, endocarditis. Multiple microabscesses, however, can result in a diffuse encephalopathy similar to that seen in sepsis. Such lesions may escape detection on CT scan and are not amenable to surgical drainage. Antibiotic treatment of the primary disease is indicated. The CSF is abnormal in 70% of cases and may be the same as with purulent meningitis (polymorphonuclear predominance, elevated protein level, and low glucose level) or with a parameningeal infection (lymphocytic predominance, modest protein elevation, and normal glucose level).

Prion Diseases

Several human diseases have been attributed to a unique infectious protein—the prion. Prion illnesses include Creutzfeldt-Jakob disease (CJD) (also called subacute spongiform encephalopathy), kuru, Gerstmann-Straussler-Scheinker syndrome, and familial fatal insomnia. Prion-related illnesses are unique in that they may be hereditary, occur spontaneously, or may be acquired by contamination with the agent. The appearance of "variant CJD" in Great Britain, in association with the outbreak of bovine spongiform encephalopathy and the contamination of beef, has greatly increased interest in this group of illnesses.

CREUTZFELDT-JAKOB DISEASE

The illness is seen worldwide, with an incidence of 0.5 to 1.0 cases per million per year. Most cases are sporadic; 5% to 15% are inherited in an autosomal dominant pattern. Higher rates of familial disease occur in descendants of Jewish populations from Libya and North Africa, where there is an annual incidence as high as 31.3 per million. The illness may also be iatrogenic, as seen in recipients of growth hormone prepared from pooled human pituitary glands, occur after cadaver corneal and dura mater transplants, and follow use of stereotactic intracerebral depth electrodes.

CJD is frequently diagnosed incorrectly initially. Prodromal symptoms include altered sleep patterns and appetite, weight loss, changes in sexual drive, and impaired memory and concentration. Disorientation, hallucinations, and emotional lability are early signs, and the patient then develops a rapidly progressive dementia associated with myoclonus (in approximately 90% of patients). Myoclonus is generally provoked by tactile, auditory, or visual startle. CJD has an apopleptic, abrupt onset in 10% to 15% of patients. Other distinctive presentations include seizures, autonomic dysfunction, and lower motor neuron disease suggesting amyotrophic lateral sclerosis. Cerebellar ataxia occurs in one third of patients.

The clinical tetrad supporting the diagnosis of CJD consists of a subacute progressive dementia, myoclonus, typical periodic complexes on electroencephalography, and normal CSF. Brain imaging is typically normal until late in the disease when there is progressive brain atrophy. Routine CSF study is generally normal. A CSF test for the protein 14-3-3, in the appropriate clinical context, is highly specific and sensitive for CJD. There is no effective therapy. The disease is inexorably progressive. Death typically occurs within 1 year of the onset of symptoms (range, 1 to 130 months).

Although the illness is not communicable in the conventional sense, there is a risk of handling materials contaminated with the prion protein. Gloves should be worn when handling blood, CSF, and other body fluids. Instruments must be disinfected by steam autoclaving for 1 hour at 132°C, by steam autoclaving for 4.5 hours at 121°C (1.5 psi), or by immersion in 1 N sodium hydroxide for 1 hour at room temperature.

REFERENCES

Darouiche RO, Hammill RJ, Greenberg SB, et al: Bacterial spinal epidural abscess: Review of 43 cases and literature survey. Medicine 1992; 71:369.

Patel KS, Marks PV: Management of focal intracranial infections: Is medical treatment better than surgery? J Neurol Neurosurg Psychiatry 1990; 53:472.

Roder BL, Wandall DA, Espersen F, et al: Neurologic manifestations in *Staphylococcus aureus* endocarditis: A review of 260 bacteremic cases in nondrug addicts. Am J Med 1997; 102:379.

Yang SY, Zhao CS: Review of 140 patients with brain abscess. Surg Neurol 1993; 39:290.

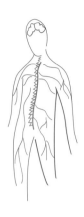

128

DEMYELINATING AND INFLAMMATORY DISORDERS

Robert C. Griggs

Demyelination refers to the process in which the myelin of central or peripheral nervous systems is injured. Diseases of peripheral nerve myelin are discussed in Chapter 129. Diseases of central nervous system (CNS) myelin are either acquired or hereditary. Multiple sclerosis (MS) is the most common acquired disease of myelin. Hereditary diseases of myelin often involve problems with formation of myelin and are sometimes referred to as *dys*myelinating as opposed to *de*myelinating. Table 128–1 lists common disorders of myelin.

Multiple Sclerosis

MS is defined clinically by typical symptoms, signs, and disease progression. The annual incidence rate for MS ranges in different populations from 1.5 to 11 per 100,000. The incidence rate may be increasing. The first symptoms of MS usually occur between the ages of 15 and 50 and the disease is more frequent in women. Individual bouts of inflammatory demyelination may be accompanied by clinical symptoms termed *relapses*, followed in most cases by some degree of recovery, producing the typical *relapsing-remitting* course seen early in the disease. Diagnosis requires intermittent or progressive CNS symptoms supported by evidence of two or more CNS white matter lesions occurring in an appropriately aged patient who lacks an alternative explanation such as recurrent strokes or systemic lupus erythematosus. The diagnosis is based on clinical features; currently available laboratory tests support the diagnosis but cannot be diagnostic.

ETIOLOGY

The initiating cause(s) of MS is unknown, but pathogenesis clearly involves autoimmune-mediated inflammatory demyelination and axonal injury. Pathologic examination of MS brain tissue shows perivascular infiltration by lymphocytes and monocytes; class II major histocompatibility complex (MHC) antigen expression by cells in the lesions; chemokines, lymphokines, and monokines secreted by activated cells; and no evidence for infection. Also present are immunologic abnormalities in blood and cerebrospinal fluid (CSF), an association with certain MHC class II allotypes, and a response of MS patients to immunomodulation. Patients may improve with immunosuppressive drugs and worsen with treatment with interferon (IFN) gamma. Moreover, there are similarities between MS and experimental allergic encephalomyelitis, which is an animal model induced by inoculating susceptible animals with myelin proteins. Both environmental and genetic factors are clearly involved. Certain populations in northern latitudes have a very high incidence of MS. No infectious cause has been found, but it is still thought that one or more ubiquitous viruses may lead to an autoimmune process in susceptible individuals. A genetic influence is well established by the higher concordance in monozygotic compared with dizygotic twins, the clustering of MS in families, racial variability in risk, and associations with class II MHC allotypes.

The earliest event in the MS lesion is breakdown of the blood-brain barrier, followed by perivenular mononuclear infiltrates, and then circumscribed areas of myelin breakdown. Macrophages are necessary for myelin loss, and B lymphocytes and plasma cells surround small CNS blood vessels. T lymphocytes and monocytes infiltrate CNS parenchyma. Products of the immune response, including immunoglobulins, interleukins, interferons, and tumor necrosis factor, accompany the acute MS lesion. There is now evidence that MS injures CNS neuronal axons; this injury may account for the brain atrophy and permanent damage that occurs as the disease progresses.

TABLE 128–1 **Demyelinating Disorders**

Unknown Cause

Multiple sclerosis
Devic's disease
Optic neuritis
Acute transverse myelopathy

Parainfectious Disorders

Acute disseminated encephalomyelitis
Acute hemorrhagic leukoencephalopathy

Viral Infections

HIV-1–associated myelopathy
Progressive multifocal leukoencephalopathy
Subacute sclerosing panencephalitis

Nutritional Disorders

Combined systems disease (vitamin B$_{12}$ deficiency)
Demyelination of the corpus callosum (Marchiafava-Bignami disease)
Central pontine myelinolysis

Anoxic-Ischemic Sequelae

Delayed postanoxic cerebral demyelination
Progressive subcortical ischemic encephalopathy

DIAGNOSIS

A diagnosis of MS must be established by clinical criteria, and laboratory tests are useful in supporting the diagnosis. Symptoms can arise from MS involvement of virtually any part of the CNS, but certain presentations are typical of the disease (Table 128–2). Sudden, unilateral visual loss, double vision, vertigo, pins and needles sensation, and loss of balance are particularly common.

TABLE 128–2 **Symptoms and Signs of Multiple Sclerosis Listed in Declining Order of Frequency**

Symptoms

Unilateral visual impairment
Double vision
Paresthesias
Ataxia or unsteadiness
Vertigo
Fatigue
Muscle weakness
Urinary disturbance
Dysarthria
Mental disturbance

Signs

Optic neuritis
Internuclear ophthalmoplegia
Nystagmus
Spasticity or hyperreflexia
Babinski sign
Absent abdominal reflexes
Dysmetria or intention tremor
Impairment of central sensory pathways
Labile or changed mood

Slight fever often worsens symptoms. The majority of patients have resolution of their initial symptoms. The criteria for diagnosis of relapsing-remitting MS (Table 128–3) are based on documentation of two or more episodes affecting two or more locations in the CNS. In younger patients, the disease usually starts with a subacute or acute onset of focal neurologic symptoms and signs, most often reflecting disease in optic nerves, pyramidal tracts, posterior columns, cerebellum, central vestibular system, or medial longitudinal fasciculus. Older individuals commonly present with insidiously progressive myelopathy, manifesting as some combination of progressive spastic leg weakness, axial instability, and bladder impairment.

LABORATORY CONFIRMATION

Neuroimaging is the first step. The computed tomographic brain scan sometimes shows hypodense regions in white matter, but computed tomography (CT) is relatively insensitive and usually shows no abnormalities. For these reasons, magnetic resonance imaging (MRI) has largely supplanted CT. Head MRI shows abnormalities in more than 85% of clinically definite MS patients. Typical lesions (Fig. 128–1) are multifocal, appear hyperintense on intermediate and T2-weighted MR images, and occur predominantly in the periventricular cerebral white matter, corpus callosum, cerebellum, cerebellar peduncles, brain stem, and spinal cord. MRI usually shows many more hyperintense lesions than were clinically anticipated. Intravenous gadolinium enhances acute lesions, which appear hyperintense on T1-weighted images. CSF examination is helpful in instances where MRI is not confirmatory. Routine analysis of CSF is usually normal except for slight elevations of protein and occasional slight pleocytosis (<50 mononuclear cells). Most MS patients have evidence of increased IgG production in the CNS: "oligoclonal" bands, increased IgG levels, and antibodies to myelin basic protein. Sensory evoked potentials, measuring conduction velocity along the optic, auditory, and somatosensory nerves, are often delayed and can confirm multifocal CNS disease.

TREATMENT

The major challenge in the treatment of MS is to halt the progressive disability that occurs with repeated acute attacks of relapsing/remitting MS or with the less common chronic progressive MS. Treatment of acute attacks with corticosteroids is of short-term benefit but has not had a major effect on long-term disability. However, three agents have recently been found to be of benefit in modifying the course of MS (Table 128–4). Two forms of recombinant IFN-β—IFN-β-1a (Avonex) and IFN-β-1b (Betaseron)—are approved for use in relapsing-remitting MS. IFN-β therapy reduces the frequency and severity of MS relapses, slows disability progression, reduces the number and volume of new MRI lesions, and slows the progressive accumulation of T2-weighted MRI lesions. Betaseron is administered at a dose of 8 million IU every other day by subcutaneous injection,

TABLE 128-3 **Washington Committee Criteria for Diagnosis of Multiple Sclerosis (MS)**

Category	Attacks	Clinical Evidence		Paraclinical Evidence*	CSF OB/IgG
Clinically definite MS					
1	2	2			
2	2	1	and	1	
Laboratory-supported definite MS					
1	2	1	or	1	+
2	1	2			+
3	1	1	and	1	+
Clinically probable MS					
1	2	1			
2	1	2			
3	1	1	and	1	
Laboratory-supported probable MS					
1	2				+

CSF = cerebrospinal fluid; IgG = immunoglobulin G; OB = oligoclonal bands.
*Magnetic resonance imaging or evoked potential studies.
From Poser CM, Paty DW, Scheinberg L, et al: New diagnostic criteria for multiple sclerosis: Guidelines for research protocols. Ann Neurol 1983; 13:227.

whereas Avonex is administered at a dose of 6 million IU weekly by intramuscular injection. Adverse effects include transient flulike symptoms after each injection with both preparations and inflammatory reactions at the injection sites with Betaseron. Glatiramer acetate (Copaxone) is also used for patients with relapsing-remitting MS. Glatiramer acetate is a myelin-like polypeptide that may inhibit cellular immune reactions to myelin. It is given daily by subcutaneous injection. It reduces the relapse rate; its principal side effect is swelling and redness at the injection sites. The effect of immunomodulatory therapy on the long-term disability of MS is unknown.

Acute attacks are treated with intravenous methylprednisolone, which shortens acute exacerbations. The dosage is 500 or 1000 mg/day for 3 days, followed by prednisone, 60 mg in a single morning dose for 3 days, tapering off over 12 days.

The differential diagnosis of MS (Table 128–5) includes a large number of diseases and is different for relapsing-remitting MS than for the less-frequent progressive disease. Alternative diagnoses must be considered initially and again with each subsequent new symptom. With the initial episode, MS is always a diagnosis of exclusion.

Neuromyelitis Optica (Devic's Disease)

Neuromyelitis optica is a syndrome characterized by partial or complete transverse myelopathy and optic neuritis. Loss of vision and paraplegia may occur, and the two major components of the disease may be widely separated in time. The syndrome of neuromyelitis optica may occur as the result of acute disseminated encephalomyelitis, systemic lupus erythematosus, or sarcoidosis, as well as during the course of typical MS or in isolation without apparent cause. In the latter case, it is considered a variant of MS.

Optic Neuritis

Optic neuritis denotes partial or complete loss of vision in one or both eyes; it is usually acute and due to inflammation. Most patients with optic neuritis have pain in, around, or behind the affected eye, followed within 1 or 2 days by visual loss that progresses for as long as a week. Optic neuritis is termed *retrobulbar neuritis* when the lesion is in the posterior two thirds of the optic nerve and *papillitis* when the lesion is in the anterior portion of the optic nerve. The ophthalmoscopic appearance of papillitis is similar to that of acute papilledema from increased intracranial pressure but differs from papilledema by markedly reduced visual acuity. Visual function almost always recovers to some degree, usually within weeks. Blindness as the result of optic nerve demyelination seldom occurs. The syndrome of optic neuritis can be caused by several diseases, of which MS is by far the most common. Other causes include tobacco-nutritional amblyopia, Leber's hereditary optic neuropathy, vasculitis, optic nerve compression on any basis, neurosyphilis, ischemic optic neuropathy, pernicious anemia, or sarcoidosis. Many patients with idiopathic isolated optic neuritis eventually develop MS; the reported frequency in several series varies from 13% to 85%, according to the length of follow-up.

More rapid but not necessarily greater total visual recovery occurs by treating optic neuritis with intravenous methylprednisolone. A 3-day course of intravenous methylprednisolone followed by a prednisone taper within 8 days of the onset appears to reduce by about

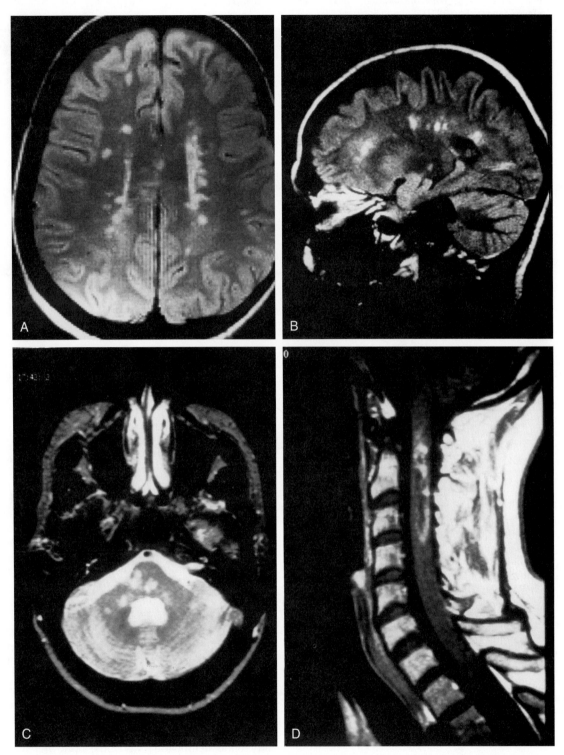

FIGURE 128–1 Magnetic resonance imaging of brain and spinal cord from a patient with multiple sclerosis. *A,* Transverse section just above the bodies of the lateral ventricles. Note the numerous high-signal lesions adjacent to the bodies of the lateral ventricles in the deep cerebral white matter. *B,* Sagittal proton-density image showing ovoid lesions extending from the lateral ventricles into the deep cerebral white matter. *C,* T2-weighted section through the brain stem and cerebellum at the level of the middle cerebellar peduncles, showing numerous high-signal lesions in the pons, cerebellar peduncles, and cerebellum. *D,* T1-weighted sagittal image through the cervical spinal cord after administration of gadolinium. Note the elongated intrinsic cervical spinal cord lesion with gadolinium enhancement as signified by high signal around the periphery of the lesion. (From Goldman L, Bennett JC [eds]: Cecil Textbook of Medicine, 21st ed. Philadelphia: WB Saunders, 2000. Courtesy of Barbara Banger, M.D., Cleveland Clinical Foundation, Department of Neuroradiology.)

TABLE 128-4   Treatment of Multiple Sclerosis

Specific
Acute exacerbations: IV methylprednisolone, 500–1000 mg/day for 3 days
Relapsing-remitting attack prevention:
Interferon β-1a
Interferon β-1b
Glatiramer acetate
Symptomatic
Antispasticity agents: baclofen, benzodiazepines
Antipyretics for intercurrent infection
Fatigue: amantadine, pemoline
Pain (uncommon): carbamazepine

50% the likelihood of conversion from idiopathic optic neuritis to MS during 2 years of follow-up.

Acute Transverse Myelitis

Acute transverse myelitis denotes rapidly developing paraparesis or paraplegia as the result of spinal cord dysfunction. If the cervical cord is involved, quadriparesis and respiratory failure can occur. Abrupt or rapidly developing back or radicular pain may be followed by ascending paresthesias and weakness that begins in the feet. Urinary and fecal retention or incontinence is common. Progression varies from minutes, resembling infarction, to steady or stepwise progression over several days. Progression over days may occur with both spinal cord compression due to a tumor and transverse myelitis. It is difficult to distinguish idiopathic transverse myelitis from compressive myelopathy; acute transverse myelitis demands immediate diagnostic evaluation.

Several disorders can produce an acute transverse myelopathy. The most important to exclude immediately are compressive lesions, including spinal or epidural abscess, tumor, herniated intervertebral disc, or injury;

TABLE 128-5   Differential Diagnosis of Multiple Sclerosis

Relapsing-Remitting
Vascular disease: strokes, vasculitis
Behçet's syndrome
Systemic lupus erythematosus
Sarcoidosis
Chronic Progressive
Vascular: multiple strokes
Degenerative: spinocerebellar ataxias, spine disease
Infections: HTLV-I–, HIV-related
Neoplastic: lymphoma
Metabolic: adrenomyeloleukodystrophy

HIV = human immunodeficiency virus; HTLV-I = human T-cell lymphotropic virus type I.

vascular occlusion due to arteritis, aortic dissection, aortic surgery, or arteriovenous malformation; varicella-zoster infection; and autoimmune disease, including MS. The evaluation must include an immediate imaging procedure such as MRI with attention to the level of involvement to rule out spinal cord compression. Cord compression from metastatic tumor may present acutely even though the tumor has been present for weeks or longer. Central herniated intervertebral discs may cause acute cord compression without producing local pain. Rapidly progressing myelopathy in a previously healthy person should always raise the question of spontaneous epidural, subdural, or intraparenchymal abscess or bleeding, the latter occurring from an arteriovenous malformation or as a complication of anticoagulation or blood dyscrasia. About one third of patients with idiopathic transverse myelitis give a history of an antecedent upper respiratory or flulike illness. Transverse myelitis may also follow several other infectious illnesses such as *Mycoplasma* infection or measles.

Transverse myelitis and slowly progressive myelopathy are common manifestations of MS, either as a first clinical manifestation or a late development. However, a syndrome suggesting complete cord transection rarely occurs. The treatment for idiopathic transverse myelitis is intravenous methylprednisolone. With severe disease, bladder catheterization, ventilatory support, and proper protection from compression neuropathies are necessary. Prognosis varies widely, with recovery ranging from almost none at all to complete, depending on the degree of acute necrosis.

Acute Disseminated Encephalomyelitis

Acute disseminated encephalomyelitis (ADEM) is a monophasic demyelinating inflammatory disorder that can appear after viral infections or immunizations. ADEM usually produces multifocal brain and spinal cord symptoms, but it may be restricted to one area, particularly the optic nerve (acute optic neuropathy) or spinal cord (acute transverse myelopathy). When related to an antecedent vitral infection, ADEM usually occurs 6 to 10 days after the appearance of systemic symptoms. When it follows immunization, it usually begins 10 days to 3 weeks after injection. ADEM can appear in the absence of any identifiable exposure. The pathogenesis is believed to comprise an antibody response, the antigen being either the injected protein or the infecting virus. Clinically, ADEM typically produces acute headache, fever, and multifocal neurologic signs. Severely affected patients may develop delirium, stupor, or coma. Seizures are relatively common. The CSF is usually abnormal, showing pleocytosis (20 to 200 lymphocytes/mm³) and an elevated gamma globulin with slight protein elevation. Glucose concentration is usually normal. The electroencephalogram is usually diffusely abnormal, with widespread slowing, but it does not have the characteristic focal slow and sharp wave activity of herpes simplex encephalitis. ADEM produces clinical and CSF manifestations similar to those of acute viral encephalitis and cannot be distinguished from that disorder by clinical findings. Despite its presumed immune mechanism, neither corticosteroids nor other immunosuppressive agents have been effective in treatment of ADEM. Anecdotal reports suggest that intravenous immunoglobulin may be of benefit. The most important similar disorder to consider is herpes simplex encephalitis (see Chapter 127).

Acute hemorrhagic leukoencephalitis is a fatal, rare variant of ADEM. The illness usually occurs after an upper respiratory tract infection and is characterized by sudden headache, seizures, and rapid progression to coma. Patients often die within a few days. The CSF often shows more polymorphonuclear leukocytes than lymphocytes. At autopsy the brain is swollen, with bilateral and asymmetric hemorrhages scattered throughout the white matter. There is no known treatment.

REFERENCES

Beck RW, Cleary PA, Trobe JD, et al: The effect of corticosteroids for acute optic neuritis on the subsequent development of multiple sclerosis. N Engl J Med 1993; 329:1764.

Rudick RA, Cohen JA, Weinstock-Guttman B, et al: Management of multiple sclerosis. N Engl J Med 1997; 337:1604–1611.

Trapp BD, Peterson J, Ransohoff RM, et al: Axonal transections in the lesions of multiple sclerosis. N Engl J Med 1998; 33:278–285.

Wingerchuk DM, Hogancamp WF, O'Brien PC, Weinshenker BG: The clinical course of neuromyelitis optica (Devic's syndrome). Neurology 1999; 53(5):1107–1114.

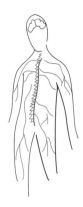

129

NEUROMUSCULAR DISEASES: DISORDERS OF THE MOTOR NEURON AND PLEXUS AND PERIPHERAL NERVE DISEASE

Robert C. Griggs

The neuromuscular diseases are disorders of the motor unit and of the sensory and autonomic peripheral nerves. Each motor unit consists of (1) the motor neuron cell body, located in either the spinal cord anterior horn (for muscles innervated by the spinal cord) or a cranial nerve nucleus (for ocular, facial, and bulbar musculature), (2) the axon of the motor neuron in the peripheral or cranial nerve, (3) the neuromuscular junction, and (4) the muscle fibers innervated by the motor neuron. The sensory peripheral nerves comprise (1) the sensory neuron cell body in the posterior (dorsal) root ganglion, (2) the central axon passing to the spinal cord in the posterior root, (3) the distal axon in the peripheral nerve, and (4) the sensory nerve terminal in skin, muscle, joint capsule, and other structures. The autonomic nerves are divided into sympathetic and parasympathetic fiber systems. The sympathetic preganglionic fibers arise from cell bodies in the intermediolateral column of the spinal cord and enter the sympathetic ganglia, where postganglionic fibers arise to innervate blood vessels or viscera. The parasympathetic preganglionic neurons lie in the brain stem and sacral portion of the spinal cord, and axons terminate in the viscera, special sensory organs, or skin, which contain the postganglionic neurons and their nerve terminals. Neuromuscular diseases are classified into four groups, according to which portion of the motor unit is involved (Table 129–1). Motor neurons and peripheral nerve diseases are considered in this chapter; myopathies are considered in Chapter 130; and neuromuscular junction diseases are considered in Chapter 131.

The symptoms and signs of the neuromuscular diseases are at times indistinguishable. However, some useful general rules apply (Table 129–2).

The peripheral nerves exiting from the spinal cord can be injured by intervertebral disk or bony compression within the spinal foramina, producing nerve root disease (radiculopathy; see Chapter 118). The roots within the cervical, lumbar, and sacral regions organize into the cervical, lumbar, and sacral plexuses before giving rise to individual peripheral nerves. Diseases of these plexuses (plexopathies) tend to be *focal* in symptoms and signs, whereas many diseases of the peripheral nerves and muscles are *generalized* and widespread in many nerves or muscles.

The major symptoms of diseases of the motor unit are muscle weakness, wasting, fatigue, cramps, pain, and stiffness. Symptoms of peripheral nerve disease also include decreased sensation (hypesthesia or hypalgesia), abnormal sensation (paresthesias), or painful sensations (dysesthesias). Symptoms and signs of autonomic nervous system disease include postural dizziness; abnormal cardiac, visceral, and ocular function; and changes in sweating. The symptoms of neuromuscular disease, particularly those of weakness or sensory disturbance, do not necessarily distinguish disorders of the peripheral nervous system from those of the central nervous system. Most neuromuscular diseases are relatively sym-

TABLE 129–1 Classification of Neuromuscular Disease

Site of Involvement	Typical Example
Anterior horn cell	
Without upper motor neuron involvement	Spinal muscular atrophy
With upper motor neuron involvement	Amyotrophic lateral sclerosis
Peripheral nerve	
Unifocal	Carpal tunnel syndrome
Multifocal	Mononeuritis multiplex (e.g., polyarteritis nodosa)
Diffuse	Diabetic neuropathy
Neuromuscular junction	Myasthenia gravis
Muscle	Duchenne dystrophy

metric, in contrast to the asymmetry of many focal central nervous system diseases.

Diagnostic Tests

BLOOD TESTS

Creatine kinase (CK) is present in high concentrations in a sarcoplasm of muscle and may leak into blood to serve as a sensitive indicator of muscle damage. In patients with active muscle destruction, the serum CK is invariably elevated, and lactic dehydrogenase (LDH), aspartate aminotransferase (AST), and alanine aminotransferase (ALT) levels are usually elevated. Because several of these enzymes are used for screening for abnormalities of organs other than muscle, it is not uncommon for a muscle disease to be first identified by an unexpected elevation in one of these enzymes. The clue to the muscle origin of the increased enzyme levels is that the degree of abnormality decreases in the order CK > LDH > AST > ALT. The serum CK level is the most sensitive indicator and may be very high (more than 10-fold above normal) in patients with diseases with muscle fiber necrosis, such as the muscular dystrophies and polymyositis. It frequently is slightly elevated in patients with spinal muscular atrophy, amyotrophic lateral sclerosis, and other motor neuron disorders but is usually normal in patients with peripheral neuropathies and neuromuscular junction disorders.

ELECTROMYOGRAPHY

The measurement of electrical activity arising from muscle fibers is performed by inserting a needle electrode percutaneously into a muscle. Normal muscle is electrically silent at rest. Spontaneous activity during complete relaxation occurs in myotonic disorders, in inflammatory myopathies, and in denervated muscles. Spontaneous activity of a single muscle fiber is called a *fibrillation*, and such activity of part of or an entire motor unit is called a *fasciculation*. In myotonia, the sarcolemma is irritable, and repeated muscle depolarization and contraction occur despite voluntary relaxation. Abnormalities in motor unit potentials occur during the course of denervation: with the development of reinnervation, the remaining motor units increase in amplitude and become longer in duration and polyphasic (Fig. 129–1). Conversely, in diseases such as polymyositis, the muscular dystrophies, and other myopathies that destroy scattered fibers within a motor unit (see Fig. 129–1), the motor unit action potentials are of lower amplitude and shorter duration and are polyphasic. A reduced recruitment (interference) pattern from maximum voluntary effort occurs in denervation. Conversely, in patients with primary muscle disease, submaximal voluntary effort produces a full recruitment pattern despite marked weakness.

Nerve conduction is studied by stimulating a peripheral nerve (e.g., the ulnar) with surface electrodes placed over the nerve. The resulting compound muscle action potential (CMAP) is recorded by electrodes placed over the nerve more proximally in the case of large sensory nerve fibers and placed over the muscle

TABLE 129–2 Presenting Clinical Features of the Neuromuscular Diseases

Clinical Feature	Anterior Horn Cell	Peripheral Nerve	Neuromuscular Junction	Muscle
Distribution of weakness	Asymmetric limb or bulbar	Symmetric distal	Extraocular, bulbar, proximal limb	Symmetric proximal limb (bulbar in some, distal rarely)
Atrophy	Marked and early	Moderate	None (or very late)	Slight early; marked later
Sensory involvement	None	Paresthesias, hypesthesia	None	None
Characteristic features	Fasciculations, cramps	Combined sensory and motor abnormality	Diurnal fluctuation	Usually painless
Reflexes	Variable (depending on degree of upper motor neuron involvement)	Decreased out of proportion to weakness	Normal in myasthenia gravis, depressed in myasthenic syndrome	Decreased in proportion to weakness

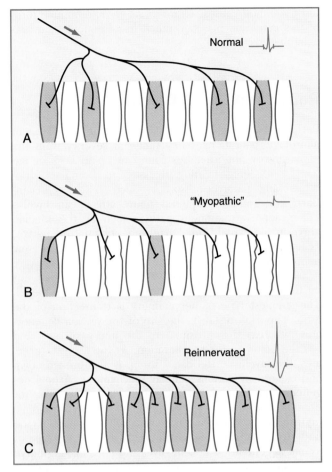

FIGURE 129-1 Motor unit potentials. The shaded muscle fibers are functional members of one motor unit; the axon, which enters from the upper left, branches terminally to innervate the appropriate muscle fibers. The motor unit action potential produced by each motor unit is seen at the upper right; its duration is measured between the two small vertical lines. The normal-appearing but unshaded fibers belong to other motor units. *A,* The normal situation, with five muscle fibers in the active unit. *B,* In this myopathic unit, only two fibers remain active; the other three (shrunken and unshaded) have been destroyed by a muscle disease. *C,* Four fibers that belonged to other motor units and had been denervated have now been reinnervated by terminal axon sprouting from the healthy motor unit. Both the motor unit and its action potential are now larger than normal. Note that only under these abnormal circumstances do fibers in the same unit lie next to one another. (From Griggs RC, Bradley WG: Approach to the patient with neuromuscular disease. *In* Isselbacher KJ, Braunwald E, Wilson JD, et al [eds]: Harrison's Textbook of Internal Medicine, 13th ed. New York: McGraw-Hill, 1994, p 2364.)

distally in the case of motor nerve fibers in a mixed motor sensory nerve.

REPETITIVE STIMULATION TESTS

In neuromuscular junction disorders, the size of the initial CMAP evoked by electrical stimulation may be normal. However, after a few stimuli at rates of 2 to 3 Hz, the amplitude of CMAP declines. It then increases again after the fourth or fifth stimulus. This pattern of decrement followed by increment is characteristic of myasthenia gravis.

Diseases of the Motor Neuron (Anterior Horn Cell) (Table 129–3)

Lower motor neurons are located in the brain stem and in the ventral spinal cord and when diseased produce decreased strength, tone, and reflexes accompanied by fasciculations and atrophy. The most common *acquired* motor neuron disease, *amyotrophic lateral sclerosis* (ALS), usually includes dysfunction of both upper and lower motor neurons. If only the lower motor neuron is affected, the term *spinal muscular atrophy* (SMA) is used. The spinal muscular atrophies are hereditary, progressive motor neuron disorders that begin in utero, infancy, childhood, or adult life. SMA types 1, 2, and 3 represent the first class of neurologic disorders in which a developmental defect in neuronal apoptosis most likely produces the disease. There are two genes involved in SMA: neuronal apoptosis inhibitor protein (NAIP) and survival motor neuron (SMN) gene. *Bulbospinal muscular atrophy* (BSMA) is a trinucleotide repeat disorder (see Chapter 1) with a CAG expansion encoding for a polyglutamine tract in the first axon of the androgen receptor gene, on chromosome Xq11–12. It is not known why disruption of the androgen receptor gene alters the function of bulbar and spinal motor neurons. BSMA is an X-linked recessive disorder. The mean age at onset of BSMA is 30 years; the range is 15 to 60 years. Gynecomastia occurs in 50% of affected individuals. Individuals present with facial, tongue, and proximal

TABLE 129-3   Diseases of the Anterior Horn Cells

Hereditary
Autosomal Dominant
Familial amyotrophic lateral sclerosis (FALS)
Amyotrophic lateral sclerosis with frontotemporal dementia (many cases are sporadic)
Autosomal Recessive
Spinal muscular atrophy
Type I: acute, infantile (Werdnig-Hoffmann disease)
Type II: late infantile
Type III: juvenile and adult types (Kugelberg-Welander disease)
X-linked
Bulbospinal muscular atrophy (Kennedy's syndrome)
Acquired
Acute: anterior poliomyelitis
Chronic:
Sporadic amyotrophic lateral sclerosis (ALS)
Postpoliomyelitis syndrome
ALS-like syndromes:
Motor neuron disease with paraproteinemia
Hexosaminidase A deficiency
Primary lateral sclerosis (rare)

weakness. Dysphagia and dysarthria are common, and fasciculations are widespread.

Sporadic ALS accounts for approximately 80% of all cases of acquired motor neuron disease; the remaining 20% of patients have either only lower motor neuron signs or a familial form of ALS (FALS). The 80% of patients that have sporadic ALS present with spasticity, hyperreflexia, and Babinski signs (upper motor neuron signs) in the setting of progressive muscle wasting and weakness (lower motor neuron signs). Autosomal dominant FALS is an adult-onset disease that is clinically and pathologically indistinguishable from sporadic ALS. FALS is caused by missense mutations in SOD1 in a sizable minority of cases. Painless, progressive weakness is the usual presenting sign of ALS. Usually focal in onset, weakness then spreads to contiguous muscle groups. Weakness is accompanied by muscle atrophy. ALS is a relentlessly progressive disease; the drug *riluzole* delays progression slightly.

Plexopathy

Brachial Plexopathy. The brachial plexus is constructed by mixed nerve roots from C5 to T1 that fuse into upper, middle, and lower trunks above the level of the clavicle and redistribute into lateral, posterior, and medial cords below that landmark. Symptoms include several patterns of weakness, as well as pain and sensory loss in structures about the pectoral girdle. Brachial plexopathy occurs with severe neck trauma, with malignant tumor invasion, as a result of radiation therapy, and most commonly with the autoimmune or postinfectious inflammatory disorder, brachial amyotrophy (brachial neuritis).

Acute Autoimmune Brachial Neuritis. This condition is characterized by the abrupt onset of severe pain, usually over the lateral shoulder but at times extending into the entire arm. Young males are predominantly affected. The acute pain generally subsides after a few days to a week; by this time, weakness of the proximal arm becomes apparent. The serratus anterior and supraspinatus are the most commonly paralyzed muscles, but other muscles of the shoulder girdle may also be paralyzed. In rare cases, most of the arm and even the ipsilateral diaphragm are paralyzed. Sensory loss is usually slight. Weakness may last weeks to months and be accompanied by severe atrophy of the shoulder girdle. Total recovery occurs in most patients within several months to 2 years. The disorder frequently follows an upper respiratory infection or an immunization, but often there is no antecedent illness. It is occasionally bilateral and may sometimes recur; in rare instances, it occurs within families.

Lumbosacral Plexopathy. The lumbosacral plexus is constructed by mixed spinal roots from T12 to S3. Predominant contributions go to femoral, sciatic, and obturator nerves. Clinical expression includes proximal pain and weakness in anterior thigh muscles (femoral) or posterior thigh muscles and the buttocks. Diabetes, malignancy, radiation therapy, and hemorrhage are the most common causes. There exists an autoimmune form of this condition but it is much less frequent than brachial neuritis.

Peripheral Nerve Disease

Peripheral neuropathies are among the most prevalent neurologic conditions. They range in severity from the mild sensory abnormalities found in up to 70% of patients with long-standing diabetes to fulminant, life-threatening paralytic disorders such as the Guillain-Barré syndrome. Peripheral neuropathies can involve single nerves (mononeuropathy), such as the median nerve in the carpal tunnel syndrome, or multiple nerves, as in metabolic neuropathies such as diabetic or uremic neuropathy.

Normal function of myelinated nerve fibers depends on the integrity of both the axon and its myelin sheath. The simplest type of nerve injury is transection of the axon. The axon distal to the site of transection degenerates, whereas that proximal to the injury survives and has the potential for regeneration. As the axon degenerates, the myelin in the distal stump is also broken down and cleared by various cellular mechanisms. Axonal degeneration caused by a focal nerve injury occurs, for example, in severe compression and in focal ischemic injury to nerves. In the symmetric polyneuropathies, the underlying pathology is usually a slowly evolving type of axonal degeneration that involves the ends of long nerve fibers first and preferentially. With time, the degenerative process involves more proximal regions of long fibers, and shorter fibers are affected. This pattern of distal axonal degeneration or "dying back" of nerve fibers results from a wide variety of metabolic, toxic, and heritable causes. The resulting clinical picture includes early loss of muscle stretch reflexes at the ankle and weakness that initially involves the intrinsic muscles of the feet, the extensors of the toes, and the dorsiflexors at the ankle; the motor signs are accompanied by distally predominant loss of large-fiber sensory modalities such as vibratory sensibility in the toes. With progression, the hands are similarly involved, and the process may spread more proximally up the legs and arms. The resulting pattern of sensory loss is frequently termed a *stocking-and-glove pattern.* Recovery from axonal degeneration requires nerve regeneration, a process that often requires 2 to 3 years.

Demyelination of a peripheral nerve at even a single site can block conduction, resulting in a functional deficit identical to that seen after axonal degeneration. In contrast to repair by regeneration, however, repair by remyelination can be quite rapid. Autoimmune attack on the myelin sheath occurs in the inflammatory demyelinating neuropathies and some neuropathies associated with paraproteinemias. Inherited disorders of myelin are the other major category of demyelinating neuropathy. Uncommon causes include some toxic, mechanical, and physical injuries to nerve. Although these examples have nearly pure demyelination, many neuropathies have an admixture of both axonal degeneration and demyelination. This mixed pathology reflects the mutual interde-

TABLE 129–4   Classification and Causes of Peripheral Neuropathy

Type of Neuropathy	Examples
Mononeuropathies	
Compression	Median carpal tunnel syndrome
Hereditary	Familial liability to pressure palsies
Inflammation; infection	Facial: Bell's palsy; herpes simplex
Multiple Mononeuropathies (Mononeuritis multiplex)	Vasculitis
Polyneuropathy	
Hereditary	Charcot-Marie-Tooth disease(s)
Metabolic	Diabetes, uremia, porphyria
Infections	Leprosy; diphtheria
Postinfectious (autoimmune)	Guillain-Barré syndrome
Toxic	Lead toxicity
Drug	Amiodarone, pyridoxine, toluene toxicity

pendency of the axons and the myelin-forming Schwann cells.

In general, axonal degeneration decreases the amplitude of the CMAP out of proportion to the degree of reduction in peripheral nerve conduction velocity, whereas demyelination produces prominent reduction in conduction velocities.

Table 129–4 gives a classification of peripheral neuropathies with many of their causes. The symptoms of peripheral neuropathies depend on their anatomic location and on their pathophysiology. *Mononeuropathies* produce sensory loss or weakness or both in the territory of the nerve. *Polyneuropathies*, if demyelinating, produce distal weakness and loss of sensation in the modalities served by large myelinated peripheral nerve fibers: vibration and proprioception. Axonal neuropathies produce distal disturbance of pain and temperature perception and may be extremely painful. Motor and sensory functions served by large myelinated fibers, including reflexes, are relatively preserved. Neuropathies generally produce distal symptoms. Exceptions include the acute and chronic inflammatory demyelinating neuropathies Guillain-Barré syndrome and chronic inflammatory demyelinating neuropathy (CIDP), which often cause proximal weakness.

Common Mononeuropathies

(Table 129–5)

Carpal Tunnel Syndrome. This syndrome is a major cause of disability claims. In classic instances, the median nerve is pathologically compressed at the wrist as it passes deep to the flexor retinaculum. Symptoms include numbness, tingling, and burning sensations in the palm and in the fingers supplied by the median nerve, including the thumb, index, middle, and medial half of the ring finger. Some patients complain that all fingers become numb. Pain and paresthesias are most prominent at night and often interrupt sleep. The pain is prominent at the wrist but may radiate to the forearm and occasionally to the shoulder. Both pain and paresthesias are relieved by loose shaking of the hand. In some patients, symptoms may persist for years without objective signs of median nerve damage. In others, sensory loss may appear over the tips of the fingers, and weakness can develop in the median nerve-innervated thumb muscles in association with atrophy of the lateral aspect of the thenar eminence. Percussion of the median nerve at the wrist often provokes paresthesias in a median nerve distribution (Tinel's sign). Flexion of the wrist for 30 to 60 seconds may provoke pain or paresthesias (Phalen's sign). Precipitating factors include activities that require repetitive wrist movements: mechanical work, gardening, house painting, meat wrapping, and typing. Predisposing causes include pregnancy, myxedema, acromegaly, rheumatoid arthritis, and primary amyloidosis.

The diagnosis is based on clinical symptoms and signs, and the demonstration of a conduction block at the wrist by motor nerve conduction velocity studies and electromyography. If rest and splinting fail, surgical treatment by section of the transverse carpal ligament decompresses the nerve. The diagnosis is often made inaccurately; neither hand and arm pain nor electrodiagnostic findings alone establish the diagnosis. Both should be present.

Ulnar Palsy. The ulnar nerve may be entrapped at the elbow (cubital tunnel) or at the wrist. Injury may also occur years after a malunited supracondylar fracture of the humerus with bony overgrowth (tardive ulnar palsy). Contrary to the findings in the carpal tunnel syndrome, muscle weakness and atrophy characteristically predominate over sensory symptoms and signs. Patients notice atrophy of the first dorsal interosseous muscle and difficulty performing fine manipulations of the fingers. There may be numbness of the small finger, the contiguous half of the ring finger, and the ulnar border of the hand.

Meralgia Paresthetica. This is the most common pure sensory mononeuropathy. It results from compression of the lateral cutaneous nerve of the thigh as it

TABLE 129–5   Common Sites of Nerve Entrapment

Median nerve
Carpal tunnel: wrist
Pronator muscle: elbow
Ulnar nerve
Elbow
Wrist
Radial nerve: humeral groove
Peroneal nerve: behind knee
Lateral femoral cutaneous nerve: inguinal ligament
Cervical and lumbar roots: intervertebral foramina

passes under or through the inguinal ligament. Numbness or burning sensations occur over the lateral thigh; sometimes prolonged standing or walking provokes the symptoms. Weight reduction may help, but in many cases the condition subsides spontaneously. A similar sensory syndrome can affect the dorsal aspect of the thumb when a tight watchband compresses a cutaneous branch of the radial nerve. If there is electrophysiologic evidence of conduction block at the inguinal ligament, surgical decompression is often helpful.

Mononeuritis Multiplex. This common syndrome is encountered in patients who almost always have an underlying symmetric peripheral neuropathy (polyneuropathy), particularly diabetes, rheumatoid arthritis, leprosy, or polyarteritis nodosa and other vasculitic disorders. There is the abrupt onset of a focal deficit such as foot drop or ulnar palsy, usually painful. Although evidence now points to ischemia of an entire cervical or lumbosacral plexus as the site of the pathology, the patient clinically appears to have two or more single nerves affected. This phenomenon reflects the fact that individual peripheral nerves are already constituted within the proximal plexuses.

Polyneuropathies

GUILLAIN-BARRÉ SYNDROME (ACUTE INFLAMMATORY DEMYELINATING POLYNEUROPATHY)

Guillain-Barré syndrome (GBS) is characterized by weakness or paralysis affecting the limbs, usually symmetrically, in association with loss of muscle stretch reflexes and with increased spinal fluid protein without pleocytosis. Since the advent of polio vaccination, GBS has become the most frequent cause of acute flaccid paralysis throughout the world.

GBS is almost certainly an immune-mediated disorder. It follows an identifiable infectious disorder in approximately 60% of cases. The best documented antecedents include infection with *Campylobacter jejuni*, infectious mononucleosis, cytomegalovirus, herpes viruses, and mycoplasma. *C. jejuni* is often associated with more severe "axonal" cases and most likely sensitizes the immune system to antigens shared between the organism and the peripheral nerve (termed *epitopic mimicry*).

Clinical Manifestations. The initial symptoms of GBS often consist of tingling and "pins-and-needles" sensations in the feet and may be associated with dull low-back pain. By the time of presentation, which usually occurs within hours to 1 to 2 days after the first symptoms, weakness has usually developed. The weakness is usually most prominent in the legs, but the arms or cranial musculature may be involved first. Muscle stretch reflexes are lost early, even in regions where strength is retained. Because the spinal roots are usually prominently involved, GBS can involve short nerves (axial and intercostal as well as cranial nerves) as well as long ones. Weakness progresses, and the nadir is reached within 30 days, usually by 14 days. Progression

can be alarmingly rapid, so that critical functions such as respiration can be lost within a few days or even a few hours. The potential for respiratory insufficiency, as well as swallowing difficulty and autonomic dysregulation, underlies the life-threatening nature of GBS.

Treatment. Two treatments are of benefit. Plasmapheresis—the exchange of the patient's plasma for albumin—was the first treatment definitively shown to shorten the time to recovery. Infusion of high doses of human immunoglobulin intravenously also produces benefit. These treatments are equally effective, and there is no added benefit to combining them. The choice of modality should be individualized. In patients with limited venous access, immunoglobulin is easier to administer.

GUILLAIN-BARRÉ SYNDROME VARIANTS

Two other acute, immune polyneuropathies resemble GBS in their relatively rapid onset, their relationship to antecedent minor illnesses, and their symmetry of involvement. Ataxic-ophthalmoplegic neuropathy (Miller-Fisher syndrome) predominantly affects oculomotor nerves, other cranial nerves, and proprioceptive sensory nerves arising from the lower limbs. The other, much more severe variant causes an acute, noninflammatory axonal neuropathy. The pattern of onset and progression of these diseases resembles that of classic GBS. Prompt immune therapy appears to halt the process, but once severe paralysis occurs, it often remains for long periods and, sometimes, permanently. Epidemiologic studies have found a close linkage to preceding *Campylobacter* infection. A particularly high prevalence of the illness has been found among children in Chinese provinces.

CIDP, sometimes referred to as chronic GBS, bears similarities to the clinical, pathologic, and laboratory pictures seen in acute GBS. It differs primarily in the time course and in the infrequency of identifiable antecedent events. The differences in response to therapy, however, suggest that the precise immunopathogenic mechanisms may differ.

Clinical Manifestations. CIDP can occur at any age. The usual picture is one of slowly evolving weakness beginning in the legs, with widespread areflexia and loss of large fiber (vibratory) sensibility on examination.

Treatment. Controlled trials have shown that, unlike GBS, most cases of CIDP respond to corticosteroids alone. Some patients with CIDP respond to plasmapheresis and intravenous gamma globulin. In most instances the first choice of therapy is with corticosteroids, at first in high doses but subsequently with the lowest dosage needed to achieve and maintain an adequate response. Plasmapheresis, although simple and safe, is expensive and usually must be repeated every several weeks to maintain a response.

MULTIFOCAL MOTOR NEUROPATHY

An uncommon related disorder, multifocal motor neuropathy, occurs as "pure motor" multiple mononeuropathy. A patient may describe, for example, development of unilateral wristdrop (radial nerve involvement) followed by footdrop on the other side (peroneal nerve involvement). In addition, muscle stretch reflexes may be lost outside the distribution of weakness, but the sensory examination is normal even in weak limbs. The pathologic characteristic, inflammatory demyelination, resembles that seen in CIDP but is highly focal and largely spares sensory nerve fibers. A characteristic electrodiagnostic feature is the presence of motor nerve conduction block, a reflection of the focal demyelination. Multifocal motor neuropathy responds favorably to intravenous immunoglobulin as well as to cytotoxic therapy but not to corticosteroids or plasmapheresis.

NEUROPATHIES ASSOCIATED WITH MONOCLONAL GAMMOPATHIES

Peripheral neuropathy occurs in some monoclonal gammopathies, both the benign type and myeloma. Monoclonal proteins of IgM, IgG, and IgA types with both kappa and lambda light chains, are all associated with neuropathy. In some instances the monoclonal protein has a role in causing the neuropathy. For example, some IgM–kappa monoclonal proteins react with sugars found on a specific Schwann cell protein, the myelin-associated glycoprotein (MAG).

The clinical picture of the neuropathy varies. The IgM-kappa monoclonal antibodies with "anti-MAG" reactivity typically produce neuropathy with prominent large-fiber sensory loss and sensory ataxia, as well as milder weakness. The electrodiagnostic tests indicate demyelination, albeit admixed with nerve fiber loss. In other cases with IgM monoclonal proteins, there is a distinctive picture that includes scleroderma-like skin changes, hepatomegaly, and endocrine abnormalities, as well as neuropathy (the POEMS syndrome, described in the next paragraph). Other patients with monoclonal proteins have a clinical picture identical to that of CIDP, and still others have distally predominant axonal degeneration.

Three disorders should be specifically sought in patients with paraproteins and neuropathy: (1) There is a special association of neuropathy with solitary plasmacytomas, often osteosclerotic. The POEMS syndrome— *p*olyneuropathy, *o*rganomegaly, *e*ndocrinopathy (hirsutism, testicular atrophy), *m*onoclonal IgM protein, and *s*kin pigmentation—is usually associated with osteosclerotic myelomas. A skeletal radiographic survey is essential in patients with monoclonal proteins and neuropathy. (2) Cryoglobulinemia, with or without monoclonal gammopathy, can produce neuropathy, and the possibility should be evaluated. (3) The monoclonal proteins may result in amyloid deposition in nerve and thus produce neuropathy indirectly.

IMMUNE-MEDIATED ATAXIC NEUROPATHIES

In this category are three disorders: carcinomatous sensory neuropathy, sensory ganglionitis associated with features of Sjögren's syndrome, and idiopathic sensory ganglionitis. All three are characterized clinically by subacute or slowly developing proprioceptive sensory loss leading to gait ataxia and inability to localize the limbs. The possibility of occult carcinoma underlying an immunogenic (paraneoplastic) ataxic neuropathy adds urgency to differential diagnosis. The most frequent associations include small cell lung, breast, and ovarian carcinomas. In addition to clinical screening for these neoplasms, there are helpful serologic tests, particularly the anti-Hu antibody.

HEREDITARY NEUROPATHIES

Heritable neuropathies are among the most prevalent inherited neurologic diseases. Because many occur in midlife, and because the family history is often previously unrecognized, the heritable disorders constitute an important aspect of differential diagnosis of any chronic polyneuropathy.

CHARCOT-MARIE-TOOTH DISEASE

The eponym, Charcot-Marie-Tooth (CMT), identifies a group of heritable disorders of peripheral nerves that share clinical features but differ in their pathology and the specific genetic abnormalities, as shown in Table 129–6. One group of disorders, classed together as CMT type I (CMT I), is characterized pathologically by abnormalities of peripheral myelination and, at a molecular level, by abnormalities of specific proteins found in the myelin sheaths or Schwann cells. The CMT II group is characterized by axonal degeneration. All forms of CMT disease tend to manifest during the second to fourth decades with insidiously evolving footdrop. Examination reveals distal weakness and wasting of the intrinsic muscles of the feet, the peroneal muscles, the anterior tibial muscles, and the calves. A variable degree of impaired large-fiber sensory function is reflected in elevated vibratory thresholds in the toes. Muscle stretch reflexes are lost, first at the ankles. Typically, a foot deformity exists, with high arches (pes cavus) and hammer toes, reflecting long-standing muscle imbalance in the feet. Most patients with CMT disease have nearly normal occupational and daily activities, and they have a normal lifespan. The footdrop can be relieved by appropriate bracing of the ankle with ankle-foot orthoses. Genetic counseling and education of affected patients and their families is important, both for reassurance and to preclude unnecessary diagnostic evaluation of affected members in future generations.

A variant of CMT is *hereditary neuropathy with liability to pressure palsies* (see Table 129–6). Recurrent mononeuropathies occur, especially in the upper limbs (particularly ulnar); the autosomal dominant hereditary pattern is seldom recognized initially.

AMYLOID NEUROPATHIES

Amyloid neuropathy is caused by extracellular deposition of the fibrillary protein amyloid in peripheral nerve and sensory and autonomic ganglia, as well as around blood vessels in nerves and other tissues. In all forms of amyloidosis, the initial and major abnormalities affect the small sensory and autonomic fibers. Involvement of small fibers responsible for pain and temperature sensi-

TABLE 129–6 **Major Hereditary Neuropathies**

Disorder	Type	Clinical Features	Pathophysiology	Inheritance	Gene Defect
Charcot-Marie-Tooth Disease					
CMT I		Slowly evolving motor-sensory neuropathies with high arches, hammertoes, hypertrophic nerves	Demyelination and re-myelination with onion bulbs		
	a			Dominant	Duplication of a segment of chromosome 17 encoding PMP-22
	b			Dominant	Point mutation in the myelin protein P_0
	x			X-linked	Mutation in connexin 32
Liability to pressure palsies			Tomaculous neuropathy	Dominant	Deletion of PMP-22 region of chromosome 17
CMT II		Similar, without hypertrophic nerves	Distally predominant axonal degeneration	Dominant	Unknown
CMT III (Dejerine-Sottas disease)		Early onset, severe motor-sensory neuropathy	Severe hypomyelination with onion bulbs	Recessive	Mutation in P_0
Familial Amyloidosis (Four Subtypes)					
Porphyria					
Others (Rare)					
Fabry's disease					
Leukodystrophies					
Refsum's disease					
Tangier disease					
Abetalipoprotein-emia					
Mitochondrial neuropathies					

bilities leads to loss of the ability to perceive mechanical and thermal injury and a risk of tissue damage. As a result, painless injuries present a major hazard of this disorder; in advanced stages they can lead to chronic infections or osteomyelitis of the feet or hands and the necessity for amputation.

DIABETIC NEUROPATHIES

Diabetes is the most frequent cause of peripheral neuropathy worldwide. Incidence figures depend on the definition used: at least some peripheral nerve abnormalities can be detected in about 70% of patients with long-standing diabetes, and symptomatic neuropathy affects 5% to 10%. The diabetic neuropathies take many clinical forms, including symmetric polyneuropathies and a variety of individual plexus or nerve injuries (Table 129–7).

Diabetic Polyneuropathy

Diabetic polyneuropathy is symmetric and usually distally predominant, beginning with sensory loss in the feet. It is the most common of the diabetic neuropathies. It is uncommon at the time of diagnosis of diabetes, but its prevalence increases with duration of diabetes. The precise pathogenesis is not defined, but, like the ocular and renal complications, diabetic neuropathy

can be reduced in incidence and in severity by maintaining blood glucose levels close to normal. This effect of tight control is consistent with the hypothesis that hyperglycemia itself contributes to nerve damage. The complications of hyperglycemia that injure nerves may include one or more of the following: abnormalities of nerve vasculature and blood flow; metabolic effects of abnormalities in polyol pathways; and nonenzymatic glycosylation of nerve proteins.

Clinical Manifestations. The neuropathy is usually asymptomatic at the onset but abnormalities in sensation and reflexes may be detected on routine examination. The symptoms usually begin insidiously, but some cases

TABLE 129–7 **Major Diabetic Neuropathies**

Diabetic mononeuropathies and plexopathies
Third nerve palsy (often spares the pupil)
Palsies of other cranial nerves
Truncal neuropathy
Lumbosacral plexopathy
Diabetic polyneuropathy
Symmetric polyneuropathy
Sensorimotor
"Small fiber": autonomic dysfunction, distal burning pain

have an abrupt onset, and in a small percentage of patients this appears to be precipitated by the institution of insulin treatment. In contrast to most other neuropathies, small-fiber sensibility as well as large-fiber sensation are typically reduced in diabetic patients, resulting in elevated pain, thermal, and vibratory thresholds. The small-fiber dysfunction is often manifested by spontaneous neuropathic pain. This includes dysesthesias, which are unpleasant sensations evoked by normally innocuous stimuli, such as the bed sheets on the toes at night. There may be continuous burning or throbbing pain, and prolonged walking is often distressing.

The diagnosis of diabetic polyneuropathy is straightforward in a patient with established diabetes with a typical clinical picture. Electrodiagnostic studies can document neuropathy, and spinal fluid protein levels frequently are moderately elevated. Conversely, diabetic neuropathy is often overdiagnosed. In general, the diagnosis of diabetic neuropathy should be made only in the setting of long-standing diabetes, usually insulin-requiring. If only mild hyperglycemia that developed recently is present, the diagnosis of diabetic polyneuropathy should be regarded as suspect. Diabetic polyneuropathy seldom causes weakness unless it is associated with the severe pain of an associated mononeuritis multiplex.

Treatment. The careful management of diabetic hyperglycemia is essential (see Chapter 68). Correction of blood sugar to as nearly normal values as possible is important for both primary prevention and slowing of the progression of diabetic neuropathy. The painful symptoms of diabetic neuropathy often respond to anticonvulsants such as gabapentin or to tricyclic antidepressants such as desipramine.

ALCOHOL-NUTRITIONAL NEUROPATHY

Polyneuropathy in persons with chronic alcoholism usually occurs in a setting of associated nutritional deficiencies. Most persons with alcoholic neuropathy have evidence of multifactorial nutritional deficiency. Occasionally, the nutritional background seems adequate, and the direct contribution of alcohol cannot be excluded. The pathology of alcohol-nutritional neuropathy is that of a "dying back" axonal disorder affecting both sensory and motor fibers. The initial symptoms are pain and paresthesias, beginning in the soles of the feet, sometimes evolving to burning sensations in the feet and severe hyperpathia and often associated with aching and tenderness of the calves. Weakness is seldom severe and invariably distal, and muscle stretch reflexes are lost first at the ankles. Treatment with nutritional supplementation, including thiamine and multivitamins, and cessation of alcohol ingestion are highly beneficial in the early stages of the disease. In advanced cases the disease may continue to progress for a period after initiation of therapy, and recovery may be incomplete.

REFERENCES

Dyck PJ, Thomas PK, Griffin JW, et al (eds): Peripheral Neuropathy, 3rd ed. Philadelphia: WB Saunders, 1993.

Feldman EL: Motor neuron diseases. In Goldman L, Bennett JC (eds): Cecil Textbook of Medicine, 21st ed. Philadelphia: WB Saunders, 2000, pp 2089–2092.

Griffin JW: Diseases of the peripheral nervous system. In Goldman L, Bennett JC (eds): Cecil Textbook of Medicine, 21st ed. Philadelphia: WB Saunders, 2000, pp 2192–2200.

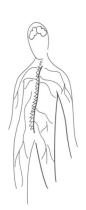

130

MUSCLE DISEASES

Robert C. Griggs

Skeletal muscle diseases (myopathies) are disorders in which there is a primary structural or functional impairment of muscle. Myopathies can be broadly classified into hereditary and acquired disorders (Table 130–1).

Organization and Structure of Muscle

Muscle comprises many motor units, each of which has four components: (1) a motor neuron in the brain stem or spinal cord; (2) its peripheral axon and terminal branches; (3) the neuromuscular junctions at each terminal nerve ending; and (4) all muscle fibers innervated by the axon. The number of muscle fibers innervated by a single motor unit varies from muscle to muscle. Muscles subserving finely coordinated movements, such as an ocular muscle, can have fewer than 10 muscles in a motor unit. Powerful proximal limb muscles have large motor units with 1000 to 2000 fibers innervated by a single motor neuron.

The muscle fibers consist of thick and thin filaments (myofibrils). The myofibrils are surrounded by the sarcolemmal membrane and basal lamina. A number of muscular dystrophies are now known to be caused by genetic defects in this region (Fig. 130–1). The sarcolemmal components are known as the dystrophin-glycoprotein complex (DGC). The DGC is a transsarcolemmal complex of proteins and glycoproteins that links the subsarcolemmal cytoskeleton to the extracellular matrix. Dystrophin was the first well-characterized protein in the DGC. Other DGC components include the dystroglycan complex (α, β), the sarcoglycan complex (α, β, γ, δ), and the syntrophin complex (α, $\beta1$, $\beta2$). Closely adherent to the extracellular portion of the sarcolemma is the basal lamina. Laminin and merosin (a collective name for similar laminins) are part of the basal lamina. Specific mutations of these various proteins are the cause of many myopathies.

Assessment

The most important aspect of evaluating a patient with a myopathy is the information obtained from the history. The most common symptom of a patient with muscle disease is weakness. If the weakness is in the legs, patients complain of difficulty climbing stairs and rising from a low chair or toilet or from the floor. When the arms are involved, patients notice trouble lifting objects (especially over their heads) and washing or brushing their hair. These symptoms point to proximal weakness, the most common site of weakness in a myopathy. In rare instances, patients first complain of poor hand grip (difficulty opening jar tops and turning door knobs) or tripping as a result of ankle weakness from distal muscle weakness, or a change in speech or swallowing, droopy eyelids, and double vision from weakness of cranial nerve–innervated muscles.

The tempo of the disease course is important. Weakness may be present all of the time (fixed) or intermittent (episodic). Myopathies can present as either fixed or episodic weakness. Muscle disorders can be *acute* (<4 weeks), *subacute* (4 to 8 weeks), or *chronic* (>8 weeks). Examples include (1) acute or subacute in inflammatory myopathies (dermatomyositis and polymyositis), (2) chronic slow progression over years (most muscular dystrophies), or (3) fixed weakness with little change over decades (congenital myopathies). Patients with channelopathies or metabolic myopathies have recurrent attacks of weakness over many years, whereas a patient with acute muscle destruction caused by a toxin such as cocaine may have a single acute episode.

Patients who complain of a generalized global "weakness" or "fatigue" seldom have a myopathy, particularly if the neurologic examination is normal. Fatigue is a complaint of the patient with myasthenia gravis but otherwise is usually a nonspecific symptom. Muscle pain (myalgia) is also a nonspecific complaint that infrequently accompanies some myopathies. Myalgias may be

TABLE 130–1 **Classification of Myopathies**

Hereditary
Muscular dystrophies
Congenital
Myotonias and other channelopathies
Metabolic
Mitochondrial
Acquired
Inflammatory
Endocrine/metabolic
Associated with systemic illness
Drug induced/toxic

episodic (e.g., metabolic myopathies) or nearly constant (e.g., occasional inflammatory myopathies). However, muscle pain is surprisingly uncommon in most muscle diseases and limb pain is more likely to be caused by bone or joint disorders. It is rare for a muscle disease to be responsible for vague aches and discomfort in muscle if strength is normal. An exception is the involuntary muscle cramp. Cramps are localized to a single muscle and last from seconds to minutes. Usually they are benign and normal; they do not reflect myopathy. Cramps occur with dehydration, hyponatremia, azotemia, and myxedema and in amyotrophic lateral sclerosis. Muscle contractures are rare and resemble a cramp. They last longer than cramps and occur with exercise in glycolytic enzyme defects. On electromyography (EMG), contractures are electrically silent whereas cramps have rapidly firing motor unit discharges. Muscle contracture should

not be confused with fixed tendon contracture. Myotonia is the phenomena of impaired relaxation of muscle after forceful voluntary contraction. Patients report muscle stiffness or persistent contraction in almost any muscle group, but particularly the hands and eyelids. Exercise-induced weakness and myalgias may be accompanied by dark or red urine—myoglobinuria. Myoglobinuria follows rapid muscle destruction.

EXAMINATION

Specific muscle function should be tested. Muscle strength is quantitated by the MRC (Medical Research Council of Great Britain) grading scale of 0 to 5:

5: Normal power
4: Active movement against gravity and resistance
3: Active movement against gravity
2: Active movement only with gravity eliminated
1: Trace contraction
0: No contraction

Muscles should be inspected for atrophy or hypertrophy. Atrophy of proximal limb muscles is usual in long-standing myopathies. Muscles can also become diffusely hypertrophic in dystrophic or myotonic conditions. In Duchenne and Becker dystrophies, the calves enlarge as a result of pseudohypertrophy from replacement with connective tissue and fat. The sensory examination should be normal in muscle disease. Reflexes are preserved early in the disease process, but when muscles become extremely weak, reflexes become hypoactive or unelicitable. Evidence of upper motor neuron damage (spasticity, Babinski signs, clonus) is only present in myopathies if there is coincidental central nervous system disease.

PATTERNS OF WEAKNESS

Six broad patterns of muscle weakness occur in myopathies:

1. The most common is in proximal muscles of the arms and legs: a limb-girdle distribution. Neck flexor and extensor muscles can also be affected. It is not known why most myopathies begin in proximal muscles.
2. Distal weakness may occur in the upper extremities (extensor muscle group) or lower extremities (anterior or posterior compartment muscle groups). Such selective distal weakness is more often a feature of neuropathies.
3. Scapuloperoneal weakness has weakness of the periscapular muscles and distal lower extremity weakness of the anterior compartment. The scapular muscle weakness is usually accompanied by scapular winging.
4. Distal upper extremity weakness in the distal forearm muscles (wrist and finger flexors) and proximal lower extremity weakness involving the knee extensors (quadriceps) may occur. This pattern is typical of inclusion body myositis and may be noted in myotonic dystrophy.

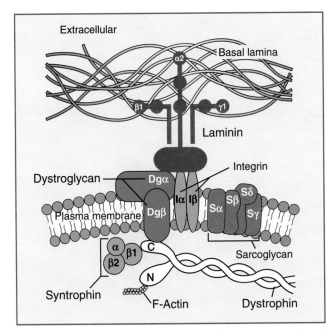

FIGURE 130–1 The dystrophin-glycoprotein complex and related proteins.

5. Involvement of ocular or pharyngeal muscles may be predominant.
6. Neck extensor weakness (the "dropped head syndrome") may be prominent.

These six patterns of myopathy are useful in differential diagnosis, but neuromuscular diseases other than myopathies can also present with one of these weakness patterns. For example, whereas proximal greater than distal weakness is characteristic of myopathies, patients with acquired demyelinating neuropathies (Guillain-Barré syndrome and chronic inflammatory demyelinating polyneuropathy) often have proximal as well as distal muscle involvement. Such neuropathies are additionally accompanied by sensory and reflex loss. Ocular, pharyngeal, and proximal limb weakness is characteristic of neuromuscular junction transmission disorders such as myasthenia gravis. However, these patients also have diplopia, weakness that fluctuates, and additional laboratory features that lead to the correct diagnosis.

MUSCLE BIOPSY

Fixed muscle is of little value for diagnosis. Muscle tissue examined under light microscopy is primarily per-formed using frozen specimens. The muscle biopsy can establish if there is evidence of either a neuropathic or myopathic disorder. It can also provide specific diagnosis of many hereditary and acquired myopathies.

Muscular Dystrophies

Muscular dystrophies are inherited myopathies characterized by progressive muscle weakness and degeneration and subsequent replacement by fibrous and fatty connective tissue. Historically, muscular dystrophies were categorized by their distribution of weakness, age at onset, and inheritance pattern. Advances in the molecular understanding of the muscular dystrophies have defined the genetic mutation and abnormal gene product for most of these disorders (Table 130–2).

Dystrophinopathies are X-linked disorders resulting from mutations of the large dystrophin gene located at Xp21. Dystrophin is a large subsarcolemmal cytoskeletal protein that along with the other components of the DGC provides support to the muscle membrane during contraction. Mutations disrupting the translational reading frame of the gene result in near-total loss of dystro-

TABLE 130–2 Major Muscular Dystrophies

Disease	Mode of Inheritance	Gene Mutation Location	Protein
X-linked			
Duchenne/Becker	XR	Xp21	Dystrophin
Emery-Dreifuss	XR	Xq28	Emerin
Limb girdle			
LGMD 1A	AD	5q22-34	Not known
LGMD 1B	AD	1q11-21	Not known
LGMD 1C	AD	3p25	Caveolin-3
LGMD 2A	AR	15q15	Calpain-3
LGMD 2B	AR	2p12	Dysferlin
LGMD 2C	AR	13q12	γ-Sarcoglycan
LGMD 2D	AR	17q12	α-Sarcoglycan
LGMD 2E	AR	4q12	β-Sarcoglycan
LGMD 2F	AR	5q33	δ-Sarcoglycan
LGMD 2G	AR	17q11	Not known
Facioscapulohumeral	AD	4q35	Not known
Oculopharyngeal	AD	14q11	Poly(A) binding protein 2
Myotonic dystrophy—type 1	AD	19q13	Myotonin-protein kinase
Myotonic dystrophy—type 2	AD	3q	Not known
Congenital			
With CNS involvement			
Fukuyama	AR	9q31-33	Fukutin
Without CNS involvement			
Merosin-deficient classic type	AR	6q2	Laminin-2 (merosin)
Merosin-positive classic type	AR	?	Not known
Integrin-deficient	AR	12q13	Integrin α7
Distal			
Late adult onset 1A (Welander)	AD	2p15	Dynactin
Late adult onset 1B (Markesbery/Udd)	AD	2p	Not known
Early adult onset 1A (Nonaka)	AR	9p1-q1	Not known
Early adult onset 1B (Miyoshi)	AR	2q12-14	Dysferlin
Early adult onset 1C (Laing)	AD	14	Not known

phin (Duchenne dystrophy), whereas in-frame mutations result in the translation of semifunctional dystrophin of abnormal size or amount (Becker dystrophy). The incidence of Duchenne dystrophy is 1 in 3500 male births; one third of the cases result from a new mutation. Duchenne dystrophy manifests as early as age 2 to 3 years as delays in motor milestones and difficulty running. The proximal muscles are the most severely affected, and the course is relentlessly progressive. Patients begin to fall frequently by age 5 to 6, have difficulty climbing stairs by age 8 years, and are usually confined to wheelchairs by age 12. Most patients die of respiratory complications in their 20s. Congestive heart failure and arrhythmias can occur late in the disease. The smooth muscle of the gastrointestinal tract is involved and causes intestinal pseudo-obstruction. The average IQ of boys with Duchenne dystrophy is low, suggesting central nervous system involvement. Becker dystrophy is a milder form of dystrophinopathy and varies in severity depending on the gene lesion. It is less common than the Duchenne form, with an incidence of 5 per 100,000.

Myotonic dystrophy is an autosomal dominant multisystem disorder that affects skeletal, cardiac, and smooth muscle and other organs, including the eyes, the endocrine system, and the brain. This is the most common muscular dystrophy, with an incidence of 13.5 per 100,000 live births. Myotonic dystrophy can occur at any age, with the usual onset of symptoms in the late second or third decade. However, some affected individuals may remain symptom-free their entire life. A severe form with onset in infancy is known as congenital myotonic dystrophy. The severity is generally worse from one generation to the next (anticipation). Typical patients exhibit facial weakness with temporalis muscle wasting, frontal balding, ptosis, and neck flexor weakness. Extremity weakness usually begins distally and progresses slowly to affect the proximal limb-girdle muscles. Percussion myotonia can be elicited on examination in most cases, especially in thenar and wrist extensor muscles.

Associated manifestations include cataracts, testicular atrophy and impotence, intellectual impairment, and hypersomnia associated with both central and obstructive sleep apnea. Respiratory muscle weakness may be severe with impairment of ventilatory drive. Cardiac conduction defects are common and can produce sudden death. Pacemakers may be necessary, and annual electrocardiograms are recommended. Chronic hypoxia can lead to cor pulmonale. The molecular defect of myotonic dystrophy is an abnormal expansion of CTG repeats in the protein kinase gene on chromosome 19q13.2. A second myotonic dystrophy locus has been mapped to chromosome 3q. Clinical features are similar to those of the 19q-linked disorder.

Proximal myotonic myopathy (PROMM) is a autosomal dominant disorder that resembles myotonic dystrophy. However, weakness is proximal and distal muscles are normal: patients usually complain of myotonia and myalgias. Patients with PROMM have less cardiac and other organ involvement, but many PROMM patients

TABLE 130–3 **Major Morphologically Distinct Congenital Myopathies**

Central core
Nemaline
Centronuclear (myotubular)
Congenital fiber type disproportion
Sarcotubular
Reducing body
Myofibrillar

develop cataracts indistinguishable from those in myotonic dystrophy. In some kindreds, PROMM has been localized to the 3q, second myotonic dystrophy locus; in others, the gene locus is unknown.

Congenital Myopathies

Congenital myopathies are defined by their appearance on biopsy (Table 130–3). They are usually present at birth with hypotonia and subsequent delayed motor development. Because most congenital myopathies are relatively nonprogressive, patients are commonly seen as adults and may not be diagnosed until the second or third decade. Clinical findings common in the congenital myopathies are reduced muscle bulk, slender body build, and a long, narrow face with skeletal abnormalities (high-arched palate, pectus excavatum, kyphoscoliosis, dislocated hips, pes cavus), and absent or reduced muscle stretch reflexes. The molecular genetic defects of many congenital myopathies are now known, and these disorders as well as the muscular dystrophies are being reclassified.

Metabolic Myopathies

Metabolic myopathies (Table 130–4) include (1) glucose/glycogen metabolism disorders, (2) lipid metabolism disorders, and (3) mitochondrial disorders.

GLUCOSE/GLYCOGEN METABOLISM DISORDERS

Glucose, and its storage form glycogen, is essential for the short-term, predominantly anaerobic energy requirements of muscle. Disorders of glucose and glycogen metabolism (called glycogenoses) have two distinct syndromes: (1) dynamic symptoms of exercise intolerance, pain, cramps, and myoglobinuria and (2) static symptoms of fixed weakness without exercise intolerance or myoglobinuria. Of the 11 glycogenoses, only glucose-6-phosphate (type I) and liver phosphorylase (type VI) deficiencies spare muscle.

TABLE 130–4 Metabolic and Mitochondrial Myopathies

Glycogen Metabolism Deficiencies

Type II	$\alpha_{1,4}$-Glucosidase (acid maltase)
Type III	Debranching enzyme
Type IV	Branching enzyme
Type V	Phosphorylase* (McArdle's)
Type VII	Phosphofructokinase* (Tarui's)
Type VIII	Phosphorylase B kinase*
Type IX	Phosphoglycerate kinase*
Type X	Phosphoglycerate mutase*
Type XI	Lactate dehydrogenase*

Lipid Metabolism Deficiencies

Carnitine palmitoyl transferase*
Primary systemic/muscle carnitine deficiency
Secondary carnitine deficiency

Mitochondrial Myopathies

Pyruvate dehydrogenase complex deficiencies
Progressive external ophthalmoplegia (PEO)
Kearns-Sayre syndrome
Myoclonic epilepsy and ragged-red fibers (MERRF)
Mitochondrial encephalopathy with lactic acidosis and stroke-like episodes (MELAS)
Mitochondrial neurogastrointestinal encephalomyopathy (MNGIE)
Mitochondrial depletion syndrome
Leigh's syndrome and neuropathy, ataxia, retinitis pigmentosa (NARP)
Succinate dehydrogenase deficiency*

* Deficiency can produce exercise intolerance and myoglobinuria.

Glycogenoses with Exercise Intolerance/Myoglobinuria

Exercise intolerance (see Table 130–4) begins in childhood with exertional muscle pain, cramps, and myoglobinuria appearing in the second or third decade. Many patients note a "second wind" phenomena after a period of brief rest so that they can continue the exercise at the previous level of activity. The muscle cramps are caused by electrically silent contractures. Strength, blood creatine kinase levels, and the EMG between attacks are usually normal early in the disease, but they may become abnormal with advancing age. After episodes of severe myoglobinuria, EMG shows myopathic units and fibrillations. EMG performed during a "cramp" (contracture) shows electrical silence. In the forearm exercise test, the venous lactate level fails to rise in myophosphorylase, phosphofructokinase, and phosphoglycerate kinase deficiencies and rises subnormally in phosphorylase b kinase, phosphoglucomutase, and lactate dehydrogenase deficiencies. Diagnosis is by muscle biopsy study of the enzymes or by definition of specific genetic mutations.

Glycogenoses with Fixed Weakness and No Exercise Intolerance

Glycogenoses with fixed weakness and no exercise intolerance (see Table 130–4) present as a syndrome of progressive proximal weakness. Diagnosis requires muscle biopsy or genetic mutation definition.

DISORDERS OF FATTY ACID METABOLISM

Lipids are essential for the aerobic energy needs of muscle during sustained exercise. Serum long-chain fatty acids are the primary lipid fuel for muscle metabolism. They are transported into the mitochondria as carnitine esters and are metabolized by means of beta oxidation. Carnitine palmitoyl transferase (CPT) I converts cytoplasmic acyl-CoA to acylcarnitine, which is then transported into the mitochondria by carnitine acyl-transferase in exchange for carnitine. CPT II on the inner mitochondrial membrane reconstitutes acyl-CoA. A deficiency of carnitine, CPT, or the enzymes of beta oxidation can lead to impaired muscle lipid metabolism.

As with glycogen pathway defects, the abnormal fatty acid metabolism causes exercise intolerance with myoglobinuria or static weakness with a lipid storage myopathy. In addition, some disorders of lipid metabolism can produce multiorgan metabolic crises with hepatic failure and altered mental status. Most lipid disorders are believed to be autosomal recessive (see Table 130–4).

MITOCHONDRIAL MYOPATHIES

Mitochondrial myopathies (see Table 130–4) produce slowly progressive weakness of proximal limbs or external ocular and other cranial muscles and abnormal fatigability on sustained exertion. Some affect multiple organs or systems, in addition to muscle. In many mitochondrial myopathies some muscle fibers contain abnormal mitochondria. These fibers appear "ragged red" on biopsy stains (trichrome) and may fail to react for cytochrome c oxidase. Serum lactic acid levels are often elevated at rest in mitochondrial myopathy. Mitochondrial diseases are caused by mutations in either nuclear or mitochondrial DNA. During fertilization, all of the mitochondria are contributed by the mother; thus, all mutations of mitochondrial DNA are either maternally transmitted or they arise de novo in the maternal ovum or in early embryonic life. However, because the majority of mitochondrial proteins (95%) are encoded from nuclear genes, mitochondrial disorders can also have autosomal dominant or X-linked heredity. Mitochondrial disorders produce biochemical defects proximal to the respiratory chain (involving substrate transport and utilization) or within the respiratory chain.

Specific Mitochondrial Disorders Affecting Muscle

PROGRESSIVE EXTERNAL OPHTHALMOPLEGIA

Severe ptosis and progressive external ophthalmoplegia (PEO) are clinical hallmarks of mitochondrial disease. Ptosis is often the presenting symptom and is generally first noted in childhood. Both ptosis and PEO (lack of eye movements) are often overlooked by patients and their physicians. Patients usually do not note double vision. Slight proximal weakness may occur. PEO caused by mitochondrial disease is associated with single or multiple mitochondrial DNA deletions. Patients with single mitochondrial deletions have the Kearns-Sayre syndrome, which presents before age 20 and includes a variety of multisystem abnormalities: retinitis pigmentosa, heart block, hearing loss, short stature, ataxia, delayed puberty, peripheral neuropathy, and impaired ventilatory drive. The Kearns-Sayre syndrome is caused by single large mitochondrial deletions; it is sporadic with no family history of the disorder. Patients with PEO who have multiple mitochondrial deletions have an autosomal dominant inheritance pattern.

MYOCLONIC EPILEPSY AND RAGGED RED FIBERS

Patients with myoclonic epilepsy and ragged red fibers (MERRF) have varying symptoms of myoclonus, generalized seizures, ataxia, dementia, sensorineural hearing loss, and optic atrophy, as well as limb-girdle weakness. Some patients also have a peripheral neuropathy, cardiomyopathy, and cutaneous lipomas. Ptosis and PEO are usually not present.

MITOCHONDRIAL ENCEPHALOMYOPATHY WITH LACTIC ACIDOSIS AND STROKE-LIKE EPISODES

Patients with mitochondrial encephalomyopathy with lactic acidosis and stroke-like episodes (MELAS) have normal early development, experience migraine-like headaches and strokes before age 40, and have chronic lactic acidosis. Other features can include dementia, hearing loss, and episodic vomiting, ataxia, and coma, as well as diabetes. Ptosis and PEO are uncommon.

Channelopathies (Nondystrophic Myotonias and Periodic Paralyses)

The myotonias are categorized into dystrophic and nondystrophic disorders. The nondystrophic myotonias and the periodic paralyses are caused by mutations of various ion channels in muscle (Table 130–5). The term *channelopathies* is often used to describe this group of disorders.

CHLORIDE CHANNELOPATHIES

Myotonia congenita is caused by point mutations in the muscle chloride channel gene. There are autosomal dominant and recessive forms that are allelic. The autosomal dominant form, (Thomsen's disease), and the autosomal recessive form (Becker myotonia congenita) are both benign and are associated with muscle hypertrophy and action, percussion, and electrical myotonia. Cold increases the myotonia, and exercise improves it. There is no involvement of the heart or other organs. Thomsen's disease patients are not weak, but Becker myotonia congenita patients have fluctuations in strength and may develop limb-girdle weakness. Many patients do not require treatment, but drugs such as quinine, procainamide, phenytoin, and mexiletine may reduce myotonia.

SODIUM CHANNELOPATHIES

Several autosomal dominant disorders are caused by point mutations in the voltage-dependent sodium channel gene. All have symptoms beginning in the first decade. Paramyotonia congenita has paradoxical myotonia in that myotonia *increases* with exercise. Myotonia is worsened by cold temperature. The myotonia can be treated with sodium channel blockers such as mexiletine.

TABLE 130–5 Channelopathies and Related Disorders

Disorder	Clinical Features	Inheritance	Chromosome	Gene
Chloride channelopathies				
Myotonia congenita				
Thomsen's disease	Myotonia	Autosomal dominant	7q35	CLC-1
Becker disease	Myotonia and weakness	Autosomal recessive	7q35	CLC-1
Sodium channelopathies				
Paramyotonia congenita	Paramyotonia	Autosomal dominant	17q13.1–13.3	SCNA4A
Hyperkalemic periodic paralysis	Periodic paralysis, myotonia, and paramyotonia	Autosomal dominant	17q13.1–13.3	SCNA4A
Calcium channelopathies				
Hypokalemic periodic paralysis	Periodic paralysis	Autosomal dominant	1q31-32	Dihydropyridine receptor
Malignant hyperthermia (some cases)	Anesthetic-induced delayed relaxation	Autosomal dominant	19q13.1	Ryanodine receptor
Rippling muscle disease	Muscle mounding/stiffness	Autosomal dominant	1q41	Unknown
Andersen's syndrome	Periodic paralysis, cardiac arrhythmia, distinctive facies	Autosomal dominant	Unknown	Unknown
Brody's disease	Delayed relaxation, no electromyographic myotonia	Autosomal recessive	16p12	Calcium-ATPase

In hyperkalemic periodic paralysis, attacks of weakness last 1 to 2 hours. Attacks are precipitated by fasting, by rest after exercise, or by ingestion of potassium-rich foods. During attacks, patients are hyporeflexic with normal sensation and there is no ocular or respiratory muscle weakness. The serum potassium level may be normal during the attack, and therefore a more appropriate term may be *potassium-sensitive periodic paralysis*. Episodes of weakness rarely necessitate acute therapy; oral carbohydrates or glucose improve weakness. Treatments to prevent attacks include thiazide diuretics, β-agonists, and a low-potassium, high-carbohydrate diet with avoidance of fasting, strenuous activity, and cold.

CALCIUM CHANNELOPATHIES

Hypokalemic periodic paralysis is an autosomal dominant condition caused by mutations in the muscle calcium channel.

Attacks begin by adolescence and are triggered by exercise, sleep, stress, or meals rich in carbohydrates and sodium. Attacks last from 3 to 24 hours. A vague prodrome of stiffness or heaviness in the legs can occur, and if the patient performs mild exercise, a full-blown attack may be aborted. Ocular, bulbar, and respiratory muscles are rarely involved. Early in the disease patients have normal interattack examinations except for eyelid myotonia (about 50%). Later, attack frequency can lessen, but many patients have proximal weakness. Preventive measures include a low-carbohydrate, low-sodium diet and drugs such as acetazolamide or dichlorphenamide. Acute attacks are treated with oral potassium.

Thyrotoxic periodic paralysis resembles hypokalemic periodic paralysis. It is most common in Asian and Latin American young male adults. β-Adrenergic blocking agents reduce the frequency and severity attacks, but the ultimate treatment is directed against the thyrotoxicosis.

Malignant hyperthermia is characterized by severe muscle rigidity, fever, tachycardia precipitated by depolarizing muscle relaxants, and inhalational anesthetic agents such as halothane. The symptoms usually occur during surgery but can first be noticed in the postoperative period. Patients may have had previous anesthesia without symptoms. During attacks the creatine kinase level is markedly elevated and myoglobinuria develops. The disorder is caused by excessive calcium release by the sarcoplasmic reticulum calcium channel, the ryanodine receptor. Some patients have mutations in the ryanodine receptor gene on chromosome 19q13, which is the same gene mutated in central core disease. The symptoms are treated with dantrolene, and at-risk patients should not be given known provocative anesthetic agents. The occurrence of malignant hyperthermia in one member of a family should prompt consideration as to whether other family members could also be at risk.

OTHER FORMS OF MUSCLE STIFFNESS

Neuroleptic malignant syndrome with muscular rigidity, altered mental status, and hyperthermia is caused by central dopaminergic blockade from neuroleptics. The muscle rigidity can produce myoglobinuria.

The stiff-person syndrome is an acquired autoimmune condition that presents as severe muscle stiffness of proximal, and especially paraspinous, muscles. The muscle spasms produce hyperlordosis, and all movements are slow and laborious. There is excess motor unit activity caused by autoantibodies to glutamic acid decarboxylase, which is a major enzyme in the synthesis of γ-aminobutyric acid, and this results in disinhibition in the central nervous system. Some patients also have antibodies to islet cells and develop diabetes mellitus. Symptomatic treatment consists of diazepam; immunosuppressive treatment can improve the condition.

Inflammatory Myopathies

Inflammatory myopathies are acquired, nonhereditary disorders (Table 130–6) that are characterized by muscle weakness and inflammation on muscle biopsy. Most have elevated creatine kinase levels, myopathic EMG, and a limb-girdle distribution of weakness. Occasionally, inflammatory myopathies have distal, focal, or other selective involvement of particular muscles.

IDIOPATHIC INFLAMMATORY MYOPATHY

The three major categories of idiopathic inflammatory myopathy are dermatomyositis (DM), polymyositis (PM), and inclusion body myositis (IBM) (Table 130–7). PM and DM are both characterized by the onset of symmetric weakness subacutely over weeks or several months. Myalgias can occur, but muscle pain and tenderness are rarely chief complaints. Patients complaining of myalgia who do not have demonstrable weakness are more likely to have polymyalgia rheumatica or fibromyalgia rather

TABLE 130–6 Major Inflammatory Myopathies

Idiopathic
Polymyositis
Dermatomyositis
Inclusion body myositis
Overlap syndromes with other connective tissue disease (e.g., systemic lupus erythematosus)
Sarcoidosis
Inflammatory myopathies with eosinophilia
Eosinophilic polymyositis
Diffuse fasciitis with eosinophilia
Myositis ossificans
Infections
Bacterial (e.g., *Staphylococcus*, *Streptococcus*, gas gangrene (*Clostridium welchii*)
Viral: acute myositis after influenza or other viral infections; retrovirus-related myopathies (HIV, HTLV-I)
Parasitic: toxoplasmosis, trypanosomiasis, cysticercosis, trichinosis
Fungal

TABLE 130–7 Idiopathic Inflammatory Myopathies: Clinical and Laboratory Features

Myopathy	Sex	Typical Age at Onset	Pattern of Weakness	Creatine Kinase	Muscle Biopsy	Response to Immunosuppressive Therapy
Dermatomyositis	F > M	Childhood and adult	Proximal > distal	Increased (up to 50× normal)	Perifascicular atrophy, MAC, immunoglobulin, complement deposition on vessels	Yes
Polymyositis	F > M	Adult	Proximal > distal	Increased (up to 50× normal)	Endomysial inflammation	Yes
Inclusion body myositis	M > F	Elderly (>50 yr)	Proximal and distal; predilection for finger/wrist flexors, knee extensors	Increased (<10× normal)	Endomysial inflammation, rimmed vacuoles; amyloid deposits; electron microscopy: 15–18 nm tubulofilaments	No

MAC = membrane attack complex.

than PM. Esophageal muscles are affected in up to 30% of both PM and DM leading to dysphagia.

The rash of dermatomyositis may accompany or precede the onset of muscle weakness: a heliotrope rash (purplish discoloration of the eyelids often associated with periorbital edema); Gotron's sign (papular, erythematous, scaly lesions over the knuckles); a macular erythematous, sun-sensitive rash on the face, neck, and anterior chest, shoulders, upper back, elbows and knees; and periungual erythema caused by dilated capillary loops with thrombi or hemorrhage.

IBM presents as an insidious onset of slowly progressive proximal and distal weakness typically after age 50. It is the most common inflammatory myopathy in the elderly. These patients have a distinctive pattern of muscle involvement with early weakness and atrophy of the quadriceps (knee extensors), volar forearm muscles (wrist and finger flexors), and tibialis anterior (ankle dorsiflexors).

Cardiac involvement, resulting in congestive heart failure and conduction defects, and interstitial lung disease, can develop in a minority of patients with PM and DM. Vasculitis of the gastrointestinal tract, kidneys, lungs, and eyes can complicate DM (but not PM), particularly in children. There is an increased incidence of malignancy in older adults with DM.

The EMG in DM, PM, and IBM demonstrates brief myopathic motor units, increased recruitment, and fibrillation potentials. The serum creatine kinase level is usually increased. The erythrocyte sedimentation rate is normal in most patients. An elevated erythrocyte sedimentation rate suggests a different or coincidental disease. A muscle biopsy should be performed in all patients with suggested inflammatory myopathy to establish the diagnosis (see Table 130–7).

Histologic features and immunologic studies suggest that DM is a humorally mediated microangiopathy. The microangiopathy leads to ischemic damage of muscle fibers. PM is likely to be a cell-mediated disorder. The cause of IBM is unknown.

Immunotherapy can improve strength and function in DM and PM. In contrast, IBM is usually refractory to immunosuppressive therapy. The first line of therapy for DM and PM patients is the corticosteroid prednisone, which reduces morbidity and improves muscle strength and function.

INFECTIOUS MYOSITIS

An acute viral myositis can occur in the setting of an influenza viral upper respiratory tract infection. In addition to typical influenza-associated myalgias, these patients develop proximal weakness, elevated creatine kinase levels, and a myopathic EMG. The disorder is self-limited, but when severe it is often associated with myoglobinuria and occasionally with renal failure. A similar syndrome can complicate infections with other viruses.

An inflammatory myopathy can occur in the setting of human immunodeficiency virus infection, either in early or later acquired immunodeficiency syndrome. The clinical presentation is similar to that of patients with PM. Patients may improve with corticosteroid therapy.

The disorder must be distinguished from the toxic myopathy caused by zidovudine, which responds to dose reduction.

Myopathies Caused by Endocrine and Systemic Disorders

Excess corticosteroids can result from endogenous Cushing's disease or can be caused by exogenous glucocorticoid administration. Iatrogenic corticosteroid myopathy (or atrophy) is the most common endocrine-related myopathy. However, muscle weakness is rarely the presenting manifestation of Cushing's disease, and in virtually all instances of corticosteroid myopathy other factors contributing to weakness are also present. Therapy consists of reducing the corticosteroid dosage to the lowest possible level. Exercise and adequate nutrition prevent and may improve weakness.

Patients with hyperthyroidism often have some degree of proximal weakness, but this is rarely the presenting manifestation of thyrotoxicosis. Hypothyroid myopathy is associated with proximal weakness and myalgias, muscle enlargement, slow relaxation of the reflexes, and marked (up to 100-fold) increase of the serum creatine kinase (CK) level.

Progressive, painless proximal weakness in a diabetic patient is seldom the result of diabetic-related myopathy. Asymmetric, usually painful proximal leg weakness can occur from an ischemic radiculoplexopathy. In rare cases, acute muscle infarction can develop in quadriceps or hamstring muscles. These patients complain of severe pain, tenderness, and swelling. Magnetic resonance imaging of the thigh shows changes consistent with a muscle infarct. The syndrome resolves spontaneously over weeks.

Toxic Myopathies

Many drugs have been associated with muscle damage; common ones are listed in Table 130–8. Most can produce proximal weakness, elevated CK, myopathic EMGs, and abnormalities on muscle biopsy. Symptoms generally improve on stopping the medication. Some

TABLE 130–8 Toxic Myopathies

Inflammatory: cimetidine, D-penicillamine
Noninflammatory necrotizing or vacuolar: cholesterol-lowering agents, chloroquine, colchicine
Acute muscle necrosis and myoglobinuria: cholesterol-lowering drugs, alcohol, cocaine
Malignant hyperthermia: halothane, ethylene, others; succinylcholine
Mitochondrial: zidovudine
Myosin loss: nondepolarizing neuromuscular blocking agents; glucocorticoids

drugs can produce acute, rapidly progressive muscle destruction and myoglobinuria, particularly the hypocholesterolemic drugs clofibrate, gemfibrozil, lovastatin, simvastatin, pravastatin, and niacin. An acute necrotizing myopathy associated with myoglobinuria occurs in chronic alcoholics after heavy drinking. Hypokalemia caused by sweating, vomiting, diarrhea, and renal wastage may be causative.

Also known as critical illness myopathy, acute quadriplegic myopathy develops in a patient in the intensive care setting and is often discovered when a patient is unable to be weaned off a ventilator. The cause of the diffuse weakness is the prolonged daily use of either (often both) high-dose intravenous glucocorticoids (usually methylprednisolone) or nondepolarizing neuromuscular blocking agents (e.g., vecuronium). Patients often have had sepsis and multiorgan failure. The diagnosis can be confirmed on muscle biopsy, which shows the loss of myosin thick filaments on electron microscopy. Treatment is supportive after discontinuing the offending agents. Strength recovers over a period of weeks or months; patients can usually be weaned off the ventilator.

Myoglobinuria

Acute muscle destruction can produce a brown discoloration of urine by myoglobin. Myoglobin, a 17,000-molecular-weight protein that contains the heme moiety, is present in muscle at a concentration of 1 g/kg. The visible discoloration of urine by myoglobin indicates both massive and acute muscle destruction and warns of impending renal damage. The pigment has to be distinguished from hemoglobin. If there is no hematuria, a positive benzidine test strongly suggests myoglobinuria.

Muscle pain, swelling, and weakness precede overt myoglobinuria by a few hours. In addition to myoglobin, phosphate, potassium, creatine, and muscle enzymes are released into the circulation. Serum CK levels can be over 1000 times normal. The heme pigment in the glomerular filtrate and casts in the tubules cause proteinuria, hematuria, and tubular necrosis. Renal failure is more likely if hypotension, acidosis, and hypovolemia coexist. With increasing renal insufficiency, hyperphosphatemia, hypocalcemia, tetany, and life-threatening hyperkalemia appear. Death may result from renal or respiratory failure.

Myoglobinuria is caused by massive ischemia of muscle from any cause, crush injuries, prolonged pressure, or persistent contraction and rigidity (such as from status epilepticus, malignant hyperthermia, neuroleptic malignant syndrome). Infectious causes include viral and bacterial infections. The acute episode is treated by rest, maintenance of adequate urine flow by hydration and diuretics, and alkalinization of the urine with sodium bicarbonate. Other measures consist of treatment of the renal insufficiency as required and removal of the offending cause if possible.

REFERENCES

Amato AA, Barohn RJ: Idiopathic inflammatory myopathies. Neurol Clin 1997; 15:615–648.

Barohn RJ: Diseases of muscle (myopathies). *In* Goldman L, Bennett JC (eds): Cecil Textbook of Medicine, 21st ed. Philadelphia, WB Saunders, 2000, pp 2201–2221.

Griggs RC, Mendell J, Miller R: Evaluation and Treatment of Myopathies. Philadelphia, FA Davis, 1995.

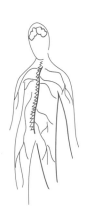

131

NEUROMUSCULAR JUNCTION DISEASE

Robert C. Griggs

Disorders of the neuromuscular junction interfere with the transmission of electrical impulses from peripheral nerve to muscle. They can be acquired or inherited and are associated with weakness and fatigability on exertion (Table 131–1). In each disorder the safety margin of neuromuscular transmission is compromised by one or more specific defects: acetylcholine (ACh) synthesis or packaging of ACh quanta into synaptic vesicles; the release of ACh quanta from the nerve terminal by nerve impulse; and the efficiency of the released ACh quanta to generate a postsynaptic depolarization.

Myasthenia Gravis

Myasthenia gravis (MG) is an acquired autoimmune disorder. Pathogenic autoantibodies induce acetylcholine receptor (AChR) deficiency at the motor end plate. Circulating AChR antibodies are present in 80% to 90% of cases, and IgG and complement components are deposited on the postsynaptic membrane. AChR deficiency results from lysis of the junctional folds and destruction of AChRs cross-linked by antibodies that block the binding of ACh to AchR. The incidence is 2 to 5 per year per million and the prevalence 13 to 64 per million. The female-to-male ratio is 6:4. The disease may present at any age, but the incidence in women peaks in the third decade and in men in the sixth or seventh decade.

CLINICAL FEATURES

MG can involve either the external ocular muscles selectively (ocular MG) or the general voluntary muscle system (generalized MG). The symptoms may fluctuate from hour to hour, from day to day, or over longer periods. They are provoked or worsened by exertion, exposure to extremes of temperature, viral or other infections, menses, and excitement. Ocular muscle in-

volvement is usually bilateral, asymmetric, and typically associated with ptosis and diplopia. Weakness of other muscles innervated by cranial nerves results in loss of facial expression, a smile that resembles a snarl, jaw drop, nasal regurgitation of liquids, choking on foods and secretions, and slurred, nasal speech. Abnormal fatigability of the limb muscles causes difficulty in combing the hair, lifting objects repeatedly, climbing stairs, walking, and running. On examination, fatigue is most reliably demonstrated in the eyes: the *curtain sign* of worsening ptosis with upgaze or asymmetric nystagmus on extremes of lateral and medial gaze. Proximal limb muscles are affected more than distal ones, but in advanced cases weakness is widespread. Initially, the symptoms are ocular in 40%, are generalized in 40%, involve only the extremities in 10%, and involve only the bulbar or bulbar and eye muscles in another 10%. Ocular muscles are affected in nearly all patients after a year of disease. The symptoms remain ocular in only 15%. When the disease becomes generalized, usually it does so within the first year of onset. Two thirds of patients with MG have thymic hyperplasia and 10% to 15% have thymoma. In about 10% the MG is associated with another autoimmune disease. Circulating AChR antibodies can be detected in most infants born to myasthenic mothers, but only 12% of such children develop MG, usually during the first few hours of life. The disease is caused by the transfer of AChR antibodies.

DIAGNOSIS

Anticholinesterase Tests. Edrophonium given intravenously acts within a few seconds and lasts for a few minutes. Two milligrams of the drug is injected intravenously over 15 seconds. If no response occurs in 30 to 45 seconds, an additional 8 mg is injected. The evaluation of the response requires objective assessment of one or more signs not easily influenced by motivation, such as degree of ptosis and range of ocular movements. Possible cholinergic side effects of the drug include fas-

TABLE 131–1 Disorders of the Neuromuscular Junction

Autoimmune

Myasthenia gravis
  Lambert-Eaton myasthenic syndrome

Congenital

Presynaptic defects in ACh resynthesis, packaging, or release
Synaptic defect: congenital end-plate AChE deficiency
Postsynaptic defects: slow-channel syndromes
Postsynaptic defects: decreased response to ACh
  Low-affinity fast channel syndromes
  Mode-switching kinetics of AChR
  AChR deficiency without kinetic abnormality
Familial limb girdle myasthenia

Toxic

Botulism
Drug-induced
Organophosphate intoxication

ACh = acetylcholine; AChE = acetylcholinesterase; AChR = acetylcholine receptor.

ciculations, flushing, lacrimation, abdominal cramps, nausea, vomiting, and diarrhea. The drug must be given cautiously to patients with cardiac disease, because it may cause sinus bradycardia, atrioventricular block, and, rarely, cardiac arrest.

Electromyography. Supramaximal stimulation of a motor nerve at 2 or 3 Hz results in a 10% or greater decrement of the amplitude of the evoked compound muscle action potential from the first to the fifth response. The test is positive in most patients with generalized MG, provided that two or more distal and two or more proximal muscles are examined.

Blood Tests. The AChR antibody test measures the binding of antibody to AChR labeled with radioactive α-bungarotoxin. The antibody binding test is positive in nearly all adults with moderately severe or severe MG, in 80% with mild generalized MG, and in 50% with ocular MG. Striated muscle antibodies also occur in MG patients. Their role is unknown, but they are often associated with thymoma.

TREATMENT

Anticholinesterases, thymectomy, alternate-day prednisone, azathioprine, cyclosporine, plasmapheresis, and intravenous immunoglobulin are used to treat MG. Anticholinesterases are useful in all forms of the disease. Pyridostigmine bromide (60-mg tablets) acts for 3 to 4 hours, and neostigmine bromide, 15 mg, acts for 2 to 3 hours. Pyridostigmine bromide has fewer muscarinic side effects and is therefore more widely used. One-half to four tablets are given every 4 hours in the daytime. This medication is also available in 180-mg "time-span" tablets for use at bedtime and as a syrup for children and patients requiring nasogastric feeding. In critically ill patients or postoperatively, intramuscularly injectable pyridostigmine bromide (the dose is one 30th of the

oral dose) and neostigmine methylsulfate (the dose is one 15th of the oral dose) can be used. Patients who have increased difficulty with respiration, feeding, or handling secretions and who are not responding to relatively high doses of anticholinesterases are best treated by drug withdrawal, tracheal intubation, and ventilator support.

In patients with generalized disease not responding adequately to anticholinesterases, other forms of therapy must be used. Thymectomy increases the remission rate and improves the clinical course of MG. Although controlled clinical studies of thymectomy have not been done, there is general agreement that the best response occurs in young women with hyperplastic thymus glands and high antibody titers. Thymoma is an indication for thymectomy because the tumor is often locally invasive. Alternate-day prednisone treatment induces remission or improves the disease in more than half the patients. Azathioprine in doses of 2 to 3 mg/kg/day also induces remissions or improvement in more than half of patients treated. The time required for improvement is 12 to 15 months. Surveillance for side effects (pancytopenia, leukopenia, and hepatocellular injury) must be maintained during therapy. Azathioprine as an adjunct to alternate-day prednisone reduces the maintenance dose of prednisone and is associated with fewer side effects. Cyclosporine and other immunosuppressants are sometimes justified. Plasmapheresis is helpful in patients with sudden worsening of MG and is indicated in severe generalized MG refractory to other forms of treatment. Three to five daily exchanges of 2 L of plasma result in objective improvement and lower the AChR antibody titer in a few days. Plasmapheresis is very expensive and not usually suitable for long-term treatment. Intravenous immunoglobulin, 2 g/kg divided over 2 to 5 days, may improve severe MG with 2 to 3 weeks of therapy. The mean duration of the response is 9 weeks in patients also treated with corticosteroids and 5 weeks in those who are not.

Lambert-Eaton Myasthenic Syndrome

Lambert-Eaton myasthenic syndrome is an acquired autoimmune disease in which pathogenic autoantibodies cause a deficiency of voltage-sensitive calcium channels at the motor nerve terminal. Among patients older than age 40 years, 70% of men and 30% of women have an associated carcinoma, usually a small cell carcinoma of the lung. Lambert-Eaton myasthenic syndrome may predate tumor detection by up to 3 years. Non-neoplastic Lambert-Eaton myasthenic syndrome has an association with other autoimmune disorders, HLA-B8 and Drw3 antigens, and organ-specific autoantibodies. Patients have weakness and fatigability of proximal limb and trunk muscles with relative sparing of extraocular and bulbar muscles. The lower limbs are more severely involved than the upper ones. On maximal voluntary contraction the force produced by a weak muscle increases for a few seconds and then again decreases. Tendon reflexes are usually hypoactive or absent. Autonomic manifestations (dry mouth, impotence, decreased sweating, orthostatic hypotension, or altered pupillary reflexes) occur in 50% of patients. On electromyography, the amplitude of the compound muscle action potential evoked by a single nerve stimulus from rested muscle is abnormally small. Repetitive stimulation at 2 Hz induces a further decrement, but stimulation at frequencies higher than 10 Hz or voluntary exercise for a brief period facilitates the response to normal amplitude. Treatment strategies include corticosteroids, azathioprine, and intravenous immune globulin. 3,4-Diaminopyridine is helpful but is not widely available in the United States; it can cause seizures and other side effects.

Drug-Induced Myasthenic Syndromes

Polymyxin and aminoglycoside antibiotics, antiarrhythmic agents (procainamide, quinidine), β-adrenergic blockers (propranolol, timolol), phenothiazines, lithium, trimethaphan, methoxyflurane, and magnesium given parenterally or in cathartics reduce the safety margin of neuromuscular transmission. However, overt myasthenic symptoms do not usually appear unless an overdose of the drug is administered or the renal or hepatic elimination of the drug is impaired. The drugs may worsen MG or Lambert-Eaton myasthenic syndrome.

Succinylcholine, a depolarizing blocking drug, is used to induce muscle relaxation during anesthesia. A single dose of the drug sufficient to cause transient apnea is eliminated by plasma pseudocholinesterase in 10 to 20 minutes. In approximately 1 in 2500 patients receiving the drug, prolonged apnea occurs and persists up to several hours. Most of these patients have an autosomal recessive abnormality of the plasma pseudocholinesterase. Curare and related agents used during surgery and in critically ill patients to induce muscle relaxation produce depolarizing blockade of the neuromuscular junction. Their use in patients with MG and other myasthenias is associated with profound and prolonged weakness.

Organophosphate Intoxication

Organophosphate insecticides irreversibly inhibit cholinesterases. Ingestion is associated with alterations in sensorium, convulsions, coma, severe muscarinic side effects, cramps, fasciculations, and muscle weakness from a depolarization block.

REFERENCES

Engel AG: Acquired autoimmune myasthenia gravis. *In* Engel AG, Franzini-Armstrong C (eds): Myology, 2nd ed. New York: McGraw-Hill, 1994, pp 1769–1797.

Engel AG: Myasthenic syndromes. *In* Engel AG, Franzini-Armstrong C (eds): Myology, 2nd ed. New York: McGraw-Hill, 1994, pp 1798–1835.

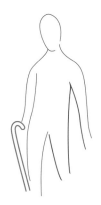

SECTION XVII

The Aging Patient

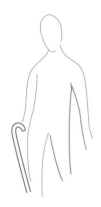

132

THE BIOLOGY OF AGING

David A. Lipschitz • Robert J. Reis
Dennis H. Sullivan

A precise definition of *normal physiologic aging* remains elusive. Although probably regulated by intrinsic cellular mechanisms, the process of aging is modulated by numerous environmental influences. Because the lifetime experiences of each person are unique and the combined effects of all environmental stimuli are impossible to calculate, differentiating whether a measured alteration noted in older persons represents an inevitable consequence of the aging process or a potentially preventable disease is frequently different. This issue has significant clinical implications. It would be important to know, for example, how much of the physiologic decline seen with advancing age could be prevented by using reasonable prophylactic measures.

The response of the whole organism to the aging process varies by organ system (Fig. 132–1 and Table 132–1). Certain organs, such as the kidneys, lungs, and immune system, develop age-related declines in basal physiologic function. Many other organs, such as the heart, bone marrow, and liver, maintain a level of basal physiologic function comparable to that of younger persons. However, the process of aging in most organ systems is characterized by a reduction in reserve capacity manifested by a blunted and more variable response to increased stimulation. This diminished reserve capacity renders older persons less able to maintain homeostasis when they are subjected to physiologic stress. As a consequence of these age-related changes, elderly persons are more susceptible to disease and are slower to recover from an injury or disease complication than are younger persons. For example, in comparison with younger persons, the elderly are more susceptible to and are less able to survive many infectious diseases because of an age-associated decline in host defense mechanisms, particularly cell-mediated immunity. The same alterations in immune function are also thought to contribute to the higher incidence of cancer seen in elderly persons.

Theories of Aging

Although the intrinsic cellular mechanisms that cause aging have yet to be identified with certainty, certain theories have been proposed, and they may be grouped into two broad categories, featuring programmed versus stochastic mechanisms.

PROGRAMMED AGING

The concept that aging may follow a genetic program, much like development, has failed thus far to explain the absence of extreme-longevity variants in most species, which would be expected to arise from disruption of such a program. The nematode *Caenorhabditis elegans* has emerged as a notable exception. Certain temperature-sensitive mutations to genes within a developmental-arrest pathway also greatly increase the longevity (by two- to fourfold) of adults that had matured at lower, permissive temperatures. This "dauer" pathway, which shows remarkable structural and functional homology to the insulin–insulin-like growth factor receptor pathway of mammals, also affects lipid (and other) metabolism, and fertility. The longevity extension arising from certain dauer-constitutive mutations may thus also support other, nonprogrammatic theories of aging (see later).

Data on telomere shortening as a function of cell proliferation thrust *telomere attrition* into the spotlight as a possible mechanism for *programmed aging*. Proliferation of diploid, untransformed mammalian cells in culture is normally limited to a fixed number of divisions characteristic of the species, cell type, and (perhaps) donor age. As a function of accrued cell divisions in such diploid cells, either in vitro or in vivo, the ends of chromosomes—comprising short-repeat DNA arrays called *telomeres*—become progressively shorter. Al-

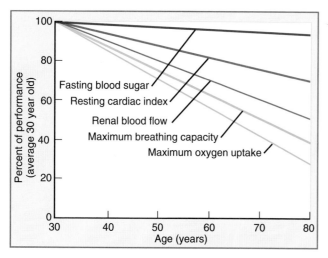

FIGURE 132–1 Percentage of decline, between the ages of 30 and 80 years, in certain physiologic functions.

though other factors are involved, it appears that this limitation in several human cell strains can be obviated by transgenic overproduction of the telomerase reverse transcriptase protein, part of the ribonucleoprotein (*telomerase*) responsible for extension of telomere ends. Moreover, inhibition of the RNA component of telomerase can terminate the otherwise unlimited proliferation of transformed, "immortal" cell lines. Although these observations are of great interest and potential utility in developing new cancer therapies and means of tissue replacement, their relevance to in vivo aging is less clear, because predominantly postmitotic animals (such as insect and nematode adults) undergo senescence, and even species such as mammals, composed of many tissues that retain proliferative capacity, do not generally exhaust that capacity during the course of normal aging.

STOCHASTIC ERROR ACCUMULATION

Aging could be a consequence of random genetic or epigenetic errors that accrue over time and result in impaired protein synthesis and a deterioration of cellular function. One member of this family of theories, *error catastrophe,* postulates that such errors occurring in the enzymes (or their genes) that govern DNA, RNA, or protein synthesis, could engender positive feedback loops leading to exponential increases in errors. This specific prediction has been found to be invalid in several animal model systems undergoing normal aging.

Free radical damage is another, more likely source of stochastic errors in which metabolic by-products of oxidative metabolism result in irreversible cellular damage. Cells normally generate free radicals such as peroxide, superoxide, and hydroxyl radicals, roughly in proportion to metabolic rate. Aging in certain animal species is characterized by a progressive decline in the levels of antioxidant defenses that are responsible for inactivating these metabolites. Although dietary supplementation with exogenous antioxidants has been widely unsuccess-

ful in delaying the declines of senescence, *caloric restriction*—typically by 25% to 35% of free intake, while maintaining nutritional sufficiency—is the one intervention that reliably extends lifespan in a wide variety of taxa, including nematodes, insects, and mammals. Although no direct evidence shows that this strategy is effective in humans, early (premortality) indices of aging are significantly retarded in calorically restricted rhesus monkeys. The most likely mechanism for caloric regulation of longevity is through attenuation of metabolic rate and hence of generation of free radicals. The accompanying reduction in core body temperature, and possible compromise of peak metabolic output, could have adverse consequences in less benign environments than the laboratory setting.

A more explicit tradeoff between longevity and reproduction, termed *antagonistic pleiotropy,* has been suggested as a rationale for the evolution of senescence and has received some support from experimental data on relatively short-lived, high-fecundity animals. In contrast, species that have attenuated fertility for other reasons (e.g., limited prey or other resources) and either have

TABLE 132–1

Organ System	Age-Related Decline in Function
Special senses	Presbyopia
	Lens opacification
	Decreased hearing
	Decreased taste, smell
Cardiovascular	Impaired intrinsic contractile function
	Decreased conductivity
	Decreased ventricular filling
	Increased systolic blood pressure
	Impaired baroreceptor function
Respiratory	Decreased lung elasticity
	Decreased maximal breathing capacity
	Decreased mucus clearance
	Decreased arterial P_{O_2}
	Impaired chemoreceptor regulation of respiration
	Increased risk of secondary infection
Immune	Decreased cell-mediated immunity
	Decreased T-cell number
	Increased T-suppressor cells
	Decreased T-helper cells
	Loss of memory cells
	Decline in antibody titers to known antigens
	Increased autoimmunity
Endocrine	Decreased hormonal responses to stimulation
	Impaired glucose tolerance
	Decreased androgens and estrogens
	Impaired norepinephrine responses
Autonomic nervous	Impaired response to fluid deprivation
	Decline in baroreceptor reflex
	Increased susceptibility to hypothermia
	Impaired gastrointestinal motility

prolonged fertile periods or care for their young may have undergone selection for increased lifespan. Possibly, longevity, a variable advantage in varying environments, may not be strictly fixed by evolution, but instead it may be allowed to change in response to levels of environmental stress, predation, and food availability.

Demographics of Aging and Implications for Health Care

As has been the case since 1900, the population of the United States is continuing to grow older. Between 1900 and 1980, the proportion of the population over the age of 65 grew from 4% to approximately 12%. By the year 2030, when most of the postwar baby boom generation will be over the age of 65, the elderly will constitute more than 20% of the population. The largest percentage of increase will occur in people over the age of 85 (Fig. 132–2). This phenomenal aging of society is the consequence of improved life expectancy and a gradually falling birth rate. Because of differences in life expectancy, by the age of 75 there are twice as many women as men.

Advancing age is associated with a higher prevalence of both acute and chronic disease and an increasing risk of becoming functionally dependent. Roughly 5.3% of adults between the ages of 65 and 75 require assistance with *basic activities of daily living* (bathing, dressing, walking, use of the toilet, and transferring from bed to chair). Slightly fewer than 6% require assistance with *instrumental activities of daily living* (cooking, shopping, use of the telephone, household chores, and handling household financial matters). By the age of 85, these numbers increase dramatically to 35% and 40%, respectively (Fig. 132–3). Functional dependence greatly increases the need for both acute and chronic health care and amplifies the risk of institutionalization.

The dramatic growth in the proportion of the United States population that is elderly has important economic

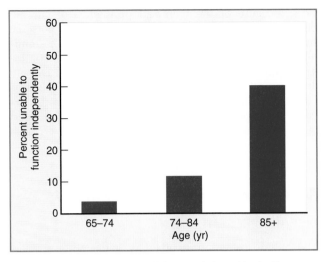

FIGURE 132–3 Percentage of the population with significant disabilities resulting in functional dependence and the need for assistance with activities of daily living.

consequences for the health care system and for the nation. Because of the increasing need for health care with advancing age, elderly persons are heavy consumers of health care resources. Although they represent only 12% of the population, the elderly account for 33% of all hospital admissions, 44% of all hospital days, and most visits to physicians. Approximately 36% of all health care dollars are spent on elderly patients. Many of these expenditures are incurred in the last year of life. Hospitalization accounts for 40% of older persons' health care costs, with visits to physicians and nursing home care each contributing 20%. In the United States, Medicare is the major provider of health care for the elderly ($70 billion), with Medicaid contributing $20 billion and third-party payers $10 billion.

Although high-technology acute care is readily available to most older persons, gross deficiencies exist in the delivery of primary and preventive care. A particular need exists for in-home care and for social support ser-

FIGURE 132–2 *A,* The absolute increase in the number of persons between the ages of 65 and 74 years and older than 75 years between 1910 and the current time. The projected increase to the year 2030 is also shown. *B,* The percentage of the population over age 65 years has significantly increased from 6% of the total population in 1940 to 11% at present. By the year 2030, it is projected that 16% of the population will be over the age of 65 years. Thus, the increase in older persons is not merely a reflection of an overall rise in the total population.

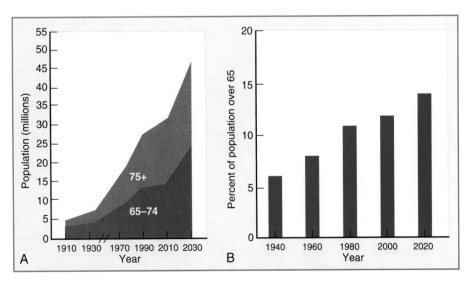

vices. Because of the increased prevalence of chronic disease and functional disability among elderly persons, such specialized supportive services are needed to minimize the risk of nursing home placement. The continued rapid increase in the older population with chronic diseases and functional dependence will contribute significantly to the current health care crisis and will certainly affect priorities and the way medicine is practiced in the near future.

Assessment of the Older Patient

DISEASE PRESENTATION

The elderly patient presenting for a diagnostic evaluation must be assessed carefully. Clinical signs and symptoms of disease in older patients are often blunted, absent, or atypical. A good example is *thyrotoxicosis.* Compared with younger patients, who typically present with a variety of classic signs and symptoms such as nervousness, weight loss, tremor, and tachycardia, elderly patients are more likely to present with cognitive dysfunction, anorexia, muscle weakness, atrial fibrillation, or congestive heart failure. Even a carefully obtained history may fail to elicit expected diagnostic clues. The older patient may not report chest pain with an acute myocardial infarction, dysuria with a urinary tract infection, or cough and shortness of breath with pneumonia. Often, only subtle and nonspecific signs and symptoms, such as a change in mental status, increased lethargy, a diminished appetite, or an increased frequency of falls, suggest that an underlying acute illness is present. Although psychiatric symptoms such as depressed mood, personality change, or inattentiveness may indicate the presence of infection, congestive heart failure, or a metabolic disorder, a true psychiatric problem such as depression may manifest with constitutional symptoms such as headache, weakness, and dizziness.

Medications often add to the diagnostic confusion. The side effects of drugs can either mimic or blunt the symptoms of acute illness. Difficulties in identifying the cause of an elderly patient's clinical deterioration can even result when the symptoms of a chronic disease mask those of a new illness. The diagnosis of acute septic arthritis may be delayed, when, for example, the patient has a history of chronic recurrent painful arthritis in the same joint. Potentially life-threatening diseases in the elderly can also present with initial manifestations that pose a diagnostic challenge for the clinician. For example, it is not uncommon for older patients with pneumonia, urosepsis, or an intra-abdominal catastrophe to present with few identifying physical signs, a blunted or absent fever response, and a white blood cell count that is mildly elevated, in the normal range, or even low. A paradoxical fall in body temperature is usually a poor prognostic sign. The likelihood that disease will manifest atypically is increased in elderly patients who are cognitively impaired, malnourished, debilitated, or suffering from multiple chronic medical conditions. For this reason, these patients often present the greatest diagnostic challenge.

ASSESSMENT OF REHABILITATION

The sequelae of disease may be particularly devastating in older persons. Even a relatively minor illness can cause a significant deterioration in the elderly patient's cognitive or physical functioning. Furthermore, compared with that in younger patients, recovery in elderly persons is likely to be slower, requiring longer and more intensive periods of recuperation and rehabilitation if return to the premorbid state is to be achieved. Loss of functional independence from either physical or cognitive disability places the elderly patient at high risk of institutionalization. For these reasons, an assessment that includes an evaluation of functional and cognitive status and the development of a treatment plan that attempts to restore independence must be included in any medical evaluation of the elderly patient. In addition, selected patients require an in-depth assessment of their social support structure (family, friends, relatives), economic status, and home environment, to determine what resources would be required to allow the patient to return to or remain at home safely. Such comprehensive assessments of the patient represent the cornerstone of geriatric care. These assessments require a *comprehensive interdisciplinary evaluation* that includes input from physicians, nurses, social workers, physical and occupational therapists, pharmacists, and, depending on the patient's needs, many other health care professionals (Fig. 132–4). In collaboration with the various team members, a treatment plan must be developed that includes optimal medical management, minimal medication use, and, as needed, a long-term strategy for physical, cognitive, or nutritional rehabilitation (Table 132–2). For elderly patients who are assessed to have a reasonable potential for rehabilitation, numerous studies have shown that such a comprehensive strategy of evaluation and care is cost effective, improves functional status, and allows many patients to return to or remain in their own homes.

Common and Often Inadequately Assessed Medical Problems of the Elderly

POLYPHARMACY

The elderly are at high risk of developing *medication-related problems.* One reason is that elderly persons tend to take multiple pharmaceutical agents. The average patient over the age of 70 takes 4.5 prescription and 3.5 over-the-counter medications. The risk of both adverse drug reactions and poor compliance increases in relation to the number of medications taken. The probability of having an adverse drug reaction, for example, increases from 2% for patients taking two or fewer medications to more than 13% for patients taking six or more. The often prohibitive cost of medications and the complexity of some treatment regimens contribute to poor compliance. The problem is compounded by the finding that elderly patients frequently see multiple physicians who are often unaware of medications prescribed

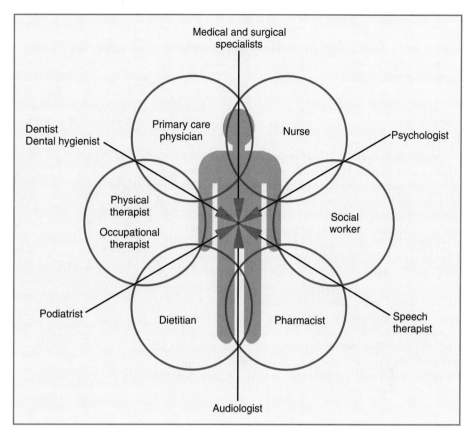

FIGURE 132-4 A diagrammatic illustration of health care professionals involved in the complex interdisciplinary assessment of frail elderly patients. The core health care team that should optimally evaluate every patient is shown *in the circles.* Consultative members of the team *(outside the circles)* contribute as needed. In many circumstances, a consultant such as a dentist, psychologist, or medical subspecialist may be critically important in the development of a treatment and disposition plan.

TABLE 132-2   Principles of Comprehensive Geriatric Assessment

1. Identify treatable medical conditions
2. Screen for depression and memory loss
3. Minimize drug use
4. Avoid restraints if possible, both chemical and physical
   a. Discuss options with family or caregivers
   b. Consider nonrestraining alternatives
5. Assess functional status
   a. Activities of daily living (bathing, dressing)
   b. Instrumental activities of daily living (shopping)
6. Set rehabilitation goals
   a. Assess rehabilitation potential with consideration of the following:
      Medical prognosis
      Cause and duration of functional debilitation
      The patient's and family's expectations or desires
   b. Develop rehabilitation program tailored to patient's needs
7. Develop a disposition plan
   a. Assess patient's ability to return to work or remain at home. Include assessment of the following:
      Family and informal community support networks
      Financial resources and availability of private community services
      Eligibility for sponsored programs or support services
   b. Evaluate need for short- or long-term placement in an institution
      Geriatric rehabilitation center
      Nursing home

by others. This lack of awareness leads to problems of overprescribing, duplicate prescriptions, and adverse drug-drug interactions.

In addition, medication-related problems often occur in elderly persons owing to age-related alterations in both pharmacokinetics and pharmacodynamics. In comparison with younger patients, elderly persons take longer to clear many medications from their systems. They also are more likely to show toxic manifestations of a drug even when the serum level is within a range considered normal for younger patients. If prescribed dosages of certain medications are not reduced appropriately, older patients can quickly develop a toxic reaction. Using drugs properly, avoiding unnecessary medications, and ensuring that medications do not aggravate existing disease are particularly important in the older patient.

FALLS AND DECREASED MOBILITY

Difficulties with walking, gait, and balance occur frequently among older persons. As a consequence, approximately 30% of people over the age of 70 fall once or more annually. This problem results in a high incidence of hip fracture and other injuries that confine patients to their beds and increase the risks of developing other medical complications, such as dehydration, pneumonia, urinary retention, and infections. Usually, the cause of falls is multifactorial and includes visual impairment, neurologic or vestibular disease, postural hypotension, decreased muscle mass, joint disease, and various foot disorders. Falls often occur at night, are more common in patients with dementia, and are increased in frequency by medication use. Reports have suggested that rehabilitation and strength training can improve muscle mass, balance, and gait and can decrease the risk of falls.

DELIRIUM

Delirium is an acute confusional state that is commonly observed in hospitalized older persons. The diagnosis, which must be made clinically, should be suspected in any older person who has confusion of recent onset and accompanied by a fluctuating level of consciousness. A decreased ability to maintain attention, daytime sleepiness, hallucinations, disorientation, and memory loss may all be part of the presenting clinical picture. Virtually any disorder can manifest with delirium in elderly patients. Common causes include dehydration, congestive heart failure, myocardial infarction, pulmonary or urinary tract infections, and numerous drugs (Table 132–3). In addition to drugs that have known central nervous system effects, delirium has been reported with use of penicillin, digoxin, cimetidine, and nonsteroidal anti-inflammatory agents such as aspirin and ibuprofen. In older persons, delirium may occur at a dose that would not usually be considered toxic.

TABLE 132–3 Causes of Delirium in the Elderly

Organ Failure
Respiratory failure
Congestive heart failure
Hepatocellular failure

Infections
Acute bronchitis
Bronchopneumonia
Bladder infections
Septicemia

Metabolic Conditions
Dehydration
Hyponatremia
Hypernatremia

Drugs
Anticholinergics
Antibiotics
Anticonvulsants
Digitalis
Alcohol
Alcohol withdrawal

Neurologic Causes
Subdural hematoma
Cerebrovascular accident
Raised intracranial pressure
Cerebral infections

Miscellaneous
Postoperative delirium
Sensory deprivation
Recent institutionalization
Change of living arrangement

Elderly patients can develop delirium even as a result of a change in their living environment, such as occurs with hospitalization or placement in a nursing home. Postoperative delirium is also extremely common in elderly patients and occurs, for example, in 50% of patients after hip surgery. In this setting, the cause is multifactorial and often includes drugs and infection. Delirium is more common in patients who have baseline disorders of cognition. Because delirium is potentially reversible, it should not be ignored as "senile dementia" or "organic brain syndrome." Management involves accurate diagnosis and treatment of underlying diseases, stopping or changing of all drugs that could be contributory, and aggressively treatment of dehydration. When agitation is severe, sedatives or tranquilizers may be required. Although neither is ideal, risperidone or haloperidol is the drug of choice. Extremely low doses must be used. The usual initial dose for both drugs is 0.5 mg administered intramuscularly or orally and repeated at 30-minute intervals as needed. Although these drugs are usually well tolerated, a rare but potentially fatal side effect is the development of the *neuroleptic malignant syndrome,* which is characterized by fever and extrapyramidal signs. For severe agitation, benzodiazepines (e.g., lorazepam) have also been recommended as therapy for delirium. However, drugs themselves are often the cause of delirium. Sedatives should be avoided in drowsy patients, and these drugs should not be given for prolonged periods. Although pharmacologic and physical restraints are used commonly in patients with delirium, they are both associated with an increased risk of morbidity and should be avoided if at all possible. For a discussion of dementia, see Chapter 115 (Fig. 132–5).

BENIGN PROSTATIC HYPERPLASIA

Age-related enlargement of the prostate gland may or may not lead to voiding problems in older persons. Anatomic irritative symptoms include nocturia, frequency, urgency, dysuria, and incontinence. Obstructive symptoms include decreased force, hesitancy, terminal dribbling, double voiding, and straining to urinate. Decisions regarding work-up and therapy depend on an evaluation of the severity of the disease. Symptom assessment by questionnaires that can be completed by the patient makes it possible to identify mild, moderate, and severe disease. A rectal examination should be performed to evaluate prostate size and to exclude the presence of nodules. Further work-up should include a urinalysis to exclude an infection and a serum creatinine determination to exclude renal impairment. Prostate-specific antigen should be obtained if a nodule is found on rectal examination. If significant obstructive symptoms are present, postvoid residual urine volume should be determined either by ultrasound or by catheterization.

Treatment options in benign prostatic hyperplasia include watchful waiting, medical therapies, or surgery. For patients with mild to moderate disease, a period of observation is often warranted. Frequently, symptoms improve without any intervention. Medical therapy is an option for the patient with moderate to severe disease who has no evidence of urinary obstruction or renal

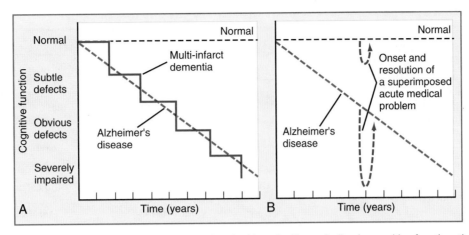

FIGURE 132-5   *A,* Normal aging is not associated with a significant decline in cognitive function; the progressive and steady decline in memory seen in patients with Alzheimer's disease is contrasted with the stepwise decreases seen in patients with multi-infarct dementia. *B,* Modest, temporary declines in cognitive function can occur in physiologically normal elderly persons during periods of acute illness. In patients with Alzheimer's disease or other disorders associated with memory loss, an acute medical illness can result in a much greater loss of cognitive function, which may or may not return to the preillness level.

impairment. α-Adrenergic receptor blockers relieve symptoms by reducing smooth muscle tone. Studies have shown significant symptomatic benefit, and these drugs are now considered the treatment of choice. Adverse effects include dizziness, postural hypotension, and fatigue. Finasteride, a 5 α$_1$-reductase inhibitor, blocks the conversion of testosterone to dihydrotestosterone and causes a 30% reduction in prostate size within 6 months of commencing therapy. The drug has been shown to relieve both irritative and obstructive symptoms. Side effects are rare and include impotence and problems with ejaculation. Patients with refractory urinary retention, an increased postvoid residual volume, recurrent or persistent gross hematuria, bladder stones, or renal insufficiency should be referred for surgical treatment.

URINARY INCONTINENCE

Incontinence is defined as loss of urine of sufficient severity to be a social or health problem. The incidence is 5% to 10% in ambulatory older persons, 30% in hospitalized geriatric patients, and 60% in nursing home residents. *Stress incontinence* is the most common cause in women under age 75, whereas *urge incontinence* is the most common cause in patients over age 75. *Overflow incontinence* is less common but must be diagnosed because of an increased incidence of urinary tract infections and impaired renal function. *Functional incontinence* is common in the nursing home and is diagnosed by exclusion. Table 132–4 lists the mechanisms, causes, and approaches to treatment of this common clinical problem. A history is important in obtaining an accurate diagnosis. Leakage with coughing or sneezing suggests stress incontinence. In urge incontinence, the patient is aware of the need to void but cannot make it to the toilet in time. Overflow incontinence should be considered in patients with neurologic deficits, including autonomic dysfunction that accompanies medication use

and diabetes. Physical examination should focus on the detection of neurologic or metabolic diseases that could result in incontinence and rectal examination as a measure of perineal floor tone and, in men, an evaluation of the prostate. Pelvic examination should be performed in women to exclude pelvic prolapse. Urinalysis is needed to screen for diabetes, hematuria, and infection. In patients with features suggestive of obstruction, postvoid residual urine volume should be measured, either by catheterization or by ultrasound. Referral for further work-up should be considered in patients with recurrent urinary tract infections, a prostatic mass, pelvic prolapse in women, a neurologic disorder that could make an accurate diagnosis difficult, hematuria, or an increased postvoid residual volume.

Initial treatment should be directed at correcting treatable conditions that can aggravate incontinence. Examples include medication use (diuretics and alcohol), fecal impaction, delirium, infections, and restricted mobility. Specific treatment for stress incontinence includes exercises to increase pelvic muscle strength (see Table 132–4). The use of biofeedback has been shown to be effective in helping women perform the exercises appropriately. Timed voiding assists in preventing the development of a full bladder. Estrogen replacement should be considered to strengthen periurethral tissues. In some patients, the use of an α-adrenergic agonist should be considered to stimulate urethral smooth muscle contraction. Exercises, biofeedback, and timed voiding should also be used in patients with urge incontinence. A bladder relaxant such as oxybutynin may also be considered. Patients with overflow incontinence are at great risk of developing infections. Mechanical obstruction should be treated surgically. Patients with neurogenic bladder require intermittent or long-term indwelling catheterization. Functional incontinence, common in the nursing home, is best treated by attempting to correct the underlying cause and by encouraging prompted voiding. Pads and external catheters should be used with

TABLE 132–4 Causes, Types, and Treatment of Urinary Incontinence

Type	Definition	Cause	Treatment
Stress	Leakage associated with increased intra-abdominal pressure (coughing, sneezing)	Hypermobility of the bladder base frequently caused by lax perineal muscles	Pelvic muscle exercise; timed voiding; α-adrenergic drugs; estrogens; surgery
Urge	Leakage associated with a precipitous urge to void	Detrusor hyperactivity (outflow obstruction, bladder tumor, detrusor instability); idiopathic (poor bladder); compliance (radiation cystitis); hypersensitive bladder	Bladder training; pelvic muscle exercise; bladder relaxant drugs (anticholinergics, oxybutynin, imipramine)
Overflow	Leakage from a mechanically distended bladder	Outflow obstruction; enlarged prostate; stricture; prolapsed cystocele; acontractile bladder (idiopathic, neurologic [spinal cord injury, stroke, diabetes])	Surgical correction of obstruction; intermittent catheter draining
Functional	Inability or unwillingness to void	Cognitive impairment; physical impairment; environmental barriers (physical restraints, inaccessible toilets); psychological problems (depression, anger, hostility)	Prompted voiding; garment and padding; external collection devices

caution because they may increase the risk of functional dependency. Long-term indwelling catheters should be used only in patients with skin disorders.

REFERENCES

Applegate WB, Blass JP, Williams TF: Instruments for the functional assessment of older patients. N Engl J Med 1990; 322:1207–1214.

Finch CE, Tanzi RE: Genetics of aging. Science 1997; 278:407–411.

Gottlieb GL, Johnson J, Wanich C, et al: Delirium in the medically ill elderly: Operationalizing the DSM-III criteria. Int Psychogeriatr 1991; 3:181–196.

Inouye SK, Charpentier PA: Precipitating factors for delirium in hospitalized elderly person: Predictive model and interrelationship with baseline vulnerability. JAMA 1996; 275:852–857.

Katzman R, Jackson JE: Alzheimer's disease: Basic and clinical advances. J Am Geriatr Soc 1991; 39:516–525.

Schneider LS, Tariot PN: Emerging drugs for Alzheimer's disease. Med Clin North Am 1994; 78:911–934.

Tinetti ME, Baker DI, McAvay G, et al: A multifactorial intervention to reduce risk of falling among elderly people living in the community. N Engl J Med 1994; 331:821–827.

Urinary Incontinence Guidelines Panel: Urinary Incontinence in Adults: Clinical Practice Guideline. AHCPR Pub No 92-0038. Rockville, MD: Agency for Health Care Policy and Research, United States Department of Health and Human Services, 1992.

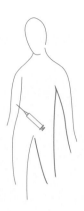

Substance Abuse

133

ALCOHOL AND SUBSTANCE ABUSE

Timothy E. Holcomb • *Jeffrey L. Clothier*

Despite educational and prevention efforts, alcohol and substance abuse remain major worldwide economic, social, and medical problems. The 1995 National Household Survey on Drug Abuse found that over 12 million Americans were currently illicit drug users. It estimated that there were 1.5 million cocaine users, 11 million heavy drinkers, and 61 million nicotine users. Most disturbing was the finding that the rate of illicit drug use among youths had doubled since 1992.

The essential features of substance abuse are compulsive self-administration, tolerance (the body's adaptation to repeated drug usage, which mitigates its pharmacologic effect), withdrawal (behavioral and physiologic changes that occur as tissue or blood levels of the substance decline) and/or a maladaptive pattern of drug usage that leads to impairment or distress.

The causes of substance abuse for an individual are multifactorial and involve a complex interplay of genetic predisposition, environmental and behavioral factors, and neurobiologic factors. Advances in the understanding of substance abuse have stressed the importance of a neuroanatomy of "reward and reinforcement," whereby stimulation in a particular area of the brain by drugs of abuse might activate certain circuits, resulting in the mediation of reward or pleasure ("brain reward mechanisms"). Key anatomic regions that appear to mediate these effects include the median forebrain bundle, nucleus accumbens, amygdala, and locus ceruleus. The median forebrain bundle houses the mesolimbic dopamine system, in which dopamine neurons arise in the ventral tegmental area and distribute axons into the nucleus accumbens and the frontal cerebral cortex. This system appears to be a major site of action for almost all abused drugs (cocaine, amphetamines, opiates, nicotine, alcohol, and cannabinoids), which stimulate the efflux of dopamine into the nucleus accumbens by many different mechanisms. Although this may play a role in compulsive drug use, the overall addiction process likely involves multiple neurotransmitters and pathways. The locus ceruleus, as the major noradrenergic cell group, plays an important role in opiate withdrawal, which indicates that the anatomic sites of compulsive use and withdrawal may be physically distinct. The amygdala, with its complex memory systems, may relate environmental cues to emotional and motivational actions and help produce a pathologic desire or craving for a specific drug.

Other advances include the elucidation of the primary neurotransmitters and molecular sites of action for most abused drugs. For example, the stimulant drugs (cocaine and amphetamine) have been shown to bind to a presynaptic dopamine reuptake transporter and block the reuptake of dopamine from the synaptic cleft. Excess dopamine and other catecholamines are left to stimulate adjacent neurons, which accounts for their physiologic responses. Amphetamines also stimulate excess release of dopamine from synaptic vesicular stores. Chronic use of these drugs can eventually lead to a decrease in dopamine stores, which indicates that other mechanisms are also important in stimulant abuse. The mechanisms of alcohol are complex; its effect appears to be mediated by multiple neurotransmitters, including activation of gamma-aminobutyric acid A (GABA) receptors, release of opioid peptides and dopamine, inhibition of glutamate receptors, and interaction of serotonin systems. Opioids act primarily at the μ receptors, whereas the sedative-hypnotic drugs (barbiturates, benzodiazepines) interact with the GABA system and the GABA-α receptor complex. Phencyclidine hydrochloride (PCP) is an antagonist of the *N*-methyl-D-aspartate (NMDA) glutamate receptor. The multiple neurotransmitters affected by recreational drugs may also explain the wide variety of psychiatric symptoms commonly seen in substance-abusing patients.

In addition, chronic exposure to drugs can produce molecular adaptations such as the upregulation of the cyclic adenosine monophosphate pathway, probably from initiation of certain transcription factors. This adaptation may be important in some withdrawal phenomena. A classic example is opiate use. Opiates acutely inhibit locus ceruleus neuron firing rates, but chronic use leads to recovery of firing rates (tolerance). Upon cessation of drug use, firing rates increase to abnormally high levels, leading to the somatic signs of opiate withdrawal.

Many of these neurobiologic discoveries offer opportunities for specific pharmacologic approaches to treating addiction. Equally important is the need for cognitive therapy to decondition the addict to environmental cues that induce relapse and for social rehabilitation to teach the addict to function in a nonaddicted society.

Screening

Physicians have the opportunity to identify patients with alcohol and substance abuse and initiate treatment before serious social, medical, or psychiatric problems develop. Historical clues to possible drug abuse include infectious processes such as endocarditis, hepatitis B or C, tuberculosis, frequent sexually transmitted diseases, recurrent pneumonias, skin abscesses, and human immunodeficiency virus (HIV) infection. Other clues include frequent emergency department visits for chest pain by young persons, insomnia, mood swings, chronic pain, repetitive trauma, and behavioral or social problems. Physical findings are usually nonspecific but may include needle marks (often obscured by tattoos), upper extremity edema, chronic sinusitis or a scarred or perforated nasal septum from cocaine use, and the presence of withdrawal symptoms. Patients with advanced alcoholic liver disease may exhibit the typical physical signs of hepatomegaly, ascites, palmar erythema, male gynecomastia and hypogonadism, spider angiomas, and jaundice.

Two effective screening tests for alcoholism include the 10-question Alcohol Use Disorder Identification Test (AUDIT) and the CAGE questionnaire. The CAGE questionnaire centers on four questions: need to *cut* down on drinking, *annoyed* by criticism of drinking, *guilty* feelings about drinking, and need for an early morning "*eye-opener*" drink; two positive answers can identify 75% of alcoholics with 95% specificity. Similar questionnaires can be used to screen for other types of substance abuse. Screening through blood and urine tests is helpful but usually cannot be obtained without consent of the patient. Urine tests can be used to screen for the presence of marijuana, cocaine, opioids, PCP, barbiturates, benzodiazepines, and amphetamines; positive screening results must be confirmed by gas chromatography–mass spectroscopy. These tests can indicate use in a specific time period but cannot disclose the pattern of use or the existence of dependence. Helpful screening blood tests for alcohol use include elevations in mean corpuscular volume and gamma glutamyl transferase.

Tobacco and Alcohol Abuse

NICOTINE

Tobacco smoking is society's greatest health burden and the most preventable cause of death in the United States. It is estimated by the Centers for Disease Control and Prevention to be responsible for about 500,000 deaths each year. It has been causally linked to lung cancer and other malignancies, cardiovascular disease, chronic obstructive pulmonary disease, complications in pregnancy, gastrointestinal disorders, and other diseases. Passive smoking is implicated in lung cancer, cardiovascular disease, and other pulmonary disorders.

Nicotine is a highly addictive stimulant that can lead to dependence, tolerance, and withdrawal. The withdrawal syndrome is highly variable but usually involves irritability, impatience, anxiety, difficulty concentrating, sleep disturbance, increased appetite, and craving. Many strategies have been advocated to promote smoking cessation, but one of the newer effective regimens includes the use of nicotine gum or patches, combined with bupropion. Bupropion is thought to increase dopamine activity in the reward centers to reduce craving. These measures should be combined with smoking cessation classes or therapy for maximal effectiveness.

ALCOHOLISM

Alcohol's toll on society is great; it causes about 100,000 deaths per year in the United States, half from trauma. Alcohol use is implicated in about half of all traffic-related deaths, and it plays a major role in homicides, suicides, domestic violence, and homelessness. Recognition of the problem is critical, because early diagnosis and treatment improve the prognosis for recovery.

Pharmacology

Alcohol is absorbed rapidly and may be detected in the blood within minutes. Ethanol is a small molecule soluble in water, readily crosses biologic membranes, and permeates all tissues of the body. It distributes in total body water. Ninety percent is metabolized by the liver, and the remainder is excreted by the kidneys, lungs, and skin. Its elimination is independent of concentration; a 70-kg man can metabolize 5 to 10 g/hr. Once drinking ceases, blood levels fall about 10 to 25 mg/dL/hr.

Metabolism

Many of the effects of chronic alcohol use result from its metabolism by the alcohol dehydrogenase pathway and the microsomal ethanol oxidizing system (Fig. 133–1). The alcohol dehydrogenase pathway metabolizes alcohol to acetaldehyde, which is then converted to acetate. In both these reactions, nicotinamide-adenine dinucleotide (NAD) is reduced to NADH. Excess NADH produces a number of metabolic problems, including elevated lactic acid and uric acid levels, hyperlipidemia, hypoglycemia (through a block in gluconeogenesis), hypoproteinemia, and increased collagen synthesis. Acetaldehyde itself has toxic effects and can promote cellular death. It can block secretion of proteins from hepatocytes; the resulting increases in proteins, lipids, and water can cause hepatocytes to swell, a finding in alcoholic liver disease. Finally, acetaldehyde can cross the pla-

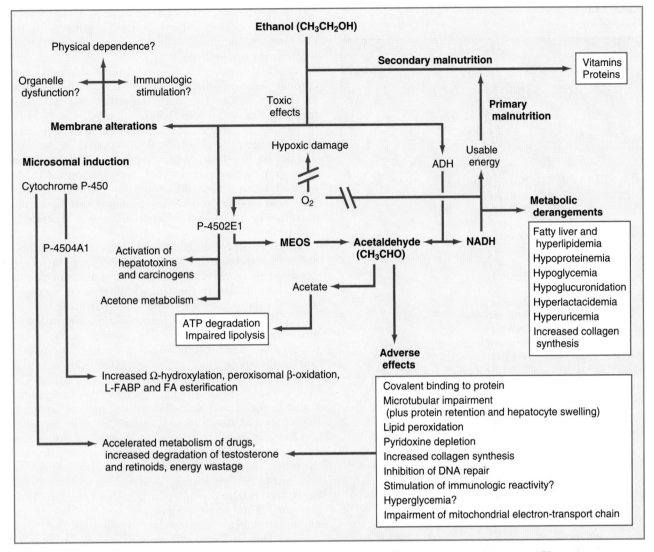

FIGURE 133–1 Toxic and metabolic effects of alcohol abuse. ADH = alcohol dehydrogenase; ATP = adenosine triphosphate; FA = fatty acids; L-FABP = liver fatty acid–binding protein; MEOS = microsomal ethanol-oxidizing system; NADH = reduced nicotinamide-adenine dinucleotide. (From Lieber CS: Medical disorders of alcoholism. N Engl J Med 1995; 333(16):1060. Reprinted with permission.)

centa and impair fetal DNA methylation, contributing to the fetal alcohol syndrome.

Long-term use of alcohol induces the microsomal ethanol oxidizing system and cytochrome P-4502E1, a key enzyme in the oxidation of ethanol. This contributes to the development of tolerance and increases the metabolism of many drugs, including pentobarbital, propranolol, tolbutamide, warfarin, and diazepam. Cytochrome P-4502E1 converts many foreign substances (solvents, anesthetic agents, cocaine, isoniazid, acetaminophen) into highly toxic metabolites. It activates carcinogens and, coupled with vitamin A deficiency and the increased mutagenicity of tobacco caused by alcohol, may increase the incidence of cancers of the gastrointestinal tract, lung, and breast. Finally, in contrast to chronic use, short-term consumption can inhibit the metabolism of many drugs as a result of direct competition for the cytochrome P-4502E1 system.

Medical Effects

The medical consequences of chronic alcohol use are listed in Table 133–1. Many of these medical problems are more severe in women and in the elderly. Blood levels tend to be higher in women because of their smaller size, higher proportion of body fat, and, in younger women, less gastric alcohol dehydrogenase activity. Liver injury, cirrhosis, and cerebral atrophy progress faster in women than in men with similar histories of alcohol use. Moderate use is now defined as no more than two drinks per day for men and one per day for women.

Many of the medical problems result from nutritional depletion. The energy content of alcohol is 7.1 kcal/g, and alcohol may account for half of an alcoholic's caloric intake. Malnutrition results both as alcohol displaces normal nutrients and from malabsorption caused by gas-

TABLE 133–1 **Alcohol-Related Medical Disorders**

Affected Organ or System	Disorder
Nutrition	Deficiencies of
	Folate, thiamine, pyridoxine, niacin, and riboflavin
	Magnesium, zinc, calcium
	Protein
Brain	Hepatic encephalopathy
	Wernicke-Korsakoff syndrome
	Cerebral atrophy
	Amblyopia
	Central pontine myelinolysis
	Marchiafava-Bignami disease
Nerve	Neuropathy
Muscle	Myopathy
Liver	Fatty liver
	Hepatitis
	Cirrhosis
	Hepatoma
Heart	Hypertension
	Cardiomyopathy
	Arrhythmia
Blood	Anemia
	Leukopenia
	Thrombocytopenia
	Macrocytosis
Gut	Esophagitis and gastritis
	Pancreatitis
Metabolites and electrolytes	Hypoglycemia
	Hyperlipidemia
	Hyperuricemia
	Ketoacidosis
	Hypomagnesemia
	Hypophosphatemia
Endocrine	Pseudo–Cushing's syndrome
	Testicular atrophy
	Amenorrhea
Bone	Osteopenia

From Diamond I: Alcoholism and alcohol abuse. *In* Wyngaarden JB, Smith LH Jr (eds): Cecil Textbook of Medicine, 18th ed. Philadelphia: WB Saunders, 1992, p 45.

trointestinal problems such as pancreatic insufficiency. Levels of folate, thiamine, and other vitamins are reduced.

Patients with chronic severe alcoholism suffer an increased incidence of optic neuropathy, a condition marked by reduced visual acuity and central or paracentral scotomas, with normal optic fundi. Dietary and vitamin therapies sometimes bring about improvement. Advanced problem drinkers can develop cerebral atrophy and signs of dementia as early as in their 40s. Abstinence may reverse the severity of these changes.

Alcohol-nutritional peripheral neuropathy usually occurs with advanced nutritional deprivation and improves only with alleviation of malnourishment. The disorder produces axonal degeneration of the small pain- and temperature-mediating fibers in the distal lower extremities. Distal motor loss also occurs. Spontaneous, often burning pain and autonomic neuropathy commonly affect persons with advanced alcoholism. Deep tendon reflexes disappear in a distal-to-proximal pattern. Recovery requires months or years of renourishment and often remains incomplete.

Alcoholic myopathy is confined to patients with chronic, severe alcoholism and can have either an acute or chronic onset. The acute form consists of sudden transient rhabdomyolysis, which often follows a cluster of seizures or trauma. It includes muscle pain, tenderness, cramping, weakness, and an elevated serum creatine kinase level. In severe cases, myoglobinuria can develop with associated renal complications. Chronic myopathy consists of diffuse proximal muscle wasting and weakness disproportional to any existing neuritic impairment. It is alleviated gradually with nutritional replacement.

Wernicke-Korsakoff disease reflects the acute and chronic central nervous system (CNS) effects of severe, sustained thiamine depletion in the presence of continued caloric intake. In the United States, severe alcoholism is the most common cause. The pathologic changes in the brain include axonal demyelination, neuronal loss, glial proliferation, endothelial thickening, and petechial pericapillary hemorrhages. The oculomotor, vestibular, and medullary autonomic nuclei, as well as the brain stem reticular formation, sustain the greatest damage. At higher levels, the mammillary bodies, the mediodorsal thalamic nuclei, and scattered cortical regions, including the hippocampus, are most affected.

Clinically, patients with acute Wernicke's disease are confused, often drowsy or semistuporous, ataxic, and dysarthric. Partial or complete external ophthalmoplegia and nystagmus are cardinal features, along with tachycardia, orthostatic hypotension, hypothermia, and diffuse analgesia. The pupils seldom are affected, but almost any motor cranial nerve can be partially paralyzed. Most patients have at least mild signs of peripheral neuropathy. Treatment consists of administering thiamine, 100 mg parenterally, upon suspicion of the diagnosis, followed by replenishment of blood volume and electrolytes. Glucose administration should not precede thiamine treatment, because its metabolic processing can precipitate acute worsening of the condition. Evidence of severe anemia, hepatic insufficiency, or infection should be corrected and the patient observed for impending seizures or delirium tremens. The response to thiamine is usually diagnostic: the ophthalmoplegia usually begins to improve within a matter of hours to a day or so.

Korsakoff's amnestic syndrome usually emerges as the acute confusional delirium of Wernicke's disease subsides. Affected patients show a profound, relatively isolated loss of memory for recent events. This, coupled with a placid lack of insight, often leads to total disorientation mixed with absurd conversations or absurd answers to questions (confabulation). Arousal, language function, and remote memories are spared. Korsakoff's syndrome arises only after either preceding attacks of Wernicke's encephalopathy or an unusually severe attack. Treatment is the same as for Wernicke's disease. About half the patients treated for the first time improve to the point of regaining independence.

Acute cerebellar degeneration occurs most often in alcoholics as a complication of an acute superimposed, severe binge. Its pathogenesis remains unclear but may reflect acute alcoholic damage to chemically vulnerable regional neurons. The symptoms reflect acute cerebellar degeneration, leading to a gradually or suddenly appearing broad-based, stiff-legged ataxia unaccompanied by incoordination in the upper extremities or nystagmus. Many patients have an associated nutritional peripheral neuropathy.

Genetics

Genetic factors play a large role in the development of alcoholism in certain people. Results of studies of siblings and adoptees suggest a genetically transmitted susceptibility for alcoholism. Earlier work implicated the gene for the dopamine D_2 receptor, but this was not confirmed in other work. The exact nature of the dopamine receptor is still unknown. Differences in the rate of ethanol metabolism and the severity of alcohol-related liver disease are also, in part, genetically determined. Levels of gastric alcohol dehydrogenase differ among ethnic groups; for example, a majority of Japanese persons lack an isoenzyme of alcohol dehydrogenase and thus can have increased blood acetaldehyde levels and an alcohol flush reaction if they drink.

Acute Alcohol Intoxication

Because there is virtually no blood-brain barrier to alcohol, uptake into the brain is rapid and is limited primarily by cerebral blood flow and capillary perfusion. Within a short time after drinking, the concentration of ethanol in the brain is nearly the same as in the blood. The blood levels correlate directly with the clinical signs and symptoms (Table 133–2). As blood levels rise, slurred speech, ataxia, incoordination, and slow or irregular eye movements may develop. At higher blood levels, CNS depression and deterioration of cerebellar and vestibular function occur. Patients may exhibit dysarthria, ataxia, nystagmus, diplopia, decreased respirations, vomiting, and pulmonary aspiration. For nondrinkers, stupor and coma may develop at blood levels of 400 mg/dL and fatalities can occur at 500 mg/dL from respiratory depression, hypotension, and acidosis. Alcoholic blackouts (amnesia) can occur after a large amount of

alcohol is consumed and are a sign of serious intoxication and probable dependence. Some younger male drinkers may develop pathologically severe aggressive and violent behavior (dyscontrol) for which they later claim no memory. This syndrome calls for total abstinence and immediate psychiatric referral.

Mild drunkenness requires no treatment other than observation. Patients with marked drowsiness or stupor require close evaluation, especially if other drugs may have been used. Other diagnostic possibilities such as hypoglycemia, acidosis, meningitis, and subdural hematomas must be considered. Evidence of head trauma or focal neurologic signs necessitate computed tomographic scanning to confirm or rule out intracranial pathology. Intubation may be necessary for severe hypoventilation or for comatose patients. Hemodialysis may be needed if the blood alcohol level exceeds 600 mg/dL.

Withdrawal Syndrome

It is apparent that a history of repeated alcohol withdrawal may sensitize a person to subsequent episodes of withdrawal. The withdrawal syndrome can be divided into several stages depending on the severity of physical dependence. Minor withdrawal symptoms may begin in 8 to 12 hours and consist of tremors, sweating, anxiety, tachycardia, nausea, diarrhea, and insomnia. These symptoms reflect a state of central adrenergic hyperexcitation that begins as the inhibitory influence of alcohol dissipates. In general, observation is sufficient management. Patients with marked alcohol dependence may develop more profound symptoms 12 to 24 hours after the last drink. These include marked tremulousness, hyperactivity, tachycardia, increased startle response, insomnia, nightmares, visual hallucinations, and alcohol craving. Withdrawal seizures (so-called rum fits) may occur 12 to 48 hours after the last drink and can be single or multiple episodes of tonic-clonic seizures. Status epilepticus is seen in less than 3% of patients. If the seizures are focal or are accompanied by a fever or status epilepticus, further evaluation is necessary.

The most severe stage is delirium tremens, which typically occurs 72 to 120 hours after cessation of drinking. It affects about 5% of patients who have been drinking fairly heavily for a decade or more. These patients have acute delirium, confusion, fear, agitation, gross tremor, insomnia, incontinence, hypertension,

TABLE 133–2   Blood Alcohol Levels and Symptoms

Level (mg/dL)	Sporadic Drinkers	Chronic Drinkers
50 (party level)	Congenial euphoria	No observable effect
75	Gregarious or garrulous	Often no effect
100	Incoordinated; legally intoxicated	Minimal signs
125–150	Unrestrained behavior; episodic dyscontrol	Pleasurable euphoria or beginning incoordination
200–250	Lethargy	Effort required to maintain emotional and motor control
300–350	Stupor or coma	Drowsy and slow
>500	Sometimes death	Coma

tachycardia, profuse sweating, and fever. Patients may be combative, destructive, and dangerous. Many patients are malnourished and may have signs of hepatic insufficiency, gastritis, dehydration, infection, polyneuropathy, or Wernicke's syndrome. Delirium tremens may last several days and is a medical emergency.

Management

Patients with mild withdrawal symptoms can be managed as outpatients. However, patients with hyperactivity, concurrent medical problems, and a history of previous withdrawal problems should be hospitalized. A typical treatment regimen is listed in Table 133–3. The adequacy of management can be judged by heart rate, blood pressure, and the degree of tremor, agitation, or insomnia. Barbiturates (phenobarbital) can be substituted for benzodiazepines.

For hallucinations or extreme agitation, haloperidol can be used cautiously but must be given with benzodiazepines because it lowers the seizure threshold. It is best used 48 hours after the last drink when the risk for seizures has lessened. Thiamine must be given before administration of a glucose load in intravenous fluids, to prevent precipitation of the Wernicke-Korsakoff syndrome. β blockers and clonidine can help reduce adrenergic signs.

Treatment of withdrawal seizures remains controversial. Although long-term use of phenytoin is not thought to be helpful, it is reasonable to consider short-term use of phenytoin for patients in withdrawal with a documented history of either non–alcohol-related seizures or withdrawal seizures.

Delirium tremens carries a mortality rate of 20% to 40% of patients who do not receive treatment. Patients with delirium tremens should be admitted to the intensive care unit, and close attention should be given to the general principles for withdrawal management. Physical restraint should be avoided, if possible, but sufficient sedation must be used to prevent self-inflicted injury. Diazepam, 5 to 10 mg, can be given every 5 to 15 minutes until the patient is calm, and maintenance therapy is continued every 1 to 4 hours as needed. Some patients may require up to 1200 mg of diazepam in the first 3 to 4 days of therapy.

TABLE 133–3   Management of Alcohol Withdrawal

Observe and normalize vital signs
Administer thiamine, 100 mg, then replace fluid and electrolytes
Sedate with chlordiazepoxide, 25 mg PO qid
Administer chlordiazepoxide, 25–50 mg IM prn for signs of withdrawal
Use haloperidol (1–2 mg PO q4h prn) or thorazine cautiously for hallucinations or agitation
Replace folic acid (1 mg/day PO) and thiamine (100 mg IM and then 100 mg/day PO)
Give multivitamin daily
Begin β-blocker (atenolol, 50 mg) or clonidine (0.2 mg PO bid) to reduce adrenergic signs

The recidivism rate for alcoholism is high. After detoxification, patients should be referred to a multidisciplinary rehabilitation program. Family members, friends, and peers must be involved, and support groups such as Alcoholics Anonymous and Al-Anon can be helpful. Comorbid psychiatric problems must be identified and treated. Problem drinkers have been shown to benefit from brief counseling sessions with their physicians, in which the physicians focus on giving feedback on health concerns, provide advice, and specify a plan of action.

Patients with alcohol problems identified through outpatient screening tests need further assessment to establish the presence of alcohol dependence. Those with moderate dependence problems should be referred to outpatient treatment facilities, whereas those with more severe dependence may need inpatient management.

Pharmacotherapies that may help include the serotonin reuptake inhibitors, which have been shown to reduce alcohol intake, probably from alleviation of depression. Other agents include the narcotic antagonists naltrexone and nalmefene, which help reduce craving and relapse. These drugs may help modulate some aspect of the mesolimbic dopamine reward circuitry. Naltrexone can be given once daily for 12 weeks but may precipitate opioid withdrawal if patients are dependent on opioids. Disulfiram is used to prevent relapse by blocking aldehyde dehydrogenase, leading to increased concentrations of acetaldehyde. Patients who drink while taking disulfiram experience flushing, nausea, tachycardia, palpitations, headache, and dyspnea. These symptoms, although uncomfortable, are self-limited and usually without risk to the patient. Alcoholics who are daily drinkers and committed to treatment are good candidates for supervised disulfiram treatment, but it should be avoided in those with heart disease, seizures, cirrhosis, diabetes, pregnancy, history of psychosis, and elevated transaminase levels.

Prescription Drug Abuse

SEDATIVE-HYPNOTICS

Benzodiazepines and barbiturates are the major sedative-hypnotic drugs. These drugs can produce physical and psychological dependence and a potentially dangerous withdrawal syndrome. The effects of these drugs are additive with other CNS depressants such as alcohol.

Benzodiazepines are available as short-acting agents such as temazepam and triazolam; intermediate-acting agents such as alprazolam, lorazepam, and oxazepam; and long-acting agents such as chlordiazepoxide, diazepam, flurazepam, and clonazepam. Flunitrazepam ("roach" or "roofies") is now a popular benzodiazepine of abuse and has been implicated in cases of date rape and gang violence. It is not legally available in the United States but is smuggled here from other countries.

Withdrawal symptoms depend on the half-life of the agent, duration of use, and dosage. In general, agents with shorter half-lives produce a more intense withdrawal syndrome. Withdrawal symptoms usually peak in 2 to 4 days for the short-acting drugs and in 5 to 6 days for the longer-acting drugs. Withdrawal is characterized by intense anxiety, insomnia, irritability, weight loss, muscle spasms, palpitations, diarrhea, hypersensitivity to light and sound, perceptual changes, tremors, and seizures. Panic attacks and disturbing nightmares may occur after long-term use and may wax and wane for months.

Detoxification requires a change to a longer-acting benzodiazepine such as clonazepam or diazepam and a tapering regimen of 7 to 10 days for short-acting drugs and 10 to 14 days for longer-acting drugs. Propranolol can be used to decrease tachycardia, hypertension, and anxiety. In acute overdose, the major danger is from respiratory depression. Flumazenil, a competitive antagonist of benzodiazepines, can be given intravenously for acute overdose but may precipitate seizures if tricyclic antidepressants or cocaine have been used.

The most commonly abused barbiturates include the short-acting drugs pentobarbital and secobarbital and the intermediate-acting drugs amobarbital, aprobarbital, butabarbital, and butalbital. Patients acutely intoxicated show sluggishness, difficulty thinking, slurred speech, poor memory and judgment, nystagmus, diplopia, and vertigo. For acute overdose, oral charcoal and alkalinization of the urine (pH > 7.5) with forced diuresis can be effective in lowering blood levels.

Withdrawal symptoms are similar to those with benzodiazepines. Psychoses and generalized seizures are rare. Treatment requires estimating the daily dose of the abused drug and using an equivalent phenobarbital dose to stabilize the patient. The dose is then tapered over 4 to 14 days, depending on the half-life of the abused drug. Benzodiazepines can also be used for detoxification, and propranolol and clonidine can help reduce symptoms.

OPIOIDS

Opioids include the natural and semisynthetic alkaloid derivatives from opium and the purely synthetic drugs that mimic heroin. Commonly abused drugs in this class include heroin, morphine, codeine, oxycodone, meperidine, and fentanyl (Table 133–4). Abuse develops as patients seek treatment for legitimate reasons and then progressively require stronger opioids for worsening pain or for addiction purposes and relief of anxiety and depression. Others intentionally misuse opioids for their euphoria-producing abilities. Intravenous heroin use, particularly when combined with cocaine ("speedball"), is increasing in the United States and represents a high-risk behavior for HIV infection.

Opioids are classified as agonists, mixed agonist-antagonists, and antagonists. They act at specific receptors that are widely distributed, but their primary action is at the μ receptor. Potency depends on receptor affinity and metabolism; for example, heroin, an agonist, has high lipid solubility and enters the brain rapidly. Mixed-action drugs act as agonists at certain opiate receptors and relieve pain but can displace morphine from other receptors and precipitate withdrawal. The pure antagonists have no opiate effect but can reverse overdose and precipitate withdrawal.

TABLE 133–4   Commonly Prescribed Opioids

Agonists
Morphine
Methadone
Meperidine (Demerol)
Oxycodone (Percodan)
Propoxyphene (Darvon)
Hydromorphone (Dilaudid)
Fentanyl (Sublimaze)
Codeine
Mixed Agonist-Antagonists
Pentazocine (Talwin)
Nalbuphine (Nubain)
Buprenorphine (Buprenex)
Butorphanol (Stadol)
Antagonists
Naloxone (Narcan)
Naltrexone (Trexan*)

* Renamed ReVia in 1995.
From O'Brien C: Drug abuse and dependence. *In* Wyngaarden JB, Smith LH Jr (eds): Cecil Textbook of Medicine, 18th ed. Philadelphia: WB Saunders, 1992, p 45.

Acute opioid overdose is marked by cyanosis, pulmonary edema, respiratory distress, and mental status changes that progress to coma. Other findings include increased intracranial pressure, seizures, fever, and pinpoint pupils. Unsterile intravenous practices can lead to skin abscesses, cellulitis, meningitis, thrombophlebitis, rhabdomyolysis, wound botulism, endocarditis, hepatitis, and HIV infection. Neurologic complications from intravenous heroin include transverse myelitis, inflammatory polyneuropathy, and peripheral nerve lesions.

For acute overdose, respiratory status must be assessed and supported. Naloxone should be administered intravenously and repeated at 2- to 3-minute intervals, often in escalating dosages. Patients should respond within minutes with increases in pupil size, respiratory rate, and level of alertness. If no response occurs, opioid overdose is excluded and other causes must be sought. Naloxone should be titrated carefully, because it can precipitate acute withdrawal symptoms in opioid-dependent patients.

Withdrawal symptoms develop 6 to 10 hours after the last injection of heroin. Feelings of drug craving, anxiety, restlessness, irritability, rhinorrhea, lacrimation, sweating, and yawning develop early and are followed by dilated pupils, piloerection, anorexia, nausea, vomiting, diarrhea, muscle spasms, abdominal cramps, bone pain, myalgias, tremors, sleep disturbance, and, in rare cases, seizures. These symptoms peak at about 36 to 48 hours and then subside over 5 to 10 days, if untreated. There can be a protracted abstinence syndrome up to 6 months, characterized by mild anxiety, sleep disturbance, bradycardia, hypotension, and decreased responsiveness. Withdrawal can be managed with methadone, a long-acting synthetic agonist drug that prevents the sudden onset of CNS effects. After test doses, methadone can be given twice daily and tapered over 7 to 10 days. L-α-acetylmethadol (L-AAM), a long-acting agonist, and buprenorphine, a partial agonist, can each be given three times a week. Clonidine can reduce autonomic hyperactivity and is especially effective if combined with a benzodiazepine.

Patients with repeated relapses can be maintained on methadone or L-AAM. Methadone has been shown to reduce opioid use and criminal behavior and to improve health and employment status. It may be used for years with appropriate supervision. Naltrexone is a long-acting opioid antagonist that blocks impulsive opioid use. It can be given daily or two to three times weekly but only after the patient is thoroughly detoxified, because it can precipitate withdrawal. Buprenorphine may also be used as maintenance therapy. Pharmacotherapies must be combined with psychotherapy and rehabilitation programs for optimal outcomes.

AMPHETAMINES

The most frequently abused amphetamines are dextroamphetamine, methcathinone, methamphetamine, methylphenidate, ephedrine, propylhexedrine, and phenmetrazine. "Ice" is a freebase form of methamphetamine that can be inhaled, smoked, or injected. Amphetamines have been used for weight reduction, attention deficit disorder, and narcolepsy, although their use is now strictly limited.

Tolerance to the stimulant effects develops rapidly, and toxic effects can occur with higher doses. Toxic effects resemble acute paranoid schizophrenia with delusions and hallucinations. Withdrawal symptoms are similar to those seen with cocaine (described in the next section).

Acute amphetamine toxicity is characterized by excessive sympathomimetic effects with tachycardia, tremors, hypertension, hyperthermia, and possible arrhythmias. There may be stereotyped compulsive behavior and tactile, visual, or auditory hallucinations. The clinical picture may be indistinguishable from that of an acute schizophrenic psychosis. There is evidence of neuronal degeneration in dopamine-rich areas of the brain, probably from formation of the neurotoxin 6-hydroxydopamine, which may increase the risk for the later development of Parkinson's disease. Treatment principles include a quiet environment and benzodiazepines for anxiety. Urine acidification with ammonium chloride may accelerate amphetamine excretion. Typical antipsychotics such as haloperidol can reduce the agitation and psychosis by blocking dopamine's effects at the receptor.

Illicit Drug Abuse

COCAINE

Cocaine is a naturally occurring alkaloid derived from the coca plant. It was introduced into the United States in the late 19th century as a local anesthetic and as an ingredient in teas, beverages, and patent medicines. Its abuse led to its ban in 1914 from proprietary use, and strict limitations were placed on its medical use.

Cocaine use has increased most dramatically among adolescents and young adults and is a frequent cause of drug-related visits to emergency rooms. During the 1990s, the use shifted from the powder form to the freebase form and the crystallized freebase form ("crack," named for the popping sound that it makes when heated). It is highly addictive.

Cocaine can be ingested orally or by snorting, injecting intravenously, or smoking (crack). The blood half-life is about 1 hour. The drug's major metabolite is benzoylecgonine, which can be detected in the urine for 2 to 3 days after a single dose. Through smoking, high brain levels are obtained within seconds, because of the vast pulmonary vascular bed. An intense, pleasurable reaction lasting about 20 to 30 minutes is followed by rebound depression, agitation, insomnia, and anorexia and later by fatigue, hypersomnolence, and hyperphagia (the "crash"). This typically lasts 9 to 12 hours but may last up to 4 days. Users repeat the sequence at short intervals to recapture the euphoric state and avoid the crash. Medical complications increase as the pattern of abuse is intensified. Alcohol and other sedatives are often used concurrently to lessen anxiety and irritability. The combination of cocaine and heroin, injected intravenously, has resulted in some deaths.

Cocaine has a powerful effect on the central and sympathetic nervous systems, resulting in tachycardia, hypertension, hyperthermia, agitation, peripheral vasoconstriction, seizures, tachypnea, pupillary dilatation, and anorexia. Medical complications are listed in Table 133–5. The most devastating medical complications are related to the cerebrovascular and cardiovascular effects of cocaine. Cocaine causes potent vasoconstriction of cerebral arteries and may result in acute stroke. It is associated with myocardial ischemia and arrhythmias and, in rare cases, with acute myocardial infarction in young people with normal or near normal coronary arteries. The principal mechanisms are coronary artery vasoconstriction, thrombosis, platelet aggregation, plasminogen-activator inhibition, increased oxygen demand, and accelerated atherosclerosis. Those with acute myocardial infarction need standard aggressive treatment with heparin, thrombolytics, or invasive procedures. Use of β blockers is controversial because the ischemia may be worsened by unopposed, α-mediated vasoconstriction. However, there are anecdotal reports of safe use of β blockers in patients with acute myocardial infarction. Benzodiazepines, nitrates, and the α antagonist phentolamine have been used successfully to treat myocardial ischemia. Patients with a normal electrocardiogram or nonspecific changes can be safely managed with observation. For those with cocaine-induced hypertension or tachycardia, metoprolol or labetalol is effective.

Immediate treatment measures for acute intoxication include obtaining vascular and airway access, if needed, and electrocardiographic monitoring. Benzodiazepines can be given intravenously and repeated at 5-minute intervals to control CNS agitation. Haloperidol or risperidone can be used for severely agitated patients. A supportive environment is needed, but detoxification is not required because there are few physical signs of true dependence. Most patients suffer psychological depen-

TABLE 133-5 Complications Associated with Cocaine Use

Cardiac	Pulmonary
Chest pain	Pneumothorax
Myocardial infarction	Pneumomediastinum
Arrhythmias	Pneumopericardium
Cardiomyopathy	Pulmonary edema
Myocarditis	Exacerbation of asthma
	Pulmonary hemorrhage
Endocrine	Bronchiolitis obliterans
Hyperprolactinemia	"Crack lung"
Gastrointestinal	**Psychiatric**
Intestinal ischemia	Anxiety
Gastroduodenal perfora-	Depression
tions	Paranoia
Colitis	Delirium
	Psychosis
Head and Neck	Suicide
Erosion of dental enamel	
Gingival ulceration	**Renal**
Keratitis	Rhabdomyolysis
Corneal epithelial defects	
Chronic rhinitis	**Obstetric**
Perforated nasal septum	Placental abruption
Aspiration of nasal septum	Low birth weight
Midline granuloma	Prematurity
Altered olfaction	Microcephaly
Optic neuropathy	
Osteolytic sinusitis	**Others**
	Sudden death
Neurologic	Sexual dysfunction
Headaches	Hyperpyrexia
Seizures	Increased risk of HIV
Cerebral hemorrhage	infection
Cerebral infarctions	
Cerebral atrophy	
Cerebral vasculitis	

HIV = human immunodeficiency virus.
From Warner E: Cocaine abuse. Ann Intern Med 1993; 119:229.

dence with intense craving for cocaine, often stimulated by conditioned cues. Personal and group therapy are important adjuncts to pharmacologic treatment. However, relapse is common and very difficult to treat. Treatment approaches developed since 1990 have centered on the short-term use of dopamine agonists (bromocriptine), tricyclic antidepressants (primarily desipramine), or the selective serotonin reuptake inhibitors (SSRIs) to decrease the severe craving for cocaine and the fatigue and depression that follow. Other early research is investigating "vaccine" strategies: injecting protein-conjugated analogues of cocaine to produce anticocaine antibodies to bind cocaine and prevent its passage across the blood-brain barrier.

CANNABIS

The cannabinoid drugs include marijuana (the dried flowering tops and stems of the resin-producing hemp plant) and hashish (a resinous extract of the hemp plant). Most of their pharmacologic effects come from metabolites of δ-9-tetrahydrocannabinol. This drug is in-

tensely lipophilic and is trapped on the surfactant lining of the lung and absorbed. Metabolites can be detected in the urine for 2 to 3 days after casual drug use and for up to 4 weeks in chronic users. Other drugs or chemicals, such as opium or cocaine paste, may be mixed with marijuana to increase its effect.

The primary mode of ingestion is smoking; mood altering and intoxicating effects can be felt within 3 minutes, with peak effects in about 1 hour. The acute physiologic effects are dose-related and may include an increase in heart rate, conjunctival congestion, decreased intraocular pressure, bronchodilation, peripheral vasodilation, dry mouth, fine tremor, muscle weakness, and ataxia. Psychoactive effects include euphoria, enhanced perception of colors and sounds, drowsiness, inattentiveness, and inability to learn new facts. Motor vehicle driving is impaired. Tolerance and physical dependence do occur, and chronic users may experience mild withdrawal with irritability, restlessness, anorexia, insomnia, or mild hyperthermia. In rare cases, acute psychosis with panic reactions can occur. Treatment is supportive and includes reassurance; benzodiazepines can be used in more severely agitated patients. Some chronic users may have poor academic performance, lethargy, poor concentration, and poor motivation (amotivational syndrome).

Medical uses of cannabinoids include antiemetic agents for cancer chemotherapy patients, weight stimulation (particularly effective in cancer and HIV patients), and treatment of glaucoma.

PSYCHEDELICS

The major psychedelic-hallucinogenic drugs include lysergic acid diethylamide (LSD), PCP, mescaline, psilocybin, 5-methoxy-3,4-methylene dioxyamphetamine (MMDA), and dimethyltryptamine. In most situations, these drugs are not truly hallucinogenic but are powerful producers of illusional and perceptual disturbances.

LSD is the most potent psychedelic drug known. It interacts with several serotonin receptors in the cortex, but the actual psychoactive mechanism is unknown. Within 20 minutes of oral ingestion, sympathomimetic effects of mydriasis, hyperthermia, tachycardia, elevated blood pressure, increased alertness, tremors, and occasional nausea and vomiting occur. Within 2 hours, psychoactive effects occur with heightened perceptions, body distortions, variable mood, and sometimes visual hallucinations. After 12 hours the syndrome starts to clear, but fatigue and tension may persist for another day. An acute panic or psychotic reaction may occur; such episodes have occasionally led to self-injury or suicide. Flashbacks, or brief reappearances of the hallucinations, may occur days or weeks after the last dose but tend to disappear without treatment. Acute panic reactions are best treated in a supportive environment; benzodiazepines can be used for severely agitated patients.

Phencyclidine is another potent hallucinogen and is now the most widely abused of this group. It was developed as an anesthetic, but its use was discontinued in 1965 because of postsurgical psychotic effects. It produces a prompt stimulant effect similar to that of amphetamines with feelings of euphoria, power, and invincibility. Patients may have hypertension, tachycardia, bidirectional nystagmus, hyperthermia, hallucinations, extreme agitation, ataxia, and slurred speech. With more severe reactions, patients may present in a comalike state with open eyes and pupils that are partially dilated, decreased pain response, brief periods of excitation, and muscle rigidity. Patients can have hypertensive crises, seizures, and bizarre, often violent behavior. Overdosing can result in death. Tolerance and mild withdrawal symptoms have been seen in daily users, but the major problem is drug craving.

Treatment entails a quiet environment, sedation with benzodiazepines, hydration, and haloperidol for terrifying hallucinations. Continuous gastric suction and acidification of the urine with intravenous ammonium chloride or ascorbic acid may aid excretion, but acidification may increase the risk of renal failure if significant rhabdomyolysis or myoglobinuria exists.

INHALANTS

The major groups of inhalants are organic solvents, organic nitrites (such as amyl nitrite or amyl butyl), and nitrous oxide. Organic solvents include toluene (airplane glue), kerosene, gasoline, carbon tetrachloride, acrylic paint sprays, shoe polish, and degreasers. These solvents, particularly toluene, are most often inhaled by children or young adolescents and can produce dizziness and intoxication within minutes. Prolonged exposure or daily use can cause bone marrow depression, cardiac arrhythmias, cerebral degeneration, and damage to the liver, kidney, and the peripheral nervous system. In rare instances, death may occur, most likely from cardiac arrhythmias. Detoxification is rarely required for the solvents, but psychiatric treatment may be needed to prevent relapse.

Amyl nitrite is a yellowish, volatile liquid that dilates smooth muscle and is used as a sexual enhancer. It is usually sprayed into the nose and can produce flushing, dizziness, and a feeling of a rush. Adverse effects include palpitations, postural hypotension, and headache, but no chronic toxicity has been reported.

DESIGNER DRUGS

The term *designer drugs* refers to illicit synthetic drugs created by slight alterations in the molecular structure of existing drugs. These compounds often have markedly increased potency over the parent compound. The most common designer drugs include analogues of fentanyl, meperidine, methamphetamines, and phencyclidine.

The major meperidine derivatives are 1-methyl-4-phenyl-4-propionoxypiperidene (MPPP) and 1-methyl-4-phenyl-1,2,3,6-tetrahydropyridine (MPTP). These drugs are capable of producing a euphoria similar to that of heroin. In some users, MPTP was found to produce an irreversible form of Parkinson's disease, which was probably related to neuronal enzyme inactivation in the substantia nigra. The best known fentanyl derivatives are α-methyl fentanyl ("China white") and 3-methyl fentanyl. These drugs are about 1000 times more potent than heroin, and fatal overdoses from respiratory depression have occurred.

The mescaline-methamphetamine analogues include 3,4-methylenedioxymethamphetamine (MDMA, or "ecstasy"), 3,4-methylenedioxyamphetamine (MDA, or "love drug"), and 3,4-methylenedioxyethamphetamine (MDEA, or "Eve"). MDMA is a CNS stimulant and produces elevated mood and increased self-esteem. However, it may cause acute panic, anxiety, paranoia, hallucinations, tachycardia, nystagmus, ataxia, and tremor. Deaths in some users have been attributed to cardiac arrhythmias, hyperthermia with seizures, or intracranial hemorrhage.

Patients often present with signs and symptoms of narcotic overdose. Management principles are identical to those for narcotic abuse except that the doses of naloxone should be much higher; some patients may require a continuous naloxone infusion. The parkinsonian symptoms can be managed with appropriate medications, but the syndrome is irreversible. The acute psychosis can be managed by a low-stimulus environment and haloperidol or benzodiazepines, if needed. Cooling blankets and ice baths can be used for hyperpyrexia, and α blockers or α/β blockers (labetalol) can be used for hypertension.

REFERENCES

Diamond I: Alcoholism and alcohol abuse. *In* Bennett JC, Plum F (eds): Cecil Textbook of Medicine, 20th ed. Philadelphia: WB Saunders, 1996, pp 47–49.

Hollander JE: The management of cocaine-associated myocardial ischemia. N Engl J Med 1995; 333:1267–1272.

Jaffe JH: Drug addiction and drug abuse. *In* Goodman and Gilman's The Pharmacological Basis of Therapeutics. Elmsford, NY: Pergamon, 1990, pp 522–573.

Lieber CS: Medical disorders of alcoholism. N Engl J Med 1995; 333:1058–1065.

Mendelson JH, Mello NK: Management of cocaine abuse and dependence. N Engl J Med 1995; 334:965–972.

O'Brien CP: Drug abuse and dependence. *In* Bennett JC, Plum F (eds): Cecil Textbook of Medicine, 20th ed. Philadelphia: WB Saunders, 1996, pp 49–56.

Warner E: Cocaine abuse. Ann Intern Med 1993; 119:226–235.

APPENDIX

COMMONLY MEASURED LABORATORY VALUES

....

This appendix lists basic serum and urinary laboratory values measured commonly in clinical medicine. The values are presented in conventional units (CUs) and standard international (SI) units. The table also includes conversion factors (CFs) for interchanging conventional and standard international units using the following formula:

$$\text{SI units} = \text{CU} \times \text{CF}$$

This collection of laboratory values is not intended to be exhaustive. Most of the laboratory values are from the following sources: Goldman L, Bennett JC (eds): *Cecil Textbook of Medicine*, 21st ed, Philadelphia, WB Saunders Co, 2000, pp 2299–2308; and Henry JB (ed): *Clinical Diagnosis and Management by Laboratory Methods*, 18th ed, Philadelphia, WB Saunders Co, 1991, pp 1366–1382. These two sources also provide more comprehensive listings of laboratory measures. Laboratory values found in this appendix but not in either of the above references are from the clinical laboratories of University Hospital, University of Arkansas for Medical Sciences, Little Rock, Arkansas.

Commonly Measured Laboratory Values

Test	Conventional Units	Conversion Factor	SI Units
Arterial Blood Gases			
pH (37°C)	—	—	7.35–7.45
Oxygen (PO_2)	83–100 mm Hg	0.133	11–14.4 kPa
Oxygen saturation	95–98%	—	Fraction: 0.95–0.98
Carbon dioxide (PCO_2)	23–29 mEq/L	1	23–29 mmol/L
Serum Electrolytes			
Sodium	136–146 mEq/L	1	136–146 mmol/L
Potassium	3.5–5.1 mEq/L	1	3.5–5.1 mmol/L
Chloride	98—106 mEq/L	1	98–106 mmol/L
Bicarbonate	18–23 mEq/L	1	18–23 mmol/L
Anion gap [Na − (Cl + HCO_3)]	7–14 mEq/L	1	7–14 mmol/L
Calcium			
Total	8.4–10.2 mg/dL	0.25	2.1–2.55 mmol/L
Ionized	4.65–5.28 mg/dL	0.25	1.16–1.32 mmol/L
Magnesium	1.3–2.1 mEq/L	0.50	0.65–1.05 mmol/L
Phosphorus	2.7–4.5 mg/dL	0.323	0.87–1.45 mmol/L
Commonly Measured Serum Nonelectrolytes			
Urea nitrogen	7–18 mg/dL	0.357	2.5–6.4 mmol/L
Creatinine	M: 0.7–1.3 mg/dL	88.4	62–115 μmol/L
	F: 0.6–1.1 mg/dL	88.4	53–97 μmol/L
Uric acid	M: 3.5–7.2 mg/dL	0.059	0.21–0.42 mmol/L
	F: 2.6–6.0 ng/dL	0.059	0.15–0.35 mmol/L
Glucose	70–105 mg/dL	0.055	3.9–5.8 mmol/L
Osmolality	—	—	275–295 mOsm/kg
Serum Endocrine Tests			
ACTH	0800 h: 8–79 pg/mL	1	8–79 ng/L
	1600 h: 7–30 pg/mL	1	7–30 ng/L
Aldosterone	Supine: 3–10 ng/dL	0.0277	0.08–0.28 nmol/L
	Upright: 5–30 ng/dL	0.0277	0.14–0.83 nmol/L
Chronic (β-hCG) gonadotropin	<5.0 mU/mL	1	<5.0 IU/L
Cortisol	0800 h: 5–23 μg/dL	27.6	138–635 nmol/L
	1600 h: 3–15 μg/dL	27.6	82–413 nmol/L
C-peptide	0.78–1.89 ng/mL	0.328	0.26–0.62 nmol/L
Estrogen	M: 20–80 pg/mL	1	20–80 ng/L
	F: Follicular phase, 60–200 pg/mL	1	60–200 ng/mL
	Luteal phase, 160–400 pg/mL	1	160–400 ng/L
	Postmenopausal, ≤130 pg/mL	1	≤130 ng/L
Follitropin (FSH)	M: 4–25 mIU/mL	1	4–25 IU/L
	F: Follicular phase, 1–9 mU/mL	1	1–9 U/L
	Ovulatory peak, 6–26 mU/mL	1	6–26 U/L
	Luteal phase, 1–9 mU/mL	1	1–9 U/L
	Postmenopausal, 30–118 mU/mL	1	30–118 U/L
Gastrin	<100 pg/mL	1	<100 ng/L
Growth hormone	M: <2 ng/mL	1	<2 μg/L
	F: <10 ng/mL	1	<10 μg/L
Hemoglobin A_{1c}	5.6–7.5% of total Hg (whole blood)	0.001	Fraction: 0.056–0.075
Insulin (12-h fasting)	6–24 μIU/mL	7.0	42–167 pmol/L
Lutropin (LH)	M: 1–8 mU/mL	1	1–8 U/L
	F: Follicular phase, 1–12 mU/mL	1	1–12 U/L
	Midcycle, 16–104 mU/mL	1	16–104 U/L
	Luteal, 1–12 mU/mL	1	1–12 U/L
	Postmenopausal, 16–66 mU/mL	1	16–66 U/L
Progesterone	M: 0.13–0.97 ng/mL	3.2	0.4–3.1 nmol/L
	F: Follicular phase, 0.14–1.61 ng/mL	3.2	0.5–2.2 nmol/L
	Luteal phase, 2–25 ng/mL	3.2	6.4–79.5 nmol/L
Prolactin	Postmenopausal, 0–20 ng/mL	1	0–20 μg/L
Renin	Supine: 1.6 ± 1.5 ng/mL/h	1	1.6 ± 1.5 μg/L/h
	Standing: 4.5 ± 2.9 ng/mL/h	1	4.5 ± 2.9 μg/L/h
Testosterone			
Free	M: 52–280 pg/mL	3.5	180.4–971.6 pmol/L
	F: 1.6–6.3 pg/mL	3.5	5.6–21.9 pmol/L
Total	M: 300–1000 ng/dL	0.035	10.4–34.7 nmol/L
	F: 20–75 ng/dL	0.035	0.69–2.6 nmol/L

Commonly Measured Laboratory Values *(Continued)*

Test	Conventional Units	Conversion Factor	SI Units
Serum Endocrine Tests *(Continued)*			
Thyrotropin (TSH)	2–10 μU/mL	1	2–10 μU/L
Thyrotropin-releasing hormone (TRH)	5–60 pg/mL	1	5–60 ng/L
Thyroxine			
Free (FT$_4$)	0.8–2.4 ng/dL	13	10–31 pmol/L
Total (T$_4$)	5–12 μg/dL	13	65–155 nmol/L
Triiodothyronine resin uptake (T$_3$RU)	24–34%	1	24–34 AU (arbitrary units)
Urine Endocrine Tests			
Catecholamines	24 h: <100 μg/d	0.059	<5.91 nmol/d
5-Hydroxyindole-acetic acid	24 h: 2–6 mg/d	5.2	10.4–31.2 μmol/d
Metanephrines	24 h: 0.5–1.2 μg/mg creatinine	0.58	0.03–0.69 mmol/mol creatinine
Vanillylmandelic acid (VMA)	24 h: 2–7 mg/d	5.05	10.1–35.4 μmol/d
17-Hydroxycorticosteroids	24 h: M: 3–10 mg/d	2.76	8.3–27.6 μmol/d
	F: 2–8 mg/d	2.76	5.5–22.1 μmol/d
17-Ketosteroids	24 h: M: 9–22 mg/d	3.44	31–76 μmol/d
	F: 6–15 mg/d	3.44	21–52 μmol/d
Serum Markers of Gastrointestinal Absorption			
β-Carotene	10–85 μg/dL	0.0186	0.19–1.58 μmol/L
Vitamin B$_{12}$	100–700 pg/mL	0.74	74–516 pmol/L
Folate			
Serum	3–16 ng/mL	2.27	7–36 nmol/L
Red blood cells (RBCs)	130–628 ng/mL packed cells	2.27	294–1422 nmol/L
Serum Lipids			
Cholesterol	Recommended: <200 mg/dL	0.026	<5.18 mmol/L
	Moderate risk: 200–239 mg/dL	0.026	5.18–6.19 mmol/L
	High risk: ≥240 mg/dL	0.026	≥6.22 mmol/L
Fatty acids, free	8–25 mg/dL	0.0356	0.28–0.89 mmol/L
HDL-Cholesterol	M: >29 mg/dL	0.026	>0.75 mmol/L
	F: >35 mg/dL	0.026	>0.91 mmol/L
LDL-Cholesterol	Recommended: <130 mg/dL	0.026	<3.37 mmol/L
	Moderate risk: 130–159 mg/dL	0.026	3.37–4.12 mmol/L
	High risk: ≥160 mg/dL	0.026	≥4.14 mmol/L
Triglycerides	M: 40–160 mg/dL	0.011	0.45–1.81 mmol/L
	F: 35–135 mg/dL	0.011	0.4–1.52 mmol/L
Serum Liver/Pancreatic Tests			
Alanine aminotransferase (ALT, SGPT)	—	—	8–20 U/L
Aspartate aminotransferase (AST, SGOT)	—	—	10–30 U/L
γ-Glutamyltransferase (GGT)	—	—	M: 9–50 U/L
			F: 8–40 U/L
Alkaline phosphatase	—	—	M: 53–128 U/L
			F: 42–98 U/L
Bilirubin			
Total	0.2–1.0 mg/dL	17.1	3.4–17.1 μmol/L
Conjugated	0–0.2 mg/dL	17.1	0–3.4 μmol/L
Amylase	—	—	25–125 U/L
Lipase	—	—	10–140 U/L
Serum Markers for Cardiac or Skeletal Muscle Injury			
Aldolase	—	—	1.0–7.5 U/L
Lactate dehydrogenase (LDH)	—	—	208–378 U/L
Isoenzymes (%)	Fraction 1: 18–33	—	0.18–0.33
	Fraction 2: 28–40	—	0.28–0.40
	Fraction 3: 18–30	—	0.18–0.30
	Fraction 4: 6–16	—	0.06–0.16
	Fraction 5: 2–13	—	0.02–0.13

Continued on following page

Commonly Measured Laboratory Values *(Continued)*

Test	Conventional Units	Conversion Factor	SI Units
Serum Markers for Cardiac or Skeletal Muscle Injury *(Continued)*			
Creatine kinase (CK)	—	—	M: 38–174 U/L
			F: 26–140 U/L
Isoenzymes (%)	Fraction 2 (MB): <4–6% of total	—	<0.04–0.06
Myoglobin	—	—	M: 19–92 μg/L
			F: 12–76 μg/L
Serum Markers for Neoplasia			
Acid phosphatase	—	—	M: 2.5–11.7 U/L
Carcinoembryonic antigen (CEA)	Nonsmokers: <2.5 ng/mL	1	<2.5 μg/L
α-Fetoprotein	<10 ng/mL	1	<10 μg/L
Prostate-specific antigen (PSA)	0–4 ng/mL	0.001	0–4 μg/L
Serum Proteins			
Albumin	3.5–5.0 g/dL	10	35–50 g/L
Immunoglobulins	IgA: 40–350 mg/dL	10	400–3500 mg/L
	IgD: 0–8 mg/dL	10	0–80 mg/L
	IgE: 0–380 IU/mL	1	0–380 KIU/L
	IgG: 650–1600 mg/dL	0.01	6.5–16 g/L
	IgM: 55–300 mg/dL	10	550–3000 mg/L
Protein			
Total	6.4–8.3 g/dL	10	64–83 g/L
Electrophoresis	α_1-globulin: 0.1–0.3 g/dL	10	1–3 g/L
	α_2-globulin: 0.6–1.0 g/dL	10	6–10 g/L
	β-globulin: 0.7–1.1 g/dL	10	7–11 g/L
	γ-globulin: 0.8–1.6 g/dL	10	8–16 g/L
Complete Blood Cell Count			
Hemoglobin (Hb)	M: 13.5–17.5 g/dL	0.155	2.09–2.71 mmol/L
	F: 12–16 g/dL	0.155	1.86–2.48 mmol/L
Hematocrit (Hct)	M: 39–49%	—	0.39–0.49
	F: 35–45%	—	0.35–0.45
Mean corpuscular Hb concentration (MCHC)	31–37% Hb/cell, or g Hb/dL TBC	0.155	481–5.74 mmol Hb/L
Mean corpuscular volume (MCV)	—	—	80–100 tL
Leukocyte count	4.5–11 × 10^3 cells/μL	—	4.5–11 × 10^9 cells/L

Differential count	%	Cells/μL		Fraction	Cells × 10^6/L
Melanocytes	0	0	—	0	0
Neutrophils—bands	3–5	150–400	—	0.03–0.05	150–400
Neutrophils—segmented	54–62	3000–5800	—	0.54–0.62	3000–5800
Lymphocytes	23–33	1500–3000	—	0.25–0.33	1500–3000
Monocytes	3–7	285–500	—	0.03–0.07	285–500
Eosinophils	1–3	50–250	—	0.01–0.03	50–250
Basophils	0–0.75	15–50	—	0–0.0075	15–50
CD_4 (T_H) count	36–54	600–1500	—	0.36–0.54	660–1500
CD_8 (T_S) count	10–33	360–850	—	0.19–0.54	360–850
T_H/T_S ratio	1.1–2.9		—	1.1–2.9	
Platelet count	150–450 × 10^3/μL (mm³)		—	150–450 × 10^9/L	

Test	Conventional Units	Conversion Factor	SI Units
Anemia Tests			
Reticulocyte count	0.5–1.5% of erythrocytes	—	0.005–0.015
Iron	M: 65–175 μg/dL	0.179	11.6–31.3 μmol/L
	F: 50–170 μg/dL	0.179	9.0–30.4 μmol/L
Ferritin	M: 20–250 ng/mL	1	20–250 μg/L
	F: 10–120 ng/mL	1	10–120 μg/L
Total iron-binding capacity	250–450 μg/dL	0.179	44.8–80.6 μmol/L
Hemoglobin electrophoresis	HbA: >95%	—	>0.95
	HbA₂: 1.5–3.5%	—	0.015–0.035
	HbF: <2%	—	<0.02
	HbS: 0%		

Commonly Measured Laboratory Values *(Continued)*

Test	Conventional Units		Conversion Factor	SI Units
Coagulation Tests				
Prothrombin time (PT)	9–13 sec		+9 sec	18–22 sec
Partial thromboplastin time (PTT)		—	—	60–85 sec
Activated PTT		—	—	25–35 sec
Bleeding time				
Ivy		—	—	Normal: 2–7 min Borderline: 7–11 min
Simplate		—	—	2.75–8 min
Clotting time (Lee-White)		—	—	5–8 min
Thrombin time		—	—	Time of control ±2 sec when control is 9–13 sec
Disseminated Intravascular Coagulation Tests				
Fibrinogen	200–400 mg/dL		0.01	2.0–4.0 g/L
Fibrin degradation products	<10 μg/mL		1	<10 mg/L
Hemolysis Tests				
Haptoglobin	26–185 mg/dL		10	260–1850 mg/L

ACTH = Corticotropin; F = female; FSH = follicle-stimulating hormone; β-hCG = β-human chorionic gonadotropin; HDL = high-density lipoprotein; LDL = low-density lipoprotein; LH = luteinizing hormone; M = male; SGOT = serum glutamic-oxaloacetic transaminase; SGPT = serum glutamate pyruvate transaminase.

INDEX

O